Principles of psychophysiology

Physical, social, and inferential elements

Edited by

JOHN T. CACIOPPO
The Ohio State University

and

LOUIS G. TASSINARY
University of Iowa

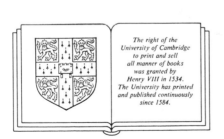

The right of the
University of Cambridge
to print and sell
all manner of books
was granted by
Henry VIII in 1534.
The University has printed
and published continuously
since 1584.

CAMBRIDGE UNIVERSITY PRESS

Cambridge
New York Port Chester Melbourne Sydney

Published by the Press Syndicate of the University of Cambridge
The Pitt Building, Trumpington Street, Cambridge CB21RP
40 West 20th Street, New York, NY 10011, USA
10 Stamford Road, Oakleigh, Melbourne 3166, Australia

First published 1990

Printed in the United States of America

Library of Congress Cataloging-in-Publication Data
Principles of psychophysiology: physical, social, and inferential
elements / edited by John T. Cacioppo and Louis G. Tassinary.

    p. cm.
Includes bibliographies.

ISBN 0-521-34432-8 hardback
1. Psychophysiology. I. Cacioppo, John T. II. Tassinary,
Louis G.
QP360.P7515 1990
    90-655

British Library cataloguing-in-publication data applied for

ISBN 0-521-34432-8 hardback

Contents

vi   *Contents*

Contributors

Erling A. Anderson
Department of Anesthesia
College of Medicine
University of Iowa

Robert E. Bohrer
Department of Mathematics
University of Illinois

John T. Cacioppo
Department of Psychology
The Ohio State University

Michael G. H. Coles
Department of Psychology
University of Illinois

Michael E. Dawson
Department of Psychology
University of Southern California

Donald D. Dorfman
Department of Psychology
University of Iowa

Douglas N. Dunham
Department of Psychology
Washington University

Monica Fabiani
Department of Psychology
University of Illinois

Diane L. Filion
Department of Psychology
University of Southern California

Alan J. Fridlund
Department of Psychology
University of California at Santa Barbara

James H. Geer
Department of Psychology
Louisiana State University

Ronald Glaser
Department of Medical Microbiology and
Immunology
The Ohio State University

John Gottman
Department of Psychology
University of Washington

Gabriele Gratton
Department of Psychology
University of Illinois

Neil E. Grunberg
Department of Medical Psychology
Uniformed Services University of the
Health Sciences

Andrew Harver
Department of Psychology
State University of New York at
Stony Brook

Susan Head
Department of Psychology
Louisiana State University

Howard C. Hughes
Department of Psychology
Dartmouth College

Alan Kim Johnson
Department of Psychology
University of Iowa

Edward S. Katkin
Department of Psychology
State University of New York at
Stony Brook

Susan Kennedy
Department of Medical Microbiology and
Immunology
The Ohio State University

vii

Janice Kiecolt-Glaser
Department of Psychiatry
The Ohio State University

Kenneth L. Koch
Division of Gastroenterology
Department of Medicine
Pennsylvania State University

Tyler S. Lorig
Department of Psychology
Washington and Lee University

Beverly S. Marshall-Goodell
Department of Psychology
University of Iowa

Rae Matsumoto
Department of Psychology
Brown University

James F. Papillo
Department of Psychology
University of California at Los Angeles

James W. Pennebaker
Department of Psychology
Southern Methodist University

Stephen W. Porges
Institute for Child Study
University of Maryland

William J. Ray
Department of Psychology
Pennsylvania State University

Sheila D. Reed
Department of Psychology
University of Wyoming

Daniel W. Russell
Hospital Health Administration
University of Iowa

Anne M. Schell
Department of Psychology
Occidental College

Gary E. Schwartz
Department of Psychology
University of Arizona

David Shapiro
Department of Psychiatry
University of California at Los Angeles

Jerome E. Singer
Department of Medical Psychology
Uniformed Services University of the
  Health Sciences

Cecile Elise E. Sison
Department of Psychology
Pennsylvania State University

J. A. Skelton
Department of Psychology
Dickinson College

John A. Stern
Department of Psychology
Washington University

Robert M. Stern
Department of Psychology
Pennsylvania State University

Michael J Strube
Department of Psychology
Washington University

Louis G. Tassinary
Department of Psychology
University of Iowa

Michael W. Vasey
Department of Psychology
Pennsylvania State University

Barbara B. Walker
Department of Psychiatry
Mirian Hospital

J. Michael Walker
Department of Psychology
Brown University

Preface

Investigations of elementary physiological events in normal thinking, feeling, and interacting individuals are now quite feasible, and these investigations provide the potential for comprehensive accounts of human nature. This approach to the study of human behavior defines the discipline of psychophysiology. More specifically, psychophysiology represents the scientific study of cognitive, emotional, and behavioral phenomena as related to and revealed through physiological principles and events. The possibility that important aspects of human nature might be discovered by focusing on the interaction between environmental stimuli and an information-processing organism was recognized more than 2,000 years ago. Only recently, however, have technological advances and scientific reasoning begun to enable investigators to use physiological principles and measures to address fundamental questions about the organization and governance of human nature and behavior.

With these developments, psychophysiology has become an important scientific approach in studies ranging from sleep to motivation, from normal to psychopathological personalities, from sensory isolation to social interactions, and from infant development to the process of aging. The appeal of a physiologically realistic theory of cognition, the return to favor of the concept of emotion, and the emerging emphasis on preventive medicine (including social and behavioral issues related to health) have further stimulated interest among behavioral, cognitive, and social scientists in physiological concepts and techniques. For instance, psychophysiology is increasingly of interest to health psychologists because the development of symptoms or changes in behavior due to changes in health tend to lag in time changes in physiology; and the observation or prediction of the loss of health (and its consequent effects on behavior) does not constitute an adequate explanation of these changes. An explanation of the mechanisms underlying these changes, whether in behavioral or physiological terms, is thus important from both applied and theoretical points of view.

Paralleling the growth in interest in the concepts and methods of psychophysiology are technological developments in signal acquisition and analysis and efforts in recent years to articulate standards for psychophysiological recording. As a result, psychophysiological analyses have never before been more powerful, accessible, or comparable. These developments have facilitated problem-oriented research in psychophysiology, and consequently, exciting advances are being made in bridging the gap between physiological data and psychological, behavioral, and health constructs. Many of these advances are summarized in this book.

Despite important advances in and growing applications of psychophysiology, there has existed no single book that covers the diverse elements of psychophysio-

ix

logy at a level of scholarship that is informative to the specialist while also covering these topics at a level of discourse that is accessible to the nonspecialist. A major objective in creating this book, therefore, was to provide sufficiently comprehensive discussions of physical, social, and inferential elements of psychophysiology to interest and inform the specialist; and sufficiently clear and explicit coverage that the potential and excitement of psychophysiology becomes apparent, and its principles and methods become more accessible, to graduate students and scientists interested but not yet well-versed in psychophysiology. The present book, therefore, is designed to fill the gap between recent undergraduate primers (e.g., Andreassi, 1989; Grings & Dawson, 1978; Hassett, 1978; Stern, Ray, & Davis, 1980) and available, excellent technical sourcebooks (e.g., Coles, Donchin, & Porges, 1986; Martin & Venables, 1980). As such, this book could be used in advanced undergraduate or graduate courses in psychophysiology; or various combinations of chapters from this book could be used in conjunction with additional readings or texts in any number of topical graduate courses or seminars.

The book is divided into four parts: (1) foundations, (2) general concepts, (3) systemic psychophysiology, and (4) issues in the analysis of psychophysiological data. As in any advanced field, time, study, and experience are required to become familiar and proficient with the various concepts and techniques of psychophysiology. A concerted effort has been made, however, to minimize the complexities of the field by parsing the coverage of the field into small, more readily comprehensible discussions and to avoid minutiae while also trying to avoid oversimplification. The balance we have sought to achieve is reflected in the selection and sequence of the chapters in the book, the organization and systematic coverage of topics within chapters, the use of figures to illustrate laboratory observations, the references within chapters to technical sourcebooks for details on more advanced or esoteric issues, and the inclusion of an extensive glossary to make even the most recondite discussions understandable to nonspecialists.

Part I is divided into two sections. It begins with a description of the psychophysiological enterprise, a brief history of the field, and conceptual frameworks for linking psychophysiological data and psychological/behavioral constructs. Since the ascription of psychological meaning to physiological responses ultimately resides in the logical and empirical relationships among the theoretical constructs and operationalizations, this section ends with a chapter reviewing how psychometric principles can aid the transition from physiological data to psychological constructs. The assignment of psychological meaning to a physiological response can nevertheless be advanced by an understanding of the physiological basis of the response. Hence, chapters are included in the second section of Part I to provide contemporary reviews of concepts, principles, and methods from the general areas of neuroscience, bioelectronics, biochemistry, and psychoneuroimmunology – all of which have significant impact on basic conceptual and technical developments in psychophysiology.

The chapters in Part II elaborate upon these foundations by highlighting principles of human behavior that have emerged from psychophysiological analyses. Included in this section are discussions of theories of arousal, somatovisceral sensation and perception, and orchestrated response patterns characterizing organismic – environmental transactions.

The chapters in Part III provide detailed overviews of the major physiological systems that are currently actively investigated in the psychophysiological literature. Included are discussions of the physiological basis of the system and the responses of interest in psychophysiology, the technical issues involved in the recording and quantification of these physiological events, and the theory underlying psychological inferences based on these physiological events. How each area of inquiry has provided conceptual insight into interesting social, psychological, and health/disease processes is also addressed in these chapters.

Although each chapter on physiological systems discusses issues related to the extraction, analysis, and interpretation of physiological data, there are several important issues in psychophysiology that are sufficiently complex and general that they warrant tutorials of their own. Part IV, on issues in the analysis of psychophysiological signals, is included for this purpose. The discussion begins with chapters on descriptive statistical analyses, which are designed to reduce large quantities of data – such as that obtained from the voltage–time functions signifying psychophysiological activity – to more manageable representations that retain as much of the information from the original function as possible. A chapter on periodic processes provides a tractable discussion of Fourier analyses, including discussions of topics ranging from autocorrelation within a given response to coherence across responses. A companion chapter on time-series analysis in psychophysiological research elaborates on these discussions and illustrates the application of readily available software for implementing time-series analyses of psychophysiological signals. Many psychophysiological signals are nonrhythmic, however, as are the power spectral density functions that one obtains from Fourier analyses of physiological signals. A chapter on nonrhythmic responses is included to illustrate an alternative, complementing analysis for waveform representation. Part IV ends with a chapter on inferential statistical analysis of multivariate data.

On a more personal note, we owe thanks to a number of people for the existence of this book. First, the contributors to this book, all of whom are active researchers and scholars, graciously consented to take time from their own research to prepare general and comprehensible reference chapters for other working scientists. We deeply appreciate the cooperation of the authors and offer our sincere thanks to all for the time and care expended in preparing their chapters. The continued support by the National Science Foundation and the personal encouragement and support of Jean Intermaggio and Richard Loutitt within the National Science Foundation have been of the utmost importance. We would like to take this opportunity to thank them formally as well.

The format for this book was developed while preparing for and during discussions with Fellows and Consultants in the first four years of our program for advanced study and research in psychophysiology and social psychology, and we thank these individuals for their invaluable input (alphabetically): Robert S. Baron (University of Iowa), Lee A. Becker (University of Colorado at Colorado Springs), James H. Blascovich (State University of New York at Buffalo), Gordon H. Bower (Stanford University), Daphne B. Bugental (University of California at Santa Barbara), Michael G. H. Coles (University of Illinois), Richard J. Davidson (University of Wisconsin), W. Jackson Davis (University of California at Santa Cruz), Michael E. Dawson (University of Southern California), Emanuel Donchin (University of Illinois), Paul Ekman (University of San Francisco), Nancy H. Eisenberg (Arizona State University), Alan J. Fridlund (University of California at Santa Barbara), John J. Furedy (University of Toronto), Russell G. Geen (University of Missouri), Gerald P. Ginsburg (University of Nevada at Reno), Ronald Glaser (Ohio State University), John M. Gottman (University of Washington), Anthony G. Greenwald (University of Washington), Neil E. Grunberg (Uniformed Services University), Christine E. Hansen (Oakland University), Ronald D. Hansen (Oakland University), Elaine Hatfield (University of Hawaii), William Iacono (University of Minnesota), William Ickes (University of Texas at Arlington), Alice M. Isen (Cornell University), J. Richard Jennings (University of Pittsburgh), Russel A. Jones (University of North Florida), Edward S. Katkin (State University of New York at Stony Brook), Janice Kiecolt-Glaser (Ohio State University), Peter J. Lang (University of Florida), John T. Lanzetta (Dartmouth College), Randy J. Larsen (University of Michigan), Diane M. Mackie (University of California at Santa Barbara), Robert Mauro (University of Oregon), Gregory McHugo (Dartmouth College), Norman Miller (University of Southern California), Clifford I. Notarius (Catholic University), Richard E. Petty (Ohio State University), Stephen W. Porges (University of Maryland), Willian J. Ray (Pennsylvania State University), Martin A. Safer (Catholic University), Gary E. Schwartz (University of Arizona), David Shapiro (University of California at Los Angeles), Stephanie A. Shields (University of California at Davis), Roxane C. Silver (University of Waterloo), Cookie W. Stephen (New Mexico State University), Walter G. Stephan (New Mexico State University), John A. Stern (Washington University), Robert M. Stern (Pennsylvania State University), Jerry Suls (State University of New York at Albany), Abraham Tesser (University of Georgia), Dianne M. Tice (Case Western Reserve University), Michael W. Torello (Ohio State University), Rebecca M. Warner (University of New Hampshire), Robert B. Zajonc (University of Michigan), and Dolf Zillmann (Indiana University). We have learned much from each.

We would also like to thank our colleagues and students at the University of Iowa and the Ohio State University for their questions and assistance. These include Lisa Alter, Barbara L. Andersen, Gary G. Berntson, Steplen Crites, Donald D. Dorfman, Edwin Dove, John Folkins, Don C. Fowles, I. Gormezano, John H. Harvey, Melanie M. Ihrig, A. Kim Johnson, Gerhard Loewenberg, Douglas K. Madsen, Barry Markovsky, Beverly S. Marshall-Goodell, Alan Randich, Daniel Russell, Fuchih Chen, Thomas R. Geen, Lisa Keyes, Kristen Klaaren, Mary E. Losch, Jeffery S. Martzke, Kathlene Merendo, Cindi Mull, Karen Quigley, Patricia A. Rourke, Stacy Siegel, Greg Smith, Mary Snyder, Bert Uchino, Eric J. Vanman, and Jon Winjum; and special thanks to Vice President Duane C. Spriestersbach for his support and encouragement.

We are especially indebted to Barbara and Melanie, and to all the members of our families, for their questions, suggestions, patience, support, and good humor. We spend all too little time with them, but they should know we love them dearly. One of us (LGT) would like to extend a special thanks to Alexas and Damien Ihrig. Their acceptance and friendship has been and will continue to be invaluable.

Finally, as good fortune would have it, the birth of this book and of Christina Elizabeth Cacioppo coincided. Among the joys she has brought are repeated demonstrations during the years we worked on this book that there is a great deal to human nature that is shaped by biological forces, driven by bodily processes, and manifest in physiological events – only occasionally and only a subset of which are articulated verbally and overtly. As she has grown, we have also seen the development of reciprocal influences between social and physiological events, and we have watched her develop a keen faculty to comment on events, both internal and external, and to construe these events in terms of a coherent scenario complete with likely causes, effects, and implications. It seems not unlike historians who render accounts of times present and past; and like contesting historians, Christina and others can view the same events and disagree sharply on accounts and actions. This can also result if there are small differences in what events are noticed or in the context in which these events are noticed. The litmus test for these scenarios (models) clearly must not be the prerequisite condition that they organize the events observed to date but rather that they generalize, stimulate, and withstand repeated attempts to disconfirm their predictions.

Although people routinely develop explanatory scenarios, only the attentive and systematic observer tries also to disconfirm these accounts, to extend beyond commonsense observation and reasoning to do so, and to discover something about the governance of the world and of ourselves in doing so. We, therefore, dedicate this book to the tradition of the attentive and systematic observer, without which this book would have neither basis nor purpose.

John T. Cacioppo
Louis G. Tassinary
October, 1989

REFERENCES

Andreassi, J. L. (1989). *Psychophysiology: Human behavior and physiological response* (2nd ed.). New York: Oxford University Press.
Coles, M. G. H., Porges, S. W., & Donchin, E. (1986). *Psychophysiology: System, processes, and applications.* New York: Guilford.
Grings, W. W., & Dawson, M. E. (1978). *Emotions and bodily responses: A psychophysiological approach.* New York: Academic Press.
Hassett, J. (1978). *A primer of psychophysiology.* San Francisco: W. H. Freeman and Company.
Martin, I., & Venables, P. H. (1980). *Techniques in psychophysiology.* Chichester: Wiley.
Stern, R. M., Ray, W. J., & Davis, C. M. (1980). *Psychophysiological recording.* New York: Oxford University Press.

PART I

Foundations

Section A: Conceptual foundations
Section B: Biological foundations

1 *Psychophysiology and psychophysiological inference*

JOHN T. CACIOPPO AND LOUIS G. TASSINARY

> Nothing could be more obvious than that the earth is stable and unmoving, and that we are the center of the universe. Modern Western science takes its beginning from the denial of this commonsense axiom...Common sense, the foundation of everyday life, could no longer serve for the governance of the world. When "scientific" knowledge, the sophisticated product of complicated instruments and subtle calculations, provided unimpeachable truths, things were no longer as they seemed.
> (Boorstin, 1983, p. 294)

1.1   INTRODUCTION

Psychophysiology concerns the study of cognitive, emotional, and behavioral phenomena as related to and revealed through physiological principles and events. As a discipline, psychophysiology not only addresses fundamental questions regarding human processes (e.g., mind–body relationships, organismic–environmental transactions, psychosomatic disorders), but also provides a conceptual perspective and a methodological armamentarium that cuts across aspects of the biological, behavioral, and social sciences.

Two cardinal postulates underlying the discipline are that physiological processes, subjective experience, and overt actions all harbor information about human nature and each of these domains also contains irrelevant data, artifacts, and misinformation. Consequently, knowledge regarding physiological mechanisms, biometric and psychometric properties, and experimental design is important in extracting veridical information about human nature. Consistent with this perspective, verbal reports as the standard of validity are challenged, reductionism as being the idealized endpoint in studies of human nature is rejected, and overt behavior as the optimally sensitive or discriminable measure of underlying processes is questioned.

Consider, for instance, the human eye – a sensory receptor that is sensitive to only a narrow band of the electromagnetic spectrum. One *could* refer to this limited band of electromagnetic energy as the "psychological" domain since electromagnetic phenomena falling within this band have clear and obvious effects on human experience. However, the visible light band is but a small part of a broader, coherent spectrum of electromagnetic energy that can also influence human experience and behavior and can be revealed through the use of specialized equipment to extend the reaches of the human senses. Reference to the portion of the electromagnetic spectrum to which our eyes respond as "visible" rather than "psychological," therefore, more accurately denotes the existence of a broader electromagnetic spectrum and the interaction between this stimulus and a

3

particular information detection and processing mechanism. Note, too, that the existence and broader organization of the electromagnetic spectrum and its various effects on the behavior of humans and animals would not be comprehensible if observations were limited to the band of visible light.

Similarly, psychophysiologists often utilize specialized equipment to study the spectrum of physiological events that allow functional descriptions and, in some instances, influence the operation of systems underlying human experience and behavior. To illustrate, consider the following sampler of psychophysiological research.

A neonate too young to comprehend or control purposeful behavior nevertheless exhibits heart rate responses when new or significant stimuli are presented; variations in this procedure reveal the attentional processes of neonates can be tracked using tracings produced by an electrocardiogram (Graham & Jackson, 1970).

A young individual sleeping quietly with eyes closed periodically shows extended sequences of rapid eye movements, as assessed by electrooculography; awakening the individual during this period usually reveals the person was dreaming (Foulkes, 1962).

A student sits quietly as auditory tones are presented through headphones; averaging of the electroencephalographic recordings time-locked to these tones reveals a larger brain potential is evoked approximately 300 ms following unexpected tones, in contrast to those expected (Squires, Wickens, Squires, & Donchin, 1976).

A college student, during a moment of self-disclosure, reflects briefly on an unpleasant experience; minute muscle action potentials, detectable using electromyography, mark this emotional event despite the person neither speaking about nor showing visible signs of the unpleasant thought or feeling (Cacioppo, Martzke, Petty, & Tassinary, 1988).

A suspect in a criminal case is questioned about evidence found at the scene of the crime; although the suspect denies knowing anything about the crime, physiological reactions are repeatedly more pronounced when information associated with the crime is presented than when equally provocative information not associated with the crime is presented (Lykken, 1981).

Married couples engage in a conflict conversational interaction while general autonomic activity is monitored; the higher the autonomic responses observed in this conflict interaction, the lower the marital satisfaction three years later (Levenson & Gottman, 1985).

An elderly individual who has bilateral occipitotemporal brain damage no longer seems to recognize her spouse or other familiar people; yet electrodermal activity is heightened when their pictures are presented (Tranel & Damasio, 1985).

An underlying theme in each of these studies is that the stimuli, thoughts, emotions, and experiences that are apparent to or can be articulated by the individual may represent but a narrow band of influences relevant to the governance of human experience and behavior. It should not be surprising, then, that psychophysiological research has provided insights into almost every facet of human nature, from the attention and behavior of the neonate to memory and emotions in the elderly. This book is about these insights and advances – what they are, the methods by which they came about, and the conceptualizations that are guiding progress toward future advances in the discipline.

Historically, the study of psychophysiological phenomena has been susceptible to "easy generalizations, philosophical pitfalls, and influences from extrascientific quarters" (Harrington, 1987, p. 5). Our objectives in this chapter, therefore, are to define the area of research and theory referred to as psychophysiology, review briefly major historical events in the evolution of psychophysiological inference, outline a taxonomy of logical relationships between psychological constructs and physiological events, and specify a scheme for strong inference within each of the specified classes of psychophysiological relationships. Additional information about the history, foundations, principles, techniques, and theories of psychophysiology is provided in the subsequent chapters of this book.

1.2   THE CONCEPTUALIZATION OF PSYCHOPHYSIOLOGY

> The body is the medium of experience and the instrument of action. Through its actions we shape and organise our experiences and distinguish our perceptions of the outside world from sensations that arise within the body itself. (Miller, 1978, p. 14)

Anatomy, physiology, and psychophysiology are all branches of science organized around bodily systems whose collective aim is to elucidate the structure and function of the parts of and interrelated systems in the human body in transactions with the environment. Anatomy is the science of body structure and the relationships among structures. Fields of study within this discipline include surface anatomy (the study of the form and markings of the surface of the body), gross anatomy (the study of structures that can be examined without a microscope), systemic anatomy (the study of specific systems of the body such as the nervous or cardiovascular systems), and developmental anatomy (the study of structural development from the fertilized egg to the adult form) (Solomon & Phillips, 1987).

Physiology concerns the study of bodily function or how the parts of the body work. What constitutes a body part in physiology varies with the level of bodily organization going from the chemical (e.g., actin, myosin) to cellular (e.g., muscle fiber) to tissue (e.g., striated muscle) to organ (e.g., biceps) to body system (e.g., muscular system) to the human organism (Figure 1.1). Thus, the anatomy and physiology of the body are intricately interrelated.

Fundamental to the conceptualization of psychophysiology are the assumptions that (1) human perception, thought, emotion, and action are embodied phenomena and (2) the responses of this corporeal body can help reveal the mechanisms underlying human nature. Psychophysiology, therefore, is also intimately related to anatomy and physiology but is concerned with what might be termed supraphysiological or psychological phenomena – the experience and behavior of organisms in the physical and social environment – rather than with the structure or function of body parts per se (see Figure 1.1). Among the complexities added when moving from physiology to psychophysiology are the capacity by symbolic systems of representation (e.g., language, mathematics) to communicate and to reflect upon history and experience and the social and cultural influences on physiological response and behavior. Both of these contribute to plasticity, adaptability, and variability in behavior (Cacioppo, 1982; Gale & Edwards, 1983). And although psychology and psychophysiology share the goal of explaining human experience and behavior, physiological constructs and processes are an integral component of theoretical thinking in psychophysiology.

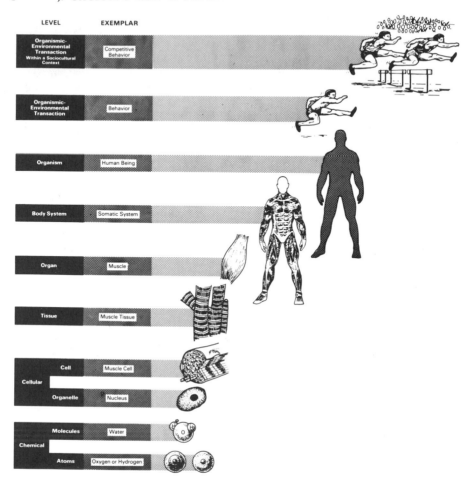

LEVEL   EXEMPLAR

Organismic-
Environmental
Transaction   Competitive
Within a Sociocultural   Behavior
Context

Organismic-
Environmental   Behavior
Transaction

Organism   Human Being

Body System   Somatic System

Organ   Muscle

Tissue   Muscle Tissue

Cell   Muscle Cell
Cellular
Organelle   Nucleus

Molecules   Water
Chemical
Atoms   Oxygen or Hydrogen

Figure 1.1. Levels of structural organization underlying human behavior.

1.2.1   *Psychophysiology as a scientific field of study*

Psychophysiology is still quite young as a scientific discipline although the concept of such a discipline dates back at least 150 years (Adams, 1839). Studies conducted around the turn of the century can be found involving the manipulation of a psychological factor and the measurement of one or more physiological responses (e.g., Berger, 1929; Darrow, 1929; Eng, 1925, Jacobson, 1930; Mosso, 1896; Peterson & Jung, 1907; Sechenov, 1878; Tarchanoff, 1890; see also, Troland, 1929–1932; Woodworth, 1938/1947), and such studies would now be considered as falling squarely under the rubric of psychophysiology. Chester Darrow (1964), in the inaugural Presidential Address of the Society for Psychophysiological Research, identified Darwin (1872/1873), Vigoroux (1879), James (1884), and Féré (1888/1976) as among the Field's earliest pioneers. Yet the first scientific periodical devoted exclusively to psychophysiological research, *Psychophysiology Newsletter*, was not begun until 1955 as an outgrowth of *Polygraph Newsletter* (Ax, 1964a). The Society for

Psychophysiological Research was formed 5 years later, and the first issue of the scientific journal *Psychophysiology* was published but a quarter century ago. When precisely psychophysiology emerged as a discipline, therefore, is difficult to specify, but it is usually identified with the formation of the Society for Psychophysiological Research in 1960 or with the publication of the first issue of *Psychophysiology* in 1964 (Fowles, 1975; Greenfield & Sternbach, 1972; Sternbach, 1966). Scientific organizations for psychophysiological research have since been established around the world, including Great Britain, Japan, Australia, and West Germany.

The formation of this international society and journal brought together scientists from diverse fields including physiology, neurology, electrical engineering, experimental psychology, clinical psychology, neurophysiology, psychiatry, and social and developmental psychology (e.g., Cacioppo & Petty, 1981; Kaplan & Bloom, 1960; Porges & Coles, 1976). The diverse goals and interests of these individuals, the technical obstacles confronting the early investigators, and the importance of understanding the physiological systems underlying their observations fostered a partitioning of the discipline into physiological measurement areas.

The organization of psychophysiology in terms of underlying physiological systems, or what can be called *systemic psychophysiology*, remains important today both for theoretical and pedagogical reasons. Physiological systems provide the foundation for information processing and behavior and are often the target of systematic observation. Hence, an understanding of the physiological system(s) under study and the biological principles underlying the responses being measured is important not only for the discrimination of signal from artifact, the safety of the individuals involved, and the acquisition and analysis of digital arrays and descriptive parameters that are reliable and valid representations of the physiological events of interest, but also for the stimulation of plausible hypotheses, the development of appropriate operationalizations, the guidance of inferences based on physiological data, and consequently, the advancement of theory regarding human nature.

Like anatomy, physiology, and psychology, however, psychophysiology is a broad science organized in terms of a *thematic* as well as a *systemic* focus. For instance, *cognitive psychophysiology* concerns the relationship between elements of human information processing and physiological events. *Social psychophysiology* concerns the study of the cognitive, emotional, and behavioral effects of human association as related to and revealed through physiological measures, including the reciprocal relationship between physiological and social systems. *Developmental psychophysiology* deals with developmental changes in psychophysiological relationships as well as the study of psychological development and aging through noninvasive physiological measurements. *Clinical psychophysiology* concerns the study of disorders in the organismic–environmental transactions and ranges from the assessment of disorders to interventions and treatments of the disorders. And *applied psychophysiology* deals with the implementation of psychophysiological principles in practice, such as operant training ("biofeedback"), desensitization, relaxation, and lie-detection procedures.

In each of these areas, the focus of study draws on but goes beyond the description of the structure or function of cells or organs to investigate the organism in transactions with the physical or sociocultural environment. Some of these areas, such as developmental psychophysiology, have counterparts in anatomy and physiology but refer to complementary empirical domains (see Figure 1.1). Others, such as social psychophysiology, have no direct counterpart in anatomy or physiology because the focus begins beyond that of an organism in isolation; yet the influence of social and cultural factors on physiological structures and functions, and their influence as moderators of the effects of physical stimuli on physiological structures and functions, leaves little doubt as to the relevance of these factors to anatomy and physiology as well as to psychophysiology (e.g., see Barchas, 1976; Cacioppo & Petty, 1983, Cacioppo, Petty, & Andersen, 1988; Waid, 1984). In sum, whether organized in terms of a systemic or a thematic focus, psychophysiology can be conceptualized as a natural extension of anatomy and physiology in the scientific pursuit of understanding human nature.

1.2.2   *Physiological and psychological perspective*

We have suggested that psychophysiology is intimately related to anatomy and physiology, and further that knowledge of the physiological systems and responses under study contributes to both theoretical and methodological aspects of psycho-physiological research (see also, Coles, Donchin, & Porges, 1986; Parts II and III of this volume). Physiological or technical expertise alone, however, is no substitute for a well-conceived experimental design. As Coles, Gratton, and Gehring (1987) noted, knowledge of the physiological systems, although contributory, is logically neither necessary nor sufficient to ascribe psychological meaning to physiological responses. The ascription of psychological meaning to physiological responses ultimately resides in the quality of the experimental design and the psychometric properties of the measures (see Strube, chapter 2). For instance, although numerous aspects of the physiological basis of event-related brain potentials remain uncertain, functional relationships within specific paradigms have been established between elementary cognitive operations and components of these potentials by systemati-cally varying one or more of the former and monitoring changes in the latter (see Coles, Gratton, & Fabiani, chapter 13).

The point is not that either the physiological or the psychological perspective is preeminent, but rather that both are fundamental to psychophysiological inquiries; more specifically, that physiological and psychological perspectives are com-plementary. Inattention to the logic underlying psychophysiological inferences simply because one is dealing with observable physiological events is likely to lead either to simple and restricted descriptions of empirical relationships or to erroneous interpretations óf these relationships (e.g., see reveiw by Cacioppo, Petty, & Tassinary, 1989). Similarly:

an aphysiological attitude, such as is evident in some psychophysiological research, is likely to lead to misinterpretation of the empirical relationships that are found between psychophy-siological measures and psychological processes or states. (Coles et al., 1986, p. ix–x)

Thus, the joint consideration of physiological and functional perspectives reduces errors of operationalization, measurement, and inference, and, hence, enriches theory and research on human processes and behavior.

1.2.3   *Definitions of psychophysiology*

Thus far, we have discussed the major assumptions, levels of analysis, and goals of psychophysiology, and we have traced briefly the history of the field as a scientific discipline. Specifying a formal definition of psychophysiology is more difficult. Some of the initial definitions of psychophysiology were in operational terms such as research in which the polygraph was used, research published by workers in the field, and research on physiological responses to behavioral manipulations (cf. Furedy, 1983). Other early definitions were designed explicitly to differentiate psychophysiology from the older and more established field of physiological psychology by designating what was unique at that time about psychophysiological inquiries, such as the use of humans in contrast to animals as subjects, the manipulation of psychological or behavioral constructs rather than anatomical structures or physiological processes, and the measurement of physiological rather than behavioral responses (Stern, 1964). Illustrative definitions offered over the past several decades follow:

Psychophysiology...is our name for the science which starts with the facts learned by introspection, and seeks their determinants in the physical structures and processes of biological organisms. Its problem is solely that of determining the formal laws, or mathematical functions which hold between curious respective aspects of consciousness and of living matter. (Troland, 1929, p. 144)

Psychophysiology is the science which concerns the physiological activities which underlie or relate to psychic events. (Darrow, 1964, p. 4)

Psychophysiology is best defined by its goals and methods as they are described in the reports published by its research workers....The general goal of psychophysiology is to describe the mechanisms which *translate* between psychological and physiological systems of the organism....The progressive theme of psychophysiological method has been to extend measurement to more covert behavior with decreasing interference with the organism. (Ax, 1964b, p. 8)

Any research in which the dependent variable (the subject's response) is a physiological measure and the independent variable (the factor manipulated by the experimenter) a behavioral one. (Stern, 1964, p. 90)

Psychophysiology is the study of the interrelationships between the physiological and psychological aspects of behavior. It typically employs human subjects, whose physiological responses are usually recorded on a polygraph while stimuli are presented which are designed to influence mental, emotional, or motor behavior; and the investigator need not be a psychologist. (Sternbach, 1966, p. 3)

The field of psychophysiology is concerned with the measurement of physiological responses as they relate to behavior. (Andreassi, 1980, p. 3)

Psychophysiology is the study of psychological processes in the intact organism as a whole by means of unobtrusively measured physiological processes. (Furedy, 1983, p. 13)

Psychophysiology is the study of mental or emotional processes as revealed through involuntary physiological reactions that can be monitored in an intact subject. (Lykken, 1984, p. 175)

Psychophysiology as a scientific discipline is concerned with the theoretical and empirical relationships among bodily processes and psychological factors. (Ackles, Jennings, & Coles, 1985, p. ix)

In general terms, psychophysiology is the scientific study of the relationship between mental and behavioral activities and bodily events. (Surwillo, 1986, p. 3)

Psychophysiology...is characterized by an emphasis on human behavior as a complex system in which physiological responses, subjective experiences and overt behavior interact in complex ways such that to separate out any one of these aspects from the others is to severely limit the theoretical or practical value of any explanatory models that are developed. (Christie & Gale, 1987, p. 8)

As is apparent, there is disagreement regarding the definition of psychophysiology. A major problem in reaching a consensus has been the need to give the field direction and identity by distinguishing it from other scientific disciplines while not limiting its potential for growth. Operational definitions are unsatisfactory for they do not provide long-term direction for the field. Definitions of psychophysiology as studies in which psychological factors serve as independent variables and physiological responses serve as dependent variables distinghish it from fields such as physiological psychology but have been criticized for being too restrictive (Furedy, 1983; cf. Coles, 1988). For instance, such definitions exclude noninvasive studies of higher order mental processes in which physiological events serve as the independent/blocking variable and human experience or behavior serves as the dependent variable (e.g., the sensorimotor behavior associated with operantly conditioned or endogenous changes in cardiovascular or electroencephalographic activity), and studies comparing changes in physiological responses across known groups (e.g., the cardiovascular reactivity of offspring of hypertensive vs. normotensive parents). Moreover, psychophysiology and physiological psychology/psychobiology share goals, assumptions, experimental paradigms, and in some instances, databases but differ primarily in terms of the level of analysis (e.g., organismic–environmental vs. organ–cellular level) and, consequently, the experimental strategy *typically* employed (e.g., noninvasive–reversible vs. invasive–irreversible experimental procedures). These fields clearly have a great deal to contribute to one another, and ideally this complementarity should not be masked in their definition by the need to distinguish these fields (e.g., see Johnson & Anderson, chapter 8).

The emergence of areas of research in psychoneuroendocrinology (e.g., Baum, Grunberg, & Singer, 1982; Frankenhauser, 1983; Mason, 1972), behavioral neurology (e.g., Lindsley, 1951; Tranel & Damasio, 1985; Tranel, Fowles, & Damasio, 1985; see Matsumoto, Walker, Walker, & Hughes, chapter 3), and psychoneuroimmunology (e.g., Ader, 1981; Henry & Stephens, 1977; Jemmott & Locke, 1984; Kiecolt-Glaser et al., 1984; see Kennedy, Glaser, & Kiecolt-Glaser, chapter 6) raises additional questions about how to define the discipline of psychophysiology. Importantly, anatomy and physiology encompass the fields of neurology, endocrinology, and immunology due both to their common goals and assumptions and to the embodiment, in a literal sense, of the nervous, endocrine, and immunological systems within the organism. Given the parallels among anatomy, physiology, and psychophysiology outlined in the preceding, however, psychophysiology should be defined in terms that accommodate its early focus on the actions of the nervous system as well as more recent psychological and behavioral studies involving neural, endocrinological, and immunological systems and the interactions among these systems.

To summarize, psychophysiology is based on the assumptions that human perception, thought, emotion, and action are embodied phenomena and that the physical responses of the corporeal body, in an appropriate experimental design, can shed light on human nature. The level of analysis in psychophysiology is not on isolated components of the body, but rather on organismic–environmental transactions, with reference to both physical and sociocultural environments.

Psychophysiology can therefore be defined as the scientific study of social, psychological, and behavioral phenomena as related to and revealed through physiological principles and events. In this way, a hierarchy is formed in which anatomy is concerned with bodily structure, physiology with bodily functions, and psychophysiology with organismic–environmental transactions (see Figure 1.1).

In the following section, we review some of the major historical developments that have contributed to contemporary thought in psychophysiology. As might be expected from the discussion thus far, many of these early developments have stemmed from studies of human anatomy and physiology.

1.3 HISTORICAL DEVELOPMENT

We often think, naively, that missing data are the primary impediments to intellectual progress – just find the right facts and all problems will dissipate. But barriers are often deeper and more abstract in thought. We must have access to the right metaphor, not only the requisite information. Revolutionary thinkers are not, primarily, gatherers of facts, but weavers of new intellectual structures. (Gould, 1985, Essay 9)

Although psychophysiology as a formal discipline is only about 30 years old, awareness of and interest in interrelationships between psychological and physiological events can be traced as far back as the early Egyptians and Greek philosopher-scientists. The Greek philosopher Heraclitus (c. 600 B.C.) referred to the mind as an overwhelming space whose boundaries could never be fully comprehended (Bloom, Lazerson, & Hofstadter, 1985). Plato suggested that rational faculties were located in the head; passions were located in the spinal marrow and, indirectly, the heart; and instincts were located below the diaphragm where they influenced the liver. Plato also believed the psyche and body to be fundamentally different; hence, observations of physiologial responses provided no grounds for inference about the operation of psyche (Stern, Ray, & Davis, 1980). Thus, despite the fact that the peripheral and central nervous system, brain, and viscera were known to exist as anatomical entities by the early Greek scientist-philosophers, human nature was dealt with as a noncorporate entity unamenable to empirical study. The classification of observations instead tended to be along qualitative lines without measurement, empirical assessment, or validation.

In the second century A.D., Galen (c. 130–200) formulated a theory of psychophysiological function that would dominate thought well into the eighteenth century (Brazier, 1959, 1961; Wu, 1984). Hydraulics and mechanics were the technology of the times, and aqueducts and sewer systems were the most notable technological achievements during this period. Bloom et al. (1985, p. 13) suggest: "It is hardly by accident, then, that Galen believed the important parts of the brain to lie not in the brain's substance, but in its fluid-filled cavities." Based on his animal dissections and his observations of the variety of fluids that permeated the body, Galen postulated that humors (fluids) were responsible for all sensation, movement, thoughts, and emotion; and that pathologies – physiological or behavioral – were based on humoral disturbances. The role of bodily organs was to produce or process these humors, and the nerves, although recognized as instrumental in thought and action, were assumed to be part of a hydraulic system through which the humors traveled. Galen's views became so deeply entrenched in Western thought that they went practically unchallenged for almost 1500 years.

In the sixteenth century, Jean Fernel (1497–1558) published the first textbook on physiology, *De Naturali Parte Medicinae* (1542). According to Brazier (1959), this book was well received, and Fernel revised and expanded the book across numerous editions. The ninth edition of the book was retitled *Medicina*, and the first section was entitled "Physiologia." Although Fernel's categorization of empirical observations was strongly influenced by Galen's theory, the book "shows dawning recognition of some of the automatic movements which we now know to be reflexly initiated" (Brazier, 1959, p. 2). This represented a marked departure from traditional views that segregated the control of human action and the affairs of the corporeal world.

Studies of human anatomy during this period in history also began to uncover errors in Galen's descriptions (e.g., Vesalius, 1543/1947), opening the way for questions of his methods and of his theory of physiological functioning and symptomatology. Within a century, two additional events occurred that had a profound impact on the nature of inference in psychophysiology. In 1600, William Gilberd (1540 or 1544–1603) recognized a difference between electricity and magnetism and, more importantly, argued in his book, *Magnete*, that empirical observations and experiments should replace "the probable guesses and opinions of the ordinary professors of philosophy." Francis Bacon (1561–1626) took the scientific method a step further in *Novum Organum* (1620/1889), adding induction to observation and adding verification to inference. Brazier (1959) summarized the importance of this work as follows:

Scientists before him were content with performing an experiment in order to make an observation; from this observation a series of propositions would follow, each being derived from its predecessor, not by experiment but by logic. Bacon's contribution to scientific method was to urge, in addition, the rigorous application of a special kind of inductive reasoning proceeding from the accumulation of a number of particular facts to the demonstration of their interrelation and hence to a general conclusion. (p. 3)

Francis Bacon's formulation and subsequent work on the logic of scientific inference (cf. Platt, 1964; Popper, 1959/1968) led to the now familiar sequence underlying scientific inference: (1) devise alternative hypotheses; (2) devise a crucial experiment, with alternative possible outcomes, each of which will disfavor, if not exclude, one or more of the hypotheses; (3) execute the experiment to obtain a clean result; and (4) recycle to refine the possibilities that remain. Such a scheme was accepted quickly in the physical sciences, but traditional philosophical and religious views segregating human existence from worldly events slowed its acceptance in the study of human physiology, experience, and behavior (Brazier, 1977; Harrington, 1987; Mecacci, 1979).

William Harvey's (1578–1657) *De Motu Cordis* (1628/1941), not only represented the first major work to use these principles to guide inferences about physiological functioning, but it also disconfirmed Galen's principle that the motion of the blood in the arterial and venous systems ebbed and flowed independent of one another except for some leakage in the heart. Pumps were an important technological development during the seventeenth century, and Harvey perhaps drew on his observations of pumps in positing that blood circulated continuously through a circular system, pushed along by the pumping actions of the heart, and directed through and out of the heart by the one-way valves in each chamber of the heart. Galen, in contrast, had posited that blood could flow in either direction in the veins. To test these competing hypotheses, Harvey tied a tourniquet above the elbow of his arm just tight enough to prevent blood from returning to the heart through the veins but not so tight as to prevent blood from entering the arm through the arteries. The veins swelled below but not above the tourniquet, implying that the blood could be entering only through the arteries and exiting only through the veins (Miller, 1978). A variation on Harvey's procedure is used in contemporary psychophysiology to gauge blood flow to vascular beds (see Johnson & Anderson, chapter 8; Papillo & Shapiro, chapter 14).

During this period, which coincided with a burgeoning world of machines, the human eye was conceived as functioning like an optical instrument whose image was projected onto the sensory nerves of the retina; movement was thought to reflect the mechanical actions of passive balloonlike structures (muscles) inflated or deflated by the nervous fluids or gaseous spirits that traveled through canals in the nerves; and higher mental functions were still considered by many to fall outside the rubric of the physical or biological sciences (Bloom et al., 1985; Brazier, 1959; Harrington, 1987). The writings of René Descartes (1596–1650) reflect the presumed division between the mind and body. The actions of animals were viewed as reflexive and mechanistic in nature, as were most of the actions of humans. But humans alone, Descartes argued, also possess a consciousness of self and of events around them, a consciousness that, like the body, was a thing but, unlike the body, was not a thing governed by material principles or connections. This independent entity called mind, Descartes proposed, resides over volition from the soul's control tower in the pineal gland located at the center of the head:

The soul or mind squeezed the pineal gland this way and that, nudging the animal fluids in the human brain into the pores or values, "and according as they enter or even only as they tend to enter more or less into this or that nerve, they have the power of changing the form of the muscle into which the nerve is inserted, and by this means making the limbs move." (Jaynes, 1973, p. 172, paraphrasing and quoting from Descartes)

Shortly following Descartes' publication of *Traite de l'Homme* (c. 1633), Steno (1638–1686) noted several discrepancies between Descartes' dualistic and largely mechanistic characterization of human nature and the extant evidence about animal and human physiology. For instance, Steno noted that the pineal gland (the purported bridge between the worlds of the human mind and body) existed in animals as well as humans, that the pineal gland did not have the rich nerve supply implied by Descartes' theory, and that the brain was unnecessary for many animal movements (cf. Jaynes, 1973). Giovanni Borelli (1608–1679) disproved the notion that movement was motivated by the inflation of muscles by a gaseous substance in experiments in which he submerged a struggling animal in water, slit its muscles, and looked for the release of bubbles (Brazier, 1959). These observations were published posthumously in 1680, shortly after the suggestion by Francesco Redi that the shock of the electric ray fish was muscular in origin (Basmajian & DeLuca, 1985; Wu, 1984).

Despite the prevalent belief during this period that the scientific study of animal and human behavior could apply only to those structures they shared in common (Bloom et al., 1985; Harrington, 1987), the foundations laid by the great seventeenth-century scientist-philosophers encouraged students of anatomy and physiology in the subsequent century to discount explanatory appeals to the human soul or mind (Brazier, 1959). Consequently, experimental analyses of physiological events and psychological constructs (e.g., sensation, involuntary and voluntary action) expanded and inspired the application of technological advances to the study of psychophysiological questions. For instance, the microscope was employed (unsuccessfully) in the late seventeenth century to examine the prevalent belief that the nerves were small pipes through which nervous fluid flowed, and by 1849 Du Bois-Reymond provided evidence using the galvanometer of electrical charges from human muscles as a result of volitional muscle contraction.

According to Brazier (1959, 1977), that electricity might be the transmitter of nervous action was initially seen as unlikely because, drawing upon the metaphor of electricity running down a wire, there was believed to be insufficient insulation around the nerves to prevent a dissipation of the electrical signal. Luigi Galvani's (1737–1798) experiments on the effects of electricity on muscle contraction and the work that followed (see Cacioppo, Tassinary, & Fridlund, chapter 11) ultimately verified that neural signals and muscular actions were electrical in nature, that these electrical signals were the result of biochemical reactions within specialized cells, and that there was indeed some dissipation of these electrical signals through the body fluids that could be detected noninvasively at the surface of the skin. Specific advances during the nineteenth and twentieth centuries in psychophysiological theory and research are discussed in the remainder of this book. However, the stage had been set by these early investigators for the scientific study of psychophysiological relationships.[1]

1.4   PSYCHOPHYSIOLOGICAL RELATIONSHIPS AND
       PSYCHOPHYSIOLOGICAL INFERENCE

> We praise the "lifetime of study," but in dozens of cases, in every field, what was needed was not a lifetime but rather a few short months or weeks of analytical inductive inference.... We speak piously of taking measurements and making small studies that will "add another brick to the temple of science." Most such bricks just lie around the brickyard. (Platt, 1964, p. 351)

The importance of the development of more advanced recording procedures to scientific progress in psychophysiology is clear as previously unobservable phenomena are rendered observable. Less explicitly studied, but no less important, is the structure of scientific thought about psychophysiological phenomena. For instance, Galen's notions about psychophysiological processes persisted for 1500 years despite the availability for several centuries of procedures for disconfirming his theory in part because the structure of scientific inquiry had not been developed sufficiently (Brazier, 1959).

One important form of psychophysiological inference to emerge from the work of Francis Bacon (1620/1889) involves the identification of two or more hypotheses about some phenomenon, devising a set of conditions with alternative possible outcomes that will exclude one or more of the hypotheses, and establishing the conditions and collecting the observations while minimizing measurement error (cf. Platt, 1964; Popper, 1959/1968). If the data are consistent with only one of the theoretical hypotheses, then the alternative hypotheses with which the investigator began become less plausible. With conceptual replications to ensure the construct validity, replicability, and generalizability of such a result, a subset of the original hypotheses can be discarded, and the investigator recyles through this sequence. One weakness of this procedure is the myriad sources of variance in psychophysiological investigations and the stochastic nature of physiological events and, consequently, the sometimes poor replicability or generalizability of the results (cf. O'Connor, 1985). A second is the intellectual invention and omniscience that is required to specify *all* relevant alternative hypotheses for the phenomenon of interest. Because neither of these can be overcome with certitude, progress in the short term can be slow and uncertain. Adherence to this sequence provides grounds for strong inference in the long term, however (Platt, 1964).

Importantly, physiological responses are often of interest only to the extent that they allow one to index a psychological process or state. This is an important endeavor, but the sequence underlying psychophysiological inferences often violates the logic of hypothetico-deductive research because inferences about events in the psychological domain are not based so much on the exclusion of alternative hypotheses as on reasoning by analogy. In a typical example, a physiological response is identified that is affected by variations in the psychological process of interest. This physiological response is subsequently monitored, perhaps in yet a different assessment context, in an effort to determine the likely presence or extent of the psychological process of interest (see review by Cacioppo & Petty, 1986). In an illustrative study, subjects were exposed to moderately or highly counterattitudinal assertions while electrodermal activity was monitored (Cooper, 1959). Results revealed greater changes in electrodermal activity following exposure to the highly counterattitudinal assertions. Based on prior research showing that emotionally arousing stimuli are associated with increased electrodermal activity, the higher electrodermal responding to highly rather than moderately counterattitudinal assertions was interpreted as meaning that more extreme attitudes were imbued with greater emotion. That is, electrodermal activity appeared *as if* an emotionally arousing stimulus had been presented. The problem with this form of psychophysiological inference is that knowledge that a statement is true (e.g., the manipulation of a psychological factor leads to a change in some target physiological response) does *not* imply that the converse is true. For instance, the prior research showing that factors other than emotional arousal can influence electrodermal activity (e.g., novelty stimulus significance; see Dawson, Schell, & Filion, chapter 10) was not considered. The logical flaw in this form of psychophysiological inference is termed the affirmation of the consequent (Runes, 1961; cf. Cacioppo, Petty, & Losch, 1986).

This need not be the case, however. In this section, we present a general framework for thinking about relationships between psychological concepts and physiological events, and we discuss the rules of evidence for and the limitations to inference in each (see also, Cacioppo & Tassinary, 1989).

1.4.1 *A simple taxonomy of psychophysiological relationships*

1.4.1.1 *Elements in the psychological and elements in the physiological domains*

A useful way to construe the potential relationships between psychological events and physiological events is to consider these two groups of events as representing independent sets (domains), where a set is defined as a collection of elements who together are considered a whole. Psychological events are conceived as constituting one set, which we shall call set Ψ, and physiological events are conceived as constituting another, which we shall call set Φ (Troland, 1929, p. 144–145).[2] Inspection of Figure 1.2 (upper left panel) reveals that all elements in the set of

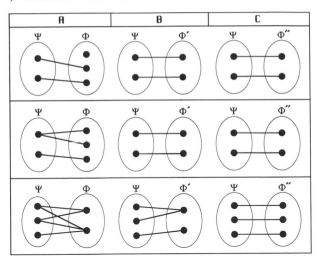

Figure 1.2. Depiction of logical relations between elements in the psychological (Ψ) and physiological (Φ) domains. *Panel A:* Links between psychological elements and individual physiological responses. *Panel B:* Links between psychological elements and physiological response patterns. *Panel C:* Links between psychological elements and profile of physiological responses across time.

psychological events are assumed to have some physiological referent, reflecting our adherence to the monistic identity thesis (i.e., the first assumption underlying psychophysiology).[3]

Focusing first on the top row of Figure 1.2, the existence of psychologically irrelevant physiological events (e.g., random physiological fluctuations; increased electrodermal activity due to minor variations in body temperature) is of importance in psychophysiology for purposes of artifact prevention or elimination. However, such elements within the physiological domain can be ignored if nonpsychologic factors have been held constant, their influence on the physiological responses of interest has been identified and removed, or it does not overlap with the physiological event of interest. These objectives are achieved through the application of proper psychophysiological recording techniques (which are discussed in detail in part III of this book). The important point here is that the achievement of these objectives simplifies the task of specifying psychophysiological relationships, in the ideal case, by eliminating physiological events that have no direct relevance to psychological events (e.g., see Figure 1.2, top row of panel B).

We can now state five general relations that might be said to relate the elements within the domain of psychological events, Ψ, and elements within the domain of physiological events, Φ (see Figure 1.3). These are as follows:

1 A one-to-one relation, such that an element in the psychological set is associated with one and only one element in the physiological set, and vice versa.
2 A one-to-many relation, meaning that an element in the psychological domain is associated with a subset of elements in the physiological domain.
3 A many-to-one relation, meaning that two or more psychological elements are associated with the same physiological element.

Psychophysiological   Domain
Relationship   Ψ   Φ

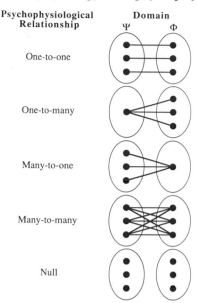

One-to-one

One-to-many

Many-to-one

Many-to-many

Null

Figure 1.3. Possible relationships between elements in the psychological domain (Ψ) and elements in the physiological domain (Φ).

4 A many-to-many relation, meaning two or more psychological elements are associated with the same (or an overlapping) subset of elements in the physiological domain.

5 A null relation, meaning there is no association between an element in the psychological domain and that in the physiological domain.[4]

Of these possible relations, only the first and second allow a formal specification of psychological elements as a function of physiological elements (cf. Coombs, Dawes, & Tversky, 1970, pp. 351–371). This is important because, as we have noted, psychophysiological research typically involves the manipulation of (or blocking on) elements in the psychological domain and the measurement of elements in the physiological domain. The grounds for inductive reasoning in psychophysiology, therefore, can be strengthened if a way can be found to specify the relationship between the elements within Ψ and Φ in terms of a one-to-one relationship. Although somewhat involved, this is often possible.

1.4.1.2 *Physiological elements as spatial and temporal response profiles*

First, a one-to-one relation can exist, such that an element in the psychological set is associated with one and only one element in the physiological set. Such relationships provide strong grounds for inference but are not common cross-situationally at present in psychophysiology (e.g., see Coles et al., 1987; Donchin, 1982). The functional opposite of the one-to-one relation is the null relation, which means that the element in the physiological domain is unrelated to and, hence, harbors no information about the element in the psychological domain.

  A third form of relation between elements in the psychological and physiological domains is the one-to-many, meaning that an element in the psychological domain is associated with a subset of elements in the physiological domain. Importantly, one-to-many relations between sets of psychological and physiological elements can be simplified greatly, reducing them to one-to-one relations, in the following fashion: Define a second set of physiological elements, Φ', such that any subset of physiological elements associated with the psychological element is replaced by a single element in Φ', which now represents a physiological syndrome or response pattern. Thus, one-to-one and one-to-many relations between elements in the psychological domain, Ψ, and the elements in the physiological domain, Φ, both become one-to-one relations between Ψ and Φ' (see Figure 1.2, middle row).

The remaining relations that can exist between elements in these domains are the many-to-one, meaning that two or more psychological elements are associated with the same physiological element; and the many-to-many, meaning two or more psychological elements in Ψ are associated with two or more of the same elements in Φ (see Figure 1.2, lower row of panel A). These relations can also be simplified with a few changes in how one conceptualizes an element in the physiological domain.

As before, a new set of physiological elements, Φ', is defined such that any subset of physiological elements associated with one or more psychological elements is replaced by a new element representing a profile of physiological responses. Thus, the elements in Φ' again represent a specific pattern or syndrome of physiological events, and many-to-many relations between elements in Ψ and Φ can be reduced to many-to-one (or, in some cases, to one-to-one) relations by viewing elements within the physiological domain as representing singular physiological responses and physiological response syndromes.

Such a reconceptualization may not be sufficient to cast *all* of the psychophysiological relations of interest in terms of one-to-one or many-to-one relations, however. This may still not be a problem because the set of physiological elements Φ' can be redefined again such that the *forms* of physiological events as they unfold over time are also considered to yield yet another set of physiological elements, Φ'' (see Figure 1.2, panel C; cf. Cacioppo, Marshall-Goodell, & Dorfman 1983). By including temporal (as well as spatial) information regarding the physiological events in the definition of the elements in Φ'', many complex psychophysiological relationships can be reduced to one-to-one or many-to-one relations (cf. Davis, 1957).[5]

1.4.1.3   *An illustration*

Consider the relationship between the orienting, defense, and startle responses as elements within the psychological domain, and changes in skin conductance response (SCR) and heart rate response (HRR) as elements within the physiological domain (see Stern & Sison, chapter 7, for a discussion of the constructs of orienting, defense, and startle). For illustrative purposes, we have simplified the elements within Ψ to include only the constructs of orienting, defense, and startle, and we have simplified the elements with Φ to include only SCR and HRR (Figure 1.4, upper panel). Even with these simplifications, the illustration clearly reveals the obstacles to strong psychophysiological inference. All three elements within Ψ are associated with changes in skin conductance and heart rate. Thus, if elements in the physiological domain are defined as changes from basal levels of activity, then the relationship is many-to-many, and physiological events cannot be specified as a

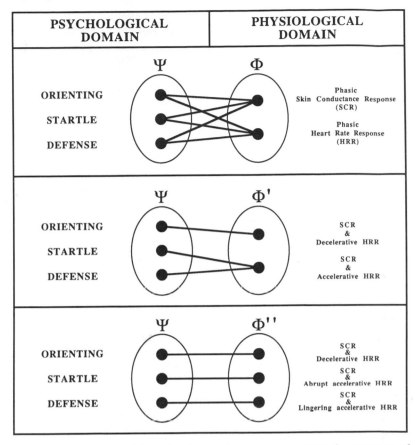

Figure 1.4. Depiction of logical relations between psychological constructs of orienting, startle, and defense and physiological measures of heart rate (HR) and skin conductance response (SCR). *Top panel:* Links between psychological elements and individual physiological responses. *Middle panel:* Links between psychological elements and physiological response pattern. *Bottom panel:* Links between psychological elements and profile of physiological responses across time.

function of psychological process (cf. Coombs et al., 1970). Accordingly, events in the physiological domain provide no basis for strong inferences about events in the psychological domain. For instance, although manipulations that are known to affect the intensity of the orienting reaction have differentiable effects on SCRs, it can be seen in Figure 1.4 that the SCR alone does not provide strong grounds for inferring an orienting response in this assessment context.

As noted, the grounds for psychophysiological inference are strengthened considerably if the spatial and temporal pattern of physiological events are considered. First, the set of physiological elements Φ is redefined such that any subset of physiological elements reliably associated with one (or more) psychological elements is replaced by a single, unique, element in Φ'. This reconceptualization of the elements constituting the physiological domain results in a one-to-one relation between the orienting reaction and physiological events; and a many-to-one relation between the concepts of startle and defense reactions and physiological events (see Figure 1.4, middle panel). The physiological events in this context can now be specified as a function of psychological elements, although the grounds for inference remain weak even in this simplified example when both increased HRR and SCR are observed.

Next, the set of physiological elements, Φ', are again redefined such that the form of the physiological responses as they unfold across time is considered. Returning to the example in Figure 1.4, both defense and startle are reliably associated with increased HRR and SCR (middle panel), but the HRR acceleration peaks and returns to normal within approximately 2 seconds in the case of startle but does not begin to rise for several seconds and peaks much later following the stimulus in the case of the defense response (Turpin, 1986). With this additional refinement in the conceptualization of psychophysiological relationships, strong inferences about which of these three psychological processes is operative can now be drawn from the associated physiological events (see Figure 1.4, bottom panel).

1.4.2   *Four categories of psychophysiological relationships*

Another complication in specifying psychophysiological relationships arises because relations between elements in the psychological and physiological domains cannot be assumed to hold across situations and individuals. This is simple to see in Figure 1.4. The elements in the psychological domain were delimited in part by holding constant other factors, such as wakefulness, general somatic activity, and the prestimulus level of physiological activity. Such a procedure is not unique to psychophysiology, as both psychological and medical tests can involve constructing specific assessment contexts in order to achieve interpretable results. The interpretation of a blood glucose test, for instance, can rest on the assumption that the individual fasted prior to the onset of the test. Only under this circumstance can the amount of glucose measured in the blood across time be used to index the body's ability to regulate the level of blood sugar (Guyton, 1971). The relationship between the physiological data and theoretical construct is said to have a *limited range of validity* because the relationship is clear only in certain well-prescribed assessment contexts (Cacioppo & Petty, 1985; Donchin, 1982). The notion of limited ranges of validity, therefore, raises the possibility that a wide range of complex relationships between psychological and physiological phenomena might be specifiable in simpler, more interpretable forms within specific assessment contexts (cf. Cacioppo et al., 1989).

To clarify these issues, it is useful to conceptualize psychophysiological relationships generally in terms of their *specificity* (one-to-one vs. many-to-one) and *generality* (context-bound vs. context-free) with the cells depicted in Figure 1.5 representing the four quadrants within this dimensional space. Causal attributes of these relationships, and whether the relationships are naturally occurring or artificially induced, constitute yet other orthogonal dimensions and are explicitly excluded here for didactic purposes. For instance, the quadrant in Figure 1.5 labeled "concomitant" refers only to the conditions and implications of covariation and is not intended to discriminate between instances in which the psychological factor is causal in the physiological response, vice versa, or a third variable causes both. In the sections that follow, each category of psychophysiological relationship and the nature of the inferences that each suggests are outlined.

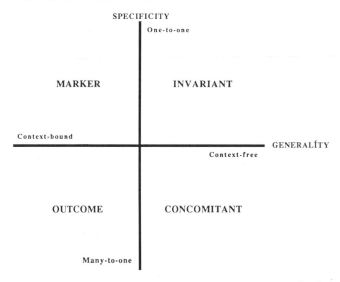

Figure 1.5. Dimensions and families of psychophysiological relationships.

1.4.2.1 *Outcomes*

In the idealized case, an outcome is defined as a many-to-one, situation-specific (context-bound) relationship between Ψ and Φ″ (see Figures 1.3 and 1.5). Establishing that a physiological response (i.e., an element in Φ″) varies as a function of a psychological change (i.e. an element in Ψ) means one is dealing at the very least with an outcome relationship between these elements. This is often the first attribute of a psychophysiological relationship that is established in laboratory practice. Whether the physiological response follows changes in the psychological event across situations (i.e., has the property of generality) or whether the response profile follows only changes in the event (i.e., has the property of specificity) is typically not possible to address initially. Hence, a given psychophysiological relationship may appear to be an outcome but subsequently be identified as being a marker as the question of specificity is examined; a relationship that appears to be an outcome may subsequently be reclassified as being a concomitant once the range of validity is examined; and a relationship that appears to be a marker (or concomitant) may emerge as an invariant upon studying the generalizability or specificity of the relationship. This progression is not problematic in terms of causing erroneous inferences, however, because any logical inference based on the assumption one is dealing with an outcome relationship holds for marker, concomitant, or invariant psychophysiological relationships as well.

This is because although the outcome is the most elemental psychophysiological relation, it can nevertheless provide the basis for strong inferences. Specifically, when two psychological models differ in predictions regarding one or more physiological outcomes, the logic of the experimental design allows theoretical inferences to be drawn based on psychophysiological outcomes alone. That is, a psychophysiological outcome enables systematic inferences to be drawn about psychological constructs and relationships based on hypothetico-deductive logic. Of course, no single operationalization of the constructs in a crucial experiment is likely to convince the adherents of both theories. If multiple operationalizations of the theoretical constructs result in the same physiological outcome, however, then strong theoretical inferences can be justified (Cacioppo & Petty, 1986).

Although the identification of a physiological response profile that is an outcome of the psychological element of interest is sufficient to infer the *absence* of this psychological element, it does not provide logical grounds to infer anything about the *presence* of the psychological element. Hence, the identification of psychophysiological outcomes can be valuable in disproving theoretical predictions, but this is insufficient when one aspires to physiological *indices* of elements in the psychological domain. This caveat is often noted in discussions of the scientific method and is perhaps equally often violated in scientific practice (Platt, 1964). Skin conductance, for instance, has been a major dependent measure in psychological research because emotional arousal is thought to lead to increased skin conductance (e.g., see Prokasy & Raskin, 1973). Similarly, electromyographic (EMG) activity over the forehead region has been a frequent target measure in relaxation biofeedback because tension has been found to increase EMG activity over this region (e.g., see Stroebel & Glueck, 1978). As noted in the previous section, however, simply knowing that manipulating a particular element in the psychological domain leads to a particular response in the physiological domain does not logically enable one to infer anything about the former based on observations of the latter because one does not know what other elements or events might bear an outcome relationship to the observed physiological response. Procedures such as holding constant and variations in the elements in the psychological domain that are not of interest, measuring these elements in addition to those of immediate theoretical interest to determine to which the observed changes in physiological response are likely to be attributable, and excluding those physiological responses believed to covary with these irrelevant elements all represent attempts to reduce many-to-one relationships to one-to-one relationships (i.e., going from psychophysiological outcomes to psychophysiological markers; see Figure 1.5). Such procedures clearly strengthen the grounds for psychophysiological inference, but they do not assure that all relevant factors have been identified or controlled, nor do they provide a means of quantifying the extent of other influences on psychophysiological responding.

These limitations can be further diminished by conceptualizing psychophysiological relationships in terms of conditional and joint probabilities (Cacioppo et al., 1988; Cacioppo & Tassinary, 1989). To illustrate, let Ψ represent the specific element of interest in the psychological domain (e.g., an emotional report) and Φ'' represent the physiological profile (e.g., facial EMG activity) of interest. It is clear from probability theory that $P(\Phi''/\Psi)$ could differ dramatically from $P(\Psi/\Phi'')$; perhaps less obvious is that this asymmetry is the root of many of the problems in psychophysiological inference outlined in the preceding. An outcome relation establishes $P(\Phi''/\Psi)$ (or, at least, that such a probability is nonzero); physiological indices of psychological events (i.e., markers, invariants), on the other hand, can be conceptualized rigorously as a statement about $P(\Psi/\Phi'')$, where

$$P(\Psi/\Phi'') = P(\Psi, \Phi'')/P(\Phi'') \qquad (1)$$

or, equivalently,

$$P(\Psi/\Phi'') = P(\Psi, \Phi'')/[P(\Psi, \Phi'') + P(\text{Not}-\Psi, \Phi'')] \qquad (2)$$

Although it is not possible to specify all relevant factors that might affect the element in the physiological domain one wishes to use to index an element in the psychological domain, it *is* possible to determine (both) the extent to which changes in the physiological element covary with changes in the psychological element of interest and the probability that changes in the physiological response occur in the absence of changes in the psychological construct of interest. As can be seen in equations 1 and 2, the utility of Φ'' to serve as an index of Ψ is weakened by the occurrence of Φ'' in the absence of Ψ. Conversely, the refinement of measures of Φ'' (e.g., through greater spatial and temporal resolution or through technological advances) is of scientific value to the extent that by doing so one reduces the likelihood of its observation in the absence of the psychological element of interest while leaving its observation in the presence of the psychological element of interest generally intact.

Consider, for example, what can be expected if the probability of a physiological element $\{P(\Phi'')\}$ is greater than the probability of the psychological element of interest $\{P(\Psi)\}$. Since this implies that $P(\Psi, \Phi'')/P(\Psi) > P(\Psi, \Phi'')/P(\Phi'')$, it can be seen from equation 1 that $P(\Phi''/\Psi) > P(\Psi/\Phi'')$ and, consequently, that research based only on outcome relationships leads to an overestimation of the presence of the psychological element.

We should emphasize that these probabilities are simply a way of thinking more rigorously about psychophysiological relations; one still needs to be cognizant that these relationships (e.g., probabilities) may vary across situations (e.g., assessment contexts). Indeed, comparisons of these probabilities across assessment contexts can provide a means of determining the generality of a psychophysiological relation. Before proceeding to this dimension of the two-dimensional space depicted in Figure 1.5, however, we elaborate further on psychophysiological relations within a specific assessment context when viewed within the framework of conditional and joint probabilities. In particular, as $P(\Psi, \Phi'')$ approaches 1.0 and $P(\text{Not}-\Psi, \Phi'')$ approaches 0.0 within a specific assessment context, the element in the physiological domain can be described as being an ideal marker of the element in the psychological domain.

1.4.2.2 *Markers*

In its idealized form, a psychophysiological marker is defined as a one-to-one, situation-specific (i.e., context-bound) relationship between abstract events Ψ and Φ'' (see Figures 1.3 and 1.5). The psychophysiological marker relation implies that the occurrence of one (usually a physiological response, parameter of a response, or profile of responses) predicts the occurrence of the other (usually a psychological event) within a given context. Thus, markers are characterized by limited ranges of validity. Such a relationship may reflect a natural connection between psychological and physiological elements in a particular measurement situation or it may reflect an artificially induced (e.g., classically conditioned) association between these elements (e.g., see Cacioppo & Sandman, 1981; Petty & Cacioppo, 1983; Tursky & Jamner, 1983). Importantly, minimal violations of isomorphism between Ψ and Φ'' within a given assessment context can nevertheless yield a useful (although imperfect) marker when viewed in terms of conditional probabilities.

Markers, like concomitants and invariants, can vary in their specificity. The more distinctive the form of the physiological response and/or the pattern of associated physiological responses, the greater is the likelihood of achieving a one-to-one relationship between the physiological events and psychological construct and the wider may be the range of validity of the relationship thereby achieved. This is because the utility of an element in Φ'' to index an element in Ψ is generally strengthened by defining the physiological element so as to minimize its occurrence in the absence of the element in the psychological domain.

In addition, a psychophysiological marker may simply signal the occurrence or nonoccurrence of a psychological process or event, possessing no information about the temporal or amplitude properties of the event in a specific assessment context. At the other extreme, a psychophysiological marker may be related in a prescribed assessment context to the psychological event by some well-defined temporal function such that the measure can be used to delineate the onset and offset of the episode of interest and/or it may vary in amplitude such that it emulates the intesnity of the psychological event.

In sum, markers represent a fundamental relationship between elements in the psychological and physiological domains that enables an inference to be drawn about the nature of the former given measurement of the latter. The major requirements in establishing a response as a marker are to (1) demonstrate that the presence of the target response reliably predicts the specific construct of interest, (2) demonstrate that the presence of the target response is insensitive to (e.g., uncorrelated with) the presence or absence of other constructs, and (3) specify the boundary conditions for the validity for the relationship. The term *tracer* can be viewed as synonymous with marker, for each refers to a measure so strictly associated with a particular organismic–environmental conditon that its presence is indicative of the presence of this condition. We turn next to a description of concomitants.

1.4.2.3   *Concomitants*

A psychophysiological concomitant (or correlate), in its idealized form, is defined as a many-to-one, cross-situational (context-free) association between abstract events Ψ and Φ'' (see Figures 1.3 and 1.5). That is, the search for psychophysiological concomitants assumes there is a cross-situational covariation between specific elements in the psychological and physiological domains. The assumption of a psychophysiological concomitant is less restrictive than the assumption of invariance in that one-to-one correspondence is not required, although the stronger the association between the elements in the psychological and physiological domains, the more informative tends to be the relationship.

Consider, for instance, the observation that pupillary responses vary as a function of individuals' attitudes toward visually presented stimuli, an observation that was followed by the conclusion that pupillary response is a *correlate* or *bidirectional index* of people's attitudes (Barlow, 1969; Hess, 1965; Metalis & Hess, 1982). However, evidence of variation in a target physiological response as a function of a manipulated psychological event establishes an outcome relation, which is necessary but insufficient for the establishment of a psychophysiological concomitant or correlate.

First, the manipulation of the same psychological element (e.g., attitudes) in another context (e.g., using auditory rather than visual stimuli) may alter or eliminate the covariation between the psychological and physiological elements because the latter is evoked either by a stimulus that had been fortuitously or intentionally correlated with the psychological element in the initial measurement context or by a noncriterial attribute of the psychological element that does not generalize across situations. For instance, the attitude–pupil size hypothesis has not been supported using nonpictorial (e.g., auditory, tactile) stimuli, where it has been possible to control the numerous light-reflex-related variables that can confound studies using pictorial stimuli (Goldwater, 1972). It is conceivable, therefore, that in several of the studies showing a statistical covariation between attitudes and pupillary response, the main luminance of subjects' selected fixations varied inversely with their attitudes toward the visual stimulus (see Janisee, 1977; Janisee & Peavler, 1974; Stern & Dunham, chapter 15; Woodmansee, 1970).

Second, the manipulation of the same psychological element in another situation may alter or eliminate the covariation between the psychological and physiological elements because the latter is evoked not only by variations in the psychological element but also by variations in one or more additional factors that are introduced in (or are a fundamental constituent of) the new measurement context. Tranel et al. (1985), for instance, recently demonstrated that the presentation of familiar faces (e.g., famous politicians, actors) evoked larger SCRs than did the presentation of unfamiliar faces. This finding and the procedure and set of stimuli employed were subsequently used in a study of patients with prosopagnosia (an inability to recognize visually the faces of persons previously known) to demonstrate that the patients can discriminate autonomically between the familiar and unfamiliar faces despite the absence of any awareness of this knowledge. Thus, the first study established a psychophysiological relationship in a specific measurement context, and the second study capitalized on this relationship. To conclude that a psychophysiological concomitant had been established between familiarity and SCRs, however, would mean that the same relationship would hold across situations and stimuli (i.e., relationship would be context independent). Yet ample psychophysiological research has demonstrated the opposite psychophysiological outcome specified by Tranel et al. (1985); that is, novel or unusual (i.e., unfamiliar) stimuli evoke larger SCRs than familiar stimuli (e.g., see Landis, 1930; Lynn, 1966; Sternbach 1966). Hence, the relation between stimulus familiarity and skin conductance does not constitute a psychophysiological concomitant.[6]

Unfortunately, evidence of faulty reasoning based on the premature assumption that one is dealing with a true psychophysiological concomitant (or invariant) is all too easy to find. Over half a century ago, Landis commented in his review of the psychological factors associated with electrodermal changes that:

I find in going through the literature that the psychogalvanic reflex has been elicited by the following varieties of stimuli ... sensations and perceptions of any sense modality (sight, sounds, taste, etc.), associations (words, thoughts, etc.), mental work or effort, attentive movements or attitudes, imagination and ideas, tickling, painful or nocive stimuli, variations in respiratory movements or rate, suggestion and hypnosis, emotional behavior (fighting, crying, etc.), relating dreams, college examinations, and so forth .... Forty investigators hold that it is specific to, or a measure of, emotion of the affective qualities; ten others state that it is not necessarily of an emotional or affective nature; twelve men hold that it is somehow to be identified with conation, volition, or attention, while five hold very definitely that it is nonvoluntary; twenty-one authorities state that it goes with one or another of the mental processes; eight state that it is the concomitant of all sensation and perception; five have called it an indicator of conflict and suppression; while four others have used it as an index of character, personality, or temperament. (Landis, 1930, p. 391)

The hinderances to scientific advances, it would seem, stem not only from obscure psychophysiological relationships, but also from difficulties in recognizing order and limitations to induction in complex psychophysiological relationships.

As in the case of a psychophysiological marker, the establishment of a psychophysiological concomitant logically allows an investigator to make a probability statement about the absence or presence (if not the timing and magnitude) of a particular element in the psychological domain when the target physiological element is observed. However, the strength of the inference in this case will be theoretically limited by the actual number and nature of elements in the psychological domain. In addition, it is important to emphasize that the estimate of the strength of the covariation used in such inferences should not come solely from evidence that manipulated or planned variations of an element in Ψ are associated with corresponding changes in an element in Φ''. Measurements of the physiological response each time the psychological element is manipulated (or changes) can lead to an overestimate of the strength of this relationship and, hence, to erroneous inferences about the psychological element based on the physiological response. As can be seen in equations 1 and 2, this overestimation occurs to the extent that there are changes in the physiological response not attributable to variations in the psychological element of interest. Hence, except when one is dealing with an invariant relationship, establishing that the manipulation of a psychological element leads cross-situationally to a particular physiological response or profile of responses is not logically sufficient to infer that the physiological event will be a strong predictor of the psychological element of interest; base rate information about the occurrence of the physiological event across situations must also be considered. This can be done in practice by quantifying the natural covariation between elements in the psychological and physiological domains and by examining the replicability of the observed covariation across situations.

1.4.2.4   *Invariants*

The idealized invariant relationship refers to a one-to-one (isomorphic), context-free (cross-situational) association (see Figures 1.3 and 1.5). To say that there is an invariant relationship, therefore, implies that (1) a particular element in Φ'' is present if and only if a specific element in Ψ is present, (2) the specific element in Ψ is present if and only if the corresponding element in Φ'' is present, and (3) the relation between Ψ and Φ'' preserves all relevant arithmetic (algebraic) operations. Moreover, only in the case of invariants does $P(\Psi/\Phi'') = P(\Phi''/\Psi)$, and $P(\text{Not} - \Psi, \Phi'') = P(\text{Not} - \Phi'', \Psi) = 0$. This means that the logical error of affirmation of the consequent is not a problem in psychophysiological inferences based on an invariant relation. Hence, the establishment of an invariant relationship between a pair of elements from the psychological and the physiological domains provides a strong basis for psychophysiological inference. Unfortunately, invariant relationships are often assumed rather than formally established, and as we have seen, such an approach leads to erroneous psychophysiological inferences and misleading theoretical "advances."

It has been suggested occasionally that the psychophysiological enterprise is, by its very nature, concerned with invariant relationships (e.g., see review by Cacioppo, Petty, & Tassinary, 1989). The search to establish one-to-one psychophysiological relationships is clearly important. As S. S. Stevens (1951) noted:

> The scientist is usually looking for invariance whether he knows it or not. Whenever he discovers a functional relation between two variables his next question follows naturally: under what conditions does it hold? In other words, under what transformation is the relation invariant? The quest for invariant relations is essentially the aspiration toward generality, and in psychology, as in physics, the principles that have wide application are those we prize. (p. 20)

It should be emphasized, however, that evidence for invariance should be gathered rather than assumed and that the utility of psychophysiological analysis does not rest entirely with invariant relationships. Without this recognition, the establishment of *any* dissociation between the physiological measure and psychological element of interest invalidates not only the purported psychophysiological relationship but also the utility of a psychophysiological analysis. However, as outlined in the preceding sections of this chapter and in the chapters that follow, psychophysiology need not be conceptualized as offering only mappings of context-free, one-to-one relationships to advance our understanding of human nature.

To summarize, the minimum assumption underlying the psychophysiological enterprise is that psychological and behavioral processes unfold as organismic–environmental transactions and, hence, have physiological manifestations, ramifications, or reflections. Although invariant psychophysiological relationships offer the greatest generality, physiological concomitants, markers, and outcomes also can provide important and sometimes otherwise unattainable information about elements in the psychological domain. In laboratory practice, the initial step is often to establish that variations in a psychological element are associated with a physiological change, thereby establishing that the psychophysiological relationship are, at least, an outcome. Knowledge that changes in an element in the psychological domain is associated with changes in a physiological response/profile assures neither that the response will serve as a marker for the psychological state (since the converse of a statement does not follow logically from the statement) nor that the response is a concomitant or invariant of the psychological state (since the response may occur in only certain situations or individuals or may occur for a large number of reasons besides changes in the particular psychological state). Nonetheless, both hypothetico-deductive reasoning and Bayesian analyses can provide a strong foundation for psychophysiological inferences about human nature.

1.5   CONCLUSION

Psychophysiology is based on the assumptions that human perception, thought, emotion, and action are embodied phenomena and that bodily responses contain information that in an appropriate experimental design can shed light on human nature. The level of analysis in psychophysiology is not on isolated components of the body but rather on organismic–environmental transactions, with reference to both physical and sociocultural environments. Psychophysiology, therefore like anatomy and physiology, is a branch of science organized around bodily systems whose collective aim is to elucidate the structure and function of the parts of and interrelated systems in the human body in transactions with the environment. Like psychology, however, psychophysiology is concerned with a broader level of inquiry than anatomy and physiology and can be organized in terms of both a thematic as well as a systemic focus. For instance, the social and inferential elements as well as the physical elements of psychophysiology are discussed in the chapters that follow.

The development of more advanced recording procedures is important to scientific progress, as previously contested predictions are resolved, previously unobservable phenomena are rendered tangible, and previously accepted conclusions are called into question. However, advanced recording procedures are not sufficient. The theoretical specification of a psychophysiological relationship necessarily involves reaching into the unknown and, hence, requires intellectual invention and systematic efforts to minimize bias and error. Psychological theorizing based on known physiological and anatomical facts, exploratory research and pilot testing, and classic biometric and psychometric approaches can each contribute in important ways by their generation of testable hypotheses about a psychophysiological relationship. It should be equally clear, however, that the scientific effectiveness of psychophysiological analyses does not derive logically from physiologizing or from the measurement of organismic rather than (or in addition to) verbal or chronometric responses. Its great value stems from the stimulation of interesting hypotheses and from the fact that when an experiment agrees with a prediction about orchestrated actions of the organism, a great many alternative hypotheses are usually excluded. There is little to be gained, for instance, by simply generating an increasingly lengthy list of "correlates" between psychological and physiological variables. To further theoretical thinking, therefore, we have outlined a taxonomy of psychophysiological relations, and we have suggested a scheme for strong inference based on these relationships. Among the questions this formulation can help to address are (a) how does one select the appropriate variable(s) for study, (b) how detailed or refined should be the measurement of the selected variables, (c) how can situational and individual variability in psychophysiological relationships be integrated into theoretical thinking about psychophysiological relationships, and (d) how can physiological measures be used in a rigorous fashion to index psychological factors. The ultimate value of the proposed way of thinking about psychophysiological relationships rests on its effectiveness in guiding psychophysiological inference, for as Leonardo Da Vinci (c. 1510) noted:

Experience does not ever err, it is only your judgment that errs in promising itself results which are not caused by your experiments.

NOTES

1 For additional detail, readers may also wish to consult the interesting historical accounts by Brazier (1959, 1977), Wu (1984), Jaynes (1973), Mecacci (1979), and Fulton (1926, ch. 1).
2 To simplify the illustration of how physiological responses can be used as a basis for strong inferences about elements in psychological domain, the physiological domain is co-extensive with the empirical domain and the psychological domain co-extensive with the theoretical domain in our discussions here. It should be emphasized, however, that which of these is the conceptual domain and which is the empirical may vary across psychophysiological inquiries. The relationships and formulas outlined in the text are based on the assumption that physiological measures are serving as indices of psychological elements. If the situation were reversed, then so, too, would be the relationships and formulas.

3 Briefly, the identity thesis states that there is a physical counterpart to every subjective or psychological event of (cf. Smart, 1959). Thus, the identity thesis is fundamental to tractable monistic philosophical solutions to the mind–body problem as well as to the scientific discipline of psychophysiology. Importantly, the identity thesis does *not* imply that the relationship between physical and subjective events is one-to-one (i.e., invariant). For example, with the context of psychophysiology, the identity thesis does not necessarily imply that the physiological representation will be one-to-one in that (a) there will be one and only one physiological mechanism able to produce a given psychological phenomenon; (b) a given psychological event will be associated with, or reducible to, a single isolated physiological response rather than a syndrome or pattern of responses; (c) a given relationship between a psychological event and a physiological response is constant across time, situations, or individuals; (d) every physiological response has specific psychological significance or meaning; or (e) the organization and representation of psychological phenomena at a physiological level will mirror what appears subjectively to be elementary or unique psychological operations (e.g., beliefs, memories, images). Given invariance cannot be assumed, psychophysiological inferences based on analogy can involve the commission of affirming the consequent (Cacioppo & Tassinary, 1989).

4 Both the many-to-many and the null relation may result in random scatterplots when measuring the natural covariation between elements in the psychological and physiological domains. These relations can be distinguished empirically, however, by manipulating the psychological factors and quantifying the change in physiological response (and vice versa). The scatterplot between this psychological factor and physiological response should remain random in the case of a null relation between them, but not if they are part of a many-to-many relation.

5 For the sake of brevity, the focus here is on reconceptualizing elements in the physiological domain to achieve a one to one psychophysiological relation. One can also consider analogous ways of reconceptualizing the elements in the psychological domain. In addition, measurement error and stochastic properties of physiological responding have been ignored for didactic purposes. Their inclusion does not change the framework outlined in the text but rather results in the fuzzy sets Ψ_F and Φ_F'', where elements (e.g., physiological response profiles) are defined in stochastic terms.

6 Nevertheless, the application of the psychophysiological outcome and assessment context developed by Tranel, Fowles, and Damasio (1985) in the study of prosopagnosics by Tranel and Damasio (1985) illustrates the scientific value of psychophysiological inquiries even when the relationship between elements in the psychological and physiological domains hold only within highly circumscribed assessment contexts.

REFERENCES

Ackles, P. K., Jennings, J. R., & Coles, M. G. H. (1985). *Advances in psychophysiology* (Vol. 1). Greenwich, CT: JAI Press.

Ader, R. (1981). *Psychoneuroimmunology.* New York: Academic Press.

Adams, S. (1839). Psycho-physiology, viewed in connection with the mysteries of animal magnetism and other hindred phenomena. *American Biblical Repository* (Second series, no. 2; whole no. 34), 362–382.

Andreassi, J. L. (1980). *Psychophysiology: Human behavior and physiological response.* New York: Oxford University Press.

Ax, A. F. (1964a). Editorial. *Psychophysiology, 1,* 1–3.

Ax, A. F. (1964b). Goals and methods of psychophysiology. *Psychophysiology, 1,* 8–25.

Bacon, F. (1889). *Novum organum* (T. Fowler, Trans.). (Originally published in 1620.)

Barchas, P. R. (1976). Physiological sociology: Interface of sociological and biological processes. *Annual Review of Sociology,* 299–333.

Barlow, J. D. (1969). Pupillary size as an index of preference in political candidates. *Perceptual and Motor Skills, 28,* 587–590.

Basmajian, J. V., & De Luca C. J. (1985). *Muscles alive: Their functions revealed by electromyography* (5th ed.). Baltimore: Williams & Wilkins.

Baum, A., Grunberg, N. E., & Singer, J. E. (1982). The use of psychological and neuroendocrinological measurements in the study of stress. *Health Psychology, 1,* 217–236.

Berger, H. (1929). Uber das elektrenkephalogramm des menschen [On the electroencephalogram of man]. *Archiv fur Psychiatrie und Nervenkrankheiten, 87,* 551–553. Reprinted in English in S. W. Porges & M. G. H. Coles (Eds.), *Psychophysiology.* Stroudsburg, PA: Dowden, Hutchinson, & Ross.

Bloom, F. E., Lazerson, A., & Hofstadter, L. (1985). *Brain, mind, and behavior.* New York: W. H. Freeman.

Boorstin, D. J. (1983) *The discoverers: A history of man's search to know his world and himself.* London: J. M. Dent & Sons.

Brazier, M. A. (1959). The historical development of neurophysiology. In J. Field (Ed.), *Handbook of physiology. Section I: Neurophysiology* (Vol. I, pp. 1–58). Washington DC: American Physiological Society.

Brazier, M. A. (1961). *A history of the electrical activity of the brain.* London: Pitman Medical Publishing.

Brazier, M. A. (1977). *Electrical activity of the nervous system* (4th ed.). Baltimore: Williams & Wilkins.

Cacioppo, J. T. (1982). Social psychophysiology: A classic perspective and contemporary approach. *Psychophysiology, 19,* 241–251.

Cacioppo, J. T., Marshall-Goodell, B. S., & Dorfman, D. D. (1983). Skeletal muscular patterning: Topographical analysis of the integrated electromyogram. *Psychophysiology, 20,* 269–283.

Cacioppo, J. T., Martzke, J. S., Petty, R. E., & Tassinary, L. G. (1988). Specific forms of facial EMG response index emotions during an interview: From Darwin to the continuous flow hypothesis of affect-laden information processing. *Journal of Personality and Social Psychology, 54,* 592–604.

Cacioppo, J. T., & Petty, R. E. (1981). Electromyograms as measures of extent and affectivity of information processing. *American Psychologist, 36,* 441–456.

Cacioppo, J. T., & Petty, R. E. (1983). *Social psychophysiology; A sourcebook.* New York: Guilford Press.

Cacioppo, J. T., & Petty, R. E. (1985). Physiological responses and advertising effect; Is the cup half full or half empty? *Psychology and Marketing, 2,* 115–126.

Cacioppo, J. T., & Petty, R. E. (1986). Social processes. In M. G. H. Coles, E. Donchin, & S. Porges (Eds.), *Psychophysiology: Systems, processes, and applications* (pp. 646–679). New York: Guilford Press.

Cacioppo, J. T., Petty, R. E., & Andersen, B. L. (1988). Social psychophysiology as a paradigm. In H. Wagner (Ed.), *Social psychophysiology: Theory and clinical applications* (pp. 273–294). London: Wiley.

Cacioppo, J. T., Petty, R. E., & Losch, M. E. (1986). Attributions of responsibility for helping and harmdoing: Evidence for confusion of responsibility. *Journal of Personality and Social Psychology, 50,* 100–105.

Cacioppo, J. T., Petty, R. E., & Tassinary, L. G. (1989). Social psychophysiology: A new look. *Advances in Experimental Social Psychology, 22,* 39–91.

Cacioppo, J. T., & Sandman, C. A. (1981). Psychophysiological functioning, cognitive responding, and attitudes. In R. E. Petty, T. M. Ostrom, & T. C. Brock (Eds.), *Cognitive responses in persuasion* (pp. 81–104). Hillsdale, NJ: Erlbaum.

Cacioppo, J. T., & Tassinary, L. G. (1989). The concept of attitude: A psychophysiological analysis. In H. Wagner & A. Manstead & Wagner (Eds.), *Handbook of psychophysiology: Emotion and social behaviour* (pp. 309–346). Chichester: Wiley.

Christie, B., & Gale, A. (1987). Introduction. In A. Gale & B. Christie (Eds.). *Psychophysiology and the electric workplace* (pp. 3–15). Chichester: Wiley.

Coles, M. G. H. (1988). Editorial. *Psychophysiology, 25,* 1–3.

Coles, M. G. H., Donchin, E., & Porges, S. W. (1986). *Psychophysiology: Systems, Processes, and applications.* New York: Guilford Press.

Coles, M. G. H., Gratton, G., & Gehring, W. J. (1987). Theory in cognitive psychophysiology. *Journal of Psychophysiology, 1,* 13–16.

Coombs, C. H., Dawes, R. M., & Tversky, A. (1970). *Mathematical psychology: An elementary introduction.* Englewood Cliffs, NJ: Prentice-Hall.

Cooper, J. B. (1959). Emotion and prejudice. *Science, 130,* 314–318.

Darrow, C. W. (1929). Differences in the physiological reactions to sensory and ideational stimuli. *Psychological Bulletin, 26,* 185–201.

Darrow, C. W. (1964). Psychophysiology, yesterday, today and tomorrow. *Psychophysiology, 1,* 4–7.

Darwin, C. (1873). *The expression of the emotions in man and animals.* New York: D. Appleton. (Original work published in 1872.)

Davis, R. C. (1957). Response patterns. *Transactions of the New York Academy of Science, 19,* 731–739.

Donchin, E. (1982). The relevance of dissociations and the irrelevance of dissociationism: A reply to Schwartz and Pritchard. *Psychophysiology, 19,* 457–463.

Eng, H. (1925). *Experimental investigation into the emotional life of the child compared with that of the adult.* London: Oxford University Press.

Féré, C. (1976). Notes on changes in electrical resistance under the effect of sensory stimulation and emotion. *Comptes Rendus des Séances de la Société de Biologie, 5,* 217–219 [Reprinted in English in S. W. Porges & M. G. H. Coles (Eds.), *Psychophysiology.* Stroudsburg, PA: Dowden, Hutchinson, & Ross]. (Original work published in 1888.)

Fernal, J. (1542). *De naturali parte medinae.* Paris: Simon de Colies. Cited in Brazier (1959).

Foulkes, D. (1962). Dream reports from different stages of sleep. *Journal of Abnormal and Social Psychology, 65,* 14–25.

Fowles, D. C. (1975). *Clinical applications of psychophysiology.* New York: Columbia University Press.

Frankenhauser, M. (1983). The sympathetic-adrenal and pituitary–adrenal response to challenge: Comparison between sexes. In T. Dembroski, T. Schmidt, & G. Blumchen (Eds.), *Biobehavioral bases of coronary heart disease* (pp. 91–105). Basel: Karger.

Fulton, J. F. (1926). *Muscular contraction and the reflex control of movement.* Baltimore: Williams & Wilkins.

Furedy, J. J. (1983). Operational, analogical and genuine definitions of psychophysiology. *International Journal of Psychophysiology, 1,* 13–19.

Gale, A., & Edwards, J. A. (1983). *Physiological correlates of human behaviour: Vol. 10. Basic issues.* London: Academic Press.

Goldwater, B. C. (1972). Psychological significance of pupillary movements. *Psychological Bulletin, 77,* 340–355.

Gould, S. J. (1985). *The flamingo's smile: Reflections in natural history.* New York: Norton.

Graham, F. K., & Jackson, J. C. (1970). Arousal systems and infant heart rate responses. In H. W. Rees & L. P. Lipsitt (Eds.), *Advances in child development and behavior.* New York: Academic Press.

Greenfield, N. S., & Sternbach, R. A. (1972). *Handbook of psychophysiology.* New York: Holt, Rinehart, & Winston.

Guyton, A. C. (1971). *Textbook of medical physiology* (4th ed.). Philadelphia: W. B. Saunders.

Harrington, A. (1987). *Medicine, mind, and the double brain: Study in nineteenth-century thought.* Princeton, NJ: Princeton University Press.

Harvey, W. (1941). *Exercitatio anatomica de motu cordis et sanguinis in animalibus.* Frankfurt: Fitzeri [Translated into English by Willius & Keys, Cardiac Classic. (Original work published in 1628.)

Henry, J. P., & Stephens, P. M. (1977). *Stress, health, and the social environment.* New York: Springer-Verlag.

Hess, E. H. (1965). Attitude and pupil size. *Scientific American, 212,* 46–54.

Jacobson, E. (1930). Electrical measurements of neuromuscular states during mental activities: III. Visual imagination and recollection. *Amercian Journal of Physiology, 95,* 694–702.

James, W. (1884). What is an emotion? *Mind, 9,* 188–205.

Janisee, M. P. (1977). *Pupillometry: The psychology of the pupillary response.* Washington, DC: Hemisphere.

Janisee, M. P., & Peavler, W. S. (1974). Pupillary research today: Emotion in the eye. *Psychology Today, 7,* 60–63.

Jaynes, J. (1973). The problem of animate motion in the seventeenth century. In M. Henle, J. Jaynes, & J. J. Sullivan (Eds.), *Historical conceptions of psychology* (pp. 166–179). New York: Springer.

Jemmott III, J. B. & Locke, S. E. (1984). Psychosocial factors, immunologic mediation, and human susceptibility to infectious diseases: How much do we know? *Psychological Bulletin, 95,* 78–108.

Kaplan, H. B., & Bloom, S. W. (1960). The use of sociological and social-psychological concepts in physiological research: A review of selected experimental studies. *Journal of Nervous and Mental Disease, 131,* 128–134.

Kiecolt-Glaser, J. K., Graner, W., Speicher, C. E., Penn, G. M., Holliday, J. E., & Glaser, R. (1984). Psychosocial modifiers of immunocompetence in medical students. *Psychosomatic Medicine, 46,* 7–14.

Landis, C. (1930). Psychology and the psychogalvanic reflex. *Psychological Review, 37,* 381–398.

Levenson, R. W., & Gottman, J. M. (1985). Physiological and affective predictors of change in relationship satisfaction. *Journal of Personality and Social Psychology, 49,* 85–94.

Lindsley, D. B. (1951). Emotion. In S. S. Stevens (Ed.), *Handbook of experimental psychology* (pp. 473–516). New York: Wiley.

Lykken, D. T. (1981). *A tremor in the blood: Uses and abuses of the lie detector.* New York: McGraw-Hill.

Lykken, D. T. (1984). Psychophysiology. In R. J. Corsini (Ed.), *Encyclopedia of psychology* (Vol. 3, pp. 175–179). New York: Wiley.

Lynn, R. (1966). *Attention, arousal, and the orientation reaction.* Oxford: Pergamon Press.

Mason, J. W. (1972). Organization of psychoendocrine mechanisms: A review and reconsideration of research. In N. S. Greenfield & R. A. Sternbach (Eds.), *Handbook of psychophysiology* (pp. 3–124). New York: Holt, Rinehart, & Winston.

Mecacci, L. (1979). *Brain and history: the relationship between neurophysiology and psychology in Soviet research.* New York: Brunner/Mazel.

Metalis, S. A., & Hess, E. H. (1982). Pupillary response/semantic differential scale relationships. *Journal of Research in Personality, 16,* 201–216.

Miller, J. (1978). *The body in question.* New York: Random House.

Mosso, A. (1896). *Fear* (E. Lough & F. Riesow, Trans.). New York: Longrans, Green.

O'Connor, K. (1985). The Bayesian-inferential approach to defining response processes in psychophysiology. *Psychophysiology, 22,* 464–479.

Peterson, F., & Jung, C. G. (1907). Psychophysical investigations with the galvanometer and pneumograph in normal and insane individuals. *Brain, 30,* 153–218.

Petty, R. E., & Cacioppo, J. T. (1983). The role of bodily responses in attitude measurement and change. In J. T. Cacioppo & R. E. Petty (Eds.), *Social psychophysiology: A sourcebook* (pp. 51–101). New York: Guilford Press.

Platt, J. R. (1964). Strong inference. *Science, 146,* 347–353.

Popper, K. R. (1968). *The logic of scientific discovery.* New York: Harper & Row. (Original work published in 1959.)

Porges, S. W., & Coles, M. G. H. (1976) *Psychophysiology.* Stroudsburg, PA: Dowden, Hutchinson, & Ross.

Prokasy, W. F., & Raskin, D. C. (1973). *Electrodermal activity in psychological research.* New York: Academic Press.

Runes, D. D. (1961). *Dictionary of philosophy: Ancient-Medieval-Modern. Patterson, NJ:* Littlefield, Adams.

Sechenov, I. M. (1965). *Elements of thought.* In R. J. Herrnstein & E. G. Boring (Eds.), *A source book in the history of psychology.* Cambridge MA: Harvard University Press. (Original work published in 1878.)

Smart, J. J. C. (1959). Sensations and brain processes. *Philosophical Review, 68,* 141–156.

Solomon, E. P., & Phillips, G. A. (1987). *Understanding human anatomy and physiology.* Philadelphia: Saunders.

Squires, K. C., Wickens, C. D., Squires, N. K., & Donchin, E. (1976). The effect of stimulus sequence on the waveform of the cortical event-related potential. *Science, 193,* 1142–1146.

Stern J. A. (1964). Toward a definition of psychophysiology. *Psychophysiology, 1,* 90–91.

Stern, R. M., Ray, W. J., & Davis, C. M. (1980). *Psychophysiological Recording.* New York: Oxford.

Sternbach, R. A. (1966). *Principles of psychophysiology.* New York: Academic Press.

Stevens, S. S. (1951). *Handbook of experimental psychology.* New York: Wiley.

Stroebel, C. F., & Glueck, B. C. (1978). Passive meditation: Subjective, clinical, and electrographic comparison with biofeedback. In G. E. Schwartz & D. Shapiro (Eds.), *Consciousness and self-regulation* (Vol. 2, pp. 401–428). New York: Plenum Press.

Surwillo, W. W. (1986). *Psychophysiology: Some simple concepts and models.* Springfield. Il: Charles C. Thomas.

Tarchanoff, J. (1976). Galvanic phenomena in the human skin during stimulation of the sensory organs and during various forms of mental activity. *Pflugers Archive Für die gesamte Physiologie des Menschen und der Tiere, 46,* 46–55. [Reprinted in English in S. W. Porges & M. G. H. Coles (Eds.), *Psychophysiology.* Stroudsburg, PA.: Dowden, Hutchinson, & Ross.] (Original work published in 1890.)

Tranel, D., & Damasio, A. R. (1985). Knowledge without awareness: An autonomic index of facial recognition by prosopagnosics. *Science, 228,* 1453–1454.

Tranel, D., Fowles, D. C., & Damasio, A. R. (1985). Electrodermal discrimination of familiar and unfamiliar faces: A methodology. *Psychophysiology, 22,* 403–408.

Troland, L. T. (1929). *The principles of psychophysiology: A survey of modern scientific psychology.* Vol. 1. *The problems of psychology and perception.* New York: D. Van Nostrand.

Troland, L. T. (1929–1932). *The principles of psychophysiology: A survey of modern scientific psychology* (vols 1–3). New York: D. Van Nostrand.

Turpin, G. (1986). Effects of stimulus intensity of autonomic responding: The problem of differentiating orienting and defense reflexes. *Psychophysiology, 23,* 1–14.

Tursky , B., & Jamner, L. D. (1983). Evaluation of social and political beliefs: A psychophysiological approach. In J. T. Cacioppo & R. E. Petty (Eds.), *Social psychophysiology: A sourcebook* (pp. 102–121). New York: Guilford Press.

Vesalius, A. (1947). *De humani corporis fabrica.* Basle: Oporinus. [Translated into English by J. B. de C. M. Saunders & C. D. O'Malley. New York: Schuman.] (Original work published in 1543.)

Vigoroux, R. (1879). Sur le rôle de la resistance électrique des tissues dans l'électro-diagnostic. *Comptes Rendus des Séances de la Société de Biologie, 31,* 336–339. Cited in Brazier (1959).

Waid, W. M. (1984). *Sociophysiology.* New York: Springer-Verlag.

Woodmansee, J. J. (1970). The pupil response as a measure of social attitudes. In G. F. Summers (Ed.), *Attitude measurement.* Chicago: Rand McNally.

Woodworth, R. S. (1947). *Experimental psychology.* New York: Henry Holt. (Original work published in 1938.)

Wu, C. H. (1984). Electric fish and the discovery of animal electricity. *American Scientist, 72,* 598–607.

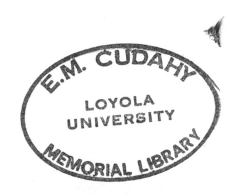

2 Psychometric principles: from physiological data to psychological constructs

MICHAEL J STRUBE

2.1 INTRODUCTION

One important use of physiological measures is to allow the linking of physical processes to psychological constructs. The theoretical and applied significance of this psychophysiological partnership has been amply demonstrated in such diverse research areas as coronary-prone behavior (for reviews, see Contrada, Wright, & Glass, 1985; Krantz, Glass, Schaeffer, & Davia, 1982; see also Krantz & Manuck, 1984; Matthews et al., 1986), low back pain (Dolce & Raczynski, 1985), the investigation of schizophrenia (Pritchard, 1986), the influence of perceived control and predictability on the experience of stress (e.g., Abbott & Badia, 1986; Abbott, Schoen, & Badia, 1984; Arthur, 1986; Miller, 1981; Thompson, 1981), individual and situational moderators of medical compliance (Cox, Taylor, Nowacek, Holley-Wilcox, Pohl, & Guthrow, 1984; Davis, Hess, Harrison, & Hiss, 1987), learning (Grossberg, 1982), and the investigation of numerous social and cognitive phenomena (e.g., Beatty, 1982; Cacioppo & Petty, 1981, 1983; Johnson, 1986; Näätänen, 1982; Pritchard, 1981). The full utility of physiological measurement for uncovering and clarifying important psychological processes rests, however, on careful attention to a number of psychometric issues. The purpose of this chapter is to provide a guide to the issues requiring attention when inferences about psychological constructs are based on collection of physiological data. In the discussion that follows, the core psychometric issues relevant to measurement in any area will be outlined, but with an emphasis on their psychophysiological application.

Before proceeding, some remarks may help place what is to follow in context. Physiological measurement, like all other forms of measurement, is the replicable assignment of numbers to represent properties (cf. Campbell, 1957). In that regard, basic psychometric principles (e.g., reliability, validity) are as relevant to psychophysiological assessment as they are to the measurement of intelligence, the assessment of job performance, or the self-report of emotion. To be sure, there are important differences across measurement domains. The point is that most able researchers have been exposed to the important principles that will be outlined here, although their direct relevance may not have been appreciated fully. The purpose of this chapter then will be to underscore the relevance of psychometric principles to psychophysiological assessment.

This chapter will not attempt to provide comprehensive coverage of the vast area encompassed by the term *psychometric principles*. Instead, discussion will focus on key issues, with references to more extensive treatments (e.g. Anastasi, 1976; Carmines & Zeller, 1979; Carnap, 1966; Cronbach, 1971; Ghiselli, Campbell, & Zedeck, 1981; Guilford, 1950; Loevinger, 1957; Nunnally, 1978) noted for readers who wish to pursue specific topics in more detail. The reader should also recognize that a discussion of psychometric principles cannot be separated completely from issues relevant to research design and statistics. Accordingly, basic training in research methodology (e.g., Cook & Campbell, 1979; Crano & Brewer, 1986; Neale & Liebert, 1980) and elementary statistics (e.g., Cohen & Cohen, 1975; Hays, 1980; Kirk, 1968; Myers, 1972; Winer, 1971) will help the reader appreciate more fully the utility of the information that follows. Finally, problems specific to particular modes of measurement will not be discussed. The number of physiological systems now measured is so numerous, and the technological advances so rapid, that focus on specific measurement procedures in this chapter would be futile (for reviews of specific measures, see, e.g., Brown, 1967; Coles, Donchin, & Porges, 1986; Gazzaniga & Blakemore, 1975; Greenfield & Sternbach, 1972; Martin & Venables, 1980; Venables & Christie, 1975; chapters 10–19, this volume). This chapter will focus instead on principles general to all psychophysiological measurement.

2.2 THE BASIC INFERENTIAL TASK

The scientific inference process is guided by a clear and carefully derived statement about constructs and construct relations (i.e., a conceptual *model*, *framework*, or *theory*). Both the ability to plan quality research and the ability to make clear inferences based on that research depend on the clarity of the guiding conceptual model. The importance of this initial step cannot be overemphasized. The most conscientious attention to the psychometric principles to be discussed will be wasted if those principles are applied to a poorly defined conceptual hypothesis.

The basic inferential task is depicted in Figure 2.1. Typically, a researcher wishes to make inferences about *hypothetical constructs* (e.g., stress, compliance, reactivity, attention, memory). To do so requires operationalizing those constructs so that numbers can be attached to them in a meaningful way that can be replicated by others.[1] This allows the logic and power of research design and inferential statistics to be brought to bear on the problem. It is this operationalization stage that also makes necessary the careful attention to psychometric principles because inferences about the hypothetical constructs and construct relations will be based on the data and data relations. Ultimately, the ability to make accurate and complete descriptive statements about the constructs (e.g., how much stress a sample of subjects is experiencing) and the ability to make logically justified inferences about construct relations (e.g., the degree to which stress is caused by a lack of control) depend on the extent to which the data possess desirable psychometric qualities.

As an example (Figure 2.2), suppose that an investigator posed the hypothesis that perceived loss of control is stressful. This implies a causal relation between two constructs. The testing of this hypothesis, however, requires the operational definition of *perceived loss of control* and *stress*. One possible set of operational definitions would be to use induced failure on an experimental task (e.g., anagrams or arithmetic problems) as the operational definition of perceived loss of control and to use physiological reactivity (perhaps systolic blood pressure, heart rate, skin conductance) as the measure of stress.

Two inferential problems become immediately clear. First, under what conditions can we safely infer that a causal relation exists between failure on the anagram task and increases or decreases in physiological indicators? Second, given that such an empirical inference is warranted, under what conditions can we make the more

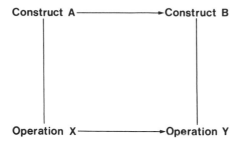

Figure 2.1. Basic conceptual model indicating relations among constructs and operational definitions.

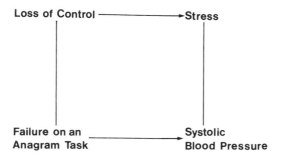

Figure 2.2. Example of simple conceptual model.

desired inference that perceived loss of control is causally antecedent to the experience of stress? As will be shown, the answers to both questions rely very heavily on the application of psychometric principles.

2.3   TWO ESSENTIAL INGREDIENTS: RELIABILITY AND VALIDITY

The ability to move from data and data relations to constructs and construct relations relies on the psychometric principles of reliability and validity. Although these two principles can be related in complex ways (e.g., see Loevinger, 1954; Nicewander & Price, 1983; Zimmerman & Williams, 1986), a simple generalization is useful: Reliability is a necessary but not a sufficient condition for validity (Nunnally, 1978). Accordingly we begin with a discussion of reliability.

2.3.1   *Reliability*

Reliability is a generic term that is used to refer to a measure's stability, repeatability, generalizability, dependability, or homogeneity. Rather than attempting to define each of these characteristics (indeed, their definitions vary considerably from author to author), a better starting point is to consider a statistical definition. In assigning numbers or scores to some phenomenon, the obtained scores (x) can be thought of as containing two major components: (1) a true score component, t, that corresponds to the score the respondent would obtain under ideal measurement conditions and (2) a component that corresponds to positive or negative score increments due to conditions present during a particular measurement occasion for a particular person (i.e., measurement error, e): $x = t + e$.[2]

The true score component, t, need not be a fixed "trait" in the usual sense. Indeed, very few human characteristics are completely stable. It is more appropriate to think of true scores as having relative stability within a certain time period. Error represents any factor not related to the variable in question that is allowed to contribute to the obtained score. Such an artifact is ubiquitous and can arise in a number of ways. In psychophysiological recording, inconsistency in the placement of electrodes, random movements by subjects, and ambient room temperature or humidity can contribute to physiological indices in ways independent of the phenomenon being studied. An artifact due to the operating characteristics of instruments may also arise and should not be routinely ignored because of the advanced technology. Indeed, the mere act of measurement itself may introduce error. As will be demonstrated shortly, the assessment and interpretation of reliability requires a very clear understanding of both a construct's relative stability and the potential sources of error that may contaminate measurement.

An important assumption in traditional reliability theory is that measurement errors are randomly and independently distributed, uncorrelated with true scores, and uncorrelated with errors or true scores on a subsequent testing (the role of *systematic* error will be discussed later). Given this assumption, the variability of obtained scores is a function of true score variability and error variability: $\sigma_x^2 = \sigma_t^2 + \sigma_e^2$. Reliability can then be defined as the relative amounts of random measurement error and true score variability: $r_{xx} = \sigma_t^2 / (\sigma_t^2 + \sigma_e^2)$. This formula indicates that a reliability coefficient is the proportion of obtained score variance that is accounted for by true score variance. The square root of a reliability coefficient estimates the correlation of obtained scores with true scores: $r_{xt} = (r_{xx})^{1/2}$. Accordingly, the more reliable a measure, the more the obtained scores reflect the true scores.

Earlier we noted that reliability is an essential requirement for making sound inferences at the level of operational definitions and consequently has important implications for making inferences about construct relations. This dependence can now be demonstrated more formally using a well-known equation indicating the degree to which a correlation between two variables is attenuated by lack of reliability: $r_{xy} = \rho_{xy} (r_{xx} r_{yy})^{1/2}$, where r_{xy} is the correlation between two different operational definitions (x and y), ρ_{xy} is the relation between the two variables under conditions of perfect reliability, and r_{xx} and r_{yy} are the reliabilities associated with measurement of x and y, respectively. The formula makes one point very clear: If either x or y is measured unreliably (i.e., $r_{xx} = 0$ or $r_{yy} = 0$), then r_{xy} will be zero regardless of whether any real relation exists (i.e., $\rho_{xy} > 0$). Consequently, the ability to detect empirical relations, upon which inferences about construct relations are based, depends upon reliability (for a discussion of other factors that can threaten *statistical conclusion validity*, see Cook & Campbell, 1979).

The attenuation formula underscores an additional point that is often ignored in experimental research: The reliability of *both* the independent variable and the dependent variable is important. In experimental research, emphasis is usually placed on ensuring the reliable measurement of the dependent variable (i.e., physiological reactivity in the example). It is just as important, however, to ensure the reliable manipulation of the independent variable (i.e., inducement of uncontrollable failure on anagrams). The ability to detect an empirical relation between the two variables depends on *both* being reliable.

Reliability of the independent variable is a deceptively complex issue (see Strube, 1989). Typically, when subjects are assigned to experimental conditions, researchers assume that the reliability of the manipulation is perfect. This is an incorrect assumption because it is not the reliability of the assignment procedure that is critical (despite the fact that everyone within an experimental condition receives the same "score" on the independent variable). Rather, the degree to which subjects within a given experimental condition are brought to the same psychological state is of most importance (Strube, 1989). In our example, some subjects exposed to the failure condition may experience the psychological state more profoundly than others. For instance, the experimenter may exhibit subtle vocal differences across subjects when delivering the feedback message so that it is stronger for some subjects than others. Some subjects in the control group may even have the subjective experience of failure because they have momentary high expectations (perhaps they just received an A on an exam) and the "success" feedback does not exceed them. These types of factors, and many others, create random variability in the psychological experiences within conditions, introducing error into the manipulation.

In developing reliable manipulations, researchers must bear in mind that manipulations have two basic features: (1) structural and (2) psychological (Strube, 1989). The structural aspects of a manipulation refer to the mechanics of carrying out the manipulation and can be made more reliable via standardization (e.g., training of experimenters or computer-driven delivery of stimuli). The psychological features of the manipulation refer to the meaning of the manipulation as perceived by the subjects. Manipulations should be constructed so that their impact is psychologically pervasive and likely to influence all subjects. Moreover, because this induced psychological state is the mediator through which the manipulation acts to influence outcome, it is critical to *demonstrate* (rather than assume) that the intended state is induced reliably. Otherwise, interpretation of the manipulation at the outcome phase is clouded. The relevance of these issues for psychophysiology cannot be ignored. Because physiological measures are used in the context of investigating relations with other variables, the failure to ensure reliability of all components will doom attempts to make inferences about empirical and construct relations.

To this point we have defined reliability, indicated its crucial role in making inferences about empirical relations, and underscored the importance of ensuring the reliability of all variables in a hypothesized relation. We have ignored, however, three important issues: (1) how is reliability assessed, (2) what is the standard for calling a measure "reliable," and (3) how can reliability be enhanced? Each of these issues will be dealt with in turn.

The assessment of reliability has itself become a rather large theoretical enterprise (e.g., Cronbach, Gleser, Nanda, & Rajaratnam, 1971). Many different kinds of reliability coefficients have been proposed with varying numbers and levels of assumptions (e.g., see Nunnally, 1978). One important general requirement, however, is that reliability must be assessed under the same conditions in which the measure will be used in practice (e.g., same subject population, same situational characteristics) because interpretation of a reliability coefficient depends on the assessment conditions. Given this general requirement, there are three basic, somewhat overlapping approaches to reliability assessment: internal consistency, test–retest, and parallel forms. All of these approaches have in common the assumption that reliability reflects consistent or replicable findings across repeated assessments (whether the repeated assessment is across items, time periods, or parallel forms). To the extent this replicability is absent, error of measurement is assumed to contaminate assessment.

If we have multiple indicators (or "items") that are to be combined into a composite, then the *internal consistency* approach (e.g., calculation of coefficient α, see Nunnally, 1978) is appropriate because we are assuming that the composite is composed of items from the same domain. This type of reliability problem arises in psychophysiological assessment, for example, when multiple indicators like systolic blood pressure, diastolic blood pressure, and heart rate are combined to create a general measure of "arousal." In addition, repeated measures on a single physiological dimension over a brief time period may be combined to represent the state of the organism during that period. For example, during a stressful task several measures of physiological response (e.g., pulse transit time computed on 10 successive heart beats) may be collected and combined to provide a single index (e.g., Goldband, 1980). Despite the apparent "test–retest" nature of the data collection, the brief time period and combination of indicators make it more similar to the internal consistency approach. In essence, because we are assuming that the composite represents one construct, we assess the homogeneity of the individual indicators.

When single indicators are not combined into composites but are instead used alone, the *test–retest* approach may be appropriate. However, test–retest reliability must be used cautiously in psychophysiological applications because of the transitory nature of many physiological phenomena. When it is used, it is absolutely critical to choose the time period with great care. The time period chosen must be short enough so that the phenomenon in question cannot reasonably be expected to change (or will change only in a constant fashion for all subjects). The key is to have a clear conceptualization of the relative stability of the construct and an understanding of the conditions under which it is expected to change. The assessment of test–retest reliability is then restricted to time periods that do not include such transition points. Otherwise, test–retest correlations may reveal more about the instability of the phenomena being measured, or the inappropriate choice of time periods, than it does about detection of true score. It is also important that reactivity or carryover effects are unlikely, otherwise the estimation of reliability may be contaminated.

Despite its limitations, there are occasions when the test–retest approach provides valuable information. For example, in establishing the reliability of the electromyogram, it is possible to demonstrate that when muscles are used in the same way (i.e., organism is "constant" across test sessions), the assessments are reliable (Gans & Gorniak, 1980; see also Cacioppo, Marshall-Goodell, & Dorfman, 1983). In addition, the test–retest method might provide crucial evidence for evaluating proposals such as Lykken, Rose, Luther, and Maley's (1966) range correction procedure. Lykken et al. argue that error due to individual differences can be reduced by adjusting responses relative to the maximum and minimum responses that can be evoked. A key question with this procedure is whether these

Table 2.1. *Calculation of the intraclass correlation coefficient*

1. Summary statistics

	Systolic blood pressure				
	Mean	Standard deviation	Variance–covariance matrix		
Time 1	119.25	9.32	86.86	100.70	98.75
Time 2	116.65	11.47		131.56	115.04
Time 3	118.85	11.32			128.14

2. ANOVA summary table

Source	df	MS	F
Between subjects (BMS)	19	325.28	30.37
Within subjects			
Between judges (JMS)	2	39.20	3.66
Residual (EMS)	38	10.71	

3. ICC Equations

$$ICC(2, 1) = \frac{BMS - EMS}{BMS + (k-1)\ EMS + k(JMS - EMS)/n} = .90$$

$$ICC(2, k) = \frac{BMS - EMS}{BMS + (JMS - EMS)/n} = .96$$

$$ICC(3, 1) = \frac{BMS - EMS}{BMS + (k-1)\ EMS} = .91$$

$$ICC(3, k) = \frac{BMS - EMS}{BMS} = .97$$

4. Parallels with coefficient α

$$r_{11} = \frac{\overline{COV}}{\overline{VAR}} = \frac{104.83}{115.52} = .91$$

$$r_{kk} = \alpha \frac{k r_{11}}{1 + (k-1)\ r_{11}} = .97$$

Note: Model designations follow Shrout and Fleiss (1979) and Lahey, Downey, and Saal (1983).

maximum and minimum responses can be evoked reliably. The test–retest approach is quite appropriate in this case.

A third approach to reliability assessment with physiological data is similar to *parallel-form* procedures used in traditional testing. In this case, human judgment plays a key role in measurement. For example, measurements that rely on careful calibration or are based on interpretation of physiological recordings are subject to error due to changes in the human part of the measurement instrument that occur from measurement occasion to measurement occasion. Although no longer commonly used in physiological research, manual measurement of blood pressure (requiring auditory detection of Korotkoff sounds) is a clear instance where error

Table 2.2. *Calculation of* κ *for two judges*

| | | Judge 1 | | | |
		Internal	External	Neither	Marginal
Judge 2	Internal	4	0	1	5
		(.2)	(0)	(.05)	(.25)
	External	0	2	1	3
		(.00)	(.10)	(.05)	(.15)
	Neither	2	0	10	12
		(.10)	(.00)	(.50)	(.60)
	Marginal	6	2	12	
		(.30)	(.10)	(.60)	

$p_0 = .2 + .1 + .5 = .8$
$p_c = (.25 \times .30) + (.15 \times .10) + (.60 \times .60) = .45$
$\kappa = (p_0 - p_c)/(1 - p_c) = (.80 - .45)/(1 - .45) = .64$

Note: Values in parentheses of classification table are proportions.

due to human judgment is quite salient. A more contemporary example is research on the psychophysiology of emotion where the coding of affect in facial expressions requires reliable scoring by human observers [e.g., use of Ekman and Friesen's Facial Action Coding System (Ekman & Friesen, 1978; see also Ekman, 1982)]. Assessing reliability in this case should be accomplished by comparing the measurements of two or more judges (e.g., see Lahey, Downey, & Saal, 1983; Schouten, 1986; Spray, 1982; Uebersax, 1987).

In summary, the choice of a reliability assessment procedure depends on the structure of the measure (multiple or single item, presence of human judgment), assumptions about the relative stability of true scores, and the kind of setting and sample for which the measure will be used (so "error" is the same in both assessment and application). Careful attention to these decisions will ensure that inferences about reliability of a measure will in fact generalize to the use of that measure in research. When more than one reliability coefficient is computed on the same operational definition, interpretation of the different reliability coefficients must proceed with careful attention to the different sources of error that can contribute to each. For example, the internal consistency of a group of indicators and the stability of that composite over time might be assessed. The stability estimate may reflect important changes in the organism or differences in testing conditions that would not be present in the internal consistency estimate.

The two most common aproaches to reliability assessment are illustrated in Tables 2.1 and 2.2. If interval level data can be assumed, then the most appropriate reliability estimate is provided by the intraclass correlation coefficient (ICC). The ICC is actually a family of statistics with selection of the proper formula dependent on the assumptions one is willing to make about the data. In all cases, however, the ICC is calculated based on the results of an analysis of variance. For example, in Table 2.1 are summary statistics for an analysis of 20 subjects whose systolic blood pressure was assessed at three time points. The four most common equations for calculating the ICC are also listed in Table 2.1. Choosing among the four equations requires two decisions. First, the researcher must decide whether a fixed-effects or random-effects model is being assumed. A fixed-effects model is appropriate when the time periods are the only ones of interest and generalization to other time periods is not pertinent. A random-effects model is appropriate when time periods represent a random sampling of time periods. Second, the unit of analysis may be the single assessment or a composite of all measures. The random-effects model estimate for a single measure is provided by equation ICC(2, 1) whereas the estimate or a composite (of k measures) is provided by equation ICC(2, k). Likewise, the fixed-effects model single-assessment estimate is provided ICC(3, 1) and the composite estimate is provided by ICC(3, k) [the designation of models follows Shrout and Fleiss (1979) and Lahey et al. (1983) for easy comparison]. For example, if we wished to combine the three assessments into a single composite (e.g., they might be the last three baseline measures) and we assumed a fixed-effects model, our estimate would be .97.

The formulas and calculations obscure several features of the ICC that bear mention. First, the time variable in the example could be replaced by any other interval-level assessment unit (e.g., judges, parallel forms, alternative testing conditions). Thus the ICC provides a general framework for assessing reliability [see Cronbach et al. (1971) for an extensive treatment of more specialized models]. Second, there is a direct relation between the fixed-effects model and coefficient α that makes clear that the ICC is an internal consistency approach. If we calculate the average of the covariances and divide that average by the average of the variances, we arrive at the average reliability of a single item (the average intercorrelation between time periods), .91. This is the same value produced by the fixed-effects model for a single assessment, ICC (3, 1). If we apply the Spearman–Brown formula to this value to estimate the reliability of a "test" of length k ($k = 3$ in the example), we arrive at coefficient α. This also happens to be the fixed-effects composite estimate of reliability, ICC(3, k). In other words, the assessment units (e.g., time periods) are analogous to items on a test; the specific nature of those units is free to vary. Note that when the items are time periods, the average single-item reliability is the average test-rest reliability. When the items are judges or alternate testing conditions, the ICC is a parallel-forms estimate. The ICC model underscores the basic commonality among different reliability assessment procedures. Finally, note that there are several reasons why an ICC may appear to indicate low reliability (e.g., insufficient variability, judge baseline differences, judges × subjects interactions). Lahey et al. (1983) provide a useful discussion of the interpretation of the ICC under these conditions.

If the data are categorical, then a different approach to reliability assessment must be taken. In this case, agreement in classification by judges must be determined. The correct estimate is provided by Cohen's (1960) κ statistic, which is illustrated in Table 2.2. Cohen's κ is a chance-corrected estimate of agreement. For example, in Table 2.2 are hypothetical data from a study where two judges are asked to classify the verbal protocol responses of 20 subjects into three categories. The responses were obtained during a challenging task and are classified as reflecting internal attributions for performance, external attributions for performance, or no clear attributional content. This "degree of self-blame" index might be associated with physiological measures of arousal. Table 2.2 indicates the classifications of each judge and a simple observed proportion of agreement (p_0) of .8. This estimate, however, does not take into account the proportion of agreement expected by chance (p_c), which is estimated by summing the products of corresponding marginal proportions in the classification table. The expected agreement is .45. When the observed agreement is adjusted for chance agreement, the resulting value is κ, which in the example is equal to .64. Additional modifications to the basic κ statistic have been developed to handle more than two judges (e.g., Conger, 1980; Fleiss, 1971; Uebersax, 1982), weighting for partial agreement (Cohen, 1968), and nonexclusive categories (Fleiss, Spitzer, Endicott, & Cohen, 1972; Kraemer, 1980). Depending on one's application, a more specialized form may be appropriate.[3] An extensive example of the calculation and interpretation of the ICC and κ can be found in Strube (in press).

Once a reliability estimate is obtained, how is it to be evaluated? One approach to answering this question is inferential. That is, reliability coefficients can be tested for significance (see, e.g., Feldt, Woodruff, & Salih, 1987). But given even modest sample sizes and modest numbers of items, most reliabilities will differ significantly from zero. As a consequence, simple rules of thumb have emerged and guide most decisions regarding achievement of "adequate reliability." For most basic research purposes, reliabilities of .80 are adequate. Naturally, the more reliable a measure is, the better it is from a validity standpoint. However, the gains in uncovering empirical relations that accrue from achieving reliabilities greater than .80 usually do not justify the extraordinary effort required to achieve such precision (Nunnally, 1978).[4] Although reliance on any rule of thumb is necessarily arbitrary (indeed, reliability is a matter of degree), consideration of practical and statistical issues as well as past convention makes .80 a reasonable choice (see Nunnally, 1978). First, when reliabilities approach .8, correlations are attentuated very little by measurement error. Second, the efforts needed to increase reliabilities beyond .8 may not be justifiable. For example, to increase the reliability of a test from .65 to .80 requires increasing its length by a factor of 2.15. But to increase reliability from .80 to .95 requires lengthening the test by a factor of 4.75. Of course, investigators are free to use *and justify* their own standards.

Given low reliability, what options does the investigator have? Actually, one answer to this question has been alluded to throughout this discussion. Reliable measurement arises from the identification and control of possible sources of extraneous variability. This, of course, identifies the sine qua non of testing, standardization, as a key component of achieving high reliability. Errors are reduced to the extent that operational definitions are clear, precise, specific, and implemented consistently. It is noteworthy in this regard that published guidelines exist for the measurement of heart rate (Jennings et al., 1981), electrodermal activity (Fowles et al., 1981), and electromyographic activity (Fridlund & Cacioppo, 1986). This kind of activity can only enhance the reliability of measurement within studies and increase comparability across studies. Investigators should, however, consider such guidelines to be minimum requirements and strive to increase standardization in their studies beyond such general recommendations.

It is also crucial that there be sufficient variability to allow detection of reliability (see, e.g., Lahey et al., 1983). It may be that apparently low reliability stems from lack of variability in the sample being investigated (i.e., restricted range), not from limitations in the measurement instrument. However, in striving to assure an adequate range for reliability assessment purposes, the researcher must not artificially create variability that exceeds the typical or natural variability of the sample (e.g., by using only the most extreme ends of the distribution or creating extreme cases that are atypical). Artificially inflated variability will lead to incorrect inferences regarding the reliability of the measure that can be expected in typical use. Likewise, sufficiently large samples need to be used to reduce the sampling error due to individuals (indeed, reliability theory is a *large-sample* theory). Where large samples are inconvenient or costly to collect (as in much psychophysiological research), replications within or across samples are desirable (e.g., Cacioppo & Dorfman, 1987; Cacioppo, Petty, Losch, & Kim, 1986).

Aside from standardization of measurement and sufficient variability, investigators can rely on one other psychometric principle to enhance reliability: aggregation. As is well known in test construction, the more items a measure has, the higher its reliability and the more precise is that estimate (provided the items are not independent). This principle underlies the previous discussion of internal consistency. With regard to physiological measures, the implication is to use multiple-item composites when they are appropriate and available (e.g., collection and averaging of repeated measures during a baseline period). Other types of composites are also possible (other than simple summation of single items), but certain limitation must be recognized. The increased reliability of a measure as the number of items increases holds only when the items are positively correlated on the average, the items are summed, and the inclusion of additional items does not substantially reduce the average interitem correlation. Other types of item combinations may produce composites of lower reliability than the individual components. One clear example is the simple difference score. As the correlation between two measures approaches the average of their reliabilities, the reliability of the difference score approaches zero:

$$r_{(a-b)(a-b)} = \frac{[(r_{aa} + r_{bb})/2] - r_{ab}}{1 - r_{ab}} \tag{1}$$

Given that one usually wants to examine change on variables that are related, there is a very real danger that difference scores will contain mostly measurement error and thus not correlate highly with anything (Cohen & Cohen, 1975). This type of situation can be anticipated and avoided by carefully considering the nature of planned composites and the characteristics of the individual components [see Nunnally (1978) and Ghiselli et al. (1981) for a more extensive treatment of reliability of composites]. In their zeal for obtaining high reliability, researchers should also be wary of combining measures that may in fact assess different constructs. Empirical solutions include the use of factor analysis (Gorsuch, 1974) to examine the viability of the assumption that several measures tap a single dimension. If they do not, derivation of principal component scores provides a means of ensuring that composites are internally consistent, although cross-validation then becomes important due to the post hoc nature of the solution (Cohen & Cohen, 1975).

Four additional comments are pertinent. First, reliability of measurement does not ensure sensitivity of measurement. A poor choice of measurement instrument may preclude detecting the phenomenon of interest even though what is detected is done so reliably. This is a matter of the resolving power of the instrument and needs to be considered carefully. For example, verbal reports are notoriously insensitive to specific visceral reactions (Pennebaker, 1982). Likewise, although the Facial Action Coding System is a reliable procedure for scoring facial expressions, an apparent absence of facial action may still be accompanied by reliable EMG signals (see Ekman, Schwarz, & Friesen reported in Ekman, 1982).

Second, to return to the example in Figure 2.2, reliable measurement alone will not allow a *causal* inference to be made. As pointed out previously, as reliability increases, the magnitude of the maximum possible correlation that can be detected between two variables increases. But this enhanced ability to detect a correlation may not imply causation. Additional considerations for inferring causality must also be considered (i.e., internal validity, e.g., Cook & Campbell, 1979).

Third, a common practice in physiological assessment is the calculation of within-subject correlations, that is, calculating a correlation for a single subject based on repeated measurement under several conditions. Most commonly, within-subject correlations examine the covariation of two different variables (e.g., heart rate and systolic blood pressure) over time or across tasks. The intent is to examine the magnitude of the correlation at the individual level (i.e., a *P*-type analysis, see Lykken, 1975; see also Cook & Campbell, 1979, for a discussion of cross-correlation analyses). One interest might be to explore moderators of correlation variability across subjects (see Strube, Lott, Heilizer, & Gregg. 1986). The two variables that are correlated could also be the same measure repeated over tasks. For example, systolic blood pressure might be examined under 10 different task conditions varying in their level of difficulty. Then the tasks could be repeated and the individual-level correlations computed to determine if there is consistency in the tasks that produce the greatest blood pressure responses at the individual level. In this way we might identify subjects who respond to challenge manipulations more consistently than others (cf. stable reactivity, Krantz & Manuck, 1984). Using within-subject correlations as a basis for reliability inferences, however, one must proceed with caution because they contain a different kind of information than ordinary reliability coefficients. Within-subject correlations index the degree of consistency in a single subject's rank ordering of responses, not the consistency of rank ordering multiple subjects. Accordingly, within-subject correlations are informative about reliability only if within-subject regressions are homogeneous across a representative sample (within-subject correlations estimate the between-subject correlation when within-subject regressions are equal, Lykken, 1975).

Finally, all that has been discussed about reliability concerns the influence of random errors on measurement. It is also possible, however, for measurement to be contaminated by systematic errors. These serve to influence obtained scores consistently in one direction. In one sense, systematic error masquerades as true score variability and clouds the meaning or interpretation of the measure. Systematic error thus challenges the validity of the interpretation attached to a measure, a topic to which we now turn.

2.3.2 *Validity*

Validity is the extent to which a test measures what it purports to measure. The basic problem of *in*validity can be demonstrated by expanding our previous definition of an obtained score to include an additional component that represents systematic error(s) $x = t + s + e$. This additional systematic component could represent a constant bias for all subjects (as when an investigator consistently reads an instrument incorrectly) or it could represent a relatively stable component at the individual level (with variation across individuals). In fact, the systematic error component can be thought of as being a true score for a different construct: $x = t_1 + t_2 + e$. Consequently, the interpretation of an obtained score becomes ambiguous because any given score can arise from more than one combination of the two (or more) systematic components (note also that true score components may be correlated and may differ in their stability). For example, heart rate would be considered a relatively poor measure of sympathetic nervous system influence because it is affected by both sympathetic and parasympathetic systems (Furedy & Heslegrave, 1983).

Strictly speaking, one does not validate a test or measure, but instead validates the interpretation or purpose for which the test is used (Ghiselli et al., 1981). Accordingly, any measure can be thought of as having as many validities as it has discrete uses or applications, and these validities can vary considerably (see, e.g., Fahrenberg, Foerster, Schneider, Müller, & Myrtek, 1986). Although validity is a unitary concept, it has been found useful to distinguish between three approaches to validation: content validity, criterion-related validity, and construct validity.

2.3.2.1 *Content validity*

Content validation is a consensual approach that relies on expert agreement as to what constitutes the content universe or domain, the degree to which a given indicator or item represents that domain, and the degree to which the collection of indicators adequately represents all facets of the domain. For some psychophysiological measures, biophysics, or physiology might define clearly the measurement needed (e.g., blood pressure), but the conditions under which it is obtained might be subject to wide variation and debate. Accordingly, the content domain might include testing conditions as important features of representativeness. For more abstract domains (e.g., arousal), demonstrating representativeness relies more heavily on judgment and a consideration of content validation becomes even more crucial.

There are actually two distinct types of content validation. The first and more common approach is to assess expert agreement after the item pool has been developed. For example, if our intent were to assess cardiovascular function, we could propose a set of indicators (e.g., systolic blood pressure, diastolic blood pressure, pulse-transit time, forearm blood volume, heart rate, etc.) and measure expert agreement concerning the suitability of each indicator and the representativeness of any set of indicators. This might be accomplished by having a group of experts rate each indicator (on a 7-point scale) according to its appropriateness given the construct definition and then assessing expert agreement with the intraclass correlation (e.g., Lahey et al., 1983). A similar approach could be taken with regard to judgments of representativeness for the set of indicators.

A second and more preferred approach is to make use of expert opinion in the item generation phase. Each expert would generate indicators believed to be appropriate given the construct definition, and then those indicators generated by a sizeable majority of the judges would be selected for inclusion (cf. parallel-panels approach, Ghiselli et al., 1981). For example, this approach was used to generate separate tests of physical function in the recently developed Objective Low Back Evaluation System (NIOSH, in press). As another example, experts could be queried as to the times of day, testing conditions, and other situational factors that should be covered to ensure adequate sampling of the blood pressure domain (cf. Pickering, Harshfield, Kleinert, Blank, & Laragh, 1982). In these cases, it is more appropriate to speak of content-oriented test development than content validation (Guion, 1978).

Not surprisingly, the content validation approach is easiest when constructs are simple and well-defined. In this case the body of content is clear and there is a greater likelihood of agreement among experts. But even for relatively concrete constructs the content validation approach is not without problems. One crucial decision is selection of judges. They should possess technical competence, have adequate knowledge of the field, and be unbiased in their research or theoretical orientations. An aggressive attempt should be made to prevent the kind of confirmatory bias that can so easily enter into validation attempts as a function of the critical choices made in structuring the research setting (e.g., Greenwald, 1975; Greenwald, Pratkanis, Leippe, & Baumgardner, 1986). Selection of judges is one such critical choice (for a different approach to defining judges in content validation, see Rose, Shulman, & Strube, 1986).

Content validation is easiest when the "distance" from the construct to the operation is fairly short. When the construct is more abstract, the identification of an adequate sample is more difficult. In this case, the content validation approach can be thought of as an initial quality check on the operational definition with the need for additional construct validation an absolute requirement.

2.3.2.2 *Criterion-related validity*

Validation by the criterion–related approach is essentially based on a desire for a measure that can "substitute" for the criterion. This type of approach arises for at least three major reasons: (1) the criterion is too difficult or costly to assess and an alternate means of detection is desired (i.e., concurrent validity; e.g., surgical detection of tumors is more costly than x-ray detection), (2) the criterion has not yet occurred but a measure that can predict its likely occurrence is desired [i.e., predictive validity; e.g., the search for cardiovascular response markers of future hypertension and coronary (CHD) onset, Krantz & Manuck, 1984], and (3) the criterion has occurred in the past but is no longer directly accessible [i.e., postdictive validity; e.g., use of electrocardiography (EKG) to determine the past occurrence of myocardial infarction]. This approach is almost entirely empirical, relying on achievement of an adequately large relation between measurement operation and criterion.

The criterion-related approach is common in the psychophysiological literature due to the cost, invasiveness, and difficulty of measuring physiological variables for certain samples or under specific conditions. Contemporary examples include the substitution of self-reported sleep for physiologically documented sleep (Hoch et al., 1987), development of an efficient measure of sleep parameters for use in the home (Helfand, Lavie, & Hobson, 1986), investigation of an indirect measure of beat-to-beat changes in blood pressure (Shapiro, Greenstadt, Lane, & Rubinstein, 1981), and development of a measure of neonatal blood pressure (Hall, Thomas, Friedman, & Lynch, 1982).

In choosing the criterion-related approach to validation, researchers need to be aware of some potential dangers. First, the selection of a criterion may be quite arbitrary and no more representative of the construct than the proposed predictor. The criterion is ideally the most appropriate operational definition from a theoretical standpoint, and its use requires theoretical and empirical justification. Second, the criterion-related approach is susceptible to mindless empiricism or "shotgun research" whereby nearly any measure is correlated with the criterion in order to find a suitable substitute but without any regard for the theoretical appropriateness or meaning of the predictor. Indeed, in the criterion-related approach there is often little interest in the nature of the predictor just as long as it provides a statistically reliable means of assessing past, present, or future presence of the criterion. This is not necessarily inappropriate if one's interests are purely functional, but more care is needed if advances in conceptual understanding are to be gained. Note also that this atheoretical approach may place one at the mercy of correlations that are inflated due to chance or dependent on unknown moderator variables.

The practical utility of the criterion-related approach is also limited in that it presupposes that a carefully validated and reliable criterion has already been established (cf. Cole, Howard, & Maxwell, 1981). In one sense, then, the criterion-related approach to validation represents a somewhat later phase in a complete validation program: (1) an important construct is identified and defined, (2) an operational definition of that construct is developed (perhaps via the content validation approach), (3) the link between construct and operational definition is validated (via construct validation), and (4) a decision is made to find additional operational definitions that are easier to obtain than the original and can be used in future theory-based and applied research. The validity of these additional operational definitions is examined via the criterion-related approach with the original operational definition as criterion (see Ghiselli et al., 1981, for a discussion of additional statistical problems that can arise with the criterion-related approach). A good example for a criterion-related substitute measure is the use of glycosylated hemoglobin (HbA1) as an indicator of recent compliance with a blood glucose control regimen (e.g., Bann, 1981; Kennedy & Merimec, 1981; for a recent debate about the validity of a biochemical index of smoking behavior, see Bliss & O'Connell, 1984).

2.3.2.3   Construct validity

Although content and criterion-related approaches to validation are useful, the most convincing evidence for an operational definition's interpretation derives from construct validation. The hallmark of the construct validation process is the placement of a construct within a network of logically and theoretically justified constructs and construct relations with specifications as to how these translate into observable operational definitions (i.e., a nomological network, Cronbach & Meehl, 1955; cf. Messick, 1981). The validation of a construct then entails the validation of the multiple operation-level relations that are derived. The network or theory surrounding the construct informs or guides the researcher as to the operational definitions that should and should not be related and the direction and magnitude of such relations. For example, if we were attempting to validate systolic blood pressure as a measure of stress, our "theory" might dictate that stress occurs in response to a perceived threat to control (see Figure 2.2). Accordingly, establishing an empirical relation between control threat and systolic blood pressure provides *partial* validation of systolic blood pressure as a measure of stress. Other empirical relations (e.g., correlations with other validated measures of stress) would add to or detract from our confidence in this interpretation.

Demonstrating construct validity is typically hampered by two common charac-teristics of operational definitions: (1) any one operational definition may capture only part of the underlying construct and (2) operational definitions are multi-dimensional and may represent two or more constructs. These relations are depicted graphically in Figure 2.3 (see also Cook & Campbell, 1979; Fiske, 1987). Note

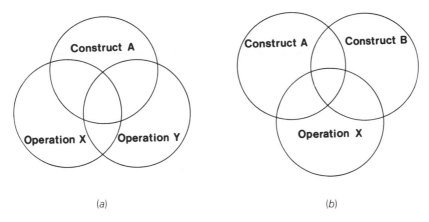

Figure 2.3. Two problems with operational definitions: (*a*) underrepresentativeness and (*b*) overrepresentativeness.

that the claim that a construct is either underrepresented or overrepresented at the operational level assumes that the construct is clearly defined in the first place. Consequently, construct invalidity can be seen to arise from problems with methods or operations (this point is argued in a very compelling fashion by Fiske, 1987).

The dangers of incomplete representation are twofold. First, it is possible that a particularly crucial aspect of the construct has been missed. For example, the full range of a construct may not be included in an experimental manipulation. Failure to find an empirical relation between operational definitions might then lead to the inference that the constructs are not related when in fact an adequate test has not been performed. In psychophysiology, exclusive use of verbal reports to measure stress or emotion may lead to the conclusion that a stimulus has no long-lasting effects on behavior. But this may be incorrect, as Zillmann (1978) has demonstrated in his work on excitation transfer. Zillmann has found that residual arousal from a prior stimulus (e.g., physical exercise) can influence later behavior (e.g., aggression) despite the report by subjects that they are no longer aroused. Second, if only part of the construct has been tested and an empirical relation is found, then there is no guarantee that the results generalize to the more complete construct. Perhaps, in fact, the need for a narrower construct or subconstruct is indicated (cf. Fiske, 1987).

Despite the best efforts to ensure complete representation for an operational definition, it is also possible that the operation will represent more than one construct (see Figure 2.3*b*). This situation often reflects the actual state of affairs: Most behaviors are multiply determined and can be expected to be influenced by more than one source of variance. Indeed, the ease with which researchers can come up with alternative explanations for internally valid empirical relations speaks to the complex and multiple constructs tapped to varying degrees by incomplete or inaccurate operational definitions. An example is the skin conductance response, which has long been recognized as being affected by widely varying stimulus conditions, across sense modalities, with interpretations including an index of specific emotions, a measure of motivation, a measure of attention, and a personality index.

The underrepresentation and overrepresentation problems indicate that reliance

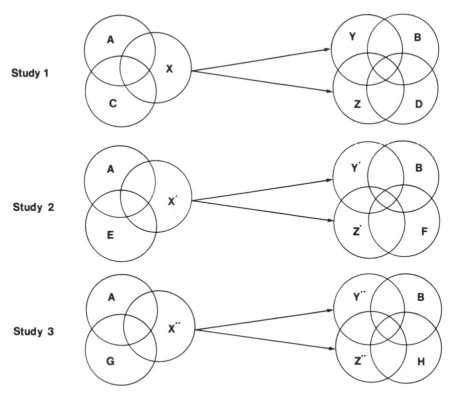

Figure 2.4. Example of multiple operationism.

on any one operation could lead to seriously distorted conclusions. The solution to both the overrepresentation and underrepresentation problems is *multiple operationism*, that is, to specify a set of correspondence rules that serve to associate a single concept with multiple operations. Only when empirical relations replicate across multiple operations can any confidence in construct relations be attained. The logic of multiple operationism (which is based on the simultaneous collection of convergent and discriminant validation evidence) is depicted in Figure 2.4. In each study, a different set of operations is used, each of which is overrepresented and underrepresented. But, across studies, the "excess" representation varies, while the relation between constructs *A* and *B* is constant. Based on supportive and consistent empirical relations, the most parsimonious explanation for the entire set of results is that *A* is causally related to *B*. Although it is not possible to rule out entirely the conclusion that, for example, *C* caused *D* in study 1, *E* caused *F* in study 2, and *G* caused *H* in study 3, such a complex model is less parsimonious and becomes less plausible as additional supportive studies are added.

Multiple operationism actually refers to two distinct tasks. First, any one construct will give rise to many possible operational definitions (e.g., the many ways that "arousal" can be operationalized physiologically). The relations among these operations must be examined for their *internal consistency*. This *monoconstruct* multiple operationism provides information about the validity of interpreting any given operation as representing the construct. Second, relations between constructs must be tested by examining the interrelatedness of different sets of operations. For example, if we investigate the hypothesis that arousal increases vigilance, we would want to examine the relations between multiple measures of arousal (e.g., heart rate and skin conductance) and multiple measures of vigilance (e.g., reaction time and event-related potential). This *multiconstruct* multiple operationism speaks to the validity of the proposed construct linkages. Both validation tasks are crucial to model testing, and both are represented in Figure 2.4 (monoconstruct multiple operationism is represented within each study for dependent variables; multiconstruct multiple operationism occurs across studies as well).

An additional word of caution regarding multiple operationism is in order. The power of using multiple operations is greatest when they diverge substantially from each other. There is little to be gained from using two self-report measures, or two nearly identical modes of physiological assessment. Any correlation between the operations might reflect their similarity in method rather than any common underlying construct. A construct should not be method bound (unless one is taking a particularly narrow view of a construct). The only way to demonstrate the independence of method and construct is through multiple operationism. The importance of avoiding method artifact has led to the development of the multiattribute–multimethod matrix procedure (Campbell & Fiske, 1959; Fiske, 1987; Hammond, Hamm, & Grassia, 1986), a technique for identifying the degree to which operational relations are contaminated by method artifact.

A concrete example might make some of the preceding discussion clearer. Expanding our previous example, we might propose that the following conditions are representative of "threat" and will bring about an increase in "stress": (1) loss of control, (2) uncertainty about possession of an important ability, (3) threat to self-esteem, (4) exposure to noxious stimuli, and (5) threat of physical harm. In successive investigations we could devise operational definitions of each of these constructs and examine their relations to our operational definition of stress: systolic blood pressure. We could also include in each study additional measures of stress (e.g., circulating catecholamines). Taken together, this type of evidence would provide convergent validation that systolic blood pressure measures stress. On the other hand, our model might also predict that stress is not related to (1) simple physical exertion or (2) chemical stimulation. Accordingly, we would not predict empirical relations between operational definitions of these variables (e.g., treadmill test, ingestion of caffeine) and systolic blood pressure. That these relations would most assuredly be found speaks to the lack of discriminant validity.

2.3.2.4 *The process of construct validation*

Although it may not be obvious, construct validation is an iterative, evolving, programmatic process. This can be highlighted by examining more closely the logic involved in making inferences based on data-level relations (see also, Nunnally, 1978). Consider again our original diagram of the inferential task (see Figure 2.1). All that we have to base our inferences on is a relation between operational variables X and Y (perhaps a causal relation, $X \rightarrow Y$). Any inference we make, however, involves three other relations: (1) the extent to which X is a valid representation of construct A, (2) the extent to which Y is a valid representation of construct B, and (3) the extent to which A is causally related to B. In any one study we cannot simultaneously make inferences about all three of these relations. Rather, we must first assume two of them to be true, and then allow the empirical relation $X \rightarrow Y$ to inform us about the plausibility of the remaining relation. For example, if our intent were to make inferences about $A \rightarrow B$, then we have to assume that X and Y are valid representations of constructs A and B, respectively. In other words, if we wish to make inferences about construct relations, then we must assume that the operational definitions have construct validity. Likewise, if we wish to make inferences about the construct validity of Y, then we must assume A and B are causally linked, and X is a valid representation of A. Our assumptions about the "truth" of the relations in our conceptual model is based on research (our own or previous research conducted by others). If our ultimate goal is making causal inferences, then we must proceed by first generating empirical evidence for the construct validity of our measures. This is a necessary first step because we must assume construct validity is present when causal hypotheses are tested; without such evidence, lack of empirical support for the causal hypothesis is uninterpretable. Furthermore, past research must be able to support considerable confidence in such assumptions because the appropriate interpretation of positive and negative empirical results hinges on the validity of those assumptions. An incorrect assumption can alter the direction of subsequent research and make the construct validation process inefficient if not completely misleading. This incremental view of construct validation returns us to the point made at the beginning of this chapter: Research must be guided by a very clear view of what one intends to infer from the data.

Several final comments about construct validation are in order. First, as with reliability, the construct validity of both independent and dependent variables requires equally careful attention. Much confusion in psychophysiological research stems from an overemphasis on the construct validity of dependent measures. A clear example exists in the Type A behavior pattern literature. Although it appears that Type As respond physiologically to "threat" or "challenge" differently than do Type Bs, it is not at all clear what most researchers mean by threat or challenge (see Strube, 1987). Second, conceptual models should be responsive to empirical findings. A conceptual hypothesis is only an educated guess about how things work. If the evidence indicates a need for revision, it behooves researchers to let their models evolve rather than fall prey to confirmatory bias (although it may be obvious, it is important that model revisions be tested on new samples). In a similar fashion, researchers should test their models "aggressively," that is, provide empirical tests of hypotheses that are not immune to falsification. Finally, researchers should realize that construct validation is a "slow," methodical process. The building of a conceptual model should be taken one sure-footed step at a time.

2.4   CONCLUSION

The psychometric principles discussed in this chapter lie at the very heart of scientific progress. Although most researchers have a rudimentary understanding of these principles, their importance and specific application are often ignored. This arises, perhaps, because psychometric principles are most often associated with the classic psychometric traditions of intelligence, ability, and personality testing. Yet, as has been stressed throughout this chapter, attention to psychometric principles is crucial no matter what form measurement takes. Whether one is attempting to map the physiological structure of mood, to identify stable physiological markers of future disease risk, to develop procedures for determining the physiological concomitants of cognitive function, or to demonstrate the practical utility of physiologically based lie detection, psychometric principles provide the essential "rules of evidence" that are used to judge the adequacy of our conceptual and applied conclusions.

NOTES

1 The term *operational definition* will be used in this chapter to mean the manner in which the construct is represented at the level of research operations (cf. Bergman, 1951; Bridgman, 1927). Naturally, a construct can be so specific and well defined that a single operational definition can represent it completely with no debate. However, this narrow sense of operationism is generally not common in psychology, giving rise to the important emphasis placed on validity to be detailed in this chapter.
2 This discussion is based on the classical test theory view. Other measurement models (e.g., the domain-sampling model, item response theory) are more complex to describe but arrive at essentially similar conclusions regarding reliability. The differences between the models are described elsewhere (see Birnbaum, 1968; Ghiselli, Campbell, & Zedeck, 1981; Hambleton, 1979; Nunnally, 1978; Weiss & Davison, 1981).
3 It is possible to calculate standard errors for both ICC (e.g., Shrout & Fleiss, 1979) and κ (e.g., Fleiss, Cohen, & Everitt, 1969). These are useful for small samples where there is concern over the stability of the reliability estimate.
4 Exceptions, of course, can be identified. Whenever important practical decisions are to be made about individuals, then much higher reliabilities are absolutely essential (e.g., .95, see Nunnally, 1978).

REFERENCES

Abbott, B. B., & Badia, P. (1986). Predictable versus unpredictable shock conditions and physiological measures of stress: A reply to Arthur. *Psychological Bulletin, 100*, 384–387.

Abbott, B. B., Schoen, L. S., & Badia, P. (1984). Predictable and unpredictable shock: Behavioral measures of aversion and physiological measures of stress. *Psychological Bulletin, 96*, 45–71.

Anastasi, A. (1976). *Psychological testing* (4th ed.). New York: Macmillan.

Arthur, A. Z. (1986). Stress of predictable and unpredictable shock. *Psychological Bulletin, 100*, 379–383.

Bann, H. F. (1981). Evaluation of glycosylated hemoglobin in diabetic patients. *Diabetes, 30*, 613–617.

Beatty, J. (1982). Task-evoked pupillary responses, processing load, and the structure of processing resources. *Psychological Bulletin, 91*, 276–292.

Bergman, G. (1951). The logic of psychological concepts. *Philosophy of Science, 18*, 93–110.

Birnbaum, A. (1968). Some latent trait models and their use in inferring an examinee's ability. In F. M. Lord and M. R. Novick (Eds.), *Statistical theories of mental test scores.* Reading, MA: Addison-Wesley.

Bliss, R. E., & O'Connell, K. A. (1984). Problems with thiocyanate as an index of smoking status: A critical review with suggestions for improving the usefulness of biochemical measures in smoking cessation research. *Health Psychology, 3*, 563–581.

Bridgman, P. W. (1927). *The logic of modern physics.* New York: Macmillan.

Brown, C. C. (Ed.) (1967). *Methods in psychophysiology.* Baltimore: Williams & Wilkins.

Cacioppo, J. T., & Dorfman, D. D. (1987). Waveform moment analysis in psychophysiological research. *Psychological Bulletin, 102*, 421–438.

Cacioppo, J. T., Marshall-Goodell, B., & Dorfman, D. D. (1983). Skeletal muscular patterning: Topographical analysis of the integrated myogram. *Psychophysiology, 20*, 269–283.

Cacioppo, J. T., & Petty, R. E. (1981). Electromyograms as measures of extent and affectivity of information processing. *American Psychologist, 36*, 441–456.

Cacioppo, J. T., & Petty, R. E. (1983). *Social psychophysiology: A sourcebook.* New York: Guilford Press.

Cacioppo, J. T., Petty, R. E., Losch, M. E., & Kim, H. S. (1986). Electromyographic activity over facial muscle regions can differentiate the valence and intensity of affective reactions. *Journal of Personality and Social Psychology, 50,* 260–268.

Campbell, D. T., & Fiske, D. W. (1959). Convergent and discriminant validation by the multitrait-multimethod matrix. *Psychological Bulletin, 56,* 81–105.

Campbell, N. R. (1957). *Foundations of science: The philosophy of theory.* New York: Dover.

Carmines, E. G., & Zeller, R. A. (1979). Reliability and validity assessment. In J. L. Sullivan (ed.), *Quantitative applications in the social sciences.* Beverly Hills, CA: Sage.

Carnap, R. (1966). *Philosophical foundations of physics: An introduction to the philosophy of science.* New York: Basic Books.

Cohen, J. (1960). A coefficient of agreement for nominal scales. *Educational and Psychological Measurement, 20,* 37–46.

Cohen, J. (1968). Weighted kappa: Nominal scale agreement with provision for scaled disagreement or partial credit. *Psychological Bulletin, 70,* 213–220.

Cohen, J., & Cohen, P. (1975). *Applied multiple regression/correlation analysis for the behavioral sciences.* Hillsdale, NJ: Erlbaum.

Cole, D. A., Howard, G. S., & Maxwell, S. E. (1981). Effects of mono- versus multiple-operationalization in construct validation efforts. *Journal of Consulting and Clinical Psychology, 49,* 395–405.

Coles, M. G. H., Donchin, E., & Porges, S. W. (Eds.). (1986). *Psychophysiology: Systems, processes, and applications.* New York: Guilford Press.

Conger, A. J. (1980) Integration and generalization of kappas for multiple raters. *Psychological Bulletin, 88,* 322–328.

Contrada, R. J., Wright, R. A., & Glass, D. C. (1985). Psychophysiologic correlates of Type A behavior: Comments on Houston (1983) and Holmes (1983). *Journal of Research in Personality, 19,* 12–30.

Cook, T. D., & Campbell, D. T. (1979). *Quasi-experimentation: Design and analysis issues for field settings.* Chicago: Rand McNally.

Cox, D. J., Taylor, A. G., Nowacek, G., Holley-Wilcox, P., Pohl, S. L., & E. Guthrow (1984). The relationship between psychological stress and insulin-dependent diabetic blood glucose control: Preliminary findings. *Health Psychology, 3,* 63–75.

Crano, W. D., & Brewer, M. B. (1986). *Principles and methods of social research.* Boston: Allyn & Bacon.

Cronbach, L. J. (1971) Test validation. In R. L. Thorndike (Ed.), *Educational measurement* (2nd ed.), Washington, DC: American Council on Education.

Cronbach, L. J., Gleser, G. C., Nanda, H., & Rajaratnam, N. (1971). *The dependability of behavioral measurements.* New York: Wiley.

Cronbach, L. J., & Meehl, P. E. (1955). Construct validity in psychological tests. *Psychological Bulletin, 52,* 281–302.

Davis, W. K., Hess, G. E., Harrison, R. V., & Hiss, R. G. (1987). Psychological adjustment to and control of diabetes mellitus: Differences by disease type and treatment. *Health Psychology, 6,* 1–14.

Dolce, J. J., & Raczynski, J. M. (1985). Neuromuscular activity and electromyography in painful backs: Psychological and biomechanical models in assessment and treatment. *Psychological Bulletin, 97,* 502–520.

Ekman, P. (1982). Methods for measuring facial action. In K. R. Scherer & P. Ekman (Eds.), *Handbook of methods in nonverbal behavioral research* (pp. 45–90). New York: Cambridge University Press.

Ekman, P., & Friesen, W. V. (1978). *The Facial Action Coding System: A technique for the measurement of facial movement.* Palo Alto, CA: Consulting Psychologists Press.

Fahrenberg, J., Foerster, F., Schneider, H. J., Müller, W., & Myrtek, M. (1986). Predictability of individual differences in activation processes in a field setting based on laboratory measures. *Psychophysiology, 23,* 323–333.

Feldt, L. S., Woodruff, D. J., & Salih, F. A. (1987). Statistical inference for coefficient alpha. *Applied Psychological Measurement, 11,* 93–103.

Fiske, D. W. (1987). Construct invalidity comes from method effects. *Educational and Psychological Measurement, 47,* 285–307.

Fleiss, J. L. (1971). Measuring nominal scale agreement among many raters. *Psychological Bulletin, 76*, 378–382.

Fleiss, J. L., Cohen, J., & Everitt, B.S. (1969). Large sample standard errors of kappa and weighted kappa. *Psychological Bulletin, 72*, 323–327.

Fleiss, J. L., Spitzer, R. L., Endicott, J., & Cohen, J. (1972). Quantification of agreement in multiple psychiatric diagnoses. *Archives of General Psychiatry, 26*, 168–171.

Fowles, D. C., Christie, M .J., Edelberg, R., Grings, W. W., Lykken, D. T., & Venables, P. H. (1981). Publication recommendations for electrodermal measurements. *Psychophysiology, 18*, 232–239.

Fridlund, A. J., & Cacioppo, J. T. (1986). Guidelines for human electromyographic research. *Psychophysiology, 23*, 567–589.

Furedy, J. J., & Heslegrave, R. J. (1983). A consideration of recent criticisms of the T-wave amplitude index of myocardial sympathetic activity. *Psychophysiology, 20*, 204–211.

Gans, C., & Gorniak, G. C. (1980). Electromyograms are repeatable: Precautions and limitations. *Science, 210*, 795–797.

Gazzaniga, M., & Blakemore, C. (Eds.). (1975). *Handbook of psychobiology.* New York: Academic Press.

Ghiselli, E .E., Campbell, J. P. & Zedeck, S. (1981). *Measurement theory for the behavioral sciences.* New York: Freeman.

Goldband, S. (1980). Stimulus specificity of physiological response to stress and the Type A coronary-prone behavior pattern. *Journal of Personality and Social Psychology, 39*, 670–679.

Gorsuch, R. I. (1974). *Factor analysis.* Philadelphia: Saunders.

Greenfield, N. S., & Sternbach, R. A. (Eds.). (1972). *Handbook of psychophysiology.* New York: Holt, Rinehart, and Winston.

Greenwald, A. G. (1975). Consequences of prejudice against the null hypothesis. *Psychological Bulletin, 82*, 1–20.

Greenwald, A .G., Pratkanis, A. R., Leippe, M. R., & Baumgardner, M. H. (1986). Under what conditions does theory obstruct research progress? *Psychological Review, 93*, 216–229.

Grossberg, S. (1982). Processing of expected and unexpected events during conditioning and attention: A psychophysiological theory. *Psychological Review, 89*, 529–572.

Guilford, J. P. (1950). *Psychometric methods.* New York: McGraw-Hill.

Guion, R. M. (1978). Scoring of content domain samples. *Journal of Applied Psychology, 63*, 449–506.

Hall, P. S., Thomas, S. A., Friedman, E., & Lynch, J. J. (1982). Measurement of neonatal blood pressure: A new method. *Psychophysiology, 19*, 231–236.

Hambleton, R. K. (1979). Latent trait models and their applications. In R. Traub (Ed.). *New directions for testing and measurement: Vol. 4. Methodological developments* (pp. 13–32). San Francisco: Jossey-Bass.

Hammond, K. R., Hamm, R. M., & Grassia, J. (1986). Generalizing over conditions by combining the multitrait-multimethod matrix and the representative design of experiments. *Psychological Bulletin, 100*, 257–269.

Hays, W. L. (1980). *Statistics* (3rd ed.). New York: Holt, Rinehart and Winston.

Helfand, R., Lavie, P., & Hobson, J. A. (1986). REM/NREM discrimination via ocular and limb movement monitoring: Correlation with polygraphic data and development of a REM state algorithm. *Psychophysiology, 23*, 334–339.

Hoch, C. C., Reynolds, C. F. III, Kupfer, D. J., Berman, S. R., Houck, P. R., & Stack, J. A. (1987). Empirical note: Self-report versus recorded sleep in healthy seniors. *Psychophysiology, 24*, 293–299.

Jennings, J. R., Berg, W. K., Hutcheson, J. S., Obrist, P., Porges, S., & Turpin, G. (1981). Publication guidelines for heart rate studies in man. *Psychophysiology, 18*, 226–231.

Johnson, R., Jr. (1986). A triarchic model of P300. *Psychophysiology, 23*, 367–384.

Kennedy, A. L., & Merimec, P. J. (1981). Glycosylated serum protein and hemoglobin A_1 levels to measure control of glycemia. *Annals of Internal Medicine, 95*, 56–58.

Kirk, R. E. (1968). *Experimental design: Procedures for the behavioral sciences.* Belmont, CA: Brooks/Cole.

Kraemer, H. C. (1980). Extension of the kappa coefficient, *Biometrics, 36*, 207–216.

Krantz, D. S., Glass, D. C., Schaeffer, M. A., & Davia, J. E. (1982). Behavior patterns and coronary disease: A critical evaluation. In J. T. Cacioppo & R. E. Petty (Eds.), *Perspectives on cardiovascular psychophysiology* (pp. 315–346). New York: Guilford Press.

Krantz, D. S. & Manuck, S. B. (1984). Acute psychophysiologic reactivity and risk of cardiovascular disease: A review and methodological critique. *Psychological Bulletin, 96,* 435–464.

Lahey, M. A., Downey, R. G., & Saal, F. E. (1983). Intraclass correlations: There's more there than meets the eye. *Psychological Bulletin, 93,* 586–595.

Loevinger, J. (1954). The attenuation paradox in test theory. *Psychological Bulletin, 51,* 493–504.

Loevinger, J. (1957). Objective tests as instruments of psychological theory. *Psychological Reports, 3*(Supp. 9), 635–694.

Lykken, D. T. (1975). The role of individual differences in psychophysiological research. In P. H. Venables and M. J. Christie (Eds.), *Research in psychophysiology* (pp. 3–15). New York: Wiley.

Lykken, D. T., Rose, R. Luther, B., & Maley, M. (1966). Correcting psychophysiological measures for individual differences in range. *Psychological Bulletin, 66,* 481–484.

Martin, I., & Venables, P. H. (Eds.). (1980). *Techniques in psychophysiology.* New York: Wiley.

Matthews, K. A., Weiss, S. M., Detre, T., Dembroski, T. M., Falkner, B., Manuck, S. B., & Williams, R. B., Jr. (Eds.) (1986). *Handbook of stress, reactivity, and cardiovascular disease.* New York: Wiley.

Messick, S. (1981). Constructs and their vicissitudes in educational and psychological measurement. *Psychological Bulletin, 89,* 575–588.

Miller, S. M. (1981). Predictability and human stress: Towards a clarification of evidence and theory. In L. Berkowitz (Ed.), *Advances in experimental social psychology* (Vol. 14., pp. 203–256). New York: Academic Press.

Myers, J. L. (1972), *Fundamentals of experimental design* (2nd ed.). Boston: Allyn & Bacon.

Näätänen, R. (1982). Processing negativity: An evoked-potential reflection of selective attention. *Psychological Bulletin, 92,* 605–640.

National Institute of Occupational Safety and Health (NIOSH). (in press). *The objective low back evaluation system.* Morgantown, WV: NIOSH.

Neale, J. M., & Liebert, R. M. (1980). *Science and behavior* (2nd ed.). Englewood Cliffs, NJ: Prentice-Hall.

Nicewander, W. A., & Price, J. M. (1983). Reliability of measurement and the power of statistical tests: Some new results. *Psychological Bulletin, 94,* 524–533.

Nunnally, J. C. (1978). *Psychometric theory.* New York: McGraw-Hill.

Pennebaker, J. W. (1982). *The psychology of physical symptoms.* New York: Springer–Verlag.

Pickering, T. G., Harshfield, G. A., Kleinert, H. D., Blank, S., & Laragh, J. H. (1982). Blood pressure during normal daily activities, sleep, and exercise. *Journal of the American Medical Association, 247,* 992–996.

Pritchard, W. S. (1981). Psychophysiology of P300. *Psychological Bulletin, 89,* 506–540.

Pritchard, W. S. (1986). Cognitive event-related potential correlates of schizophrenia. *Psychological Bulletin, 100,* 43–66.

Rose, S. J., Shulman, A. D., & Strube, M. J. (1986). Functional assessment of patients with low back syndrome. *Topics in Geriatric Rehabilitation, 1,* 9–30.

Schouten, H. J. A. (1986). Statistical measurement of interobserver agreement. *Psychometrika, 51,* 453–466.

Shapiro, D., Greenstadt, L., Lane, J. D., & Rubinstein, E. (1981). Tracking-cuff system for beat-to-beat recording of blood pressure. *Psychophysiology, 18,* 129–136.

Shrout, P. E., & Fleiss, J. L., (1979). Intraclass correlations: Uses in assessing rater reliability. *Psychological Bulletin, 86,* 420–428.

Spray, J. A. (1982). Effects of autocorrelated errors on intraclass reliability estimation. *Research Quarterly for Exercise and Sport, 53,* 226–231.

Strube, M. J. (1987). A self-appraisal model of the Type A behavior pattern. In R. Hogan & W. H. Jones (Eds.), *Perspectives in personality* (Vol. 2, pp. 201–250). Greenwich, CT: JAI Press.

Strube, M. J. (1989). Assessing subjects' construal of the laboratory situation. In N. Schneiderman, S. M. Weiss, & P. Kaufman, (Eds.), *Handbook of research methods in cardiovascular behavioral medicine* (pp. 527–542). New York: Plenum Press.

Strube, M. J. (in press). Statistical analyses of therapist reliability in the NIOSH Objective Low Back Evaluation Project. In *The objective low back evaluation system,* Morgantown, WV: NIOSH.

Strube, M. J., Lott, C. L., Heilizer, R., & Gregg, B. (1986). Type A behavior pattern and the judgment of control. *Journal of Personality and Social Psychology, 50,* 403–412.

Thompson, S. C. (1981). Will it hurt less if I can control it? A complex answer to a simple question. *Psychological Bulletin, 90,* 89–101.

Uebersax, J. S. (1982). A generalized kappa coefficient. *Educational and Psychological Measurement, 42,* 181–183.

Uebersax, J. S. (1987). Diversity of decision-making models and the measurement of interrater agreement. *Psychological Bulletin, 101,* 140–146.

Venables, P. H., & Christie, M. J. (Eds.). (1975). *Research in psychophysiology.* New York: Wiley.

Weiss, D. J., & Davision, M. L., (1981). Test theory and methods. In M. R. Rosenzeig & L. W. Porter (Eds.), *Annual review of psychology* (Vol. 32, pp. 629–658). Palo Alto, CA: Annual Reviews.

Winer, B. J. (1971). *Statistical principles in experimental design.* New York: McGraw-Hill.

Zillmann, D. (1978). Attribution and misattribution of excitatory reactions. In J. H. Harvey, W. Ickes, & R. F Kidd (Eds.), *New directions in attribution research* (Vol. 2, pp. 335–368). Hillsdale, NJ: Erlbaum.

Zimmerman, D.W., & Williams, R. H. (1986). Note on the reliability of experimental measures and the power of significance tests. *Psychological Bulletin, 100,* 123–124.

3 *Fundamentals of neuroscience*

RAE MATSUMOTO, BARBARA B. WALKER,
J. MICHAEL WALKER, AND HOWARD C. HUGHES

3.1 INTRODUCTION

The human brain contains approximately one trillion nerve cells (10^{12}), and each of them may communicate with between 10 and 10,000 other nerve cells. The messages transmitted between cells may involve the secretion of one or many chemical secretory messengers, and the nature of this chemical message is alterable. With a "wet weight" of only about 3 pounds, the human central nervous system is undoubtedly the most complex structure known to exist in the universe.

In spite of its complexity, a considerable understanding of the brain has been achieved through both reductionistic and organismic approaches. The actual term *neuroscience* originated with a group of "systems" and "components" scientists committed to the notion that any comprehensive understanding of the nervous system must include both molar and molecular concepts. This perspective has encouraged the conceptualization that the brain is composed of functional subsystems, and the principles governing one system frequently operate in others. The discoveries of general principles of interneuronal architecture and communication have been encouraging signs that we are beginning to understand some of the fundamental mechanisms of the brain. Central to these discoveries has been the application of modern biobehavioral technologies; these methods have accounted for much of the knowledge about the brain that has emerged over the last 100 years. Armed with such heuristics, neuroscience has made great strides in understanding what appears at first sight to be a hopelessly complex gelatinous mass.

A tremendous growth of knowledge about the basic anatomical and neurochemical mechanisms of the brain has occurred in the last 25 years. With this new knowledge has come a greater need to integrate these two aspects of the nervous system. A central tenet of this chapter is that the structure, neurochemistry, and physiology of the nervous system must be considered together to understand brain organization and function. Further, many areas of cross-fertilization between psychophysiology and neuroscience can emerge from interdisciplinary studies, but this can occur only if workers are familiar with both fields. It is our hope the new student of psychophysiology finds this chapter to be a foundation and a beginning toward this goal.

Complete coverage of the field of neuroscience cannot be achieved in one chapter, and our difficulty has been to select the areas to be covered and to provide an appropriate depth. The following is a combination of subjects from classical neuroscience and a selected set of more detailed descriptions of systems that may illustrate important principles or add specific information that is applicable to psychophysiology. Further, an attempt is made to identify important recent developments in the field. The chapter makes no pretense of being a sufficient source of information, even for the beginning psychophysiologist. The interested reader is encouraged to pursue more extensive treatments found in many excellent texts on physiological psychology, psychopharmacology, and neuroscience. Four excellent sources are *Physiology of Behavior*, by N. Carlson (1986), *Fundamentals of Neuropsychopharmacology*, by R. S. Feldman and L. F. Quenzer (1984), *Principles of Neural Science*, edited by E. R. Kandel and J. H. Schwartz (1985), and *Medical Physiology*, edited by U. Mountcastle (1980). We begin our treatment by considering the general structure of the human nervous system. This is followed by an examination of the electrochemical basis of neuronal excitability and intercellular communication. Finally, we outline some of the major subsystems of the nervous system.

3.2 ANATOMY OF THE CENTRAL NERVOUS SYSTEM

3.2.1 *Neuroembryology*

Knowledge of the development of the nervous system can provide a conceptual framework for understanding the regional anatomy of the central nervous system (CNS). We therefore briefly consider the anatomy of the developing nervous system before examining the endpoint of that development, the regional anatomy of the adult human CNS.

The human embryo consists of three distinct layers of cells: the *endoderm* (inner layer), the *mesoderm* (middle layer), and the *ectoderm* (outer layer). The central nervous system derives from a specialized portion of the ectoderm called the *neural plate*. The neural plate lies on the dorsal (back) surface of the embryo and runs along the midline.

As development proceeds, the neural plate first invaginates and eventually closes to form an elongated tube called the *neural tube*. The neural tube is hollow, and the lumen is called the *central canal*. The central canal persists throughout development and eventually forms the *ventricular system* of the brain. The inner wall of the neural tube is lined with a thin layer of cells called epithelial cells. Through repeated mitotic cell divisions, the epithelial layer of the neural tube generates virtually all of the nerve cells (*neurons*) and supporting cells (*glia*) that form the adult nervous system. The generation of neurons is not uniform along the length of the neural tube; the rostral (toward the head) portion of the neural tube generates many more neurons than the caudal part (toward the "tail"). Consequently, as development proceeds, several enlargements in the neural tube form along its rostral end. These enlargements, called vesicles, develop into the brain. The caudal part of the neural tube, which retains its tubelike appearance throughout development, becomes the spinal cord. Initially, only three cephalic ("head") vesicles are present (Figure 3.1). The most rostral is called the *prosencephalon* (forebrain), the middle is called the *mesencephalon* (midbrain), and the most caudal is called the *rhombencephalon* (hindbrain). Later, five vesicles can be seen: the prosencephalon develops into two subdivisions, the *telencephalon* and the *diencephalon*, and rhombencephalon develops into the *metencephalon* and the *myelencephalon* (see Figure 3.1). The mesencephalon remains one vesicle throughout development. With these rudimentary aspects of the developing brain in mind, we turn to a consideration of the major derivatives of each vesicle in the adult brain.

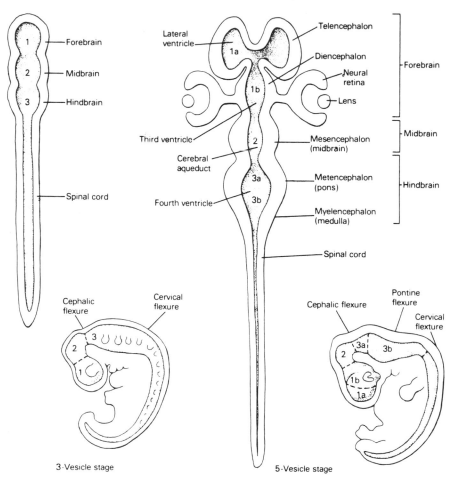

Figure 3.1. The brain and spinal cord develop from the neural tube. The brain arises from several enlargements, called vesicles, in the rostral portion of the neural tube. Early in development, three cephalic vesicles are present; later five cephalic vesicles differentiate into the various parts of the brain. In *Principles of neural science* (E. Kandel and J. Schwartz, Eds.), p. 246. Copyright 1985 by Elsevier Science.

3.2.2   Telencephalon

Major structures found in the telencephalon include the *lateral ventricles* (derived from the embryonic central canal), the *cerebral cortex*, the *basal ganglia* (which consist of the caudate, putamen, and globus pallidus), the *olfactory bulbs*, the *hippocampus*, the *fornix*, and the *amygdala*. Because of the great proliferation of neurons in the frontal and temporal lobes of the cerebrum, many of the forebrain structures are C-shaped; these include the lateral ventricles, the caudate nucleus, the hippocampus, and the fornix.

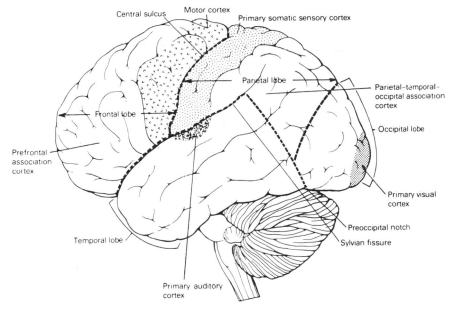

Figure 3.2. Lateral view of the brain showing major divisions of the cerebral cortex. (Reprinted by permission of the publisher from J. P. Kelly, Principles of the functional and anatomical organization of the nervous system, in *Principles of neural science*, E. Kandel and J. Schwartz, Eds., p. 214. Copyright 1985 by Elsevier Science.)

3.2.2.1   Cerebral cortex

The cerebral cortex covers most of the cerebrum and consists of two hemispheres interconnected by the *corpus callosum*. The cortex can be grossly subdivided into the frontal, parietal, temporal, and occipital lobes (Figure 3.2). Parts of the *frontal lobes* are involved in the generation of certain emotional states, motor functions, oculomotor control, speech production (Broca's area), and foresight (e.g., Kolb & Whishaw, 1980). The *temporal lobes* are associated with audition, auditory and visual recognition (e.g., Gross, Rocha-Miranda, & Bender, 1972; Iwai & Mishkin, 1968; Mishkin, 1979), and some of the perceptual aspects of language (comprehension and syntax). The *parietal cortex* contains the somatosensory projection fields (cortical representation of the skin senses and kinesthesia) as well as some areas related to visual processing and convergence of visual with somesthetic information. The parietal cortex may also play a role in some aspects of sensorimotor processing and visual attention (e.g., Lynch, Mountcastle, Talbot, & Yin, 1977; Posner, Walker, Friedrich, & Rafal, 1984; Robinson, Goldberg, & Stanton, 1978). The occipital lobes are associated with vision.

3.2.2.2   Subcortical structures

Telencephalic structures that lie beneath the cerebral cortex are often referred to as subcortical structures. These include the *caudate, putamen,* and *globus pallidus,* which lie below the corpus callosum and follow the course of the lateral ventricles

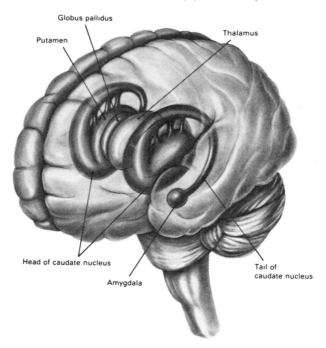

Figure 3.3. Subcortical telencephalic and diencephalic structures of the human brain. (Reprinted by permission of the publisher from N. R. Carlson, *Physiology of behavior*, p. 102. Copyright 1986 by Allyn and Bacon, Needham Hts., MA.)

(Figure 3.3). Collectively, these structures comprise the basal ganglia, a system involved in motor processing. The hippocampus, another subcortical structure, is part of an interconnected system of forebrain structures called the limbic system. Like the caudate, the hippocampus has a C shape because it follows the course of the lateral ventricles. The hippocampus is heavily interconnected with other limbic structures such as the *septal nuclei*, the amygdala, and the *mammillary bodies*. Many of the afferent and efferent connections of the hippocampus lie within the fornix, a large fiber bundle that arches from the hippocampus past the septal area and terminates within the hypothalamus. Limbic structures, such as the hippocampus, the mammillary bodies, and the amygdala, play an important role in memory (Olton, 1984; Squire, 1982; Zipser, 1985). The septum and parts of the amygdala appear to be involved in the elaboration of certain emotional states (especially fear and rage). Thus, lesions of the basolateral division of the amygdala produce docility, whereas stimulation produces affective attack (Hilton & Zbrozyna, 1963).

3.2.3   Diencephalon

The diencephalon derives primarily from a secondary vesicle of the prosencephalon. Major structures of the diencephalon include the *third ventricle*, the *thalamus*, and the *hypothalamus* (Figure 3.4). These structures lie below the hippocampus,

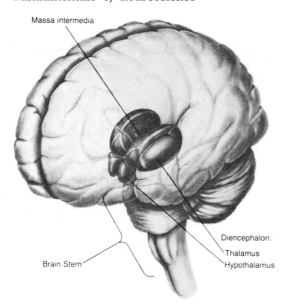

Figure 3.4. The location and structures of the diencephalon (thalamus and hypothalamus) of the brain. The massa intermedia connects the two thalami. (Reprinted by permission of the publisher from N. R. Carlson, *Physiology of behavior*, p. 103. Copyright 1986 by Allyn and Bacon, Needham Hts., MA.)

fornix, and caudate of the telencephalon. The thalamus can be regarded as the "gateway" to the cerebral cortex; almost all of the input to the cerebral cortex gains access via a synaptic relay in the thalamus. The thalamus actually consists of a number of identifiable nuclei, each of which projects to a fairly well-defined "cortical field" and has specific patterns of afferent (input) connections. This is most clearly seen in the *specific relay nuclei* of the thalamus. Each relay nucleus processes modality-specific sensory or motor information and transmits that information to the corresponding cortical projection field.

In contrast to the thalamus, the hypothalamus has no direct cortical connections. Lying beneath the thalamus (*hypo* = under), the hypothalamus is involved in homeostasis and related motivational states (e.g., hunger, thirst, and reproduction). The hypothalamus can also be viewed as an interface between sensory inputs and motor outflow for emotional and motivational behavior. Hypothalamic afferents (inputs) originate from the retina, frontal cortex, limbic structures such as the amygdala, septum, cingulum, and hippocampus, certain thalamic nuclei, and a variety of brainstem afferents including the solitary nucleus (which receives primary gustatory afferents). In addition, there are a variety of receptors that provide information concerning blood chemistry (e.g., glucose concentration) and osmolarity (associated with thirst). Some hypothalamic neurons clearly respond to a variety of sensory inputs arising both from internal sensory receptors (e.g., Anand & Brobeck, 1951) and exteroceptors such as vision and taste (e.g., Rolls, 1982).

Hypothalamic efferents are distributed to (1) parts of the thalamus, which in turn project to the frontal lobes as well as to the cingulate gyrus (providing feedback pathways to the already described fronto-hypothalamic and cingulo-hypothalamic projections), (2) the posterior lobe of the pituitary, and (3) a variety of zones within the midbrain, pons, and medulla. These latter areas in turn send projections to moto neurons of the somatic and autonomic motor systems. Not surprisingly, then, much of the hypothalamic output is directed toward regulation of the viscera and the endocrine system.

The *pituitary gland*, which is suspended by the infundibular stalk immediately below the hypothalamus, serves as a connection between the hypothalamus and the endocrine system. The pituitary is sometimes referred to as the "master gland" because it aids in the coordination of brain and bodily functions through the regulation of many other glands in the head and trunk. However, later it will become clear that the pituitary is really a mere storage and transducing mechanism since the brain dictates its activities; for this and other reasons, which will become clear later, the brain may be more deserving of the title "master gland."

3.2.4   Mesencephalon

The mesencephalon, or midbrain, can be divided into two general areas: the dorsal portion (called the *tectum, "roof"*) and the ventral portion (called the *tegmentum, "floor"*). A small canal that comprises the midbrain's portion of the ventricular system courses through the center of the midbrain and demarcates the boundary between tectum and tegmentum. This canal is known as the *cerebral aqueduct*, or the *aqueduct of Sylvius*. Surrounding the cerebral aqueduct is the *periaqueductal gray* (PAG), an important area for the central inhibition of pain that operates through the release of opioid neurosecretory products. Two main structures comprise the tectum: the *superior colliculi*, which lie rostrally and play an important role in vision (especially with respect to eye movements), and the *inferior colliculi*, which lie behind the superior colliculi and play an important role in audition. From the cerebral aqueduct to the ventral surface of the midbrain is the midbrain tegmentum, sizable structure containing many nuclei including the *red nucleus* and *substantia nigra* (two nuclei involved in motor functions), the *midbrain reticular formation* (clusters of cells with varied functions, including control of arousal), the *oculomotor nucleus* (motoneurons for extra- and intraocular muscles), and the *cerebral peduncles* (a large bundle of fibers originating in the cortex and terminating in the midbrain, pons, medulla, and spinal cord; it is involved in the cerebral control of movement and in the modulation of incoming sensory information).

3.2.5   Metencephalon

Major structures in the metencephalon include the *fourth ventricle*, the *pons*, and the *cerebellum* (see Figure 3.5.). The pons contains several cranial nerve nuclei (both sensory and motor), the *pontine reticular formation* (again, involved in regulation of consciousness and sleep), and the *pontine nuclei* (which project to the cerebellum). The cerebellum overlies the pons and is involved in motor coordination and the control of posture. It is especially important in the control of ballistic movements and in the sensory control of motor output.

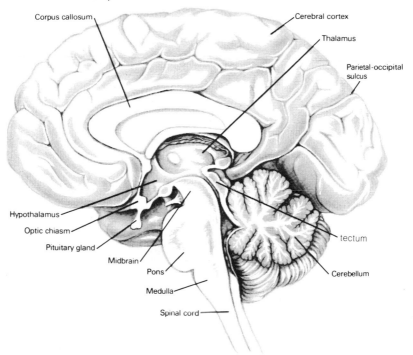

Figure 3.5. Sagittal section of the brain showing mesencephalic, metencephalic, and myelencephalic structures of the brain. The mesencephalon, or midbrain, includes the tectum (or roof) and tegmentum (or floor, which is the site labelled midbrain in the figure). Structures of the metencephalon include the cerebellum and pons. The myelencephalon is represented in the figure by the medulla. (Reprinted by permission of the publisher from J. P. Kelly, Principles of the functional and anatomical organization of the nervous system, in *Principles of neural science*, E. Kandel and J. Schwartz, Eds., p. 213. Copyright 1985 by Elsevier Science.)

3.2.6   *Myelencephalon*

The myelencephalon is the most caudal part of the brain and is usually referred to as the *medulla* (see Figure 3.5). A large portion of the medulla is comprised of the caudal portion of the reticular formation, called the *medullary reticular formation*, which receives inputs from interoceptors such as baroreceptors and chemoreceptors in the vasculature. Medullary reticular efferents project largely to the spinal cord (i.e., reticulo-spinal tracts). Thus, areas within the medullary reticular formation play an important role in the control of respiration, blood pressure, and maintenance of posture. In addition, there are a number of sensory and motor cranial nerve nuclei within the medulla. The *pyramidal tract*, a caudal extension of the cerebral peduncles, lies at the ventral surface of the medulla. It represents a subset of descending cortical fibers specifically destined for the spinal cord to control movement.

3.3   ANATOMY AND PHYSIOLOGY OF THE AUTONOMIC NERVOUS SYSTEM

Generally, a distinction is made between the *central nervous system* (CNS), comprised of the brain and spinal cord, and the *peripheral nervous system*, comprised of all the other nerve fibers. The peripheral nervous system is usually subdivided into two divisions: the *somatic nervous system* and the *autonomic nervous system*. The somatic nervous system consists of the nerves to and from motor and sensory organs whereas the autonomic nervous system innervates the viscera.

The autonomic nervous system regulates internal states. Emotions, cognitive activity, responses to environmental changes, and disease all involve complex regulation of internal activity; this is accomplished through interactions between the autonomic nervous system and the CNS. These interactions have been the focus of many psychophysiological studies and have illuminated some of the contributions of the autonomic nervous system to behavior.

The integrative mechanism in the autonomic nervous system serves a critical purpose for the maintenance of life by keeping the body's internal states within acceptable ranges. The principle governing this regulatory system is a process Walter B. Cannon (1935) called *homeostasis*. Homeostasis is often understood in the context of control theory (the systematic use of feedback to maintain a system at a desired state or set point). Thus, the essential elements of a controlled system are (1) feedback pathways that provide information about the state of the system, (2) a mechanism that defines the set point, (3) a comparison between the state of the system (as reflected in the feedback) and the desired state (as reflected by the set point), and (4) effectors that can modify systems parameters so as to minimize the difference between the set signal and the feedback signal. As described in what follows, the autonomic nervous system uses each of these components to set an appropriate internal state for each of life's varying circumstances. Certain areas of the brain, including many brainstem nuclei and the hypothalamus, play a crucial role in this process.

For a long time, the operation of the automatic nervous system and the attendant smooth muscles was thought to be "involuntary." This contrasted with the view of the "voluntary" control of the striate or skeletal muscles by the CNS. This distinction is less clear today due to demonstrations that visceral learning can take place (Miller, 1969); the underlying mechanisms for these effects remain controversial.

3.3.1   *Sympathetic and parasympathetic nervous system*

The autonomic nervous system can be divided into a *sympathetic division* (or thoracolumbar) and a *parasympathetic division* (or craniosacral). These antagonistic branches of the autonomic nervous system differ structurally, functionally, and chemically but work together to maintain homeostasis.

The major function of the sympathetic nervous system is to prepare the body for action, and each visceral change elicited by this system can be viewed as a step toward adapting to the action requirements of a situation. Stimulation of the sympathetic fibers, for instance, leads to dilation of the bronchioles and pupils, constriction of blood vessels supplying the skin, inhibition of the gastrointestinal system, and increases in blood pressure, stroke volume, cardiac output, and sweating. These are all physiologically compatible responses that are observed in organisms that are either stressed or challenged. Cannon termed this the "fight-or-flight" response, an idea that has had enormous impact on the field of psychophysiology.

In contrast to the quick diffuse actions of the sympathetic nervous system, the parasympathetic nervous system works to restore and maintain bodily resources. Stimulation of parasympathetic fibers leads to decreases in heart rate and blood pressure, constriction of the bronchioles and pupils, and increases in digestive functions. Whereas the sympathetic nervous system often discharges as a whole, components of the parasympathetic division typically operate more independently and are less diffuse. There seems little reason, from an adaptive point of view, for the parasympathetic nervous system to discharge all at once as the sympathetic nervous system does in an emergency.

These functional differences between the sympathetic and parasympathetic divisions of the autonomic nervous system are supported by very clear anatomical differences between the two divisions (Figure 3.6). In both divisions, neurons exit the brain or spinal cord and make connections with other neurons in *ganglia*, collections of neuronal cell bodies outside the central nervous system. The first-order neuron is called the *preganglionic fiber*; the neuron connecting the ganglia to the organ is called the *postganglionic fiber*. Preganglionic fibers of the sympathetic nervous system emerge from the first thoracic to the third lumbar level of the spinal cord and are carried to a vertically oriented collection of ganglia called the *sympathetic chain*. Since the sympathetic chain is close to the spinal cord, the preganglionic sympathetic fibers are short and the postganglionic fibers are long. As the preganglionic fibers leave the spinal cord, they diverge considerably; some of them make connections with ganglia several segments above and/or below their point of origin. Thus, a single ganglion in the sympathetic chain receives input from several segments of the spinal cord. A number of ganglia fuse to produce large numbers of postganglionic neurons that travel to the visceral organs they innervate. With this diverging structural organization, one can see how an impulse from any portion of the sympathetic nervous system could potentially activate a large portion of the visceral system.

The fibers of the parasympathetic nervous system emerge either from cranial nerves or the sacral division of the spinal cord, but there are no interactions between the two. As a result, the parasympathetic nervous system produces more specific visceral changes than the sympathetic nervous system. The preganglionic fibers of the parasympathetic nervous system make connections in ganglia very close to or within the organs they innervate. Thus, in contrast to the sympathetic nervous system, the preganglionic fibers of the parasympathetic nervous system are long and the postganglionic fibers are short.

The details of the anatomy of the parasympathetic nervous system are shown in Figure 3.6. Note the major role played by the vagus nerve (cranial nerve X), which innervates nearly all the organs and glands of the trunk. The exceptions are the bladder, lower bowel, and genitalia, which are innervated by the pelvic nerve. The parasympathetic nerves arising from the oculomotor (III), the facial (VII), and the glossopharyngeal (IX) cranial nerves control the glands of the head.

Not only are the parasympathetic and sympathetic divisions structurally different, they release different chemical messengers as well. When preganglionic fibers

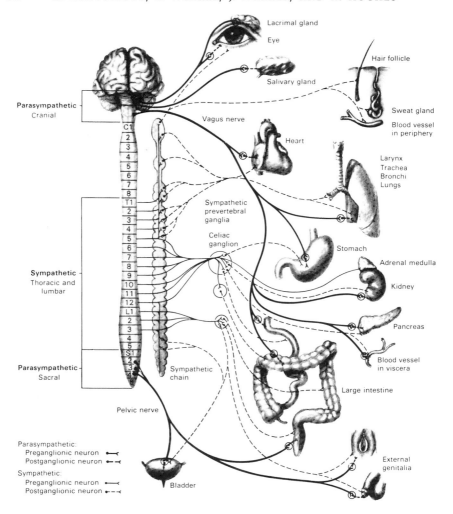

Figure 3.6. Target organs innervated by the parasympathetic and sympathetic divisions of the autonomic nervous system. (Reprinted by permission of the publisher from N. R. Carlson, *Physiology of behavior*, p. 117. Copyright 1986 by Allyn and Bacon, Needham Hts., MA.)

make connections with postganglionic fibers, they secrete acetylcholine (ACh) in both the sympathetic and the parasympathetic nervous system. Acetylcholine is also secreted by the postganglionic parasympathetic neurons. Postganglionic neurons in the sympathetic nervous system, however, secrete norepinephrine (NE), a substance similar to that secreted by the adrenal medulla. Thus, there is a chemical as well as a structural basis for diffuse sympathetic nervous system effects as opposed to more localized parasympathetic effects.

The considerable regularity in the particular chemical messengers used by different branches of the autonomic nervous system is not without exceptions, however. The sweat glands, for instance, are innervated almost exclusively by the sympathetic nervous system, and acetylcholine, rather than NE, is the predominant chemical messenger. However, a minor adrenergic innervation is present (Shields, MacDowell, Fairchild, & Campbell, 1988). Hair follicles receive only sympathetic nervous innervation, and almost all blood vessels are innervated exclusively by the sympathetic division. Note, also, that the nature of chemical transmission in the autonomic nervous system is more complex than this overview would imply; details are provided after further discussion of chemical communication between neurous.

3.3.2 *Sympathetic–parasympathetic interactions*

The parasympathetic and the sympathetic divisions of the autonomic nervous system differ structurally, functionally, and chemically, and they often operate antagonistically. However, it is important to realize that both the sympathetic and parasympathetic divisions are always active. One is not "on" when the other is "off." The interactions are complex, and it is therefore not usually possible to ascertain which branch is responsible for a change in a particular visceral response from the response itself. Heart rate acceleration, for instance, may be attributed to an increase in sympathetic activation, a decrease in parasympathetic activity, or both. Generalizing about the sympathetic nervous system as a whole from a change in electrodermal activity (EDA; see Dawson, Schell, & Filion, chapter 11) is also difficult since the sweat glands are innervated primarily by atypical cholinergic sympathetic fibers.

Psychophysiologists have begun to outline ways to differentiate between the parasympathetic and sympathetic contributions to visceral change (e.g., Porges Bohrer, chapter 21), but at this point, it is difficult to do so using most non-invasive psychophysiological measures. To add further to the complexity, in some systems there is a clear lack of antagonism between the sympathetic and parasympathetic nervous system. Although very clear antagonistic relations are seen in the heart and lungs, supplementary interactions between sympathetic and parasympathetic nerves occur in the control of salivation and sexual reflexes.

The autonomic nervous system typically has direct effects on smooth muscles. However, those interested in the gut should note that an *enteric nervous system* also exists (cf. Costa, Furness, & Gibbins, 1986). The enteric nervous system is an extensive plexus of nerves within the bowel that is modulated by the autonomic nervous system. Costa et al. (1986) assert that there are more neurons in the enteric nervous system than in the spinal cord. This implies that understanding the neural control of the gut requires understanding the interplay between sympathetic and parasympathetic influences, the spontaneous activity of smooth muscle, and the physiology of the enteric nervous system (see Stern, Koch, & Vasey, chapter 16).

Any tendency to think of the autonomic nervous system as mostly motor output is to be avoided. Afferent neurons comprise at least half of the autonomic nervous system; the cell bodies of these autonomic afferents are found in the dorsal root ganglia along with those of sensory neurons arriving from the somatic nervous system (see Truex & Carpenter, 1969). These pathways provide information for autonomic reflexes, which perform complex regulatory functions in the autonomic nervous system. An excellent description of these reflexes may be found in Koizumi and Brooks (1980).

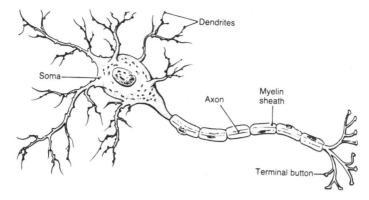

Figure 3.7. Morphology of a neuron. (Reprinted by permission of the publisher from N. R. Carlson, *Physiology of behavior*, p. 18. Copyright 1986 by Allyn and Bacon, Needham Hts., MA.)

3.4   NEURONAL EXCITABILITY AND SYNAPTIC TRANSMISSION

3.4.1   *Cell morphology*

Information is conveyed between nerve cells through chemical and electrical signals. This process of information transfer is called synaptic transmission. In order to understand how information is transferred between cells in the nervous system, some basic morphological features of nerve cells must be described. This review is by no means comprehensive and focuses on those aspects of the nerve cell that are important for cellular signaling.

The nerve cell, or *neuron,* is the fundamental unit of the nervous system (Figure 3.7). Neurons, like all cells, are closed bags with walls made out of proteins and lipids; the cell wall is called the *membrane.* The nerve cell membrane is much more than a wall, however; it has extraordinary electrochemical properties that are described in what follows. All nerve cells have a cell body, or *soma,* where energy is generated and other life-sustaining functions of the cell occur. Secretory products called *neurotransmitters* or *neuromodulators* are often, but not invariably, synthesized in the soma. Arborizations called *dendrites* extend from the cell body and receive signals from other neurons; these signals regulate the electrical state of the cell. Most neurons in the central nervous system have many dendrites, but some neurons have only a few or just one. The *axon* of a neuron is a stalklike structure that extends from the cell body for distances ranging from several micrometers to about a meter in the human adult. Each neuron has only one axon, but many axons send out branches (called *collaterals*) and arborize extensively at their ends. At the tips of these branches are bulbous structures called *terminal butons,* which form attachments with other neurons. A gap of approximately 200 Å, called the *synapse,* occurs between the terminal buton and the adjoining cell's membrane (Figure 3.8). The secretory products of the neuron (e.g., neurotransmitters) remain stored within the terminals in packets called *vesicles* until they are released as cellular signals. When released, the chemicals affect the electrochemical properties of the

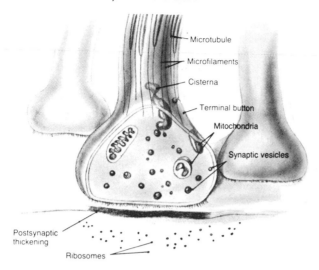

Figure 3.8. Details of a pre- and postsynaptic neuron at a synapse. The terminal button of the presynaptic neuron is shown above the postsynaptic cell. Microtubules and microfilaments form an internal network of tubes that interconnect various regions of the cell. Mitochondria provide energy for cellular functions. Neurotransmitters are synthesized and transported to the terminals through microtubules; in the terminals, neurotransmitters are stored in synaptic vesicles. The membrane of the postsynaptic cell is thicker at a synapse; this portion of the neuron is called the postsynaptic thickening. Ribosomes, which assist in protein synthesis, are shown in the postsynaptic neuron. (Reprinted by permission of the publisher from N. R. Carlson, *Physiology of behavior*, p. 53. Copyright 1986 by Allyn and Bacon, Needham Hts., MA.)

membrane of the adjacent cell. Synapses are found on dendrites, cell bodies, and axon terminals. An important morphological feature of the neuron is the *axon hillock*, which is located at the junction of the cell body and axon. The summation of information received from other cells at this site on the neuron determines whether or not that neuron will pass on a message to other cells.

3.4.2   *Electric and ionic mechanisms of nerve conduction*

3.4.2.1   *Generation of electrical potentials by ions*

A neuron may be thought of as one link in a vast communication network. In terms of its communicative functions, a neuron can be in one of three states: (1) at rest, neither receiving nor conveying a signals; (2) receiving a signal from another neuron or sensory receptor; or (3) conveying a signal to another neuron. These activity states can be described in terms of the electrical and chemical signals that are used by cells when they receive input from and pass on information to other cells.

Electrical signals in nerve cells are generated by *ions* (electrically charged atoms) that flow into and out of neurons. The generation of electricity results simply from the movement of these ions. Three ions are especially important in generating

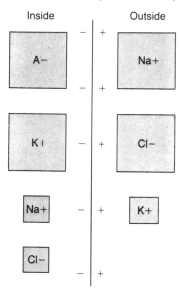

Figure 3.9. Distribution of important ions inside and outside of a model cell. Na^+ = sodium, K^+ = potassium, Cl^- = chloride, A^- = large anions. The vertical line in the center represents the neuronal membrane. (Reprinted by permission of the publisher from N. R. Carlson, *Physiology of behavior*, p. 36. Copyright 1986 by Allyn and Bacon, Needham Hts., MA.)

electrical signals in nerve cells: sodium (Na^+), potassium (K^+), and chloride (Cl^-). These ions are differentially distributed inside and outside of neurons (Figure 3.9), and ions move across the membrane through small pores called *ion channels* (cf. Hille, 1984). Ion channels are sometimes called *ionic gates* to indicate their function of determining whether or not an ion can cross the membrane. When the gate for a particular ion is closed, the membrane is impermeable to that ion. When the gate is open, ions of that type may move freely across the membrane. Given that the ion channel is open, whether an ion moves into or out of a cell depends largely on one of two passive physical forces; a diffusional force and an electrochemical force. The diffusional force, called the *concentration gradient*, operates upon each type of ion *independently*, favoring the flow of an ion from regions of high concentration to regions of low concentration. For example, since K^+ is found in high concentrations inside the neuron, the concentration gradient tends to move K^+ out of the cell. The electrochemical force, the *electrical gradient*, favors the attraction of oppositely charged species (e.g., + and −) and the repulsion of like-charged species (e.g., − and −, + and +), a process that maintains electrical neutrality in most physical systems. Since large negatively charged proteins are trapped inside neurons, electrochemical forces favor the flow of positively charged ions, such as K^+, from outside to inside the cell to neutralize the electrical imbalance. This however, opposes the concentration gradient, which tends to push K^+ out of the cell. A compromise condition (*equilibrium*) occurs such that neither force "wins": Neither electrical neutrality nor total diffusion of ions occurs.

It should be noted that in addition to the influence of physical forces, ions may move through the cell membrane at random due to the leaky nature of the porous cell wall. To compensate for the leakiness of the cell membrane to Na^+ and K^+, neurons actively control ionic movement through a mechanism referred to simply as a pump. Unlike diffusional and electrochemical forces that are passive, the pump requires energy from the neuron to operate. Thus, passive physical forces and a cellular pump control the flow of ions across the cell membrane, which in turn generates electrical potentials. These forces are summarized in Figure 3.9.

When the gates for a particular ion are open, the membrane potential moves toward a particular voltage specific to that ion (*equilibrium potential*) that balances out the various forces described in the preceding paragraphs. The equilibrium potential for an ion can be calculated from the *Nernst equation* if the concentration of the ion inside and outside the cell is known (Koester, 1985; cf. Kuffler, Nicholls, & Martin, 1984). The values for particular ions have been calculated and compared to experimentally measured values during different activity states of neurons (e.g., when the neuron is at rest). This line of investigation is important because when the predicted and measured values are comparable, one can conclude that (1) the membrane is likely to be permeable to that ion during that activity state and (2) that ion may be important in generating the observed electrical potential. Conversely, if there is a discrepancy between the predicted and measured values, the membrane is probably not permeable to that ion and that ion probably is not responsible for the electrical potential.

3.4.2.2   *Types of electrical potential in neurons*

Resting potential. Three types of electrical signals are generated by neurons, each corresponding to one of the three activity states of a neuron (receiving, sending, or resting). The potential that can be measured across the cell membrane when the neuron is at rest is called the *resting potential*. The value of the resting potential (about -70 mV) is close to the K^+ equilibrium potential predicted by the Nernst equation, and experimental studies have confirmed that alterations in K^+ are followed by changes in the resting potential. The small discrepancy between the K^+ potential and the resting potential is due to a small leakage of Na^+. This illustrates that the membrane potential is the result of the combination of the equilibrium potentials for each ion and the permeability of the membrane to each ion. This relationship is formally described in the Goldman–Hodgkin–Katz equation (see DeVoe & Maloney, 1980; cf. Hille, 1984). Thus in a resting state, the membrane potential is largely governed by K^+, reflecting the permeability of the membrane to K^+.

Graded potential. A second type of electrical potential is associated with cells when they are receiving information. This type of electrical potential is called a *graded potential*. Graded potentials can be subdivided into two types: synaptic potentials and receptor potentials. *Synaptic potentials* are generated when a neuron receives signals from other cells. Synaptic potentials are normally referred to as *inhibitory postsynaptic potentials* (IPSPs) or *excitatory postsynaptic potentials* (EPSPs), depending on whether the chemical input tends to inhibit or excite the cell on which it acts. Electroencephalograms, potentials that are commonly recorded from the scalp by psychophysiologists, are the sum of synaptic potentials from all of the neurons in the vicinity of the electrode (cf. Thompson & Patterson, 1974). *Receptor potentials* are generated when first-order sensory neurons (*primary afferents*) receive input from sensory receptors.

Graded potentials spread from their point of origin, acting at a distance to control the state of the neuron. Therefore, understanding synaptic physiology requires an appreciation of the properties of graded potentials. First, the initial size of a graded potential is proportional to the size of the triggering stimulus. Second, as graded potentials spread away from their point of origin, they decrease in strength due to the cable properties of neurons (e.g., the presence of leakage, resistance, and capacitance). Finally, graded potentials are summed over both space and time at the axon hillock. Thus, at this junction of the soma and the axon, the overall effect of all the messages being received by the cell are weighed to determine the type of signal the neuron will pass on to other cells. If many more excitatory than inhibitory inputs are received by the cell (due to many excitatory inputs at different locations on the cell or to a fast sequence of excitatory inputs), the neuron passes on a message. On the other hand, if many more inhibitory than excitatory inputs are received by the cell, the cell will be inhibited and thus prevented from sending a chemical signal. It should be recognized that cellular inhibition is itself a form of communication, one that is primary in the regulation of many neuronal systems.

Action potentials. When neurons are excited into sending a message, a third type of electrical potential can be measured, the *action potential*. During an action potential, the membrane voltage swing from -70 mV to approximately $+40$ mV and back again over a period of time that ranges from 0.5 to 5 msec for different cells. The action potential is sometimes called "spike" because of its appearance on an oscilloscope. Figure 3.10 illustrates the characteristic waveform of an action potential. The initial rising portion of the waveform is carried mainly by the influx of sodium ions (Na^+); the falling portion of the waveform is associated with the efflux of potassium ions (K^+). When an action potential occurs, the cell is said to discharge, fire, or produce an impulse.

Action potentials are generated when the sum of graded potentials drives the resting membrane potential positive by about 15 mV. Although action potentials occur when the cell is more positive, the membrane voltage (having a resting value that is negative) is decreased; hence, the neuron is excited when it is *depolarized*. For a particular neuron, an action potential occurs at a specific membrane voltage called the *threshold voltage*. When the threshold is crossed, an action potential is generated; when the membrane potential is more negative than the threshold, no action potential is generated. Unlike the amplitude of a graded potential, the size of an action potential is not affected by the amplitude of the triggering stimulus, although the latency of the action potential is proportional to the size of the excitatory stimulus once the threshold is reached. Thus, in a given cell, a stimulus just over threshold will generate the same size action potential as a stimulus much over threshold. Therefore, action potentials are said to be *all or none*: Action potentials either occur (when the membrane voltage is above threshold) or they do not occur (when the membrane voltage is below threshold).

Action potentials travel from the cell body to the terminals, a process called *propagation*. Unlike graded potentials, which "fade" as they spread away from the point of origin, action potentials exhibit no decrement as they move down an axon

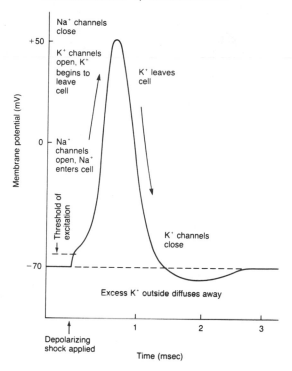

Figure 3.10. A typical action potential and the ionic fluxes associated with various components of the waveform. (Reprinted by permission of the publisher from N. R. Carlson, *Physiology of behavior*, p. 42. Copyright 1986 by Allyn and Bacon, Needham Hts., MA.)

toward the nerve terminals. This movement is really the generation of successive action potentials along the length of an axon. This occurs through the electrical current spread during an action potential that depolarizes the adjacent membrane.

Many axons are sheathed with a lipid insulator called myelin, which is interrupted at regular intervals to expose the axon. At these gaps, the *nodes of Ranvier*, the axon is susceptible to depolarization. Because the sheathed part of the axon is insulated, action potentials jump from one node to the next, a process called *saltatory conduction*. This jumping action greatly increases propagation velocity, the rate of which ranges from about 3 to 120 m/s. Two factors largely determine the speed of propagation: the diameter of the axon and whether or not it is myelinated. Myelinated axons with wide diameters conduct the fastest, whereas fine caliber unmyelinated axons conduct the slowest.

Action potentials are followed by refractory periods during which the membrane becomes electrically unresponsive. At first, the membrane cannot generate another action potential at all (*absolute refractory period*); later, a greater than normal positive change in membrane voltage is required to generate another action potential (*relative refractory period*).

(a)

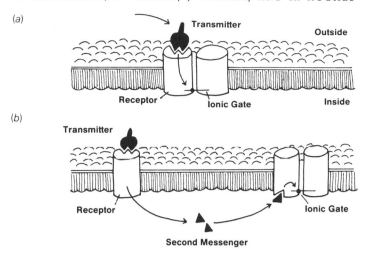

(b)

Figure 3.11. Activation of ion channels by neurotransmitters. Panel *a* shows direct activation of an ion channel by the binding of a transmitter, such as acetylcholine, to the receptor; panel *b* shows indirect activation of an ion channel by a transmitter. In the latter case, second messenger molecules serve as the connection between the actions of the neurotransmitter (primary messenger) and activation of the ion channel.

3.4.3   *Neurotransmission*

Action potentials lead to the release of neurotransmitters from the cell. When action potentials propagate down the axon, they cause voltage-sensitive Ca^{2+} channels at the nerve terminals to open. Calcium ions rush into the terminal, where they bind with the enzyme, calmodulin. This enzyme facilitates the release of neurotransmitters from the terminal (*exocytosis*) into the synaptic cleft. In this context, the cell releasing the transmitter is called the *presynaptic* cell, and the cell upon which the transmitter acts is called the *postsynaptic* cell.

Transmitters affect the membrane voltage of the postsynaptic neuron by binding to receptor molecules, specific proteins that span the postsynaptic cell membrane. Neurons generally possess many different types of receptors so that they may respond to each of the possible transmitters released from the many synapses usually present. The receptor molecules have a three-dimensional structure that matches the three-dimensional structure of the transmitter molecule, much like the three-dimensional structure of a lock matches the three-dimensional structure of a key. Thus, different types of neurotransmitters interact with different classes of receptor. For instance, dopamine molecules fit into certain receptor proteins (dopamine receptors) that are different in three-dimensional structure from the receptor proteins for other neurotransmitters. When binding occurs, the neurotransmitter alters the three-dimensional structure of the receptor, which leads to a series of events inside the postsynaptic neuron, resulting in alterations in ionic conductance. Although the typical description of the action of transmitters is postsynaptically on the soma or dendrites, transmitters may also bind to receptors on the presynaptic cell (*autoreceptors*), a form of neuronal feedback control.

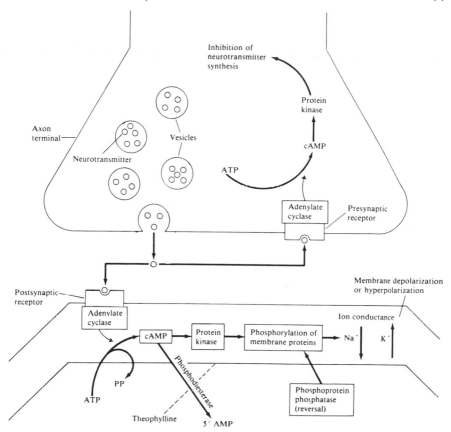

Figure 3.12. Chemical reactions involved in the activation of an ion channel by cyclic AMP. (Reprinted by permission of the publisher from R. S. Feldman and L. F. Quenzer, *Fundamentals of neuropsychopharmacology*, p. 109. Copyright 1984 by Sinauer Associates, Sunderland, MA.)

The binding of a transmitter to a postsynaptic receptor results in the generation of graded potentials (IPSPs and EPSPs) through the opening and closing of particular ion channels. Some transmitters, such as acetylcholine, directly activate ion channels when they bind to receptors (Karlin et al., 1983). This occurs because the ion channel and the receptor are part of the same protein. Some ion channels, however, are located on a separate part of the cell membrane, away from the receptor protein. In these instances, intracellular chemical signals coordinate the functioning of the two (see Figure 3.11). The intermediary molecules used for this purpose are called *second messengers*. Thus, when receptor proteins spanning the cell membrane are bound by the appropriate transmitters, second messengers on the inside of the cell are activated and go through a series of chemical reactions that eventually lead to the opening or closing of an ion channel. Two second messenger systems have been well characterized. They are cyclic adenosine monophosphate (cAMP) and phosphoinositol (PI).

The activation of an ion channel via cAMP involves several steps (Greengard, 1976, 1979) (Figure 3.12). First, a neurotransmitter or hormone binds to a receptor on the extracellular side of the cell membrane. This frees the catalytic subunit of adenylate cyclase inside the cell, thus forming the active state of the enzyme. The activated adenylate cyclase than catalyzes the formation of cAMP from adenosine triphosphate (ATP). Cyclic AMP then activates a cAMP-dependent protein kinase (protein kinase A) that can catelyze the phosphorylation of an ion channel, which alters its conformation and opens or closes the channel (see the bottom portion of Figure 3.12).

The PI system (Berridge, 1987; Berridge & Irvine, 1984) is somewhat more complex because at least two molecules carry out the transduction. One of these is diacylglycerol, which activates protein kinase C, which then can phosphorylate an ion channel as in the cAMP system. The second transducing molecule in the PI system is inositol triphosphate. Inositol triphosphate is involved in a number of receptor-mediated events such as mobilization and release of intracellular Ca^{2+} from nonmitochondrial stores (a process associated with Ca^{2+}-sensitive processes such as secretion and muscle contractions).

Recently, G proteins, another group of modulatory chemicals, have been found to link some receptors to a second messenger system (Gilman, 1987; Stryer & Bourne, 1986). Two types of proteins are particularly important: G_s stimulates adenylate cyclase activity, while G_i inhibits the enzyme. Recent evidence shows that these G proteins can affect the transduction of cAMP-dependent signals to ion channels (Hescheler et al., 1986, 1987). Other G proteins transduce signals between receptors and ion channels via intermediaries in the PI system (Ewald et al., 1988, Brown et al., 1984). Although G Proteins usually indirectly modify ion channels through second messengers, they apparently directly activate some K^+ and Ca^2+ channels (Brown & Birnbaumer, 1988).

The interaction between transmitter and receptor does not involve a long-lasting covalent bond; rather it involves an ionic bond, and after a time, the transmitter dissociates from the receptor and returns to the extracellular space. At that time, the transmitter may be taken into the presynaptic terminal for recycling and reuse or it may be broken down by enzymes and excreted. In either case, the synaptic action of the transmitter is terminated.

3.4.4   Summary

After a transmitter is released from a presynaptic cell, it binds to a receptor protein on the postsynaptic neuron. This leads to the opening or closing of ion channels, either through a direct coupling between the receptor and the ion channel or through the activation of a second messenger. The flow of ions into and out of the cell causes the voltage across the cell membrane to either increase or decrease. These changes in membrane voltage are measured as graded potentials. Graded potentials (IPSPs and EPSPs) are summed at the axon hillock. If the overall input onto that cell is inhibitory, the cell will be prevented from passing on a chemical message to other cells. If the overall input, however, is both excitatory and exceeds the critical firing threshold, an action potential is generated and propagates down the axon. When the action potential reaches the terminals, voltage-sensitive calcium channels are opened. Calcium ions in the extracellular space enter the terminal and bind calmodulin. Transmitter is then released from the cell through a process called exocytosis. The transmitter molecules released into the synaptic cleft can then bind to receptor proteins on the postsynaptic membrane and the process repeats itself.

3.5 THE SYNAPTIC MESSAGE

Only recently have we begun to understand the complexity of the synaptic message and how it applies to function. As we discuss in what follows, relatively recent discoveries about synaptic messages blur the previous simple conception of synaptic signaling. Although these findings have complicated matters, they have led to a better understanding of the fundamental properties of brain function. The analysis of synaptic messages has become an important new way of studying the nervous system and moves us away from a purely connectionistic/electronic-circuit view. We now know that a neuron may secrete many messenger molecules, and it may alter the mix of secretory products as a result of experience. You might say that we used to think that neurons speak in words, but now we know they speak in sentences. Further, we now know that the brain responds as a target organ for certain hormones; and some neuronal release products act more like hormones than the electronically fast neurotransmitters we tend to think of in the nervous system. These findings have profoundly altered the way we think about the nervous system and therefore have important implications for research in psychophysiology.

3.5.1 *Classes of neurotransmitters*

Let us begin the discussion of neurotransmitters with a current list of the classes of chemicals thought to be released from neurons (cf. Feldman and Quenzer, 1984; see Table 3.1). Acetylcholine was the first substance shown to mediate chemical transmission across the synapse (Loewi, 1921). Subsequently, several monoamines were identified: norepinephrine, epinephrine, dopamine, and serotonin (5-hydroxytryptamine). Some neurons use amino acids as transmitters. Some of these amino acids, such as glycine and glutamate, are found in all cells for use in protein synthesis, while others, such as gamma-aminobutyric acid (GABA), are modified from one of the 20 or so standard amino acids. In recent years, investigators have increasingly recognized the importance of polypeptide neurotransmitters (or simply peptides, or neuropeptides). Peptides are cleaved from proteins into products; thus peptides are in fact small proteins. Close to 100 such substances have been discovered and postulated to be transmitters. Several other substances such as adenosine and several purines including the ubiquitous ATP have also been postulated to act as neurotransmitters.

In a few cases, the discovery of specific receptors for a drug led to the implication that an endogenous ligand (or transmitter) for the receptor must be present. This logic led to the discovery of the opioid peptides or endorphins (cf. Akil et al., 1984). Currently, the most prominent example of a receptor in search of a neurotransmitter is the benzodiazepine receptor (cf. Tallman & Gallager 1985). This receptor apparently mediates the actions of valiumlike anxiolytic drugs and a remarkable class of opposite-acting compounds (β-carbolines) that elicit reports of feelings of panic in humans (Dorow, Horowski, Paschelke, Amin, & Beastrup, 1983) and learned helplessness in rats (Drugan, Maier, Skolnick, Paul, & Crawley, 1985). More than six endogenous substances have been proposed as the putative endogenous ligand for benzodiazepine receptors, but a definite role as a neurotransmitter has not been established for any of them (e.g. Ferrero, Guidotti, Conti-Troconi, & Costa, 1984; Skolnick & Paul, 1982). Another receptor in search of a transmitter is the so-called haloperidol-sensitive σ receptor (cf. Walker et al., 1988). This receptor binds many antipsychotic drugs and a variety of $(+)$-morphinans and $(+)$-benzomorphans,

Table 3.1. *Major neurotransmitters and neuromodulators*

Acetylcholine (ACh) Monoamines
Dopamine (DA)
Norepinephrine (NE noradrenalin)
Epinephrine (E, adrenalin)
Serotonin (5-hydroxytryptamine, 5HT)

Amino acids
Aspartic acid
Glutamic acid
Homocysteic acid
β-Alanine
Gamma-aminobutyric acid (GABA)
Taurine

Peptides
Alpha-neoendorphin
Alpha-melanocyte stimulating hormone (α-MSH)
Angiotensin II
Cholecystokinin (CCK)
Corticotropin-releasing factor
Dynorphin
β-endorphin
Enkephalin
Leutinizing hormone-releasing hormone
Neuropeptide Y (NPY)
Somatostatin
Substance P
Vasoactive intestinal polypeptide
Vasopressin (antidiuretic hormone, ADH)

Other
Histamine
Adenosine
Various purines

---

some of which produce psychosislike effects in humans. Recent evidence suggests that this system may mediate some of the antipsychotic actions or motor side effects of neuroleptic drugs. Presumably, certain neurons in the brain release transmitters for these receptors (Contreras, DiMaggio, & O'Donohue, 1987).

3.5.2   *Complex synaptic messages*

3.5.2.1   *Neuromodulation*

A "wiring diagram" of nervous structures can no longer be considered sufficient to make inferences about function because the message at the synapse is much more complex than previously assumed. In recent years, the term *neuromodulator* has come into increasing use for neuronal release products that do not fit the standard definition of short-acting, hyper-, or depolarizing neurotransmitters.

The term neuromodulator is sometimes used to refer to compounds that modify the actions of other secretory products (Barker, 1976; Barker, Neale, Smith, & MacDonald, 1978). Neuromodulators of this sort do not exert direct effects on the postsynaptic membrane but alter the efficacy of another substance. For example, enkephalin (an opioid peptide) applied iontophoretically to mouse spinal neurons depresses glutamate-evoked responses. This action is unusual because the inhibition of glutamate occurs independently of any direct effect of enkephalin on membrane conductance. Although in some cells, enkephalin directly alters ionic gates like a typical neurotransmitter, in this case, it acts as a neuromodulator by altering conductance changes associated with the actions of another transmitter.

The term neuromodulator is also used to refer to substances that show an unusually long time course. For example, β-endorphin is a very potent opioid peptide that produces long-lasting cellular and behavioral effects (e.g., Walker et al., 1977). This substance is directly relevant to psychophysiological work because it is released from neurons arising in two important centers of autonomic integration, the hypothalamus and the nucleus tractus solitarius (cf. Akil et al., 1984). Very low doses of the substance can cause alterations in pain sensitivity that last an hour or more. In view of its distinctly hormonelike action in the central nervous system, perhaps it is not surprising that β-endorphin is also released as a hormone from the pituitary gland. Indeed, some development studies indicate that hormone-producing endocrine cells and peptide-secreting neurons have a common embryonic origin (Pearse, 1976).

In related research, Sandman et al. (1971) demonstrated long-lasting EEG effects of analogs of alpha-melanocyte-stimulating hormone, a further indication that some neuronal products exert potent long-term actions characteristic of hormones. A number of other centrally acting peptides also exert unusually long-lasting effects including substance P, cholecystokinin, vasopressin, and others (e.g., Krnjevic & Morris, 1974; Meck, Church, & Wenk, 1986; Mueller & Hsiao, 1978; cf. Sandman et al., 1971). These hormonelike neuromodulatory effects suggest that certain functions in the nervous system that exhibit long time constants (e.g., mood shifts) may be mediated by hormonelike neuromodulators rather than ill-defined and yet to be identified reverberating circuits frequently postulated in the past.

One unexpected finding from studies of the relationship between hormones and neurotransmitters was that the brain sometimes reverses roles with the glands. In other words, the brain becomes the target organ under the command of the glands. For example, the work of Lewis, Tordoff, Sherman, and Liebeskind (1982) suggests that opioids released along with catecholamines from the adrenal gland may then be transported to the brain via the blood to produce analgesia. This conclusion is based on studies that showed that opioid stress-induced analgesia depends upon the integrity of the adrenal medullary axis. Further support that the brain is sometimes the target organ derives from studies of angiotensin II (Severs & Daniels-Severs, 1973) and cholecystokinin (CCK; see Mueller & Hsiao, 1978), two peripheral hormones that may enter the brain from the systemic circulation and affect behavior upon commands from peripheral organs.

3.5.2.2 *Multiple release of transmitters*

At one time, most introductory neuroscience courses taught a rule called Dale's Principle. Dale's Principle asserts that each neuron secretes one and only one neurotransmitter. The principle is wrong on two counts. First, Dale never postulated this principle; Dale thought that all branches of the same neuron have the same secretary product(s) (Dale, 1935). Second, many (perhaps most) neurons secrete many substances (cf. Hokfelt et al., 1986). The evidence for multiple release is practically indisputable, and the new principle (multiple release) has important ramifications because the proportions of the release products can vary as function of experience.

The earliest clear sign of multiple neuromodulators per cell came from studies of neurons that produce opioid peptides. Biochemists and molecular biologists (Nakanishi et al., 1979) found that the potent opioid peptide β-endorphin was derived from a protein precursor that produced a whole array of interesting peptides. The entire molecular structure of this precursor (called proopiomelanocortin, POMC) was eventually determined, and we now know a good deal about the products that are released from neurons that use β-endorphin. In particular, we know that neurons that secrete β-endorphin also secrete α-melanocyte-stimulating hormone (referred to previously), gamma-melanocyte-stimulating hormone, and several other peptides.

In the case of β-endorphin, the functional significance of multiple release has been determined to at least some extent (Akil, Young, Walker, & Watson, 1986; Walker et al., 1987). These studies used analgesia as a dependent measure because β-endorphin apparently serves naturally to modulate pain sensitivity. Studies of the behavioral properties of other products of the β-endorphin precursor show that they too affect pain sensitivity (e.g., Walker, Akil, & Watson, 1980). Some products act as analgesics but do not have an opiate pharmacology (Walker, Berntson, Sandman, Kastin, & Akil, 1981). Other products are potentiators; they have no analgesic properties of their own but enhance the analgesia produced by other products. At least one of the release products may act as an antagonist; this peptide (β-endorphin$_{1-27}$, the first 27 amino acids of β-endorphin) significantly reduces the analgesia produced by β-endorphin.

The significance of these findings for behavior was further suggested by studies of stress-induced analgesia (Akil et al., 1986). Uncontrollable footshock under appropriate conditions causes animals to become analgesic. However, with repeated administration the animal shows behavioral tolerance, and the analgesic effect of stress is diminished. Biochemical studies have shown that this alteration in stress-induced analgesia is accompanied by a change in the chemical release patterns of β-endorphin-containing neurons. These neurons normally secrete little of the opiate-attenuator molecule (β-endorphin$_{1-27}$). However, after repeated stresses, the neurons switch to producing little β-endorphin and much more of the attenuator substance. These findings indicate that the synaptic message is modifiable in terms of the transmitter products released. The words of the synaptic sentence have been changed.

3.5.2.3 *Autonomic nervous system: differential release as a function of firing rate*

The multiple-release phenomenon is not limited to the central nervous system. This mode of synaptic transmission occurs widely in the autonomic nervous system as well. In fact, studies of chemical transmission in the autonomic nervous system have substantially clarified our understanding of multiple release. This is not surprising; historically, the autonomic nervous system has provided a model for the central nervous system because it is much easier to isolate secretory products and analyze their actions in the autonomic nervous system. These studies indicate a frequency-dependent release of different transmitters that sometimes exert opposite effects postsynaptically.

DeGroat and colleagues (1985, 1984) suggested such a frequency-dependent release of different transmitters from studies of the preganglionic innervation of the urinary bladder. In these neurons, acetylcholine is colocalized with enkephalin and the other half dozen or more products of the enkephalin precursor. They found that the usual postganglionic discharge elicited by stimulation of a branch of the pelvic nerve is inhibited by repetitive (20–30 Hz, 3–5 sec) stimulation of another branch of the same nerve. This effect is blocked by naloxone, a specific opiate antagonist, suggesting that at low stimulation frequencies acetylcholine is preferentially released and at higher frequencies enkephalin (which is sensitive to naloxone) is released. Since enkephalin and acetylcholine exhert opposite effects on the bladder, the chemical mix released at a given frequency is an important source of information beyond the electrical activity alone.

Another example of frequency-dependent release of different transmitters in the autonomic nervous system derives from the studies of Lundberg and Hokfelt (1986; see also Lundberg, Rudehill, Sollevi, Theodorsson-Norheim, & Hamberger, 1986). They demonstrated that low-frequency stimulation of the splenic nerve (sympathetic postganglionic) results in the release of NE. At higher frequencies of stimulation, a peptide (neuropeptide Y) that is costored with NE is preferentially released. Psychophysiologists may take additional interest in the vasoconstrictor responses produced by neuropeptide Y and the observation that burstlike firing in these nerves produces a greater vasoconstrictor response than the same number of action potentials in regular firing nerve. These studies suggest that higher frequency bursts may normally be associated with the preferential release of peptide products, many of which exert hormonelike actions.

We tend to associate a state of rest with the parasympathetic division of the autonomic nervous system and a state of emergency, the "fight or flight" responses, with the sympathetic division of the autonomic nervous system. Clearly, the data described in the preceding paragraphs indicate that the postsynaptic actions of autonomic nerves may change as a function of firing rate through the release of opposite-acting transmitters. These observations would thus appear to be applicable to psychophysiological models of the autonomic nervous system, especially if measures of burst firing in autonomic nerves can be developed.

3.5.2.4 *Multiple release and the vascular system*

The experiments described in the previous section further imply that some release products regulate blood flow. Indeed, the vasculature in the brain responds to increased neuronal firing by increasing blood flow to the local area (e.g., Lassen, Ingvar, & Skinhoj, 1978). Increasingly, it appears that this change in local blood flow is mediated by chemical products released from nerve cells that leave the synapse and bind to receptors or the vascular walls. Many vasoactive peptides are present in neurons, and biochemists have demonstrated the presence of receptors for these substances on vascular membranes. Some release products from neurons may accomplish a vascular function secondary to a postsynaptic action, whereas others may serve only a vascular function. In addition, vascular effects of some breakdown products of neuromodulators suggest that release products may convey a synaptic message while metabolites convey a corresponding vascular message. These findings suggest that we should look outside the synapse as well as at the postsynaptic membrane when considering the functions of multiple release.

3.6   ORGANIZING PRINCIPLES OF THE CENTRAL NERVOUS SYSTEM

Undoubtedly, the case for a neurochemical understanding of the nervous system cannot be isolated from the elegant wiring of the nervous system. Indeed, it may be self-evident that chemical transmitters and neuroanatomical connections must be considered together to understand neural mechanisms. Thus, the afferent (input) and efferent (output) connections of neurons provide important clues to the functional organization of neural systems. A great deal of anatomical order exists within many levels of analysis, ranging from major axonal pathways between nuclei down to specific patterns of synaptic contacts on individual neurons. In this section, we describe some of the general principles of anatomical organization. Here we delineate some of the major systems and discuss patterns of organization found within them. We will divide the central nervous system into (1) sensory systems, (2) motor systems, and (3) integrative systems. We hasten to note, however, that there exists a great deal of anatomical and functional interplay between these divisions, and many structures lie along the interfaces of these divisions.

3.6.1   Sensory systems

An important division between sensory systems is based on the orgin of the stimulus. The five special senses are called *exteroceptive* because the driving energy arrives from the outside world. However, anyone who has suffered from appendicitis can confirm that we have many sensors that report the state of our internal environment (*interoceptors*). These include not only pain sensors (nociceptors) but also baroreceptors, CO_2 receptors, joint position detectors, muscle spindles, and others. Many of these latter receptors apparently do not receive representations in the cerebral cortex, which is presumably why their activity does not reach subjective consciousness (see Reed, Harver, & Katkin, chapter 9).

3.6.1.1   Sensory transduction, receptive fields, and lateral inhibition

Several common features of all sensory systems have been discovered. Sensory systems always involve a transducer function that selectively converts a form of energy into electrochemical currents in the transducing cell. This function can occur either in specialized receptor cells (e.g., photoreceptors, haircells) or in distal processes of primary sensory neurons. The connections between the set of these receptor cells and the set of primary afferents are spatiotopically precise. That is to say, individual nerve cells only receive inputs from a small and usually contiguous subset of sensory receptors. As a result, individual sensory neurons will only respond to stimulation of a particular region of receptor surface (e.g., a particular portion of the skin). This small region of the receptor surface that elicits some response when stimulated is called the neuron's *receptive field*. The concept of the receptive field is central to any understanding of sensory systems. Indeed, the discipline of sensory physiology has as its principal concern the development of accurate descriptions of receptive fields of sensory neurons, since such a description is a prerequisite to understanding how the brain encodes, processes, and interprets sensory inputs.

One universal feature of receptive fields is termed *lateral inhibition*: The effects of activity in one sensory receptor are usually opposed by simultaneous stimulation of the surrounding receptors. Lateral inhibition was first described by H. K. Hartline

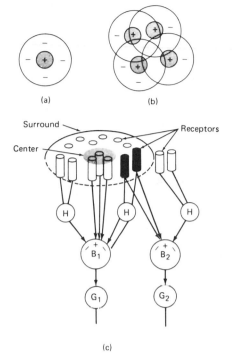

Figure 3.13. The center–surround receptive field organization of retinal ganglion cells. Note that regions in the center of a receptive field and in the surrounding doughnut-shaped area exert opposing influences as in *a*. This is accomplished as shown in the bottom panel. Inhibition by the surround region occurs in the retina through the interactions of horizontal cells (labelled *H*) that inhibit the bipolar cells (labelled *B*). (Reprinted by permission of Kurt Schlesinger, University of Colorado, Boulder.)

(1949) in the compound eye of the primitive invertebrate *Limulus* (the horseshoe crab). In this species, the receptor cells are directly interconnected via a fiber plexus, and Hartline's early work clearly showed that the light-induced activity in a receptor was attenuated by stimulation of an adjacent receptor via these lateral connections (Hartline & Ratliff, 1957). In vertebrate systems, this inhibition usually is mediated by an interneuron. The basic circuit that produces lateral inhibition in the vertebrate retina is schematically illustrated in Figure 3.13.

A general characteristic of all sensory (and probably nonsensory) neural systems, lateral inhibition has the important consequence of *accentuating differences* in stimulus intensity in adjacent areas while simultaneously attenuating responses to spatially uniform stimuli. In the case of vision, lateral inhibition enhances sensitivity to contours (see Figure 3.13) while it reduces sensitivity to gradual changes in luminance. The importance of lateral inhibition can be inferred from its occurrence at the first opportunity in retinal processing: the second-order neuron (bipolar cell; see Figure 3.13). Indeed, sensory systems generally implemented some form of lateral inhibition at the level of the first synaptic station (which is, of course, the first opportunity to include interneurons); lateral inhibition therefore characterizes all second-order sensor cells (e.g., cells in the cochlear nucleus in the auditory system and dorsal column nuclei in the somesthetic system). Techniques exactly analogous to the center–surround antagonism first described in the vertebrate eye by Kuffler (1953) are now routinely used to enhance contrast in digital image processing.

We have seen how lateral inhibition sharpens the spatial profile of sensory activity produced by stimulation of adjacent regions of the receptor surface. Despite the obvious differences between sensory systems, the consequence of these lateral interactions is always to enhance the system's ability to discriminate sites of activity within the mosaic of sensory receptors. For example, in the auditory system, tonal frequency is largely encoded by the place of activity on the basilar membrane (the receptor surface of the auditory system). Therefore, lateral inhibition results in what is known as *two-tone inhibition* (Greenwood & Maruyama, 1965). The important point to recognize is that two-tone inhibition enhances tonal discrimination capacity in the same manner that center–surround antagonism enhances spatial resolution in vision.

The central connections of primary afferents always preserve the topology of the receptor mosaic. As a result, neurons with nearby receptive fields also tend to be in close spatial proximity. When we consider the three-dimensional structure of a sensory nucleus within the brain, we find that the distribution of receptive fields within the nucleus recapitulates (often with astonishing precision) the receptor mosaic. This property is called receptotopic organization. We will have more to say about these receptotopic patterns shortly. For now we simply point out that the *locus* of activity within a nucleus is in fact part of the neural code for stimulus quality.

We should make one more point with respect to the organization of receptive fields. It is often the case that as we examine the response characteristics of progressively higher order sensory neurons, the receptive field characteristics become increasing more specific with respect to the spatio-temporal distribution of effective stimuli. When studying the highest levels of sensory systems, the cells often become very difficult to "drive" with sensory inputs, making it difficult to address the issue of how higher order percepts are encoded by individual neurons or by ensembles of neurons. Eventually, this increase in receptive field complexity is accompanied by an increase in receptive field size. Thus the receptotopic order described in the preceding paragraph ultimately gives way to representations that are not closely tied to the particular location of the eliciting stimulus. This is apparently a consequence of progressive convergence and is often regarded as evidence that the processing has gone from a strict receptor-based coordinate system to a nonreceptotopic system that one usually associates with higher order percepts (i.e., components of the system respond to intrinsic features of a given stimulus regardless of its position on the receptor surface).

3.6.1.2 *Central distribution of sensory inputs*

The central distribution of sensory inputs can be generally characterized as taking three specific routes. First, all primary sensory afferents contribute to reflex pathways that are localized in the spinal cord and brainstem. Second, sensory pathways influence the cerebellum, which has motor functions. Third, sensory afferents form multisynaptic pathways that synapse in the thalamus, which then projects to specific sensory areas of the cortex.

Reflex pathways. Reflexes involve relatively stereotyped sensorimotor behavioral patterns that are supported by specific neuronal pathways. Reflexes vary in complexity from the simplest direct connections between sensory and motor neurons to multisynaptic circuits involving many interneurons. Both exteroceptive and interoceptive reflexes are commonplace. Examples of exteroceptive reflexes include the monosynaptic myotatic reflex (described in more detail in what follows), the constriction of the pupil of the eye in response to light (the pupillary light reflex), and the contraction of the tensor tympani and stapedius muscles (which protect the cochlea by dampening the motion of the middle ear ossicles) in response to intense auditory inputs. Interoceptive examples include the baroreceptor reflex (which controls vasoconstriction and heart rate in response to changes in blood pressure) and changes in respiration resulting from chemoreceptors that sample CO_2 concentration in the blood. Reflexes are by definition relatively simple sensorimotor pathways; yet even the simplest of these circuits is subject to a variety of modulating influences. The monosynaptic stretch reflex, for example, is subject to modulatory influences based on adaptive constraints such as body posture and center of gravity (Nashner, 1976).

Cerebellar pathways. The cerebellum ("little brain") receives information from virtually all sensory systems. In general, these cerebellar circuits lie in parallel with the reflex pathways previously discussed and, in some cases, modulate reflex activity in important ways. For example, consider the vestibulo-ocular reflex (VOR). The afferent limb of this reflex originates in the semicircular canals of the inner ear, which sense acceleration of the head in any plane. These pathways terminate on second-order neurons in the vestibular complex of the medulla. The second-order neurons project in turn onto motoneurons that control eye position through their connections on the extraocular muscles. Through these connections, this reflex produces compensatory changes in eye position in response to angular rotation of the head, so that the visual image on the retina remains stable during head movements.

The VOR is a marvelous feat of nature's engineering. One of the most interesting aspects of this reflex is its remarkable degree of plasticity. If a person wears left–right inverting prisms, the world is turned backward and the old movements of the eyes from the reflex are likewise backward. However, after a time, the relationship between the motion of the head and the movements of the eyes is somehow reversed, restoring the adaptive value of the reflex. Remarkably, this "plasticity" of the VOR is dependent on a particular region of the cerebellum that receives primary afferent input from the semicircular canals and projects in turn to vestibular nuclei of the medulla. Lesions of this "vestibulo-cerebellum" result in a reversal of the reflex in adapted animals back to the unadapted state and prevent any further adaptation from occurring (Robinson, 1976).

Thalamocortical projection systems. All of the exteroceptive sensory afferents contribute to pathways whose ultimate destination is the cerebral cortex. These cortical pathways are associated with the conscious perception of sensory events, and the associated circuits are important to the processes of recognition and discrimination and to the perception of the external environment. Indeed, a substantial domain of neuroscience is concerned with the cortical mechanisms subserving the sensory and motor functions of the cerebral cortex.

Most of the inputs to the cerebral cortex originate in the thalamus of the diencephalon. Every sensory modality except smell (touch, taste, audition, balance, and vision) projects to a specific thalamic nucleus, which in turn projects to relatively specific cortical targets or "projection fields." As a result, each sensory modality has a specific cortical representation (i.e., visual cortex auditory cortex, somatosensory cortex; see Figure 3.2). There have been dramatic advances in our understanding of the general organization of sensory areas of the cortex over the past 10–15 years. We now turn to a brief consideration of these advances.

The traditional view of the cortical organization of sensory systems was that each modality gained access to the cerebral cortex through its representation in one particular thalamic relay nucleus. For example, in vision, the retinal ganglion cells project to the lateral geniculate nucleus of the thalamus (LGN). The dorsal division of this nucleus (LGNd) in turn projects to a cortical area variously known as area 17, striate cortex, or visual cortical area 1 (V1). Some readers may be familiar with the general organization of this geniculo-striate system as it has been delineated primarily through the classic work of Hubel and Wiesel (1977); space does not allow us to present their findings here. Also note that the designation "area 17" originates from studies by the German neuroanatomist Brodmann (1909), who designated different areas of cortex with numbers based upon the pattern of distribution of morphologically distinct neurons (Figure 3.14). Area 17 contains a complete representation of the contralateral visual field, so that visually responsive neurons are laid out on the cortex in a spatial pattern that corresponds to the spatial pattern of visual space at the eye. The term V1 refers to this so-called visuotopic organization, whose boundaries correspond exactly with cytoarchitectural boundaries.

In primates (presumably including humans), the vast majority of geniculate projections are confined to this cortical target (V1). However, surrounding area 17 is another cytoarchitecturally defined cortical field called area 18, and for many years area 18 was known to also contain a representation of the contralateral visual hemifield. For this reason, area 18 is often referred to as V2 (visual area 2). Beyond area 18 is a third cortical field, area 19. The conceptualization of area 19 has changed dramatically in the last 10 years, however, and these later developments in many ways serve to illustrate new insights into the cortical organization of sensory systems more generally.

3.6.1.3 *Parallel thalamocortical pathways*

As indicated in the preceding section, the geniculo-striate system was regarded at one time to be the sole route through which visual information could reach the neocortex. This view is implicit in the term *primary visual cortex*. In fact, this notion was not restricted to visual cortex, but to somatosensory and auditory cortices as well. The cortical fields surrounding the primary sensory fields were thought to depend on the primary fields for their principal inputs and were therefore regarded as "higher order" stages in sensory processing. Thus, with respect to visual processing, areas 18 and 19 were regarded as visual association cortex and were thought to subserve more "perceptual" functions. The association cortex was classically defined as lacking a thalamic input: It simply processed the inputs from the primary projection areas. Thus, the cortical processing of sensory information was viewed very much in terms of serial processing. When anatomists discovered that in fact all neocortex receives a

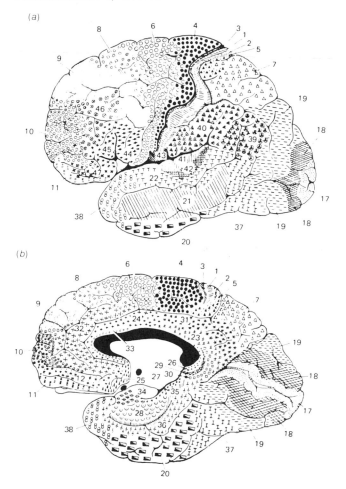

Figure 3.14. Lateral view of the cerebral cortex showing Broadmann's divisions. The areas outlined by Broadmann are based on differences in cytoarchitecture, the typical morphological features of the neurons found in a region. (Reprinted by permission of the publisher from J. Kelly, Anatomical basis of sensory perception and motor coordination, in *Principles of neural science*, E. Kandel and J. Schwartz, Eds., p. 237. Copyright 1985 by Elsevier Science.)

thalamic projection, the definition of association areas was simply extended to include those thalamic nuclei that were known to project to association areas, and these were referred to as *association nuclei of the thalamus*. The defining characteristic of association areas (either cortical or thalamic) was that the afferents depended on the primary visual cortex for their inputs. Areas 18 and 19 receive a thalamic input from a massive nucleus called the pulvinar; so when it was discovered that the pulvinar received a projection from the superior colliculus (a major visual structure in the midbrain that receives direct input from the retina), it was recognized that even the modified definition of association cortex was no longer tenable. Thus, areas 18 and 19 were recognized as receiving visual information via at least two parallel pathways; first via the geniculo-striate system and second via the newly discovered pathway from the retina to the colliculus, thence to the pulvinar (cf. Diamond & Hall, 1969). This parallel thalamocortical organization is now recognized as a ubiquitous feature of cortical systems (Woolsey, 1982).

3.6.1.4   *Multiplicty of visual cortical areas*

Following these developments, physiological studies revealed a previously unrecognized complexity in the visuotopic order of cortical areas surrounding area 17. Rather than consisting of one representation of the visual hemifield that was coexistensive with the cytoarchitectural field of area 19, it was discovered that area 19 actually consisted of nine or more discrete representations of the visual field (cf. Van Essen, 1979; Woolsey, 1982)! A great deal of recent work has focused on the functional properties of cells in these different regions as well as the specific afferent and efferent patterns that exist. Not surprisingly, there appears to be some degree of functional specialization between these areas (some areas seem specialized for color or movement; see Livingstone, 1988). Moreover, this multiplicity of representation is a general feature of the cortical organization of all sensory systems (Woolsey, 1982).

3.6.1.5   *Some functional considerations*

As previously indicated, the cerebral cortex is often regarded as essential to processes such as recognition, discrimination, and conscious awareness of sensory events. Here, we briefly point out two phenomena that support this position. First, based on studies using an evoked response technique (see Coles, Gratton, & Fabani, chapter 13), Libet and colleagues (Libet, Alberts, Wright, & Feinstein, 1967) assert that the cortex is necessary for conscious awareness. Evoked responses are alterations in the electroencephalogram (EEG) that are locked to stimuli. Typically, the EEG is averaged using a computer, and the averaging is time locked to the onset of the stimulus. Components of the EEG that are consistently elicited by the stimulus "grow", whereas random components average to zero. In the work reported by Libet et al. (1967), however, this averaging was not necessary as the evoked responses were recorded with fine electrodes that were actually implanted in the cortex itself. These workers show that a specific component of the evoked response in primary somatosensory cortex (S1) correlates with conscious awareness of a cutaneous sensation. Following an initial biphasic wave, this component occurs relatively late (approximate latency of 300 ms), and it invariably happens when a detectable stimulus (in these experiments, a mild electric shock) is applied to the skin. If, however, an electrical pulse is delivered to the somatosensory thalamic relay nucleus, the early components of the cortical evoked response occur, but the later components may not be present (their occurrence depends on the duration of the electrical pulse train to the thalamus). Libet et al. (1967) report that human subjects experience a conscious sensory event that is referred to a specific portion of the body (entirely predictable based on the receptotopic order) only when the late component of the evoked response is present, indicating that a substantial amount of neural processing must occur in the somatosensory cortex in order to produce a conscious cutaneous sensation (a process he refers to as achieving neuronal adequacy).

A second example of the role of sensory cortex in conscious awareness derives from the work of Wieskrantz and colleagues (Weiskrantz, Warrington, Sanders, & Marshall, 1974) on visual discrimination performance in human patients following removal of primary visual cortex. These surgeries are sometimes performed to remove life-threatening brain tumors. Damage in the primary visual cortex in humans produces a dramatic decrease in visual sensitivity in the contralateral visual field, a condition referred to as a scotoma or cortical blindness. This blindness is, from the point of view of the patient, quite dense: Such patients fail to report visual events that occur in the affected portion of the visual field. However, Weiskrantz et al. (1974) report that if forced to make binary choices concerning the identity of visual stimuli presented within this area of blindness (e.g., to guess whether a luminous bar was horizontal or vertical), such patients are correct on as many as 90 percent of the trails despite their insistence that they are unaware that a stimulus was presented at all! Not surprisingly, Weiskrantz has called this phenomenon "blind sight." While some have raised the possibility that these demonstrations of residual capacity within a cortical scotoma are artifactual (Campion, Latto, & Smith, 1983), others have countered with demonstrations of blind sight when the potential for such artifacts had presumably been eliminated (Stoerig, Huber, & Poppel, 1985). In any case, since these residual capacities are clearly not possible with more extensive damage to the visual areas of the neocortex, these findings illustrate the importance of cortex for conscious sensory processing. The important remaining issue is the location (striate or extrastriate?) and nature of the neural mechanisms that support residual vision.

3.6.2   *Motor systems*

As early as 1906, Sherrington proposed that simple movements beginning with reflexes serve as building blocks that are sequentially executed to form complex motor acts. Other early theorists recognized that the activity of many muscles must be coordinated to accomplish a particular task. We know today that voluntary movements require coordination of many levels of the neural axis. The first portion of this section outlines some basic properties of muscles and how they interact with the central nervous system to elicit basic movements. Later sections describe supraspinal mechanisms that are involved in the control of movement.

3.6.2.1   *Motoneurons*

Motoneurons are neurons that innervate muscles. Two types of motoneurons, alpha- and gamma-motoneurons, project from the ventral horn of the spinal cord to muscles. These neurons release the neurotransmitter acetylcholine, which produces muscular contractions (Dale et al., 1936).

Alpha- and gamma-motoneurons innervate different types of muscle fibers and are thus associated with different functions. *Alpha-motoneurons* are very large myelinated neurons that innervate extrafusal fibers. *Extrafusal fibers* are the large muscle fibers that do the bulk of the work. Thus, alpha–motoneurons are important in regulating contractions in the muscle bulk responsible for most of the work under a load. A *motor unit*, the smallest functional unit controlled by the nervous system, is comprised of one alpha-motoneuron and all the muscle fibers it innervates.

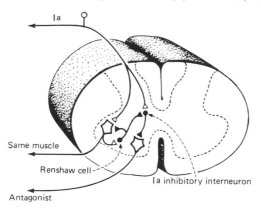

Figure 3.15. Schematic showing the neural basis for recurrent collateral inhibition involving Renshaw cells. (Reprinted by permission of the publisher from T. Carew, The control of reflex action, in *Principles of neural science*, E. Kandel and J. Schwartz, Eds., p. 459. Copyright 1985 by Elsevier Science.)

Since alpha-motoneurons are constantly receiving inputs, they are in danger of overstimulation. However, overstimulation does not occur because alpha-motoneurons have axon collaterals that terminate on interneurons called Renshaw cells. These Renshaw cells synapse on the same alpha-motoneuron and inhibit it (Figure 3.15). This arrangement, called recurrent collateral inhibition, results in a sharing of the load among all the motor units. This concept is similar to that of a refractory period in an axon, the period immediately following an action potential during which no other action potentials can propagate. Both arrangements protect neurons from overstimulation; Renshaw inhibition additionally protects muscle fibers from overstimulation.

In contrast to alpha-motoneurons, which innervate extrafusal fibers, *gamma-motoneurons* innervate *intrafusal muscle fibers,* which work together to set the position of a limb under varying loads. Through spinal reflex mechanisms, gamma-motoneurons and stretchreceptors use feedback control to maintain the extrafusal muscle at a present length. Gamma-motoneurons, through reflex circuity (involving 1a afferents), can also indirectly activate extrafusal (load-bearing) muscle fibers. The synaptic arrangement is diagrammed in Figure 3.16.

3.6.2.2   *Coding*

When a motoneuron fires, it releases acetylcholine, which binds to receptors on muscle cell membranes. Muscle cells are very similar to nerve cells in their electrical properties, and when the transmitter binds, the muscle is depolarized. With sufficient depolarization a *muscle action potential* is produced; this results in the contraction of the muscle fiber. The force of a muscular contraction is governed by recruitment and firing rate. The more motoneurons that are active during a contraction (*recruitment*), the greater the force of the muscle contraction. Also, the faster the motoneurons fire, the greater the force. Changes in the force of muscle contraction through either recruitment or firing rate are associated with changes in the electrical activity of the muscle. These voltage fluxes, called *electromyograms*, or

(a)

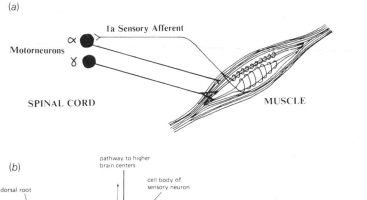

(b)

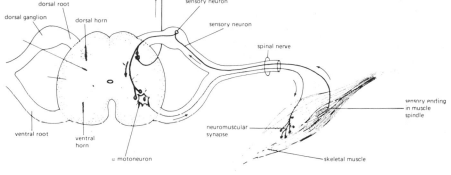

Figure 3.16. (a) Synaptic connections allowing for interactions between extrafusal and intrafusal muscle fibers. (b) Synaptic connections involved in the myotactic or stretch reflex. Stretching of a sensory ending in the muscle spindle causes the sensory neuron to fire. This activates a monosynaptic pathway that releases an excitatory transmitter onto an alpha-motoneuron. Activation of the motoneuron causes all of the muscle fibres of the motor unit to contract. Although gamma-motoneurons are also present in the spinal cord (see panel a), they are not mono-synaptically activated by the sensory afferents. (Panel b reprinted by permission of the publisher from F. L. Strand, *Physiology: A regulatory systems approach,* 2nd ed. Copyright 1983 by Macmillan.)

EMGs, may be recorded using either needle electrodes inserted near the muscle itself or surface electrodes attached to the skin (see Cacioppo, Tassinary, & Fridlund, chapter 11). Electromyograms are useful in determining whether a particular muscle is active during a task and yield useful information about the relative timing between muscle groups.

3.6.2.3 *Muscle receptors*

Muscle receptors convey information about the state of the muscles to the nervous system. They provide important feedback to the central nervous system that is used to coordinate movements. Two main types of receptors are found within muscle fibers: *Golgi tendon organs* and *muscle spindles.*

Golgi tendon organs are found near the junction of the muscle and tendon. Activation of afferents in Golgi tendon organs conveys information to the spinal cord about the amount of force being generated by the muscle. In addition, when Golgi tendon organs are stretched, a protective reflex is activated to prevent damage to the tendon.

Muscle spindles are the second major type of muscle receptor. Muscle spindles are stretch receptors found within intrafusal muscle fibers. They signal to the spinal cord information about the length of the muscle and the rate at which the length of the muscle is changing.

3.6.2.4 *Spinal reflexes*

We have discussed autonomic reflexes and the vestibulo-ocular reflex. Now we turn to a discussion of some spinal reflexes that form the basis for more complex movements. As discussed, reflexes are modulated by higher structures, and they may be "chained" to form a more complex series of movements. The circuitry underlying all spinal reflexes involves three components: (1) a sensor such as a sensory receptor that receives input about environmental conditions, (2) a spinal neuron such as a motoneuron in the ventral horn of the spinal cord, and (3) an effector such as a muscle fiber that contracts in response to appropriate stimuli.

One important reflex based on the muscle spindle feedback to the spinal cord is the *myotatic,* or *stretch, reflex.* If the reader has ever observed the knee-jerk reflex, then he or she has observed the stretch reflex in action. The neuronal circuitry of the myotatic, or stretch, reflex is shown in Figure 3.16. Stretch of a sensory ending in the muscle spindle activates an afferent from the muscle. The afferent makes a monosynaptic *excitatory* connection with an alpha-motoneuron controlling synergist muscles (see figure) and an *inhibitory* connection via an interneuron with an alpha-motoneuron to antagonist muscles (interneuron and antagonist muscle not shown in diagram). The myotatic reflex controls load management by causing contraction of extrafusal muscles to relieve the stretch on intrafusal muscle fibers. This has the effect of maintaining a constant length (and position) under varying load. This happens quite quickly and unconsciously because only one synapse is involved. During voluntary movement *coactivation* occurs such that both the alpha- and gamma-motoneurons fire simultaneously. This serves to maintain the sensitivity of the gamma/spindle (stretch reflex) length control system.

The circuitry of the *flexor reflex* is outlined in Figure 3.17. This reflex is responsible for withdrawal from noxious stimuli. For example, when one touches a hot stove, nociceptive receptors in the skin activate neurons in the dorsal horn of the spinal cord. These sensory connections synapse onto motoneurons in the ventral horn of the spinal cord, which leads to contraction of fibers in the flexor muscle. Due to the protective nature of the flexor–withdrawal reflex, it is noteworthy that it will override any other reflex that happens to be active at the same time.

The *crossed extensor reflex* is basically the flexor reflex already described plus the contralateral half of the same reflex. The crossed reciprocal innervation that is characteristic of the crossed extensor reflex is diagrammed in Figure 3.18. Basically, the connections of the crossed reciprocal innervation are such that on one side are flexor excitation and extensor inhibition whereas on the other are extensor inhibition and flexor excitation. This combination is important for postural stability. For example, if one steps on a hot coal at a barbecue, the withdrawal of the burnt limb is accompanied by extension of the contralateral limb helping to maintain balance. Note that the reciprocal flexion–extension pattern coded in the crossed extensor

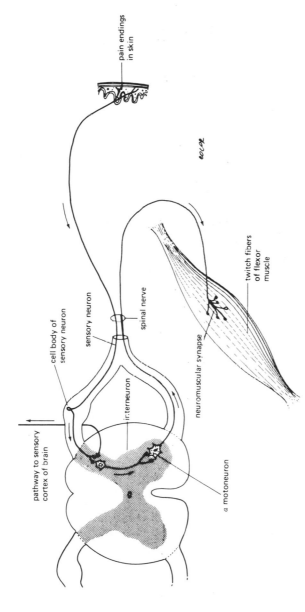

Figure 3.17. Disynaptic connections of the flexor reflex. Stimulation of pain endings in the skin activates an interneuron in the dorsal horn of the spinal cord. The interneuron then stimulates an alpha-motoneuron in the ventral horn, which produces a contraction of twitch muscle fibers. All the synapses in this pathway are excitatory. (Reprinted by permission of the publisher from F. L. Strand, *Physiology: A regulatory systems approach*, 2nd ed. Copyright 1983 by Macmillan.)

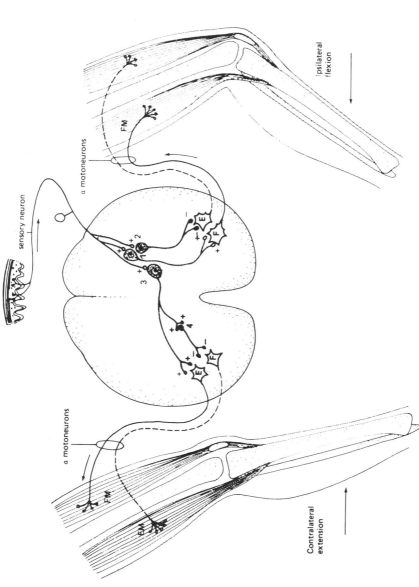

Figure 3.18. Circuitry underlying the crossed extensor reflex. When sensory endings in the skin are stimulated, the reciprocal innervation present in this reflex allows ipsilateral flexion and contralateral extension to occur simultaneously. E = extensor, F = flexor, open nerve terminals release excitatory (+) substances, closed nerve terminals release inhibitory (−) substances. (Reprinted by permission of the publisher from F. L. Strand, *Physiology: A regulatory systems approach*, 2nd ed. Copyright 1987 by Macmillan.)

reflex is the basic spinal pattern associated with locomotion. Thus, the crossed extensor reflex is the first reflex described thus far that clearly illustrates Sherrington's idea that complex motor acts may be built from elementary reflex actions. It is notable that spinal animals make reasonably good bilateral stepping movements, supporting the idea that much locomotor activity derives its basic patterning from spinal mechanisms.

A set of reflexes called *long spinal reflexes* is another example of how fairly complex patterns of movement can be coded at the spinal level. These reflexes involve relatively long interneuronal connections running up and down the spinal cord. The best examples of long spinal reflexes are the Magnus reflexes. These reflexes allow for postural adjustments of the body during natural head movements. For example, several patterns of postural adjustments have been described in the cat that involve receptors associated with the cervical vertebrae: (1) when the neck is extended, the hindlimbs flex and the forelimbs extend (similar to the posture of a cat looking up at a fishbowl); (2) when the neck is flexed, the forelimbs flex and the hindlimbs extend (similar to the posture of a cat looking down a hole); and (3) when the head is turned to one side, the forelimb on that side extends and the contralateral forelimb flexes.

3.6.2.5 *Cortical mechanisms of movement*

The spinal reflexes form a basis for complex movements and relieve the brain from having to carry out the most basic regulation of posture and tone of the muscles. The messages sent to the cord from higher levels may take a simpler form, serving in part to modulate reflex circuitry to produce the desired movements. We now turn to the role of various brain structures in coordinating motor control.

Many areas of the cerebral cortex are involved in the regulation of movement. Voluntary movement is preceded by increased activity in the *primary motor cortex*, a strip of cortex just anterior to the central sulcus (Evarts, 1968). This strip of cortex projects directly to alpha- and gamma-motoneurons in the spinal cord through the pyramidal tract; it also influences interneurons that are involved in reflex control. The primary motor cortex is organized topographically so that discrete regions of the cortex influence discrete body parts on the contralateral side (Foerster, 1936; Penfield & Jasper, 1954; Woolsey et al., 1950). Stimulation of the motor cortex causes movements in corresponding regions of the body; conversely, lesions to the motor cortex lead to weakness (*paresis*) or paralysis of discrete areas. Recordings of the activity of single cells in the motor cortex of awake primates suggest that neurons in the motor cortex encode the force (Evarts, 1968) and direction (Georgopoulos, Schwartz, & Kettner, 1986) of movement of a particular body part.

While the primary motor cortex has direct influences on motoneurons, the programming required for complex, goal-oriented movement is accomplished in the other areas of the cortex: the supplementary motor area, the premotor area, the primary somatosensory area, and the posterior parietal cortex. Although the precise roles of each of these cortical regions are not fully understood, certain clear divisions of functions have been identified. Stimulation of either the *premotor* or the *supplementary motor cortex* produces complex movements (Penfield & Welch, 1951; Woolsey et al., 1950). The *posterior parietal cortex* and the *primary somatosensory cortex* participate in cortical motor control, apparently by integrating sensory spatial maps with motor spatial maps (Lynch et al., 1977; Robinson et al. 1978). Lesions to the posterior parietal cortex result in an inability to learn complex movements (apraxia) and a profound neglect of "sensory space" on the contralateral side (cf. Denny-Brown & Chambers, 1958).

Whereas the cortical control of movement is of great importance, large subcortical structures play important roles in the generation and patterning of movement. In this respect it is interesting that primary motor cortex neurons become quiescent during some types of movements, especially for movements occurring during emotional outbursts and rhythmical movements such as chewing (e.g., Fetz, Cheney, & German, 1976). These findings reflect the ability of different parts of the brain to independently control the motor system and to suppress the other circuitry that generates movement. This redundancy in the motor system, along with its hierarchical organization, appears to be a general feature of the nervous system. As Hughlings Jackson, the father of modern neurology, noted in the last century, functions are represented and re-represented in the nervous system. Nowhere is the general principle of multiple representation of function more clear than in motor systems.

3.6.2.6   *Subcortical mechanisms of movement: the basal ganglia*

The basal ganglia include several telencephalic subcortical structures (caudate, putamen, globus pallidus, and claustrum). Some investigators also include certain thalamic nuclei and the substantia nigra. These structures are highly interconnected and influence movement by direct connections to brainstem premotoneurons and the motor cortex.

Previously, the basal ganglia were thought to have generalized, diffuse effects on movement. However, it has become increasingly apparent that the basal ganglia are highly organized, both in terms of specific body loci and in terms of zones of inputs and outputs within various structures. A central role is played by the substantia nigra and the caudate. These structures are interconnected by two pathways: the nigrostriatal pathway from the substantia nigra to the caudate/putamen and a return connection, the striatonigral pathway. This core loop has been the source of considerable interest, in part because perturbations of this system profoundly disturb movement as in Parkinson's disease, Huntington's chorea, and extrapyramidal side effects of antipsychotic drugs (neuroleptics).

Many investigators view the striatum (caudate, putamen, and globus pallidus) as a receptive zone because it receives inputs from all areas of the cortex and from the substantia nigra pars compacta (the dorsal, dopaminergic part of the nigra). The striatum integrates the incoming information and relays it to so-called output structures, particularly the substantia nigra pars reticulata (the nondopaminergic, ventral aspect of the nigra) and the globus pallidus. Neurons in these output areas then synapse on *premotoneurons* (neurons that project to motoneurons). For example the neurons in the substantia nigra pars reticulata project to the superior colliculus, which gives rise to the tectospinal tract. This pathway regulates eye and head movements, especially orienting responses to novel stimuli (Hikosaka & Wurtz, 1983a,b). Regulation of movement by the basal ganglia also occurs via pathways connecting in the thalamus and thence back to the motor cortex.

Recent work (cf. Alexander, DeLong, & Strick, 1986) suggests considerable specificity in the basal ganglia. To begin with, cortical projections to the striatum are highly organized. Different areas of the caudate and putamen in primates and man receive inputs from different areas of the cortex such that inputs from motor areas of the cortex (e.g., motor cortex, supplementary motor cortex, somatosensory cortex, and arcuate premotor area) all terminate in the same region.

Alexander et al. (1986) propose a model of the basal ganglia that extends beyond simple motor functions or sensorimotor integration. They suggest that at least five parallel functionally segregated pathways form closed loops: beginning with a discrete cortical region, each pathway projects to a circumscribed area of the basal ganglia, then to a thalamic area, and then back to the cortex. Although the regions of termination of different classes of inputs overlap, a reasonable degree of topographic specificity is retained at the level of the basal ganglia. Clear motor functions are associated with at least two of these loops. However, limbic cortical areas (e.g., anterior cingulate cortex, entorhinal cortex, inferior temporal gyrus) also project to particular zones in the caudate/putamen, which are separable from the inputs from motor areas. Although the functions of this limbic input are unknown, their presence suggests that the basal ganglia subserve functions beyond those of simple motor output. These findings also reflect on the high degree of anatomical organization present within the basal ganglia.

3.6.2.7 *Subcortical mechanisms of movement: cerebellum and associated circuits*

The cerebellum regulates movement through its interactions with spinal, cortical, and brainstem structures (see Ghez & Fahn, 1985; Ito, 1984). The cerebellum is unique in its highly regular synaptic architecture and connections. Principal sources of inputs are the cortex, inferior olive, and several brainstem nuclei that are influenced by cortical and spinal inputs. Monoaminergic systems, particularly serotonergic raphe neurons and noradrenergic locus coeruleus neurons, exert inhibitory influences over wide regions of the cerebellum.

Outputs from the cerebellum all derive from one of the deep nuclei: lateral, fastigial, interpositus, and dentate. Functional segregation occurs within these nuclei so that different deep nuclei project to separate brain regions subserving either different body parts (e.g., distal vs. proximal muscles) or functions (e.g., movement initiation). Three important functional divisions of the cerebellum are the *vestibulocerebellum*, discussed previously in the section on eye movements and head position, the *spinocerebellum*, which participates in the feedback regulation of movement, and the *cerebrocerebellum*, which may help to maintain a match between planned motor acts and ongoing movements. These functional divisions correspond anatomically to different regions of the cerebellum.

Whereas traditionally regarded as a center for motor coordination, there is an increasing appreciation that cerebellar functions go beyond the coordination of movement. For example, we know that the cerebellum and related circuits such as the red nucleus play an important role in the classically conditioned nictitating membrane withdrawal response studied in rabbits (Thompson, McCormick, Lavond, Clark, Kettner, & Mauk, 1983). These studies and others (e.g., Bernston & Hughes, 1976; Berntson & Micco, 1976; Brooks & Thach, 1981) have advanced our understanding of the cerebellum beyond the original conception that it is a circuit that patterns coordinated movement, an idea that was based mostly on the effects of cerebellar disease in humans.

3.6.3   *Central integrative systems*

Most of the structures of the central nervous system are neither clearly motor nor sensory. Here, we discuss the major systems that fall in this domain. In general, these systems process interoceptive afferents, integrate this information with higher order (cognitive) processes, control autonomic functions to maintain homeostasis, and regulate emotion and memory. Although an exhaustive treatment would be impossible here, we consider the major brain structures that mediate these actions.

3.6.3.1   *Hypothalamus*

The hypothalamus is a walnut-sized collection of at least nine identifiable nuclei that lie at the base of the forebrain (see Figure 3.19). Although the hypothalamus represents only 1 percent of the total volume of the brain, it is directly involved in what sometimes seems a bewildering array of essential body functions. When it comes to packing a variety of functions into a small package, the hypothalamus has no rival.

Much of the data indicating the importance of the hypothalamus in mediating overt behavior comes from experiments in which electrical stimulation of localized regions of the hypothalamus produces changes in an animal's behavior. W. R. Hess made the original observations, for which he won the Nobel Prize in 1949. Hess (1954) observed that the behavioral changes induced by hypothalamic stimulation are not disorganized. Rather, hypothalamic stimulation produces complex species-specific behavioral patterns characteristic of particular emotional or motivational states (e.g., anger, hunger, sexual activity). In addition, there is a great deal of functional localization within the hypothalamus: Different behaviors can be elicited preferentially by stimulating different parts of the hypothalamus.

One reason for the great interest in Hess's findings is the remarkable similarity between hypothalamically induced behaviors and their naturally occurring counterparts (e.g., Bernston, Hughes, & Beattie, 1976). Some evidence indicates that stimulation of the hypothalamus elicits specific constellations of somatic and autonomic activity because the stimulation produces a motivational state. For example, animals will perform work, such as pressing a lever, in order to get access to the object of the motivated behavior (e.g., food if the animal eats in response to the stimulation; Roberts & Carey, 1965; Roberts & Kiess, 1964); Moreover, it is clear that hypothalamic stimulation [or, for that matter, stimulation in the brainstem (Berntson & Hughes, 1976)] does not simply elicit motor automatisms, as the occurrence of particular behaviors depends on the availability of an appropriate goal object as well the stimulation itself (cf. Berntson & Micco, 1976). The detailed topology of the elicited behaviors is also dependent on environmental features, emphasizing the "appropriateness" of the elicited motor sequence. Further, under natural conditions, species-typical motivated behaviors and emotional states are accompanied by changes in the autonomic and somatic motor systems as well as in the endocrine system. Hypothalamic stimulation likewise induces consistent patterns of behavioral, autonomic, and endocrine changes (Hess, 1954).

On the other hand, there is evidence of a lack of complete determinism produced by brain stimulation that is inconsistent with the notion that hypothalamic stimulation induces motivational states. Occasionally, stimulation of one site produces more than one class of responses. In such situations, the availability of suitable goal objects can alter the probability that one or the other behavior occurs

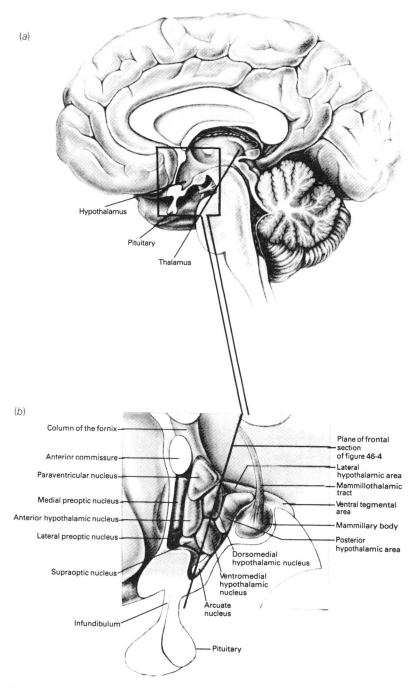

(a)

Hypothalamus

Pituitary

Thalamus

(b)

Column of the fornix

Anterior commissure

Paraventricular nucleus

Medial preoptic nucleus

Anterior hypothalamic nucleus

Lateral preoptic nucleus

Supraoptic nucleus

Infundibulum

Plane of frontal section of figure 46-4

Lateral hypothalamic area

Mammillothalamic tract

Ventral tegmental area

Mammillary body

Posterior hypothalamic area

Dorsomedial hypothalamic nucleus

Ventromedial hypothalamic nucleus

Arcuate nucleus

Pituitary

Figure 3.19. (*a*) Location of the hypothalamus within the diencephalon in relation to the pituitary gland and the thalamus. (*b*) Detail of the hypothalamus and the structures around it. (Reprinted by permission of the publisher from I. Kupfermann, Hypothalamus and limbic system I: peptidergic neurons, homeostasis, and emotional behavior, in *Principles of neural science*, E. Kandel and J. Schwartz, Eds., p. 615. Copyright 1985 by Elsevier Science.)

(Valenstein, Cox, & Kakolewski, 1970). Perhaps the best way to view the effects of hypothalamic stimulation on behavior is to suggest that the hypothalamus, through its descending connections to the brainstem, can facilitate sensorimotor reflex mechanisms that are important in the actual execution of particular classes of motivated behaviors (Flynn, Vanegas, Foote, & Edwards, 1970; Roberts, 1970). This can account for the dependence of stimulation-produced behaviors on the presence of appropriate goal objects. The occurrence of more than one type of response upon stimulation of the same hypothalamic site might be attributed to simultaneous facilitation of more than one class of reflexes, which might reasonably be expected given the number of cells influenced by brain stimulation. This suggestion has received some empirical support (Flynn et al., 1970; MacDonnell & Flynn, 1966a, b). Of course, this suggestion begs the question as to whether naturally induced hypothalamic activity can in any way be regarded as a sine qua non of motivated states.

Intertwined with its role in the organization of life-sustaining motivated behavior, the hypothalamus plays a crucial role in maintaining homeostasis by coordinating the somatic, autonomic, and endocrine systems. As one would expect, the afferent and efferent organization of the hypothalamus can be understood in these terms. Hypothalamic afferent sources are widespread and include massive indirect projections from autonomic afferents as well as inputs from interoceptors located within the hypothalamus (e.g., receptors for blood glucose and blood osmolarity). In addition, many hypothalamic neurons possess receptors for a variety of endocrine hormones, emphasizing again the growing appreciation that the brain is itself a target organ of the endocrine system. Many exteroceptive afferents also send collaterals into the hypothalamus. Perhaps the most noteworthy of these is the direct connections between the retina and the hypothalamic suprachiasmatic nucleus, a pathway involved in phase locking the circadian rhythm with the light-dark cycle (Moore & Eichler, 1972; Stephen & Zucker, 1972). Finally, many limbic structures that are intimately involved in emotional states project to the hypothalamus. Indeed, many limbic functions depend on these hypothalamic connections for their expression (e.g., Vergnes, 1976).

The efferent (output) connections of the hypothalamus exerts control over four systems: (1) the autonomic nervous system (via multisynaptic pathways within the brainstem reticular formation, described in what follows) (2) the endocrine system (both directly by secreting neuroendocrine hormones and indirectly through the pituitary gland), (3) the somatic motor system (again via multisynaptic pathways within the brainstem and spinal cord), and (4) the limbic system (described in more detail in the next section).

Hypothalamic control over the endocrine system deserves special mention. As indicated, there are two modes of control. First, neurosecretory cells in two hypothalamic nuclei (the paraventricular and supraoptic nuclei) project to the posterior pituitary where they secrete two neurohormones (oxytocin and vasopressin) directly into the bloodstream. These neurohormones are then carried via the blood supply directly to target organs. Second, a variety of hypothalamic cells release various neuropeptides into the portal vasculature of the pituitary. These peptides are carried in the blood to the anterior pituitary where they control the secretion of various hormones from pituitary cells. These pituitary hormones in turn circulate in the bloodstream and control the secretions of the other endocrine glands. This, then, represents the indirect mode of endocrine control, as it is

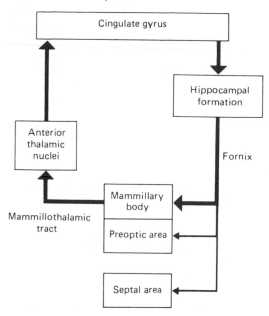

Figure 3.20. A schematic of Papez's circuit, which has been shown to be involved in the regulation of emotional states, showing the interconnections between various limbic system structures. (Reprinted by permission of the publisher from *Hypothalamus and limbic system I: peptidergic neurons, homeostasis, and emotional behavior,* in *Principles of neural science,* E. Kandel and J. Schwartz, Eds., p. 615. Copyright 1985 by Elsevier Science.)

mediated via intermediary *hypothalamic hormones* that regulate the secretion of anterior pituitary hormones.

3.6.3.2 *Limbic system*

The term *limbic system* refers to a highly interconnected set of subcortical structures located primarily in the forebrain (telencephalon). These structures include the cingulate gyrus of the neocortex, the hippocampus, the amygdala, the septum, and the medial nucleus of the thalamus. Many investigators would also include portions of the midbrain reticular formation due to its intimate anatomical connections with other limbic structures. Classical wisdom had it that much of the limbic system was related to the sense of smell, but this is no longer tenable. Considerable evidence now supports the idea that the limbic system subserves emotional responses.

Papez (1937) was the first to suggest that a specific circuit interconnecting various limbic structures represented the neuronal substrates of emotion (Figure 3.20). Although the details of his conceptualization are almost surely inadequate, both the connections of the limbic system and a great deal of neuropsychological work support the general proposition that the limbic system plays an important role in the modulation and expression of emotional states. Particularly important in this respect are the extensive interconnections between limbic structures and the hypothalamus. Based in part on these limbic–hypothalamic connections, the limbic system is thought to exert modulatory influences over the hypothalamus and, consequently, over the expression of emotional states. Consistent with the suggestions derived from these anatomical considerations are the findings that damage to or stimulation of different limbic structures produces dramatic alterations in the emotional states of both humans and animals. Lesions of the septum, for example, result in extreme expressions of rage, whereas lesions of the amygdala produce a taming effect. Interestingly, the influences of both the septum and amygdala appear to be mutually antagonistic. Thus, bilateral amygdalectomy eliminates the rage response produced by lesions of the septum (Jonasson & Enloe, 1971). Many of these effects have been noted in humans as well as in animals. Electrical stimulation of these same structures has the expected complementary effects. Thus, electrical stimulation of the septum reportedly produces intensely pleasurable effects, including an increased libido (cf. Lindsley & Holmes, 1984).

Perhaps the most well-known syndrome associated with damage to the temporal lobe of the cerebrum (which includes several important limbic structures) is the *Kluver–Bucy syndrome*. The syndrome is characterized by certain forms of visual agnosia (impairments in visual recognition), dramatic reductions in fear, docility, and increased sexual activity (Kluver & Bucy, 1939). Similar symptoms have occasionally been described in the human neurological literature and result from very extensive bilateral damage to the temporal lobe, the neocortex, the amygdala, and the hippocampus. More restricted damage to the hippocampus produces another classic neuropsychological syndrome known as *anterograde amnesia*. In this form of amnesia, long-term memories formed prior to the surgery are largely unaffected; the memory loss is specific to the long-term retention and/or retrieval of postsurgical memories (Scoville, Band, & Milner, 1975).

As is the case in many conceptualizations of nervous control, emotional states can fruitfully be regarded as a hierarchy in which higher level processes influence emotional states via descending projections. The lowest level of this hierarchy is the constellation of motoric responses associated with the emotional state, which derives from activity in both the somatic and autonomic motor systems. These responses must be integrated with each other and with sensory inputs if they are to be goal directed. These later processes appear to depend on mechanisms in the brainstem and hypothalamus. Finally, the occurrence of emotional displays is influenced by situational variables that may "gate" or modulate the display via connections between the cerebral cortex and the limbic system. Note, however, that the limbic structures described previously are interconnected and linked to relevant structures such as the hypothalamus and cerebral cortex. They therefore do not conform to a hierarchical system in a literal way. Nevertheless, to think of the neural control of emotional states in hierarchical terms has had heuristic value and empirical support.

3.6.3.3   *The reticular formation*

Throughout the central core of the brainstem, extending from the midbrain rostrally to the medulla caudally, lies the reticular formation. Once thought to be both functionally and anatomically amorphous, there is now a greater appreciation for both the anatomical specificity and functional diversity of this complex region of the central nervous system.

The reticular formation contains a great variety of nuclei defined according to

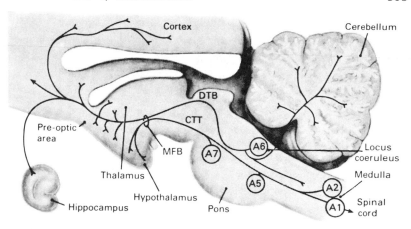

Figure 3.21. Sagittal section showing the noradrenergic pathways in the the brain. Nuclei giving rise to these neurons are labelled using the terminology of the original histochemists who mapped noradrenalin: A2, A5, A6, A7. Note that A6 corresponds to the locus coeruleus, a major source of forebrain noradrenalin. CTT = central tegmental tract, DTB = dorsal tegmental bundle, MFB = medial forebrain bundle. (Reprinted by permission of the publisher from *Physiology of Behavior* by N. R. Carlson, p. 524. Copyright 1986 by Allyn and Bacon, Needham Hts., MA.)

their cytoarchitecture and histochemistry (the distribution of neurotransmitters). Thus, the collection of serotonergic neurons that lie along the midline of the reticular formation is collectively referred to as the raphe complex. In addition, a variety of NE-containing cell groups lie within the reticular formation. The best known of these is the locus coeruleus, a small pigmented nucleus at the base of the cerebellum that is thought to have diverse and powerful effects on behavior through its widespread connections to the forebrain, cerebellum, brainstem, and spinal cord (Figure 3.21).

The reticular formation receives inputs from a diverse array of sensory modalities, including both exteroceptive and interoceptive systems. Many reticular neurons represent interneuronal links in a wide variety of reflex pathways, and much of the sensory input to the reticular formation represents the afferent limbs of these reflex pathways. These sensory inputs are also viewed as being important in controlling the level of arousal, a second major function of this region.

There are two major classes of efferent projections from the reticular core: those that ascend to the forebrain and those that descend to the spinal cord. The descending reticular projections originate in the medullary and pontine reticular formation and terminate on interneurons in the spinal cord. They are collectively referred to as the reticulo-spinal pathways. These descending projections are of two basic classes: those that modulate the tone of the proximal musculature and those that influence sensory transmission within the spinal cord. The former are involved in the regulation of posture and the control of locomotion. Much of this control is mediated via gamma-motoneurons. Some studies have shown that reticular cells increase their firing rates prior to very specific patterns of movement (e.g., turning of the head, protruding of the tongue, specific vectors of saccadic eye movements). Others have shown that electrical stimulation of a particular reticular nucleus induces locomotion even in decerebrate animals that cannot otherwise walk on their own. This "locomotor region" appears to participate in the initiation of walking as well as in the control of velocity (Shik, Severin, & Orlofsky, 1966). The descending sensory influences of the reticular formation appear to modulate the responsiveness of spinal cord cells that respond to painful stimulation and are an important part of the analgesic effects of exogenous opiates and endogenous opioid peptides (Basbaum & Fields, 1984).

Various regions within the reticular formation project to a wide variety of forebrain structures including the thalamus, cerebral cortex, limbic system, and hypothalamus. The functions of these ascending projections are undoubtedly diverse but have often been associated with the control of sleep, wakefulness, and levels of arousal (cf. Carlson, 1988, chapter 9). Thus, the NE-containing neurons in the locus coeruleus are implicated in wakefulness, in part because many drugs that enhance arousal (e.g., amphetamine) cause the release of NE (Carlson, 1988, chapter 9). Conversely, serotonergic neurons within the raphe complex are associated with the onset of sleep because drugs that enhance serotonergic activity promote sleep.

There is also good evidence that ascending reticular projections may play a role in phasic changes in alertness and attention. Electrical stimulation of the midbrain reticular formation enhances excitability of thalamocortical projection neurons and has similar effects on the excitability of cortical cells. Singer, Tretter, and Cynader (1976) have shown that reticular stimulation increases both spontaneous discharge as well as visually induced activity in striate cortex. It is interesting to note that although the visual responses are enhanced, this is achieved at the cost of decreased selectivity in cortical responsiveness. So, for example, whereas striate cells generate enhanced responses to normally effective stimuli following reticular stimulation, they also generate responses to stimuli to which they would not normally respond at all. Thus, it is possible that reticular stimulation does not enhance signal-to-noise ratios, as many current views of attention suggest.

There is also evidence that cortical NE plays an important role in certain forms of cortical plasticity. Thus, the changes in connections between the geniculate and cortex that normally accompany monocular deprivation in developing kittens appear to require the presence of cortical NE: The application of neurotoxins specific to NE blocks the occurrence of these developmental changes (Kasamatsu & Pettigrew, 1979). The major source of NE in the cortex comes from the reticular formation.

3.7   CONCLUDING REMARKS

We have discussed many areas of neuroscience – from studies conducted in the 1800s to the present. Most importantly, we discussed concepts that have general applicability across neural systems. Some of these concepts or modes of discussion have not changed much; for example, many anatomical structures still bear the names that Vesalius assigned in 1543 in his work *De Fabrica Corporis Humani*. Perhaps more difficult are the new ways of thinking about the nervous system that have emerged; we have tried to identify trends that will continue to bear fruit. Prominent among these have been molecular processes that have proven to have considerable power in explaining basic brain functions and have enriched our understanding of synaptic transmission. Psychophysiological investigations of the systemic bodily processes involved in cognition, emotion, and behavior will continue to provide an organismic framework necessary for the comprehensive understanding of the nervous system envisioned by the modern founders of neuroscience.

NOTE

We dedicate this chapter to Donald R. Meyer and Patricia M. Meyer, Emeritus Professors of Psychology at The Ohio State University. We acknowledge that most of the important concepts in this chapter came to us (BBW, JMW, and HCH) under their tutelage. These ideas have withstood the test of time for us, and we expect that they will for the readers as well.

REFERENCES

Akil, H., Watson, S. J., Young, E. A., Lewis, M. E., Khachaturian, H., & Walker, J. M. (1984). Endogenous opioids: Biology and function. *Annual Review of Neuroscience, 7*, 223–255.

Akil, H., Young, E., Walker, J. M., & Watson, S. J. (1986). The many possible roles of opioids and related peptides in stress-induced analgesia. *Annals of the New York Academy of Sciences: Stress-Induced Analgesia, 467*, 140–153.

Alexander, G. E., DeLong, M. R., & Strick, P. L. (1986). Parallel organization of functionally segregated circuits linking basal ganglia and cortex. *Annual Review of Neuroscience, 9*, 357–381.

Anand, B. K., & Brobeck, J. R. (1951). Hypothalamic control of food intake in rats and cats. *Yale Journal of Biology and Medicine, 2*, 123–140.

Barker, J. L. (1976). Peptides: Roles in neuronal excitability. *Physiological Reviews 56*, 435–452.

Barker, J. L., Neale, J. H., Smith, T. G., & MacDonald, R. L. (1978). Opiate peptide modulation of amino acid responses suggests novel form of neuronal communication. *Science, 199*, 1451–1453.

Basbaum, A. I., & Fields, H. L. (1984). Endogenous pain control systems: Brainstem spinal pathways and endorphin circuits. *Annual Review of Neuroscience, 7*, 309–338.

Berntson, G. G., & Hughes, H. C. (1976). Behavioral characteristics of grooming induced by hindbrain stimulation in the cat. *Physiology and Behavior, 17*, 165–168.

Berntson, G. G., Hughes, H. C., & Beattie M. S. (1976). A comparison of hypothalamically induced biting attack with natural predatory behavior in the cat. *Journal of Comparative and Physiological Psychology, 90*, 167–178.

Berntson, G. G., & Micco, D. J. (1976). Organization of brainstem behavioral systems. *Brain Research Bulletin, 1*, 471–483.

Berridge, M. J. (1987). Inositol triphosphate and diacylglycerol: Two interacting second messengers. *Annual Review of Biochemistry, 56*, 159–193.

Berridge, M. J., & Irvine, R. F. (1984). Inositol triphosphate, a novel second messenger in cellular signal transduction. *Nature, 312*, 315–321.

Brodmann, K. (1909). *Vergleichende Lokalisationslehre der Grosshirnrinde*. Leipzig: Barth.

Brooks, V. B., & Thach, W. T. (1981). Cerebellar control of posture and movement. In V. B. Brooks (Ed.), *Handbook of physiology* (pp. 877–946). Bethesda, MD: American Physiological Society.

Brown, A. M., & Birnbaumer, L. (1988). Direct G protein gating of ion channels. *American Journal of Physiology, 254*, H401–H410.

Brown, J. E., Rubin, L. J., Ghalayini, A. J., Tarver, A. P., Irvine, R. F., Berridge, M. J., & Anderson, R. E. (1984). Myo-inositol polyphosphate may be a messenger for visual excitation in *Limulus* photoreceptors. *Nature, 311*, 160–163.

Campion, J., Latto, R., & Smith, Y. M. (1983). Is blindsight due to scattered light, spared cortex and near threshold effects? *Behavioral and Brain Sciences, 6*, 423–486.

Cannon, W. B. (1935). Stresses and strains of homeostasis. *American Journal of Medicine, 189*, 1.

Carew, T. J. (1985). Posture and locomotion. In E. R. Kandel & J. H. Schwartz (Eds.), *Principles of neural science*. New York: Elsevier.

Carlson, N. R. (1986). *Physiology of behavior*. Boston: Allyn & Bacon.

Carlson, N. R. (1988). *Foundations of physiological psychology*. Boston: Allyn & Bacon.

Contreras, P. C., DiMaggio, D. A., & O'Donohue, T. L. (1987). An endogenous ligand for the sigma opioid binding site. *Synapse, 1*, 57–61.

Costa, M., Furness, J. B., & Gibbins, I. L. (1986). Chemical coding of enteric neurons. *Progress in Brain Research, 68*, 217–239.

Dale, H. (1935). Pharmacology and nerve-endings. *Proceedings of the Royal Society of Medicine (London), 28*, 319–332.

Dale, H. H., Feldberg, W., & Vogt, M. (1936). Release of acetylcholine at voluntary motor nerve endings. *Journal of Physiology, 86*, 353–380.

DeGroat, W. C., & Kawatani, M. (1985). Neural control of the urinary bladder. Possible relationship between peptidergic inhibitory mechanisms and detrusor instability. *Neurourology and Urodynamics, 4*, 285–300.

DeGroat, W. C., Kawatani, M., Booth, A. M., & Whitney, T. (1984). Enkephalinergic modulation of cholinergic transmission in parasympathetic ganglia of the urinary bladder of the cat. *Abstr. Conf. Dynamics of Cholinergic Function*, Ogleby.

Denny-Brown, D., & Chambers, R. A. (1958). The parietal lobe and behavior. *Research Publications (Association for Research in Nervous and Mental Disease), 36*, 35–78.

DeVoe, R. D., & Maloney, P. C. (1980). Principles of cell homeostasis. In V. Mountcastle (Ed.). *Medical physiology* (14th ed.). St. Louis: Mosby.

Diamond, I. T., & Hall, W. C. (1969) Evolution of neocortex. *Science, 164*, 251–262.

Dorow, R., Horowski, R., Paschelke, G., Amin, M., & Braestrup, C. (1983). Severe anxiety induced by FG-7142, a β-carboline ligand for benzodiazepine receptors. *Lancet, 2*, 98–99.

Drugan, R. C., Maier, S. F., Skolnick, P., Paul, S. M., & Crawley, J. N. (1985). An anxiogenic benzodiazepine receptor ligand induces learned helplessness. *European Journal of Pharmacology, 113*, 453–457.

Evarts, E. V. (1968) Relation of pyramidal tract activity to force exerted during voluntary movement. *Journal of Neurophysiology, 31*, 14–27.

Ewald, D. A., Sternweis, P. C., & Miller, R. J. (1988). Guanine nucleotide-binding protein G_o-induced coupling of neuropeptide Y receptors to Ca^{2+} channels in sensory neurons. *Proceedings of the National Academy of Sciences of the United States of America, 85*, 3633–3637.

Feldman, R. S., & Quenzer, L. F. (1984) *Fundamentals of neuropsychopharmacology*. Sunderlan, MA: Sinauer.

Ferrero, P., Guidotti, A., Conti-Tronconi, B., & Costa, E. (1984). A brain octadecaneuropeptide generated by tryptic digestion of DBI (diazepam binding inhibitor) functions as a proconflict ligand of benzodiazepine recognition sites. *Neuropharmacology, 23*, 1359–1362.

Fetz, E. E., Cheney, P. D., & German, D. C. (1976). Corticomotorneuronal connections of precentral cells detected by postspike averages of EMG activity in behaving monkeys. *Brain Research, 114*, 505–510.

Flynn, J. P., Vanegas, H., Foote, W., & Edwards, S. (1970). Neural mechanisms involved in a cat's attack on a rat. In R. E. Whalen, R. F. Thompson, M. Verzeano, & N. M. Weinberger (Eds.), *The neural control of behavior*. New York: Academic Press.

Foerster, O. (1936). Motor cortex in man in the light of Hughlings Jackson's doctrines. *Brain, 59*, 135–159.

Georgopoulos, A. P., Kalaska, J. F., Caminiti, R., & Massey, J. T. (1982). The relations between the direction of two-dimensional arm movements and cell discharge in primate motor cortex. *Journal of Neuroscience, 2*, 1527–1537.

Georgopoulos, A. P., Schwartz, A. B., & Kettner, R. E. (1986). Neuronal population coding of movement direction. *Science, 233*, 1416–1419.

Ghez, C., & Fahn, S. (1985). The cerebellum. In E. R. Kandel & J. H. Schwartz (Eds.), *Principles of neural science*. New York: Elsevier, pp. 502–522.

Gilman, A. G. (1987). G Proteins: Transducers of receptor-generated signals. *Annual Review of Biochemistry, 56*, 615–649.

Greengard, P. (1976). Possible role for cyclic nucleotides and phosphorylated membrane proteins in postsynaptic actions of neurotransmitters. *Nature, 260*, 101–108.

Greengard, P. (1979). Cyclic nucleotides, phosphorylated proteins, and the nervous system. *Federation Proceedings, 38*, 2208–2217.

Greenwood, D. D., & Maruyama, M. (1965). Excitatory and inhibitory response areas of auditory neurons in the cochlear nucleus. *Journal of Neuro Physiology, 28*, 863–883.

Gross, C. G., Rocha-Miranda, C. E., & Bender, D. B. (1972). Visual properties of neurons in inferotemporal cortex of the macaque. *Journal of Neurophysiology, 35*, 96–111.

Hartline, H. K. (1949). Inhibition of activity of visual receptors by illuminating nearby retinal areas in the *Limulus* eye. *Federation Proceedings, 8,* 69.

Hartline, H. K., & Ratliff, F. (1957). Inhibitory interaction of receptor units in the eye of *Limulus*. *Journal of General Physiology, 40,* 357–376.

Hartline, H. K., Wagner, H. G., and Ratliff, F. (1956). Inhibition in the eye of *Limulus*. *Journal of General Physiology, 40,* 357–376.

Hescheler, J., Kameyama, M., & Trautwein, W. (1986). On the mechanism of muscarinic inhibition of cardiac Ca current. *Pfluger's archives, 407,* 182–189.

Hescheler, J., Tang, M., Jastorff, B., & Trautwein, W. (1987). On the mechanism of histamine induced enhancement of the cardiac Ca^{2+} current. *Pfluger's archives, 410,* 23–29.

Hess, W. R. (1954). *Diencephalon: Autonomic and extra-pyramidal functions.* New York: Grune & Stratton.

Hikosaka, O., & Wurtz, R. H. (1983a). Visual and occulomotor functions of monkey substantia nigra pars reticulata. I. Relation of visual and auditory responses to saccades. *Journal of Neurophysiology, 49,* 1230–1253.

Hikosaka, O., & Wurtz, R. H. (1983b). Visual and occulomotor functions of monkey substantia nigra pars reticulata. II. Visual responses relate to fixation of gaze. *Journal of Neurophysiology, 49,* 1254–1267.

Hikosaka, O., & Wurtz, R. H. (1983c). Visual and occulomotor functions of monkey substantia nigra pars reticulata. III. Memory-contingent visual and saccade responses. *Journal of Neurophysiology, 49,* 1268–1284.

Hikosaka, O., & Wurtz, R. H. (1983d). Visual and occulomotor functions of monkey substantia nigra pars reticulata. IV. Relation of substantia nigra to superior colliculus. *Journal of Neurophysiology, 49,* 1285–1301.

Hille, B. (1984). *Ionic channels of excitable membranes.* Sinauer: Sunderland.

Hilton, S. M., & Zbrozyna, A. W. (1963). Amygdaloid region for defence reactions and its afferent pathway to the brainstem. *Journal of Physiology 165,* 160–173.

Hokfelt, T., Lundberg, J. M., Schulteberg, M., Johansson, O., Ljungdahl, A., & Rehfeld, J. (1986). Coexistence of peptides and putative transmitters in neurons. In E. Costa & M. Trabucchi (Eds.), *Neural peptides and neuronal communication.* New York: Raven, pp. 1–23.

Hubel, D. H., & Wiesel, T. N. (1977). Functional architecture of macaque monkey visual cortex. *Proceedings of the Royal Society of London B, 198,* 1–59.

Ito, M. (1984). *The cerebellum and neural control,* New York: Raven Press.

Iwai, E., & Mishkin, M. (1968). Two visual foci in the oral lobe of monkeys. N. Yoshii & N. A. Buchwald (Eds.), *Neuropsychological basis of learning and behavior.* Osaka: Japan: Osaka University Press.

Jonasson, K. R., & Enloe, L. J. (1971). Alterations in social behavior following septal and amygdaloid lesions in the rat. *Journal of Comparative and Physiological Psychology, 75,* 286–301.

Kandel, E. R., & Schwartz, J. H. (1985). *Principles of neural science.* Amsterdam: Elsevier.

Karlin, A., Holtzman, E., Yodh, N., Lobel, P., Wall, J., & Hainfeld, J. (1983). The arrangement of the subunits of the acetylcholine receptor of *Torpedo californica. Journal of Biological Chemistry, 258,* 6678–6681.

Kasamatsu, T., & Pettigrew, J. (1979). Preservation of binocularity after monocular deprivation in the striate cortex of kittens treated with 6-hydroxydopamine. *Journal of Comparative Neurology, 185,* 139–161.

Kluver, H., & Bucy, P. C. (1939). Preliminary analysis of functions of the temporal lobes in monkeys. *Archives of Neurology and Psychiatry (Chicago), 42,* 979–1000.

Koester, J. (1985). Resting membrane potential and action potential. In E. R. Kandel and J. H. Schwartz (Eds.), *Principles of neural science.* Amsterdam: Elsevier.

Koizumi, K., & Brooks, C. M. (1980). The autonomic system and its role in controlling body functions. In V. Mountcastle (Ed.) *Medical physiology* Vol. 1. St. Louis: Mosby.

Kolb, B. B., & Whishaw, I. (1980). *Fundamental of human neuropsychology.* San Francisco: Freeman.

Krnjevic, K., & Morris, M. E. (1974). An excitatory action of substance P on cuneate neurons. *Canadian Journal of Physiology and Pharmacology, 52,* 736–744.

Kuffler, S. W., Nicholls, J. G., & Martin, A. R. (1984). *From neuron to brain.* Sinauer: Sunderland.

Lassen, N. A., Ingvar, D. H., & Skinhoj, E. (1978). Brain function and blood flow. *Scientific American, 239,* 62–71.

Lewis, J. W., Tordoff, M. G., Sherman, D. E., & Liebeskind, D. C. (1982). Adrenal-medullary enkephalin-like peptides may mediate opioid stress analgesia. *Science, 217*, 557–559.

Libet, B., Alberts, W. W., Wright, E. W., Jr., & Feinstein, B. (1967). Response of human somatosensory cortex to stimuli below threshold for conscious sensation. *Science, 158*, 1597–1600.

Lindsley, D. H., & Holmes, J. E. (1984). *Basic human neurophysiology*. New York: Elsevier.

Livingstone, M. S. (1988). Art, illusion and the visual system. *Scientific American, 258*, 1–22.

Loewi, O. (1921). Ueber Humorale Uebertragbarkeit der Herznervenwirkung. *Pflugers Archives, 189*, 239–242.

Lundberg, J. M., & Hokfelt, T. (1986). Multiple co-existence of peptides and classical transmitters in peripheral autonomic and sensory neurons – functional and pharmacological implications. *Progress in Brain Research, 68*, 241–261.

Lundberg, J. M., Rudehill, A., Sollevi, A., Theodorsson-Norheim, E., & Hamberger, B. (1986). Frequency- and reserpine-dependent chemical coding of sympathetic transmission: Differential release of noradrenaline and neuropeptide Y from pig spleen. *Neuroscience Letters, 63*, 96–100.

Lynch, J. C., Mountcastle, V. B., Talbot, W. H., & Yin, T. C. T. (1977). Parietal lobe mechanisms for directed visual attention. *Journal of Neurophysiology, 40*, 362–389.

MacDonnell, M. F., & Flynn, J. P. (1966a). Control of sensory fields by stimulation of the hypothalamus. *Science, 152*, 1406–1408.

MacDonnell, M. F., & Flynn, J. P. (1966b). Sensory control of hypothalamic attack. *Animal Behavior, 14*, 399–405.

Meck, W. H., Church, R. M., & Wenk, G. L. (1986). Arginine vasopressin innoculates against age-related increases in sodium-dependent high affinity choline uptake and discrepancies in the content of temporal memory. *European Journal of Pharmacology, 130*, 327–331.

Miller, N. E. (1969). Learning of visceral and glandular responses. *Science, 163*, 434–455.

Mishkin, M. (1979). Analogous neural models for tactile and visual learning. *Neuropsychologia, 17*, 139–152.

Moore, R. Y., & Eichler, V. B. (1972). Loss of circadian adrenal corticosterone rhythm following suprachiasmatic lesions in the rat. *Brain Research, 42*, 201–206.

Mountcastle, V. (Ed.). (1980). *Medical physiology* (14th ed.). Louis: Mosby.

Mueller, K., & Hsaio, S. (1978). Current status of cholecystokinin as a short-term satiety hormone. *Neuroscience Behavior Reviews, 2*, 79–87.

Nakanishi, S., Inoue, A., Kita, T., Nakamura, M., Chang, A. C. Y., Cohe, S. N., & Numa, S. (1979). Nucleotide sequence of cloned cDNA for bovine corticotropin-β-lipotropin precursor. *Nature, 278*, 423–427.

Nashner, L. M. (1976). Adapting reflexes controlling the human posture. *Experimental Brain Research, 26*, 59–72.

Olds, M. E., & Fobes, J. L. (1981). The central basis of motivation: Intracranial self-stimulation studies. *Annual Review of Psychology, 32*, 523–574.

Olton, D. S. (1984). Animal models of human amnesia. In L. K. Squire & N. Butters (Eds.), *The neuropsychology of memory*. New York: Guildford Press.

Papez, J. W. (1937). A proposed mechanism of emotion. *Archives of Neurology and Psychiatry, 38*, 725–743.

Pearse, A. G. E. (1976). Peptides in brain and intestine. *Nature, 262*, 92–94.

Penfield, W., & Jasper, H. H. (1954). *Epilepsy and the functional anatomy of the human brain.* Boston: Little, Brown.

Penfield, W., & Welch, K. (1951). The supplementary motor area of the cerebral cortex, a clinical and experimental study. *Archives of Neurology and Psychiatry, 66*, 289–317.

Posner, M. I., Walker, J. A., Friedrich, F. J., & Rafal, R. D. (1984). Effects of parietal injury on covert orienting of visual attention. *Journal of Neurophysiology, 4*, 1863–1874.

Roberts, W. W. (1970). In R. E. Whalen, R. F. Thompson, M., Verzeano, & N. M. Weinberger (Eds.), *The neural control of behavior.* New York: Academic Press.

Roberts, W. W., & Carey, R. J. (1965). Rewarding effect of performance of gnawing aroused by hypothalamic stimulation in the rat. *Journal of Comparative and Physiological Psychology, 59*, 317–324.

Roberts, W. W., & Kiess, H. O. (1964). Motivational properties of hypothalamic aggression in cats. *Journal of Comparative and Physiological Psychology, 58*, 187–193.

Robinson, D. A. (1976). Adaptive gain control of vestibulocular reflex by the cerebellum. *Journal of Neurophysiology, 39*, 954–969.

Robinson, D. L., Goldbert, M. E., & Stanton, G. B. (1978). Parietal association cortex in the primate: Sensory mechanisms and behavioral modulations. *Journal of Neurophysiology, 41,* 910–932.

Rolls, E. T. (1982). Feeding and reward. In B. G. Hobel & D. Norin (Eds.), *The neural basis of feeding and reward.* Brunswick, ME: Haer Institute.

Sandman, C. A., Denman, P. M., Miller, L. H., Knott, J. R., Schally, A. V., & Kastin, A. J. (1971). Electroencephalographic measures of melanocyte stimulating hormone activity. *Journal of Comparative and Physiological Psychology, 76,* 103.

Schmitt, F. O., & Melnechuk, T. (1966). *Neurosciences research symposium summaries: Vol. 1. An anthology from the Neurosciences Research Program Bulletin.* Cambridge, MA: MIT Press.

Scoville, W., Band, W., & Milner, B. (1957). Loss of recent memory after bilateral hippocampal lesions. *Journal of Neurology, Neurosurgery and Psychiatry, 20,* 11–21.

Severs, W. B., & Daniels-Severs, A. E. (1973). Effects of angiotensin on the central nervous system. *Pharmacological Reviews, 25,* 415–449.

Sherrington, C. S. (1906). *The integrative of the nervous system.* New Haven: Yale University. Press.

Shields, S. A., MacDowell, K. A., Fairchild, S. B., & Campbell, M. L. (1987). Is mediation of sweating cholinergic, adrenergic, or both? A comment on the literature. *Psychophysiology, 24,* 312–319.

Shik, M. L., Severin, F. V., & Orlovsky, G. N. (1966). Control of walking and running by means of electrical stimulation of the midbrain. *Biophysics, 11,* 756–765.

Singer, W., Tretter, F., & Cynader, M. (1976). The effect of reticular stimulation on spontaneous and evoked activity in the cat visual cortex. *Brain Research, 102,* 71–90.

Skolnick, P., & Paul, S. M. (1982). Benzodiazepine receptors in the central nervous system. *International Review of Neurology, 23,* 103–140.

Squire, L. R. (1982). The neuropsychology of human memory. *Annual Review of Neuroscience, 5,* 241–273.

Stephan, R. K., & Zucker, I. (1972). Circadian rhythms in drinking behavior and locomotor activity of rats are eliminated by hypothalamic lesions. *Proceedings of the National Academy of Sciences of the United States of America, 69,* 1583–1586.

Stoerig, P., Huber, M., & Poppel, E. (1985). Signal detection analysis of residual vision in a field defect due to a post-geniculate lesion. *Neuropsychologia, 23,* 589–599.

Strand, F. L. (1983). *Physiology: A regulatory systems approach* (2nd ed.) New York: Macmillan.

Stryer, L., & Bourne, H. R. (1986). G Proteins: A family of signal transducers. *Annual Review of Cell Biology, 2,* 391–419.

Tallman, J. F., & Gallager, D. W. (1985). The Gaba-ergic system: A locus of benzodiazepine action. *Annual Review of Neuroscience, 8,* 21–44.

Thompson, R. F., McCormick, D. A., Lavond, D. G., Clark, G. A., Kettner, R. E., & Mauk, M. D. (1983). The engram found? Initial localization of the memory trace for a basic form of associative learning. In J. M. Sprague & A. E. Epstein (Eds), *Progress in psychobiology and physiological psychology,* (Vol. 10, pp. 167–196). New York: Academic Press.

Truex, R. C., & Carpenter, M. B. (1969). *Human neuroanatomy.* Baltimore: Williams & Wilkins.

Valenstein, E. S., Cox, V. C., & Kakolewski, J. W. (1970). Re-examination of the role of the hypothalamus in motivation. *Psychological Review, 77,* 16–31.

Van Essen, D. C. (1979). Visual areas of the mammalian cerebral cortex. *Annual Review of Neuroscience, 2,* 227–263.

Vergnes, M. (1976). Controle amygdalien de comportements d'aggression chez le rat. *Physiology and Behavior, 17,* 439–444.

Walker, J. M., Akil, H., & Watson, S. J. (1980). Evidence for homologous action of pro-opiocortin products. *Science, 210,* 1247–1249.

Walker, J. M., Berntson, G. G., Sandman, C. A., Kastin, A. J., & Akil, H. (1981). Induction of analgesia by central administration of ORG 2766, an analog of $ACTH_{4-9}$. *European Journal of Pharmacology, 69,* 71–79.

Walker, J. M., Ghessari, A., Peters, B. A., Watson, S. J., Seidah, N., Chretien, M., & Akil H. (1987). Functional aspects of multitransmitter neurons: Studies of interactions among pro-opiomelancortin (POMC) products. In J. Lewis & J. Akil (Eds.), *Neurotransmission and pain* (pp. 160–177). Berlin: Karger.

Walker, J. M., Matsumoto, R. R., Bowen, W. D., Gans, D. L., Jones, K. D., & Walker, F. O. (1988).

Evidence for a role of haloperidol-sensitive "opiate" receptors in the motor effects of antipsychotic drugs. *Neurology, 38,* 961–965.

Walker, J. M., Sandman, C. A., Berntson, G. G., McGivern, R., Coy, D. H., & Kastin, A. J. (1977). Endorphin analogs having potent and long lasting analgesic effects. *Pharmacology Biochemistry and Behavior, 7,* 543.

Weiskrantz, L., Warrington, E. K., Sanders, M. D., & Marshall, J. (1974). Visual capacity in the hemianopic field following restricted occipital ablation. *Brain, 97,* 709–723.

Woolsey, C. N. (Ed.). (1982). *Cortical sensory organization* (Vols. 1 & 2). Clifton, NJ: Humana Press.

Woolsey, C. N., Settlage, P. H., Meyer, D. R., Sencer, W., Hamuy, T. P., & Travis, A. M. (1950). Patterns of localization in precentral and "supplementary" motor areas and their relation to the concept of a premotor area. *Association for Research in Nervous and Mental Disease, 163,* 763–778.

Zipser, D. (1985). A computational model of hippocampal place fields. *Behavioral Neuroscience, 99,* 1106–1018.

4   *Principles of bioelectrical measurement*

BEVERLY S. MARSHALL-GOODELL, LOUIS G.
TASSINARY, AND JOHN T. CACIOPPO

4.1   INTRODUCTION

> The most significant functions of laboratory instruments are measurement and control. Since the scientist's principal activities are observations under controlled conditions, one index of the usefulness of instruments to experimenting psychologists is the extent to which they facilitate the observation, quantification and control of variables relevant to the psychological situation.
>
> (Grings, 1954, p. 2)

Parallels in the development of science and technology have been observed in both the physical and the biobehavioral sciences. Technological advances supply the scientist with progressively better tools for measurement and control. Within the phsysical sciences, for example, the development of the radio telescope allowed astronomers to detect and examine starlike quasars at a level beyond the range of optical imaging (Schmidt, 1963). Brown and Saucer (1958) noted several examples within the behavioral sciences in which technological advances facilitated scientific progress. For example, development of the vacuum tube oscillator greatly improved stimulus control within the study of audition, and the development of suitable amplifiers and display devices (described later in this chapter) enabled the reliable detection and quantitative description of subtle bioelectrical signals as brief as a single action potential (Erlanger & Glasser, 1937). More recently, technological advances permitting detection of weak magnetic fields led to the discovery and quantification of event-related magnetic activity in the brain (Beatty, Barth, Richer, & Johnson, 1986).

Although technological advances may permit scientists to venture into frontier areas of research, inadequate or incomplete technical knowledge may lead to serious errors of inference. For example, soon after the discovery of X-rays, numerous scientists employing the technology for observing the effects of X-rays reported a related phenomenon called *N*-rays (Rostron, 1960, cited in Barber, 1976). The effects misattributed to *N*-rays were later shown to be the result of difficulties involved in estimating by eye the brightness of faint objects (Wood, 1904). In addition, soon after the birth of experimental psychology, the reaction times being measured in Wilhelm Wundt's laboratory at the University of Leipzig were discovered by James Cattell to be in error because of asymmetries in the time required for the magnet in the chronoscope to attract and release the armature (Schal, Davis, & Merzbach, 1976). More recently, Jonides (1982) reported a surprising effect involving temporal integration of a sequence of two very briefly presented visual patterns. It was later determined that the method for presentation of the visual patterns failed to properly account for the decay time of the phosphor on the display screen, so that the patterns actually overlapped in time (Jonides, Irwin, & Yantis, 1983).

The field of psychophysiology is, at present, highly dependent on electronic instrumentation for detection, amplification, recording, and quantification of physiological processes. Numerous texts on techniques in psychophysiology attest to the fact that the establishment and maintenance of any psychophysiology laboratory requires certain technical expertise (e.g., Brown, 1967; Coles, Donchin, & Porges, 1986; Greenfield & Sternbach, 1972; Martin & Venables, 1980; Stern, Ray, & Davis, 1980; Venables & Martin, 1967). Although a psychophysiologist need not become a bioelectrical engineer, an understanding of some fundamentals of electricity and electrical circuits, the unique properties of bioelectrical signals, and the principles of physiological measurement can guide the researcher in the proper application of existing and yet to be developed instruments.

This chapter begins with a description of the physical properties of electricity and electrical transmission. Next, the unique properties of bioelectrical signals are described and related to techniques for detection of bioelectrical signals. Afterward, both the essential and optional components of sensor systems for detecting, amplifying, and storing physiological responses are described.

4.2   BASICS OF ELECTRICITY

All electrical phenomena[1] are traceable to an intrinsic property of matter called charge. The exact nature of electrical charge is understood only in terms of the behavior of particles. The fundamental particles of electrical charge are protons and electrons. Protons, located in the nucleus of all atoms, possess a unit positive charge and electrons, located in planetarylike orbits about the nucleus of an atom, possess a unit negative charge. The simplest molecular structure is that of a hydrogen atom, with one proton in the nucleus and one orbiting electron. The electrical charge of a single electron is quite small, and the coulomb, the physical unit for electrical charge, was developed before discovery of the electron. One coulomb is the charge of 6.2×10^{18} electrons.

Electrons are maintained in orbit about the nucleus of an atom by a mechanical force of attraction that exists between particles of opposing charges. This force, called *electrical potential*, measured in volts (V), is the force underlying all electrical signals. Although electrical potential can .be a measure of force of attraction between any two locations, measures of voltage at a particular location are most often reported relative to an electrically neutral location. Such an electrically neutral location is called electrical or earth *ground*. The electrical potential within and surrounding atoms is best described as a spherical *electrical field* centered about the nucleus. The strength of the electrical potential within this field is inversely proportional to the square of the distance from the center of mass. Consequently, electrons, particularly those most distant from the nucleus of an atom, can move more freely than protons and neutrons. The movement of charged particles through an electrical field is called an *electrical current* and is measured in amperes (A). Within a vacuum electrical current can travel almost as fast as light, but within all other media speeds of conduction are somewhat slower.

Electrons that orbit atomic nuclei are located within nested energy levels, called shells, each with a limited capacity for electrons. The innermost shells are filled in succession as the number of electrons increases across elements, and the number of electrons in the outermost shell of an atom determines the chemical and electrical

1a																	0
1 H	2a											3a	4a	5a	6a	7a	2 He
3 Li	4 Be											5 B	6 C	7 N	8 O	9 F	10 Ne
11 Na	12 Mg	3b	4b	5b	6b	7b	8		1b	2b		13 Al	14 Si	15 P	16 S	17 Cl	18 Ar
19 K	20 Ca	21 Sc	22 Ti	23 V	24 Cr	25 Mn	26 Fe	27 Co	28 Ni	29 Cu	30 Zn	31 Ga	32 Ge	33 As	34 Se	35 Br	36 Kr
37 Rb	38 Sr	39 Y	40 Zr	41 Nb	42 Mo	43 Tc	44 Ru	45 Rh	46 Pd	47 Ag	48 Cd	49 In	50 Sn	51 Sb	52 Te	53 I	54 Xe
55 Cs	56 Ba	57 La	72 Hf	73 Ta	74 W	75 Re	76 Os	77 Ir	78 Pt	79 Au	80 Hg	81 Tl	82 Pb	83 Po	84	85 At	86 Rn
87 Fr	88 Ra	89 Ac															

LANTHANIDES

58 Ce	59 Pr	60 Nd	61 Pm	62 Sm	63 Eu	64 Gd	65 Tb	66 Dy	67 Ho	68 Er	69 Tm	70 Yb	71 Lu

ACTINIDES

90 Th	91 Pa	92 U	93 Np	94 Pu	95 Am	96 Cm	97 Bk	98 Cf	99 Es	100 Fm	101 Mv	102 No	103 Lw

Figure 4.1. Periodic table of elements.

reactivity of that element. Atomic elements that appear in the same row of the periodic table (Figure 4.1) have differing numbers of electrons in the same outermost shell, whereas elements in the same column have the same number of electrons in different outermost shells. Elements in the last column of the periodic table, such as neon, are chemically stable and electrically uncharged because the outermost electron shell is full and the number of protons and electrons remains equal.

Electrically charged atoms are called *ions*. Elements in the first column, such as sodium, or the seventh column, such as chlorine, are chemically reactive and are rarely found in the electrically uncharged state. Sodium, for example, which has only one electron in its outermost shell, tends to lose one electron, eliminating the outermost shell and forming a *cation*, an atom with a net positive charge. Chlorine, on the other hand, which has seven electrons in its outermost shell, tends to gain one electron, completing the outermost shell and forming an *anion*, an atom with a net negative charge. Chemically reactive elements tend to form *ionic* chemical bonds by actual transfer of electrons from one atom to another. Atoms of less reactive elements, such as carbon, with four electrons in the outermost shell, form *covalent* chemical bonds by sharing electrons among atoms rather than actually transferring electrons from one atom to another.

In sum, the electrical and chemical properties of matter are integrated and inseparable. One of the most familiar sources of electrical voltage, a carbon-zinc (dry-cell) battery, relies on a chemically generated electrical potential between a carbon rod and a zinc plate when separated by an *electroyte* medium, a paste containing free ions. The electrolyte in a dry-cell battery is composed of zinc chloride, ammonium chloride, and manganese dioxide. Chemical generation of an electrical potential is based on the production of separate concentrations of cations and anions. Inside the carbon-zinc battery, zinc atoms are dissolved into the electrolyte solution, forming doubly charged zinc ions and leaving behind two free electrons. At the same time, the ammonium ions and the manganese dioxide work together to withdraw electrons from the carbon rod, leaving it positively charged. The negatively charged zinc plate is called the *negative terminal*, or *anode*, and the positively charged carbon rod is called the *positive terminal*, or *cathode*. When the positive and negative terminals of the battery are connected externally as through an electrical circuit, free electrons flow from the zinc plate through the circuit to the carbon rod, generating electrical current in the circuit. As long as the circuit is continuous, current continues to flow until the ionic supply within the battery is exhausted.

The voltage provided by a battery is unidirectional and relatively stable in amplitude throughout the effective life of the battery and thus provides a unidirectional current referred to as *direct current* (DC). The amplitude of DC potential at either terminal of a battery is generally referenced to 0 V. A typical dry-cell battery provides an electrical potential of about 1.5 V DC. In *storage batteries* such as those used in automobiles, the chemical reactions that produce the separate ionic concentrations can be reversed by an external energy source, and potentials of 6, 12, or 25 V DC are common.

The nature of the atomic structure within a material determines the extent to which that material will support the movement of charged particles. Solid materials high in unbound electrons, such as metals, and ionic solutions such as saline are classified as *conductors*, or carriers, of electrical current. Materials low in unbound electrons, such as rubber, paper, and glass, do not carry electrical current, and are used as electrical *insulators*. Materials with an intermediate level of unbound electrons such as carbon, silicon, and germanium, called *semiconductors*, are used in production of solid-state electronic components such as transistors and integrated circuits.

The extent to which a material impedes the flow of a unidirectional electrical current between two points of unequal electrical potential is quantified as *resistance*, measured in ohms. The commonly accepted symbol for ohms is the Greek letter omega, Ω. An ohm is a very small unit, and practical resistances within physiological systems range from kilohms to megohms. Conductors are low in resistance; insulators are high in resistance. Even the best conductors provide some resistance to flow of current. However, conductors with a large cross-sectional area provide many more current paths than those with a small cross-sectional area and thus provide a lower resistance to current flow. It is often useful to describe the ability to conduct current in terms of the reciprocal of resistance, called *conductance*, reported in siemens, S (1 siemen = 1/ohm).

The relationship between electrical potential V, current I, and resistance R is described mathematically as Ohm's Law, $V = I \times R$. An analogy to fluid systems helps to clarify this mathematical relationship. Electrical potential is a force similar to the pressure at a water faucet. The forces of both hydraulic pressure and electrical potential are present even in the absence of water and of current flow, respectively. When a valve in a hydraulic system is closed, the pressure is present, but the resistance offered by the valve prevents the flow of water. Opening the valve reduces this resistance, permitting water to flow. The flow of water is analogous to electrical current. A large-diameter hose attached to the valve provides less resistance to the flow of water than a small-diameter hose. Thus, one can increase the water flow by increasing the water pressure or by decreasing the resistance with

a) Sine wave voltage signal

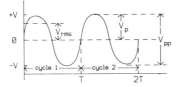

b) 90° phase shift, positive DC offset

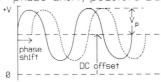

c) 180° phase shift, negative DC offset

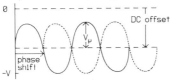

Figure 4.2. Quantification of component parts of simple sine wave voltage signals as function of time. Peak voltage V_p, peak-to-peak voltage V_{pp}, rms voltage V_{rms}, and period T for two-cycle sine wave (*a*). Sine wave voltage signals with positive and negative DC offsets in (*b*) and (*c*), respectively. A second sine wave voltage phase shifted from the original in (*a*) by 90° and 180° is shown in (*b*) and (*c*), respectively.

larger valves and hoses. Likewise, electrical currents are greatest when electrical potentials are high and electrical resistances are low.

The fluid analogy given here may give the false impression that electrical currents and voltages are always unidirectional and remain fixed at a constant level determined by the electrical resistance present.[2] Although DC sources such as batteries do provide unidirectional, steady-state potentials, the voltages provided by the electrical wall outlets available in a laboratory are not steady but vary regularly with time. Assuming for the moment that electrical resistances remain fixed, Ohm's Law indicates that periodically changing voltages must produce periodically changing currents. *Alternating currents* (AC) periodically vary in both amplitude and direction of flow.

A sine wave, one of the simplest of periodic waveforms, along with several standard measures of change in the time and amplitude dimensions, is illustrated in Figure 4.2 (top panel). The time interval required for one cycle is called the *period* (*T*). The reciprocal of the period is the *frequency* (*f*), typically reported as the number of cycles per second, or *hertz* (Hz). The relationship between period and frequency for selected values is shown in Table 4.1. For a sinusoidal potential signal that is symmetrical about 0 V, the peak voltage V_p is the maximum voltage observed, and the peak-to-peak voltage V_{pp} is twice V_p. Likewise, for a sinusoidal current, symmetrical about 0 A, the maximum current observed is called the peak current I_p, and the peak-to-peak current I_{pp} is twice I_p. Because the amplitude of an AC signal

Table 4.1. *Relationship between period and frequency*

Period(s)	Frequency (HZ)
1.0	1
0.5	2
0.1	10
0.05	20
0.001	100
0.0001	1,000
0.00001	10,000

changes across time, the peak value is not the best indicant of the average effective amplitude. The *root-mean-square* (rms) *value* for an alternating current or voltage provides a time-averaged amplitude that quantifies variations across time. The general formula for calculation of the rms value for a set of sampled voltages containing n different values $V_1 \ldots v_n$ is given by

$$V_{\text{rms}} = \sqrt{\frac{1}{n} \sum_{i=1}^{n} V_i^2}$$

This formula can be used with any voltage or current signal that changes with time, including complex physiological signals described later. However, the rms value of a pure sine wave voltage or current V_{rms} or I_{rms} can be reduced to the peak value V_p or I_p divided by the square root of 2. Instruments for measuring AC potentials and currents are universally calibrated in terms of rms values. Unless stated otherwise, it is generally understood that AC potentials and currents are characterized by their rms values. Laboratory AC power lines operate at frequency of 60 Hz in the United States and 50 Hz in Europe with rms amplitudes of 117 and 220 V, respectively. As we shall see, these frequencies overlap with those present in some biopotentials, and the voltages are considerably higher than physiological levels.

In addition to frequency and amplitude, AC signals can be compared in terms of *phase shift* and *DC offset*. Phase shift refers to displacement along the time dimension, and DC offset refers to displacement along the amplitude dimension. Although phase shifts represent temporal displacements, they are generally reported as a *phase angle*, where the period T corresponds to an angle of 360°. When two identical sine wave signals are phase shifted by 0°, 360°, or multiples of 360° (or 2π radians), they appear synchronized in time and are called "in phase." When one of two identical sine wave signals is phase shifted by 90°, the peaks and valleys of one signal correspond in time to the median amplitude level for the other signal. When the peaks of one sine wave signal correspond in time to the valleys of the other signal, the signals are completely out of phase, and the phase angle is 180°. Two identical sine waves that are 90° and 180° out of phase are illustrated in the middle and bottom panels of Figure 4.2.

When the median level of an AC signal is displaced above or below the 0 V level, the waveform can be described as the sum of two waveforms, one AC signal symmetrical about zero plus one constant DC offset signal, either positive or negative, which accounts for the constant displacement from zero. Positive and negative DC offsets are shown in the middle and bottom panels of Figure 4.2, respectively. It is often useful to be able to separate the slow DC-like and fast AC-like components of a single bioelectrical signal. For example, sensor systems for detection of cyclic respiration rate often include an uninteresting DC offset in the signal. Compensatory circuitry that effectively removes the DC offset in the signal can allow selective amplification of the AC signal of interest. However, it is not always appropriate to disregard the DC offset. In particular, some electrical properties of the skin discussed later in this chapter include discrete responses superimposed on a DC offset, the latter of which reflects the basal level of electrodermal activity (see Dawson, Schell, & Filion, chapter 10).

It is important to note that current, the amount of flow of electrical charges, not voltage, is what poses a risk for electrocution. Thus, although *static electricity*, the separation of charged ions due to friction, is characterized by high voltages, the currents associated with static discharge are minute and pose no risk to subjects. The main sources of tissue-damaging currents are AC power lines and devices attached to them. The typical current flow through a 100-W light bulb attached to an AC power line is about 1 A. However, currents in the milliampere (10^{-3} A) range are hazardous to living organisms. The threshold for detection of current is about 1 mA, and currents of 10 mA are painful. At about 20 mA the muscles exhibit tetanic contraction, making it impossible to let go of a wire that may have been grasped. Muscle damage can occur at 50 mA, and at 100 mA disorganized contractions of the heart, called *fibrillation*, occur. Procedures designed to prevent placing the subject at risk from electrical hazard are discussed in detail in Section 4.6.

4.3   SIMPLE CIRCUITS

An *electrical circuit* consists of a complete conductive path that permits the flow of current. The simplest DC circuit is a single conductive wire connecting the anode and cathode of a battery. The true direction of electron flow is from anode (negative) to cathode (positive). The convention for the direction of current in electronics, however, is based on the direction of movement of a positive charge, which is from positive to negative. Using Ohm's Law, the amount of current flow within the wire can be computed as $I = V/R$, where V is the battery voltage and R is the resistance of the wire. Since R for most conductors is small, such a simple circuit would permit rapid current flow and would quickly deplete the battery potential.

Most practical electrical circuits include components that have more resistance than a single conductive wire. Increasing the electrical resistance within a DC circuit reduces the current flow. For circuits using batteries as the DC potential source, greater resistance means longer life for the battery. It is often useful to add components of known resistance, called *resistors*, to a circuit to control current flow. When voltage is constant, as in DC circuits, increasing circuit resistance also serves to reduce power consumption. Specifically, when voltage is constant, power P, computed as $P = I^2R$, can be reduced to $P = V^2/R$ by substitution of V/R for I (Ohm's Law). The unit of measurement for power is the watt (W).

An electrical circuit that provides a single current path between the positive and negative potential source is called a *series circuit*. A simple series circuit consisting of a potential source such as a battery or an AC wall outlet, a switch, a fuse, an indicator lamp, and a box used to designate a circuit complex within some laboratory instrument is illustrated in Figure 4.3 (top panel). The circuit components

a)   Series Circuit

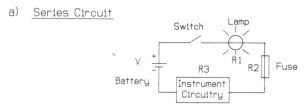

b)   Parallel Circuit

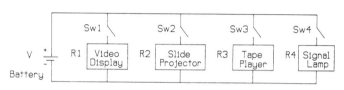

Figure 4.3. Series circuit (a) and parallel circuit (b).

are all connected end-to-end to form a single loop. Each component has an associated internal resistance, designated as R_1, R_2, R_3, and R_4. Closing the single switch would supply electrical power to all four circuit components. It is common practice to connect fuses and power (on–off) indicator lamps in series with all other internal circuitry within an instrument. A lighted power lamp then verifies the continuity of the internal circuitry, and a single fuse can disconnect all internal components from the power source when rendered discontinuous (blown) by a current surge. The current in this simple circuit is given by the voltage V divided by the total resistance encountered in the current loop. Stated another way, the equivalent resistance of resistors in series is a simple sum of the individual resistances, or $R_{series} = R_1 + R_2 + \cdots + R_n$. Thus, each component added to series circuit reduces the current flow through all components. Furthermore, a breakdown of the conducting path through any component in such a series circuit would disrupt the single current path and prevent the equipment from operating.

A simple *parallel circuit* for four independent pieces of laboratory equipment plus four separate switches and a potential source is illustrated in the bottom panel of Figure 4.3. In this parallel circuit each piece of equipment and its associated resistance is connected to both sides of the potential source. One familiar example of a parallel circuit is the separate sockets on a multitap AC wall outlet or a power strip. Most electrical circuits contain some components connected in series with the voltage source and some components connected in parallel with the voltage source, but separate examination of the embedded series and parallel circuits can provide useful information such as the current flow through each component. Connecting resistance in parallel to a voltage source provides multiple current paths for current to flow from the voltage source. Each resistance added to a parallel circuit increases the total current flow through the voltage source without reducing or disrupting current flow through the other components. One hydraulic model for resistors in parallel is a closed water system consisting of a large tank of water and multiple water outlets that convey the water along hoses or pipes before returning the water

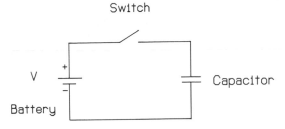

Figure 4.4. DC circuit to charge capacitor.

to the original tank. The amount of water flow from the tank is the lowest when only one outlet is opened, and as more water outlets are opened, the addition of more paths for the water to follow permits a greater flow of water. The equivalent resistance of resistors in parallel is always smaller than the smallest of the resistors, and resistors in parallel add as reciprocals. That is, the equivalent resistor for resistors in parallel is given by $1/R_{\text{parallel}} = 1/R_1 + 1/R_2 + 1/R_3 + \cdots + 1/R_n$.

For the series and parallel circuits illustrated in Figure 4.3, it was assumed that the potential source could be either DC or AC. There are, however, many circuits that react differently to AC compared to DC potentials. These differences are quantified by Ohm's Law for AC circuits in which the resistance term R for DC circuits is replaced by a term for resistance to alternating currents, called *impedance* (Z). Impedance, measured in ohms, includes DC resistance plus two forms of resistance specific to alternating currents, *capacitive reactance* and *inductive reactance*, both described later in this chapter. An understanding of *reactance* (X) is facilitated by an examination of some simple circuits that react differently to AC compared to DC potentials.

One unique feature of AC potentials is the ability to conduct electrical current across thin, nonconductive barriers that cannot be crossed by DC potentials. Consider a simple series circuit consisting of a source of DC potential such as a battery, a switch, and conducting plates separated by a thin insulator, as illustrated in Figure 4.4. Closing the switch connects the positive and negative terminals of the battery to different plates. The potential difference between the two plates causes positive and negative charged particles, attracted to each other across the thin insulating gap, to line up along the opposing plates. When this occurs, the plates are said to be *polarized*, that is, one plate contains a matrix of positively charged particles and the other a matrix of negatively charged particles. The amount of charge that can be stored on either side of such a gap is called *capacitance* (C). The unit for capacitance, the farad, is very large, and typical capacitances are in the range of picofarads (pF) to microfarads (μF). Capacitance has a special significance to the psychophysiologist because, as will be described later, the detection of many bioelectrical potentials requires a capacitive connection between the laboratory data collection equipment and the subject at the electrode interface.

Capacitance depends upon the size of the conductive plates and the size of the gap. The highest capacitances are found with large plates and small gaps since these conditions maximize the concentrated attractive force between opposing charges on the two plates. With DC potentials, current (i.e., movement of charged particles) flows in the circuit for the brief instant after closure of the switch during which the plates of the capacitor are polarized. Once the plates are fully polarized, also called charged, the potential across the gap would be equal and opposite to the DC source potential, and current would no longer flow (Figure 4.4). By reversing the connections to the battery, the plates can be discharged and polarized in the opposite direction, and another brief current flow can be detected. If the battery were replaced with a laboratory source of AC potential (e.g., 60 Hz, 117V), the polarity of the plates would be reversed 60 times per second, producing an effective current that alternated in direction. The process of charging and discharging the plates of a capacitor requires time, and the resulting current is phase shifted from the input potential by $+90°$.

The amplitude of current flow across a capacitive gap increases with increases in the frequency of alternation of the AC potential. The extent to which a capacitive gap impedes current flow, termed capacitive reactance (X_c) is inversely related to capacitance C and the frequency of the AC potential (ω) as given by $X_c = 1/\omega C$. Thus, a capacitor appears like an *open switch* to DC signals, and as the frequency of the signal is *increased*, the amount of current flow through a capacitor *increases*. Connecting capacitors in a parallel circuit is analogous to increasing the area of the plates, thus increasing the effective capacitance, and capacitances in a parallel circuit add directly (i.e., $C_{parallel} = C_1 + C_2 + ... + C_n$). Connecting capacitors in a series circuit can be compared to increasing the effective size of the gap to be crossed, thus decreasing the effective capacitance, and capacitances in series add as reciprocals (i.e., $1/C_{series} = 1/C_1 + 1/C_2 + \cdots + 1/C_n$).

A second unique property of AC compared to DC potentials results from the magnetic field that exists surrounding the current in any conductor. The lines of force of the magnetic field produced by an electrical current in a straight wire are circular and perpendicular to the current flow. The orientation of the magnetic field surrounding a conductive wire is conventionally described by the "right-hand rule." That is, when grasping the wire with the right hand so that the thumb points toward the anode, the fingers will point in the direction of the magnetic field. The strength of an electrically produced magnetic field can be concentrated in one region by looping conductive wire into a coil and adding conductive material such as iron in the center of the coil, as is done in most electromagnets. Many instruments used in the psychophysiology laboratory operate on electromagnetic principles, including the physical displacement of pens on an ink-writing chart recorder, galvanometers on biofeedback display equipment, and mechanical relay switches used to gate stimulus events. Furthermore, the electrical activity of the brain produces corresponding low-intensity magnetic fields, and localized changes in neuromagnetic activity have been elicited by visual, auditory, and somatosensory stimuli (Beatty et al., 1986).

Not only does any electrical current generate a surrounding magnetic field, but also the force of any *changing* magnetic field will induce an electrical current in any nearby conductors. The strength of the induced current is directly proportional to the rate of change of the magnetic field affecting the conductor. Regardless of the orientation of the conductor, the induced current is always oriented to produce a magnetic field that directly opposes the original changing magnetic field. Thus, at any instant in time, the induced current in a conductive wire placed parallel to a wire conducting an alternating current is opposite in direction to the direction of the original alternating current. The strength of this magnetic opposition to changes in current is quantified as *inductance*, abbreviated L and measured in *henries* (H). The opposition to changes in current offered by inductance in electrical systems has been likened to the resistance to motion in mechanical systems, called inertia (DeMarre, Kantrowitz, Zucker, & Simmons, 1979).

The principles of inductance are uniquely linked to AC as compared to DC potentials in two important ways. First, the common method for generating alternating currents relies on inductance. Typically, a large coil of wire wound around a soft iron core is placed near a pivoted magnet that is mechanically forced to rotate by means of water, steam, or wind. The fluctuations in the magnetic field surrounding the coil of wire produced by the rotating magnet induce a current that changes in amplitude and direction with each half rotation of the magnet. Second, any conductor that carries an alternating current is surrounded by a changing magnetic field capable of inducing current in other nearby conductors. The concentrated magnetic field produced by an *inductor* such as a coil of wire resists the passage of alternating current by inducing a current opposite in direction to the applied current. The resulting alternating current through an inductor is phase shifted by $-90°$ relative to the input potential. It is the principle of inductance that makes electromagnetism a mixed blessing for the psychophysiologist. Specifically, the amplitude and frequency of current induced by AC power lines is sufficient to mask many biopotential signals, and psychophysiological laboratories should be designed or selected to isolate sources of magnetic fields from physiological signals.

Inductive coils conduct direct current without distortion, since the magnetic field produced by direct current is constant and no opposing currents are induced. The extent to which an inductor impedes the flow of alternating current, termed *inductive reactance* (X_L) is directly related to inductance (L) and the frequency of the AC potential, ω, as given by $X_L = \omega L$. Thus, an inductor appears as a *closed switch* to a DC signal, and current flow *decreases* as the signal frequency *increases*. Connecting inductors in series has the same effect as increasing the number of turns on the coil of a single inductor, increasing the effective inductance, and inductances in series add directly (i.e., $L_{series} = L_1 + L_2 + ... + L_n$). Connecting inductances in parallel permits multiple current paths, reducing the effective inductance, and inductances in parallel add as reciprocals (i.e., $1/L_{parallel} = 1/L_1 + 1/L_2 + ... + 1/L_n$). Inductors are used in many laboratory instruments, particularly as voltage transformers. A voltage transformer operates on the principle of *mutual inductance*, in which the changing magnetic field around one multiturn coil induces current in an adjacent coil that in turn generates a magnetic field in opposition to the initial field. The strength of magnetic fields, like that of electrical fields, decreases as the square of the distance from the source, and thus the amplitude of induced currents is highly dependent on the distance between the two coils. Mutual inductance is maximized when the two coils are wound around the same iron core, as shown in Figure 4.5. Voltage transformers can be designed to step up (increase) or step down (decrease) the input voltage, depending on the ratio of the number of turns on the primary coil (n_1) generating the magnetic flux and that on the secondary coil (n_2) intercepting the magnetic flux as current. The oldest means for administration of controlled electrical current (shock), the *inductorium*, is based on mutual inductance between coupled coils (Grings, 1954, p. 269).

4.4   TOOLS FOR BIOELECTRICAL MEASUREMENT

The techniques of electrical measurement were developed to permit unobtrusive observation of local electrical activity, that is, observation that does not in itself

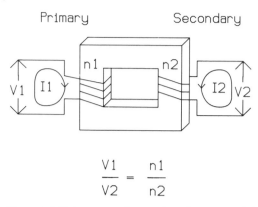

Primary   Secondary

$$\frac{V1}{V2} = \frac{n1}{n2}$$

Figure 4.5. Voltage transformer based on mutual inductance.

perturb the activity being measured. Although electrical measurement can be seen as a tool for design and repair of electrical instruments, the principles of electrical measurement provide the psychophysiologist with useful tools for assessing physiological responses. The three most common tools for electrical measurement are the *multimeter*, the *oscilloscope*, and the *bridge circuit*. Each of these tools can be extremely valuable in the psychophysiology laboratory, and the principles for their use generalize to all types of psychophysiological measurement.

Typical multimeters include separate internal circuits for measuring current (*ammeter*), potential (*voltmeter*), and resistance (*ohmmeter*). The appropriate use of each of these three meter circuits is illustrated in Figure 4.6. A very simple electrical circuit that includes a potential source V and an attached load resistance R_{load} is shown in panel *a* of Figure 4.6. To measure the current passing through R_{load}, the ammeter circuit is attached anywhere in the current loop in series with R_{load}. This requires that the existing current loop be opened (physically separated) and the meter circuit inserted in the opening to complete the loop, as shown in panel *b* of Figure 4.6. Because resistances in series add directly, it is important for the internal resistance of an ammeter circuit to be low relative to R_{load} so that addition of the ammeter to the circuit will not substantially reduce the current in the loop being measured.

To measure the electrical potential across R_{load}, the voltmeter circuit is connected in parallel with R_{load}, as shown in panel *c* of Figure 4.6. Note that connecting a meter in parallel need not disrupt the existing circuit loop. Voltmeter circuits are designed with high internal resistance so that the amount of current diverted from the circuit element being measured is minimal. The ability to measure voltage without disruption of the circuitry generating the signal makes measurement of bioelectrical potentials possible at the skin surface, where direct measurement of bioelectrical currents is difficult.[3]

It is possible to compute the resistance of R_{load} in Figure 4.6 using an ammeter to measure the current through R_{load} and a voltmeter to measure the voltage across R_{load} and then applying Ohm's Law. However, an ohmmeter circuit can be used to measure resistances directly. The ohmmeter circuit must be connected in parallel with the resistance being measured, as shown in panel *d* of Figure 4.6.

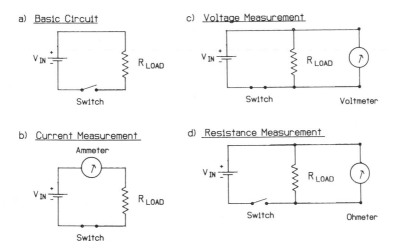

Figure 4.6. Simple circuit consisting of voltage source and load resistance (*a*) and appropriate circuit for measurement of current with ammeter (*b*), voltage with voltmeter (*c*), and resistance with ohmmeter (*d*).

Because most ohmmeter circuits measure resistance by applying a potential and assessing current, it is important that potential sources outside the ohmmeter circuit be switched off when using the ohmmeter. Thus, in Figure 4.6*d* the switch that completes the circuit loop containing the potential source and the load resistance is in the open position. The ohmmeter is also a useful tool for assessing the integrity of electrical connections, since the resistance between two unconnected conductors approaches infinity and the resistance between two connected conductors approaches zero.

Most multimeters can accurately measure both AC and DC currents and potentials but generally measure only resistance. Measurement of impedance (resistance and reactance) requires a specialized form of an ohmmeter that uses AC test currents rather than DC test potentials. The ability to measure resistance and impedance is useful in psychophysiology because the amplitude and integrity of the bioelectrical potentials detected from surface electrodes increases as the resistance/ impedance at the electrode interface decreases. More specifically, the skin-electrode barrier acts as if a resistor were placed in series between the biopotential source and the amplification circuitry, thus potentially altering the measurable amplitude and frequency of the voltage signal. In selecting commercial *impedance meters* for psychophysiological applications, it is important that the amplitude of the test currents be well below 100 μA, preferably below 10 μA, and that the frequency range of the test currents be matched to the frequency range of the physiological signals to be measured. Circuit diagrams for two simple impedance meters can be found in Dunseath (1982) and in Loeb and Gans (1986, p. 192).

A multimeter measures instantaneous amplitude and polarity of potentials and currents but provides no information about phase or variation with time. Most bioelectrical signals, however, vary almost continuously with time. The *cathode-ray oscilloscope* is an instrument used to simultaneously quantify the amplitude and time components of an electrical signal. An electron gun in the oscilloscope directs a high-velocity focused beam of electrons onto a phosphor-covered glass faceplate.

When the phosphor is struck by an electron, it fluoresces, emitting light visible on the $X-Y$ grid coordinates of the faceplate display screen. The beam of electrons can be deflected both vertically and horizontally by pairs of deflecting plates that flank the electron beam. The amount and direction of deflection depend on the voltage applied across the pairs of plates.

Changes in a voltage signal across time can be traced on the oscilloscope display screen by applying the input voltage across the vertical deflection plates and an internal timing voltage across the horizontal deflection plates. Internal timing voltages, also called *horizontal-sweep voltages*, are oscillating ramp signals that show linear increases in amplitude for a selected duration followed by rapid decreases to zero. During each cycle of the horizontal-sweep voltage the electron beam moves across the oscilloscope display screen from left to right, tracing any corresponding changes in the input voltage along the vertical axis. Calibrated vertical and horizontal gain and DC offset controls permit measurements of voltage and time components to be made directly from the display screen. Although the oscilloscope is basically a voltage-sensitive device, current can be indirectly assessed as a voltage change across a fixed resistance or measured directly with a specialized input to the oscilloscope called a *current probe* positioned to encircle the conducting cable and measure the magnetic field produced by the current. Most oscilloscopes can be set to display continuously or to begin displaying when a trigger voltage is detected. Triggering the oscilloscope display from an electrical event can be useful in measurement of event-locked activity. Some oscilloscopes have the capacity to simultaneously display multiple signals as separate channels, and some *storage oscilloscopes* can temporarily fix a tracing on the display screen to facilitate measurements.

When very accurate measurements of resistance/conductance, capacitance, or inductance are required, an instrument with a *bridge circuit* is frequently used. For example, one class of psychophysiological signals, that of electrodermal activity (EDA), results from changes in the resistivity/conductivity of the skin. In addition, bridge circuits are central to many transducer circuits for detection of physiological signals such as respiration and blood volume. Although bridge circuits can be built using resistors, capacitors, or inductors and can be driven by DC potentials or AC currents, all bridge circuits work on the same principle, that of balance. The Wheatstone bridge circuit for measurement of resistance, consisting of a potential source, four resistors, and an ammeter, is illustrated in panel *a* of Figure 4.7. Two of the resistors, R_1 and R_2, have resistances that are known and fixed, one, $R_{variable}$, can be adjusted, and the fourth, $R_{unknown}$, is the resistance to be measured. When all four resistances are equal, the current through each resistor is the same, no potential difference exists between points A and B in the circuit, and thus no differential current flows through the ammeter. When no differential current is present at the ammeter, the bridge is said to be balanced.

To better understand the conditions under which points A and B in panel *a* of Figure 4.7 will be equipotential, the Wheatstone bridge circuit is redrawn in the bottom panels of Figure 4.7 as two separate series circuits. Within each of these two series circuits the same current passes through both of the resistors. The current is determined by Ohm's Law to be V_{in}/R_{total}. Thus, the current through R_1 and R_{var}, called I_1, equals $V_{in}/(R_1 + R_{var})$, and the current through R_2 and $R_{unknown}$, called I_2, equals $V_{in}/(R_2 + R_{unknown})$. Circuits with resistors in series are sometimes called *voltage dividers* because the voltage measured across any one resistor such as R_1

a) Wheatstone Bridge

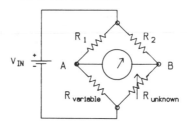

b) Two Voltage Dividers

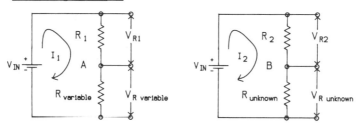

Figure 4.7. Wheatstone bridge circuit (a) and same circuit redraw as two voltage-divider circuits (b).

is a fraction of the total input voltage V_{in} determined by the ratio of R_1 to the total resistance $R_1 + R_{var}$, or $V_{R1} = R_1 / (R_1 + R_{var})$. Likewise, the voltage across R_2 is computed as $V_{R2} = R_2 / (R_2 + R_{unknown})$. In order for point A and B in the circuit to be equipotential, it is not necessary for I_1 to equal I_2, but it is necessary for the voltage across R_1 to equal the voltage across R_2. Setting $V_{R1} = V_{R2}$ gives $R_1 / (R_1 + R_{var}) = R_2 / (R_2 + R_{var})$. By cross multiplying and subtracting R_1R_2 from both sides of this equation, the balance conditions for the bridge can be reduced to $R_1 R_{unknown} = R_2 R_{var}$, or the equivalent expression, $R_1 / R_{var} = R_2 / R_{unknown}$.

In most applications of the Wheatstone bridge R_1 and R_2 are fixed resistances either of equal value or switch selectable in ratios differing by powers of 10. In the simplest case where R_1 and R_2 are equal, the bridge will only be balanced when $R_{variable}$ is adjusted to equal $R_{unknown}$. If a calibrated scale for $R_{variable}$ is provided that accounts for changes in R_1/R_2, the value of $R_{unknown}$ can be read from the calibrated scale at the balance point. Similar bridge circuits using two fixed and one variable capacitor or inductor can be used to measure unknown capacitances and inductances, respectively.

The Wheatstone bridge circuit is commonly used in the measurement of skin resistance. With this procedure, the subject contributes the unknown resistance. Baseline (tonic) skin resistance levels are measured by adjusting the variable resistance, either manually or automatically, until the voltage (and thus the current) between A and B, often monitored with a voltage-activated pen recorder, is zero. Once adjustments to offset the baseline skin resistance level have been made, phasic skin resistance responses can be measured as calibrated changes in the voltage between A and B. Skin conductance, the reciprocal of skin resistance, can be measured directly with a variation of the basic bridge circuit (see Dawson et al., chapter 10).

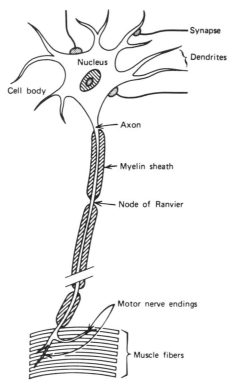

Figure 4.8. Schematic of motor neuron. (Reprinted with permission from J. R. Cameron & J. G. Skofronick, *Medical Physics*, © John Wiley & Sons, Inc., New York, 1978.)

4.5   BIOPOTENTIALS

Bioelectrical signals[4] generated inside the body control, either directly or indirectly, all functions and activities of the brain, muscles, and organs (see Matsumoto, Walker, Walker, & Hughes, chapter 3). These bioelectrical signals are the result of sudden, reversible changes in the distribution of ions within and outside of specialized cells. Nerve cells, or *neurons* (Figure 4.8), are the major source of biopotentials, but other sources include muscle and cardiac cells. When a neuron is at rest, the cell membrane is differentially permeable to positively charged potassium, K^+, and negatively charged chlorine, Cl^-, ions compared to positively charged sodium, Na^+. The Na^+ and Cl^- ions are more concentrated outside the cell whereas K^+ ions are more concentrated inside the cell. In addition, neurons contain concentrations of negatively charged protein molecules too large to pass through the cell membrane. This concentration of protein molecules inside the cell is normally too high to be balanced by the resting distribution of the K^+, Na^+, and Cl^- ions. As a result, when a neuron is at rest, the potential inside the cell is more negative, about -70 mV, than the potential outside the cell.

Neurons receive electrical signals from sensory receptors or other neurons

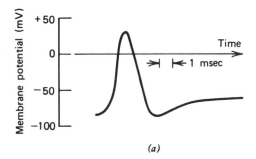

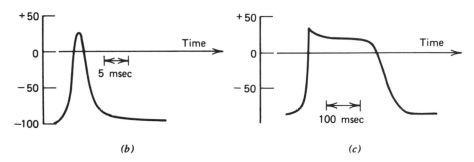

Figure 4.9. Waveform of action potentials from (a) nerve axon, (b) skeletal muscle cell, and (c) cardiac muscle cell. Note different time scales. (Reprinted with permission from J. R. Cameron & J. G. Skofronick, *Medical Physics*, © John Wiley & Sons, Inc., New York, 1978.)

through contacts called *synapses* located on the *dendrites* or the *cell body* (see Figure 4.8). When a neuron is sufficiently stimulated, the cell membrane rapidly increases in permeability to Na^+ ions, permitting the temporary influx of Na^+ ions followed by an efflux of K^+. This migration of charges produces a temporary increase in the potential inside versus outside the neuron, termed *depolarization*, and a subsequent return to the resting potential due to a compensatory *repolarization*, which are together measured as an *action potential*. Action potentials are then transmitted along a fiber called an *axon* to muscles, glands, or other neurons. The amplitude of a single action potential is less than 100 mV, and the duration ranges from a few milliseconds in the case of nerve axon to 150–300 ms for cardiac muscle cells (Figure 4.9). Immediately after an action potential, a neuron is initially incapable of carrying another action potential and hence is temporarily less excitable, for a period 1 to 3 times the duration of the action potential. The duration of this *"refractory time"* appears to vary randomly and permits some, but not all, Na^+ ions to be pumped out of the cell and be replaced by K^+ ions.

Figure 4.10 is a schematic representation of the transmission of a wave of depolarization along an axon and the corresponding potential observed at point *P* on the axon as a function of time. The velocity of conduction of action potentials varies as a function of the axon diameter, the presence or absence of myelin, and the type of cell. First, as with any conductor, the internal resistance of an axon decreases with increases in diameter, and large-diameter axons tend to conduct action

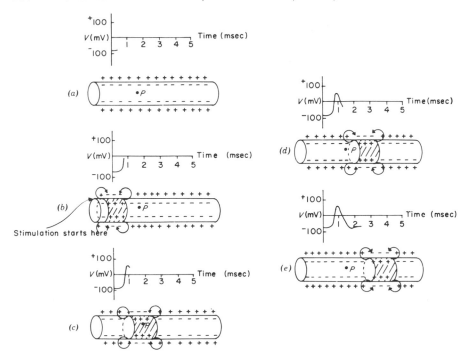

Figure 4.10. Transmission of nerve impulse along axon. Graphs show potential at point *P*. (*a*) axon has resting potential of about −80 mV. (*b*) Stimulation on left cause Na^+ ions to move into cell and depolarize membrane. (*c*) Positive current flow on leading edge, indicated by arrows, stimulates regions to right so that depolarization takes place and potential change propagates (*d, e*). Meanwhile K^+ ions move out of core of axon and restore resting potential (repolarize membrane). Voltage pulse moving along nerve is action potential. (Reprinted with permission from J. R. Cameron & J. G. Skofronik, *Medical Physics,* © John Wiley & Sons, Inc., New York, 1978.)

potentials faster than small-diameter axons. In addition, the membranes of some nerve axons are covered with a fatty insulating layer (*myelin*) that has small uninsulated gaps (*nodes of Ranvier*) every few millimeters (see Figure 4.8). The insulating properties of myelin reduce the capacitive charge stored on the axon membrane. Lower stored charge means faster depolarization, since fewer ions must be moved, and results in correspondingly faster conduction velocities. Action potentials traveling along myelinated fibers appear to jump from one node to the next due to faster conduction velocities between nodes, where myelin is present, compared to within nodes, where no myelin is present. Myelinated human nerve fibers exhibit propagation rates of around 100 m/s, compared to velocities of 0.3 m/s in unmyelinated axons (Curtis, Jacobson, & Marcus, 1972). Much slower transmission rates, in the range of 30–45 cm/s, have been observed in human cardiac tissue where transmission delays on the order of 100 ms may be implicated in the synchronization of the action of the upper and lower chambers.

The occurrence of an action potential is an all-or-none event, but subthreshold levels of stimulation can affect the threshold for elicitation of an action potential in a given cell by altering the cell's resting potential. The changes in the resting potential of cell bodies and dendrites, called *synaptic potentials*, can be graded rather than all or none. An *excitatory postsynaptic potential* (EPSP) lowers the threshold for an action potential by raising the resting potential, and an *inhibitory postsynaptic potential* (IPSP) raises the threshold by lowering the resting potential. Almost all interactions among neurons in the mammalian nervous system occur at synapses, and the EPSP and IPSP are the major kinds of synaptic processes demonstrated in mammals (Thompson, 1975). Another type of synaptic interaction known to occur in the mammalian brain, *presynaptic excitation* and *inhibition*, alters synaptic transmission by modulating the axonal output before it reaches its target cell body or dendrite. Specifically, a modulating axon terminal ends on another axon terminal instead of on a cell body or dendrite and either excites or inhibits the effect of the axonal output of the target cell.

The bioelectrical potentials studied by psychophysiologists are typically not single action potentials like those shown in Figure 4.9. One reason for this is that isolation of single nerve and muscle cells is difficult and invasive. A second and more important reason is that the electrical activity of a single cell may not be representative of the activity of a system of interacting cells. Psychophysiologists interested in monitoring the activity of a physiological system (e.g., central nervous system, skeletomuscular system) often measure the combined electrical activity of groups of cells located at varying distances from the site of interest. As a result, biopotential signals have waveforms much more complex than the sine waves shown in Figure 4.2. These complex waveforms can be decomposed into a set of sine waves of various amplitudes and frequencies. A Fourier series is a weighted sum of sine waves varying in frequency, amplitude, and phase that characterizes a complex waveform (see Dorfman & Cacioppo, chapter 20; Gottman, chapter 22; Porges & Bohrer, chapter 21).

The amplitude and frequency ranges for several biopotentials of interest to the psychophysiologist are shown in Figure 4.11. Note that the amplitude and frequency axes are scaled logarithmically, but the corresponding physical units of millivolts and hertz are also provided. Many of the biopotentials included in Figure 4.11 are described at length in other chapters of this volume. However, a brief description of each source of biopotentials is also provided here.

Electroencephalography (EEG) is the measurement of low-level aggregate electrical activity of the brain, most often detected using sensors placed at specific scalp locations. At present it is widely accepted that the EEG biopotential includes changes in presynaptic and postsynaptic potentials rather than primarily action potentials (Elul, 1972; Li & Jasper, 1953). Typical human EEG signals range in amplitude from 1 to 100 μV and range in frequency from 0.005 to 100 Hz. Note that this is at least 10^6 times smaller than the voltage in a 60-Hz laboratory AC power line. More detailed information on the origin and characteristics of the EEG can be found in Cooper, Osselton, and Shaw (1980) and Ray (chapter 12).

Electromyography (EMG) is the measurement of the electrical activity of a muscle or muscle fiber that is related to muscle contraction. Electromyography can be detected with sensors placed on the skin over a muscle site or from needle or fine-wire electrodes inserted directly into the muscle. The aggregate EMG signal ranges in frequency from 1 to 2000 Hz. Signal amplitudes for the EMG are higher than that for EEG, ranging from fractions of 1 μV to over 2 mV. With surface electrodes the median frequency is approximately 30–140 Hz, a frequency range that spans the 60 Hz frequency for laboratory AC power lines, but as is true of the EEG, at a much lower voltage. More detailed information on specific recording

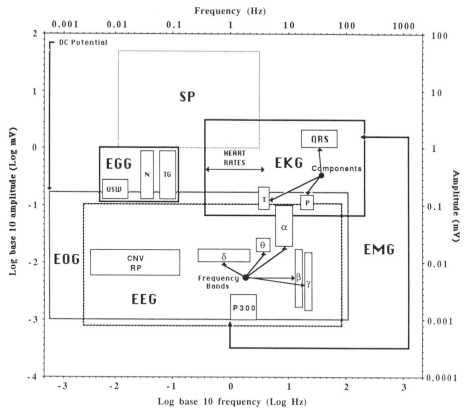

Figure 4.11. Schematized quantitative representation of frequency–amplitude characteristics of major biopotential signals recorded directly from skin surface in humans. Both axes are logarithmically scaled (base 10) and upper and right-hand scales are expressed in corresponding original physical units of hertz and millivolts, respectively. Abbreviations: SP, skin potential; EGG, electrogastrogram; USW, ultraslow wave; N, normal; TG, tachygastria; EKG, electrocardiogram; EEG, electroencephalogram; CNV, contingent negative variation; RP, readiness potential; ERP, event-related potential; EMG electromyogram.

techniques and quantification procedures can be found in Basmajian and Deluca (1985), Cacioppo, Tassinary, and Fridlund (chapter 11), and Loeb and Gans (1986).

Electrocardiography (EKG) is measurement of the electrical activity of the beating heart. The changing electrical potential resulting from propagation of an action potential along the wall of the heart is conducted through the torso and can be detected at the skin surface. The distribution of electrical potential over the entire heart approximates that of an *electric dipole* in which equal positive and negative charges are separated from each other. The instantaneous amplitude and orientation of the heart's dipole potential can be measured as it projects along any axis of the heart. When measured at the skin surface, the heart wave potential is less than 5 mV in amplitude and ranges from 35 to 200 beats per minute. See Papillo and Shapiro (chapter 14) for more information on recording and quantifying cardiac activity.

Electrooculography (EOG) is measurement of the dipole potential of the eye. The EOG can provide an index of eye movements in both the horizontal and vertical planes. The electropotential of the cornea is positive with respect to the retina, and movement of the eye changes the orientation of the eye's dipole field. As is the case with the heart dipole potential, these changes can be detected at the skin surface. The frequency component of EOG signals may be quite slow, at times approximating a DC signal. Amplitudes are generally lower than that of the heart wave potential, in the microvolt to millivolt range. See Oster and Stern (1980), Stern and Dunham (chapter 15), and Young and Sheena (1975) for further information on recording and quantifying the EOG.

Other methods for assessing biopotentials in psychophysiology include *electrogastrography* (EGG), measurement of the electrical activity accompanying gastric contractility (see Stern, Koch, & Vasey, chapter 16), and *skin potential* (SP), measurement of biopotential differences between electrodermally active sites such as the fingers, palm of hand, or sole of foot and an inactive site (see Dawson, Schell, & Filion, chapter 10).

4.6   INSTRUMENTATION FOR PSYCHOPHYSIOLOGICAL DATA COLLECTION

Before beginning any discussion of instrumentation for the psychophysiology laboratory, it is important to make some general suggestions regarding electrical safety. Two primary concerns in the design of a psychophysiological data collection system are the safety of the subject and the integrity of the data. Fortunately many of the procedures essential for the subject's safety from electrical hazard also help reduce the level of electrical noise (unwanted components in the recorded signal). As mentioned earlier, it is the level of current flow through the body that determines the amount of damage to an organism caused by electricity. Recall that with a regulated voltage source the level of current flow is governed by the resistance of the attached load.

Alternating current sources and AC-powered equipment pose a particular risk because they provide a high-current source. Two procedures are routinely used to protect subjects from dangerous currents, isolation and grounding. Within the psychophysiology laboratory the subject should be physically isolated from all AC sources and, whenever possible, all AC-powered equipment. Many commercial laboratory instruments use optically or magnetically coupled power supplies that transfer power to the instrument without a direct current path to the AC power source to help isolate the operator from hazardous currents. The use of low-current, battery-operated lighting is both safer for the subject and less electrically noisy than using nearby AC-powered lamps. When overhead AC-powered lighting is desirable, grounded wire mesh shields can be placed around the lights to minimize the spread of electrical noise.

Since it is not always possible to completely isolate a subject from high-current sources, it is essential that the subject and all high-current equipment close to the subject or attached to the data collection system be properly grounded. A single ground lead is attached to the subject, and all electrode connections are protected from any current flow above 10 μA by a current-limiting device that automatically interrupts the connection between the subject and the recording system when higher currents are detected or that simply does not conduct higher currents. Only triple conductor power extension cords should be used, and all AC-powered

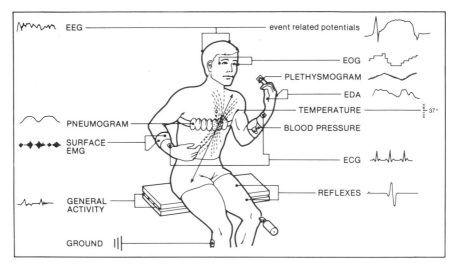

Figure 4.12. Commonly used measures in psychophysiological research. (Adapted with permission from J. Pillard, *Psychophysiologie du comportement*, Vol. 3, © Presses Universitaires de France, 1966, and reprinted in C. H. M. Brunia, *Activation*. In J. A. Michon, Eg G. J. Eijkman, & Len F. W. Klkerk (Eds.), *Handbook of psychonomics*, Vol. 1, © Amsterdam, North-Holland, 1979.)

equipment with a three-prong AC plug must be properly attached to the building power ground rather than attached to ungrounded two-prong adaptors. For additional information on electrical safety precautions, see Spooner (1980).

4.6.1   *Detection of physiological signals*

The psychophysiologist categorizes physiological signals according to the physiological system of origin. A representative sample of response systems monitored by psychophysiologists along with sample tracings of the amplitude by time recordings is provided in Figure 4.12. The systems illustrated include, for example, the nervous system, the skeletomuscular system, the cardiovascular system, the respiratory system, the gastrointestinal system, and the endocrine system. The nervous system is often further subdivided into central and peripheral, autonomic and somatic, sympathetic and parasypathetic (see Matsumoto, Walker, Walker, & Hughes, chapter 3). However, when discussing instrumentation for the detection of physiological signals, it is more useful to group signals according to electrical and physical properties. By describing physiological signal detection according to the properties of the signal rather than according to the site of origin, it is possible to derive appropriate detection procedures for physiological responses not specifically described here. Three categories of detection procedures are described here: (1) measurement of biopotentials originating in body tissue (e.g., EEG, EMG), (2) measurement of bioelectrical phenomena other than potentials (e.g., skin resistance/conductance), and (3) measurement of physical (nonelectrical) change (e.g., blood pressure or volume, respiration, temperature).

When directly sensing biopotentials such as the EEG and EMG, some form of *electrode* is used to detect potential differences between two body (usually skin or scalp) locations. Detection of physiological signals other than potential (e.g, skin conductance, blood pressure) requires a *transducer* to convert the form of energy produced by the body to an electropotential analog of the desired signal. This is because most electronic recording and storage equipment respond only to voltage changes. The transduction of bioelectrical phenomena other than potential, such as measurements of electrical properties of the skin (resistance, conductance, impedance, etc.) and changes in impedance that accompany respiration (*impedance pneumography*), peripheral blood volume (*impedance plethysmography*), cardiac stroke volume (*impedance cardiography*), and brain blood volume (*impedance rheoencephalography*) is based on Ohm's Law relating resistance and impedance to voltage. Specialized transduction systems have been developed for nonelectrical phenomena such as blood pressure, blood flow, respiration rate or flow, cardiac sounds (*phonocardiography*), volume or girth plethysmography, tissue temperature, gastric motility, and body and limb movement.

The selection of specific *biosensors*, whether electrodes or transducers, should be guided by the desired application including not only the frequency and amplitude characteristics of the physiological signals of interest, but also such factors as the placement site on the body, the duration of the recording session, and the amount of subject movement required during recording. Six important design parameters of all dynamic sensors are (1) sample loading, (2) output impedance, (3) damping, (4) frequency response, (5) linearity, and (6) noise (DeMarre & Michaels, 1983). All six parameters are interrelated, and most sensor systems fall short of the ideal on one or more of them. Each is discussed here in turn.

Sample loading, the effect of the sensor on the system it is measuring, should be minimized to avoid distortion of the process of interest. For example, electrodes for detection of facial muscle movements need to be small and lightweight so that they do not restrict or inhibit movement.

The *output impedance* of a sensor is the combined DC and AC resistances measured between the two output leads of the sensor. For electrode systems, this includes the impedance of the body tissue between the two electrodes. In most electronic applications it is desirable to match the output impedance of each component in the system to the input impedance of the next component in the circuit for maximum power transfer. However, with sensors attached to living organisms, matching the output impedance of the sensors with the input impedance of the signal amplifier maximizes the level of current allowed to pass between the subject and the amplifier. To prevent damaging current flow between the subject and the amplifier, it is recommended that electrode output impedances be at least 10^6 times less than the input impedance of the amplifier. Because the resistance of the skin imposes a lower limit on output impedance for surface electrodes of $10^2–10^4\Omega$, bioelectrical amplifiers are generally designed with input impedances on the order of $10^{10}\Omega$ (range $10^7–10^{12}\Omega$). Electrode output impedance also acts as a barrier to the transmission of biopotentials, so further reduction in electrode output impedance is desirable to increase sensitivity to the physiological signal. When reduction of electrode output impedance is not possible, as is sometimes the case with subdermal microelectrodes, high-impedance couplers can be placed between the electrode and the amplifier to prevent excess electrode currents and minimize distortion of low-frequency signals.

Damping refers to the extent to which a sensor faithfully reproduces the frequency components of the input physiological signal. In transducers of physical movement, damping may result from inertia, producing a slowed response to rapid initiation and cessation of movement. A critically damped sensor neither overreacts (the underdamped state) nor underreacts (the overdamped state) to the input signal. The *frequency response* of a sensor is related to the damping and refers to the range of frequencies to which it will respond. The effective bandwidth of frequencies for a sensor should be selected to approximate the frequency range of the event being measured.

The ideal relationship between the amplitude of physiological input to a sensor and the amplitude of the electrical output to the amplifier is a linear one. Although obtaining *linearity* within restricted amplitude and frequency ranges is not typically a problem with bioelectrode systems, it is important that the range of input amplitudes and frequencies over which a transducer provides linear output be matched to the range of physiological input amplitudes and frequencies.

The last design parameter, that of *noise*, refers to the extent to which a sensor either produces or conducts undesired signals. Noise is any unwanted signal and may arise from the sensor itself, from physiological sources such as limb movement, and from ambient electrical noise generated by the proximity of necessary AC-powered equipment such as lighting, video display monitors, and so on. Ambient electrical noise may be impossible to eliminate, but it can be attenuated using grounded shielding on all power sources to reduce magnetic flux, and pickup of ambient noise can be reduced using grounded shields on all signal cables. In addition, the use of twisted pairs of sensor leads that are then exposed to the same ambient electrical noise can be applied to differential amplifiers, described later, which magnify the difference between the two signals, attenuating the noise component common to both leads.

4.6.1.1   *Electrode systems*

Biopotential electrodes may be separated into three categories based on their physical construction: (1) microelectrodes, (2) needle or fine-wire electrodes, and (3) skin surface electrodes. Microelectrodes for recording from a single cell have a fine point in the micrometer range and can be constructed from a micropipette and filled with a conductive electrolyte. The use of microelectrodes is most common in physiology, and their use in psychophysiology is quite limited. Stainless steel or platinum needle and fine-wire electrodes are sometimes used for human EEG and EMG recording and are used frequently in animal research. Skin surface electrodes, the most prevalent type in human psychophysiology, pose the least risk to the subject but are the most distant from the signal source(s) and are separated from the source(s) by the skin, which acts as an electrical insulator.

The ideal biopotential electrode is a perfect conductor that provides a stable current path between the source of the desired physiological signal and the laboratory data collection system. The conducting material must be inert to the chemicals on or in the body to prevent polarization, an accumulation of ions on the electrode surface that blocks conduction of the signal due to capacitive reactance as well as reducing the possibility of toxic reactions. For this reason, less chemically active metals such as silver and platinum are preferable over active metals such as zinc and nickel. Although more reactive metals such as copper tend to be electrically consistent over time, *generating* less irrelevant electrical potentials than

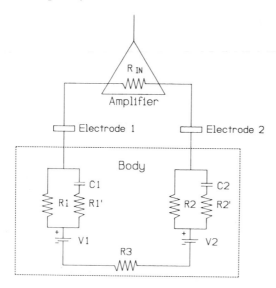

Figure 4.13. Equivalent circuit for pair of surface electrodes. (Adapted with permission from J. J. Carr & J. M. Brown, *Introduction to biomedical equipment technology*, © John Wiley & Sons, Inc., New York, 1981.)

the less reactive metals, their use is limited to very short term exposures (DeMarre & Michaels, 1983). Silver–silver chloride (Ag–AgCl) surface electrodes are highly recommended because they provide good current transfer with minimum polarization. Typical silver–silver chloride electrodes consist of circular disks of silver electroplated with silver chloride or of cylindrical blocks of sintered particles of silver and silver chloride.[5]

When using surface electrodes to measure low-level biopotentials (EEG, EMG), it is important to reduce the natural insulating properties of the skin by thoroughly cleansing it with alcohol to remove any dirt or oils and lightly abrading to remove the surface layer of dead skin cells. In addition, an electrolyte paste or gel is used between the skin and the surface of the electrode to improve the conductive path from underlying tissues to the external electrode and to maintain a stable electrode interface. Some of the electrolyte penetrates the skin at the electrode site, and the remaining electrolyte forms a conductive bridge between the electrode surface and the skin surface that is not easily disrupted by bodily movements. When measuring higher amplitude biopotentials (EKG), abrading the skin is not necessary.

The equivalent circuit for a pair of biopotential electrodes is shown in Figure 4.13. The biopotential electrode surface and the skin surface form a chemical half-cell (battery) between the metal in the electrode and the electrolytic fluid beneath the electrode, capable of developing an electrical potential at each electrode. The electrode offset potential observed at the amplifier is the difference between V_1 and V_2. The amplitude and stability of this electrode potential depends mainly on the metallic content of the electrode. The electrode potential in series with the biopotential being measured adds DC offset to the biopotential signal. Large and variable DC offset potentials can mask the characteristics of the biopotential and may need to be removed from the signal at the time of signal conditioning. When

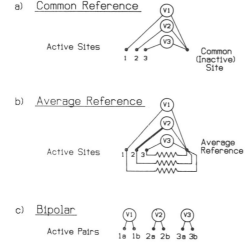

Figure 4.14. Common reference (*a*), average reference (*b*), and bipolar (*c*) placement patterns for electrodes.

the electrodes are identical and differential amplifiers are used, electrode offset potential does not pose a problem to detection of physiological signals. In addition to the signal distortion produced by electrode potentials, the insulating properties of the skin that are not fully overcome by cleaning and abrading at each electrode site add resistances R_1 and R_2 in series with the electrodes that attenuate the level of the output signal. The body fluids and tissue under the skin between the two electrodes adds an additional resistance, R_3. Finally, a double layer of ionic charges may develop at the electrode interface, producing an effective capacitance, C_1 and C_2, and a corresponding capacitive reactance, R'_1 and R'_2. Capacitive reactance is also called the polarization impedance. Recall that capacitors appear as open circuits to DC signals, and current flow increases directly with increases in signal frequency. Thus, fast AC-like biopotentials produce greater current flow across the electrode interface than slower DC-like signals. What is not clear from Figure 4.13 is that the resistances and capacitances are not stable either between subjects or within a single subject across time. However, since the electrical parameter of interest is voltage and not current, it is neither necessary nor desirable to maintain high current flow at the interface between the electrode and the skin. Amplifiers with high input impedance, R_{IN}, minimize the current flow between the electrode and thus attenuate the variable effects of electrode polarization.

Three types of placement patterns are used with biopotential electrodes: common reference, average reference, and bipolar (Cooper, Osselton, & Shaw, 1980). All three techniques compare the potential between a set of electrodes. With common reference placements, one electrode is placed over an electrically active site, and the other is placed over an electrically inactive site (see Figure 4.14, panel *a*). The output of common reference electrodes yields information about the absolute level of electrical activity at the active site. For example, in EEG recording, each individual active scalp placement may be compared to one electrode placed at a relatively inactive site such as the mastoid area.

With average reference placements, the activity at each electrically active site is compared to the average of the activity at all electrode sites used. The average reference signal is generated by connecting each active signal electrode through equal resistors to a single point (see Figure 4.14, panel *b*). If the potentials at the active sites are unrelated, the average reference potential tends toward zero as the number of active electrode sites increases. However, widespread synchronous activity that affects many active sites or large-amplitude artifacts at a single site will raise the amplitude of the reference potential. The output of average referenced electrodes yields information about the level of electrical activity unique to each active site relative to the level of overall activity.

With bipolar placements, the two electrodes are placed close together over an active site (see Figure 4.14, panel *c*). This placement pattern is particularly sensitive to localized changes in electrical activity. Bipolar placements are common in EMG recording, with the two electrodes positioned parallel to the muscle fibers close to the middle of the muscle. When a series of electrodes is placed in a straight line across an electrically active site, montages formed from the potential between adjacent pairs of electrodes yield information about the gradient of the electrical potential across the active site. In EKG recording, a variety of bipolar placements are possible, ranging from a simple two-electrode arrangement using sites on the right arm and the left leg or the right collarbone and left lower rib when only heart rate is required, to more complex three- and five-electrode arrangements when time and amplitude components of the complete cardiac waveform are required. Each pair of EKG electrodes spans a different axis of the heart, and in clinical settings the type and site of cardiac disorders can be diagnosed from the resulting pattern of waveform anomalies.

In addition to the detection of biopotentials, electrode systems are used to detect other electrical properties such as resistance and impedance. The electrodes used for detection of skin conductance/resistance and for low-frequency (less than 5 Hz) skin impedance changes require the same characteristics as biopotential electrodes. That is, they should be electrochemically stable and nonpolarizable. The measurement of DC resistance (and its reciprocal, conductance) and/or impedance (and its reciprocal, admittance) at the skin's surface requires the application of known signals between two surface sites. Most often a constant (low) voltage is applied and changes in current are monitored, but the reverse is also possible. However, for impedance measurements using high-frequency AC signals (greater than 10 kHz), such as impedance pneumography, plethysmography, cardiography, and rheoencephalography, the speed at which the direction of current flow changes eliminates the polarization problem. Both copper and aluminum electrodes can be used for impedance plethysmography. Though nonpolarizable electrodes are not necessary with high-frequency measurements, they can be used as well.

The detection of skin conductance/resistance is described in detail elsewhere (see Dawson, Schell, & Filion, chapter 10), but the general procedure is described briefly here to illustrate the application of electrical principles to detection of bioelectrical responses other than potentials. It is generally agreed that electrodermal activity is related to eccrine sweat gland activity, and it is affected by the level of hydration of the skin (Fowles, 1986; Venables & Christie, 1973). Since hydration of the skin is the peripheral physical parameter of interest, a special-purpose electrolyte is used that closely approximates the ionic concentrations in the body fluids and thus does not hydrate the skin (Fowles et al., 1981; Schneider & Fowles, 1978). The electrode site is cleansed with soap and water to remove surface dirt and oil, but procedures that might alter the inherent conductive/resistive properties of the skin are avoided. Specifically, cleansing with alcohol, which causes drying, and abrading the skin, which removes an insulating layer of skin, are not recommended. Two identical electrodes on electrodermally active sites (bipolar) can be used or one electrode at an active site such as the palm can be compared to another electrode at an inactive site such as the earlobe (common reference). Either a constant current (e.g., 8 $\mu A/cm^2$) or a constant voltage (e.g., 0.5 V) is applied across the two electrodes, and a type of bridge circuit is used to quantify changes in resistance or conductance.

Two additional electrode systems for bioelectrical responses also merit discussion here: impedance pneumography and impedance plethysmography. In impedance pneumography, a low-voltage 50–500 kHz AC signal is applied to the subject via a pair of surface electrodes on the chest (Carr & Brown, 1981). Large fixed resistors are connected in series with each electrode, creating a constant-current source. The voltage drop across these fixed resistors represents the thoracic impedance. Without respiration the current through the subject's chest is nearly constant, but it changes with respiration. The impedance pneumograph is a reliable and valid indicator of respiration rate and relative amplitude; however, absolute measures of respiration amplitude are possible over only a limited portion of the range of observed tidal volumes (see Lorig & Schwartz, chapter 17).

In impedance plethysmography, changes in the instantaneous blood volume of the whole body or selected limbs are inferred from changes in impedance between pairs of surface electrodes. Impedance cardiography is a special case of plethysmography for cardiac stroke volume. Impedance rheoencephalography is a special case of plethysmography for cranial (forehead or mastoid) sites. Detection of whole-body and single-limb blood volume changes typically use pairs of band electrodes that encircle the site of interest such as the neck or the abdomen and thorax. With whole-body and limb measurements, a typical applied current is a 100-kHz, 6-mA signal (DeMarre & Michaels, 1983). Circular disk electrodes are common for cranial sites, with applied currents of 1–10 mA at 30–70 kHz (Geddes & Baker, 1975). Although absolute blood volume measurements are possible, percentage or ratio change measurements are more common in psychophysiological research.

4.6.1.2   Transducer systems

Geddes and Baker (1975, p. 3) describe a transducer as a "sense organ for the electronic processing equipment." The meaning conveyed by this statement is that organisms as well as laboratory equipment only process information of a specific type, and both require peripheral preprocessors to convert incoming signals from various physical forms to an interpretable signal. The range of nonelectrical physiological changes of interest to the psychophysiologist include but are not restricted to blood pressure and flow, respiration rate and flow, skin or core temperature, and body or limb movements.

Transducers are by necessity specialized for detection of distinct types of physical change, so that some are useful for measurement of variation in pressure whereas others are sensitive to changes in temperature or mechanical displacement. In addition, any electrical parameter (most often resistance) may be made to vary as a function of the signal of interest. As is the case with measurement of any resistive properties (e.g., resistance/conductance, impedance), most transducers require some type of bridge circuit such as the Wheatstone bridge described earlier for accuracy at low levels and often require a coupler capable of offsetting changes in DC potential. In addition, in order for the absolute amplitude of the transducer output to be meaningful, it must be calibrated to some physical or physiological standard.

Two general guidelines for transducer selection are offered (Seippel, 1983). First, when measuring effort or potential variables like pressure, force, or voltage, select a transducer that greatly impedes motion or flow. For example, a simple transducer system for momentary blood pressure (cuff ascultation) uses an inflatable cuff to temporarily occlude arterial blood pressure. The pressure in the cuff can be adjusted until it matches the pulsatile systolic blood pressure indicated by disappearance of the pulse sound and then reduced until it matches the arterial pressure indicated by Korotkoff sounds. Likewise, voltmeters and oscilloscopes, both voltage-sensitive devices, are designed with high input impedance to minimize the level of current diverted from the circuit of interest. More generally, when measuring voltage, it is important to minimize the current through the measurement device. Second, when measuring motion or flow, select a transducer that readily allows motion. Thus, for example, proper use of the chest strain gauge for detection of respiration rate requires that the chest band not restrict movement. The nasal thermistor method for respiration detection is another example of a low-resistance transducer.

A wide variety of resistive transducers are available. The simplest ones use linear or rotary *potentiometers*, variable resistors that change resistance with mechanical movement or rotation. Volume controls and dimmer switches are common types of potentiometers. In psychophysiology rotary potentiometers have been used to quantify movements such as eyeblinks (e.g., Braff et al., 1978). For measurement of very small movements, resistive changes due to physical distortion of the metal within a *strain gauge* can be used. For example, one method for transduction of respiration uses a mercury strain gauge attached to a chest band. The band is adjusted so that movement of the chest cavity associated with respiration produces corresponding changes in the length of a flexible tube filled with mercury. The resistance of the mercury increases as the tube lengthens and reduces the cross-sectional area. Because the resistivity of metals exhibits a considerable degree of temperature dependence, metallic *resistance thermometers* and metal–metal oxide *thermistors* are also effective transducers for core and skin temperature. These devices change in resistance as a function of changes in temperature. For example, nasal thermistors can be used to detect respiration rate based on the cyclic cooling and heating that results from the movement of air during nasal breathing (see Lorig & Schwartz, chapter 17).

Three additional types of transducers deserve mention here because of their uses in psychophysiological research: photoelectric, magnetic, and ultrasonic transducers. Each of the three transducer types employ an energy source or transmitter, an energy receiver, and a medium through which the energy must travel. In psychophysiological applications the medium is the body. For example, a light source and a photoconductive cell placed on opposite sides of a finger or an earlobe can transduce changes in blood volume as the reciprocal of light energy reaching the receiver. Likewise, magnetic and ultrasonic sources and receivers can be used to transduce changes such as blood volume in larger body regions not penetrable by light, such as the brain.

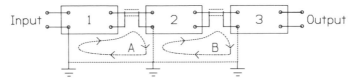

Figure 4.15.Ground-loop circuits resulting from use of multiple grounds in multiple-stage signal-processing system.

4.6.2   *Bioelectrical amplifiers and signal conditioners*

Following the detection of the physiological signal of interest, it is necessary to selectively magnify and shape the electrical signal to permit display, quantification, and storage. A variety of *signal processors* are used in psychophysiological research that perform mathematical transformations on the detected signal. Signal processors are attached in parallel with the two signal leads of the electrode or transducer and typically provide a single-ended (zero-referenced) output of the transformed signal. In the event that multiple stages of signal processing are required, as is often the case in psychophysiological research, all grounded components of a given stage should be returned to a single ground point, preferrably at the initial input stage. If multiple grounds are used, so-called *ground loops*, or current paths through the metal chassis, are formed (Figure 4.15). Large ground loop currents introduce *cross-talk* (undesired signal coupling between stages) that can mask the desired signal.

One essential signal processor for physiological signals of psychological interest is an *amplifier* that increases the amplitude (voltage) of the signal. Other special-purpose signal processors include *filters* that selectively pass or prevent passage of certain frequencies of the input signal, *integrators* that average input amplitudes over a selected time period, and *amplitude-sensitive rate devices* that are triggered when the input signal exceeds a preset threshold. The characteristics and applications for these four signal processors are described in turn.

The low voltage levels for all biopotentials makes amplification the first and most crucial of all signal processing. In addition to the initial or *preamplification* stage, other amplifiers and signal conditioners may be chained in parallel with the input to further magnify and shape the signal. The critical design parameters for pre-amplifiers (and to some extent, all signal processors) are (1) input impedance, (2) output impedance, (3) gain, (4) common-mode rejection ratio, (5) bandwidth, (6) power distribution, (7) distortion, and (8) noise (DeMarre & Michaels, 1983).

The need for amplifiers with extremely high (10–50 MΩ) *input impedance* was pointed out in the earlier section on detection methods. This is because the electrical parameter of interest is voltage, not current. To maximize sensitivity to changes in voltage, current flow through the measurement instrumentation must be minimized. Minimizing current levels also poses less risk to the subject, since it is current, not voltage, that can damage tissue. Amplifier *output impedance* should be selected to produce an output signal that is an exact amplified replica of the input signal of interest while remaining 10 times less than the input impedance of the next stage of signal processing or recording. Note that successive stages of signal amplification and other processing are chained together in parallel, and each stage is designed to be sensitive to changes in voltage. Thus, the output impedance of each signal processor in the chain is maintained at a level lower than that of the

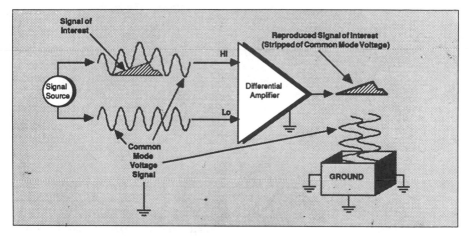

Figure 4.16. Differential amplifier used to reject voltage signal common to two electrode sites. (Reprinted with permission from *Codas analog to digital converter selector guide: application note 4,* © Dataq Instruments, Inc.)

following stage for the same reasons input impedance is maintained at a higher level than the preceding stage, to produce a maximum sensitivity to changes in voltage rather than changes in current. If one stage in the signal-processing sequence is a device with a naturally low input impedance, an additional stage of amplification with high input impedance and low output impedance, called buffering, is used to adjust impedances.

The *gain* of a signal processor is the ratio of signal input to signal output for voltage, current, or power and can be (1) fractional, indicating a reduction in the signal level; (2) 1, indicating no change in the signal level; or (3) greater than 1, indicating an increase in signal level. Fractional gains are also called negative gains. Bioelectrical amplifiers typically have positive voltage gain, negative current gain, and negative power gain. In practice, several positive voltage gains may be switch selectable. Gain factors are typically categorized as low $(10^0–10^1)$, medium $(10^1–10^3)$, and high $(10^3–10^6)$.

Differential amplifiers are signal-processing devices that selectively magnify the potential difference between two inputs and are extremely useful when the signal amplitude is small relative to the ambient electrical noise. The quality of differential amplifiers is rated by the extent to which they reject or attenuate signals common to both inputs. The effect of differential amplification is illustrated in Figure 4.16. It is not possible for a differential amplifier to completely eliminate common inputs, and the *common-mode rejection ratio* (CMRR), computed as the output amplitude divided by the common input amplitude, is a dimensionless index of the level of attenuation achieved. For measurement of EEG, EMG, and EKG, common-mode rejection ratios of 90–130 dB are recommended.

Amplifiers can effectively process only a limited range of input frequencies. *Bandwidth* and *power distribution* together quantify the frequency response of an amplifier. The bandwidth is the effective range of input frequencies the amplifier is capable of boosting, and the power distribution is a function of the gain at each frequency in the bandwidth. The gain rating provided for an amplifier is the amount of amplification for most input frequencies in the middle of the bandwidth. Because amplifier gain drops off gradually rather than completely at frequencies above and below those frequencies for which the amplifier is maximally responsive, specification of an amplifier bandwidth requires selection of a criterion for the minimum-gain acceptable percentage of the rated (peak) gain. Two common criteria for amplifier bandwidth specification are ±3 and ±6 dB, which include those frequencies where the gain is no less than 70.7 and 50 percent of the rated (peak) gain respectively. Bandwidths of 0.01 Hz–20 kHz are common for bioelectrical amplifiers.

Bioelectrical amplifiers are either DC and AC coupled. Thus, for purposes of signal amplification and processing it is useful to divide bioelectrical signals into two general categories, fast-wave signals and slow-wave signals. Some of the biopotentials shown in Figures 4.11 and 4.12 such as EOG and EEG can include both fast-wave and slow-wave components, and separate but parallel DC-coupled and AC-coupled amplification and processing may be required to detect both signal components from a single set of electrodes. When the input signal to the amplifier remains constant for long periods of time or changes very slowly, as with EGG and electrodermal activity, some form of DC coupling is required. When the input signal changes at frequencies of 0.05 Hz or higher, AC coupling is recommended to eliminate DC offset potentials at the sensors. Fast-wave signals include EMG and EKG.

Regardless of the techniques used, all signal processing introduces some *distortion*. However, the most noticeable distortions of a processed signal occur at the sensor and at the display rather than at the amplifier. If the amplifier is distorting the signal more than 1 percent, it is often traceable to improper impedance matching between two of the stages of amplification. With commercial modular signal-processing equipment using integrated circuitry, amplifier-induced distortion is not a problem. What is a problem is amplification of ambient electrical noise detected at the sensor or induced through unshielded leads. Precautions such as removal of unnecessary AC equipment near the subject, shielding of necessary equipment, use of grounded shields on signal lines from the sensor to the preamplifier, and differential amplification will help, but some signal conditioning to remove noise may also be necessary.

Electronic *filters* are used to selectively attenuate unwanted frequency components of signals. Filters are characterized by the frequency range they pass or reject. Thus, *high-pass filters* selectively attenuate frequencies below a selected cutoff frequency, and *low-pass filters* selectively attenuate frequencies above a selected cutoff frequency. With EEG recording it is often useful to use a low-pass filter cutoff of 30 Hz to reject high-frequency signals above the physiological range for beta waves. Restricted-range *band pass* and *band reject filters* are also available.

A particularly useful band reject filter known as a *notch filter* selectively attenuates signals in the frequency range of 58–62 Hz, the band surrounding 60-Hz AC noise. However, as was noted earlier in the section on biopotentials, 60-Hz filtering is not always appropriate. A major part of EMG signals is in this frequency range, and 60-Hz filtering of AC ambient noise will also remove 60-Hz frequency components of the EMG signal.

When recording psychophysiological signals that include very high frequency components, such as the EMG, it can be useful to electronically time average the input signal prior to display or storage of the signal. *Integrators* are a special type of low-pass filter that rectify the input (invert the negative components of the signal) and store a cumulative sum of the resulting positive amplitudes for selected periods of time. The storage of these signals decays exponentially with time, and the time taken for the output to decay to approximately 67 percent of the input amplitude is known as the *time constant*. *Amplitude-sensitive rate devices* are also useful for high-frequency signals when the amplitude components of the signal are not required. The output for rate devices is typically a state change (stepwise low to high or high to low voltage) or a brief pulse of fixed duration. The Schmitt trigger is an example of a rate device used for determination of heart rate. The trigger threshold is adjusted so that only the occurrence of the *R*-spike component of the heart wave is detected, and heart rate is either computed from the time between state changes or read directly as the calibrated amplitude of the output signal (see Papillo & Shapiro, chapter 14).

4.6.3   *Display and storage systems*

Once the psychophysiological signal of interest has been detected and amplified, it is necessary to display and store a representation of the data to permit inspection for artifacts, examination of the topographical features, and extraction of dependent variable measures. For some applications such as stimulus-evoked muscle action potentials, the display screen of a storage oscilloscope may be sufficient to permit detection of the presence or absence of component reflexive responses. When a permanent record of the signal is required, a special oscilloscope camera can be used to photograph the display in single frames or as a continuous-motion picture. For many psychophysiological applications in which multiple physiological response systems are monitored for periods of from several seconds to an hour or more, an analog recorder is particularly useful. The two more common analog recording systems used in psychophysiology are graphic recorders and magnetic tape recorders. Other types of storage systems for physiological data include card and tape punches, videotape recording, and transient recorders with digital memory. For more information on these systems, the reader is referred to Goovaerts, Ross, and Schneider (1979).

All graphic recorders include an electromechanically controlled stylus that converts a voltage input to mechanical movement and a paper drive assembly to move the chart paper past the stylus at a constant speed. Graphic recorders differ in the number of signals that can be simultaneously recorded and in the method of transcription (e.g., ink writing, pressure writing, thermal writing, photographic writing, electrostatic writing). Both ink and pressure writing systems severely attenuate high-frequency inputs (over 100 Hz for ink writing systems, over 250 Hz for pressure writing systems). This limitation does not significantly affect recording of slower frequency signals such as EEG or EDA, but does affect recording of the nonintegrated EMG. Ink-jet recorders can accurately reproduce frequencies up to about 1 kHz, and photographic and electrostatic recorders are accurate to about 5 kHz. To overcome this limitation, some graphic recorders now include memory modules that permit brief data sampling followed by data recording at a slower rate, resulting in undistorted reproduction of higher frequencies.

Magnetic tape recording systems continuously store coded patterns on a moving magnetic tape. These patterns can be reproduced later at a different speed, allowing time expansion or compression. The magnetic code cannot be visually inspected during recording, and simultaneous monitoring of the input signal with an oscilloscope or graphic recorder is recommended. Three types of recording techniques are available: direct recording, frequency modulation, and pulse-code modulation.

In *direct recording*, the signal voltage is superimposed on a 70–100 kHz bias signal to increase the magnetizing force of the signal. The recording head converts the electrical input to a varying magnetic flux that changes the residual magnetism on the tape as it moves past the recording head. The frequency response of direct recording is poor for frequencies less than 100 Hz, and thus direct recording is not appropriate for most psychophysiological signals. With *frequency modulation* (FM) recording, the input signal is used to modulate the frequency of a carrier signal before storage. The bandwidth for FM recording is proportional to the tape speed and can range from DC to 108,000 Hz at speeds of 60 revolutions per second. In *pulse-code modulation* (PCM) the input signal is converted to a digital signal representing the momentary signal amplitude. The amplitude resolution of PCM recording with a 12-bit analog-to-digital converter (ADC) provides a better signal-to-noise ratio than FM recording.

4.7   SUMMARY AND CONCLUSIONS

This tutorial on bioelectrical measurement began with the basics of electricity and electrical conduction. It was noted that electrical charge is a fundamental property of all matter that is intrinsically associated with chemical reactivity. The relationship between electrical potential, current, and resistance described by Ohm's Law was elaborated as the basis for explanations of the properties of simple circuits and the use of tools for electrical measurement. The distinctive properties of DC and AC signals were delineated and related to capacitance and inductance. The appropriate uses of the three most common tools for electrical measurement – the multimeter, oscilloscope, and bridge circuit – were described and related to measurement of bioelectrical signals. The sources and the frequency and amplitude ranges for illustrative biopotential signals were surveyed.

Some general guidelines for sensor systems were provided, and the detection of physiological signals was subdivided into electrode systems for biopotentials and impedance and transducer systems for nonelectrical physiological changes. Within electrode systems, the electrical properties of the subject–electrode interface were discussed. Within transducer systems, it was noted that transducers are by necessity specialized for distinct types of physical change, and the role of the bridge circuit in transduction was described. The necessity for signal amplification and conditioning was noted, and the application of three types of special-purpose signal processors (filters, integrators, and amplitude-sensitive rate devices) in psychophysiology was presented. Finally, the prototypic systems for display and storage of voltage signals and their application in psychophysiology were described.

Progress in science is limited by the integrity of scientific observations. Whereas technology provides the tools for scientific observation, it is the responsibility of the observer to apply the tools appropriately. Failure to do so can result in a faulty data base and erroneous inferences. With all the sciences, development and distribution of technical tools will expand the ability of the psychophysiologist to observe, to quantify, and to control (Tassinary, Marshall-Goodell, & Cacioppo, 1985). Because it is difficult to anticipate future advances in technology, the psychophysiologist who learns only to apply existing technology may be at a disadvantage when the inevitable technological advances occur. On the other hand, the psychophysiologist who understands the principles underlying the procedures for bioelectrical measurement will be in a much better position to incorporate and apply new technologies.

NOTES

1 Additional information on the physical and chemical properties of electricity can be obtained from most introductory physics or physical chemistry textbooks. However, for information on the behavior of simple circuits, an electronics textbook such as Brophy (1983) or a self-teaching guide such as Kybett (1986) is recommended.
2 Conceptualizing resistors as impediments can be confusing because of the implicit assumption that the more resistors in the circuit, the less the overall flow. As elaborated in section 4.3, adding resistors in parallel actually increases flow rather than decreases flow (see Gentner & Gentner, 1983, for a useful discussion on the limitations of heuristic models of electricity).
3 Ionic current flow through a cell membrane can be assessed using voltage clamp techniques that apply controlled currents across the membrane while maintaining a constant membrane potential. Under voltage clamp conditions, the current required to maintain the membrane potential must be equal and opposite any membrane current (see Kandel & Schwartz, 1985, for a more detailed description of voltage clamp techniques).
4 See Brazier (1977) for a more detailed description of the sources and properties of bioelectrical activity.
5 When electrodes must be implanted or attached for more than a few days, the chemical stability of platinum makes it the best choice.

REFERENCES

Barber, T. X. (1976). *Pitfalls in human research.* New York: Pergamon.
Basmajian, J., & Deluca, C. J. (1985). *Muscles alive: Their functions revealed by electromyography* (5th ed.). Baltimore: Williams & Wilkins.
Beatty, J., Barth, D. S., Richer, F., & Johnson, K. A. (1986). Neuromagnetometry. In M. G. H. Coles, E. Donchin, & S. W. Porges (Eds.), *Psychophysiology: Systems, and applications* (pp. 26–40). New York: Guilford Press.
Braff, D. L., Stone, C., Callahan, E., Geyer, M., Glick, I., & Bali, L. (1978). Prestimulus effects on human startle reflex in normals and schizophrenics. *Psychophysiology, 15,* 339–343.
Brazier, M. A. B. (1977). *Electrical activity of the nervous system* (4th ed.). Baltimore: Williams & Wilkins.
Brophy J. J. (1983). *Basic electronics for scientists* (4th ed.). New York: McGraw-Hill.
Brown, C. C. (1967). *Methods in psychophysiology.* Baltimore: Williams & Wilkins.
Brown, C. C., & Saucer, R. T. (1958). *Electronic instrumentation for the behavioral sciences.* Springfield, IL: Charles C. Thomas.
Carr, J. J., & Brown J. M. (1981). *Introduction to biomedical equipment technology.* New York: Wiley.
Coles, M. G. H., Donchin, E., & Porges, S. W. (Eds.). (1986). *Psychophysiology: Systems, processes, and applications.* New York: Guilford Press.
Cooper, R., Osselton, J. W., & Shaw, J. C. (1980). *EEG technology* (3rd ed.). London: Butterworths.
Curtis, B. A., Jacobson, S., & Marcus, E. M. (1972). *An introduction to the neurosciences.* Philadelphia: Saunders.
DeMarre, D. A., Kantrowitz, P., Zucker, L., & Simmons, D. (1979). *Applied biomedical electronics for technicians.* New York: Marcel Dekker.
DeMarre, D. A., & Michaels, D. (1983). *Bioelectronic measurements.* Englewood Cliffs, NJ: Prentice-Hall.
Dunseath, W. J. R. (1982). A low-cost precision electrode impedance meter. *Psychophysiology, 19,* 117–119.
Elul, M. R. (1972). The genesis of the EEG. *International Review of Neurobiology, 15,* 227–272.

Erlanger, J., & Glasser, H. S. (1937). *Electrical signs of nervous activity.* Philadelphia: University of Pennsylvania.

Fowles, D. C. (1986). The eccrine system and electrodermal activity. In M. G. H. Coles, E. Donchin, & S. W. Porges (Eds.), *Psychophysiology: Systems, processes, and applications* (pp. 51–96). New York: Guilford Press.

Fowles, D. C., Christie, M. J., Edelberg, R., Grings, W. W., Lykken, D. T., & Venables, P. H. (1981). Committee report: Publication recommendation for electrodermal measurement. *Psychophysiology, 18,* 232–239.

Geddes, L. A., & Baker, L. E. (1975). *Principles of applied biomedical instrumentation* (2nd ed.). New York: Wiley.

Gentner, D., & Gentner, D. R. (1983). Flowing waters or teaming crowds: Mental models of electricity. In D. Gentner & A. L. Stevens (Eds.), *Mental models.* New York: Erlbaum.

Goldman, D. (1950). The clinical use of the "average" reference electrode in monopolar recording. *Electroencephalography and Clinical Neurophysiology 39,* 526.

Goovaerts, H. G., Ross, H. H., & Schneider, H. (1979). Storage systems. In R. S. Reneman and J. Strackie (Eds.), *Data in medicine: Collection, processing, and presentation* (pp. 181–205). The Hague: Martinus, Nijhoff.

Greenfield, N. S., & Sternbach, R. A. (Eds.). (1972). *Handbook of psychophysiology.* New York: Holt, Reinhart and Winston.

Grings, W. W. (1954). *Laboratory, instrumentation in psychology.* Palo Alto, CA: National.

Jonides, J. (1982). Integrating visual information from successive fixations. *Science, 215,* 192–194.

Jonides, J., Irwin, D. E., and Yantis, S. (1983). Failure to integrate information from successive fixations. *Science, 222,* 188.

Kandel, E. R., & Schwartz, J. H. (1985). *Principles of neural science.* New York: Elsevier.

Kybett, H. (1986). *Electronics: A self-teaching guide* (2nd ed.). New York: Wiley.

Lambert, E. H. (1962). Electromyography. In O. Glasser (Ed.). *Medical physics* (Vol. 3). Chicago: Year Book Medical.

Li, C. L., & Jasper, H. H. (1953). Microelectrode studies of the electrical activity of the cerebral cortex in the cat. *Journal of Physiology, 121,* 117.

Loeb, G. E., & Gans, C. (1986). *Electromyography for experimentalists.* Chicago: University of Chicago.

Martin, I., & Venables, P. H. (Eds.). (1980). *Techniques in psychophysiology.* Chichester: Wiley.

Oster, P., & Stern, J. (1980). Measurement of eye movement: Electrooculography. In I. Martin and P. H. Venables (Eds.), *Techniques in psychophysiology.* Chichester: Wiley.

Rostron, J. (1960). *Error and deception in science.* New York: Basic Books.

Schmidt, M. (1963). A star-like object with large red-shift. *Nature, 197,* 1040.

Schneider, R. E., & Fowles, D. C. (1978) A convenient, non-hydrating electrolyte medium for the measurement of electrodermal activity. *Psychophysiology, 15,* 483–486.

Seippel, R. G. (1983). *Transducers, sensors, and detectors.* Reston, VA: Reston.

Sokal, M. M., Davis, A. B., & Merzbach, U. C. (1976). Laboratory instruments in the history of psychology. *Journal of the History of the Behavioral Sciences, 12,* 59–64.

Spooner, R. B. (1980). *Hospital electrical safety simplified.* Research Triangle Park, NC: Instrument Society of America.

Stern, R. M., Ray, W. J., & Davis, C. M. (Eds.). (1980). *Psychophysiological recording.* New York: Oxford University Press.

Tassinary, L. G., Marshall-Goodell, B., & Cacioppo, J. T. (1985). Microcomputers in social psychophysiological research: An overview. *Behavioral Research Methods, Instruments, and Computers, 17,* 532–536.

Thompson, R. F. (1975). *Introduction to physiological psychology.* New York: Harper & Row.

Venables, P. H., & Christie, M. J. (1973). Mechanisms, instrumentation, recording techniques and quantification of responses. In W. F. Prokasy & D. C. Raskin (Eds.), *Electrodermal activity in psychological research.* New York: Academic.

Venables, P. H., & Martin, I. (Eds.). (1967). *A manual of psychophysiological methods.* New York: Wiley.

Wood, R. W. (1904). The n-rays. *Nature, 70,* 530–531.

Young, L., & Sheena, D. (1975). Survey of eye movement recording methods. *Behavior Research Methods and Instruments, 7,* 397–429.

5 *Biochemical measurement*

NEIL E. GRUNBERG AND JEROME E. SINGER

5.1 INTRODUCTION

At the end of the nineteenth century, disciplinary lines did not pose restrictive boundaries to scientists and academicians. James's (1890/1950) *Principles of Psychology* clearly illustrates willingness to draw from philosophy and biological sciences to try to understand behavior. Darwin's (1872/1965) work on emotions provides another striking example of a multidisciplinary approach to psychology as he drew on cross-species facial responses, skeletal muscle wiring, and observational behavioral studies to investigate emotions.

With the proliferation of scientific activity in the first half of this century also came increased specialization. This development followed logically from increased knowledge and the demands of mastering vast amounts of information as well as a large array of technical and procedural skills. Unfortunately, increased specialization narrowed the perspective of many scientific disciplines to a degree that trivialized the questions under examination.

For example, in the late 1950s and early 1960s, conventional learning theory, whether of Hullian, Spencerian, or other variety, had strayed from its original conceptions. Framed as general sets of principles applicable across species to all behaviors, specific studies were instead concerned with minutiae of rats' performance in extraordinarily restricted and controlled environments. Generalizability to problems of larger interest was virtually nonfeasible. In social psychology, very wide-ranging theories of cognitive consistency, foreshadowing the cognitive psychology emphasis of recent years, degenerated to theme and variation, showing or not showing the same effect in often highly contrived situations.

Over the past 20 years psychology has again widened its intellectual and technological domains to address questions and problems of behavior and thought. Developments in psychophysiology, for example, have addressed topics in attention, arousal, emotions, stress, cardiovascular function, and health (cf. Cacioppo & Petty, 1983). Many of these topics are considered or are alluded to in this volume. The value of this approach is clear.

A different multidisciplinary approach is to integrate biochemical measures with behavioral and psychological assessments. This chapter addresses this particular marriage and reviews some ways in which biochemical measures can be effectively used by psychologists.

Many psychologists express a phobia to chemistry that is reminiscent of computer phobias of the 1970s. As a result of this condition, biochemical measures either are avoided or are approached on a contractual basis, conceptually as well as financially. That is, many of those psychologists who do use biochemical measures

149

in their work simply ship the biological samples to an appropriate laboratory for analysis and expect numbers by return mail. Frequently, there is little understanding of what the numbers represent, how they were determined, and whether the study was designed appropriately for the values to be meaningful.

For those psychologists working in human experimentation, especially in social, personality, and developmental psychology, there was another, historically based, avoidance of biological considerations. The often glib and unconvincing reductionism of some of the biologically oriented psychologists of the post–World War II era brushed aside major problems in human psychology and suggested that biological concerns, at least in theory, would make all these "softer" areas of psychology unnecessary. If the social and personality people could only put their problems into stimulus–response terms, it was claimed, the difficulties would disappear. To many of that era, the incorporation of biological considerations represented an acceptance of a reductionist framework, which, by explaining everything, explained little in particular cases.

The purpose of this chapter is to present our views on how biochemical measures should be used in psychological research. We do not expect readers of this chapter to become experts in analytical chemistry but believe they can become adept in incorporating biochemical concepts and assays into their research. As an analogy, many psychologists study computer programming although they do not become programmers. They do, however, learn the strategy of programming and its utility and to productively communicate and collaborate with programmers. We hope that readers will gain an increased understanding of how to use biochemical measurement and will be thoughtful in the use and interpretation of the "soft" numbers of this so-called hard-science discipline.

5.2   USES OF BIOCHEMICAL MEASURES IN PSYCHOLOGICAL RESEARCH

There are three different ways in which biochemistry can be used in psychological research: (1) as a direct measure, (2) as an index of a process, and (3) as a mechanism of action.

5.2.1   *Direct measure*

Biochemical measures can be used as "direct measures" in psychology research to check the functioning of a particular physiological system. For example, in studies of diabetics, insulin and glucose could be measured to determine the status of patients. As another example, patients with a genetic abnormality such as pheochromocytoma (a tumor of the adrenal gland) could be biochemically evaluated in a study of psychology and health in this population to assess adrenal function. Patients who are being screened for starvation–amenorrhea (anorexia nervosa) could have measurements of pituitary hormones (including growth hormone and thyroid-stimulating hormone) to confirm the diagnosis and to determine whether there is pituitary disease (such as Simmonds disease). Female sex hormones (e.g., progesterone and estrogen) can be measured to determine phase of the menstrual cycle. All of these examples measure biochemical levels to directly assess a physiological function relevant to a psychological study. In many ways, although they are not always independent variables, the use of analytical chemical measurements is equivalent to a social psychologist checking on the effectiveness of a manipulated variable.

5.2.2   *Index of a process*

A second way in which biochemical measures are valuable in psychological research is as an index of a psychological construct or process. Just as polygraphic measures of blood pressure do not directly measure arousal but instead can be used as an index of arousal, measures of biochemicals are not direct measures of stress but rather are indices of this process. The most widely used biochemical measures to index a process in psychological research are catecholamines and corticosteroids in studies of stress. Baum, Grunberg, and Singer (1982) provide a detailed discussion of biochemical measures in the study of stress. For a more detailed discussion of the psychophysiological aspects of stress, see chapter 8, by Johnson and Anderson. The theories and investigations they use as examples relate cognitive and environmental events to other cognitive and environmental events with the biochemical measurements used as markers to verify that the process is occurring. This use of these particular measures is probably the most common use of biochemical measures by psychology researchers. Therefore, this approach is discussed here in more detail.

5.2.3   *Mechanism of action*

A third way in which biochemical measures can be used in psychological research is to assess potential mechanisms of action. We believe that the most useful biosocial research is that which combines both biological and social variables rather than defining one in terms of the other. In order to have a composite theory or model, social factors must be shown to have an effect on biological ones and vice versa, and both must fit into an explanation. For example, it has been suggested that cigarette smoking decreases preference for and consumption of sweet-tasting foods by acting on circulating insulin, which in turn changes glucose availability (Grunberg, 1986b). In this case, the measurement of insulin is used to assess this presumed mechanism of action that mediates behavioral and psychological processes. Another example of this category is the measurement of catecholamines (most often epinephrine and norepinephrine) in studies of stress or individual differences (e.g., Type A pattern of coronary-prone behavior, hostility) to assess whether stress acts to increase risk of cardiovascular pathophysiology (Krantz & Manuck, 1984). In this latter example, catecholamines are measured not as an index of stress but as a biological mechanism through which psychological experiences may affect physical health.

Clearly, biochemical measures can be used in more than one way simultaneously. For example, urinary catecholamines may be measured in a given study as a biochemical index of stress and as a measure of the mechanism by which stress causes cardiovascular disease. In fact, in this example catecholamines serve as a validation check of the independent variable (assuming stress was manipulated), as a dependent variable in response to the stress, and as an independent variable for endpoint cardiovascular function (e.g., blood pressure responses) or cardiovascular pathology. Recognition of this multipurpose role of these measures is important in interpreting and analyzing data.

5.3   TECHNOLOGICAL ADVANCES RELEVANT TO BIOCHEMISTRY IN
         PSYCHOLOGY

Until relatively recently, techniques and methodologies for measuring chemicals in biological fluids were not available to most psychologists. The pioneering work of physiologists and endocrinologists, from Walter Cannon (1929) to John Mason (1968), on psychological phenomena revealed valuable ways in which biobehavioral approaches could include biochemical measures. But in general, as recently as the early 1970s, biochemical changes were the stuff that theories were made of for psychologists and not a readily accessible tool. Physiological psychologists certainly talked about the hypothalamic–pituitary–adrenal axis, and many of these researchers studied the brain. But even this central nervous system (CNS) work usually involved electrical stimulation or ablations of central brain structures coupled with behavioral measures (Miller, 1961; Olds & Milner, 1954; Thompson, 1962, 1965). Many psychologists measured changes in peripheral physiological function (e.g., Glass & Singer, 1972; Lacey, 1956; Obrist 1976; Schachter & Singer, 1962). It was rare for the first group of psychologists, who worked with central mechanisms, and the second group, who worked with peripheral mechanisms, to incorporate each other's work into their discussions. And neither group used biochemical measurements.

Advances in the instrumentation and techniques for the measurement of biochemical variables in the 1960s and 1970s began to make these measures available. By the late 1970s psychologists not only could access these measures, but also could learn to make the measurements. Today, a psychologist can use many biochemical measures as readily as we use psychophysiological measures. Of course, substantial training is required to become expert in this approach. But, as in psychophysiology, certain measures (blood pressure and heart rate) are easily learned, whereas others [contingent negative variation (CNV), evoked potentials] require increased sophistication and knowledge.

The major biochemical techniques currently available to psychology research are (1) radioenzymatic assays (REAs); (2) radioimmunoassays (RIAs); (3) chromatography, including gas chromatography (GC) and high-performance liquid chromatography (HPLC); (4) automatic sampling systems (e.g., sugar or alcohol analyzer).

1. Radioenzymatic assay is a measurement technique (*assay*) that exposes chemicals of interest to enzymes (chemicals that break down those target chemicals) in the presence of radiation-emitting materials (*radioisotopes*). The radioisotopes attach to "label" the target chemicals so that the amount of the target chemicals that is present in a biological fluid (urine, blood, tissue, or cerebrospinal fluid) can be quantified by measuring the amount of radiation emitted. The greater the amount of target chemical present, the greater the amount of radioactive label that attaches to it. The amount of radioactivity indicates how much unknown target was originally there – hence the name *radioenzymatic assay*, a measurement that relies on radioisotopic labeling during enzymatic action on target chemicals. We shall discuss more of REAs in describing the measurement of catecholamines in the study of stress.

2. Radioimmunoassay is a measurement technique that uses radiation-emitting chemicals with principles of immune function. Basically, target chemicals of interest are exposed to substances (*antisera*) that recognize these target chemicals. Radioisotopes are used either to label the target chemicals of interest for

quantification (single-antibody RIA) or to compete for binding with the target chemicals before quantification (single- or double-antibody competitive binding RIA).

All of these strategies rely on the fact that antibodies are very specific in the chemicals to which they bind. Although various assays differ in how direct the binding agents are (e.g., some bind to the target chemical , others to an intermediate agent), they all employ the same basic principle; if a known amount of labeled reagent that has a specific amount of radioactivity is added at some stage in the assay, it will bind to a target. When the unbound reagent is washed away or removed, the radioactivity of the bound fraction reveals how much has bound. This in turn reveals how much of the target there was. Two points should be noted. First, even though the concept is simple, the mechanics of the assay and the calculations to convert from radioactivity measurements to amounts of one or another chemical may be detailed and involve a good deal of practice. Second, the ability to create or use an assay depends upon the availability of a labeled reagent. Even so, kits that package the reagents and provide algorithms for the calculations are most often worth the premium they command over just the reagents. We comment more on this in what follows.

3. Chromatography refers to a wide array of techniques that rely on chemical movement in various media depending on the physical, chemical, and electrical properties of the target chemicals, "carrier" chemicals, and media. The word *chromatography* is derived from *chromos* and *graph*, or "picture of color." This phrase is derived from an early version of the technique that was used to separate chemical constituents of plants in a manner that produced bands of color on paper (paper chromatography) or on a silica gel-coated glass plate (thin-layer chromatography, TLC). In effect, chromatography can be likened to a paper towel commercial for displaying the absorbance of a towel. Basically, the towel is held in a plane perpendicular to the spill with one edge of the paper towel immersed a half inch or so in the spilled fluid. By capillary action, the pool of spilled fluid disappears from the surface and travels up the paper towel, defying gravity. The denser the fluid, the slower and less far it will travel. Paper chromatography and TLC essentially rely on this principle. Increased sensitivity of separation comes as the "spilled" fluid (carrier solvent) and the "towel" (medium) are changed to differentially affect the migration of different chemical constituents in the fluid along the medium. Lighter constituents will travel faster and go farther in migrating than heavier ones. The chemicals that were mixed all together in the fluid can thereby be separated by cutting apart strips of paper or scraping off sections of material (e.g., silica gel) and then measuring the contents of these sections in various ways. Column chromatography separates chemicals from a fluid or biological sample by placing the sample on top of a column of materials (usually silica or glass beads) so that chemicals of different size come off ("elute" off) the column at different times. (Think of pinballs of various sizes cascading down the face of an elaborate pinball machine with mazes, bumpers, and traps of different sizes. The pinballs will reach the bottom at different times, according to size.) Gas chromatography (GC or gas–liquid chromatography) builds on the principles of column and paper chromatography by forcing carrier gases (in place of liquid solvent carriers in paper chromatography or TLC) through a narrow column to separate chemicals. High-performance liquid chromatography (HPLC) is similar to GC, except that high pressures are used to further improve the separation capacities of the system.

Table 5.1. *Assay equipment*

Assay	Equipment	Personnel
REA	Refrigerated centrifuge, shaking water bath, liquid scintillation (β) counter, lyophylizer, thin-layer chromatography developing jars, chemical fume hood, oscillating shaker,	Experienced technician required; others can easily learn to assist to increase number of samples assayed
RIA kits	Refrigerated centrifuge, gamma-counter, shaking water baths, refrigerator	Technician required; individual can run large numbers of samples
Chromatography	Refrigerated centrifuge, chromatography apparatus with accessories (GC, HPLC, etc.), oscillating shaker	Experienced technician with specialized training required; machinery requires careful attention
Automatic samplers	Refrigerated centrifuge, sampling machine with accessories (e.g., glucose analyzer)	Some training and experience necessary to use

4. Automatic sampling machines are another type of machine that has recently undergone major changes to become increasingly "user friendly." There are now machines available for measuring glucose, fructose, lactose, galactose, starch, and alcohol in samples that are simply injected into the machine. In addition, there are nutrient analyzers, amino acid analyzers, cholesterol, and lipoprotein automatic analyzers. The term *automatic sampler* is simply a name for a machine that performs a particular type of assay. Some automatic samplers are densitometers that measure how much light goes through a fixed amount of sample. Others are fluorometers that measure how much fluorescence is emitted when a sample is excited by light energy of a particular wavelength. Still others work on different chemical and physical principles. Each of these functions could be performed by a less automated, more general-purpose instrument that does not include internal reference standards or a processor that transforms the measurements from physical to functional units. It has proven useful to construct machines that are single-purpose analyzers for one particular type of compound, such as sugars. All the machinery is in a black box, and the mechanism and physical basis of the assay are not apparent to the user. Microcircuits report one type of result. Consequently, the user places a sample in the instrument and receives "automatically" information about how much of a particular chemical was in the sample.

The current technological and methodological state of these four types of assays opens up the world of biochemistry to the psychologist. Biochemists who have the appropriate machinery (Table 5.1) can easily perform numerous assays relevant to our work in a time-efficient manner. They do not need to devote all of their laboratory time and energy for weeks or months to assay a dozen or so samples. Instead, 100 samples can be assayed for catecholamines by REA in a week or two, 100 samples can be assayed by RIA (e.g., for insulin, sex hormones, cortisol) in 2 days, 100 samples can be assayed by GC or HPLC equipped with an automatic injection system in a week or two, and 100 samples can be assayed for sugars or alcohol in 2 days. This efficient assay schedule makes collaborations worthwhile from the point of view of some biochemists because they can readily work a few hundred samples into their schedule and provide an additional level of analysis for the research psychologist.

Besides collaborating to get this chemistry done, you could do it yourself either in a collaborating laboratory (to gain access to necessary equipment) or in your own biochemistry laboratory designed to support psychology research. Clearly, how much you do yourself depends on knowledge and willingness to learn the theory and techniques as well as your ability to acquire facilities, technical assistance, and instrumentation.

Radioenzymatic assay requires relatively sophisticated supervision and quality control because so many steps are involved and because of the risks associated with working with radioisotopes and toxic materials. However, the techniques themselves mostly require careful work and can be readily learned. Therefore, one can operate a laboratory to perform REAs with one experienced technician who can perform the difficult steps of the assay and who can supervise students or other technicians in the more time-consuming steps.

Radioimmunoassays are a different story. Many RIAs are now commercially available as "kits." If you have some familiarity with chemistry laboratory procedures, can read, and are not overly clumsy, you can use an RIA kit. Because of competition in the RIA kit market, kits are beautifully packaged, with antisera, reagents, and solvents clearly labeled and often color coded. Therefore, procedural instructions read like a cookbook: Take x amount of the red liquid and add it to y amount of the blue liquid, and so on. These kits involve handling radioactive materials, so a laboratory must be authorized by the institution and Nuclear Regulatory Commission to handle radioisotopes. However, assuming proper procedures are followed to avoid absorption or ingestion of any of the radioisotopes, the amount of radiation exposure in processing 100 samples using an RIA kit is a small fraction of natural background radiation and poses minimal risk. There are, of course, many RIAs that are not currently available by kit and that, therefore, require enormous energy, time, and expertise. We think of the kits as analogous to modern cake mixes – just add packets 1 and 2, water, and eggs – whereas other RIAs are like making a cake or bread from scratch – including milling the flour.

Gas chromatography and HPLC require sophisticated equipment and an experienced operator. Again, one knowledgeable technician can run samples, but this equipment usually requires excessive care and attention. We do not recommend this approach to the casual or part-time user. In the hands of an expert, however, these approaches provide tremendous amounts of information about chemicals and their metabolites.

Automatic samplers are the easiest of all to use. Literally, you just squirt in your sample, run some controls for comparison, and within a minute the value of each sample is provided. The only problem is getting access to the appropriate machine.

5.4   BIOCHEMICAL MEASURES IN SERVICE OF A PSYCHOLOGICAL QUESTION

As mentioned earlier, biochemical measures can be valuably used to assess a physiological function. However, we believe that the more interesting use is in service of a psychological question. This use includes measures as indices of a process and as mechanisms underlying a process. One use of biochemical measures that has proven valuable and that is gaining increased use is obtaining biochemical measures in the study of stress (Baum et al., 1982). To illustrate the use of biochemistry in the study of stress, a brief digression is necessary.

Stress refers to the reaction of an organism, human or animal, to impending threats, challenges, or dangers. The stress response is a mixture of an environmental event or its perception and appraisals of the aspects of its potential harm. The triggering event is called the stressor. According to Selye (1956), stressors result in an alarm response, a phase of resistance, and then exhaustion. This General Adaptation Syndrome (GAS) is a nonspecific response to different stressors. *Nonspecific* does not mean that the response cannot be described or specified; instead it means that a similar response occurs to different stressors. Stressors (physical and psychological) cause responses of the autonomic nervous system and the hypothalamic–pituitary–adrenal cortical axis. Stressors act to increase release of catecholamines (norepinephrine and epinephrine) from the adrenal medulla (primarily epinephrine, or adrenalin) and from nerve terminals (primarily norepinephrine). In addition, there is a release of corticosteroids from the adrenal cortex (stimulated by adrenocorticotropic hormone, ACTH, from the brain). The catecholamines act to increase blood pressure, heart rate, respiration, peripheral vasoconstriction, and blood flow to active muscles whereas the corticosteroids increase energy mobilization.

The stress response, however, is not simply a lightswitch response to a stressful stimulus. Lazarus (1966), for example, argues that a stimulus must be appraised as stressful to generate a stressful response. A stressor can occur because some event in the outside world presents itself, because our cognitions raise threats or potential threats, or because some unnoticed threat (e.g., a microbe or pollutant) begins to affect us. In order for such events to be stressful, most theorists agree that some series of appraisal processes must occur. The potential of the event to be damaging, the ability of the person to cope with the threat, the success of the coping strategy chosen, and the accuracy of judgments about the severity of the situation and its consequences are all factors that come into play. In brief, however, the conjunction of an event (a stressor) and an appropriate appraisal trigger off the stress response. It is thought that these stress reactions include biochemical responses that, in turn, affect pathophysiology and immune function. Catecholamines can increase the risk of developing cardiovascular problems whereas corticosteroids can be immunosuppressive. Therefore, the measurement of catecholamines and corticosteroids in stress research can serve as an index of this process (Is it occurring? How much?) and can help to explicate a mechanism underlying the translation of psychological experience to physical health problems.

Let us digress for a moment to consider an important issue. If you are studying some psychological aspect of stress, such as, for example, how different means of perceived control moderate a stressor's effect, biochemical measures might prove extremely helpful in tracking the process. But which ones should be used? Cortisol measurements can effectively monitor the steroid output of the adrenal cortex. However, cortisol is the most common of one type of steroid called a glucocorticoid. Other steroids of a different type, called mineralocorticoids, could also be assayed. The hormone from the pituitary gland that stimulates the adrenal cortex (ACTH) or the hormone that stimulates the pituitary to secrete ACTH could be measured. And this list of stimulating agents is just the surface of the problem. There is seemingly no limit to the number of chemicals that have a part in the stress reaction. As has been attributed to David Krech (cited in Gazzaniga, 1988), there is no phenomenon, no matter how complex, that after careful examination does not turn out to be more complex.

How is the psychologist to choose the level of sophistication in biochemical measurement that is appropriate for her or his psychological investigation? There is no pat answer to this question. Our suggested approach is drawn from a parallel with the application of statistics to experimental design and data analysis. We advise our students to choose the most technically correct and advanced procedures that they can understand and explain on their own. This same general principle should hold for biochemical measurement. What you assay should be consistent with what you understand of the process. If your understanding is that cortisol is part of the stress response, then measure cortisol. If you are familiar and comfortable with precursors, metabolites, blockers, inhibitors, receptors, and so on, then measure them as needed.

Invariably, researchers learn as they do research, and you usually wish at the end of the study that you had included more or different measures when you started. With the ongoing explosion in neuroscience and psychobiology it seems that every week a new substance is implicated in every process, particularly in the stress response. How can you incorporate these new chemicals into your study to guard against alternative explanations hinging on the "peptide of the month." One possibility is to save or extract an extra amount of fluid from each subject; save some of the urine or take an extra vial of blood. If freezer or storage space is available, label and store these materials. The odds are not great that these extras will prove useful, but under some circumstances, they can be assayed for still other biochemicals, and a retrospective experiment, with dependent measures not present in the original design, can be run. Depending on storage costs, this process can be a very inexpensive gamble for high payoff. A related aspect of the storage process will be discussed later.

We advocate the use of several levels of analysis in the study of stress: self-reports, behavioral, psychophysiological, and biochemical. Interestingly, there can be changes in some but not all of these levels in response to stressors; the stress response in these systems does not necessarily move in parallel. Therefore, it is important to use multilevel assessment simultaneously.

Self-reports [e.g., histories, or self-completed paper and pencil instruments, such as psychiatric outpatient mood scale (POMS), mood adjective checklist (MACL), and perceived stress scale (PSS)], provide information about experiences, affect, and so on. Behavioral measures (e.g., performance on proofreading or embedded figures tasks) provide another level of analysis. These three domains of stress responses – attitudinal, behavioral, and physiological – are loosely linked. They co-occur with enough frequency and probability to verify their interconnections, but they are not in one-to-one correspondence. They sometimes all arise; other times only one or two will appear. For example, Glass and Singer (1972) report a series of laboratory studies using noise as a stressor. Peoples' irritation with the noise was a function of its intensity: They were more upset with 105 dBA noise than with 55 dBA noise. Performance deficits, however, did not vary with noise intensity but were a function of whether or not the noise was predictable. Unpredictable 55 dBA noise resulted in greater performance effects than predictable 105 dBA noise. Further, although the noise produced changes in electrodermal conductivity (psychophysiological) effects at first, there was rapid adaptation no matter what the noise level or its predictability status. Both the behavioral and attitudinal reports are necessary to describe the phenomenon; psychophysiological measures (e.g., blood pressure, muscle tension, heart rate, respiration, skin conductance) add to the picture. Biochemical measures provide additional information that is valuable in interpreting the other measures. For example, both epinephrine and norepinephrine stimulate the sympathetic nervous system to increase blood pressure. Yet they differ in signaling perceived uncertainty (cf. Levine, 1988).

The biochemical measures that have been most useful in the study of stress are the catecholamines norepinephrine and epinephrine and corticosteroids (primarily cortisol in humans). Any biological sample (blood, urine, tissue, cerebrospinal fluid) can be assayed for these chemicals. Which type of sample is collected depends on practical and conceptual issues. Practically, urine samples are easiest to gather in psychology research with human subjects because this sampling is not invasive. Few normal volunteers would agree to provide tissue or cerebrospinal (CSF) samples, and the potential dangers of collecting these samples often exceed the potential value of the information. Blood sampling requires, at a minimum, trained and credentialed personnel (phlebotomy training), and many institutions require a supervising physician; many subjects do not want to have venipuncture performed or indwelling catheters inserted. [The worry about acquired immune deficiency syndrome (AIDS) has increased this concern.] In addition, blood draws become impractical in field research for two additional reasons: (1) subjects frequently are left with questionnaires to fill out and asked to collect their own samples for later biochemical analyses, a procedure that is simple for urine but not for blood, and (2) even if blood were drawn, it needs to be processed (usually by centrifugation) to separate serum or plasma from whole blood and transferred quickly to cold storage areas to preserve the chemicals of interest before they deteriorate. Therefore, in general, we advocate the collection of urine samples in human psychology research on stress in circumstances other than well-controlled and equipped laboratory settings.

The use of urine samples in the study of stress is not solely a matter of convenience. Many people assume that blood samples are better than urine samples. It is not that simple. Plasma levels of catecholamines, for example, are extremely reactive to stressful stimuli. Therefore, venipuncture itself will increase circulating catecholamines. If you are interested in a rapid and short-lived response to a stressful stimulus, blood samples are the way to go. But if this is the case, one must insert a venous catheter and allow the subject to sit quietly for at least 20 min before drawing a meaningful blood sample. Even then, movement (standing up or moving the arms) can affect the catecholamine levels. Blood draws via an indwelling catheter are an excellent approach to measure acute stress (e.g., Glass et al., 1980). However, this approach is not the best way to biochemically assess chronic stress. It is also more expensive. Not only do blood draws require more time from highly trained personnel, but the expense of the supplies, such as nonreusable catheters, can be considerable.

If chronic stress, such as that produced by urban hassles, work, or other environmental and life stressors, is the focus of the study, then urine samples collected over time (8–24 hr) are more informative than blood samples to measure catecholamines and corticosteroids. Urinary levels of these *stress hormones* reflect the amount of these chemicals excreted over an extended period of time. Concurrent information gathered from other levels of analyses (self-reports of mood, perceived stress; performance assessments; psychophysiological measurements) can provide a thorough profile of responses to the stressful stimuli or environment. This approach of gathering urine samples is invaluable in field research of stress (e.g., Baum, Gatchel, & Schaeffer, 1983; Fleming, Baum, Reddy, & Gatchel, 1984) and also is valuable in laboratory studies in which the experimenter cannot or chooses not to collect blood (Frankenhaeuser, 1976).

5.5 THE USE OF URINE SAMPLES IN FIELD RESEARCH OF STRESS

One excellent example of the use of this approach is in field studies of chronic stress. For example, Baum and co-workers (Baum, Fleming, & Singer, 1983; Baum et al., 1983) have integrated the measurement of urinary catecholamines into field studies of chronic stress connected with man-made disasters [the nuclear accident at Three Mile Island (TMI); toxic waste dump sites] and to life events (work stress; unemployment). These events and experiences are clearly different from the acute stress of a short-duration loud noise or burst of light. In the cases of the acute stressors, blood sampling would be the best approach to assess biochemical responses. In contrast, for the chronic stressors, urine sampling provides a more meaningful picture of the state of the individual.

Acute versus chronic stress can be distinguished in terms of duration of the stressor, whether there is a remaining threat, and duration of the response (Baum, 1986a). In order to assess the magnitude of chronic stress, Baum and co-workers took a variety of measures from subjects, including urine samples for biochemical analysis. The samples taken were 18-hr urine collections. (Because most of the biochemicals measured vary over a 24-hr cycle, a 24-hr collection would be better to eliminate diurnal variability from the samples. When this is not feasible, the investigator should make sure, as Baum did, that the same shorter time period is used for each subject; e.g., they should all run from 6:00 a.m. to midnight.) The results of the assay of the urine samples can then be interpreted together with the information in the other measures. In a series of studies of chronic stress at TMI, Baum and co-workers have found that compared to control subjects living near an undamaged nuclear plant, a coal-fired plant, or not near a power plant, persons living near the failed nuclear reactor show more somatic complaints and self-reports of anxiety, worse performance on performance tasks, and higher levels of excreted norepinephrine, epinephrine, and cortisol. Similarly, biochemical indices of stress in people living near toxic waste dumps also show increases in catecholamines and corticosteroids (Baum, 1986b).

This approach, of course, can also be used in other chronic studies of stress. In the case of the TMI studies, subjects may have reason to report more somatic complaints and problems than they are experiencing in order to explain away other personal problems or to increase their chances at litigation against the power company. Whether intentional or not, such concerns cast some question on self-report measures. The biochemical analyses provide useful complementary data. In contrast, in studies of individuals dealing with chronic illness of a loved one (e.g., chronic cancer patients or AIDS victims), self-reports may put on a strong face and thereby hide the real stress being experienced. Together, psychological and biological measures provide more complete and useful information. Neither approach suffices alone.

Another recent application of this approach is in studies of individuals living in isolated and confined environments (ICEs), such as in the Antarctic. Carrere et al. (Carrere, Evans, & Stokols, 1987; Evans, Stokols, & Carrere, 1987) have reported that catecholamines are elevated when people first arrive at these ICEs and decrease over time until a new team arrives just before the residents are about to return home. The use of biochemical indices of stress have allowed these investigators to better understand the stress experienced by people who "winter over" in the Antarctic.

5.6   THE USE OF URINE SAMPLES IN LABORATORY RESEARCH OF STRESS

Frankenhaeuser and her colleagues (e.g. Frankenhaeuser, 1973; Frankenhaeuser & Gardell, 1976) have analyzed catecholamines and cortisol from urine samples in laboratory studies using a double-voiding technique in contrast to the extended hour collection. This enables the use of noninvasive collections in controlled experiments. When subjects first arrive at the experimental session, they are asked to void their urine. They are then put through the appropriate experimental procedures and, at the session's conclusion, are asked to provide a second urine sample. Because the second sample was deposited in each subject's bladder during the experiment, the levels and concentrations of catecholamines and cortisol it contains reflect responses to the conditions of the experiment. If subjects in one experimental condition have higher levels than subjects in another experimental condition, then one may infer that the first condition was more stressful. The use of double voiding in experimental sessions offers the possibility of greater precision but needs to be carefully administered.

There are several procedural and interpretive difficulties with a double-voiding technique. First, subjects' production of catecholamines and cortisol is still subject to diurnal variation. Therefore, a subject's excretion of these chemicals during a 60- to 120-min session depends not only on the experimental circumstances but also on what particular time of day – morning, afternoon, evening – the study is run. Care must be used to either hold time of day constant or counterbalance it so as to get comparable results. Second, double voiding works only to the extent that subjects are able to double void. Quite often subjects will not be able to produce a large enough volume of urine during the experiment to be able to void at its conclusion. Helping strategies, such as providing the subjects with supplies of water to drink or padding the experimental procedures to lengthen the time between the first and second voids, can sometimes be used, but they often run the risk of interfering with the study. Consequently, it may not be possible to get data from all subjects with this technique. Third, the interpretations of the concentrations and amounts of each chemical are not as simple as it would seem at first glance. The stress response and its associated biochemical events, as with most human phenomena, exhibit individual differences of considerable magnitude. With the rather small sample sizes of laboratory research, between-subject variability may overshadow differences produced by experimental differences. One way to control for this possibility is to assay the first-void urine (the one provided at the start of the session) and use its values as within-subject baselines for interpreting the values from the second-void urine. This procedure needs further caution. Most psychological experiments are not stress neutral for the subjects no matter how benign they may seem to the experimenter. It is usually the case that the first-void urine, collected before the experiment starts, has a higher concentration of stress marker chemicals than the second-void urine, collected at the conclusion of the experiment. This is true even when the experiment includes stressful and stress-inducing procedures. Baseline adjustments have to be made in careful fashion, such as a covariance, and then stress will have to be inferred indirectly. For example, intuition would suggest that if condition *A* is more stressful than condition *B*, subjects in *A* would excrete more catecholamines than subjects in *B*. With the double-void procedure, the greater stress in condition *A* would be inferred if subjects in *A* showed a smaller drop in catecholamines over the course of the study than did those in *B*.

Even with all these restrictions, double voiding is less invasive than venipuncture and less demanding of personnel than an indwelling catheter. Unlike blood sampling, it does not provide moment-to-moment information on catecholamine and cortisol levels but rather gives information on the amount produced over the course of the study. The technique has been very useful and has potential for wide use. In some cases, the double-voiding procedure has been incorporated into field studies (cf. Singer, Lundberg, & Frankenhaeuser, 1978) under circumstances where other methods of biochemical assessment would not be appropriate or feasible.

Two further points need emphasis. First, when urine is collected for short time periods and complicated procedures are used to assay some of its biochemical constituents, the numbers produced by the assays are often difficult to interpret as absolute values. That is, they do not provide a definitive measure of the physiological level of those substances in the subject's blood. These measures are best used when they are compared to similar measures from the same subjects from a different time or times or when they are contrasted to similarly obtained measures from subjects in other groups or other experimental conditions.

Second, the biochemicals in urine are subject to degradative changes between the time of collection and when they are assayed. Some means must be employed to preserve them during this interval. Low-temperature refrigeration, usually at $-20°C$ but in some cases down to $-70°C$, is the best preservative, but it is expensive and not usually available. In some cases, as when a subject is given a container for an 18- or 24-hr collection, the interim refrigeration depends on the subject's ability and willingness to comply with the refrigeration instructions, a point that cannot be taken for granted. A more feasible way to preserve samples is to place a chemical preservative in the collection container itself. Each of the substances to be analyzed has its own optimal preservative. Nevertheless, usually compromises must be made in what to add to the container. Chemicals that best preserve catecholamines, for example, may interfere with the cortisol assay, so the less efficient preservatives may be best for both assays. Or the optimal preservative may be highly corrosive or dangerous, and ethics and prudence may advise against leaving it with a subject. The point is that the preservatives used must be carefully considered and well planned with the collaboration of someone familiar with all the assays to be utilized. Earlier, we suggested that extra samples of fluids be collected for retrospective assays of biochemicals not part of the original study. The success of these retrospective assays will depend on fortuitous inclusion of preservatives well suited to prevent the degradation of the unknown chemical.

5.7   BLOOD SAMPLES IN HUMAN STUDIES OF STRESS

Some laboratory studies of social and personality variables have used assays of blood samples for various biochemical constituents. The information contained in these assays was useful despite the extraordinary constraints posed by the blood draw methodology. It should be noted that blood assays are quite common in the biological literature and in many of the comparative and physiological psychology studies that usually employ animal subjects. Animals that are naive do not have apprehension and learned fear of hypodermic needles used to extract blood samples; consequently, their levels of circulating hormones are less reactive to the blood-drawing procedure. It is also procedurally easier to surgically implant an indwelling catheter in an animal at some time prior to the experimental session so that blood samples can be obtained concurrently with behavioral measurements without repeated needle insertions. And finally, blood can be obtained from animals that are sacrificed.

Even so, there remain difficulties. Animal use review boards require justification for surgery and sacrifice; associative learning may cause changes in circulating hormone levels in animals repeatedly sampled; indwelling catheters may cease to be patent over time; some small animals such as mice may not have enough blood so that samples of sufficient volume to be assayed can be drawn in a short time. Yet enough of these studies have been conducted so that the procedures for the preparation of the blood for assays is well documented.

When blood is drawn from humans for adjunctive biochemical measurements in psychological studies, two sources of problems arise. One is the reactivity of the human subject to the blood draw itself. Venipunctures are a form of stress that, for some subjects, is quite aversive and, for all subjects, probably increases the transient blood level for a spectrum of endogenous biochemicals. Insertion of a catheter is equally reactive; a waiting period of 20 min to an hour will probably restore the subject to precatheter baselines. In order to be successful, the waiting period must be soothing, restful, and nonanxious. The subjects' cognitions about the catheter, physical restraints on the subjects' movements to keep the catheter in place and to prevent movement artifacts, and apprehensions about catheter removal and other experimental procedures made salient by the catheter all add to the reactivity.

In addition, taking blood samples from volunteers is not a simple procedural matter. Subjects must give voluntary consent. Not all subjects will do so. This selectivity may limit the study's generalizability. The procedures for drawing the blood will require clearance by an Institutional Human Subjects Review Board. At the least, the board will insist that the actual puncture, whether by venipuncture or catheterization, be done by a trained and certified phlebotomist. In our experience, the board will often require the general supervision of a collaborating physician as well. Sometimes, the presence of a cardiovascular "crash cart" for emergency situations is also mandated. And because human blood is being collected from an unspecified group of subjects in an era when the HIV (AIDS) virus in human blood poses risks to laboratory personnel, the Center for Disease Control guidelines in blood handling must be followed by all those participating in the study.

The point is not to paint the use of blood samples as impossible or not achievable, but rather to highlight that preparation and careful planning are necessary to manage them fruitfully. For social psychologists used to staging elaborate scenarios in order to circumvent parallel problems with human cognitions and expectations, these precautions represent another layer of constraints to challenge their experimental ingenuity.

In spite of these considerations, some studies have profitably used blood samples and subsequent assays to complement social and personality explorations. Glass and his associates (1980) used indwelling catheters to repeatedly sample Type A and Type B subjects' reactivity in the face of challenge and competition. Similar uses could be made in any experiment in which the value of the information – acute changes in circulating levels of hormones and other chemicals – justified the effort required to secure the permission, personnel, and costs of the procedure. Depending on what is to be assayed, the investigator must make a series of decisions. How are the samples to be obtained; by venipuncture, by repeated draws from a catheter, or from a continuous flow from a slow-acting pump? How is the blood to be treated? Is it to be centrifuged, frozen, heparinized? Each study has its own requirements. The decisions will differ, but they must be stated well in advance and thoroughly incorporated into the experimental plans.

5.8 OTHER EXAMPLES OF BIOCHEMISTRY IN PSYCHOLOGY RESEARCH

Most of the preceding discussion emphasized the use of biochemical measures as an index of stress. In addition, many of these investigations include these measures to explore mechanisms that may underlie effects of stress on the development of cardiovascular pathology. The points to be made are not uniquely applicable to the study of stress or the measurement of catecholamines and cortisol.

These same methods also are relevant, for example, to studies of energy expenditure and metabolism. For example, Grunberg (1986a, b) has reported that nicotine (the drug of addiction in tobacco products) causes decreased preference and consumption of sweet-tasting high-carbohydrate foods, which in turn affects body weight. Grunberg et al. (1988) have reported that nicotine decreases circulating insulin and have suggested that this biochemical change accounts for the changes in sweet food preferences and increases in fat utilization. Further, Grunberg (1986b; Grunberg et al., 1988) has suggested that effects of nicotine on serotonin in the body account for changes in carbohydrate cravings and mood changes. Other psychologists (e.g., Pomerleau & Pomerleau, 1984) have found that smoking increases plasma levels of endogenous opioid peptides and have speculated that this effect is responsible for effects of nicotine on pain and anxiety.

Other examples of biochemical measures in psychology research can, of course, be cited, but our main purpose is to encourage other psychologists to learn about and to incorporate this level of analysis into their work. Therefore, to provide a more detailed understanding of a commonly used assay that many psychologists find useful, we discuss the REA for catecholamines. This discussion is meant to provide an example of just one available assay but with enough detail to alert readers to the type of theory and methods involved. It is beyond the scope and length of this chapter to discuss all of the potentially relevant assays in detail. The discussion of the catecholamine REA is meant to illustrate the concerns and level of knowledge necessary to understand a biochemical assay. We do not expect all psychologists to perform assays themselves, but we believe that researchers should understand what is involved in a given assay to ensure that samples are being appropriately collected, processed, and stored and that data are being appropriately analyzed and interpreted. After discussing the REA for catecholamines in some detail, we address issues that affect the samples. It is not necessary for psychologists to become biochemists in order to incorporate these data into their studies. They should

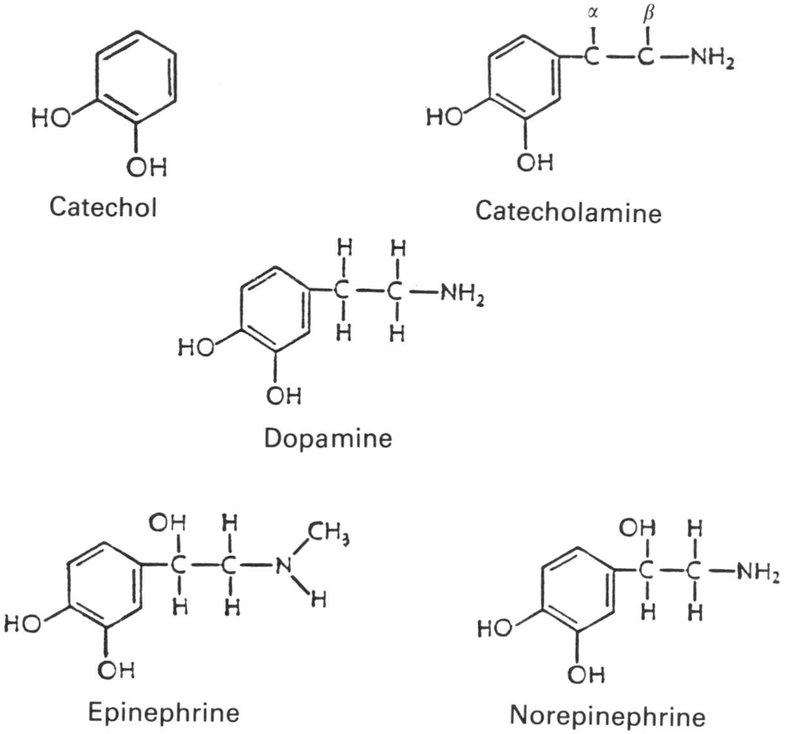

Figure 5.1. Chemical structures of major catecholamines.

realize, however, that they will be ultimately responsible for the reports they generate. They must learn enough about what is actually done in the assay so that they can respond intelligently to reasonable questions about methods and procedures used in their work. Biological scientists who are collaborating with psychologists will be more sophisticated in assay methods than the psychologist and may use some methods that the psychologist does not understand. We repeat our earlier advice that when psychologists incorporate these data into their reports, they should do so at a level they are comfortable with and could explain to both a technical and nontechnical audience.

5.9   AN EXAMPLE OF HOW AN ASSAY WORKS: REAs FOR
       CATECHOLAMINES

There are three major catecholamines that are of interest to many psychologists: norepinephrine, epinephrine, and dopamine (Figure 5.1). These three chemicals have similar structures. A ring of six carbons, called a benzene ring, is extremely stable and occurs throughout nature. When the benzene ring has two hydroxyl groups (oxygen plus hydrogen) attached to two adjacent carbons, the structure is called a *catechol* ring. When a catechol ring is connected to a *side chain* consisting of two carbons and a nitrogen-based complex (an amino group), such as NH_2, the structure is called a catechol amine.

Epinephrine (adrenaline) and norepinephrine are chemically similar, and the names of these chemicals indicate exactly how they differ. Norepinephrine, or "nor epinephrine," is epinephrine without (*ohne*, German for *without*) the radical group (i.e., the CH_3 side group: *radikal* in german) on the nitrogen. *Nor* is an acronym for *n*itrogen *o*hne *r*adikal. Both norepinephrine and epinephrine have an OH group on the first carbon of the amine chain, that is, the carbon that attaches to the catechol. Dopamine is similar to norepinephrine except that there are no hydroxyl groups on either carbon of the amine chain. There are also precursors of catecholamines (e.g., tyrosine) and metabolites of catecholamines (e.g., homovanillic acid) that may be of interest to some investigators. We shall not discuss them here.

We spend some time on this basic chemical structure because it is important to be alert to similar chemicals and how a given assay deals with chemicals that look alike. Some assays have high *cross-reactivity*; that is, they measure the chemical of interest and anything that resembles it. Low cross-reactivity is important if specific, similar chemicals must be distinguished. In the working example, there are assays that measure "catecholamines" and that do not easily distinguish one catecholamine from another. In fact, most psychology research that reported catecholamine values before the 1970s did just this.

Of the various biochemical assays being used by psychologists today, the REA for catecholamines is probably the most complex to perform and involves the greatest number of steps. Therefore, we describe this assay in some detail. Our purpose is to provide an example of what issues arise and what the analytical chemist is doing. The other assays (e.g., RIAs, GC, HPLC) involve fewer steps and are relatively simpler, except that some require sophisticated machines (e.g., GC, HPLC) that a skilled technician must operate. Some also take substantially more time and cannot handle as large a number of samples simultaneously.

The first decision to be made is what source of specimen to use: blood, tissue, CSF, urine, saliva. The biological fluid collected depends on the question being addressed. For example, are the biochemicals to be measured involved in an acute stimulus and response situation (then use blood) or a more chronic stimulus and response (urine is best)? It also depends on the subject: healthy human volunteer, human patient undergoing other procedures (e.g., spinal tap), animal model. Human volunteers readily provide urine samples and often will allow blood to be drawn. The human patient in the hospital to undergo surgical or other procedures certainly can provide urine and blood samples and may provide other samples (e.g., fat tissue, muscle punch biopsy, CSF). Saliva can be readily taken from a human volunteer or patient, but values assayed on saliva must be carefully interpreted. Many chemists, when asked, will assay saliva and will assure the psychologist that the assays are sensitive and not cross-reactive. However, few chemists or psychologists attend to the fact that stimuli and conditions of interest (e.g., stress) markedly alter salivary flow. We are all familiar with "dry mouth" under stress. If a salivary sample is taken, the chemist can provide assays of many materials and the values will reflect *concentration*, that is, chemical per unit volume. However, without measuring salivary flow per unit time (something that is rarely if ever done), the *values* (i.e., concentration) are dramatically altered by volume of saliva. It is difficult to know if numbers gathered in this way reflect changes in biochemical levels, changes in volume, or both. Further, many people dislike spitting into a tube or putting dry cotton or gauze in their mouths to gather a saliva sample. Some chemicals can be measured in saliva meaningfully (e.g., cotinine, the primary metabolite of nicotine, can be valuably measured in saliva to indicate qualitatively whether an individual smoked a cigarette recently) whereas others become questionable as salivary volume is affected by stimuli of interest. Because salivary volume is so low, small changes in volume can profoundly change concentrations.

For chronic stress studies and when a noninvasive sample is preferred, urine samples are the best way to go. When urine is collected, it is important to collect the sample, measure the volume of urine collected, and record the amount of time over which the sample is collected. For urine samples to measure catecholamines in a chronic stress study, collect the samples in a specimen jar and transfer it to a collection jar (large enough to gather total volume over the period of interest). The collection jar should be kept in a refrigerator to slow down metabolism (breakdown) of the catecholamines to be measured. Addition of a preservative (e.g., hydrochloric acid or sodium metabisulfite) is also useful to decrease oxidation of the catecholamines. If subjects are collecting the samples themselves and are storing the collected samples before bringing them to the researcher, sodium metabisulfite is preferred because it is not a dangerous material itself. To collect a long-term sample (e.g., 14 hr), subjects can collect their urine at home from the time they get home until they go to work the next day. They can bring the urine container (a plastic container with a lid) to the laboratory on their way to work or school or first thing in the morning. The researcher should measure and record volume and can then take a small aliquot (sample) of 5 ml from the well-mixed sample. The aliquot can be transferred to a test tube (labeled with some sample number code) and frozen at $-20°C$ or below. (This temperature is sufficient to preserve urinary catecholamines for at least 6 months. Blood, tissue, or CSF should be stored at $-70°C$ or below.)

When it is time to assay for catecholamines, the samples are thawed. They should not be refrozen because multiple thawing can destroy biochemicals. So one freezing and thawing cycle is best. If different assays are to be performed on the same sample, multiple aliquots should be stored in different test tubes initially.

The first step in the REA for catecholamines is to add to each sample the enzyme COMT, catechol-O-methyltransferase. This enzyme catalyzes the transfer of a methyl group (CH_3) in the presence of a methyl donor to an oxygen on the catechol ring. This enzyme does no good if no CH_3 group is available. Further, it does not help just to break down catecholamines unless they can be measured somehow. Remember, the purpose is to count (quantify) the amount of different catecholamines present in the biological fluid samples (e.g., urine from subjects). Something must be done to allow catecholamines to be counted.

As a digression, let us say that we wanted to know how many books were in an office, but we could not see books to count unless they were colored red. Then we might pour red paint all over our office, literally covering everything with the paint. We would use a special red paint that sticks particularly well to books. After pouring the paint everywhere to be sure that no books were missed, we would wait (to let the paint stick) and then hose the office down with water. The red paint would continue to stick to the books but the extra paint would be washed away. Now, we are ready to count red objects, which, indirectly, would indicate how many books were present.

In a sense, this is how the REA works. But instead of using red paint, we use radioisotopes to attach to (label) the materials of interest (i.e., catecholamines) for counting. More specifically, we take an aliquot of urine (0.1 ml) and add COMT and a compound that supplies methyl groups that contain a radioactive hydrogen (tritium). The catecholamines contained in the sample are broken down by the COMT and the radioactive methyl groups are added to these metabolites (normetanephrine, metanephrine, and 3-methoxytyramine). Then these labeled metabolites are separated from the surrounding liquid and the amount of radioactivity emitted is positively related to the amount of catecholamine present. After labeling catecholamines, most of the steps of the REA are designed to "clean up," or separate, the catecholamines to increase the sensitivity and accuracy of the quantification. Remember, at this point all of the catecholamines ("books") are similarly labeled ("painted red"). We can measure radiation emitted, but we cannot distinguish one catecholamine type (e.g., epinephrine) from another (norepinephrine) simply by counting radiation. So the REA involves labelling catecholamines, separating them from each other, isolating them to get rid of noise (other materials), and counting radiation in portions of the original samples separated into the individual types of catecholamines of interest.

Back to the steps of the assay, the first step is to introduce COMT in the presence of ^{3}H–SAM (tritiated S-adenosylmethionine), a compound that donates tritiated methyl groups (tritium is a form of radioactive hydrogen). Other chemicals also are added (e.g., coenzymes, buffers) to the mixture that increase the likelihood of radioactive methyl groups attaching to the catecholamines present. This first step in the REA is called methylation.

As an aside, we find that most psychologists assume that biochemistry assays provide "hard" objective numbers. From this one step alone, readers should realize that our ability to count "red books" relies on procedures that we cannot verify completely. For example, was every catecholamine thoroughly exposed to the COMT and were plenty of tritiated methyl groups available? Radioenzymatic assay procedures are refined to a point that we can include multiple aliquots from single samples to check for reliability and to infer validity. However, this first step involves imperfect procedures. Quality control can certainly be performed, but is that information gathered in a laboratory to which you subcontract?

The next step in the REA is extraction. We now have primary metabolites of three catecholamines of interest. We assume that there is a one-to-one correspondence between these primary metabolites and their parent chemicals. Now we need to get rid of all the other materials in the urine that will obscure the sensitive measurement of radioactivity from these metabolites. It is a basic problem of signal-to-noise ratio. Decrease the noise and refine the signal to improve measurement of the signal.

Basically, the extraction procedures make use of physical properties of insolubility or organic and inorganic liquids, differential freezing points, and different densities of molecules. Think of the difference between adding water to soda pop (they mix) and adding gasoline to water (they do not mix). Also, other physical conditions, such as temperature, alter solubility (the ability of a material to dissolve in a liquid). For example, add lots of table sugar to iced tea, and the sugar collects at the bottom of the glass. Add the same amount of sugar to hot tea, and it disappears; it dissolves. These types of physical phenomena are used in the extraction procedures of the REA to separate the catecholamines.

After the methylation step and a measured amount of time, we add chemicals (a high pH borate buffer and boric acid) to stop the breakdown of the catecholamines. We then add toluene and isoamyl alcohol (two liquids). The catecholamines migrate to these organic solvents; other substances in our samples do not. Next, we freeze this mixture because the aqueous ("water") portion freezes (without catecholamines) whereas the organic liquid portion (containing the catecholamines) does not. The organic liquid is poured off from the frozen portion. (Think of putting freshly made chicken soup into a refrigerator. The fat rises to the surface and solidifies. Low-fat chicken stock can be easily separated.) We have now dramatically concentrated the catecholamines, but we may have lost some in the freezing and pouring.

Our new saved liquid includes catecholamines plus other chemicals that stayed in the organic layer. Now we add acetic acid because catecholamines have a particular affinity for acid media. Therefore, the catecholamines leave the organic layer and move into the acetic acid, an aqueous medium. The samples are shaken and centrifuged to separate materials based on density as well as on differential solubility. The unwanted materials in the organic layer sit on top of the acetic acid (like an oil slick on the ocean). The undesired organic layer can be aspirated off (pulled by a vacuum through a pipette; think of a miniature straw) to further concentrate the portion of the sample that contains the catecholamines. Extraction procedures are repeated several times to isolate the catecholamines more and more. Of course, any "errors" introduced by each procedure add up. So, each time we lose a little bit of the desired material.

After the extraction steps, the samples are put into a lyophilizer (a freeze dryer) to remove aqueous liquid while leaving the catecholamines in the test tubes. When these test tubes are taken out of the lyophilizer, we cannot see the catecholamines. We are left with the catecholamines and little else, which may look at most like a speck of dust. Because we are interested in distinguishing among the catecholamines, we need to separate these molecules from each other. Remember, all are "painted red" similarly; that is, they all are radioactively labeled.

The step to separate the three major catecholamines uses TLC. Different physicochemical properties of molecules affect the movement of the chemicals along solid media in the presence of specific solvents (see previous TLC description). The dried test tubes containing the three major catecholamines have HCl and alcohol added.

The solution plus catecholamines is transferred ("spotted") by capillary tube to a TLC plate coated with a silica-based material (Figure 5.2). The spotted TLC plate is placed vertically in a glass container ("developing jar") containing a small amount of solvent. The solvent will move up the TLC plate (like water moving up a paper towel) carrying the three types of catecholamines with it. However, the three types of catecholamines will migrate to different positions on the TLC plate based on molecular size (i.e., heavier, bigger molecules do not move as far up). The TLC plate silica coating also contains a fluorescent material that appears purple under ultraviolet (UV) light. Because the fluorescent material is covered by the catecholamines, their location on the plate appears dark under UV light. Therefore, plates can be marked with a pencil under UV illumination to indicate where the "bands" of catecholamines are sitting. Three nonfluorescent (dark) bands appear on the TLC plates corresponding to the three major catecholamines: epinephrine, norepinephrine, and dopamine.

Next, a razor blade or scalpel is used to scrape off the spot on the TLC plate corresponding to each catecholamine type for each sample. This scraped sample (a bit of dust containing concentrated catecholamines of one type) is brushed gently into a vial. There will be a separate vial for each scraping. If you started with N subjects and were assaying for three catecholamines, with two replicates per subject

19-channel TLC plate

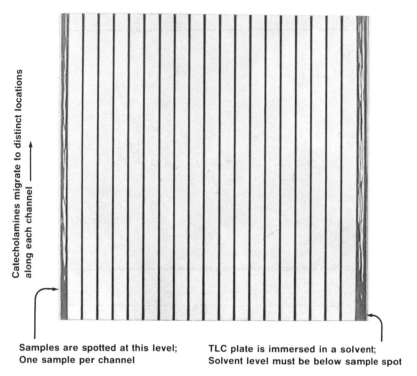

Catecholamines migrate to distinct locations along each channel ⟶

Samples are spotted at this level; One sample per channel

TLC plate is immersed in a solvent; Solvent level must be below sample spot

Figure 5.2. Thin-layer chromatography plate used in catecholamine assays.

for quality control and reliability, you will have $6 \times N$ vials to count. So, for example, 20 subjects will result in approximately 140 vials to count; 120 will be unknowns from the subjects' urines and the rest will be "standard" or known amounts of the relevant chemical for calibration purposes.

A small amount of liquid scintillation cocktail is added to each vial. This "cocktail" includes liquid solvents plus a chemical that is excited to release photons of light in the presence of radioactive materials (i.e., the tritium on the methylated chemicals). In a sense, this step serves to amplify the signal. The "signal" is measured on a particular machine, a liquid scintillation (or beta-) counter.

The numbers provided by the beta-counter are used to calculate the concentration of each catecholamine type in each sample. The numbers measured are not the actual concentrations of catecholamines in the original samples. Instead, one has to include "standard curves" and calculate concentration. To do this, a series of samples of known concentration are included in this entire assay run and are treated in identical manner as are unknown samples. The radiation emissions measured by the beta-counter are compared to the known concentrations of the standards to generate a function that is used, in turn, to convert radiation emission from the unknowns to a concentration value.

In the case of beta-counting and catecholamines assayed by REA, the *standard curves* are close to linear. This is not the case with all chemicals and assays (see following). Therefore, the values given to the psychologist are indirect *calculations*. The amount of error in these calculations includes the error introduced throughout the steps of the assay plus the care taken in constructing standard curves and fitting the curves with appropriate mathematical functions. For example, interpolated values are better than extrapolated values, so that concentrations in the standards should bracket those in the samples. Also, standard curves differ if they are included at the beginning or end of a "run" of unknowns because there is some radiation and metabolic decay while sitting in the counter waiting to be measured. Therefore, it is best to include and average at least two standard curves at the beginning and end of each assay to more accurately compare unknown sample values.

With respect to calculations based on curve fitting, how is the algorithm computed? One can fit a line in several ways, each introducing different amounts of error. There are substantial differences of error generated by different techniques of curve fitting. If you contract to a chemist to assay for catecholamines (or other assays), do you know how many standard curves they include, how curves are fit, or how quality control is performed? Do they throw out bad duplicates based on intuition or some standard procedure? Many chemists perform assays the way they learned and are not sensitive to statistical and mathematical issues that affect their "hard numbers." Remember that most chemical assays are indirect; the numbers are not as hard and objective as you may assume. More about this later.

5.10   CAUTIONS AND PROBLEMS

Although we advocate the use of biochemical measures in psychological research, there is a variety of potential problems that may make biochemical values meaningless. None of these problems is insurmountable, but the researcher must be alert to them. The cautions and problems addressed in this section are relevant to the psychologist even if a chemist is performing the assays. That is, these concerns are separate from the quality control issues involved in a given assay.

5.10.1   *Sampling*

As already discussed, the type of sample (blood, urine, saliva, CSF, time) must be determined initially based on theoretical (e.g., acute vs. chronic response; hypothesized mechanism under study) and practical issues. In addition, when to sample must be determined in advance. It is relevant to consider daily circadian rhythms that may affect the values as well as weekday versus weekend effects resulting from sleep patterns, physical activity, diet, and stress. It is best to draw samples at the same time each day and to avoid a nadir or crest of a natural cycle.

5.10.2   *Processing*

Once the sample is taken, the subject (if self-collecting) and experimenter must know how to process the sample. Should it be measured in any way (e.g., volume or pH) before storing? Should it be diluted or not? For blood, should it be treated with heparin to avoid clotting, should it be centrifuged to separate plasma or serum from whole blood, or should it be treated in other chemical or physical ways to avoid degradation of the chemical of interest? How much time can elapse from collection to processing? There are clear answers to each of these questions based on the assays that will be performed. For example, for catecholamines in urine to be assayed by REA, the total volume excreted must be measured and recorded before sample aliquots of urine are taken and frozen. This volume is necessary to calculate total amount of catecholamines excreted per unit time. The processing differs for different assays and must be performed correctly for the assays to be meaningful. Therefore, decisions about which assay will be performed must be established before samples are collected.

5.10.3 *Storage*

In some cases samples will go directly from processing to assay. It is more usual to collect and store many samples before assaying them. Therefore, storage techniques become an issue. What preservatives should be used? What temperature freezer (e.g., -20 or $-70°C$) is best? What material should be used for the storage containers (e.g., glass or plastic)? How many aliquots should be stored separately per sample? Again, there are answers to these questions, but they differ depending on the type of sample and assay to be performed. For our example REA, aliquots are stored at $-20°C$ or below in plastic tubes that resist cracking at low temperatures. Preservatives are frozen with each aliquot. The volume of each aliquot should be sufficient to allow multiple assays of each sample; 5 ml should be plenty. This type of information must be known before gathering samples.

5.10.4 *Interfering variables*

It is also important to consider what variables, separate from the independent variables under investigation, affect the biochemical measures. For example, foods (e.g., coffee, certain cheeses), physical activity and position (e.g., exercise vs. standing vs. lying down during sampling), and drugs (including tobacco, alcohol, and medications) can all affect many biochemicals of interest. These "interfering" variables can be dealt with in some studies by controling them. However, for some variables this control (e.g., smoking abstinence for smokers) also may induce biochemical changes. Alternatively, measurement of relevant interfering variables can be used to statistically control for these influences. How to deal with these variables depends on the questions addressed, sample size, and so on. It is critical to recognize that if a chemist doing assays for you answers the question "Can you assay for x?" with a yes, he or she probably has not considered that your subjects may be eating different foods, drinking or not, or smoking or not. It is up to you to raise the question of potential interfering variables.

5.10.5 *Assay procedures*

There are, of course, many concerns and issues in the assay procedures that must be addressed by the investigator who performs the assays. However, our intention here is to highlight the concerns of the researcher who is *not* performing the assays per se. With respect to the assay procedures, is your chemist running more than one aliquot per sample, running individual or pooled samples, computing and reporting to you mean values of all aliquots per sample or ignoring what looks wrong in computing values, basing averaged versus single values on some predetermined criterion for classifying an outlier, including one or more standard curves, curve-fitting with linear models or more sophisticated curvilinear equations, interpolating or extrapolating values from standard curves, or performing quality control procedures? These are legitimate questions to ask. Consider, for example, a psychologist conducting a simple two-group experiment. Some treatment is applied and some behavior of interest is noted for subjects in both the experimental and the control groups. In addition, a blood sample is taken from each subject to be assayed for some chemical, Q. The psychologist would expect to receive a value of Q for each subject so that the biochemical information could be combined with the behavioral data for each individual subject. When group differences are to be assessed, for either kind of data, the psychologist would look at the mean group differences with respect to within-group variability. If a chemist were conducting the study, particularly if the assay for Q is expensive, laborious, or time consuming, the chemist might use a different strategy. The chemist is likely to take an aliquot from each subect in the experimental groups and pool them (i.e., place them together) in one container; then the chemist would do the same thing for the control groups. The assay would yield two values, one for the experimental group and the other for the control group. A careful chemist might do this three times, so there would be three replicates for each group, and test group differences against the variability in the replicates. It is imperative that the psychologist make certain that the chemist is clear about what the psychologist wishes to be assayed and that the chemist understands how much work will be involved if pooled group samples are not to be used.

Often in chemical techniques each sample is varied in a number of ways, so that the basic two pooled samples may each be measured a number of times, such as after serial dilutions. This opens up the possibility for a major misunderstanding between chemist and psychologist. The psychologist, receiving a measurement mean with a standard error based on a large number of values, assumes each subject has been individually assayed. The chemist, if asked casually, will report that this value is representative of variation within each group. A more careful dialogue reveals there are no data at the individual subject level.

At the time the collected samples are given to a chemist, he or she will commonly ask to know which samples are from which group. Their purpose is not to capitalize on experimenter bias, but instead to appropriately group the samples in preparation for a pooled assay. This is not inappropriate per se and may be a cost-saving step to determine the utility of individual assays. Our goal is to alert people to the need to be very precise in exactly what is to be done. It reinforces our contention that even if assays are to be done by collaborators, psychologists must know enough of the procedures to make sure that they meet their needs.

5.10.6   *Effects of some chemicals on others*

When a biochemical value is measured, it is also important to consider whether different biochemicals are independent. Psychologists may inadvertently interpret biochemical results as independent findings either when they affect each other or when they are indices of a single process. For example, if two chemicals are both products of the same precursor, their values will be correlated. Treating related variables as independent will lead to false statistical power and potential misinterpretation of findings.

5.11 CONSIDERATIONS BEFORE USING BIOCHEMICAL ASSAYS

The most important consideration for a psychologist before using biochemical assays is what biochemical measure is relevant to the question being addressed. Certainly, biochemical measures can add a valuable level of analysis to studies, but it is important, as with any measure, to have specific reasons and hypotheses that point to specific biochemicals to measure. A fish net approach is rarely worthwhile and usually provides reams of uninterpretable data. To decide what biochemicals are relevant to a particular investigation (e.g., catecholamines, corticosteroids, sex hormones, endogenous opioid peptides) may be obvious (e.g., sex hormones to assess menstrual cycle; catecholamines in stress studies) or may require library research and discussions with physiological psychologists, neuroendocrinologists, and biochemists.

Once specific biochemicals are identified, one must decide whether appropriate sample collection is practical. One also must decide a priori how the samples will be assayed (i.e., what specific assays) and who will perform the assays to determine the costs and logistics of every step from sample collection through final data analysis. The basic options are contracting to private laboratories; contracting to academic-based laboratories; collaborations; or doing the assays "yourself" or in your department. The option chosen is based on pragmatic concerns and cost-effectiveness.

We find that many psychologists are reluctant to set up a biochemistry laboratory in their psychology departments. There certainly are many problems to be solved, including finding a knowledgeable supervisor, training technicians, handling radiation, disposing of radioactive wastes, and handling toxic chemicals. However, there are psychologists being trained with this knowledge, and it can be extremely cost-effective to set up individual or departmental biochemistry laboratories. For example, costs for supplies and other consumables for catecholamine REA are currently roughly $15 per sample (excluding personnel). Yet private laboratories charge as much as $100 per sample. (This difference in costs is not just profit for the private laboratory. A beta-scintillation counter can cost upward of $25,000 and must be amortized. So too with expensive glass jars to hold the chromatography plates. These jars cost several hundred dollars each. The assay requires other equipment such as centrifuges, analytical balances, and freeze-driers. And private labs, unlike university departments, have rent and utility costs.) For one or two studies, it may be best to contract out. But if three or more investigators plan to incorporate biochemical measures into their work, it may be best (for cost-effectiveness and quality control) to hire a chemist for the psychology department. In addition, a departmental laboratory allows consultation for investigators and another means of education for students.

5.12 A NOTE ON COLLABORATION

At several points throughout this chapter, we have referred to a collaboration with a biochemist as a way to do assays or obtain technical information. The advice is still valid, but the collaboration need not be a one-way street with the chemist helping the psychologist and getting nothing in return. There are important ways in which psychologists can assist chemists.

Assays are a form of measurement. As with any set of measurements, the concepts of reliability and validity are applicable. Psychologists, grounded in psychometrics, can formalize these and related issues in ways that are not usually done for biochemical assays. Earlier we discussed pooled samples. If a chemist is given N samples from each of two groups, but pools the samples, with three replicates, only six composite samples need be tested. If the samples are kept distinct, with the same three replicates, $6 \times N$ samples need to be tested for group differences. The pooled samples have only between-replicate variance; the individual samples have both between-replicate and between-subject variances. The group means will be the same, but the standard errors will be very different. Psychologists should have no particular difficulty analyzing this type of data, and their analysis can add to the understanding of the phenomenon.

Assays such as REA and RIA rely on a count of radioactivity. Specifically, the counters keep track of how many radioactive disintegrations occur in a fixed period of time. Radioactive disintegrations are truly random events. The number that occur in a particular sample, in, say 60 s, will vary from one minute to the next. If each sample is counted for 5 min, the resulting measure will be an average (or possibly a sum) of 5 min-long counts. Modern machines (beta- or gamma-counters) will report not only each sample's count but a measure of variability, reflecting the differences from one 60-s count (or whatever measure is used as an internal time standard) to another. This additional source of variability is usually ignored and not reported in research reports; yet it can be very useful in assessing the reliability of an assay. It is yet another source of data that a psychologist, by training, can easily handle but is not part of the usual chemist's research repertoire.

The point is that psychologists' professional training has a contribution to make to the assay process. The points we have called cautions are as appropriately labeled opportunities. They are places where quantitative analytical skills can be applied to produce better data and data that are less ambiguous.

5.13   CONCLUSIONS

To understand behavior and thought requires multilevel assessment including sociology, epidemiology, social psychology, individual behavioral assessment, self-report measures, physiological responses, and biochemistry. Although biochemical measures are foreign to many psychologists, they should not be. The value of this level of analysis is unquestionable and the techniques are now available.

Because we are scientists and not mystics we share in the belief that behaviors and thoughts have associated biological and physiological events. As a profession we have argued against a simplistic reductionism that would convert all behavior and cognition to mere biological description. Now that modern theories and techniques enable us to measure a wide variety of biochemicals, we can incorporate biological and psychological information and begin to redeem the promise of an integrated biopsychological study of the human being.

REFERENCES

Baum, A. (1986a). *Chronic and extreme stress: Psychobiological mechanisms.* APA, Division of Health Psychology Research Award Lecture, American Psychological Association Annual Meeting, Washington, DC.

Baum, A. (1986b). Toxins, technology, and national disasters. In G. R. VandenBos & B. K. Bryant

(Eds.), *Cataclysms, Crises, and Catastrophes* (pp. 5–53). Washington, DC: American Psycholgical Association.

Baum, A., Fleming, R., & Singer, J. E. (1983). Coping with victimization by technological disaster. *Journal of Social Issues, 39*, 117–138.

Baum, A., Gatchel, R. J., & Schaeffer, M. A. (1983). Emotional, behavioral, and physiological effects of chronic stress at Three Mile Island. *Journal of Consulting and Clinical Psychology, 51*, 565–572.

Baum, A., Grunberg, N. E., & Singer, J. E. (1982). The use of psychological and neuroendocrinological measurements in the study of stress. *Health Psychology, 1*, 217–236.

Cacioppo, J. T., & Petty, R. E. (Eds.) (1983). *Social Psychophysiology: A Sourcebook*. New York: Guilford Press.

Cannon, W. B. (1929). *Bodily changes in pain, hunger, fear, and rage*. New York: Appleton-Century-Crofts.

Carrere, S., Evans, G., & Stokols, D. (1987). *Winter-over stress*. Paper presented at the NASA-NSF Conference: The human experience in Antarctica: Applications to life in space. Sunnyvale, CA. August.

Darwin, C. (1965). *The expression of the emotions in man and animals*. Chicago: University of Chicago Press. (Original work published 1872.)

Evans, G., Stokols, D., & Carrere, S. (1987). *Human Adaptation to Isolated and Confined Environments*. NASA Technical Report for NASA Grant NAG2-387.

Fleming, R., Baum, A., Reddy, D. M., & Gatchel, R. J. (1984). Behavioral and biochemical effects of job loss and unemployment stress. *Journal of Human Stress, 10*(1), 12–17.

Frankenhaeuser, M. (1973). *Experimental approaches to the study of catecholamines and emotion*. Reports from the Psychological Laboratories, University of Stockholm (392).

Frankenhaeuser, M., & Gardell, B. (1976). Underload and overload in working life: Outline of a multidisciplinary approach. *Journal of Human Stress, 2*, 35–46.

Gazzaniga, M. S. (1988). *Mind matters* (p. 175). Boston: Houghton Mifflin.

Glass, D. C., Krakoff, L. R., Contrada, R., Hilton, W. F., Kehoe, K., Manucci, E. G., Collins, C., Snow, B., & Elting, E. (1980). Effects of harrassment and competition upon cardiovascular and plasma catecholamine responses in Type A and Type B individuals. *Psychophysiology, 17*, 453–463.

Glass, D. C., & Singer, J. E. (1972). *Urban stress: Experiments on noise and social stressors*. New York: Academic Press.

Grunberg, N. E. (1986a). Behavioral and biological factors in the relationship between tobacco use and body weight. In E. S. Katkin & S. B. Manuck (Eds.), *Advances in behavioral Medicine* (Vol. 2, pp. 97–129). Greenwich, CT: JAI Press.

Grunberg, N. E. (1986b). Nicotine as a psychoactive drug: Appetite regulation. *Psychopharmacology Bulletin, 22*(3), 875–881.

Grunberg, N. E., Popp, K. A., Bowen, D. J., Nespor, S. M., Winders, S. E., & Eury, S. E. (1988). Effects of chronic nicotine administration on insulin, glucose, epinephrine, and norepinephrine. *Life Sciences, 42*, 161–170.

James, W. (1950). *The principles of psychology*. New York: Dover. (Original work published 1890.)

Krantz, D. S., & Manuck, S. B. (1984). Acute psychophysiologic reactivity and risk of cardiovascular disease: A review and methodologic critique. *Psychology Bulletin, 96*, 435–464.

Lacey, J. I. (1956). The evaluation of autonomic responses: Toward a general solution. *Annals of New York Academy of Sciences, 67*, 123–164.

Lazarus, R. S. (1966). *Psychological stress and the coping process*. New York: McGraw-Hill.

Levine, S. (1988). Stress and performance. In D. Druckman & J. Swets (Eds.), *Enhancing human performance: Issues, theories and techniques: Vol. 2. Background papers*. Washington, DC: Academy Press.

Mason, J. W. (1968). A review of psychoendocrine research on the sympathetic-adrenal medullary system. *Psychosomatic Medicine, 30*, 631.

Miller, N. E. (1961). Learning and performance motivated by direct stimulation of the brain. In D. E. Sheer (Ed.) *Electrical stimulation of the brain* (pp. 387–396). Austin: University of Texas Press.

Obrist, P. A. (1976). The cardiovascular-behavioral interaction – as it appears today. *Psychophysiology, 13*, 95–107.

Olds, J. & Milner, P. (1954). Positive reinforcement produced by electrical stimulation of septal area and other regions of rat brain. *Journal of Comparative Physiological Psychology, 47,* 419–427.

Pomerleau, O. F., & Pomerleau, C. S. (1984). Neuroregulators and the reinforcement of smoking: Towards a biobehavioral explanation. *Neuroscience & Biobehavioral Reviews, 8,* 503–513.

Schachter, S., & Singer, J. E. (1962). Cognitive, social, and physiological determinants of emotional state. *Psychological Review, 69,* 379–399.

Selye, H. (1956). *The stress of life.* New York: McGraw-Hill.

Singer, J. E., Lundberg, U., & Frankenhaeuser, M. (1978). Stress on the train: A study of urban commuting. In A. Baum, J. E. Singer, & S. Valins (Eds.), *Advances in environmental psychology; Vol. 1. The urban environment.* Hillsdale, NJ: Erlbaum.

Thompson, R. F. (1962). Role of the cerebral cortex in stimulus generalization. *Journal of Comparative Physiological Psychology, 55,* 279–287.

Thompson, R. F. (1965). The neural basis of stimulus generalization. In D. J. Mostofsky (Ed.) *Stimulus generalization* (pp. 154–178). Stanford, CA: Stanford University Press.

6 *Psychoneuroimmunology*

SUSAN KENNEDY, RONALD GLASER, AND
JANICE KIECOLT-GLASER

6.1 INTRODUCTION

During the last several years, empirical evidence has begun to accumulate
supporting the notion that psychological factors may significantly affect the body's
ability to combat or succumb to infection or disease. Moreover, the complex
interactions between the immune, nervous, and endocrine systems are just now
being realized. Although still in its infancy, psychoneuroimmunology has begun to
unravel some of these intricate interactions and has led to a clearer understanding
of the ways in which they operate.

As its name suggests, psychoneuroimmunology is a multidisciplinary science and,
as such, is both unique and important, enabling the amalgamation of several
seemingly diverse, yet intimately linked areas of study.

This chapter will attempt to provide an overview of some recent developments in
the field of human psychoneuroimmunology. Beginning with a summary of the
major cells of the human immune system and their functions, a general
examination of neuroendocrine–immune interactions will be presented; finally,
data implicating psychological and psychosocial factors in immunomodulation will
be discussed.

Although this chapter focuses on human psychoneuroimmunology, the reader
should be aware of the rather extensive animal literature (e.g., Borysenko &
Borysenko, 1982; Justice, 1985) and should consult this literature for any questions or
interest that may arise in this regard while reading this review.

6.2 THE HUMAN IMMUNE SYSTEM: BASIC ELEMENTS AND MECHANISMS

The human immune system is comprised of a variety of different cell types, each
having its own function, yet all highly interrelated and orchestrated with each other.
Although an in-depth view of the immune system is beyond the scope of this
chapter, a general overview will be presented that will serve as the basis for
understanding many concepts and empirical findings that follow.

Classically, the immune system has been functionally divided into two general
categories: nonspecific responses and specific responses (see Roitt, Brostoff, & Male,
1985). Nonspecific responses refer to the general bodily defenses that follow initial
contact with a pathogen and include the activation of phagocytic cells that engulf
and destroy the invading agent as well as the activation of Natural Killer (NK) Cells,
which continually monitor the body for infectious agents. If these nonspecific
responses fail to prevent infection, more specific immune responses are activated.
These responses include those mediated by lymphocytes, namely, antibody

Table 6.1. *Major cells of the human immune system*

Cell type	Origin	Primary functions
1. Helper/inducer T-lymphocytes	Thymus	Initiation of immune response; replicates upon contact with antigen; releases lymphokines that stimulate T-cell replication; activates antibody production by B-lymphocytes
2. Suppressor/cytotoxic T-lymphocytes	Thymus	Inhibition of immune responses, primarily by suppressive effects on B-cell antibody production
3. B-lymphocytes	Bone marrow (?)	Production of antibody that binds to antigen
4. Natural Killer Cells	?	Surveillance and destruction of virally infected and tumor cells; activated by interferon
5. Macrophages	Bone marrow	Phagocytosis and destruction of foreign substances; produce IL-1 that stimulates T-helper lymphocytes; presents antigens to T-lymphocytes

production by B-lymphocytes (referred to as humoral immunity) as well as responses mediated by T-lymphocytes (cellular immunity).

An important distinction between the two types of immune responses is that lymphocyte-mediated responses may involve "immunological memory." That is, initial contact with a pathogen may induce a memory for that pathogen, such that reexposure results in a less severe disease or no disease at all.

A more detailed description of the cells of the immune system and their functions follows; Table 6.1 summarizes each cell type, its origin, and function.

6.2.1   *Lymphocytes*

Lymphocytes constitute those cells of the immune system that originate in the thymus (thymus derived; T-lymphocytes). They also include mononuclear cells of the avian bursa of Fabricius (B-lymphocytes). Although the human equivalent of the bursa is unknown, one postulated site is the bone marrow. T-lymphocytes manufacture several important chemical substances that serve to initiate immune responses following initial contact with a foreign substance (antigens, pathogens, and other substances that elicit antibody formation). In addition, T-lymphocytes help activate the production of antibody from B-lymphocytes.

T-lymphocytes are further subdivided on the basis of their function. T-helper/ inducer cells, for example, are critical for the immune response, in that they assist in the production of antibody by B-lymphocytes. Helper/inducer cells also produce several important substances called lymphokines, each with diverse, yet crucial immunoenhancing properties. One such lymphokine is interleukin-2, a protein that promotes the replication of T-helper cells (and is sometimes referred to as T-cell growth factor), as well as T-lymphocytes destined to become killer cells (cytolytic T-lymphocytes). Gamma-interferon is a glycoprotein released from T-helper/inducer cells following initial contact with a virus or antigen. Its primary functions include increasing the lytic ability of tumor-destroying cells (NK cells) as well as the protection of cells from virus infection.

In addition to helper cells, one subclass of T-lymphocytes has the role of inhibiting or down regulating the immune response, primarily by effects on T-helper cells. These cells, termed T-suppressor/cytotoxic cells, inhibit B-lymphocytes primarily by the inhibition of antibody production.

It is possible to experimentally quantify the percentages of various kinds of blood cells by the use of commercially available monoclonal antibodies. Monoclonal antibodies are produced by the fusion of antigen-primed spleen cells and myeloma cells and are used for the identification of certain "markers" on the cell surface. For example, the CD4 marker indentifies helper/inducer lymphocytes; CD8 indentifies suppressor/cytotoxic cells.

In addition to quantification methods, T-lymphocytes are also widely studied from a functional perspective through the use of mitogens, substances that can induce lymphocyte proliferation. Mitogens are thought to represent a valid in vitro model of how cells might respond to antigens that are encountered naturally. The most commonly used mitogens include concanavalin A (Con A) and phytohemagglutinin (PHA), which can stimulate T-lymphocytes, and pokeweed mitogen (PWM), which can stimulate B-lymphocytes.

In contrast to T-cells, B-lymphocytes mature into plasma cells, whose primary function is the synthesis and secretion of antibody molecules that bind to specific antigens. In addition, B-cells are characterized by the presence of surface immunoglobulin (Ig), which can be detected by the use of flourescent antibodies. In one widely used immunological assay, indirect immunoflourescence, for example, serum or plasma to be tested is absorbed to antigen-producing cells. Antibody present in the serum will bind to a given specific antigen; identification and quantification of the antibody is revealed after absorption with a flourescent antibody complex to an immunoglobulin (e.g., to the IgG, IgA, or IgM). In this way, antibody levels (titers) in serum or plasma can be assessed.

6.2.2 *Natural Killer Cells*

Natural Killer Cells (NK cells) are cells whose primary function appears to be the surveillance and destruction of certain tumor cells and virally infected cells; they are believed to have a role in tumor surveillance. The lytic capacity of NK cells is significantly enhanced by gamma-interferon, primarily by the development of mature NK cells from progenitors; furthermore, NK cells are believed to produce interferon. In order to experimentally study the lytic ability of NK cells, peripheral blood lymphocytes are typically incubated with "target" cells (e.g., tumor cells) that are made radioactive using a label (e.g., 51Cr). Following incubation, cell supernatants are harvested, and the percentage of lysis of targets from cells is determined by the amount of radioactivity released from the lysed cells.

6.2.3 *Macrophages*

Macrophages are large, nonlymphoid cells whose primary function is the ingestion and degradation of foreign matter. In addition, macrophages may also present antigens to T-helper cells and may thereby initiate the cascade of events involved in the immune response (i.e., T-cell replication and lymphokine production, antibody stimulation from B-cells, etc.). This latter function appears to be related to the release of a chemical, interleukin-1 (IL-1), which upon release stimulates T-cells and triggers their replication.

6.3   NEUROENDOCRINE–IMMUNE INTERACTIONS

The cells of the immune system are now recognized as interacting not only with one another, but also with the nervous and endocrine systems. This complex neuroendocrine–immune network has prompted several investigations into the mechanisms that govern such interactions and has led to a clearer understanding of the ways in which these systems may communicate. Some of these possible communicative channels will be described in what follows, including the immune system's interaction with the hypothalamic-pituitary axis, the existence of receptors on lymphoid tissue, and neurotransmitter innervation of certain lymphoid organs.

One of the primary mechanisms by which the nervous system interacts with the immune system is by the release of neurohormones, such as ACTH (adrenal corticotrophic hormone) from the pituitary.

Specifically, the hypothalamus, via corticotrophic releasing factor (CRF), triggers the release of pituitary ACTH, which subsquently signals the release of cortisol and other corticosteroid hormones from the adernal cortex. Levels of ACTH have been found to be sensitive to a variety of immune challenges, including psychological stress (e.g., Hennessy & Levine, 1979; Rose, 1980). Moreover, increased cortisol levels have been reported following prolonged strenuous physical activity as well as during biopsy and during or prior to surgery (see Rose, 1980, for a critical review).

Recently, Blalock and his colleagues (Blalock, Harbour-McMenamin, & Smith, 1985) have modified the "classic" concept of the hypothalamic–pituitary axis to include immune mechanisms. This modification is based primarily on the finding that ACTH is manufactured by lymphocytes and has immunosuppressive effects via the inhibition of gamma-interferon production by T-helper lymphocytes (Johnson, Torres, Smith, Dion, & Blalock, 1984). Blalock et al. (1985) have speculated that when the immune system encounters a viral agent or other antigen, hypothalamic CRF signals lymphocytes to produce ACTH. In this way, neural signaling by the hypothalamus is thought to represent one mechanism of communication with the neuroendocrine and immune systems.

In addition to interactions with the neuroendocrine system, lymphocytes have recently been found to express surface receptors for several neuroendocrine and neurotransmitter substances (Blalock, Bost, & Smith, 1985; O'Dorisio, Wood, & O'Dorisio, 1985; Pert, Ruff, Weber, & Herkenham, 1985; Russell et al., 1985; Wybran, Appelboom, Famaey, & Govaerts, 1979). For example, cholinergic receptors have been identified on lymphocytes (Lopker, Abood, Hoss, & Lionetti, 1980). In addition, lymphocytes possess surface receptors for several neuropeptides, including vasoactive intestinal peptide (VIP) and somatostatin (Bhathena, Schecter, Gazdan, Louie, & Recant, 1980; O'Dorisio et al., 1985; Pert et al., 1985; Recant, Voyles, Luciano, & Pert, 1981).

The opiate peptides (enkephalins, endorphins) have been targeted by investigators because of their influence on the immune system. In addition to their widespread distribution in both the central nervous system and in the periphery, lymphocytes appear not only to bear receptors for these neuropeptides, but also to produce substances similar to β-endorphin following certain viral infections (Smith & Blalock, 1981).

Functionally, the endorphins have been studied with respect to their effects on mitogen-stimulated lymphocytes and on the activity of NK cells. McCain and his colleagues (McCain, Lamster, & Bilotta, 1986), for example, have reported an inhibition of blastogenesis when β-endorphin was added to cultures containing phytohemagglutinin. However, since the inhibition was not blocked by the opiate antagonist naloxone, the authors concluded that the effects of β-endorphin were probably mediated by a nonopiate receptor. Other studies, however, have reported opposite effects. Thus, Weber and Pert (1984) have found enhancing effects of β-endorphin on lymphocyte proliferation to PHA as well as on the production of IL-2 from a mouse-derived T-cell line. Both of these effects were reversed by naloxone. Similarly, Plotnikoff and Miller (1983) reported enhanced blastogenesis with PHA with both leu- and met-enkephalin.

The ability of NK cells to lyse targets is also affected by opiates. Lysis has been found to increase significantly when β-endorphin is added to cultures of human lymphocytes and target cells (Kay, Allen, & Morley, 1984; Mathews, Froelich, Sibbit, & Bankhurst, 1983); similar results are obtained with met-enkephalin (Mathews et al., 1983).

Quite recently, Pert and her colleagues (1985) have demonstrated that human monocytes (progenitors of macrophages) will chemotax toward opiates. That is, monocytes will migrate toward opiates (as well as toward other neuropeptides) when placed in an experimental chamber. Importantly, chemotaxis is blocked when the specific antagnoist to the neuropeptide is added. Pert et al. suggest that the existence of opiate receptors on immune cells may represent a communication medium between the central nervous system and the immune system.

Finally, the nervous and immune systems may communicate by way of direct neurotransmitter innervation of lymphoid tissue. For example, immune tissue receives input from the sympathetic autonomic nervous system (Besedovsky, del Rey, Sorkin, Da Prada, & Keller, 1979), as evidenced by altered immune responses following pharmacologic manipulation of the innervating fibres. In a recent report, Felten and his colleagues (Felten, Felten, Carlson, Olschowka, & Livnat, 1985) have demonstrated noradrenergic nerve terminals on several lymphoid structures, including the thymus, bone marrow, and spleen. Terminal endings were located close to lymphocytes and macrophages as well as other cell types. Felten et al. suggest that the presence of noradrenergic nerve terminals may serve to communicate with receptors located on adjacent cells (e.g., on lymphocytes).

In addition to noradrenergic innervation, lymphoid tissue may be innervated by neuropeptides, including VIP and met-enkephalin (Felten et al., 1985). Such innervation may serve as a communicative link with neuropeptide receptors on the surface of lymphocytes and demonstrates another potential mechanism by which the nervous, endocrine, and immune systems are intricately orchestrated.

Given these mechanisms, it now becomes important to examine the ways in which psychological stressors may influence immune function.

6.4   PSYCHOLOGICAL AND PSYCHOSOCIAL FACTORS AND IMMUNITY: LINKS
       BETWEEN STRESS AND HEALTH

The notion that psychological stress may increase an individual's susceptibility to infection or disease has, until quite recently, been highly speculative. Over the last several years, however, an impressive amount of empirical data has begun to accumulate suggesting the link between psychological/psychosocial factors and immune competence.

6.4.1   Major life events and immune function

In an early study of the effects of psychological stress on immunity, Bartrop and his colleagues (Bartrop, Luckhurst, Lazarus, Kiloh, & Penny, 1977) examined lymphocyte function in bereaved individuals subsequent to the death of a spouse. Relative to controls, lymphocytes from the bereaved subjects showed depressed responses to the mitogens Con A and PHA 6 weeks following the spouse's death. Because these changes occurred despite no differences in T-cell or B-cell number, immunoglobulins, or serum concentrations of several hormones, they are presumed to reflect *functional* alterations in lymphocytes rather than quantitative changes.

Using a prospective design, Schliefer and his associates (Schliefer, Keller, Camerino, Thornton, & Stein, 1983) investigated lymphocyte responses to mitogens in bereaved men both prior to and following the death of their wives from advanced breast cancer. Depressed responses to Con A, PHA, and PWM were found following the loss of the spouse relative to prebereavement levels. Because the same subjects were studied both during baseline and postbereavement, the depression in cell function is assumed to reflect the psychological stress associated with spousal death rather than an already existing depression resulting from the stress of terminal illness of a loved one. Importantly, as the authors note, stress associated with the spouse's terminal illness did not result in recovery of normal lymphocyte function (i.e., habituation) prior to the death of the spouse, indicating that the observed immune responses were a direct consequence of the stressful event.

One important question regarding stress-related immune changes involves the extent to which individuals may adapt to more chronic stressors in their environments; that is, when confronted with a stressor over relatively long time periods, does the immune system adapt and subsequently resume "more normal" levels of function? In order to assess this possibility, Kiecolt-Glaser and her colleagues (1987) have examined immune function in recently divorced or separated women. Marital satisfaction has been shown to be one of the most important contributors to an individual's overall happiness and psychological well-being (Glenn & Weaver, 1981); indeed, increases in illness and medical problems as well as increased mortality from infectious disease are reliably reported following the disruption of a marriage (Lynch, 1977; Somers, 1979; Verbrugge, 1979).

Kiecolt-Glaser et al. (1987) analyzed responses from separated or divorced (S/D) women and married controls on several psychological inventories, including the Brief Symptom Inventory (BSI; Derogatis & Spencer, 1982), the UCLA Loneliness Scale (Russell, Peplau, & Cutrona, 1980), Kitson's attachment scale (Kitson, 1982), and the Dyadic Adjustment Scale (Spanier, 1976), an index of marital quality. Lymphocyte function and numbers were assessed using several immunological assays. Separated or divorced women who had been more recently separated

Table 6.2. *Mean[a] for 16 women who were separated 1 year or less and 16 matched married controls*

	Separated-divorced women	Married women
EBV VCA[b]	520.50 (706.84)	147.12 (191.88)
Percentage of helper T-lymphocytes[b]	26.43 (7.59)	32.91 (7.03)
Percentage of suppressor T-lymphocytes	20.01 (6.70)	22.66 (7.76)
Helper-suppressor ratio	1.49 (0.66)	1.69 (1.47)
Percentage of NK cells[b]	7.50 (5.05)	12.79 (8.05)

[a] Plus or minus standard deviation, in parentheses.
[b] $p < 0.05$
Source: From "Marital quality, marital disruption, and immune function," by J. K. Kiecolt-Glaser, L. D. Fisher, P. Ogrocki, J. C. Stout, C. E. Speicher, and R. Glaser, *Psychosomatic Medicine*, Vol. 49, pp. 13–34. (Reprinted by permission of Elsevier Science Publishing Co., Inc. Copyright 1987 by the American Psychosomatic Society, Inc.)

(within 1 year of testing) were found to have significantly poorer immune function than married controls; specifically, lymphocytes from the S/D women showed poorer blastogenic responses to the mitogens Con A and PHA, indicating a deficit in the potential of cells to respond to naturally occurring antigens. Moreover, as shown in Table 6.2, separated women had significantly lower percentages of T-helper lymphocytes as well as lower percentages of NK cells. In addition, S/D women were found to have higher antibody titers to the Epstein–Barr Virus (EBV) virus capsid antigen (VCA), a human herpes virus that causes infectious mononucleosis. Elevated antibody titers to EBV are found in individuals undergoing chemotherapy as well as in persons with certain immunosuppressive disorders and are thought to reflect poorer cellular immune competence in holding the virus in check.

These data are in accord with epidemiological studies linking marital disruption to increased health risks (Verbrugge, 1979). It is noteworthy that the degree of attachment to the (ex)husband was found to be a significant indicator of psychological state, as well as immune function, with greater attachment predicting greater depression and compromised immune function. Previous studies have also pointed to the importance of healthy interpersonal relationships for both psychological and immunological well-being (e.g., Glaser, Kiecolt-Glaser, Speicher, & Holliday, 1985; Kiecolt-Glaser et al., 1984a, b) and suggest that such relationships may have health-related consequences.

In a follow-up study (Kiecolt-Glaser et al., 1988), S/D men and married controls were studied on several psychological and immunological measures. Separated or divorced men were found to have significantly higher antibody titers to EBV VCA as well as higher titers to herpes simplex virus. Moreover, S/D men were significantly more depressed than their matched controls and reported significantly more illness in the 2 months preceding the test session.

In a related study assessing chronic stressors and immune function, family caregivers of victims of Alzheimer's disease were studied (Kiecolt-Glaser et al., 1987). Alzheimer's disease is an irreversible degenerative disease of the central nervous system characterized in later stages by severe memory loss, incontinence, and an inability to care for oneself (Heckler, 1985; Reisberg, 1983). Because the time course of the disease is lengthy, with a modal survival time of 8 years after onset, caregiving by family members may well be considered a chronic stressor. Caring for a victim of Alzheimer's has been reported to be associated with clinical depression (Eisdorfer, Kennedy, Wisnieski, & Cohen, 1983); in addition, self-report data from caregivers has suggested that as the afflicted family member becomes progressively more impaired, there is a corresponding decrease in life satisfaction on the part of the caregiver as well as increases in their psychiatric symptoms (George & Gwyther, 1984).

In our study, psychological and immunological data from 34 caregivers and 34 sociodemographically matched control subjects were assessed. Caregiving time in the study ranged from 9 months to 16 years, with mean caregiving time of 5.45 years. Consistent with previous studies (Eisdorfer et al., 1983; George & Gwyther, 1984), caregivers reported greater psychological distress and greater loneliness than controls; in addition, caregivers had significantly lower percentages of total lymphocytes, lower percentages of T-helper cells, and higher antibody titers to EBV VCA.

Collectively, these data suggest that there is not measurable immunological or psychological adaptation to the level of well-matched comparison subjects to two long-term stressors. An important question that arises when one considers the existing literature on chronic stressors and immune competence is whether such stressors are associated with changes in health status (e.g., frequency of illness throughout the course of a divorce,). Unfortunately, there are no data at present that are sufficient to answer this question. What is clearly needed in the area of human psychoneuroimmunology are studies aimed at following the same individuals over long periods of time, with psychological and immunological assessments made at various points. In addition, these studies must include medical examinations and neuroendocrine assessments in order to provide a complete health profile on the individuals being studied.

In the two sections that follow, data will be presented suggesting that more short-term, acute stressors may also have adverse effects on T-lymphocyte function as well as on the ability of NK cells to monitor that body for potentially carcinogenic cells.

6.4.2   Stress and cancer

Carcinogens are present in various forms in the environment. For example, many foods, such as meat, are processed with nitrites, and pesticide residues exist on fresh fruits and vegetables. Sunlight emits potentially harmful radiation while industrial by-products provide carcinogenic chemicals to the air (Miller, 1978). Although ubiquitous, however, exposure to carcinogens is usually limited or at levels below that which is cancer producing.

The mechanism by which carcinogenic agents produce cancer is believed to be via damage to cellular DNA. Once altered, the DNA may either undergo repair or remain impaired, thereby producing a mutant (cancerous) cell that subsequently proliferates (Setlow, 1978). Once transformed, the mutant cells may be destroyed by immune surveillance, for example, by NK cells (Herberman, 1982; Herberman et al., 1982). Hence, the body may respond to carcinogen exposure both by activation of an intracellular repair process and by the surveillance and destruction of tumors by NK cells.

To examine a possible direct relationship between psychological stress and carcinogenesis, 28 newly admitted, nonpsychotic, nonmedicated psychiatric patients were divided into high- and how-distress subgroups based on their responses to the Depression Scale of the MMPI (Minnesota Multiphasic Personality Inventory; Kiecolt-Glaser, Stephens, Lipetz, Speicher, & Glaser, 1985). Lymphocytes from both groups were exposed to X-irradiation in order to damage cellular DNA. High distress was found to be associated with poorer DNA repair, whereas better DNA repair was associated with low distress. These stress-related deficits in DNA repair may have critical implications in terms of the etiology of cancer cells. In addition, when lymphocytes are confronted with an antigen, they typically respond by increases in cellular DNA and subsequent proliferation. These responses aid in attacking the foreign invader and thereby in warding off disease. Impairments in DNA may therefore limit the cell's ability to divide and combat infection.

In a similar vein, it has been found that psychiatric patients may be more susceptible to cancer (Ernster, Sacks, Selvin, & Petrakis, 1979; Fox, 1979) and that high MMPI depression scores are associated with a higher incidence of cancer (Shekelle et al., 1981).

As previously mentioned, impaired cellular DNA may result in the transformation of cells to a mutant state, which may involve subsequent destruction by NK cells. Recent data suggest that the ability of NK cells to destroy tumors may be adversely affected by psychological stress (Aarstad, Gaundernack, & Seljelid, 1983; Herberman, 1982; Kiecolt-Glaser et al., 1984a,b; 1986; Shavit, Lewis, Terman, Gale, & Liebeskind, 1984). In one such study, for example (Locke, Kraus, & Leserman, 1984), college students reporting limited psychological distress despite high levels of life change stress had higher NK cell activity than students reporting high psychological stress. More recently, Glaser and his colleagues (Glaser, Rice, Speicher, Stout, & Kiecolt-Glaser, 1986) examined NK activity and total NK in second-year medical students during final examinations as well as 6 weeks before exams. As shown in Figure 6.1, NK cell lysis significantly decreased during examinations relative to baseline at all effector-to-target-cell ratios. In addition to the impaired NK lysis, the percentage of NK cells (as determined by using a monoclonal antibody) decreased during examinations. Concomitant with deficits in NK cell number and activity, interferon levels produced by mitogen-stimulated lymphocytes were also found to decrease significantly during examinations (Table 6.3). Interferons are glycoproteins that are produced by cells upon viral infection or antigenic or mitogenic stimulation. Upon release from a stimulated cell, interferon binds to surface receptors on adjacent cells, thereby triggering the synthesis of proteins aimed at destroying the virus. One well-documented function of interferon is its enhancement of NK cell lysis (e.g., Herberman et al., 1982) by activation of NK precursors into a lytic state. Stress-associated decreases in interferon levels, therefore, may clearly have adverse consequences for immune competence via effects on NK cells.

Self-report data confirmed that examinations were more stressful as compared to baseline. These data imply that relatively commonplace stressful events may have serious effects for immune function. Stress-induced deficits in NK cells may ultimately result in poorer surveillance and destruction of transformed cells. Collectively, the data suggest that psychological stress and its concomitant alterations in cellular immunity may increase the susceptibility of individuals to

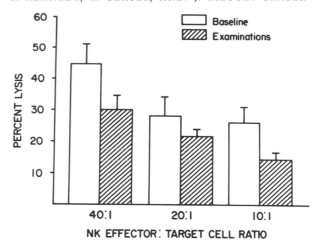

Figure 6.1. Means (plus or minus SEM) for percent lysis of MOLT-4 cells for three NK effector-to-target-cell ratios at baseline and during examinations. (Copyright 1986 by the American Psychological Association. Reprinted by permission of the publisher and author.)

Table 6.3. *Means^a of IFNs produced by PBLs stimulated with Con A and plasma IFN levels at baseline and during examinations*

Sample	Leukocyte IFNs (U/ml)	Plasma IFNs (U/ml)
Basline		
M	2,003.03	0
SE	179.13	0
Examination		
M	80.00	0
SE	17.99	0

^{a} Plus or minus standard error (SE); *M*, mean.
Note: Abbreviations: IFN, interferon; PBL, peripheral blood leukocytes. Reprinted by permission of the publisher and author. Copyright 1986 by the American Psychological Association.

infection or to malignant disease either via faulty repair of cellular DNA or by impairments in NK cells to monitor and destroy mutant cells.

6.4.3   *Minor life events and immunity*

In the preceding section on psychological factors and immunity, recent findings were documented that support the link between major stressful life events and suppressed immune function. Fortunately, such major life events are generally not encountered with any regularity throughout the course of one's lifetime; rather, smaller scale "minor" stressors are far more common. Given the frequency with

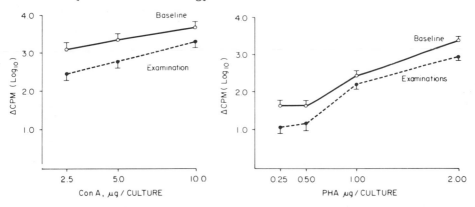

Figure 6.2. Mean (Plus or minus SEM) T-lymphocyte response to mitogen stimulation at baseline and during examinations. (Reprinted by permission of Elsevier Science Publishing Co., Inc., from "Stress-Related Impairments in Cellular Immunity," by R. Glaser, J. K. Kiecolt-Glaser, K. L. Tarr, C. E. Speicher, J. E. Holliday, *Psychiatry Research*, Vol. 16, pp. 233–239, Copyright 1985 by Elsevier Science Publishers, B. V.)

which minor stressors are encountered, it is important to examine their influence on the immune system and on health.

For the last several years, our laboratory has been involved in the study of one commonplace stressor, academic examinations and their impact on immune function (e.g., Glaser et al., 1986; Kiecolt-Glaser et al., 1986). Medical students at Ohio State take examinations concurrently as a group, making for ideal experimental conditions.

Psychological and immunological data are obtained from 30 first-year medical students at six sample points over the course of the academic year. The first, third, and fifth of these samples occur approximately 1 month prior to exams (baseline), whereas the second, fourth, and sixth occur during examinations (stress). Such a design enables data from the same students to be compared in pairs (i.e., in three sets of baseline–stress dyads) over relatively long periods of time (one academic year).

In addition to the aforementioned deficits in NK cell activity associated with examinations (see section 4.2), several other indices of immunosuppression have reliably been documented in our medical student population during exams. For example, lymphocyte responses to two mitogens (Con A and PHA) are consistently and significantly lower relative to baseline tests (Glaser et al., 1985; see Figure 6.2). Furthemore, percentages of T-helper and T-suppressor cells are often found to be lower during exams, which may indicate a functional deficit in these cell types. Importantly, although these changes are not associated with any *major* illnesses in the students, there are self-reported increases in upper respiratory tract infections during exams. Concomitant with these immune changes, responses on psychological inventories support the stressful nature of the exams.

These data are important, as they demonstrate that the immune system is sensitive to relatively minor life events and the psychological stress associated with these events may ultimately result in an immunocompromised state. Moreover, it is critical to keep in mind that medical students are quite adept at test taking and yet are significantly immunosuppressed. Given a not-so-healthy population, however (e.g., the elderly), such minor life stressors and the psychological and immune changes associated with them might, in fact, result in increased incidence of overt physical illness, infectious disease, or cancer (Glaser et al., 1985).

6.5   CONCLUDING COMMENTS

Although a relatively new discipline, psychoneuroimmunology has already begun to shed light on the complex interactions between the nervous, endocrine, and immune systems. This multifaceted approach is long overdue and promises to increase our knowledge as to how these systems work together in health and in disease.

For example, the links between psychological distress and suppressed immune function are becoming well recognized. What remains to be learned, however, are the mechanisms that operate in individuals during long periods of stress: These mechanisms may include neuroendocrine changes, changes in lymphocyte receptor number or sensitivity, or alterations in lymphokine levels that have feedback consequences on levels of circulating neuroendocrines. Clearly, the need for such longitudinal studies is imperative to understand the effects of chronic stressors on immune function.

In addition to the need for longitudinal efforts, other important questions remain unanswered. These include how individual "coping" mechanisms are manifested in immune function, how neurotransmitters interact with lymphocytes and lymphokines in both acute and chronic stress, and how stress that is experienced early in development affects later immune function.

REFERENCES

Aarstad, H. J., Gaundernack, G., & Seljelid, R. (1983). Stress causes reduced NK activity in mice. *Scandinavian Journal of Immunology, 18*, 461–464.

Bartrop, R. W., Luckhurst, E., Lazarus, L., Kiloh, L. G., & Penny, R. (1977). Depressed lymphocyte function after bereavement. *Lancet, 1*, 834–836.

Basedovsky, H. O., Del Rey, A., Sorkin, E., Da Prada, M., & Keller, H. H. (1979). Immunoregulation mediated by the sympathetic nervous system. *Cellular Immunology, 48*, 346–355.

Bhathena, S. J., Louie, J., Schecter, P. P., Redman, R. S., Wahl, L., & Recant, L. (1980). Identification of human mononuclear leukocytes bearing receptors for somatostatin and glucagon. *Diabetes, 30*, 127–131.

Blalock, J. E., Bost, K. L., & Smith, E. M. (1985). Neuroendocrine peptide hormones and their receptors in the immune system. *Journal of Neuroimmunology, 10*, 31–40.

Blalock, J. E., Harbour-McMenamin, D., & Smith, E. M. (1985). Peptide hormones shared by the neuroendocrine and immunologic systems. *Journal of Immunology, 135*, 858–861.

Borysenko, M., & Borysenko, J. (1982). Stress, behavior, and immunity: Animal models and mediating mechanisms. *General Hospital Psychiatry, 4*, 59–67.

Derogatis, L. R., & Spencer, P. M. (1982). *The Brief Symptom Inventory (BSI), administration, scoring, and procedures manual I.* Baltimore: Clinical Psychometrics Research.

Eisdorfer, C., Kennedy, G., Wisnieski, W., & Cohen, D. (1983). Depression and attributional style in families coping with the stress of caring for a relative with Alzheimer's Disease. *Gerontologist, 23*, 115–116.

Ernster, V. L., Sacks, S. T., Selvin, S., & Petrakis, N. L. (1979). Cancer incidence by marital status: U.S. Third National Cancer Survey. *Journal of the National Cancer Institute, 63*, 567–585.

Felten, D. L., Felten, S. Y., Carlson, S. L., Olschowka, J. A., & Livnat, S. (1985). Noradrenergic and peptidergic innervation of lymphoid tissue. *Journal of Immunology, 135*, 755–765.

Fox, B. H. (1978). Cancer death risk in hospitalized mental patients. *Science, 201,* 966–967.

George, L. K,. & Gwyther, L. P. (1984). *The dynamics of caregiver burden: Changes in caregiver well-being over time.* Paper presented at the annual meeting of the Gerontological Society of America, San Antonio.

Glaser, R., Kiecolt-Glasser, J. K., Speicher, C. E., & Holliday, J. E. (1985). Stress, loneliness, and changes in herpesvirus latency. *Journal of Behavioral Medicine, 8,* 249–260.

Glaser, R., Kiecolt-Glaser, J. K., Stout, J. C., Tarr, K. L., Speicher, C. E., & Holliday J. E. (1985). Stress-related impairments in cellular immunity. *Psychiatry Research, 16,* 233–239.

Glaser, R., Rice, J., Speicher, C. E., Stout, J. C., & Kiecolt-Glaser, J. K. (1986). Stress depresses interferon production by leukocytes concomitant with a decrease in natural killer cell activity. *Behavioral Neuroscience, 100,* 675–678.

Glenn, N. D., & Weaver, C. N. (1981). The contribution of marital happiness to global happiness. *Journal of Marriage and Family, 43,* 161–168.

Heckler, M. M. (1985). The fight against Alzheimer's disease. *American Psychologist, 40,* 1240–1244.

Hennessy, J. W., & Levine, S. (1979). Stress, arousal and the pituitary-adrenal system: A psychoendocrine hypothesis. *Progress in psychobiology and physiological psychology, 8,* 133–178.

Herberman, R. B. (1982). Possible effects of central nervous system on natural killer (NK) cell activity. In S. M. Levy (Ed.), *Biological mediators of behavior and disease: Neoplasia* (pp. 235–248). New York: Elsevier.

Herberman, R. B., Ortaldo, J. R., Riccardi, C., Timonen, T., Schmidt, A., Maluish, A., & Djeu, J. (1982). Interferon and NK cells. In T. C. Merigan & R. M. Friedman (Eds.). *Interferons* (pp. 278–294). London: Academic Press.

Johnson, H. M., Torres, B. A., Smith, E. M., Dion, L. D., & Blalock, J. E. (1984). Regulation of lymphokine (γ-interferon) production by corticotropin. *Journal of Immunology, 132,* 246–250.

Justice, A. (1985). Review of the effects of stress on cancer in laboratory animals: Importance of time of stress application and type of tumor. *Psychological Bulletin, 98,* 108–138.

Kay, N., Allen, J., & Morley, J. E. (1984). Endorphins stimulate normal human peripheral blood lymphocyte natural killer activity. *Life Sciences, 35,* 53–59.

Kiecolt-Glaser, J. K., Fisher, L. D., Ogrocki, P., Stout, J. C., Speicher, C. E., & Glaser, R. (1987). Marital quality, marital disruption, and immune function. *Psychosomatic Medicine, 49,* 13–34.

Kiecolt-Glaser, J. K., Garner, W., Speicher, C. E., Penn, G. M., Holliday, J. E., & Glaser, R. (1984a). Psychosocial modifiers of immunocompetence in medical students. *Psychosomatic Medicine, 46,* 7–14.

Kiecolt-Glaser, J. K., Glaser, R., Shuttleworth, E. C., Dyer, C. S., Ogrocki, P., & Speicher, C. E. (1987). Chronic stress and immunity in family caregivers of Alzheimer's disease victims. *Psychosomatic Medicine, 49,* 523–535.

Kiecolt-Glaser, J. E., Glaser, R., Strain, E. C., Stout, J. C., Tarr, K. L., Holliday, J. E., & Speicher, C. E. (1986). Modulation of cellular immunity in medical students. *Journal of Behavioral Medicine, 9,* 5–21.

Kiecolt-Glaser, J. E., Kennedy, S., Malkoff, S., Fisher, L., Speicher, C. E., & Glaser, R. (1988). Marital discord and immunity in males. *Psychosomatic Medicine, 50,* 213–229.

Kiecolt-Glaser, J. K., Ricker, D., Messick, G., Speicher, C. E., Garner, W., & Glaser, R. (1984b). Urinary cortisol, cellular immunocompetency and loneliness in psychiatric inpatients. *Psychosomatic Medicine, 46,* 15–24.

Kiecolt-Glaser, J. K., Stephens, R. E., Lipetz, R. D., Speicher, C. E., & Glaser, R. (1985). Distress and DNA repair in human lymphocytes. *Journal of Behavioral Medicine, 8,* 311–320.

Kitson, G. C. (1982). Attachment to the spouse in divorce: A scale and its application. *Journal of Marriage and Family, 44,* 379–393.

Locke, S. E., Kraus, L., & Leserman, J. (1984). Life change, stress, psychiatric symptoms and natural killer cell activity. *Psychosomatic Medicine, 46,* 441–453.

Lopker, A., Abood, L. G., Hoss, W., & Lionetti, F. J. (1980). Stereoselective muscarinic acetylcholine and opiate receptors in human phagocytic leukocytes. *Biochemical Pharmacology, 29,* 1361–1365.

Lynch, J. (1977). *The broken heart.* New York: Basic Books.

Maclean, D., & Reichlin, S. (1981). Neuroendocrinology and the immune response. In R. Ader (Ed.), *Psychoneuroimmunology.* New York: Academic Press.

Mathews, P. M., Forelich, C. J., Sibbit, W. L., & Bankkhurst, A. D. (1983). Enhancement of natural cytotoxicity by B-endorphin. *Journal of Immunology, 130,* 1658–1662.

McCain, H. W., Lamster, I. B., & Bilotta, J. (1986). Immunosuppressive effects of the opiopeptins. In N. P. Plotnikoff, R. E. Faith, A. J. Murgo & R. A. Good (Eds.), *Enkephalins and endorphins: Stress and the immune system.* New York: Plenum Press.

Miller, E. C. (1978). Some current perspectives on chemical carcinogenesis in humans and experimental animals: Presidential address. *Cancer Research, 38,* 1479–1496.

O'Dorisio, M. S., Wood, C. L., & O'Dorisio, T. M. (1985). Vasoactive intestinal peptide and neuropeptide modulation of the immune response. *Journal of Immunology, 135,* 792–796.

Pert, C. B., Ruff, M. R., Weber, R. J., & Herkenham, M. (1985). Neuropeptides and their receptors: A psychosomatic network. *Journal of Immunology, 135,* 820–826.

Plotnikoff, N. P., & Miller, G. C. (1983). Enkephalins as immunomodulators. *International Journal of Immunopharmacology, 5,* 437–444.

Recant, L., Voyles, N. R., Luciano, M., & Pert, C. B. (1981). Naltrexone reduces weight gain, alters "B-endorphin" and reduces insulin output from pancreatic islets of genetically obese mice. *Peptides, 1,* 309–313.

Reisberg, B. (Ed.). (1983). *Alzheimer's disease: The standard reference.* New York: Free Press.

Roitt, I., Brostoff, J., & Male, D. (1985). *Immunology.* St. Louis: Mosby.

Rose, R. M. (1980). Endocrine responses to stressful psychological events. *Psychiatric Clinics of North America, 3,* 251–276.

Russell, D., Peplau, L. A., & Cutrona, C. B. (1980). The revised UCLA loneliness scale: Concurrent and discriminant validity evidence. *Journal of Personality and Social Psychology, 39,* 472–480.

Russell, D. H., Kibler, R., Matrisian, L., Larson, D. F., Poulos, B., & Magun, B. E. (1985). Prolactin receptors of human T and B lymphocytes: Antagonism of prolactin binding by cyclosporine. *Journal of Immunology, 134,* 3027–3031.

Schliefer, S. J., Keller, S. E., Camerino, M., Thornton, J. C., & Stein, M. (1983). Suppression of lymphocyte stimulation following bereavement. *Journal of the American Medical Association, 250,* 374–377.

Setlow, R. B. (1978). Repair deficient human disorders and human cancer. *Nature* (London), *271,* 713–717.

Shavit, Y., Lewis, J. W., Terman, G. W., Gale, R. P., & Liebeskind, J. C. (1984). Opioid peptides mediate the suppressive effect of stress of natural killer cell cytotoxicity. *Science, 223,* 188–190.

Shekelle, R. B., Raynor, W. J., Ostfeld, A. M., Garron, D. C., Bieliauskas, L. A., Liv, S. C., Maliza, C., & Paul, O. (1981). Psychological depression and the 17 year risk of cancer. *Psychosomatic Medicine, 43,* 117–125.

Smith, E. M., & Blalock, J. E. (1981). Human leukocyte production of ACTH and endorphin-like substances: Association with leukocyte interferon. *Proceedings of the National Academy of Sciences, USA, 78,* 7530–7534.

Somers, A. R. (1979). Marital status, health, and use of health services. *Journal of the American Medical Association, 241,* 1818–1822.

Spanier, G. B . (1976). Measuring dyadic adjustment: New scales for assessing the quality of marriage and similar dyads. *Journal of Marriage and Family, 38,* 15–28.

Verbrugge, L. M. (1979). Marital status and health. *Journal of Marriage and Family, 41,* 267–285.

Weber, R. J., & Pert, C. B. (1984). Opiatergic modulation of the immune system. In E. E. Miller & A. R. Ganazzani (Eds.), *Central and peripheral endorphins: Basic and clinical aspects.* New York: Raven Press.

Wybran, J., Appelboom, T., Famaey, J., & Govaerts, A. (1979). Suggestive evidence for receptors for morphine and methionine-enkephalin on normal human blood T lymphocytes. *Journal of Immunology, 123,* 1068–1070.

PART II

General concepts

7 *Response patterning*

ROBERT M. STERN AND CECILE ELISE E. SISON

> Our knowledge of somatic patterns is very meager indeed. I think we do know
> enough of them, however, to say that earlier guesses of one, two, or three modes of
> variation are a long way short of the facts. Tangled as the relations are, there is an
> assuring hope for us in their very complexity. The peripheral patterns may provide
> us with a way of exposing to direct light the wealth of intermediate processes that we
> can suspect in a person, but cannot otherwise see. (Davis, 1957, p. 738)

An understanding of the principles that contribute to the spatial and temporal
responses patterning within and across neural, muscular, and humoral systems is
vital in order to interpret properly the results of psychophysiological studies and to
begin to uncover the intermediate processes referred to by Davis. In the first part of
this chapter we highlight some of the principles the contribute to the patterning of
bodily responses, with a special emphasis on the patterning that is observed within
the autonomic nervous system (ANS). In the latter portion of the chapter we discuss
tendencies to respond that are idiosyncratic to the individual and, therefore, of
particular relevance to the understanding of research in the areas of personality,
psychopathology, and behavioral medicine.

7.1 TYPES OF PSYCHOPHYSIOLOGICAL RESPONSES

Research involving psychophysiological responding primarily consists of discrete
responses to a specific stimulus, *phasic responses.* However, background electrical
activity – *tonic activity* – is always present, and *spontaneous responses or nonspecific*
responses occasionally appear even when it may seem that the subject is relaxing or
asleep.

7.1.1 *Tonic activity*

Tonic activity is often referred to as the background level or resting level of activity
of a particular physiological measure. However, resting level is not a good
description of tonic activity because what is really being discussed is the level of
activity when a subject is (1) not making a spontaneous response and (2) not making
a discrete response to a known stimulus. The subject might be very highly aroused
and certainly not resting. For example, the tonic level of one individual's heart rate
while waiting in the dentist's office for a root canal procedure might be 130 beats per
minute. Another subject, perhaps not so anxious about dental work, might have a
tonic level of heart rate in the same situation of 80 beats per minute. Thus, tonic

193

level is simply the level of activity of some response measure at a particular point in time prior to stimulation.

There are two separate reasons for determining tonic level. In the first place, tonic level is of interest in its own right as a measure of the activity of physiological systems when the subject is not responding to a specific stimulus. In such cases, the level is a complex result of many factors, including central nervous system (CNS) reactions to environmental and internal stimuli and the delicate balance between the sympathetic nervous system (SNS) and the parasympathetic nervous system (PNS). People with essential hypertension and tension headaches are examples of individuals who may have extremely high tonic levels. Individuals with essential hypertension may have high blood pressure due to elevated levels of SNS activity (Schneiderman & Hammer, 1985). Muscle potential recordings from some individuals who suffer from frequent tension headaches reveal that even when they do not have headaches, the muscles of their head and/or neck show higher levels of activity than those of people who do not have tension headaches (Malmo & Shagass, 1949).

The second reason tonic level is of interest is that in some cases the size of a response to a specific stimulus (the phasic response) depends upon the tonic level as measured immediately prior to the stimulus. This relationship is referred to as the law of initial values and is discussed later in this chapter.

7.1.2   Phasic activity

Phasic activity is a discrete response to a specific stimulus – an evoked response. Phasic activity can be an increase or decrease in frequency or amplitude or a change in waveform.

The most important factor to consider when quantifying phasic activity is that the subject's response is not being made against a background of zero activity. If the subject is alive, he or she is constantly responding to internal as well as external stimuli. Three difficulties that sometimes occur are (1) determining the magnitude of a subject's phasic response to a specific stimulus and separating it from other phasic responses and from spontaneous activity; (2) attempting to introduce a correction factor for the magnitude of the phasic activity as a function of the preceding tonic activity, that is, the law of initial values; and (3) identifying a common measure across systems and individuals, for example, range corrections, autonomic lability scores, and standardized scores.

7.1.3   Spontaneous or nonspecific activity

A spontaneous psychophysiological response to an unknown stimulus looks the same as a response to a known stimulus such as a tone, a shock, or a snake. It may take the form of, for example, a change in heart rate or skin conductance in the palm of the hand. Spontaneous activity is a name given in ignorance to what may be several different types of responses. What is referred to as spontaneous activity is in reality a change in activity that occurs in the absence of any known stimulus. For example, the subject might have just had an anxious thought about what the experimenter was going to do. However, unless the subject is asked immediately following the psychophysiological response what he or she was thinking about (and even that would be admittedly shaky data), the experimenter would not know the cause of the so-called spontaneous activity. Changes in heart rate, skin conductance, and/or other bodily responses that follow a deep breath, movement, or a cough are phasic responses and are not considered to be spontaneous responses.

Spontaneous psychophysiological responses are of interest because it is important to be aware of their existence in order to avoid misinterpreting the data from a study on the effects of some known stimulus on bodily activity. An obvious example would be the presentation of a stimulus to the subject while he or she is making a spontaneous response. The net effect might be a response greater than normal, but then again, it might be smaller if the spontaneous response is in the opposite direction. In either case, quantification of the stimulus-contingent response will be difficult. Spontaneous responses are also of interest because sometimes they can be used to index tonic levels (e.g., nonspecific skin conductance responses).

7.2 SOME GENERAL PRINCIPLES OF PSYCHOPHYSIOLOGY

7.2.1 *Activation, habituation, and rebound*

7.2.1.1 *Activation*

The concept of activation has its roots in Cannon's (1915) notion of the unified body preparing for fight or flight. Duffy (1957) extended this concept to include the intensity aspect of all behavior. Duffy hypothesized an inverted U-shaped curve relating level of activation and performance. (This U-shaped function was first suggested by Yerkes & Dodson, 1908.) If the measure of performance is how fast subjects can run the 100-m dash and the measure of level of activation is their heart rate, we might well obtain an inverted U-shaped curve. Those who were too lowly aroused started slowly, and those who were too highly aroused committed false starts and had to hold themselves back in order to achieve even minimal success at the task. For a more detailed account of Duffy's theory, we refer the interested reader to her book *Activation and Behavior* (1962) and a more recent chapter (Duffy, 1972). Lindsley (1952) related the concept of unidimensional activation continuum to EEG data, and Malmo (1959) supported both the theory of the unidimensional activation continuum and the hypothesized inverted U-shaped curve. Duffy's activation theory accounts for the data from many experiments and has received support in terms of hypothesized physiological mechanisms such as the reticular activating-system (RAS).

Lacey (1967) and others have criticized the one-dimensional activation theory of Duffy (1972) and Lindsley (1952). Lacey suggested that there are at least three different forms of activation or arousal: cortical, autonomic, and behavioral. He pointed out that each is very complex, not a simple continuum. Lacey and other investigators have presented evidence showing that one form of arousal cannot always be used as a valid measure of another form of arousal. However, Brunia (1979), in a critique of the concept of activation, points out that both Duffy and Lindsley, in addition to postulating a single continuum of activation status, also discuss the existence of activation patterns of individual subsystems of the organism. Thus, Brunia states that the activation theories of Lacey, Duffy, and Lindsley are not as different as Lacey believes. The difference may be one of emphasis: Duffy and Lindsley emphasize a unidimensional continuum of activation, whereas Lacey emphasizes the dissociation of the activation of subsystems of the organism.

Major criticism of unidimensional activation theory can be found in the principle of stimulus–response specificity, to be discussed more completely later in this chapter. Basically, this principle states that specific stimulus situations – for example, noticing that your wallet or purse is missing – bring about certain patterns of responding, not just an increase or decrease in a unidimensional activation continuum. The pattern might include an increase in muscle tension, skin conductance, and respiratory amplitude but a decrease in respiratory rate and heart rate.

As a final point in his criticism of activation theory, Lacey (1967) referred to a special case of stimulus–response specificity that he termed directional fractionation. Imagine the following scenario: A soldier is on guard duty while his three comrades sleep. They are in enemy territory, and it is late at night. Suddenly there is an approaching noise heard in the darkness. What happens to the arousal level of the soldier? If we measured his EEG, we would conclude that he showed cortical arousal. If we measured skin conductance and heart rate as autonomic indices, however, we would probably find that his skin conductance increased but his heart rate decreased. This is what Lacey meant by directional fractionation. And if we observe the soldier's behavior, we see that he is probably standing very still, looking toward the source of the noise and trying to determine if it is being made by friend or foe. It does not appear that a concept of activation based on a unidimensional continuum (or tridimensional, for that matter) can deal adequately with such complexities.

7.2.1.2   *Adaptation*

The concept of adaptation is just as basic to psychophysiology as the concept of activation. They are in a sense complementary. Whereas activation suggests responding to a stimulus, adaptation describes the cessation or diminution of responding that occurs to the repeated presentation of the same stimulus.

Adaptation always occurs to the repeated presentation of the same stimulus, except in cases of unusually intense stimulation. (See the discussion of defensive responses that follows.) Adaptation will be slower the greater the intensity of stimulation, the more unique the stimulus, and the more complex the stimulus. Adaptation will also be affected by the rate of presentation of the stimuli and the duration of each presentation. If the subject is required to make a behavioral response – for example, to rate the subjective intensity of the stimuli – adaptation will be somewhat inhibited. To summarize, anything that draws a subject's attention for one reason or another – such as intensity, surprise, or uniqueness – inhibits habituation. When stimuli lose their distinctive meaning and become highly predictable, habituation ensues. The interested reader should consult the edited volume by Pecke and Petrinovich (1984) for a review of current work on the related processes of habituation and sensitization and the review by Graham (1973) for an in-depth discussion of the habituation of autonomic responses in particular.

7.2.1.3   *Rebound*

If we look at the response to one strong stimulus rather than to a repetitive stimulus, we often see that the response of interest gradually returns to its prestimulus level and may overshoot it. It is this "overshooting" that Sternbach (1966) referred to as rebound.

It is easy to see this phenomenon in the response of systems that are innervated by both the SNS and the PNS. For example, during fear or anxiety, when SNS activity is dominant, gastric activity is usually inhibited, but the period of inhibition is often followed by hyperactivity. This PNS overcompensation, or vagal rebound as it is sometimes called, can be observed in zealous eating behavior following the termination of an anxiety situation. The mechanisms involved in vagal rebound are not known but may be related to PNS activity being a response to SNS activity and still being present at high levels after SNS activity has decreased. An example of this behavior is the eating of Liddell's sheep (Liddell, James, & Anderson, 1934) immediately after being released from harnesses that restrained them during shock avoidance trials.

Interestingly, rebound is also seen in response systems that do not have dual ANS innervation. Sternbach (1966) reported seeing rebound in finger pulse volume, which is innervated only by adrenergic SNS fibers. Allen, McKay, Eaves, and Hamilton (1986) provided a good example of rebound in brain chemistry. They speculate that one reason why several astronauts suffered from space motion sickness is that they suddenly stopped exercising. Excercise increases the level of endorphins, endogenous opiates, which normally give protection from motion sickness. The authors go on to suggest that the sudden cessation of exercise causes the level of endorphins to drop below the normal resting level, thereby making the astronauts more prone to any form of exogenous emetic stimuli.

Rebound is of interest in itself. When does it occur? What is its course of action? What is the underlying physiological explanation for its presence in the various response systems? And so on. Rebound also serves as a reminder of the constantly changing, dynamic system, the human organism, upon which we impose stimuli and expect responses that lend themselves to simple quantification.

7.2.2   *Homeostasis*

The word *homeostasis* has been used to describe both a state of the organism and a process that takes place within the organism. When we refer to the homeostatic state, we are identifying equilibrium, stability, constancy, and the like. What we are really describing is a steady-state internal environment providing the right temperature, nourishment, oxygen, and fluids for optimal functioning of all cells. In our opinion, it is no more meaningful to specify the homeostatic state of the whole organism than it is to specify the stability of an entire university. In both cases, some parts (physiological systems or departments) may be very stable, whereas other are not. A typical statement appearing in the literature is "Some animals are more successful than others in maintaining homeostasis." We feel that such a statement should always be qualified. In actuality, some animals are more successful in maintaining, for example, constant temperature, whereas others are more success-ful in maintaining constant blood pressure. The mechanism that underlies the homeostatic process is negative feedback. However, the presence of the homeosta-tic state, that is, stability, is not invariably a sign of negative feedback.

Let us examine Davis's (1958) analysis of the homeostatic control of body temperature in human beings. When we become too hot, regulation is accom-plished by the evaporation of water secreted through the skin. Temperature is regulated, but what is happening to the sweating mechanism? Davis's answer was that every bit of reduced variation in temperature is brought about by increased variation in sweating.

The general concept of homeostasis as first stated by Claude Bernard—"*Le fixité du milieu interieur est la condition de la vie libre"* ("The stability of the internal environment is the condition of a healthy life") and later supported by Cannon (1939) in his book *The Wisdom of the Body* – captured the imagination of physiologists and psychologists alike. The maintenance of equilibrium was accepted by some as the unifying principle of motivation and, indeed, as a model for many other aspects of behavior.

We believe that the following quotation from Davis (1958, p. 13) puts the concept of homeostasis in better perspective:

Homeostasis exists, of course, with respect to certain variables, and one should try to find out what those are. But it is to be understood as a special case of the more general conception of the response of systems to inputs. There is no compulsion to think that the organism is an elaborate machine for the purpose of getting itself back to the status quo ante, or, indeed, for any other purpose.

A practical example of why psychophysiologists should be aware of the possible complicating effects of homeostatic mechanisms follows. Stern (1976) studied heart rate responses between the "get set" and "go" of a race. In the initial design, subjects were instructed to get down on their hands in a typical sprinter's starting position, just prior to the "get set". But the homeostatic response of the cardiovascular system to this postural change was a dramatic slowing of the heart. This effect was so great and long-lasting that it was not possible to determine the effect on heart rate of receiving the "get set" and waiting for the "go", the variable of interest in the study. To resolve this problem, in subsequent experiments subjects began from a standing position.

7.2.3   Autonomic balance

Most internal organs, such as the heart, are innervated by both branches of the autonomic nervous system: the SNS and the PNS. The rate at which the heart beats is determined by the relative excitation from the SNS and PNS, or the autonomic balance.

Eppinger and Hess (1915) were the first to classify people as vagotonics or sympathicotonics. Vagotonics (from vagus nerve, the primary parasympathetic nerve) are individuals who show unusually large responses to drugs that stimulate the PNS. Sympathicotonics are persons who show unusually large responses to drugs that stimulate the SNS. The interested reader is referred to early work on autonomic balance by Gellhorn, Cortell, and Feldman (1941) and Darrow (1943).

Wenger (1941) developed a technique for comparing an individual's resting scores on a group of ANS measures with the scores of other individuals and, in so doing, came up with an estimate of autonomic balance for each subject. The measures included dermographia persistence (23) (persistence of a red mark on the skin after being stroked with a stimulator), salivary output (25), heart period (28), palmar skin conductance (37), volar forearm skin conductance (39), respiration period (57), systolic blood pressure (76), diastolic blood pressure (77), and pulse pressure (80). The score for each measure (e.g., heart period) is converted to *t*-scores and included in a regression equation. The superscript *a* following subscripts 37 and 39 indicates that on these tests a low raw score is represented by a proportionally high standard score. One example of such an equation follows:

$$\bar{A} = .1\,(T_{23}) + .2\,(T_{28}) + .3\,(T_{37}{}^{a}) + .1\,(T_{39}{}^{a}) + .2\,(T_{80})$$

Each $\bar{A}$-score falls somewhere along a continuum, with low numbers indicating SNS dominance and high values indicating PNS- dominance. For a given group of individuals, Wenger found that the scores are normally distributed. Wenger studied autonomic balance in children, college students, military personnel, and hospitalized groups. Wenger and his associates reported a higher incidence of psychosomatic, psychotic, neurotic, and physical disorders in people with low $\bar{A}$-scores, individuals who appear to be SNS dominant. In 1971, Wineman studied autonomic balance changes during the human menstrual cycle and concluded that $\bar{A}$-scores varied with phases of the menstrual cycle. Few publications have appeared on the concept of autonomic balance since the review article of Wenger and Cullen (1972).

7.2.4   Law of initial values

Another principle that is relevant to response patterning is the law of initial values (LIV). The LIV is really a principle and not a law, but we refer to it as the LIV since this is the terminology commonly used in the literature. As was stated earlier in this chapter, tonic activity is important because it is relevant to the level that a phasic response will attain in many cases. The LIV, first formulated by Wilder in the 1930s (Wilder, 1931), states that the higher the initial value of a physiological activity, the lower the tendency of the physiological response to change (Wilder, 1967). He attributes this tendency to be a result of a "state of the organs" or "vegetative nerves." Both the magnitude and direction of change are affected by the prestimulus level. An organ at a high level of excitement would tend to have a weaker reaction because it is less susceptible to more excitation and more susceptible to inhibiting stimuli. The assumption is that the responding of an organ is subject to the negative-feedback mechanism of homeostasis. Wilder claims this law applies to a majority of vegetative functions.

Surwillo (1986) questions whether the LIV is anything more than the regression toward the mean effect that occurs in all natural phenomena. According to the regression effect, measures at the extremes of a distribution will, when they are replicated, show a tendency to be less extreme or to regress in the direction of the mean of the distribution. Stern, Ray, and Davis (1980) state that studies have found that the LIV usually applies to heart rate and skin resistance but not skin conductance. Hord, Johnson, and Lubin (1964) found that the LIV applies to heart rate and respiration rate but not to skin conductance and skin temperature.

The LIV alerts us to a serious complication in the interpretation of psychophysiological data. Because the magnitude of the response is dependent on prestimulus levels, comparability within and between subjects and even for the same subject within the same session is compromised if prestimulus levels vary. To correct for this, several methods have been proposed by Lacey (1956), Benjamin (1967), Lykken (1968), and others. Two general methods have been utilized; in both cases the level reached during each trial is corrected to take into account the prior level of functioning. Lacey (1950) introduced the term *autonomic lability score*, a measure of momentary displacement from a prestimulus level imposed by a stimulus event. It is the deviation of attained level from expected level in z-score units. The other method is the analysis of covariance. Engel (1960) and Sersen, Clausen, and Lidsky (1978) have derived standard scores using a covariance model and have used z-scores as units of analysis. We know of no studies that have compared these methods of compensating for the LIV. However, see Russell (chapter 23) for a detailed tutorial on multivariate analysis of change.

Recently Myrtek and Foerster (1986) have claimed that most physiological measures do not follow the LIV. They argue that the LIV is flawed because whenever the correlation between the initial (a) and final (b) values is less than 1.00, the negative correlation predicted by the LIV between the initial value a and the change score $a - b$ is biased by an artifactual $a(a - b)$ effect. Myrtek and Foerster describe the flaw in the LIV as follows: "The notion of the $a(a - b)$ effect suggests that for any correlation between two values that have a common term, e.g., for a and $(a - b)$...the correlation coefficient [between a and $(a - b)$] cannot be equal to zero, whenever a and b are independent" (p. 229). This statement is true. [Let a and b be independent random variables with positive variance, i.e., var(a), var(b) > 0. Then the covariance of a and $a - b$ is cov(a, $a - b$) $= E[a(a - b)] - E(a)E(a - b) = $ var(a), where E denotes expectation. Because cov(a, $a - b$) > 0, the correlation of a and $a - b$ is positive.] However, the authors go on to state: "It follows that any initial-value dependency is contaminated by the negative correlation...from the $a(a - b)$ effect whenever the correlation coefficient [between a and b] < 1.00" (p. 229). In other words, Myrtek and Foerster claim that if the correlation between the initial and final values is not 1.00 (as it almost never would be), then the correlation between the initial value a and the change score $a - b$ cannot be zero. This statement is not correct. A counterexample is easily given. By definition corr(x, y) $= [E(xy) - E(x)E(y)]/[$var(x)var(y)$]^{1/2}$.   Suppose $E(a) = E(b) = 0$,   corr(a, b) $= \frac{1}{2}$, var(a) $= 1$, var(b) $= 4$. A straightforward calculation shows cov(a, $a - b$) $= 0$; hence corr (a, $a - b$) $= 0$ but corr(a, b) $= \frac{1}{2} < 1$, a result that Myrtek and Foerster claim is impossible. The point is that in general nothing can be said about the consequences of the correlation between a and b not being zero and how this nonzero correlation relates to the correlation of a and $a - b$. Because of this flaw in reasoning, we must question the later developments and recommendations in their paper.

In summary the LIV has been found to apply to many psychophysiological responses. Statistical methods exist for dealing with the influence of prestimulus level on magnitude of responses. However, it should be mentioned again that the "law" is really a principle and does not hold for all subjects and all response systems. We suggest that investigators compute the correlation between pre- and poststimulus parameters in order to determine whether the LIV is operative.

7.3   SPECIFICITY

A person's physiological responses could be described as being constituted of components arising from the demands of the stimuli or situation, individual predispositions to respond, and the interaction of these two. Stimulus response (SR) specificity (or stereotypy) pertains to the tendency of a stimulus or situation to evoke a specific pattern of physiological response. Individual response (IR) specificity (or stereotypy) is the disposition in each individual to exhibit a particular pattern across various situations (Engel, 1960, 1972). Motivational response (MR) specificity (Ax, 1964) is the interaction of these two factors.

The concepts of IR and SR specificity represent psychophysiological parallels to idiographic and nomothetic perspectives in personality theory (Endler & Magnusson, 1976). By virtue of its focus on individual responses in treatment of data, IR specificity takes on an idiographic perspective. Stimulus response specificity takes the perspective of group mean response to specific stimulus and perceptual situations (Ax, 1953; Lacey, 1959), and as such it takes on a nomothetic perspective. This difference was first brought to attention by Lacey, Bateman, and Van Lehn (1953). They found that individuals could be differentiated in terms of rigidity of their response pattern across different stressors. In a later paper, Lacey (1959) further differentiated the concept of response stereotypy. He used the term *intrastressor stereotypy* for the tendency of an individual to exhibit reproducible patterns of response to a single stressor. Lacey (1959) also noted the tendency for different individuals to vary in degree of stereotypy of response patterns. He used the term *interstressor stereotypy* to denote this tendency in some individuals to reproduce one pattern of response to different stressors.

Engel (1960) found statistical support for the existence of both SR specificity and IR specificity. This finding at first seems to be a paradox. How could one reconcile the finding that each stimulus situation tends to evoke a specific pattern of response if, in addition, each individual tends to respond to a stressor or stimulus with her or his own idiosyncratic patterns of response? This dilemma could be resolved if we consider that whereas a certain stimulus situation could elicit a given hierarchy of responses, the extent to which a given physiological system reacts may be modulated by the individual's tendency toward her or his habitual response.

Engel and Moos (1967) used the term *individual consistency* to refer to the tendency for an individual to exhibit a consistent hierarchy of responses to a set of stimuli. This concept is identical to IR stereotypy or intrastressor stereotypy (Lacey, Bateman, and Van Lehn, 1952). Engel and Moos (1967) described another form of IR specificity called *individual uniqueness*, the concept of using a single characteristic to group individuals. The group as a whole is expected to react differently from a control group. A group of hypertensive individuals and a group of normals subjected to the cold pressor task while several physiological measures are taken is an example of an experiment that examines individual uniqueness. By proposing the concept of individual uniqueness, Engel and Moos (1967) elucidated a model by which the responses of different groups of individuals with psychosomatic and psychological disorders such as hypertension (Engel & Bickford, 1961), ulcers (Walker & Sandman, 1977), and schizophrenia (Crooks & McNulty, 1966) can be studied.

Sternbach (1966) has suggested that individual differences in degree of response pattern rigidity or stereotypy may be normally distributed. The possibility of a normal distribution of response stereotypy in the general population and its clinical implications have not been pursued as yet.

The assessment of IR specificity has been conceptualized by Averill and Opton (1968) in terms of an analysis-of-variance framework. If one were to take repeated measurements of various physiological variables under different situations, the portion due to the interaction of the response variables and individual differences, regardless of the situation, is the portion of variance one can attribute to IR specificity.

The Laceys (Lacey & Lacey, 1958) have used several methods to test the hypothesis of specificity. For example, they took several physiological measurements to several stressors over a number of days. They then made profiles of the physiological responses according to level of response and compared odd and even days of testing. Subjects would also be categorized according to number of measures that show maximal response across stressors. The probability for these groups to occur by chance would then be tested.

Engel (1960) defined IR specificity in terms of (1) maximal change in the same physiological measure within a subject across a set of stimuli, (2) consistent rank orders of responses to a set of stimuli, and (3) consistent intercorrelations within the same subject to a set of stimuli.

7.3.1   Situational or stimulus specificity and stereotypy

The classic study by Engel (1960) investigating both SR and IR specificity was referred to previously. He exposed 20 nurses to five stimulus trials: horn, mental arithmetic, proverbs, cold pressor test, and exercise. Engel took measures of blood pressure, respiration rate, skin conductance, heart rate, heart rate variability, finger temperature, and face temperature. He found that three of the stimuli – horn, mental arithmetic, and cold pressor – each evoked similar hierarchies of response from the 20 subjects.

In a more recent series of studies, Foerster and his associates (Foerster, 1985; Foerster, Schneider, & Walschburger, 1983) have shown that SR specificity accounts for a small but stable portion of the variance in response patterns of eight physiological measures to conditions of mental arithmetic, reaction time, free speech, cold pressor, and the drawing of blood from a finger. Berman and Johnson (1985) found that 25 out of 30 subjects exhibited a high degree of SR stereotypy.

7.3.1.1   Orienting, defense, and startle

Pavlov (1927) first described the pattern of response that occurs in the presence of novel stimuli. He called this the "what is it" response. Sokolov (1963) elaborated on this "reflex." He wrote that it was a nonspecific response with regard to the quality and intensity of the stimulus. With repeated presentation of the same stimulus, the orienting response (OR) habituates. However, Sokolov also wrote that the extinction of the OR is selective according to various properties of the stimulus. Any change in the intensity and magnitude of the stimulus will elicit the OR once again.

The orienting response or functional system is comprised of the following psychophysiological patterns: increased sensitivity of the sense organs, dilation of cerebral blood vessels, constriction of peripheral vessels, decreased heart rate, increased skin conductance, and increased somatic or muscular tone, a turning of the eyes toward the stimulus, and increased beta in the EEG (Cacioppo & Petty, 1983; Lynn, 1966; Sokolov, 1963; Stern, et al., 1980). Respiration also shows a delay followed by an increase in amplitude and a decrease in frequency. Graham and Clifton (1966) reviewed studies concerned with heart rate and the orienting response and proposed that the heart rate deceleration found by Lacey (1967) to occur with environmental intake should be considered part of the orienting response. The orienting response functions to enable the organism to attend to a novel stimulus and facilitates an adaptive response to it. Once the stimulus poses no threat to the organism, the OR habituates.

The defense response (DR) described by Sokolov (1963) is elicited by a strong stimulus that may be dangerous and painful. In contrast to the OR, the DR habituates very slowly. It protects the organism from intense stimulation. While the OR is associated with a dilation of cerebral blood vessels and constriction of peripheral blood vessels, the DR is associated with the constriction of both cerebral and peripheral blood vessels. Other changes associated with the defense reaction are a decrease in sensitivity of the sense organs, muscular changes that facilitate moving or turning away from the stimulus, and increases in heart rate (Cacioppo & Petty, 1983; Lynn, 1966; Stern et al., 1980).

The startle response is a response pattern that arises from sudden stimulation. According to Turpin (1986), this pattern consists of heart rate acceleration, peak latency around 4 s; digital vasoconstriction, habituation rate dependent upon intensity; and cephalic vasodilation. Many of the studies on the startle response have been done with animal subjects. With humans, stimuli commonly employed have been auditory tones of varying intensities and white noise. For example, Oster, Stern, and Figar (1975) found that subjects show a cephalic dilation response to fast rise time tones of 90 dB within one to two heart beats after stimulus onset, compared to a cephalic dilation response of 3–5 s after stimulation onset in an orienting situation.

The elicitation of either the DR or the OR has been found to be related to the level of fear a person may experience in response to a particular stimulus. For example, Hare (1973) found that subjects high in fear of spiders showed heart rate acceleration and vasoconstriction of cephalic vessels (DR) when shown pictures of spiders. Subjects low in spider fear, on the other hand, showed HR deceleration and cephalic vasodilation associated with the OR. In 1977, Klorman, Weissberg, and Weisenfeld divided undergraduates into groups of high and low in terms of fear of mutilation. They showed the subjects slides depicting mutilation, neutral, and humorous scenes. Klorman et al. (1977) found that subjects high in fear of mutilation exhibited heart rate acceleration, and low-fear subjects showed heart rate deceleration in response to the mutilation slides. In terms of skin conductance, the mutilation stimuli evoked more activity compared to the other stimuli, but the level did not vary with level of fear. Thus, at least for the preceding studies, it seems that elicitation of a DR versus an OR may depend on the subjective set of the individual. High-fear subjects may show a DR whereas low-fear subjects tend to orient and attend to the same fear-relevant stimuli.

7.3.1.2 *Emotion-specific response patterning*

In 1884, William James proposed a view of the role of physiological activities in emotional experience. His thesis was that "bodily changes follow directly the perception of the exciting fact, and that our feeling of the same changes as they occur is the emotion." Thus it follows that every emotion emerges from a specific configuration of bodily response. At the same time Lange (1885/1922) attempted to describe the bodily changes that accompany sorrow, joy, and anger.

In 1915 and 1928 Cannon described bodily changes that occur in the gastrointestinal and cardiovascular systems as a result of SNS action during experiences of intense fear and rage. According to him, these changes serve to prepare the organism to be mobilized for "fight or flight."

Gellhorn (1953, 1970; Gellhorn, et al., 1941) also studied physiological changes in emotion. He argued that behavior in general and emotions in particular depend on the balance of the trophotropic and ergotropic systems. The trophotropic system refers to the PNS and its related somatic processes, whereas the ergotropic system refers to the SNS and its related somatic processes. Gellhorn focused on the role of the PNS, in contrast to Cannon's emphasis on the SNS. Thus Gellhorn was able to illuminate the changes in the vago-insulin system that accompany emotional experience.

Magda Arnold (1970) stated that, in contrast to Cannon's emergency theory of emotion that assumes that all emotions involve SNS excitation, different emotions have different physiological states. She cites the example of lust as a PNS phenomenon and goes on to say that the parasympathetic system is active whenever we appraise something as good and enjoy it. Arnold stresses the importance of phenomenological analysis of the psychological activities from perception to emotion to action.

Funkenstein (1955) investigated the biochemical correlates of two emotional states, anxiety, or anger in, and anger out. He found the state of anxiety to be associated with a discharge of adrenaline and the state of anger to be associated with increased levels of norepinephrine. However, subsequent studies with humans (e.g., Levi, 1965) failed to support the assumption that adrenaline and norepinephrine are selectively released in different emotional states. Frankenhaeuser (1974, p. 81) summarized the state of research in this area as follows:

Later studies, however, lend no support to the assumption that adrenaline and noradrenaline would be selectively released in different emotional states. Instead, the general picture indicates that adrenaline is secreted in a variety of affective states, including both anger and fear. Similarly, a rise in noradrenaline secretion may occur in different affective states, but the threshold for noradrenaline release in response to psychosocial stimulation is generally much higher than for adrenaline secretion.

The application of multiple measures of autonomic functions in the differentiation of emotions was initiated by Ax in 1953. He found that in 7 out of 14 measures, fear could be differentiated from anger. Joseph Schachter (1957) applied this methodology to the study of hypertensive individuals. He took measures of 12 specific functions and found that based on their configurations, fear gave rise to an adrenalinelike effect; pain, to a norepinephrinelike effect; and anger showed a mixed picture. In addition, he found that hypertensives tended to show greater rises in blood pressure in these emotions compared to normotensives. These two studies were conducted in the tradition of James (1884), in that an association was sought between specific patterns of bodily changes and various emotional states.

Aside from the emotions mentioned in the preceding, other investigators have studied the feelings of sadness and happiness. Sternbach (1962) found that children watching a movie showed greater skin resistance and lacrimation during sad scenes and a slower gastric peristaltic rate during happy scenes. He interpreted the former as an inhibition of SNS activity and the latter as a decrease in vagal activity. However, Averill (1969) found that in his subjects sadness led to higher blood pressure, which he took as a rise in SNS activity. Mirth was found to be characterized by increases in respiratory measures.

Some of the more recent studies in this area of emotional differentiation have used the technique of imagery to induce emotion, and they have tended to concentrate on cardiovascular variables. For example, Weerts and Roberts (1976) found that diastolic blood pressure distinguished between the emotions of fear and anger during the imagery of emotion-related scenes. Schwartz, Weinberger, and Singer (1981) used an imagery and nonverbal expression task for six emotions. They also asked subjects to do an exercise task. Cardiovascular measures of diastolic and systolic blood pressure and heart rate were taken. Schwartz et al. found that blood pressure differentiated between fear and anger. They also found that the patterning of the three variables was different for anger and fear versus happiness and sadness, whereas happiness and sadness were different from relaxation and the control condition. These studies of fear and anger are of interest to clinicians because of their application to the development of different imagery-based relaxation techniques for the treatment of emotional disorders.

Ekman, Levenson, and Friesen (1983) investigated the question of emotional specificity using facial expressions and the reliving of emotional experiences as inductions. Six emotions of anger, fear, sadness, happiness, surprise, and disgust were studied. The results indicated that there were ANS differences among the six emotions. For example, heart rate and finger temperature were found to increase more with anger than with happiness. The results of the preceding studies tend to support James's (1884) theory that emotional experience reflects concomitant patterns of autonomic change.

7.3.2 Individual response specificities

Habitual tendencies by individuals to show specific patterns of autonomic responses have been studied by several investigators. As mentioned previously in this chapter, Eppinger and Hess (1915) conceptualized the SNS and PNS as two opposing forces regulated by the secretion of hormones. The tonic state of the organism is established by the balance of these forces. Abnormally strong or weak tone in either system could lead to a pathological condition. For Eppinger and Hess, individuals who show high degree of tonic level and irritability in the PNS are vagotonics. Individuals who show a dominance of SNS functioning are sympatheticotonics. As mentioned previously, Wenger (1941) undertook a research program to investigate SNS/PNS balance.

7.3.2.1 History of the concept of individual response specificity

The principle of individual patterns of responding to stress or stimulation has its origins in both the clinical and experimental traditions of psychology. Franz Alexander (1943) attempted to explain the variety of psychosomatic disorders in psychoanalytic terms. He proposed that different symptoms represent an attempt on the part of the individual to resolve a deep psychological conflict. For example, in gastrointestinal disorders, gastric disorder reflected a wish to receive, colitis a wish to give, and constipation a wish to retain.

Other writers attempted to classify types of bodily reactions to stress. Cameron (1944) noted that these patterns tended to fall into three groups depending on the system involved: the skeletal musculature, the smooth musculature, and a group with equal involvement of both. Wolf and Wolff (1946) noted that real-life situations associated with such emotions as anxiety, anger, guilt, and tension tended to be associated with different reactions such as dyspnea, palpitation, heart pain, faintness, and fatigue. Furthermore, Wolf and Wolff observed that individuals differ in terms of the intensity and duration of these cardiovascular and respiratory symptoms.

7.3.2.2   Symptom specificity

Malmo and Shagass (1949) were interested in the physiological effects of adverse environmental situations or emotional disturbance in groups of psychiatric patients complaining of physical disturbances such as head and neck problems. Malmo and Shagass exposed these subjects to a thermal stressor and took measures of heart rate and muscle potential. By comparing head and heart complainers and patients with both head and heart complaints as well as noncomplainers, Malmo and Shagass found that the patients responded most with the system involved in their complaints: Head complainers showed higher muscle potentials whereas heart complainers showed higher and more variable heart rate. These findings led Malmo and his co-workers (Malmo & Shagass, 1949; Malmo, Shagass, & Davis, 1950) to formulate the principle of symptom specificity: "In psychiatric patients presenting a somatic complaint, the particular physiologic mechanism of that complaint is specifically susceptible to activation by stressful experience." However, one limitation to the generalizability of the principle was the use of a single stressor.

7.3.2.3   Individual responses specificity in the laboratory

During the time Malmo and his co-workers were studying psychiatric patients, Lacey (1950) and other investigators were interested in the issue of differential responding in the normal population. Lacey et al. (1952, 1953) exposed healthy subjects to four different stressors. They found that their subjects tended to display maximal activation in the same physiological measure under different stress conditions. This research extended the concept of symptom specificity to a normal population, and the findings were referred to as relative response specificity. In addition, Lacey et al. (1953) found that individuals tended to vary in the degree to which a certain pattern was fixed across stressors. Some individuals displayed the same pattern through all stressors, whereas others were not as fixed.

Subsequent investigators have obtained results supporting the principle of relative IR specificity from other organ systems. Schnore (1959) found that the concept of IR specificity generalized to the muscular system. Other investigators have expanded studies in this area to include other tasks or stressors and methods of analysis (Engel, 1960; Sersen, Clausen, & Lidsky, 1978; Wenger, Clemens, Coleman, Cullen, & Engel, 1961). Although the results of these studies generally supported the principle of IR specificity, other factors that must be taken into consideration include resting level of autonomic functions, similarity and variety of chosen stimuli or stressors, and method of score standardization and analysis.

In this decade, attention has continued to be given to the principle of IR specificity along with stimulus and motivation specificities. Foerster et al. (1983) and Foerster (1985) found that a quarter to half of their subjects showed stable response patterns. However, these numbers tended to decrease with time. Berman and Johnson (1985) found that the stability of response patterns depend on the type of experimental task.

7.3.2.4   Stability of individual response specificity and stereotypy

The question of the stability of IR specificity has been addressed by several investigators. Lacey (1950) found that females subjected to a single word-naming task exhibited characteristic patterns that were reproducible over 9 months. In another paper, Lacey (1959) mentioned a study in which children taking the cold pressor test produced stable patterns after a period of 4 years. It seems that at least to a single stressor, consistent patterns of responses tend to be seen in individuals across time.

Manuck and Schaeffer (1978) tested heart rate reactors and nonreactors performing on a concept formation task on two occasions a week apart. They found support for the stability of intrastressor stereotypy.

Oken et al. (1962) exposed healthy college students to three different stressors on three different occasions. They found that the level of the physiological measures tended to be consistent over the three sessions, but there was less consistency in terms of the variable showing maximum responding. Oken et al. concluded that IR specificity in terms of a stable hierarchy of level does seem to characterize many subjects. However, specificity in terms of a consistent pattern of change was sensitive to other factors such as stimulus-specific characteristics.

In summary, it seems that stable IR specificity patterns are more clearly seen when a single stressor is used. Once multiple stressors are utilized, the factor of the specific demands of the different stimuli may complicate the picture of stable responding. This difference suggests that the interaction of individual propensities and situational demands need to be considered in future studies

7.3.2.5 *Individual response specificity within organ systems*

Some studies in this area have had the stated objective of dealing with responsivity within specific organ systems. For example, Goldstein, Grinker, Heath, Oken, and Shipman (1964) investigated IR specificity across seven skeletal muscles under four interview conditions. They also included autonomic measures. Goldstein et al. found that most subjects showed maximal responding in a single muscle across all four interview conditions. They also found consistent hierarchies of response in most subjects. Shipman, Heath, and Oken (1970) obtained comparable results.

In terms of cardiovascular variables, Manuck and Schaeffer (1978) and Lawler (1980) studied groups of heart rate reactives and nonreactives. Group designation was determined by the change in heart rate from baseline to the first minute of a mental arithmetic task. In both studies, heart rate reactive individuals showed greater cardiovascular responses to tones and mental arithmetic compared to nonreactive individuals. In addition, Lawler (1980) found that heart rate nonreactors tended to be high-skin-conductance reactors. They tended to respond maximally with this measure.

7.3.2.6 *Individual response specificity and psychosomatic disorders*

The principle of IR specificity lent itself easily to the study of disorders involving ANS functions. Various groups of individuals with disorders such as hypertension and arthritis became subjects in studies involving several stimulus conditions and the measurement of a variety of physiological functions.

Engel and Bickford (1961) first applied the principle of IR specificity to the study of hypertensive subjects. They found that hypertensives, more than normotensives, tended to respond maximally with blood pressure across all stimuli. Hypertensives also exhibited a greater degree of IR stereotypy, or rigidity of pattern, across all stressors. In 1962, a similar study was done with hypertensives and individuals with arthritis (Moos & Engel, 1962). These investigators found that their subjects responded to a greater degree with their symptomatic system than with other ANS functions.

Hypertension has received the most attention of researchers in this area. For example, adolescents (Price, Lott, Fixler, & Browne, 1979), male military draftees (Svensson & Theorell, 1982), and factory workers age 55 and over (Steptoe, Melville, & Ross, 1984) have been screened for hypertensive tendencies, and tested with different stimuli while blood pressure measure and other ANS functions were recorded. The results showed that individuals exhibiting hypertensive tendencies produced greater blood pressure reactions. More recent studies with similar results have been conducted by Fredrickson, Dimberg, and Frisk Holmberg (1980) and Fredrickson et al. (1985). In the latter study, a subgroup of subjects was administered therapeutic doses of an adrenergic blocking agent, a common type of medication for hypertension. Fredrickson et al. (1985) found that whereas the beta blockers decreased levels of cardiovascular activity, the blockers had no effect on the degree of IR specificity.

In the area of gastrointestinal disorders, Walker and Sandman (1977) used the electrogastrogram (EGG) to study the gastric myoelectric response of individuals with ulcer or rheumatoid arthritis and normal individuals. They also took additional measures of other bodily functions. Walker and Sandman found a tendency for the ulcer patients, compared to the other subjects, to show more EGG activity when viewing autopsy slides. Patients with arthritis differed from the other groups in terms of increased muscle activity.

The condition of migraine headaches has been the object of similar studies. Cohen, Rickles, and McArthur (1978) found that individuals who have a tendency for migraine headaches, compared to controls who do not, exhibit higher head and hand temperatures and lower frontalis EMG. They also tend to be more stereotyped in their manner of physiological responding to various stimuli.

In summary, studies of IR specificity in individuals with psychophysiological disorders have supported the notion that individuals tend to respond maximally with their symptomatic function as compared to controls. There are also indications of more stereotypy or rigidity in these response tendencies across various situations in the experimental laboratory.

7.3.2.7   *Psychological correlates of individual response specificity*

Few investigators have attempted to establish links between IR specificity and psychological constructs to shed light on the question of the development of such tendencies.

Roessler, Greenfield, and Alexander (1964) attempted to relate IR specificity to ego strength. They found that subjects exposed to various intensities of tones tended to be more stereotyped in responding when they were either high or low in ego strength. Individuals of moderate ego strength did not show such stereotypy.

A unique perspective in the study of correlates of response specificity is the body image hypothesis put forward by Fisher and Cleveland (1957, 1960). According to this hypothesis, individuals with psychosomatic symptoms are classifiable in terms of their concept of body boundaries. Persons with symptoms of the exterior body layers would have a concept of their body boundaries as protective barriers compared to persons with symptoms of the internal organs. In terms of reactivity, the former group would be more reactive with the exterior organs. Fisher and

Cleveland (1960) found that individuals who had rheumatoid arthritis were more reactive in galvanic skin reflex, whereas ulcer patients were more reactive in terms of heart rate.

A similar hypothesis is the specificity of attitude theory proposed by Grace and Graham (1952). They suggested that each psychosomatic symptom is associated with an attitude toward a situation that is temporally related to the outbreak of the symptom. For example, urticaria may be associated with the feeling that the person is about to receive a blow since vasodilation is the reaction of the skin to trauma. This hypothesis was the object of several studies, most of which involved the hypnotic induction of a psychological attitude that was hypothesized to be related to a physiological reaction. For example, Graham, Stern, and Winokur (1958) and Graham, Kabler, and Graham (1962) gave their subjects suggestions of attitudes for hives, hypertension, and Raynaud's disease. Results indicated that finger temperature tended to rise in the hives condition and fall in the Raynaud's condition. Stern, Winokur, Graham, and Graham (1961) found a rise in blood pressure in response to a hypertension suggestion.

One question raised by the methodology of these studies was whether the effects were due to suggestion or to the use of hypnosis. In 1971, Peters and Stern attempted to induce hives and a Raynaud-like response with suggestions to both hypnotized and unhypnotized subjects. They found no effects for the attitude suggestions but found effects for the hypnosis condition itself. Additional research is needed to determine if a hypnotic design is an appropriate method of exploring the relationship between suggested attitudes and physiological response patterns.

Another line of research in psychophysiology that is related to IR specificity deals with the perception of autonomic responses (Katkin, Blascovich, & Koenigsberg, 1984; Pennebaker, 1982; Shields & Stern, 1979; Stern & Higgins, 1969). Shields and Stern (1979) presented a review of studies that deal with the perception of autonomic responses and concluded that IR specificity exists at the perceptual level. They indicated that persons reporting a high degree of autonomic awareness show greater autonomic reactivity than low perceivers. Also, high perceivers tend to overestimate their physiological reactivity whereas low perceivers underestimate their reactivity.

As can be seen, the study of the psychological correlates of IR specificity has been highly diverse. Hypotheses regarding psychological correlates could be categorized in terms of intensity of response, direction of response, and psychological constructs such as personality, attitude, body image, and ego strength.

7.3.3 *Motivational response specificity*

According to Ax (1964), MR specificity is defined as the psychophysiological complex that results from the interaction of the individual's "definition of the situation" with IR specificity, SR specificity, and the LIV. In 1983, Foerster et al. followed up on Ax's suggestion of investigating individual, stimulus, and motivation specific response. They operationalized MR as the three-way interaction of subject, situation, and trial, or the difference between the stimuli by subject interaction and average patterns elicited by specific stimuli. The results reflect the "disposition of an individual to react consistently under specific stimulus conditions." In their more recent investigations, Foerster and his colleagues have found that MR accounts for 17 percent (Foerster et al., 1983) and 10–11 percent (Foerster, 1985) of variance in a correlational analysis of the different specificities. In a multiple analysis of variance, MR accounted for 21 percent (Foerster et al., 1983) and 16–18 percent (Foerster, 1985) of the variance. Motivational response tended to account for more variance than stimulus-specific response, confirming the importance of the interaction of individual disposition with stimulus-specific patterns that lead to idiosyncratic rather than conforming tendencies for response.

Averill and Opton (1968) define MR as the tendency for a pattern to be specific to the subjective appraisal of a stimulus. As such, orienting, defense, startle, and emotion-specific response may be considered special cases of MR specificity.

7.4   DISCUSSION AND CONCLUSIONS

A review of the literature dealing with the sources of response patterning reveals that investigators have generally shown interest in one, and occasionally more, aspects of the transactions of the individual with the environment. Situational and stimulus properties that are usually followed by certain response patterns include experiences of orienting and defense, the taking in or rejecting of the environment; whereas individual differences in psychological variables have been conceptualized to be related to habitual tendencies to respond with specific physiological patterns.

The experimental study of IR specificity has shown that individual differences exist with regard to tendencies to respond in specific organs or groups of organs to most stresses. This tendency has been found to be more pronounced in individuals with psychosomatic disorders and physiological symptoms. However, a specific relationship between responsitivity and psychosomatic disorder has yet to be uncovered.

Gannon (1981) has suggested that aside from IR specificity, perhaps two factors may be related to the etiology of psychosomatic disease: resting levels of physiological activity and recovery rate. Awareness of the concept of resting or tonic levels forces one out of the stimulus-response model that is the basis of the experimental design of most responsivity studies and makes one consider the possible effects of physiological functioning not bound to stimulus conditions. Perhaps there are differences in the manner of the constant ebb and flow of physiological function that may place certain individuals at risk for certain symptoms. See Gottman (chapter 22) and Porges and Bohrer (chapter 21) for tutorials on techniques for quantifying rhythmicities in physiological response patterns. We believe that the future study of IR specificity, resting levels of activity, and recovery, which are undoubtedly mutually dependent, may shed light on the question of the etiology of psychosomatic diseases.

Research linking the implications of IR specificity and stereotypy with its psychological correlates has not been pursued vigorously, and therefore, no definite conclusions can be put forward regarding relationships between these two domains. Except for the classical psychoanalytic theories, the weak-organ hypothesis and common everyday notions that certain bodily symptoms tend to be associated with anxiety, the development and study of the concept of IR specificity has been relatively atheoretical. Whereas the roots of the experimental studies may have been in psychoanalytic theories, investigators have not been able to confirm or refute the presence of a nuclear conflict underlying a stereotyped response. All one can conclude at this point is that IR specificity exists to a statistically significant degree in the population. Also, results tend to support the notion of idiosyncratic physiological responding to anxiety. Some people get a stomachache, others a headache, in a stress situation. There is the suggestion that individuals who suffer from psychosomatic diosorders tend to display maximal response in the symptomatic organ and may be more stereotyped in their pattern of response compared to nonsymptomatic individuals. The important question remains whether stereotypy causes psychosomatic disorders or is the result of a disorder. However, before such studies are attempted, a tremendous challenge exists for the formulation of a theory that would provide a framework by which these different factors – individual, situational, emotion, motivation, and their interactions – could be related. It is realized that such theorizing is a rather grand undertaking; however, it may be the only way to impose order on the confusing amalgamation of experimental results and clinical findings regarding IR specificity and its psychological concomitants and correlates.

NOTE

We thank Hoben Thomas and Michael W. Vasey for their comments and suggestions for section 6.2.4.

REFERENCES

Alexander, F. (1943). The influence of psychological factors upon gastrointestinal disturbance. *Psychological Quarterly, 3,* 501.
Allen, M. E., McKay, C., Eaves, D.M., & Hamilton, D. (1986). Naloxone enhances motion sickness: Endorphins implicated. *Aviation, Space and Environmental Medicine, 57,* 647–653.
Arnold, M. B. (1970). Perennial problems in the field of emotions. In M. B. Arnold (Ed.), *Feelings and emotions.* New York: Academic Press.
Averill, J. R. (1969) Autonomic response patterns during sadness and mirth. *Psychophysiology, 5,* 399–414.
Averill, J. R., & Opton, E. M. (1968). Physiological assessment: Rationale and problems. In P. McReynolds (Ed.), *Advances in psychological assessment* (Vol. 1). Palo Alto: Science and Behavior.
Ax, A. F. (1953). The physiological differentiation between fear and anger in humans. *Psychosomatic Medicine, 15,* 433–442.
Ax, A. F. (1964). Goals and methods of psychophysiology. *Psychophysiology, 1,* 8–25.
Benjamin, L. S. (1967). Facts and artifacts in using analysis of covariance to "undo" the law of initial values. *Psychophysiology, 4,* 187–206.
Berman, P. S., & Johnson, H. J. (1985). A psychophysiological assessment battery. *Biofeedback and Self-Regulation, 10,* 203–221.
Brunia, C. H. M. (1979). Activation. In J. A. Michon, E. G. J. Eijkman, & L. F. W. deKlerk (Eds.), *Handbook of psychonomics* (Vol. 1). Amsterdam: North-Holland.
Cacioppo, J. T., & Petty, R. E. (1983). Foundations of social psychophysiology. In J. T. Cacioppo & R. E. Petty (Eds.), *Social psychophysiology.* New York: Guilford Press.
Cameron, D. E. (1944). Observations in the patterns of anxiety. *American Journal of Psychiatry, 101,* 36–41.
Cannon, W. B. (1915). *Bodily changes in pain, hunger, fear and rage.* New York: Appleton-Century-Crofts.
Cannon, W. B. (1928). The mechanism of emotional disturbance of bodily functions. *The New England Journal of Medicine, 198,* 877–884.
Cannon, W. B. (1939). *The wisdom of the body.* New York: Norton.
Cohen, M. J., Rickles, W. H., & McArthur, D. L. (1978). Evidence for physiological response stereotypy in migraine headache. *Psychosomatic Medicine, 40,* 344–354.

Crooks, R. C., & McNulty, J. A. (1966). Autonomic response specificity in normal and schizophrenic subjects. *Canadian Journal of Psychology, 20,* 280–295.

Darrow, C. W. (1943). Physiological and clinical tests of autonomic function and autonomic balance. *Physiological Reviews, 23,* 1–36.

Davis, R. C. (1957). Response patterns. *Transactions of the New York Academy of Science, 19,* 731–739.

Davis, R. C. (1958). The domain of homeostasis. *Psychological Review, 65,* 8–13.

Duffy, E. (1957). The psychological significance of the concept of "arousal" or "activation." *Psychological Review, 64,* 265–275.

Duffy, E. (1962). *Activation and behavior.* New York: Wiley.

Duffy, E. (1972). Activation. In N. S. Greenfield & R. A. Sternbach (Eds.), *Handbook of psychophysiology.* New York: Holt, Rinehart and Winston.

Ekman, P., Levenson, R. W., & Friesen, W. V. (1983). Autonomic nervous system activity distinguishes among emotions. *Science, 221,* 1208–1210.

Endler, N. S., & Magnusson, D. (1976). Toward an interactional psychology of personality. *Psychological Bulletin, 83,* 956–974.

Engel, B. T. (1960). Stimulus-response and individual-response specificity. *Archives of General Psychiatry, 2,* 305–313.

Engel, B. T. (1972). Response specificity. In N. S. Greenfield & R. A. Sternbach (Eds.), *Handbook of psychophysiology.* New York: Holt, Rinehart & Winston.

Engel, B. T., & Bickford, A. F. (1961). Response specificity: Stimulus response and individual response specificity in essential hypertensives. *Archives of General Psychiatry, 5,* 478–489.

Engel, B. T., & Moos, R. H. (1967). The generality of specificity. *Archives of General Psychiatry, 16,* 574–581.

Eppinger, H., & Hess, L. (1976). Vagotonia: A clinical study in vegetative neurology. In S. W. Porges & M. C. Coles (Eds.), *Psychophysiology.* Stroudsburg, PA: Dowden, Hutchinson, & Ross. (Originally published in 1915.)

Fisher, S., & Cleveland, S. (1957). An approach to physiological reactivity in terms of a body-image schema. *Psychological Review, 64,* 26–37.

Fisher, S., & Cleveland, S. (1960). A comparison of psychological characteristics and physiological reactivity in ulcer and rheumatoid arthritis groups. *Psychosomatic Medicine, 22,* 290–293.

Foerster, F. (1985). Psychophysiological response specificities: A replication over a 12-month period. *Biological Psychology, 21,* 169–182.

Foerster, F., Schneider, H. J., & Walschburger, P. (1983). The differentiation of individual specific response patterns in activation processes: An inquiry investigating their stability and possible importance in psychophysiology. *Biological Psychology, 7,* 1–26.

Frankenhaeuser, M. (1974). Sympathetic-adrenomedullary activity, behaviour and the psychosocial environment. In P. H. Venables & M. J. Christie (Eds.), *Research in psychophysiology.* New York: Wiley.

Fredrickson, M., Danielson, U., Engel, B. T., Frisk-Holmberg, M., Strom, G., & Sundin, O. (1985). Autonomic nervous system function and essential hypertension: Individual response specificity with and without beta blockade. *Psychophysiology, 22,* 167–174.

Fredrickson, M., Dimberg, U., & Frisk-Holmberg, M. (1980). Arterial blood pressure and electrodermal activity in hypertensive and normotensive subjects during inner and outer-directed attention. *Acta Media Scandinavica, 646,* 73–76.

Funkenstein, D. H. (1955). The physiology of fear and anger. *Scientific American. 192,* 74–78.

Gannon, L. (1981). The psychophysiology of psychosomatic disorders. In S. N. Haynes & L. Gannon (Eds.), *Psychosomatic disorders, a psychophysiological approach to etiology and treatment.* New York: Praeger.

Gellhorn, E. (1953). *Physiological foundation of neurology and psychiatry.* Minneapolis: University of Minnesota Press.

Gellhorn, E. (1970). The emotions and the ergotropic and trophotropic systems. *Psychologische Forschung, 34,* 48–94.

Gellhorn, E., Cortell, L., & Feldman, J. (1941). The effect of emotion, sham rage and hypothalamic stimulation on the the vago-insulin system. *American Journal of Physiology, 133,* 532–541.

Goldstein, I. B., Grinker, R. R., Heath, H. A., Oken, D., & Shipman, N. G. (1964). Study in psychophysiology of muscle response specificity. *Archives of General Psychiatry, 11,* 322–330.

Grace, W. J., & Graham, D. T. (1952). Relationship of specific attitudes and emotions to certain bodily diseases. *Psychosomatic Medicine, 14,* 243–251.

Graham, D. T., Kabler, J. D., & Graham, F. K. (1962). Physiological response to the suggestion of attitudes specific for hives and hypertension. *Psychosomatic Medicine, 24,* 159–169.

Graham, D. T., Stern, J. A., & Winokur, G. (1958). Experimental investigation of the specificity of attitude hypothesis in psychosomatic disease. *Psychosomatic Medicine, 20,* 446–457.

Graham, F. K. (1973). Habituation and distribution of responses innervated by the autonomic nervous system. In H. V. S. Peeke & M. J. Herz (Eds.), *Habituation: Vol 1. Behavioral studies.* New York: Academic Press.

Graham, F. K., & Clifton, R. K. (1966). Heart-rate change as a component of the orienting response. *Psychological Bulletin, 65,* 305–320.

Hare, R. D. (1973). Orienting and defensive responses to visual stimuli. *Psychophysiology, 10,* 453–464.

Hord, D. J., Johnson, L. C., & Lubin, A. (1964). Differential effect of the law of initial values (LIV) on autonomic variables. *Psychophysiology 1,* 79–87.

James, W. (1884). What is an emotion? *Mind, 9,* 188–205.

Katkin, E. S., Blascovich, J., Koenigsberg, M. R. (1984). Autonomic self-perception and emotion. In W. M. Waid (Ed.), *Sociophysiology.* New York: Springer-Verlag.

Klorman, R., Weissberg, R. P., & Weisenfeld, A. R. (1977). Individual differences in fear and autonomic reactions to affective stimulation. *Psychophysiology, 14,* 45–51.

Lacey, B. C., & Lacey, J. I. (1978). Two-way communication between the heart and the brain. *American Psychologist, 33,* 99–113.

Lacey, J. I. (1950). Individual differences in somatic response patterns. *Journal of Comparative Physiological Psychology, 43,* 338–350.

Lacey, J. I. (1956). The evaluation of autonomic responses: Towards a general solution. *Annals of New York Academy of Science, 67,* 123–163.

Lacey, J. I. (1959). Psychophysiological approaches to the evaluation of psychotherapeutic process and outcome. In E. A. Rubinstein, & M. B. Parloff (Eds.), *Research in psychotherapy.* Washington, DC: American Psychological Association.

Lacey, J. I. (1967). Somatic response patterning and stress: Some revisions of activation theory. In M. H. Appley & R. Trumbull (Eds.), *Psychological stress; Issues in research.* New York: Appleton-Century-Crofts.

Lacey, J. I., Bateman, D. E., & Van Lehn, R. (1952). Automatic response specificity and Rorschach responses. *Psychosomatic Medicine, 14,* 256–260.

Lacey, J. I., Bateman, D. E., & Van Lehn, R. (1953). Autonomic response specificity. An experimental study. *Psychosomatic Medicine, 15,* 8–21.

Lacey, J. I., & Lacey, B. C. (1958). Verification and extension of the principle of autonomic response stereotypy. *American Journal of Psychology, 71,* 51–73.

Lange, C. (1922). The emotions. In W. James & C. Lange (Eds.), *The emotions.* Baltimore: Williams & Wilkins. (Originally published in 1885.)

Lawler, K. A. (1980). Cardiovascular and electrodermal response patterns in heart rate reactive individuals during psychological stress. *Psychophysiology, 17,* 464–470.

Levi, L. (1965). The urinary output of adrenaline and noradrenaline during pleasant and unpleasant emotional states. *Psychosomatic Medicine, 27,* 80–85.

Liddell, H. S., James, W. T., & Anderson, O. D. (1934). The comparative physiology of the conditioned motor reflex, based on experiments with the pig, dog, sheep, goat and rabbit. *Comparative Psychology Monograph, 11* (51).

Lindsley, D. B. (1952). Psychological phenomena and the electroencephalogram. *EEG and Clinical Neurophysiology, 4,* 443–456.

Lykken, D. (1968). Neurophysiology and psychophysiology in personality research. In E. F. Borgatta & W. W. Lambert (Eds.), *Handbook of personality theory and research.* Chicago: Rand McNally.

Lynn, D. (1966). *Attention, arousal and the orientation reaction.* Oxford: Pergamon Press.

Malmo, R. B. (1959). Activation: A neuropsychological dimension. *Psychological Review, 66,* 367–386.

Malmo, R. B. (1975). *On emotions, needs and our archaic brain.* New York: Hold, Rinehart and Winston.

Malmo, R. B., & Shagass, C. (1949). Physiologic study of symptom mechanisms in psychiatric patients under stress. *Psychosomatic Medicine, 11,* 25–29.

Malmo, R. B., Shagass, C., & Davis, F. H. (1950). Symptom specificity and bodily reaction during interview. *Psychosomatic Medicine, 12,* 362–376.

Manuck, S. B., & Schaeffer, D. B. (1978). Stability of individual differences in cardiovascular activity. *Physiology and Behavior, 21,* 675–678.

Moos, R. H., & Engel, B. T. (1962). Physiologic reaction in hypertensive and arthritic patients. *Journal of Psychosomatic Research, 6,* 227–241.

Myrtek, M., & Foerster, F. (1986). The law of initial value: A rare exception. *Biological Psychology, 22,* 227–237.

Oken, D., Grinker, R. R., Heath, H. A., Herz, T. M., Korchin, S. J., Sabshin, M., & Schwartz, N. (1962). Relation of physiologic response to affect expression. *Archives of General Psychiatry, 6,* 20–35.

Oster, P. J., Stern, J. A., & Figar, S. (1975). Cephalic and digital vasomotor orienting responses: The effects of stimulus intensity and risetime. *Psychophysiology, 12,* 642–648.

Pavlov, I. P. (1927). *Conditioned reflexes: An investigation of the physiological activity of the cerebral cortex.* London: Oxford University Press.

Pecke, H., & Petrinovich, L. (1984). Approaches, constructs, and terminology for the study of response change in the intact organism. In H. Pecke & L. Petrinovich (Eds.), *Habituation, sensitization, and behavior.* New York: Academic Press.

Pennebaker, J. W. (1982). *The psychology of physical symptoms.* New York: Springer-Verlag.

Peters, J. E., & Stern, R. M. (1971). Specificity of attitude hypothesis in psychosomatic medicine: A reexamination. *Journal of Psychosomatic Research, 15,* 129–135.

Price, K. P., Lott, G., Fixler, D. E., & Browne, R. H. (1979). Cardiovascular responses to stress in adolescents with elevated blood pressure. *Psychosomatic Medicine, 41,* 74.

Roessler, R., Greenfield, N. S., & Alexander, A. A. (1964). Ego strength and response stereotypy. *Psychophysiology, 1,* 142–150.

Schachter, J. (1957). Pain, fear, and anger in hypertensives and normotensives: A psychophysiological study. *Psychosomatic Medicine, 19,* 17–29.

Schneiderman, N., & Hammer, D. (1985). Behavioral medicine approaches to cardiovascular disorders. In N. Schneiderman & J. J. Tapp (Eds.), *Behavioral medicine, the biopsychosocial approach.* Hillsdale, NJ: Erlbaum.

Schnore, M. (1959). Individual patterns of physiological activity as a function of task differences and degree of arousal. *Journal of Experimental Psychology, 58,* 117–128.

Schwartz, G. E. (1982). Psychophysiological patterning and emotion from a systems perspective. *Social Science Information, 6,* 781–817.

Schwartz, G. E., Weinberger, D. A., & Singer, J. A. (1981). Cardiovascular differentiation of happiness, sadness, anger, and fear following imagery and exercise. *Psychosomatic Medicine, 43,* 343–364.

Sersen, E. A., Clausen, J., & Lidsky, A. (1978). Autonomic specificity and stereotypy revisited. *Psychophysiology, 15,* 60–67.

Shields, S. A., & Stern, R. M. (1979). Emotion: The perception of bodily change. In P. Pliner, K. R. Blankstein, & I. M. Spigel (Eds.), *Perception of emotion in self and others.* New York: Plenum Press.

Shipman, N. G., Heath, H. A., & Oken, D. (1970). Response specificity among muscular and autonomic variables. *Archives of General Psychiatry, 23,* 369–374.

Sokolov, E. N. (1963). *Perception and the conditioned reflex.* Oxford: Pergamon.

Steptoe, A., Melville, D., & Ross, A. (1984). Behavioral response demands, cardiovascular reactivity and essential hypertension. *Psychosomatic Medicine, 46,* 33–48.

Stern, J. A., Winokur, G., Graham, D. T., & Graham, F. K. (1961). Alterations in physiological measures during experimentally induced attitudes. *Journal of Psychosomatic Research. 5,* 73–82.

Stern, R. M. (1976). Reaction time and heart rate between the GET SET and GO of simulated races. *Psychophysiology, 13,* 149–154.

Stern, R. M., & Higgins, J. (1969). Perceived somatic reactions to stress: Sex, age, and familial occurrence. *Journal of Psychosomatic Research, 13,* 77–82.

Stern, R. M., Ray, W. J., & Davis, C. M. (1980). *Psychophysiological recording.* New York: Oxford University Press.

Sternbach, R. A. (1962). Assessing differential autonomic patterns in emotions. *Journal of Psychosomatic Research, 6,* 87–91.

Sternbach, R. A. (1966). *Principles of psychophysiology.* New York: Academic Press.

Surwillo, W. W. (1986). *Psychophysiology.* Springfield, IL: Charles C. Thomas.

Svensson, J. C., & Theorell, T. (1982). Cardiovascular effects of anxiety induced by interviewing young hypertensive male students. *Journal of Psychosomatic Research, 26,* 359–370.

Turpin, G. (1986). Effects of stimulus intensity on autonomic responding: The problem of differentiating orienting and defense reflex. *Psychophysiology, 21,* 1–14.

Walker, B. B., & Sandman, C. A. (1977). Physiological response patterns in ulcer patients; Phasic and tonic components of the electrogastrogram. *Psychophysiology, 14,* 393–400.

Weerts, T. C., & Roberts, R. (1976). The physiological effects of imaging anger provoking and fear provoking scenes. *Psychophysiology, 13,* 174.

Wenger, M. A. (1941). The measurement of individual differences in autonomic balance. *Psychosomatic Medicine, 3,* 427–434.

Wenger, M. A., Clemens, T. L., Coleman, D. R., Cullen, T. D., & Engel, B. T. (1961). Autonomic response specificity. *Psychosomatic Medicine, 24,* 267–273.

Wenger, M. A., & Cullen, T. D. (1972). Studies of autonomic balance in children and adults. In N. S. Greenfield & R. A. Sternbach (Eds.), *Handbook of psychophysiology.* New York: Holt, Rinehart and Winston.

Wilder, J. (1931). The "law of initial value": A neglected biological law and its significance for research and practice. *Zeitschrift für die Gesamte Neurologic and Psychiatric, 137,* 317–324, 329–331, 335–338.

Wilder, J. (1967). *Stimulus and response: The law of initial value.* Bristol: Wright.

Wineman, E. W. (1971). Autonomic balance changes during the human menstrual cycle. *Psychophysiology, 8,* 1–6.

Wolf, G. T., & Wolff, H. G. (1946). Studies on the nature of certain symptoms associated with cardiovascular disorders. *Psychosomatic Medicine, 8,* 293–296.

Yerkes, R. M., & Dodson, J. D. (1908). The relation of strength of stimulus to rapidity of habit-formation. *Journal of Comparative and Neurological Psychology, 18,* 459–482.

8 *Stress and arousal*

ALAN KIM JOHNSON AND ERLING A. ANDERSON

8.1 INTRODUCTION

8.1.1 *Overview*

Characterizing the simultaneous mobilization of physiological and behavioral responses during exposure of organisms to external stimuli has been a major focus of research in psychophysiology. This has been especially true for research defining the relationship of responses to aversive or noxious stimuli. Early in its development psychophysiology adopted the concepts of *stress* and *arousal*[1] initially used in physiology and endocrinology and applied them in both theoretical and experimental analyses (see Brunia, 1979). Although, occasionally, the concepts have been employed independently in psychophysiology, they have been used more often to describe variables in the stimulus→organism→response process. That is, stress has been used to refer to a stimulus (i.e., stressor) or the physiological response of the organism to stimulation; arousal has been used to refer to the response to stimulation or the state of an organism.[2]

The primary purpose of this chapter is to provide psychophysiologists with a strategy for selecting physiological (or biochemical) parameters to be measured as dependent variable(s) associated with a manipulated or measured psychological variable(s). The concepts of stress and arousal are complex and defy simple definitions. Our approach to defining these terms will be to show how they evolved historically and how experimental findings provide pressure for their continued evolution. Since one mainstream of pschophysiology has focused extensively on the stress activation model of analysis, section 2 of this chapter will be directed at understanding the emergence and current status of stress activation research. Section 3 will discuss rationales for selecting physiological variables for psychophysiological research. Section 4 will show how judicious selection of physiological measures can be especially effective in generating important experimental findings in stress activation research. In addition, we hope to increase the awareness that applying a functionally oriented approach can present the psychophysiologist a greater opportunity to address the interests of related fields such as behavioral and psychosomatic medicine.

8.1.2 *Prefatory remarks on stress and arousal*

The terms stress and arousal are similar to the term *intelligence:* Everyone knows what it means, but it defies precise definition. Stress is defined as a response, or set of responses, to a stressor. Conversely, a stressor is that which elicits stress responses. Clearly the definitions are circular. This stems from the fact that there is

216

tremendous variability in what is perceived as a stressor as well as in the nature of stress responses. We hope to show that the heterogeneity of perceived stressors and stress responses can be resolved by considering the perceptual, sensory, and effector systems that cause organisms to respond to similar events in different ways (Anderson, 1987; Lazarus, 1966) and by considering the central nervous system's role in orchestrating response patterns (Anderson, Sinkey, & Mark, 1987b).

This chapter will begin by establishing working definitions of stress, arousal, and the stress response. *Stressors* can be defined as uncontrollable events perceived as threatening physical or psychological harm. Physical harm can range from the discomfort of receiving electric shocks to the gross bodily harm of surgery. Psychological harm can include damage to self-esteem, disruption of social relationships, or an impoverished environment. An excellent review of the literature on this topic is provided by McGrath (1970).

Stress is a set of responses elicited by the perception of facing a stressor. These responses can be physiological (e.g., increased activation of the sympathoadrenal axis), psychological (e.g., feelings of anxiety), or behavioral (e.g., verbal report of anxiety). Many measures of these three components have been developed. McGrath (1970) notes that the measures can be divided into subjective reports and observational measures.

Examples on the *physiological* level are symptom checklists (subjective) and observations of physical tension such as perspiration or changes in palmar sweat gland activity (observational). Examples on the *psychological* level are anxiety questionnaires (subjective) and observations of psychological or behavior disturbances such as stammering (observational). Examples on the *behavioral level* are questionnaires on interpersonal conflict (subjective) and evaluation of task performance (observational) (see McGrath, 1970).

Arousal is an integral part of the stressor–stress relationship. Arousal is the physiological state elicited by an organism's perceptions of its environment. Arousal is not synonymous with stress since arousal can define physiological states ranging from deep sleep to quiet sitting to extreme agitation.

Is the physiological state associated with stress or arousal at any level unidimensional? That is, does it represent a continuum? The answer to this question is almost certainly no. As reviewed in what follows, the consensus is that the stress response is highly complex and multifaceted. This complexity reflects the central nervous system's role in integrating a wide variety of variables to generate somatic and behavioral responses. These variables include such diverse factors as ongoing physiological state, psychological and environmental history, and perception of control over the environment. Further, as we shall show, integration of these factors by the central nervous system can be influenced by genetics, which may predispose an individual to a particular response pattern.

8.2 A BRIEF HISTORY OF STRESS AND AROUSAL

8.2.1 *The stress concept*

8.2.1.1 *Early developments*

Although Hans Selye (1936, 1967) is the scientist most commonly associated with the term stress, the physiologist Walter B. Cannon (1914) employed the term nearly a quarter of a century prior to Selye. In many ways it is appropriate that Cannon should have elected to use the term since he provided the major development of the principles associated with the concept of homeostasis. It is important to recognize that a stressor can only be viewed as deleterious if the concept of the optimum state of physiological condition is first defined. Cannon expanded Claude Bernard's idea that the body functioned to maintain a consistent *"milieu interieur,"* that is, a steady state maintained by coordinated physiological processes (Cannon, 1963). He defined stress as a force acting to perturb the internal homeostatic state.

While conducting endocrinological studies, Selye (1936) observed that injections of crude bovine ovarian extracts into rats produced a constellation of pathophysiological changes including increased adrenal cortical size, gastric ulcers, and alternations in immune system tissues (e.g., atrophy of thymus, lymph nodes, and spleen and reduced lymphocytes and eosinophils). Selye's critical insight was that the same changes were produced with injections of extracts from other organs (e.g., renal or spleenic). These results suggested a generalized, multisystem response to diverse classes of noxious stimuli or demands initially described as stresses and later as stressors. Selye's investigations and reflections prompted him to describe the responses of the body to prolonged stressors in terms of a cluster of signs and symptoms. He called this ongoing process the *General Adaptation Syndrome* (GAS), which consisted of three distinct sequential stages: (1) the alarm reaction; (2) the stage of resistance; and (3) the stage of exhaustion.

The *alarm reaction*, the initial responses to a stressor, actually consists of a *shock phase* and a *countershock phase* (Vingerhoets, 1985). The shock phase is characterized by increased heart rate, reduced temperature, decreased blood pressure, and loss of muscle tone. During the second phase of the alarm reaction the body responds with a "call to arms" characterized by an activation of the pituitary (adrenocorticotrophic, or ACTH, release) and adrenal (adrenocorticoid release) axis. If the challenge to the animal is so great that the acutely mobilized defenses are inadequate, it will die. On the other hand, if the animal survives, a *stage of adaptation or resistance* follows. In this second stage the adrenal cortex becomes rich in secretory granules. In the final phase, the *stage of exhaustion*, the acquired adaptation to the stressor is lost and the symptomatology resembles that of the shock phase of the alarm reaction. For example, he observed a depletion of markers of adrenal cortical hormones during this terminal period.

One question raised by Selye (1967) was how information about the presence of a stressor was conveyed to the area of the brain (hypothalamus) that controls ACTH release and, in turn, the adrenal glucocorticoid response. Because many different classes or types of stressors can evoke pituitary ACTH release, he believed that there was a common afferent signal that he termed the *first mediator*. Logically, this centripetal signal could be neural or humoral (i.e., blood borne). Selye believed that the mediator did not operate over neural channels, although he was never able to specify an "afferent" humoral change.

A second question raised by Selye dealt with the problem of predicting which organ or tissue would be damaged by a chronic stressor. He employed the concept of *conditioning* or *conditioning factors* to explain which *disease of adaptation* might ultimately manifest itself. Selye used conditioning factors (or conditions) not in the Pavlovian sense but to mean endogenous traits (e.g., sex, age, genetic predisposition) or exogenous factors (e.g., diet, environment that predisposed a vulnerability of a particular organ/system).

Methodological improvements in endocrinology and the neurosciences during the 1960s allowed more precise quantification and description of the hormonal responses for several endocrine systems and represented an important point of departure for the further theoretical development of the concept of stress. Notable among endocrinologists pursuing stress research was John W. Mason (Mason, 1968, 1971; Mason, Wool, Mougey, Wherry, Collins, & Taylor, 1968) at Walter Reed Army Institute of Research. While conducting studies on the hormonal responses of different organs, Mason was impressed that endocrine systems were exquisitely sensitive to psychological influences. Mason pointed out that most, if not all, of the stressors described by Selye included some degree of emotional response, discomfort, or pain (Mason, 1968, 1971).

Mason (1968) and Mason et al. (1968) clearly demonstrated the importance of psychological discomfort in mediating physiological stress responses with studies on food-deprived monkeys. In these studies, two monkeys housed with six others were suddenly deprived of food for several days. The food-deprived monkeys, which could observe the others being fed during this time, showed considerable agitation when others were fed. The fasting period was associated with marked increases in urinary corticosteroid levels. To determine whether this hormonal stress response was caused by fasting or the associated emotional stress, Mason reduced the emotional distress associated with food deprivation by removing food-deprived monkeys from the presence of others and by feeding them nonnutritive food pellets similar to their usual food. These procedures reduced psychological reactions and eliminated the previously observed increase in corticosteroids. Mason concluded that the fasting situation, rather than fasting per se, was the stimulus for part of the physiological stress response.

Mason made a major contribution to research on the stress response. His postulation that a psychological component was a concomitant of all effective stressors aided in solving the problem of Selye's elusive mediator. By recognizing that organisms respond to stimuli that are perceived as threatening or aversive as stressors, it is not necessary to postulate an additional afferent factor beyond classical intero- and exteroceptive sensory systems that provide the information contributing to the perception of a stimulus as a stressor.

Mason's incorporation of the psychological perspective into the study of stress represents a refinement in the specification of afferent mechanisms. Recent developments have increased our understanding of the dynamics of the physiological response systems mediating the efferent limb of the stress process. Specifically, these advances deal with the number of systems involved in the stress response and the degree of activation within a given system.

Both Cannon's and Selye's respective realizations that exogenous factors could activate the autonomic nervous system and endocrine responses led each of them to conclude there was a generalized or massive activation of a specific system. Cannon's (1939) overemphasis of the sympathetic nervous system was based upon the anatomically diffuse interconnectivity of the chain of sympathetic ganglia from which he envisioned a functional manifestation of a broad systemic response. He supported his contention by noting that cats exposed to excitement or to cold exhibit piloerection over the entire body. In a similar fashion Selye overemphasized the prominence of the pituitary-adrenocortical response to stress and neglected other hormonal systems.

An obvious explanation for what was almost certainly an unintentional distortion of the prominence of the sympathetic and ACTH-adrenal systems by the respective investigators was that they had to cope with limited methodologies. Mason (1968), in his endocrinological studies, not only enjoyed the opportunity to sample responses to different stressors but was also able to quantitatively measure many different endocrine responses. From this broader perspective he could deduce the commonality among stressors as well as determine that different stressors had the capacity to preferentially activate particular hormonal systems, that there were patterns of different hormones released, and that the endocrine release could be graded.

The second of Selye's questions, the one dealing with the specification of which symptoms develop and in which individuals, again benefited from concepts developed within a field with a behavioral perspective. The psychology of individual differences and its application to clinical psychology led to logical accounts of why different organisms show differential responses to what would appear to be identical situations. Largely through the work of Lazarus and his colleagues (Lazarus, 1966) came the appreciation that individuals' reactions to stressors are markedly influenced by their perception of the probability of disruption of well-being, that is, the capacity to deal with the situation. This ability or coping resource involves a dynamic appraisal process in which the severity of the threat is assessed and reassessed as coping techniques are developed. Clearly any predisposing factor, either genotypic or experiential, could influence the coping process and explain individual differences in the response to stressors.

8.2.1.2   *The stress response: further elaborations and a current view*

From its origins with Cannon and Selye, the concept and experimental analysis of stress has undergone an evolution. At the present time it is possible to describe more precisely the processes involved in an organism's response to stressors. Wilson and Schneider (1981, cited in Asterita, 1985) note that there are over 1,400 physicochemical changes associated with a stress response. Almost certainly, any stressor of sufficient intensity and duration will lead to perturbations of definable biochemical, physiological, or behavioral endpoints. Obviously, for stress to serve as a heuristic concept, it is necessary to identify the most salient changes in bodily responses to a stressor and to describe such changes as a function of time.

Selye's most valuable contribution to the stress concept was the idea that stress produced a syndrome with different contributing factors and manifestations as a function of time. Clearly, this syndrome can presently be considered to involve multiple systems in addition to the specific changes in the pituitary-adrenal axis noted by Selye to accompany each of the three stages of the GAS. The syndrome can best be viewed as a stress response that changes over time as a result of the sequential mobilization of different bodily defenses (see Figure 8.1).

The first-level response to a noxious stimulus is autonomic activation. Cannon's early characterization of the fight-or-flight response implicated the sympathetic nervous system, particularly the adrenal medulla (1914). Although Cannon's perception was that sympathetic activation was massive and nonspecific, current understanding of the initial response to a stressor indicates the sympathetic response is more refined, specific, and graded. Experimental results discussed in later sections of this chapter will provide examples of the exquisite sensitivity and differentiation of sympathetic control that occurs even within seconds after the onset of an evoking stimulus.

CANNON

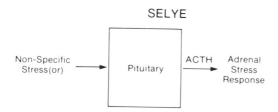

SELYE

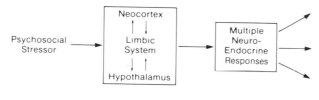

MASON

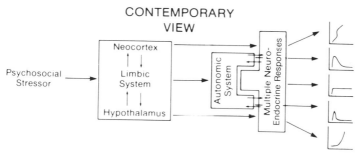

Figure 8.1. Schematic representation of progressive changes in stress concept. Original application of term began with Cannon, who spoke of "great emotional stress" or "stress of the moment." For Cannon, aversive physical and emotional stimuli disrupting homeostasis were responded to with generalized sympathetic nervous system activation. Selye first used *stress* and later *stressor* to indicate types of stimuli that gave rise to general adaptation syndrome (GAS). Selye attended to ACTH–glucocorticoid response as primary focus in response to stressor and as primary index of stages of GAS. Mason's broader endocrinological characterization of response to stressor provided insights into psychological dimension common to effective stressors and to varied and graded nature of responses in different endocrine systems. A contemporary view of the stress concept requires recognition of complexity of functional interrelationships between behavioral, hormonal, and physiological systems. These interactions vary as function of time, intensity, and nature of stressor.

Most notable among the systems activated during the alarm reaction is the adrenocortical-glucocorticoid response, but as noted, many other hormones are involved in the stress response. The actions and interrelationships of stress-related hormones are complex and occur at many different levels in the cellular biochemical events involved in hormonal regulation (e.g., see Axelrod & Reisine, 1984, for review).

The autonomic nervous system is designed to initiate almost instantaneously a corrective action at the onset of a stressor but does not provide an adequate long-term defense. For example, as shown in a control systems analysis of blood pressure by Guyton, Coleman, Cowley, Manning, Norman, & Ferguson (1974), there are rapid corrective effects of neural reflexes such as the baroreceptor reflex, but there is appreciable error in the outcome of this response in comparison to slower control mechanisms such as the ability of the kidney to excrete salt and water. The sensory components of the reflex arc have a short time constant and thus adapt quickly to any steady-state input. Therefore, one can view the activation of hormonal mechanisms, such as ACTH – glucocorticoids, during the later phase of the *alarm reaction* and throughout the stage of resistance as providing a more adequate long-term defense against the effects of the stressor.

In summary, a contemporary consideration of stress incorporates the ideas of Cannon, Selye, Mason, Lazarus, and many others. The contemporary view defines a stressor as a threat to well-being as perceived by the organism and considers the stress response as a syndrome similar to the GAS but in a broader perspective that includes an interplay over time involving neural systems, many hormones, and target tissues.

8.2.2   Activation theory

Cannon's (1939) concept that aversive stimuli produce a *global* activation of the sympathetic nervous system had a great impact on psychologists seeking a unified explanation of behavior. The idea of a mass mobilization of bodily resources coupled with the discovery of an activating system intrinsic to the brain in the late 1940s and early 1950s (Lindsley, Schreiner, Knowles, & Magoun, 1950; Moruzzi & Magoun, 1949) gave rise to the development of activation theory by Lindsley (1951), Duffy (1951, 1957, 1962, 1972), and Malmo (1959). These theorists conceived of a continuum of arousal anchored with coma and increasing to the extremes of excited, agitated behaviors.

The earliest accounts of activation theory focused on the general arousal and alerting functions. The idea that there should be a generalized activating mechanism was very consistent with the prevailing behavioral theory of the early 1950s. Specifically, Hull (1943) had proposed that although the induction of a drive state may come about by any number of antecedent conditions (e.g., food deprivation, water deprivation, electric shock), all contributed to a generalized drive referred to as "D". Drive functioned to initiate behavior and was nondirectional (i.e., not goal oriented; Logan, 1959). Later treatments of activation theory took into account central neural substrates that provided for the focusing of activity to reduce a specific drive (Grossman, 1967; Lindsley, 1957; Routtenberg, 1968).

The earliest formulations of activation theory implied there was a lawful parallelism (or at least a lawful covariation) among indices of cephalic bioelectrical potentials, autonomic activity, and somatomotor responses. This provocative idea spawned a vigorous search for empirical demonstrations of such manifestations, particularly intersystem relationships. However, the psychophysiological literature accumulated few, if any, experimental reports unequivocally supporting activation theory. Lacey's classic 1967 paper is viewed by most as the death knell for the naive line of research testing the simplified form of activation theory that predicts parallel incremental relationships among response systems. Lacey's dismissal of activation theory derived from his assembling examples showing that (1) electrophysiological and behavioral arousal were dissociable; (2) various physiological indices of activation were dissociable; (3) different stimulus situations reliably produced different patterns of physiological responses (i.e., "situational stereotypy"); and (4) afferent inhibitory feedback (i.e., buffering mechanisms) was present in the cardiovascular system.

Similar to the events that occurred during the development of the stress concept, activation theorists began to recognize that there were different patterns of responding to different arousing stimuli and individual response differences to specific stimuli (see Engel, 1983, for review). Engel (1983) has formalized this theoretical development in activation theory as *specificity theory*, which considers both stimulus–response specificity and individual–response specificity. Both types of specificity have been considered in terms of uniqueness and consistency (Engel, 1972; Engel & Moos, 1967). For example, *stimulus–response consistency* is defined as the tendency for a stimulus to elicit a consistent hierarchy of responses, whereas *stimulus–response uniqueness* is defined as the tendency for different stimuli to elicit different responses from a single group of subjects (Engel, 1983). Similarly, *individual–response consistency* is defined as the tendency for a subject to emit a consistent hierarchy of responses to a set of stimuli, whereas *individual–response uniqueness* is the tendency for one group of subjects to respond differently to a given stimulus when compared with another group. (See Stern & Sison, chapter 7.)

There are similarities in the evolution of activation theory and the development of the stress concept. In addition to an expanding data base, methodological advances in both physiology and endocrinology markedly influenced the course of thinking. As pointed out previously for stress responses, activation responses were initially conceived of as massive, nondifferentiated mobilizations of homeostatic systems. The emphasis of Cannon and Selye on the sympathetic nervous system and the pituitary–adrenal axis, respectively, was in all certainty influenced by the techniques available for their study. By necessity, Cannon had relied on distal endpoints (e.g., piloerection) as an index of autonomic activation. Selye could readily weigh the adrenal tissue glands to assess hypertrophy and thereby presumably infer "stress" (increased weight represented increased stress). The subsequent refinements in both stress and activation theory have largely derived from methodological improvements permitting more precise measurements of the autonomic and endocrine systems per se as well as the responses at the effectors. These methodological advances have involved (1) precise quantification of response magnitude of autonomically controlled effectors and of hormones; (2) advances in the simultaneous recording of multiple responses in different response systems; and (3) the characterization of multiple responses within one homeostatically regulated system.

In the subsequent sections we consider strategies to exploit such developments in the design and execution of psychophysiological experiments. In particular, we emphasize and demonstrate the value of employing measures of multiple variables or systems that regulate the endpoints for a homeostatic system.

8.3   THE SELECTION OF BIOLOGICAL ENDPOINTS FOR PSYCHOPHYSIOLOGICAL STUDIES

8.3.1   *The matching of psychological variables and physiological measures*

The idea that covert psychological processes can be tapped by physiological measurements has provided the primary motivation for the development of psychophysiology. The extent to which the psychophysiological approach has been successful has depended largely upon demonstrating reliable relationships in specific assessment contexts between psychological processes and a dependent physiological variable (see Cacioppo & Tassinary, chapter 1). With this consideration it becomes obvious that a careful scrutiny of the physiological measures to be employed may be of great significance in determining the success of a single experiment or a line of research.

To begin with, it is important to emphasize that *both* physiology and psychology are developing and complementary disciplines. Although it is easy to advise the behavioral scientist to be an expert in physiology, it must be recognized that there are lacunas in the body of biological knowledge dealing with function that are just as great as those in the behavioral sciences. In our view, real progress is made in evaluating and conducting psychophysiological research when it is understood that biological data do not constitute psychological theory and that psychological theories are fundamentally about biological events.

Given that psychophysiologists seek reliable physiological measures of a psychological process, we can examine ways to achieve this. At the outset we recognize that the physicochemical measure that "successfully" relates to a psychological variable may in fact have little apparent face validity. The field of psychological measurement abounds with examples of tests (e.g., MMPI) constructed with questions having little face validity but great construct validity. The history of psychophysiology includes many serendipitous discoveries of reliable relationship between physiological measures and psychological variables. Given the state of behavioral and physiological naivete, the bases for the relationships underlying a reliable measure may not be obvious and would never have been deduced on logical grounds. An example of the application of a physiological phenomenon used to assess a psychological process is the use of the P300 event-related evoked potential (Sutton, Braven, Zubin, & John, 1965). The magnitude of the P300 response is a reliable marker of both the occurrence and extent of expectancy-related processes and states, yet the physiological basis of this electrocortical response remains an active area of research (see Coles, Gratton, & Fabiani, chapter 13). However, given experimental constraints, it behooves the investigator to proceed with a logically developed, physiologically informed plan to increase the probability of discovering reliable psychophysiological relationships.

One maximizing strategy is to evaluate the biological relevance of a physiological variable in relation to a psychological process under study. It is reasonable to assume that the more intimately the psychological and physiological variables are mechanistically related, the greater the probability of achieving significant correlations (i.e., positive experimental outcomes). For example, as discussed previously (Lacey, 1967), it has been demonstrated repeatedly that when correlating indices of behavioral and physiological systems, "generic" measures of arousal are of little use. In contrast, if as well as specifying the type of arousal (e.g., sexual arousal) a biologically appropriate physiological measure (e.g., genital activation) is employed, it is possible to demonstrate remarkable correlations in psychophysiological experiments (Venables, 1984). Here the strategy is to precisely specify the psychological variable and to pick a logically related physiological endpoint.

It is beyond the scope of this chapter to cover all physiological systems pertinent to the field of psychophysiology. However, some especially relevant physiological concepts, largely derived from regulatory physiology, will serve the psychophysiologist well when conceptualizing the relationships of different types of physiological variables and when selecting appropriate physiological endpoints. Briefly, there are multiple mechanisms that control a single endpoint, and the framework of control theory provides a basis for studying the relationship of the controlling mechanisms with the regulated endpoint.

8.3.2 *Systems analysis: controls and regulation*

As applied by physiologists, the term *homeostasis* means the tendency toward keeping constant conditions in the body's internal environment. Multiple parameters, or endpoints, are maintained within critical limits in the healthy animal. Examples of regulated variables are body temperature, arterial blood pressure, acid–base balance, extracellular fluid osmolality, and electrolyte concentrations. It is well recognized that there is a hierarchical ordering in terms of priority and tolerance among various regulated endpoints. In effect, the maintenance of a more critical parameter may be done at the expense of another. Tissues, organs, and systems of the body function to maintain homeostasis through concerted actions and interactions. The physical distance between different tissues and organ systems requires communication to coordinate correction of perturbations in homeostatically regulated endpoints. Both the nervous and endocrine systems play this role.

The discipline of regulatory physiology focuses on the systems involved with the maintenance of a constant physicochemical environment. To help unravel the nature of the complex processes involved in homeostasis, regulatory physiologists have made considerable use of concepts derived from engineering control theory. Since the psychophysiologist frequently works at the same level of analysis and within the same systems as the regulatory physiologist, it is worthwhile examining how the latter discipline has made use of systems analysis and control theory to simplify the study of complex, interacting processes.

Since virtually any physicochemical parameter is fair grist for the psychophysiologist, considering the role of the parameter in a homeostatic or regulatory system will aid in the conceptualization of what biological significance a change in that parameter is likely to mean to the animal. Systems analysis (Brobeck, 1965; Guyton et al., 1974; Hardy, 1965; Houk, 1980, 1988) provides a strategy for determining whether a variable is (1) a regulated (homeostatic) endpoint, (2) an afferent signal involved in the activation of mechanisms involved in achieving regulation, (3) an activity of sensory elements, (4) an efferent feedback signal, or even (5) a perturbation or disturbance to a controlled system.

Figure 8.2 is a block diagram representing many of the typical components found

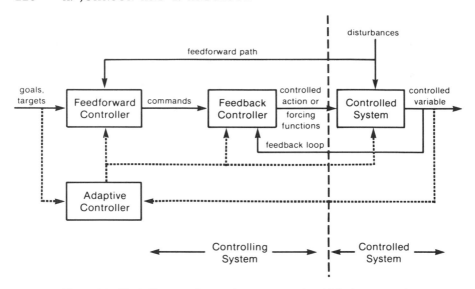

Figure 8.2. Block diagram of a regulatory system in which three control strategies, feedback, feedforward, and adaptive, are illustrated. See text for discussion of control systems and types of controlling systems. (Adapted from Hardy, 1965, and Houk, 1980, 1988.)

in a control system (Houk, 1988). A *control system* can be considered to be a set of communication channels and interconnected subsystems that processes information. A *controlled system* is one that can be manipulated through a *controller action* (also frequently called a *forcing function*) to produce a specific output that is the *controlled variable*. The other input into the controlled system is indicated as *disturbances*, which are the disruptions or perturbations produced in the controlled system.

Three organizational plans, *negative feedback*, *feedforward*, and *adaptive control*, used in automatic control processes are represented in Figure 8.2 (Houk, 1988). Negative feedback provides a closed loop of control through the action of a *feedback controller* that compares command signals with the value of the controlled variable. A *feedforward controller* derives input independent of continuous negative feedback. The input for a feedforward controller is derived from a higher element in the control system and provides the capacity to respond in anticipation of need. The central nervous system has been proposed to frequently function in *feedforward control* (see what follows). An *adaptive controller* modifies elements of the control system to alter (improve) their function rather than producing immediate changes in output.

Engineers prefer the term *control* to that of *regulation*. In contrast, many physiologists employ control to describe management and regulation to denote the preservation of a relatively constant value by means of physiological mechanisms that include a specialized sensor for the critical endpoint or some function of it (Hardy, 1965). For example, body temperature is regulated by the control actions of muscular activity (shivering), piloerection (increasing the insulating capacity of fur), vasodilation of the skin (increases radiant heat loss), evaporative cooling from the skin, and behavioral thermoregulation (i.e., movement from a cold to a warm

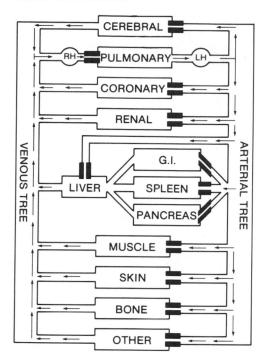

Figure 8.3. Model of circulation showing flow of blood throughout body. Filled rectangles indicate precapillary regions where locally generated factors, circulating hormones, and neurotransmitters have action on vascular smooth muscle, thereby affecting vascular tone, vessel diameter, resistance, and blood flow within a given vascular bed. Cardiac output depends on rate and force of contraction of left heart (LH). Total peripheral resistance (TPR) is the sum of resistances across all vascular beds. Arterial pressure is the product of cardiac output and TPR and represents a regulated endpoint. (RH, right heart; LH, left heart). (Adapted from Peterson, 1965.)

environment). Similarly, blood pressure is regulated by the control of heart rate, stroke volume, and regional blood flow in each vascular bed. It is reasonable to consider each critically maintained homeostatic endpoint as a regulated physiological variable.

A heuristic for classifying variables is a proximal–distal dimension. The distal variable is the regulated endpoint. Proximal variables are those involved in control of the regulated endpoint. Another way of classifying variables as proximal and distal is their "distance" from the central nervous system. For example, blood pressure is regulated by cardiac output and total peripheral resistance. Therefore, pressure is distal to the underlying proximal variables of cardiac output and peripheral resistance.

8.3.3 *The regulation of arterial blood pressure: an example of interactive multiple control systems achieving regulation*

The function of the cardiovascular system is to provide optimum perfusion of tissues. Figure 8.3 is a schematic representing the distribution of blood flow through the body. The blood pumped from the left ventricle of the heart to the arterial vascular tree passes through multiple vascular beds (e.g., cerebral and pulmonary) and returns to the left atrium. Force is generated by the muscular contraction of the heart to move blood through the resistive network comprising the systemic circulation.

Arterial blood pressure (ABP) is the product of the *cardiac output* (CO) times the *total peripheral resistance* (TPR) (ABP = CO × TPR). Cardiac output is the volume of blood ejected from the heart per unit time. Cardiac output is determined by the amount of blood returning to the heart, the strength and frequency of contraction of the heart, and the resistance against which the heart is pumping. Sympathetic and parasympathetic influences on the heart interact to determine stroke volume and cardiac rate. Since regional vascular beds are arranged in parallel, the total peripheral resistance represents the reciprocal of the sum of the conductances of all the vascular beds of the body.

Blood flow in each vascular bed can be individually adjusted. That is, the body has the capacity to "direct" blood flow away from some areas (e.g., muscles) and toward others (e.g., brain and heart). This derives from the capacity of vascular muscle located in the small arteries and arterioles to alter tone and increase or decrease vessel diameter. Contraction and relaxation of vascular muscle is influenced by both neural and humoral factors. Vasoconstrictor agents cause contraction and reduce blood flow. Vasodilator agents cause relaxation and increase blood flow.

Many substances synthesized within the body, as well as drugs, are vasoactive agents. Examples of endogenous vasoconstrictors include norepinephrine, vasopressin, and angiotensin II. Vasodilators include histamine, bradykinin, and prostaglandins of the E and A series. It should be noted that some substances (e.g., epinephrine) can produce vasoconstriction in one vascular bed and vasodilation in another by acting on different types of local receptors. Thus, the degree of vascular contraction represents the result of the integrated action of multiple constricting/dilating factors derived from local sources, from sympathetic innervation, and from the circulation as well as the intrinsic tone of the muscle.

Most likely the reader will recognize most of the agents listed in the preceding as being either hormones or neurotransmitters. This is not surprising considering the central nervous system (CNS) acts through neural as well as hormonal effectors to coordinate the simultaneous action of dilator and constrictor agents in the various vascular beds. Therefore, the CNS has the capacity to determine the pattern of blood distribution within the body (i.e, shunting it from one part to another). The ability to "direct" blood flow provides optimum perfusion of critical tissues without requiring inordinately large and grossly maladaptive blood volume. The management of blood distribution provides for increased adaptability of the animal in different behavioral and environmental settings. Flow can be increased to specific beds without a disproportionately large increase in blood pressure. The importance of redirecting flow is most obvious during exercise when skeletal muscle blood flow increases dramatically. Exercise increases blood pressure through sympathetic vasoconstriction in many vascular beds. With a pharmacologically blocked sympathetic nervous system, blood pressure actually falls during exercise.

Muscular exercise results in a specific, patterned cardiovascular response. Cardiac output and heart rate increase, blood pressure rises, blood reserves in the capacitance portions of the circulation (venous and pulmonary) are shifted to the high-pressure side, blood flow to the exercising skeletal muscle increases, and blood flow to some vascular beds (e.g, mesenteric and renal) decreases. These hemodynamic adjustments are initiated by activation of efferent pathways from the brain (i.e., the source of central command) and influenced by metabolic demands in the exercising muscle (Rowell, 1986). The feedforward mechanism of central command provides animals with the adaptive advantage of increasing perfusion of the exercising tissue in anticipation of need, that is, before it would occur as a result of a peripherally initiated reflex (Rowell, 1986). The coordination of feedforward and feedback control systems in the regulation of blood pressure during exercise is represented schematically in a control theory framework in Figure 8.4.

The integrative capacity of the CNS to process numerous afferent inputs and to orchestrate changes in regional blood flows raises the possibility that different behaviors may be associated with unique hemodynamic patterns. Each may result in a specific maximizing strategy to ensure an optimal distribution of a finite amount of blood. It is known that there can be dramatic shifts in blood flow or in cardiac function without changes in arterial pressure. Therefore, studying the proximal controlled variables (e.g., multiple regional blood flows and heart rate) in addition to the more distal, regulated variable (i.e., blood pressure) is likely to yield more information about physiological responses associated with behaviors.

8.4 EXAMPLES OF THE APPLICATION OF MULTIPLE DISTAL AND PROXIMAL
MEASURES AND METHODS: AN ANALYSIS OF THE CARDIOVASCULAR
DEFENSE RESPONSE IN ANIMALS AND HUMANS

8.4.1 *A history of the defense response*

Unrestrained animals exposed to aversive stimuli usually demonstrate either fight or flight behaviors. The aggressive or defensive responses under such conditions involve both somatic and visceral effector systems. The pioneering studies of Cannon (reviewed in Cannon, 1929) directed attention to the role of the central nervous system in initiating and controlling the behavioral, endocrine, and autonomic concomitants of affective response patterns. Continuing the work of Cannon, his student Bard (1928) implicated the hypothalamus as the critical site of integration by demonstrating that the integrity of this structure was critical for the rage response associated with "sham rage" produced by decortication. Further evidence for the role of diencephalic structures in the generation of emotion-related behavioral and physiological responses came from two subsequent lines of research employing electrical brain stimulation. Hess (1949) stimulated the hypothalamus of awake, freely moving cats and showed that responses indistinguishable from normal defensive behaviors (*Abwehrreacktion*) could be elicited. That is, the cat displayed responses comparable to those seen when confronted by a barking dog. Ranson and Magoun (1939) stimulated the hypothalamus of anesthetized cats and evoked visceral responses similar to those accompanying rage.

Later stimulation studies employing refined techniques for cardiovascular characterization culminated with the investigations of Uvnas, Folkow, Hilton, and others (Abrahams, Hilton, & Zbrozyna, 1960, 1964; Folkow, Heymans, & Neil, 1965; Uvnas, 1960). These investigators demonstrated that stimulation within a broad region of the central nervous system in anesthetized animals could elicit a cardiovascular pattern consisting of increased arterial pressure, heart rate, and

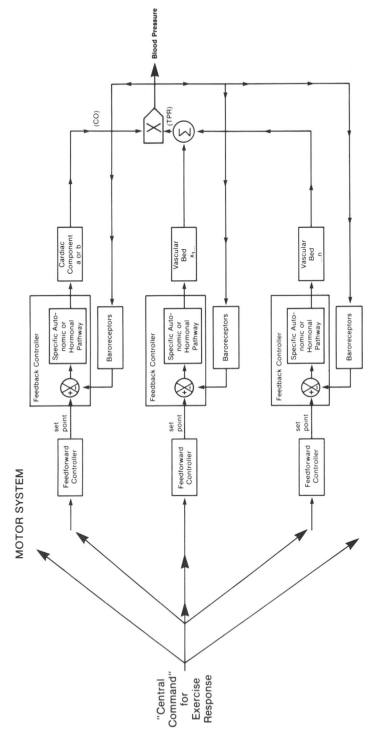

Figure 8.4. Simplified schematic from control model perspective representing interactions of control systems of cardiac output and of regional circulations. For simplification determinants of cardiac output have been lumped into a single box, and only two of the many controlled vascular beds are represented. The concept of central command to initiate cardiovascular adjustments in anticipation of need arising from behavior is incorporated into the schematic. A central command accompanying exercise has been proposed to act through the feedforward controller to raise the set point for arterial pressure. Baroreceptor reflexes (feedback) are important for maintaining blood pressure at a new set point. (Adapted from Houk, 1988.)

stroke volume; decreased blood flow to renal, intestinal, and skin vascular beds; and increased skeletal muscle blood flow.

This electrically elicited cardiovascular pattern, defined as the *defense reaction*, appeared similar to responses evoked by stressful stimuli producing arousal and increased blood flow to skeletal muscle in preparation for fighting. Fighting requires increased blood flow to skeletal muscle. The increase in skeletal muscle blood flow is supported by increases in cardiac output and blood pressure. Shunting blood from mesenteric and renal beds can be viewed as adaptive since the resulting decreased absorption of food from the intestine and reduced renal excretory function would have little effect on surviving a fight. More recently developed techniques have allowed investigators (e.g., Stock, Schlor, Heidt, & Buss, 1978) to measure multiple cardiovascular parameters in freely moving animals and to correlate visceral and behavioral responses. In these studies the brain stimulation elicited defense response (BSEDR) gives rise to behavioral and cardiovascular reactions similar to the defense response.

Compared to what is known about the BSEDR, much less is known about the hemodynamic responses and behaviors elicited by noxious external physical or psychosocial stimuli. The majority of experimental animal studies have examined cardiovascular changes accompanying conditioning. Until recently only a few studies such as those from Zanchetti's laboratory (e.g., Adams, Bacceli, Mancia, & Zanchetti, 1969) have examined cardiovascular changes in behaving animals when natural defense and aggression were elicited.

A classic hemodynamic study on the effects of an anxiety-eliciting stimulus in humans was carried out by Brod, Fencl, Hejl, & Jirka (1959). They studied hemodynamic responses during acute mental stress (performing mental mathematics under pressure). Mental stress significantly increased heart rate and blood pressure. Underlying the pressure increase was splanchnic and renal vasoconstriction and vasodilation in forearm skeletal muscle. Perhaps most importantly, Brod et al. (1959) noted that changes in total peripheral resistance during mental stress depended on the balance between simultaneous vasodilation in muscle and vasoconstriction in the viscera. Thus, total peripheral resistance was determined by the interaction of changing vascular tone in different circulatory beds.

Beyond the fact that animal and human studies employing simultaneous cardiovascular and behavioral measures are likely to generate data relevant to psychophysiologists, these studies have been particularly provocative to the investigation of cardiovascular disease. One hypothesis of the pathogenesis of hypertension is that repetitive activation of the cardiovascular defense response, especially in genetically susceptible individuals, may lead to essential hypertension (Charvat, Dell, & Folkow, 1964; Folkow & Rubenstein, 1966). Human epidemiological and experimental animal studies have led some reviewers to conclude that chronic exposure to stressors requiring continuous behavioral and physiological adjustments can contribute to the development of hypertension (Eyer, 1975; Gutman & Benson, 1971; Henry & Cassel, 1969).

Although the methodologies and studies we shall now discuss were motivated because of our interests in elucidating mechanisms in the pathogenesis of hypertension, they are presented in order to illustrate several points we believe are important for psychophysiological studies of stress and arousal. First, the studies will serve to illustrate the advantage of employing multiple proximal measures in addition to a single distal measure. Second, the studies reviewed will demonstrate

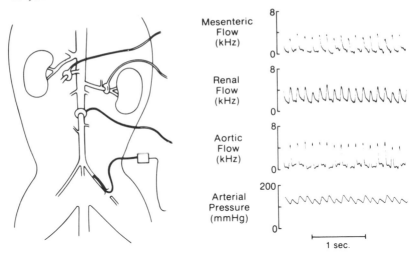

Figure 8.5. Diagram showing placement of pulsed Doppler flow probes on blood vessels in the rat. *Right:* Sample polygraph records showing phasic changes in Doppler shift, reflecting changes in blood flow through mesenteric and renal arteries and terminal aorta as a function of the cardiac cycle. Rats are also implanted with arterial catheters for blood pressure recording.

the great specificity of sympathetic nervous system responses to stress, thereby continuing the conceptual evolution away from the mass sympathetic response concept imbued by Cannon. Third, the studies will demonstrate that what appear as stereotyped cardiovascular responses are under the influence of feedback. Fourth, the experiments will emphasize the value of conducting animal studies that parallel human investigations.

8.4.2   Techniques for the mechanistic analysis of cardiovascular regulation and control

8.4.2.1   Methods: animal studies

The rat is the most widely studied experimental species in the behavioral sciences. Until recently, cardiovascular measurements made in freely moving rats have been largely limited to arterial pressure and heart rate recordings. However, Michael J. Brody and his colleagues, at the University of Iowa (e.g., see Haywood, Shaffer, Fastenow, Fink, & Brody, 1981), have modified the pulsed Doppler flowmeter described originally by Hartley and Cole (1974) to allow the direct measurement of regional blood flow in freely moving rats. This flowmeter uses a single piezoelectric crystal as both transmitter and receiver of ultrasound signals. The advantage of this flowmeter is that it is mounted in a very small silastic cuff and can be placed around arteries supplying blood to different vascular beds.

Routinely, Iowa researchers (Haywood et al., 1981) have placed flow probes on the renal and mesenteric arteries and on the lower abdominal aorta. An example of probe placements and the types of blood flow tracings that can be obtained from chronically instrumented animals is shown in Figure 8.5. In addition to the flow probes, rats are instrumented with a femoral or carotid arterial catheter that directly measures arterial pressure. Wires from the flow probes and catheter are run subcutaneously to the head and neck, respectively. These wires are soldered to a head mount plug attached to a cable, and the arterial catheter is connected to a pressure transducer. The lines exit the top of the cage and are counterweighted to allow the animal nearly unrestricted movement.

The flowmeter system determines blood flow velocity through the vessels that has been shown to be directly proportional to absolute blood flow as determined by an electromagnetic flowmeter. Although absolute blood flow cannot be determined with these flow probes, it is possible to calculate relative resistances and determine changes in vascular resistance in the vascular bed served by the artery on which the probe is placed. With this instrumentation it is possible to simultaneously record blood pressure, heart rate, and changes in blood flow in the kidney, mesentery, and skeletal muscle vascular beds in the behaving rat.

8.4.2.2 *Methods: human studies*

A variety of techniques have been developed to measure parameters of the defense response in humans. One of the most studied aspects of the defense response is skeletal muscle blood flow. Blood flow to skeletal muscle can be quantified by venous occlusion plethysmography. Plasma catecholamines, which reflect sympathetic influences on skeletal muscle blood flow, can be measured in arterial or venous blood. Further, sympathetic neural outflow to blood vessels in skeletal muscle can be recorded directly by microneurographic recording techniques.

Skeletal muscle blood flow is controlled by multiple factors. These include circulating hormones such as epinephrine as well as sympathetic neural tone (i.e., central sympathetic vasoconstrictor outflow). The factors controlling skeletal muscle blood flow can be conceptualized along a distal–proximal continuum. As noted in the preceding, distal factors (e.g., arterial blood pressure) reflect the influence of multiple underlying (or proximal) mechanisms such as regional blood flow and sympathetic nerve activity. More proximal measures reflect a specific mechanism of sympathetic nerve activity that partly controls regional blood flow. We now briefly review the techniques of plethysmography, plasma catecholamine analysis, and microneurography. Studies illustrating their use will then be reviewed as examples of how they can be applied to the study of cardiovascular responses to stress.

Venous occlusion plethysmography. Venous occlusion plethysmography is used to measure blood flow to the arm or leg as well as segments of these limbs such as the forearm, calf, or fingers. Blood flow to these regions includes skin and muscle flow, and the relative contribution of muscle and skin flow varies (Siggaard-Andersen, 1970). Forearm blood flow primarily reflects flow in skeletal muscle tissue since the proportion of muscle to skin is greater in the arm than it is in the hand. Conversely, blood flow to the hand or fingers reflects skin blood flow because of the greater proportion of skin to muscle in this extremity.

Venous occlusion plethysmography involves placing a pneumatic cuff on the bicep and briefly inflating it to 40 mm Hg, a pressure that arrests venous return from the limb (Figure 8.6). Limb volume increases during the 5–8 s of venous occlusion as arterial inflow accumulates in the venous system. This increase is measured by a

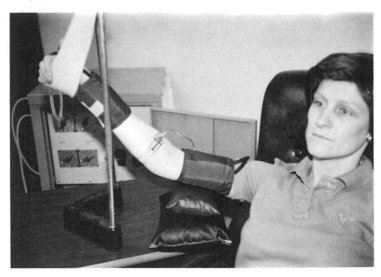

Figure 8.6. Experimental setup for recording forearm blood flow. Cuff on the bicep is inflated to 40 mm Hg. This arrests venous outflow from the arm but does not impede arterial inflow. Cuff on the wrist is inflated to 200 mm Hg to arrest blood flow to the hand, which is primarily skin blood flow. A Whitney strain gauge is placed around widest part of forearm. Mercury-filled silastic tubes (attached to strain gauge) encircle the arm. When bicep cuff is inflated for 7–8 s, the forearm expands as venous drainage is arrested. Forearm expansion during venous occlusion stretches the silastic tube which changes resistance to DC current passed through mercury. Volume changes in ml per minute per 100 ml of forearm volume can then be calculated.

plethysmographic recording device (see what follows). The cuff is then deflated for 8–10 s to allow blood to drain from the limb. A cycle of cuff inflation, measurement, and cuff deflation takes approximately 15 s allowing four measurements per minute.

Measuring skeletal muscle blood flow in the forearm or calf requires placement of a second cuff on the wrist or ankle to exclude flow to the hand or foot, respectively. Inflating this distal cuff to 200 mm Hg arrests blood flow to the hand or foot. An arresting cuff at the wrist excludes the hand circulation, which is primarily skin flow.

Three major assumptions underlie the use of venous occlusion plethysmography to measure blood flow: (1) arresting venous return does not impede arterial inflow; (2) venous return is stopped completely during measurement; and (3) the increase in venous pressure during occlusion does not alter arterial inflow. These assumptions have been widely tested and found valid (see Formel & Doyle, 1957, or Hyman & Winsor, 1961).

The strain gauge plethysmograph (introduced by Whitney, 1953, and shown in Figure 8.6) is the most commonly used plethysmographic device for measuring limb flow. This method measures changes in limb circumference and not changes in volume (Williams, 1984). Changes in circumference are measured by placing a mercury-filled silastic tube around the limb (e.g., forearm) and passing DC current through the mercury. Tube length increases as the limb expands. This produces changes in electrical resistance. Calibration is performed by shortening the silastic tubing known amounts (e.g., 1 mm) and noting the change in electrical resistance. Shortening is usually done by means of a calibration screw mounted on a Wheatstone bridge to which the silastic tube is attached (see Figure 8.6).

Circumference changes during venous occlusion are indicated by changes in resistance across the mercury-filled tube. The percentage of change in volume is twice the percentage of change in circumference, and increases in circumference can therefore be converted to volume increase in ml per minute per 100 ml of limb volume (Whitney, 1953; Williams, 1984).

Plasma catecholamines. Plasma concentrations of the catecholamines epinephrine and norepinephrine can be measured by drawing samples of arterial or venous blood. Plasma catecholamine levels are frequently used as an index of sympathetic nerve activity. They may reflect adrenal release of epinephrine or activity of sympathetic nerves in skeletal muscle that release norepinephrine. They do not reflect "overall" sympathetic activity since catecholamines from the splanchnic region are metabolized by the liver before entering accessible veins.

The use of plasma catecholamine measurements in psychological research has greatly increased since the development of assay techniques that permit accurate measurement of their plasma levels. Assay techniques include radioenzymatic assay and high-performance liquid chromatography. The former is exceedingly accurate but time consuming and expensive, whereas the latter is less expensive and more rapid. However, both techniques require considerable expertise, and analyses are frequently performed in collaboration with laboratories dedicated to such procedures. (See Grunberg & Singer, chapter 5.)

Plasma catecholamines have a very short biological half-life (90 s), and their levels change rapidly. Collecting venous blood requires a venipuncture that acutely increases sympathetic nerve activity and catecholamine levels. Thus, measurements are best made by means of an indwelling catheter with samples drawn after a waiting period following venipuncture.

Blood samples for catecholamine assays can be drawn by means of heparin lock or an automated blood withdrawal pump. Both methods are described in detail by Dimsdale (1984), who provides an excellent example of how plasma catecholamine measurements can be used to study the stress of public speaking.

Within the framework of proximal and distal measurements of sympathetic activity, plasma catecholamine assays fall between plethysmographic measurement of skeletal muscle blood flow (which is influenced by other systems as well as the sympathetic system) and direct recording of sympathetic nerve activity (which directly records sympathetic neural activity). Direct recording of sympathetic nerve activity by microneurography provides a continuous and exceedingly sensitive measure of sympathetic outflow. Further, it reflects central sympathetic outflow, whereas plasma catecholamine levels may reflect abnormalities in peripheral mechanisms (e.g., increased transmitter release, altered metabolism of catecholamines, or changes in reuptake mechanisms).

Microneurography. Microneurography involves inserting microelectrodes into peripheral nerves for directly recording sympathetic nerve activity (Figure 8.7). It is safe and tolerated well when performed properly (Hagbarth, 1979). It requires special equipment and training. Although developed by Hagbarth and Valbo in

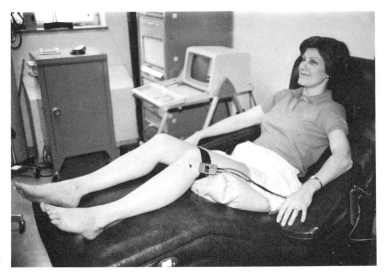

(a)

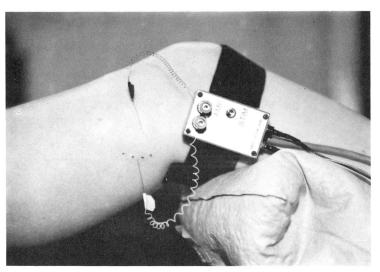

(b)

Figure 8.7. *Top:* Experimental setup for microneurographic recording from the peroneal nerve in the leg. Knee is elevated slightly and stabilized. Preamplifier is attached at the knee just proximal to recording site. *Bottom:* Close-up of microelectrode placement for measuring nerve activity. Black dots on the leg show path of personeal nerve as determined by percutaneous stimulation. Top electrode is reference electrode. Bottom electrode (white flag) is inserted into the nerve. Nerve is located by stimulating through this electrode. After entering the nerve (indicated by twitches obtained with stimulation), electrode is switched to recording mode by switching from stimulation to amplify (STIM and AMP switch on amplifier).

Sweden during the 1960s, microneurography has only recently begun to be applied systematically to the study of stress (Anderson, Wallin, & Mark, 1987c).

Microneurography is most frequently used to measure postganglionic activity in unmyelinated, efferent Type C sympathetic fibers innervating muscle and skin. This activity represents efferent vasoconstrictor activity of most interest to the study of cardiovascular responses to stressors mediated by the sympathetic nervous system.

The procedure for locating and recording from nerves involves three steps. First, percutaneous electrical stimulation is used to locate the position of the nerve. This is followed by insertion of an electrode into the nerve using weak electrical stimulation through the electrode. Finally, small adjustments of electrode position are made to obtain a satisfactory recording site. Use of this technique in psychophysiological research is described in detail by Anderson and Mark (1989).

Equipment required for microneurography includes a nerve stimulator and stimulus isolation unit, signal conditioning and amplification circuitry, a storage oscilloscope, and an audioamplifier. Tungsten wire electrodes (30–40 mm long, 0.2 mm wide, tapering to a 1–5-μm tip) are used for recording. Such small electrodes can be inserted without local anesthetic and with minimal discomfort to subjects.

Of the techniques discussed in this chapter to study autonomic reactions to stressors, microneurographic measurement of sympathetic nerve activity is the most proximal measure. Microneurography quantitates central sympathetic outflow, whereas plasma catecholamine levels, which are influenced by sympathetic outflow, are influenced by factors such as the amount of neurotransmitter released by a nerve and the efficiency of reuptake/metabolic mechanisms.

Microneurography can be used to characterize sympathetic nerve activity to both skin and muscle. Skin and muscle sympathetic nerve activity (SNA) differ both in the resting state and in the response to different interventions. Muscle SNA is primarily vasoconstrictor, whereas skin includes vasoconstrictor, sudomotor, and piloerector activity. Blood flow to skin is involved in temperature regulation, and skin SNA therefore changes with changing body temperature. When recording sympathetic nerve activity, skin and muscle sympathetic activity can be easily distinguished. Apnea increases muscle sympathetic activity as does tapping upon the innervated muscle. Skin sympathetic activity is increased by stroking the innervated skin as well as by stimuli causing a startle response.

Psychological factors have a major influence on skin SNA. Skin SNA increases during arousal and declines during relaxation. Both pleasant and unpleasant novel stimuli cause sudden increases in skin SNA (Lidberg & Wallin, 1981). In contrast, muscle SNA responds less quickly to psychological stimuli than SNA (Delius, Hagbarth, Hongell, & Wallin, 1972a). Further, there is little relationship between muscle and skin SNA at rest or in response to different interventions. Thus, skin SNA does not provide an index of muscle SNA (Delius, Hagbarth, Hongell, & Wallin, 1972b). These findings have significant implications for those studying electrodermal responses as a measure of sympathetic activation and arousal. They suggest that electrodermal responses provide a limited index of sympathetic activity. Further, they provide less information relevant to control of arterial pressure since changes in skeletal muscle blood flow are of greater importance in blood pressure regulation.

8.4.3   *Recent animal and human studies of the defense response: application of multiple proximal and distal measures of activation by stressors*

8.4.3.1   *Animal models*

The defense response in the resident–intruder paradigm. The defense response elicited by electrical brain stimulation has played a prominent role in the study of neural control of the circulation. It has been taken as the functional prototype for supporting the contention that specific behaviors are associated with specific cardiovascular patterns (e.g., increased cardiac output and skeletal muscle blood flow with decreased renal and mesenteric flow). It has also provided seminal support for the concept that the central nervous system simultaneously organizes behavioral and cardiovascular responses. There are some shortcomings with much of the research conducted in experimental animals on the defense response. First, the characterizations and analysis of behaviors that accompany electrically elicited responses have been largely anecdotal. Responses such as hissing and piloerection have been taken by investigators to be adequate indices of defensive or aggressive behaviors. Second, electrical stimulation of the brain has the strong potential to induce artifactual components in both the cardiovascular and behavioral responses. As noted in the preceding, there are only a few studies of the hemodynamic changes accompanying defense and aggression evoked by environmental stimuli. As a result, we have begun to employ techniques to quantitatively characterize multiple hemodynamic changes (i.e., cardiovascular characterization of the defense response) in the behaving rat under a variety of situations where behaviors are under the control of aversive or threatening stimuli (i.e., stressors).

The first studies were conducted by Richard J. Viken as part of his doctoral dissertation (Viken, 1984). A well-studied behavioral situation, the resident–intruder paradigm (see Grant & MacIntosh, 1963; Lehman & Adams, 1977) was employed in this research to permit the simultaneous specification of each component of agonistic exchanges between two rats along with hemodynamic changes recorded from one of the two.

The resident–intruder paradigm consists of isolating two male rats for a period of 30–60 days. At the conclusion of the isolation period one rat, the "intruder", is introduced into the home cage of the other, the "resident." Numerous studies have demonstrated that each of the two rats adopt specific roles. The resident becomes the aggressor and ultimately defeats the intruder. Conversely, the intruder demonstrates defensive behaviors and eventually submits to the resident. Both animals show a rich repertoire of behaviors during the agonistic exchange, which is videotaped, and the behaviors are scored on a second-by-second basis.

Using this paradigm, Viken studied intruders that were instrumented with renal, mesenteric, and hindlimb vascular bed flow probes and arterial catheters for recording blood pressure. Because this behavioral paradigm affords such precise specification of behaviors, an initial hypothesis we entertained was that each offensive and defensive behavior might have its own distinguishable cardiovascular "signature." Viken's studies indicated that this was not the case for each individual behavior. However, there was a cardiovascular pattern apparent in the intruder once it was attacked. The cardiovascular response of the intruder to attack by the resident was an increase in heart rate and hindquarter blood flow and a decrease in blood flow to renal and mesenteric vascular beds. Being attacked resulted in increased variability of the intruder's blood pressure, but there was no consistent, marked elevation from baseline. Thus, although a similar cardiovascular response pattern was displayed by the intruder during attack regardless of the specific defensive or offensive behavior it was displaying, only a portion of the pattern resembled the BSEDR (i.e., the classic defense response elicited by brain stimulation). Specifically, the direction of change in the blood flows are comparable for the two situations, but the marked pressor response typically described to be part of the BSEDR was absent. With the more naturalistic resident–intruder paradigm the intruder's blood pressure appears to be remarkably well maintained in spite of marked regional changes in blood flow.

Hemodynamic changes in an exogenously evoked defense response (EEDR). Although the resident–intruder paradigm proved to be a promising method for the concomitant study of behavior and cardiovascular patterning in the rat, the vigorous aggressive exchanges often induced suffcient motor artifacts to prevent continuous recording. In addition, pharmacological interventions that would be extremely valuable in analyzing the mechanisms underlying hemodynamic changes were likely to alter the overt behaviors and disrupt the dynamic interaction between resident and intruder. To allow a more thorough characterization of the mechanisms mediating the various flow changes accompanying the response to an exogenous stressor, we have studied the hemodynamic responses during the presentation of a light/tone stimulus that has previously been paired with intermittent footshock.

In these studies (Callahan, Brody, & Johnson, 1985; Callahan, Kirby, Brody, & Johnson, 1985) male Sprague-Dawley rats received miniaturized pulsed Doppler flow probes to measure hindquarter, renal, and mesenteric blood flow. After a recovery period, rats received 30 pairings of light/tone (15 s) followed by 15 s of intermittent footshock (1 mA, 0.5 s duration, delivered 1 per s) per day. We have referred to the behavioral and hemodynamic changes produced by this paradigm as an EEDR. After 2 or 3 days, the behavioral and hemodynamic changes during presentation of the light/tone became remarkably consistent. On subsequent days, animals received adrenergic receptor antagonists between trials 10 and 11, and the responses of these trials were compared.

The typical behavioral response during presentation of the light/tone signal was immobility.[3] Therefore, high-quality recordings of hemodynamic measures were readily attainable. The usual hemodynamic response (Figure 8.8) during the light/tone stimulus consists of a primary pressor response occurring at approximately 1 s, then a slight decrease, followed by a secondary pressor response that remains for the remainder of the light/tone stimulus. Analysis of flow data indicates that at 1 s after light/tone onset, there is a significant mesenteric vasoconstriction with no change in the other beds. At 8 s after light/tone stimulus onset, mesenteric resistance reaches a peak, whereas resistance in the hindquarter bed decreases significantly.

The use of pharmacological antagonists has proved to be most useful in characterizing the sympathetic mechanisms underlying the pressor response of the EEDR. Aplha-1-adrenergic receptor blockade with the antagonist prazosin (0.5 mg/kg i.v.) attenuates the pressor response to the light/tone stimulus. This occurs because prazosin attenuates an alpha-1-receptor-mediated vasoconstriction in the mesenteric bed that occurs immediately upon onset of the light/tone presentation. It

EEDR

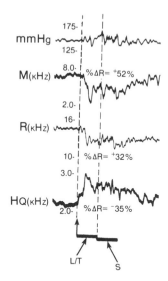

Figure 8.8. Dynograph (Beckman) record of exogenously evoked defense response (EEDR) in rat. Record shows mean arterial blood pressure (mm Hg) and mesenteric (M), renal (R), and hindquarter (HQ) blood flows. This stereotyped cardiovascular response occurs and remains remarkably consistent after first four to six pairings of 15-s of mild intermittent footshock. The EEDR, hemodynamic pattern occurring during 15-s L/T period, is comprised of slight biphasic increase in blood pressure and an increase in hindlimb blood flow (i.e., decreased hindquarter resistance and decreased mesenteric and renal blood flow. Calculated resistance changes for different vascular beds reflect changes in resistance at maximum pressure increase. Rats remain immobile during L/T presentation.

appears that because the initial rise in pressure was blunted, the hindquarter vasodilation, which is probably under baroreceptor feedback, control, is reduced. The hindquarter vasodilation itself is normally effected by the action of catecholamine on beta-adrenergic receptors since the beta-adrenoceptor antagonist, *di*–propranolol (0.1 mg/kg i.v.) blocks the dilatory response seen at 8 sec. Blocking hindlimb vasodilation produces a greater pressor response. The results of these studies demonstrate that the cardiovascular response to the light/tone stimulus consists of a complex hemodynamic pattern. First, the primary pressor response immediately after light/tone onset is mediated in part by increased sympathetic drive, causing mesenteric vasoconstriction. The magnitude of the subsequent pressor response depends upon the interaction of a mesenteric bed vasoconstriction with a skeletal muscle bed vasodilation.

The results of this experiment demonstrate several features of the EEDR. First, the EEDR has a very consistent hemodynamic pattern with many, but not all, of the components of the BSEDR (i.e., as classically described, the increase in blood pressure, heart rate, and skeletal muscle blood flow and the decrease in renal and mesenteric blood flow). Second, as in the case for the blood pressure of the intruder in the resident–intruder paradigm, mean arterial pressure is remarkably well maintained. In the EEDR, the blood pressure increased only slightly during exposure to the stressor and certainly not to the extent usually reported for the BSEDR. Third, the expression of the defense response elicited by an exogenous stressor is not a ballistic event but is subject to modification. Specifically, if the early increase in mesenteric resistance is prevented and the pressor response blunted, then subsequent normal increase in skeletal muscle blood, which would tend to offset the initial rise in pressure, is reduced. This suggests that the skeletal muscle vasodilation in the EEDR is to some extent under baroreceptor reflex control and not totally evoked by a central command.[4]

It is worthwhile noting the implications that a study that characterizes the interaction of baroreceptor feedback mechanisms with the cardiovascular response to a stressor has for the study of psychophysiology. Recall that one of Lacey's (1967) major points in his attack on the simplistic formulation of activation theory was the presence of afferent inhibitory feedback in the cardiovascular system (see section 2.2). In light of the study just discussed, it can be appreciated that although feedback mechanisms may complicate the psychophysiological analysis of responses to a stressor, they do not make such investigations impossible. An appreciation of the nature of multicomponent control systems and how they relate to the physiological response systems under investigation coupled with appropriate physiological measures can enhance psychophysiological inquiry that otherwise might be stifled.

Genetic background, hypertensive state, and the cardiovascular responses to an environmental stressor. The response to environmental stressors has been hypothesized to be a major contributing factor to the pathogenesis of hypertension. The spontaneously hypertensive rat (SHR) has been characterized as having a cardiovascular system that is hyperresponsive to stressful stimuli. We (Kirby, Callahan, & Johnson, 1987) have conducted studies to determine if SHRs show hemodynamic responses that are merely exaggerated as compared to normotensive rats (Wistar-Kyoto, WKY) or whether there are qualitative as well as quantitative response differences between the two strains. The SHRs and WKYs were subjected to 5 min of intermittent footshock (1.0 mA intensity, 0.5 s duration, once every 5 s). Mean arterial pressure and heart rate were recorded from a catheter in the common carotid artery, and changes in regional vascular resistance were obtained using Doppler flow probes.

Baseline mean arterial pressure was elevated in the SHRs compared to the WKYs (160 ± 6.5 and 119 ± 3.9, respectively) although heart rate did not differ between the two strains. In response to footshock, mean arterial pressure increased only slightly for both strains. However, heart rate was increased to a greater degree in the SHRs both immediately and 5 min after footshock (Figure 8.9). The qualitative changes in regional vascular resistance to footshock were characteristic of the BSEDR for both SHRs and WKYs, although the degree to which flow changes varied between strains. Immediately following footshock, vascular resistance increased in the mesenteric and renal beds, whereas resistance decreased in the abdominal aorta. The most pronounced change in blood flow occurred in the mesenteric artery of the SHR, where resistance increased by 54 percent over basal levels at the termination of footshock and remained elevated 5 min later. In contrast, mesenteric resistance in the WKYs was only increased by 15 percent at the termination of footshock and decreased slightly 5 min postfootshock.

Again, as in the two previous studies, the results of this study demonstrate that a

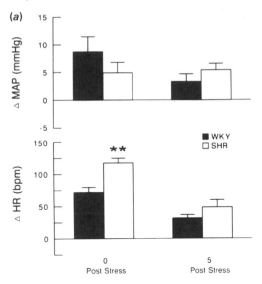

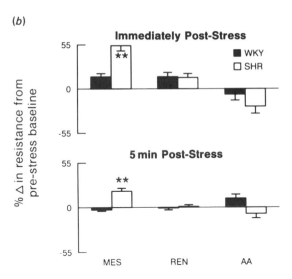

Figure 8.9, *Top:* Increase above resting baseline in mean arterial pressure (MAP) and heart rate (HR) immediately and 5 min poststress in Wistar-Kyoto, WKY (i.e., normotensive) and spontaneously hypertensive (SHR, genetic model of hypertension) rats. Note that pressor responses were comparable for hypertensive and normotensive rats (*bottom*). Changes in resistance in mesenteric (MES), renal (REN), and hindlimb (AA) vascular beds immediately and 5 min poststress. Although both strains showed similar patterns of vascular resistance changes, responses were more pronounced in SHR (p > .01). (From Kirby, Callahan, & Johnson, 1987, with permission.)

stressor (footshock in this case) had relatively little effect on arterial pressure. The slight increase in pressure was not significantly different for the two strains. In spite of this similarity in the pressor response, there were markedly different changes in the more proximal measures of heart rate and mesenteric blood flow, which indicates that the visceral response to a stressor is quite different between SHRs and WKYs. Although the index of skeletal muscle vasodilation (i.e., the change in resistance in the hindlimb supplied by the abdominal aorta) was not statistically significant, the relatively larger decrease in resistance suggests that the pressor contribution deriving from increased heart rate (and therefore probably increased cardiac output) and increase in mesenteric resistance were in all likelihood offset by a larger vasodilation in the SHRs. Again, this demonstrates the interplay of different controls of arterial pressure regulation. The appreciation of this capacity to achieve moment-to-moment pressure regulation in the rat, as we shall see, has had important implications for interpretation of human cardiovascular responses to stressors.

8.4.3.2 *Human studies*

We now review briefly three studies in humans that illustrate the use of distal and proximal measures of stress previously discussed. Perhaps more importantly, these studies demonstrate the specificity of stress responses and the influence of genetic factors.

Stress, forearm blood flow, and family history of hypertension. Recently, Anderson and colleagues (Anderson, Mahoney, Lauer, & Clarke, 1987a) compared cardiovascular responses to stress in children with and without a hypertensive parent. Blood pressure, heart rate, and forearm blood flow (measured by venous occlusion plethysmography) were measured during 10 min of verbal mental math (e.g., 1489 − 17) performed under time pressure.

Previous studies have indicated that children with a family history of hypertension may have exaggerated blood pressure and heart rate responses to mental math (Falkner, Onesto, Angelakos, Fernandes, & Langman, 1979). These findings, as well as work in animals, have led to the hypothesis that individuals with a genetic predisposition to develop hypertension have exaggerated defense response reactions to stress. It has been suggested that the repeated pressor responses to stress may contribute to the development of hypertension by injuring resistance vessels (Folkow, 1982). Findings of exaggerated blood pressure responses to stress in those with a family history of hypertension is not, however, a uniform finding. As reviewed above, studies from animal models of hypertension indicate that abnormalities in regional blood flow (e.g., skeletal muscle and splanchic) may be detected in genetically predisposed animals before the elevated blood pressure responses to stress are seen (Kirby et al., 1987).

This study comparing regional blood flow responses in the children of hypertensive versus normotensive parents was conducted to determine if children of hypertensive parents have an exaggerated defense response during stress (i.e., increased skeletal muscle blood flow). A further goal was to determine if dilation in skeletal muscle offsets constriction in other beds during stress in children of hypertensive parents. The two groups did not differ in resting blood pressure, heart rate, or forearm blood flow. Mental stress produced virtually identical blood

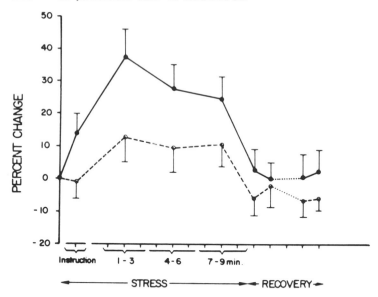

Figure 8.10. Percentage of change in forearm blood flow during 10 min of mental stress (mental arithmetic) and 5 min of recovery. Increase in forearm blood flow during stress was significantly greater in children with hypertensive parents (solid line) than in children with normotensive parents (dashed line). The two groups did not differ in their blood pressure and heart rate responses to stress. (From Anderson et al., 1987a, with permission.)

pressure and heart rate responses in the two groups of adolescents. However, the increase in forearm blood flow during stress was 3.5 times greater in children with a family history of hypertension compared with children without such a family history (Figure 8.10).

Evidence from animal studies reviewed above would suggest that increased forearm blood flow may serve to buffer greater constriction in other vascular beds. The present study in adolescents indicates that regional blood flow responses underlying similar blood pressure response increases during mental stress may be different in adolescents with and without a family history of hypertension.

Blood pressure is determined, in part, by total peripheral resistance. Thus, in this study, measuring the hemodynamics in skeletal muscle represents a more proximal measure than measuring arterial pressure alone. It was only by comparing differences in regional blood flow that the variation in response to stress in the two groups could be seen. Comparison of blood pressure and heart rate alone would not have differentiated the groups. Further, comparison of the results with animal studies suggests that a fundamental pathology in the response to stress in children with a genetic predisposition for hypertension may involve altered regional circulation in the splanchnic bed. This could lead to increased sodium retention or alterations in blood vessels.

Sympathetic nerve activity and stress. There is increasing evidence that the defense response is highly organized by the central nervous system and may vary

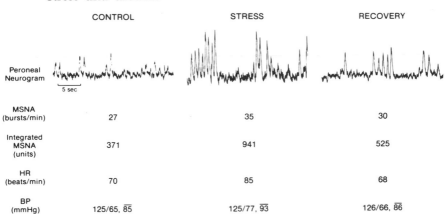

Figure 8.11. Recording of muscle sympathetic nerve activity (MSNA) in the leg (peroneal nerve) in one subject during control, stress, and recovery periods. Stress was 4 min of verbal mental arithmetic. Spikes in the neurogram represent firing of sympathetic vasoconstrictor fibers. MSNA is quantified both as bursts/min and integrated MSNA (i.e., burst frequency times mean burst amplitude). Sympathetic nerve activity in the leg increased during stress and remained elevated during recovery. Blood pressure and heart rate also increased during stress but returned quickly to control levels during recovery. (From Anderson et al., 1987c, with permission.)

depending upon the type of stressor. An increase in the blood flow to skeletal muscle has long been considered a major component of the defense response. However, Rusch, Shepherd, Webb, and Vanhoutte (1981) found evidence that there may be a regional specificity in the change in blood flow to skeletal muscle during stress. Using plethysmography, they measured blood flow to the arm and calf during stress (a delayed auditory feedback task). They reported that stress increased forearm blood flow but not calf blood flow. Thus, changes in blood flow to the same type of vascular bed (i.e., skeletal muscle) may vary depending upon where it is measured.

This regional specificity could reflect altered sympathetic outflow to these two areas of skeletal muscle. Anderson et al. (1987c) tested the hypotheses that (1) mental stress causes an increase in muscle sympathetic outflow to the calf and (2) stress causes a dissociation of muscle sympathetic outflow to the arm and the leg with leg muscle SNA increasing and arm muscle SNA remaining unchanged or decreasing.

Muscle SNA was measured by microneurographic techniques from the peroneal nerve in the leg. Muscle SNA to the leg increased during stress (Figure 8.11). This finding is especially interesting since stress is associated with an increase in blood pressure that would be expected to reflexly inhibit SNA by activation of arterial baroreceptors. Sympathetic nerve activity recorded simultaneously from the arm (radial nerve) and the leg shows a remarkable parallelism at rest. However, in this study, stress was found to cause a dissociation of muscle SNA to the arm and leg. Leg SNA increased, whereas arm SNA did not change (see Figure 8.12). Interestingly, arm SNA increased after stress, and leg SNA remained elevated. Heart rate and blood pressure returned to control levels immediately after stress.

This study is important for several reasons. First, the lack of parallelism between heart rate and muscle SNA suggests that they are controlled by different mechanisms. Second, the differences in arm and leg SNA demonstrates the great

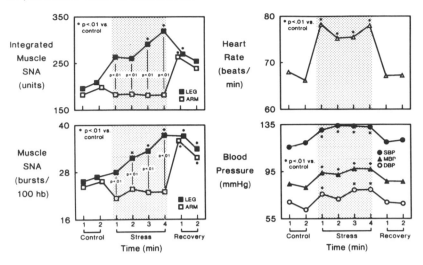

Figure 8.12. Muscle sympathetic nerve activity (SNA) recorded from the arm and leg (left panels), heart rate, and blood pressure (right panels), responses to mental stress. Heart rate and blood pressure increased during stress and returned promptly to control levels after stress. Sympathetic nerve activity in the leg (peroneal nerve) increased significantly during stress and remained elevated during recovery. In contrast, sympathetic nerve activity in the arm did not change significantly during stress. However, sympathetic nerve activity in the arm increased significantly after stress. (SBP, MAP, DBP: systolic, mean, and diastolic pressures). (From Anderson et al., 1987c, with permission.)

regional specificity in central neural outflow to similar types of vascular beds during stress. Finally, it indicates that stress might inhibit baroreflex control of SNA. Specifically, SNA is inhibited by increases in arterial pressure. However, stress increased arterial pressure but, in contrast to the expected decrease in SNA, caused an increase in SNA to the leg.

Stress, sympathetic nerve activity, and baroreceptor function. The last human study to be noted (Anderson, Sinkey, & Mark, 1987b) followed up the observation that mental stress can alter the central nervous system responses to arterial baroreceptor input. This study indicates how central nervous system responses to a wide variety of inputs can be modified by psychological stress.

In this study, arterial pressure was raised by infusing phenylephrine (which causes constriction of blood vessels). Increasing arterial pressure stimulates arterial baroreceptors and causes a marked decrease in heart rate and sympathetic neural outflow. After obtaining a stable baseline of suppressed SNA, subjects performed a mental arithmetic task. Performing this task caused a further increase in blood pressure above that previously obtained by phenylephrine infusion (Figure 8.13). Most importantly, baroreceptor suppression of SNA was inhibited and sympathetic outflow to the leg increased toward preinfusion levels. This clearly demonstrates that changing a subject's environment (e.g., by a stress task) can alter how the central nervous system integrates input from peripheral baroreceptors.

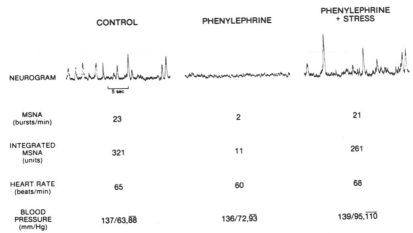

Figure 8.13. Recording of muscle sympathetic nerve activity (MSNA) from one subject during control (*left*), phenylephrine infusing (*center*), and phenylephrine infusion plus mental stress (*right*). Phenylephrine infusion raised mean arterial pressure from 88 mm Hg during control to 93 mm Hg. This was associated with marked suppression of MSNA (from 23 to 2 bursts/min) and heart rate (from 65 to 60 beats/min). Applying mental stress during phenylephrine infusion further increased mean arterial pressure (to 110 mm Hg). Despite the further elevation in arterial pressure, which would be expected to inhibit MSNA, MSNA increased during stress. This suggests that mental stress overrides or inhibits normal baroreceptor control of MSNA.

In summary, these three studies in humans have important implications for psychophysiologists. First, they show that measuring blood pressure and heart rate alone (which are determined by many "proximal" or underlying factors) may not provide sufficient sensitivity for understanding the physiology and pathophysiology of stress responses, especially when comparing groups of individuals that differ systematically (e.g., in family history of hypertension). Second, it is clear that responses to stress are remarkably complex. It is only by simultaneously monitoring both the regulated endpoints (e.g., blood pressure) and the controlling mechanisms (e.g., sympathetic nerve activity) that it is possible to understand the complex patterning of responses to stress. Finally, level of arousal or stress can markedly alter the central integration of basic cardiovascular reflexes such as baroreceptor input.

8.5   SUMMARY AND CONCLUSIONS

Although the concepts of stress and arousal had their genesis in the fields of physiology and endocrinology, they were soon adopted by psychologists and psychophysiologists as valuable concepts to describe a unique class of stimulus–response relationships. Both concepts are complex and defy simple definitions but are understood best by appreciating their historical evolution. Certain generalizations can be made about their evolution. First, both concepts were initially associated with a global activation of efferent mechanisms directed toward systemic effector systems, that is, the sympathetic nervous system and the ACTH–glucocorticoid neuroendocrine system. Methodological advances allowing more precise measurement of neural, hormonal, and effector responses have provided a clearer resolution not only of the dynamics of the processes involved in response to aversive or noxious stimuli but also of the concepts themselves. Specifically, we now have (1) a better understanding of the nature of the stimuli that are considered as stressors and produce activation and (2) a realization that we are unlikely to discover high correlations between unidimensional physiological, biochemical, or psychological variables that presumably could serve as indices of arousal.

A fundamental goal of the psychophysiologist is to obtain physiological or biochemical parameters that are significantly correlated with behavior or with related hypothetical variables that are inferred from behavior. Although it has been at times possible to discover highly correlated psychological and physicochemical variables, such discoveries have more often been the result of good fortune than good planning. In the light of this we have tried to present a strategy that may increase the probability of uncovering highly correlated psychophysiological responses while providing a mechanistic analysis of the physiological mechanisms underlying important homeostatic endpoints. This approach requires techniques that allow simultaneous measurement of variables controlling a regulated physiological endpoint and of the endpoint variable itself. These variables have been discussed in terms of being relatively proximal or distal. The assessment of multiple physiologically related measures increases the probability of demonstrating reliable relationships between physiological responses and psychological variables. In addition, this approach will enhance the understanding of basic physiological mechanisms underlying stress and arousal.

NOTES

Research of the authors cited in this chapter was supported by grants from the Public Health Service (NIH 1 RO1 HL33447, NIH HI14388, NIH 5 RO1 HL35600) and the Iowa Affiliate of the American Heart Association. Some of the studies by A. K. Johnson were supported by an NIMH Research Scientist Development Award MH0064. Studies of E. A. Anderson were supported by NRSA Awards HL07385; and HL07121 by Grant RR59 from the General Clinical Research Center's Program, Division of Research Resources, NIH; and by research grants HL24962 and HL36224 from the NHLBI. The authors express their appreciation to R. F. Kirby, N. Mottet, and L. Schenkel for their helpful comments and assistance with the manuscirpt.

1 Only occasionally in the psychophysiological literature (e.g., Pribram & McGuinness, 1975) have the terms *arousal* and *activation* been defined to have different meanings. In this chapter we follow the more common convention and use the terms arousal and activation as interchangeable and equivalent.
2 As we shall see, this imprecision of usage has constituted a major stumbling block in the effective application of these concepts.
3 This freezing response has been studied extensively and was described initially by Estes and Skinner (1941) as a conditioned emotional response (CER). We have employed the term EEDR to describe our paradigm, since we have not conducted the appropriate experiments to demonstrate that the observed hemodynamic response pattern to the light/tone stimulus is in fact conditioned.
4 See the role of central command shown in Figure 8.4.

REFERENCES

Abrahams, V. C., Hilton, S. M., & Zbrozyna, A. (1960). Active muscle vasodilation produced by stimulation of the brain stem: Its significance in the defense reaction. *Journal of Physiology, 154*, 491–513.

Abrahams, V. C., Hilton, S. M., & Zbrozyna, A. W. (1964). The role of active muscle vasodilation in the alerting stage of the defense reaction. *Journal of Physiology, 171,* 189–202.

Adams, D. B., Bacceli, G., Mancia, G., & Zanchetti, A. (1969). Cardiovascular changes during naturally elicited fighting behavior in the cat. *American Journal of Physiology, 216,* 1226–1235.

Anderson, E. A. (1987). Preoperative preparation for cardiac surgery facilitates recovery, reduces psychological distress, and reduces the incidence of acute postoperative hypertension. *Journal of Consulting and Clinical Psychology, 55,* 513–520.

Anderson, E. A., Sinkey, C. A., & Mark, A. L. (1987b). Mental stress increases sympathetic nerve activity and arterial pressure despite stimulation of arterial baroreceptors. *Circulation Monograph, 9,* IV–347.

Anderson, E. C., Mahoney, L. T., Lauer, R. M., & Clarke, W. R. (1987a). Enhanced forearm blood flow during mental stress in children of hypertensive parents. *Hypertension, 10,* 544–549.

Anderson, E. A., Mark, A. L. (1989). Microneurographic measurement of sympathetic nerve activity in humans. In Schneiderman et al. (Eds.), *Handbook of research methods in cardiovascular behavioral medicine,* p. 483. New York: Plenum, 1989.

Anderson, E. S., Wallin, B. G., & Mark, A. L. (1987c). Dissociation of sympathetic nerve activity to arm and leg during mental stress. *Hypertension, 9,* (Suppl. III), 114–119.

Asterita, M. F. (1985). *The physiology of stress.* New York: Human Sciences Press.

Axelrod, J., & Reisine, T. D. (1984). Stress hormones: Their interaction and regulation. *Science, 224,* 452–459.

Bard, P. (1928). A diencephalic mechanism for the expression of rage with special reference to the sympathetic nervous system. *American Journal of Physiology, 84,* 490–515.

Brobeck, J. R. (1965). Exchange, control, and regulation. In W. S. Yamamoto, & J. R. Brobeck (Eds.), *Physiological controls and regulations* [Bicentennial volume]. Philadelphia: Saunders.

Brod, J., Fencl, V., Hejl, Z., & Jirka, J. (1959). Circulatory changes underlying blood pressure elevation during acute emotional stress (mental arithmetic) in normotensive and hypertensive subjects. *Clinical Science, 18,* 269.

Brunia, C. H. M. (1979). Activation. In J. A. Michon, G. J. Eijkman, & F. W. de Klerk (Eds.). *Handbook of psychonomics* (Vol. 1, pp. 533–601). Amsterdam: Elsevier, North-Holland.

Callahan, M. Γ., Brody, M. J., & Johnson, A. K. (1985). Classically conditioned cardiovascular changes resembling the defense reaction in the rat. *Federation Proceedings, 44,* 1006.

Callahan, M. F., Kirby, R. F., Brody, M. J., & Johnson, A. K. (1985). Role of alpha 1–and beta adrenergic receptors in the cardiovascular responses to classically conducted defense reaction in the rat. *Neuroscience Abstracts, 11,* 1270.

Cannon, W. B. (1914). The interrelations of emotions as suggested by recent physiological researches. *American Journal of Psychology, 25,* 256–282.

Cannon, W. B. (1963). *The wisdom of the body.* New York: Norton. Reprinted from 1939 edition.

Cannon, W. B. (1929). *Bodily changes in pain, hunger, fear and rage* (2nd ed.). Boston: Charles T. Brandford.

Charvat, J., Dell, P., & Folkow, B. (1964). Mental factors and cardiovascular diseases. *Cardiologia, 44,* 124–141.

Delius, W., Hagbarth, K. E., Hongell, A., & Wallin, B. G. (1972b). Manoeuvres affecting sympathetic outflow in human skin nerves. *Acta Physiologica Scandinavica, 84,* 82–94.

Delius, W., Hagbarth, K. E., Hongell, A., & Wallin, B. G. (1972b). Manoeuvres affecting sympathetic outflow in human muscle nerves. *Acta Physiologica Scandinavica, 84,* 177–186.

Dimsdale, J. E. (1984). Techniques for collecting blood samples in the field and in the laboratory. In A. J. Herd, A. M. Gotto, P. G. Kaufman, & S. M. Weiss (Eds.), *Cardiovascular Instrumentation. National Institutes of Health* (No. 84–1654, 263–276).

Duffy, E. (1951). The concept of energy mobilization. *Psychological Review, 58,* 30–40.

Duffy, E. (1957). The psychological significance of the concept of "arousal" or "activation." *Psychological Review, 64,* 265–275.

Duffy, E. (1962). *Activation and behavior.* New York: Wiley.

Duffy, E. (1972). Activation. In N. S. Greenfield & R. A. Sternbach (Eds.), *Handbook of psychophysiology.* New York: Holt, Rinehart and Winston.

Engel, B. T. (1972). Response specificity. In N. S. Greenfield & R. A. Sternbach (Eds.), *Handbook of psychophysiology.* New York: Rinehart & Winston.

Engel, B. T. (1983). Assessment and alteration of physiological reactivity. In T. M. Dembroski, T. H. Schmidt, & G. Blumchen (Eds.), *Biobehavioral bases of coronary heart disease*. New York: Karger.

Engel, B. T., & Moos, R. H. (1967). The generality of specificity. *Archives of General Psychiatry, 16*, 574–582.

Estes, W. K., & Skinner, B. F (1941). Some quantitative properties of anxiety. *Journal of Experimental Psychology, 29*, 390–400.

Eyer, J. (1975). Hypertension as a disease of modern society. *International Journal of Health Sciences, 5*, 539–558.

Falkner, B., Onesto, G., Angelakos, E. T., Fernandes, M., & Langman, C. (1979). Cardiovascular response to mental stress in normal adolescents with hypertensive parents: Hemodynamics and mental stress in adolescents. *Hypertension, 1*, 23.

Folkow, B. (1982). Physiological aspects of primary hypertension. *Physiological Review, 62*, 347.

Folkow, B., Heymans, C., & Neil, E. (1965). Integrative aspects of cardiovascular regulation. In W. F. Hamilton & P. Dow (Eds.), *Handbook of physiology, circulation* (Section 2. Vol. 3, p. 1787). Washington, DC: American Physiological Society.

Folkow, B., & Rubenstein, E. H. (1966). Cardiovascular effects of acute and chronic stimulation of the hypothalamic defense area in the rat. *Acta Physiologica Scandinavica, 68*, 48–57.

Formel, P. F., & Doyle, J. T. (1957). Rationale of venous occlusion plethysmography. *Circulation Research, 5*, 351–356.

Grant, E. C., & MacIntosh, J. H. (1963). A comparison of the social postures of some common laboratory rodents. *Behaviour, 21*, 246–259.

Grossman, S. P. (1967). *A textbook of physiological psychology*. New York: Wiley.

Gutmann, M. C., & Benson, H. (1971). Interaction of environmental factors and systemic arterial blood pressure: A review. *Medicine, 50*, 543–553.

Guyton, A. C., Coleman, T. G., Cowley, A. W., Manning, R. D., Norman, R. A., & Ferguson, J. D. (1974). A systems analysis approach to understanding long-range arterial blood pressure control and hypertension. *Circulation Research, 35*, 159–176.

Hagbarth, K. E. (1979). Exteroceptive, proprioceptive, and sympathetic activity recorded with microelectrodes from human peripheral nerves. *Mayo Clinic Proceedings, 54*, 353–365.

Hardy, J. D. (1965). The "set-point" concept in physiological temperature regulation. In W. S. Yamamoto & J. R. Brobeck (Eds.), *Physiological controls and regulations* [Bicentennial volume]. Philadelphia: Saunders.

Hartley, C. J., & Cole, J. S. (1974). An ultrasonic pulsed Doppler system for measuring blood flow in small vessels. *Journal of Applied Physiology, 37*, 626–629.

Haywood, J. R., Shaffer, R. A., Fastenow, C., Fink, G. D., & Brody, M. J. (1981). Regional blood flow measurement with a pulsed Doppler flowmeter in the conscious rat. *American Journal of Physiology, 241*, H273–278.

Henry, J. P., & Cassel, J. C. (1969). Psychosocial factors in essential hypertension: Recent epidemiologic and animal experimental evidence. *American Journal of Epidemiology, 90*, 171–200.

Hess, W. R. (1949). *Das Zwischenhirn. Syndrome. lokalizationen, funktionen*. Basel: Benno Schwabe.

Hilton, S. M., & Zbrozyna, A. W. (1963). Amygdaloid region for defense reactions and its efferent pathway to the brain stem. *Journal of Physiology, 105*, 160–173.

Houk, J. C. (1980). Homeostasis and control principles. In V. B. Mountcastle (Ed.), *Medical physiology* (Vol. 1). St. Louis: Mosby.

Houk, J. C. (1988). Control strategies in physiological systems. *FASEB Journal, 2*, 97–107.

Hull, C. L. (1943). *Principles of behavior*. New York: Appleton-Century-Crofts.

Hyman, C., & Winsor, T. (1961). History of plethysmography. *Journal of Cardiovascular Surgery, 35*, 506–518.

Kirby, R. F., Callahan, M. F., & Johnson A. K. (1987). Regional vascular responses to an acute stressor in spontaneously hypertensive and Wistar-Kyoto rats. *Journal of the Autonomic Nervous System, 20*, 185–188.

Lacey, J. I. (1967). Somatic response patterning and stress: Some revisions of activation theory. In M. H. Appley & R. Trumbull (Eds.), *Psychological stress: Issues in research*. New York: Appleton-Century-Crofts.

Lazarus, R. S. (1966). *Psychological stress and the coping process*. New York: McGraw-Hill.

Lehman, M.N., & Adams, D.B. (1977). A statistical and motivational analysis of the social behaviors of the male laboratory rat. *Behavior, 61*, 238–275.

Lidberg, L., & Wallin, B. G. (1981). Sympathetic skin nerve discharges in relation to amplitude of skin resistance responses. *Psychophysiology, 18,* 268–270.

Lindsley, D. B. (1951). Emotion. In S. S. Stevens (Ed.), *Handbook of experiemental psychology.* New York: Wiley.

Lindsley, D. B. (1957). Psychophysiology and motivation. In M. R. Jones (Ed.), *Nebraska symposium on motivation.* Lincoln: University of Nebraska Press.

Lindsley, D. B., Schreiner, L. H., Knowles, W. B., & Magoun, H. W. (1950). Behavioral and EEG changes following chronic brainstem lesions in the cat. *EEG Clinical Neurophysiology, 2,* 483–498.

Logan, F. A. (1959). The Hull-Spence approach. In S. Koch (Ed.), *Psychology: A study of a science. Study I. Conceptual and systematic: Vol. 2. General systematic formulations, learning, and special processes.* New York: McGraw-Hill.

Malmo, R. B. (1959). Activation: A neuropsychological dimension. *Psychological Review, 66,* 367–386.

Mason, J. W. (1968). A review of psychoendocrine research on the pituitary-adrenal cortical system. *Psychosomatic Medicine, 30,* 576.

Mason, J. W. (1971). A re-evaluation of the concept of "non-specificity" in stress theory. *Journal of Psychiatric Research, 8,* 323–333.

Mason, J. W., Wool, M. S., Mougey, E. H., Wherry, F. E., Collins, D. R., & Taylor, E. D. (1968). Psychological vs. nutritional factors in the effects of "fasting" on hormonal balance. *Psychosomatic Medicine, 30,* 554.

McGrath, J. E. (1970). Setting, measures, and themes: An integrative review of some research on social-psychological factors in stress. In J. E. McGrath (Ed.), *Social and psychological factors in stress.* New York: Holt, Rinehart and Winston.

Moruzzi, G., Magoun, H. W. (1949). Brainstem reticular formation and activation of the EEG. *EEG Clinical Neurophysiology, 1,* 455–473.

Peterson, L. H. (1965). Control and regulation of the cardiovascular system. In W. S. Yamamoto & J. R. Brobeck (Eds.), *Physiological controls and regulations* [Bicentennial volume]. Philadelphia: Saunders.

Pribram, K. H., & McGuinness, D. (1975). Arousal, activation and effort in the control of attention. *Psychological Review, 82,* 116–149.

Ranson, S. W., & Magoun, H. W. (1939). The hypothalamus. *Ergebnisse der Physiologie, 41,* 56–163.

Routtenberg, A. (1968). The two-arousal hypothesis: Reticular formation and limbic system. *Psychological Review, 75,* 51–80.

Rowell, L. B. (1982). Neural control of the circulation in exercise. In O. A. Smith, R. A. Galosy, & S. M. Weiss (Eds.), *Circulation, neurobiology and behavior.* New York: Elsevier Biomedical.

Rowell, L. B. (1986). *Human circulation: regulation during physical stress.* New York: Oxford University Press.

Rusch, N. J., Shepherd, J. T., Webb, R. C., & Vanhoutte, P. M. (1981). Different behavior of the resistance vessels of the human calf and forearm during contralateral isometric exercise, mental stress, and abnormal respiratory movements. *Circulation Research 48 (Suppl. 1),* I-118–I-130.

Selye, H. (1936). A syndrome produced by diverse noxious agents. *Nature, 138,* 32.

Selye, H. (1967). *In vivo: The case for supramolecular biology presented in six informal, illustrated lectures.* New York: Liveright Publishing.

Siggaard-Andersen, J. (1970). Venous occlusion plethysmography on the cell. *Danish Medical Bulletin, 17* (Suppl. I), 1–68.

Stock, G., Schlor, K. H., Heidt, H., & Buss, J. (1978). Psychomotor behaviour and cardiovascular patterns during stimulation of the amygdala. *Pflugers Archiv: European Journal of Physiology, 176,* 177–184.

Sutton, S., Braven, M., Zubin, J., & John, E. R. (1965). Evoked potential correlates of stimulus uncertainty. *Science, 150,* 1187–1188.

Uvnas, B. (1960). Sympathetic vasodilator system and blood flow. *Physiological Reveiw, 40* (Suppl. IV), 69–76.

Venables, P. H. (1984). Arousal: An examination of its status as a concept. In M. G. H. Coles, J. R. Jennings, & J. A. Stern (Eds.), *Psychophysiological perspectives: Festschrift for Beatrice and John Lacey.* New York: Van Nostrand Reinhold.

Viken, R. J. (1984). *Blood pressure, heart rate, and regional blood flow during agonistic behavior.* Unpublished doctoral dissertation, University of Iowa.

Vingerhoets, A. (1985). *Psychosocial stress: An experimental approach. Life events, coping, and psychobiological functioning.* Lisse: Swets & Zeitlinger.

Whitney, R. J. (1953). The measurement of volume changes in human limbs. *Journal of Physiology, 121,* 1–27.

Williams, R., Lane, J., Kuhn, C., Melosh, W., White, A., & Schaneberg, S. (1982). Type A behavior and elevated physiological and neuroendocrine responses to cognitive tasks. *Science, 218,* 483–485.

Williams, R. B. (1984). Measurement of local blood flow during behavioral experiments: Principles and practice. In A. J. Herd, A. M. Gotto, P. G. Kaufman, & S. M. Weiss (Eds.), *Cardiovascular instrumentation.* National Institutes of Health (No. 84–1654, 207–217).

Wilson, E. S., & Schneider, C. (1981). The neurophysiologic pathways of distress. *Stress/Pain Manager Newsletter.* Kansas City, MO: S/P Management Group.

9   *Interoception*

SHEILA D. REED, ANDREW HARVER,
AND EDWARD S. KATKIN

Until recent times the viscera were considered remarkably insensitive, and except for the sensation of pain, it was assumed that there was little afferent input from visceral organs to higher centers. Accordingly, the study of visceral sensation traditionally attracted little interest from either physiologists or psychologists. The study of receptors residing in the internal organs (i.e., interoceptors) traditionally constituted a distinctly minor subject of study in physiology (Bykov, 1954/1957; Chernigovskiy, 1960/1967; Schmidt, 1986). Sherrington, who in 1906 organized the distribution of sensory receptors along "deep" and "surface" receptive fields, also recognized the difficulty of applying psychophysics to the field of interoception (Sherrington, 1948). Few experimental psychologists have studied visceral afferent functions, reflecting the widely held assumption that the classical laws of psychophysics were inapplicable to interoceptors (Adám, 1978).

There has, however, been a surge of scientific interest in the neurophysiological and psychological bases and mechanisms of visceral sensation during the last decade. A recent volume on neurophysiological mechanisms (Cervero & Morrison, 1986) addresses the various types of visceral receptor activation, the transmission of visceral afferent signals in the central nervous system, and the functional organization of viscerosomatic convergence in the spinal cord and brain. In psychology, too, prompted largely by research and theory on autonomic control and biofeedback (e.g., Brener, 1974a, b; Gannon, 1977), there has been renewed interest in visceral self-perception, marked by widespread attempts to demonstrate a relationship between the ability of human subjects to perceive visceral activity and their ability to control that activity (e.g., Bergman & Johnson, 1971; Blanchard, Young, & McLeod, 1972; Brener, Ross, Baker, & Clemens, 1979; Carroll, 1977; Fudge & Adams, 1985). Parallel to these developments there has been a noticeable increase in the application of sensory psychophysics to the study of visceral sensations (e.g., Harver, Baird, McGovern, & Daubenspeck, 1988; Tursky, Papillo, & Friedman, 1982; Whitehead, Engel, & Schuster, 1980).

In this chapter we review the psychology of visceral self-perception, focusing on methodologies used to quantify visceral sensation. Methods of sensory psychophysics will be summarized, and then considerable attention will be devoted to techniques designed specifically to assess cardiac self-perception. The implications of these methodologies for social behavior, for behavioral medicine, and for conceptual and theoretical controversies plaguing visceral perception will be discussed. Before considering these issues, we review the history of and physiological and neural basis for a *psychophysiology of interoception.*

253

9.1   A BRIEF HISTORY OF THE STUDY OF INTEROCEPTION

In this section we review, briefly and selectively, neurophysiological and psychological origins of a psychophysiology of interoception. Additional detail is available in Boring (1942), Bykov (1954/1957), Chernigovskiy (1960/1967), and Schmidt (1986).

9.1.1   *Neurophysiological contributions*

The special senses – vision, audition, taste, smell, and touch – were classified centuries ago and were not unknown to Aristotle (Geldard, 1972). Until the late 1800s, however, philosophers and physiologists tended to ignore sensations arising from the visceral structures because sensations, regarded as the avenue by which the mind learns about things, must normally have an object, whereas sensations such as cramps, tickle, and hunger appear to have no object (Boring, 1942). More importantly, little was known about the structure and function of sensory receptors. Nevertheless, prior to the discovery of sensory receptors, the foundation for a neurophysiology of sensation had been laid. Between 1791 and 1831, for example, Galvani, Volta, Ohm, and Faraday presented their initial findings on the electrophysiological properties of muscles and tissues (see Cacioppo, Tassinary, & Fridlund, chapter 11). Other significant historical contributions to a neurophysiology of sensation included Müller's doctrine of the specific energy of nerves in 1838 and Helmholtz's successful measurement of the velocity of nervous impulses in 1850 (Boring, 1942).

In 1826 Sir Charles Bell revealed that muscles contained both sensory and motor fibers. For many decades this discovery provided the basis for experiments surrounding a sixth sense, the "muscle sense." Sensations related to the sense of movement (i.e., kinesthesis) were subsequently shown to arise from receptors in muscles, tendons, and joints. Between 1830 and 1880 muscle spindles and Golgi tendon organs were discovered. Sherrington (1948), in 1906, called these receptors proprioceptors, and since then the term *proprioception* has generally replaced *kinesthesis.*

The identification of receptors subserving proprioception paralleled the discovery of receptors subserving vegetative functions. For example, in 1866 Cyon and Ludwig discovered the existence of sensory endings in the cardiovascular system giving rise to reflex regulation of blood pressure, and in 1868 Hering and Breuer revealed that reflexes affecting respiration originated in pulmonary mechanoreceptors (Chernigovskiy, 1960/1967). These discoveries proved that the autonomic nervous system, which was well defined by 1900, was not simply a "visceral *motor* system."

Soviet physiologists anticipated these findings. Sechenov, the founder of Russian physiology, 1866, and Pavlov, in 1911, hypothesized that sensory nerves – Pavlov's "internal analyzers" – permeated all internal tissues (Chernigovskiy, 1960/1967). Sherrington, who hypothesized that sensory nerves were activated by an "adequate stimulus," formulated the concept of the reflex arc in 1906, and Pavlov demonstrated numerous reflexive conditional responses by 1910. Individual sensory potentials were recorded subsequently from receptors in the eyes, ears, skin, and muscles, and by the 1920s and 1930s, sensory intensity was known to be a function of the number and frequency of active nerve fibers (see Boring, 1942). These observations later proved critical for the formulation of a neural basis of sensory psychophysics (Stevens, 1970).

9.1.2   Early psychological contributions

The field of sensory psychology emerged from the synthesis of sense physiology and the sensationistic psychology of the philosophers in the middle of the nineteenth century. The publication of Fechner's classic volume on psychophysics in 1860 and the establishment of the first experimental psychology laboratory by Wundt in 1879 are significant events in the history of experimental psychology. The new science of psychology defined sensation as the basic issue for study, including sensations elicited from within the body. James Mill, for example, added the "sensations of disorganization" (pain, muscular sensations, and those associated with the alimentary canal) to the five classic senses, and Alexander Bain catalogued the sensations of nerve (pain, fatigue, health), organic feelings of circulation and nutrition, feelings of respiration (relief, suffocation), and sensations of the alimentary canal (Boring, 1942). By 1896, Titchener had generated a list of 44,435 sensations including four cutaneous qualities, two qualities from muscles, one from tendon, one from joint, three more or less from the alimentary canal, one or more from blood vessels, and perhaps one from the lung (Boring, 1942).

Some of the first experiments designed to examine the ability of individuals to perceive visceral sensations were conducted by Boring in 1915 (Boring, 1915a, b). In those experiments, he examined the sensitivity of humans to pressure, temperature, and chemicals (e.g., mustard and alcohol) applied to portions of the alimentary canal and stomach. Boring found that subjects were sensitive to the distension of the alimentary canal and that warmth and cold were adequate stimuli for sensations arising from both the esophagus and stomach. For instance, raising the temperature of the contents of the stomach to 40 °C produced warm sensations, whereas cooling the contents to 30 °C produced cold sensations. At about the same time (1912), the coincidence of hunger pangs and stomach contractions was described by Cannon and Washburn (Boring, 1942).

Perhaps the most influential theoretical discussion of the role of visceral sensibility for behavior was generated by William James (1884). James suggested that when certain stimuli excited the viscera, the perception, or "feeling," of the elicited bodily changes defined an emotion. The "object-simply-apprehended" became the "object-emotionally-felt." During the century to follow, James's theory was criticized severely by Cannon, revived by Schachter and Singer (1962), and given empirical support by Katkin (1985). A preoccupation with the role of visceral sensation in human emotion, and a constant struggle to develop appropriate scientific methods to assess objectively the perception of visceral sensation, has characterized a great deal of contemporary research in emotional experience (see Harris & Katkin, 1975; Mandler, Mandler, & Uviller, 1958; Schachter & Singer, 1962).

9.1.3   Pavlovian conditioning

Until very recently, Soviet physiologists appeared to have monopolized the study of visceral afferents. Between 1900 and 1961, nearly 5,000 experiments concerned with visceral afferent processes were reported by Soviet scientists. These experiments, which document numerous visceral reflexes and conditioned visceral responses, have been reviewed extensively by Bykov (1954/1957), Chernigovskiy (1960/1967), and Razran (1961). The volume by Bykov (1954/1957) reviewed many early experiments and concluded that practically any interoceptive conditional reflex may be created. Chernigovskiy (1960/1967) cited more than 2,000 studies, and

Razran (1961) summarized a large number of investigations conducted during the 1950s that were largely unknown outside the Soviet Union. Non-Soviet contributions by Ádám (1967) and by Newman (1974) complement this enormous literature.

Many experiments reviewed in these volumes share a surprisingly similar paradigm (see Razran, 1961). The conditional stimulus or the unconditional stimulus or both are delivered to the mucosa of some specific viscus. A typical stimulus used in many experiments is the distension of the lumen of some organ by a fine-walled rubber balloon inflated with either air or water. The temperature of the water is manipulated in some cases to examine thermal sensitivity. The nature of these studies dictates that most of the data are collected on animal models, but reflex responses to visceral stimulation and conditional visceral responses also have been demonstrated in humans. To accomplish this, stimuli are applied through fistulas in patients or through swallowed balloons.

Interoceptive conditioning procedures follow patterns similar to those observed in reflexes elicited by exteroceptive environmental stimuli (Ádám, 1967). However, conditional interoceptive reflexes, though readily obtainable, are slower to acquire and more resistant to extinction than exteroceptive conditional responses (Ádám, 1967; Bykov, 1954/1957; Razran, 1961). It would be impossible to list all the reflex responses that have been examined, but they include both visceral–visceral and visceral–somatic connections. Examples include conditional skeletal and visceral activity elicited by uterine contractions, stomach distensions, and gall bladder stimulations; conditional urinary secretions, heart rate accelerations, and vascular responses; and in man, conditional gastric secretions, vasoconstriction, vasodilation, hyperventilation, and bladder fullness (Ádám, 1967; Bykov, 1954/1957; Newman, 1974; Razran, 1961).

Experiments surrounding interoceptive conditioning represent, perhaps, the most substantial coherent contribution to the psychophysiology of interoception. Repeated demonstrations of interoceptive reflexes provide irrefutable evidence for the existence of a highly organized different system that allows the transfer of interoceptive afferent signals to the central nervous system. These investigations have also provided specific information about the projection and termination of visceral afferent fibers in the central nervous system.

9.1.4   Biofeedback

Although there had been a voluminous literature on the Pavlovian conditioning of autonomic responses, virtually no research had been done on the instrumental conditioning of such responses. The absence of such reports was attributable, in part, to Skinner's (1938) assertion that such conditioning was impossible. As recently as 1961 influential texts reported that "for autonomically mediated behavior, the evidence points unequivocally to the conclusion that such responses can be modified by classical, but not instrumental, training methods" (Kimble, 1961, p. 100). Within the subsequent decade, these beliefs succumbed to an avalanche of data supporting the view that autonomic responses could, indeed, be modified by instrumental conditioning methods (see Katkin & Murray, 1968; Kimmel, 1967; Miller, 1969). More recent failures to replicate visceral learning in animal preparations are reviewed by Dworkin and Miller (1986).

These revolutionary new views on instrumental autonomic conditioning led directly to the development of biofeedback techniques, with strong emphasis on the use of augmented visceral sensory feedback as a mediator of acquired visceral self-control. The relationship between visceral perception and visceral self-control was stated clearly by Brener (1977), who asserted that persons who are trained to discriminate a visceral response should display improvement in their ability to control that response as well as improvement in their ability to identify specific occurrences of it. For these reasons there has been considerable interest among biofeedback researchers in the development of adequate means for assessing individual differences in visceral self-perception.

At about the same time as biofeedback researchers turned their attention to visceral self-perception, researchers who had an interest in the relationship of visceral perception to emotions, specifically in James's (1884) assertion that an emotion *is* the perception of physiological arousal, turned their attention to the problem (see Katkin, 1985; Schandry, 1981; Skelton & Pennebaker, chapter 19). In order to test the Jamesian hypothesis, they also found it necessary to develop methods that reliably assessed an individual's interoceptive capabilities.

9.2   PHYSIOLOGICAL AND NEURAL BASIS OF INTEROCEPTION

9.2.1   *Interoceptors*

Sensory receptors may be organized in terms of their anatomical location. The system used to characterize sensory receptors by location originated with Sherrington (1948), who organized the distribution of receptor organs into two "receptive fields," the "deep field" and the "surface field." Sherrington's deep field consists of *proprioceptors* mediating sensations arising from muscles and joints, such as position and movement; the relation of body segments to one another; and forces on the tendons and joints (Schmidt, 1986). Sherrington's surface field is comprised of the external (exteroceptive field) and internal (interoceptive field) surfaces of the body. The external field is open to the environment, and its *exteroceptors* mediate sensations that impinge on the surface of the body, such as sound and pressure on the skin (i.e., the classic and cutaneous senses). The internal field consists of all the internal bodily receptors (i.e., *interoceptors*) that reside in the walls, coverings, and attachments of the viscera, including all thoracic, abdominal, and pelvic organs, and in addition blood vessels, bone, and endocrine glands (Bykov, 1954/1957; Chernigovskiy, 1960/1967).

Sensory receptors may be classified also in terms of their function. The various sensory receptors that provide information arising from the internal organs, regardless of the type of stimuli detected, constitute the interoceptors. Mechanoreceptors signal changes in cell deformation induced by pressure, stretch, or tension. Thermoreceptors detect changes in temperature. Chemoreceptors react to various chemical substances. Nociceptors are synonymous with pain receptors. Additional specialized sensory transducers include the electromagnetic receptors of the rods and cones, osmoreceptors sensitive to the osmotic concentration of blood plasma, and volume receptors, which regulate the volume of body fluids (Chernigovskiy, 1960/1967; Guyton, 1981; Schmidt, 1986).

Information about the types and total numbers of somatovisceral receptors, and about their responses to stimuli, is still incomplete (Iggo, 1986; Schmidt, 1986). On the other hand, knowledge about the structure and function of cardiovascular, respiratory, and alimentary interoceptors and about the conscious sensations these systems elicit is increasing (e.g., Cervero & Morrison, 1986; see also Papillo & Shapiro, chapter 14; Lorig & Schwartz, chapter 17; Stern, Koch, & Vasey, chapter 16).

9.2.1.1 Cardiovascular interoceptors

The structure and function of cardiovascular interoceptors, which consist primarily of receptors that respond to mechanical distension of the heart muscle and alterations in blood chemistry, have been the focus of several recent reviews (Iggo & Ilyinsky, 1976; Malliana, Lombardi, & Pagani, 1986; Paintal, 1977, 1986). Sensory information from cardiac receptors is transmitted to the central nervous system (CNS) through both vagal and sympathetic afferent fibers. Both myelinated and unmyelinated afferent vagal fibers innervate all chambers of the heart. Atrial myelinated fibers relay information about tension in the atrial wall and about atrial volume from two receptor types. Type A receptors are sensitive to atrial systolic pressure and atrial wall tension, whereas the slowly adapting, Type B stretch receptors are sensitive to atrial filling. Ventricular myelinated fibers carry information from receptors that discharge with the rise in intraventricular pressure. Atrial and ventricular unmyelinated fibers seem to respond to both atrial filling and contraction.

Cardiac receptors that seem to display tonic impulse activity in relation to normal and specific hemodynamic events are transmitted to the CNS through both myelinated and unmyelinated afferent sympathetic fibers. In addition, ventricular mechanoreceptors with sympathetic fibers increase their discharge rate following coronary occulsion and when intraventricular pressure rises (Paintal, 1986).

Sensory information about blood pressure and blood chemistry is carried over both the vagal and glossopharyngeal nerves. The baroreceptors (situated at the origin of the internal carotid arteries and aortic arch) and the chemoreceptors (situated bilaterally in the carotid bodies and in the aortic bodies of the aortic arch) reflexively regulate, respectively, blood pressure and the chemical makeup of the blood.

The large mechanical forces associated with the filling and emptying of the chambers of the heart as well as the large pressure swings involved in heart pumping (e.g., a rise in the left ventricle of 0–120 mm Hg) probably excite many mechanoreceptors in the muscles, joints, and subcutaneous tissues of the chest and spine (Schmidt, 1986). The pulse waves also excite a large number of mechanoreceptors in the periphery of the body, most likely Pacinian corpuscles. In addition, receptors sensitive to arterial pressure are distributed throughout practically all of the vascular network (Chernigovskiy, 1960/1967).

In general, receptor information from the cardiovascular system does not appear to give rise to conscious sensations (Paintal, 1977, 1986; Schmidt, 1986). For example, none of the cardiovascular interoceptors with vagal afferents seem to be associated with sensation, although they may be involved in the conscious appreciation of arrhythmias (Malliani et al., 1986). Nonetheless, a number of cardiac sensations apparently do reach consciousness. Sensations associated with cardiac interoceptors are summarized in Table 9.1.

9.2.1.2 Respiratory interoceptors

Unlike the cardiovascular system, stimulation of lung receptors can cause a variety of sensations in man. Although the afferent pathways involved in these experiences

Table 9.1. *Sensations arising from afferent interoceptors of three physiological systems*

Physiological system	Receptor type and location	Nervous pathways	Sensations
Cardiovascular	mechanoreceptors of carotid sinus	glossopharyngeal	?
	mechanoreceptors of aortic arch	vagus	?
	chemoreceptors of carotid bodies	glossopharyngeal	probably none
	chemoreceptors of aortic arch	vagus	probably none
	mechanoreceptors of systemic circulation	sympathetic ganglia (?)	pulsatile sensations (?)
	atrial mechanoreceptors	vagus and sympathetic ganglia	abnormal cardiac motion (?)
	ventricular mechanoreceptors	vagus and sympathetic ganglia	abnormal cardiac motion (?); cardiac ischemia (?)
Respiratory	peripheral mechanoreceptors	somatosensory	pulsatile sensations (?)
	slowly adapting stretch receptors	vagus	sensitized in severe bronchoconstriction (?)
	airway irritant (rapidly adapting) mechanoreceptors	vagus	tightness in chest (?); burning sensation of endotracheal catheter; "tearing" sensation of lung reinflation
	Type J (alveolar) mechanoreceptors	vagus	tightness in chest; breathlessness in exercise; suffocation in heart failure (?)
	mechanoreceptors of chest wall and diaphragm	somatosensory	obstructed breathing
Alimentary	mechanoreceptors of upper airway	glossopharyngeal	sensations referred to throat
	mechanoreceptors and thermo-receptors of esophagus	vagus	passage of food and fluids (?); hot and cold sensations
	mechanoreceptors of stomach	vagus and splanchnic	stomach contractions; hunger and thirst (?)
	mechanoreceptors of bladder	pelvic and hypogastric	bladder fullness
	mechanoreceptors of colon and rectum	pelvic and splanchnic	rectal fullness

are not totally determined (Widdicombe, 1986), it does seem clear that sensations such as tightness in the chest and bronchial irritation result from the perception of afferent vagal activity (Fillenz & Widdicombe, 1972; Guz, 1977). Sensations elicited by stimulation of receptors of the respiratory apparatus also are summarized in Table 9.1.

There are three types of pulmonary mechanoreceptors whose impulses are transmitted to the CNS over vagal pathways: (1) slowly adapting stretch receptors, located mainly in the bronchi and small airways, which discharge in phase with inspiration; (2) rapidly adapting "irritant receptors," which are stimulated by rapid and deep inflations of the lung and are located in the mucosal layers of the trachea and airways; and (3) Type J receptor endings, which lie in the interstitium in collagen tissue. Type J receptors are stimulated by alterations in the interstitial volume following increases in pulmonary capillary pressure (pulmonary edema) and by strong irritants (Paintal, 1977, 1986).

Pulmonary mechanoreceptors may subserve sensations of pressure, flow, ventilation, and lung volume displacement, but these sensations more likely emerge from respiratory muscle afferents, particularly muscle spindles, tendon organs, and joint receptors (Guz, 1977; Widdicombe, 1986). Glaring deficiencies exist in our knowledge about other sensations arising from sensory structures of the respiratory apparatus. For example, virtually no analytic studies of temperature sensitivity have been conducted, nor have pharyngeal or laryngeal sensations been examined, despite large numbers of sensory endings among laryngeal muscles (Widdicombe, 1986).

9.2.1.3   *Alimentary interoceptors*

The alimentary interoceptors include a broad group of receptors serving the esophagus, liver, stomach, pancreas, large and small intestines, colon, and rectum. These receptors are excited by mechanical distension, temperature variations, and chemical substances, and most of their activity is carried in unmyelinated fibers of the vagus, splanchnic, and pelvic nerves. The stomach, pancreas, and liver also seem to contain "glucose-sensitive" receptors, osmoreceptors, and "polysensory" receptors sensitive to both mechanical stimulation and one or more chemical stimuli (Andrews, 1986). Most sensations from the alimentary canal, summarized in Table 9.1, arise from gastric mechanoreceptors. The abdominal viscera and their attachments are endowed with a high degree of sensitivity. The abdominal and pelvic organs are supplied with a broad spectrum of fibers ranging from large-diameter myelinated fibers to small-diameter unmyelinated fibers. Most stomach afferents are carried in the splanchnic nerves, but a high proportion of small-diameter myelinated fibers from the stomach are also found in the vagus. Gastric stretch receptors are found "in series" with contractile elements of smooth muscles, especially in the walls of the stomach and urinary bladder (Andrews, 1986; Iggo, 1986; Newman, 1974). Other gastric receptors, including mechanoreceptors of the intestines, signal the passage or presence of gastric contents (Paintal, 1986).

9.2.1.4   *Interoceptive mediation of synthetic sensations*

In addition to sensations arising from cardiovascular, respiratory, and alimentary interoceptors, many other afferent impulses give rise to more general organic, or "synthetic," sensations, including hunger, thirst, and shortness of breath. These sensations seem to result from the excitation of multiple receptors. For example, the sensation of hunger probably results from the convergence of activity from mechanoreceptors of the stomach, glucoreceptors in the liver, stomach, and small intestine, thermoreceptors, and "liporeceptors" (Schmidt, 1986).

The sensation of thirst also results from the integrated response of many types of receptors in the periphery and in the CNS. Osmoreceptors in the hypothalamus, interoceptors in the digestive tract, stretch receptors in the walls of the large veins near the heart and atria, and unspecified receptors in the oral mucosa sensitive to "dryness of the mouth" all participate in a complicated fashion to elicit thirst (Chernigovskiy, 1967; Schmidt, 1986).

Finally, the sensation of breathlessness or difficulty in the act of breathing involves events at the diaphragm, traffic up the vagus, and an abnormal drive to breathe (Guz, 1977).

9.2.2 Somatovisceral ascending pathways

Sensory information from somatovisceral afferents reaches higher nervous centers directly through glossopharyngeal and vagus nerves and indirectly through ascending spinal tracts. Sensory information from the thoracic viscera and the stomach, from the abdominal organs, and from the pelvic organs are conveyed to the brainstem primarily along the vagus, the greater and lesser splanchnic nerves, and pelvic nerves, respectively (Adám, 1967; Newman, 1974; Schmidt, 1986). The components of this network are displayed schematically in Figure 9.1, which shows afferent pathways leading to the CNS from selected internal organs. Afferent information is relayed to the CNS through cranial nerves, through sympathetic chain ganglia to thoracolumbar spinal segments, and through nerve plexuses to sacral spinal segments. Cranial and spinal afferent pathways from the viscera are listed in Table 9.2.

Sensory information from interoceptors, along with cutaneous senses and proprioceptors, enter the dorsal roots of the spinal cord and terminate on dendrites and cell bodies of the dorsal horn. Incoming afferent axons characteristically send collateral axons that both ascend and descend for one or two spinal segments above and below the incoming spinal segment (Newman, 1974). From there, signals ascend in the spinal cord along one of two projection systems. Many stimuli activate both systems, and there are many and diverse interactions between the two systems.

The primary projection system is called the lemniscal, or dorsal-lemniscal, or dorsal column-medial lemniscal system. Sensory information surrounding the innocuous distension of certain viscera, including the bladder and rectum as well as the passage of urine and feces and the completion of urination and defecation, is possibly transmitted over this tract (Willis, 1986). The dorsal-lemniscal system is comprised primarily of large, myelinated, rapidly conducting fibers that transmit information to the CNS quickly (30–110 m/s) and with a high degree of spatial orientation and organization among its terminal fibers (Guyton, 1981; Schmidt, 1986). Many terminal fibers can be traced to anatomically and neurophysiologically distinct peripheral structures.

The second projection system, the extralemniscal, or spinothalamic, or antero-lateral spinothalamic system, is comprised primarily of much smaller diameter

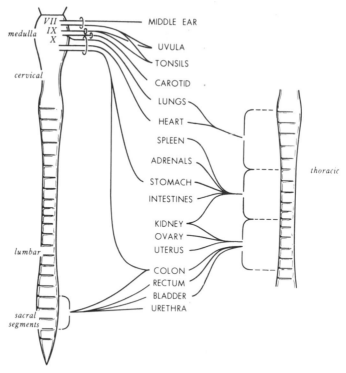

Figure 9.1. Afferent pathways leading from selected internal organs to the central nervous system. (Adapted from Adám, 1967.)

Table 9.2. *Cranial and spinal visceral afferent pathways to central nervous system*

Afferent pathways	Internal organs and tissues
Glossopharyngeal nerve	carotid sinus and carotid body, portions of throat, uvula, and tonsils; oral mucosa
Vagus nerve	common carotid and brachiocephalic artery, subclavian artery, coronary vessels, aortic arch, pericardium, epicardium, cranial and caudal vena cavae, vessels of pulmonary blood circulation, trachea, bronchi, bronchioles, alveoli, visceral pleura, esophagus, stomach, duodenum, pancreas, liver, gall bladder, small and large intestines, colon
Afferent pathways mostly through greater and lesser splanchnic nerves to thoracolumbar spinal segments	heart muscle (T1–T4), trachea, bronchi (T1–T4), visceral pleura, systemic circulation, duodenum (T3–T6), stomach (T5–L4), pylorus (T5–T12), small intestine (T5–T12), cecum (L3–L4), rectum (L1–L4), spleen (T2–L2), urinary bladder (T11–L4), uterus (T10–T12)
Afferent pathways mostly through pelvic, pudendal, and hypogastric nerves to sacral spinal segments	colon (S2–S4), rectum (S2–S4), uterus, urinary bladder (S2–S4), urethra, portions of the large intestine, genital organs

Source: Adapted from Adám (1967) and Chernigovskiy (1960/1967).

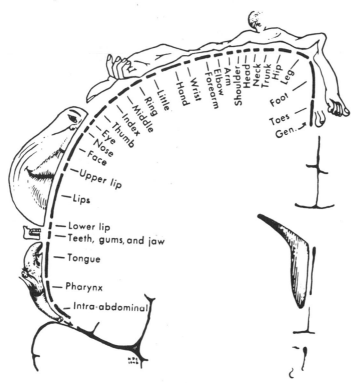

Figure 9.2. Sensory homunculus. (Reprinted with permission of Macmillan Publishing from *The Cerebral Cortex of Man*, by W. Penfield and T. Rasmussen. Copyright © 1950 by Macmillan Publishing Company, renewed 1978 by T. Rasmussen.)

myelinated fibers that transmit information to the CNS more slowly (10–60 m/s) and more diffusely (Guyton, 1981; Schmidt, 1986).

Sensory signals transmitted along the dorsal-lemniscal fibers in the spinal cord are first relayed to the medulla. Second-order neurons cross to the opposite side of the body through the thick bundle of fibers known as the medial lemniscus and project to the thalamic ventrobasal nuclear complex. From the thalamus, third-order neurons relay sensory information to specific areas of the somesthetic cortex. The somesthetic cortex has been well described and consists of two somatosensory projection areas. Somatosensory area 1 (S1) is located in the postcentral gyrus of the human cerebral cortex. Each side of the cortex receives sensory information from the opposite side of the body. Somatosensory area 2 (S2), also known as the "visceromotor cortex" (Adám, 1967), is a much smaller area that lies posterior and inferior to the lower end of the postcentral gyrus and on the upper wall of the lateral fissure. The highly spatially organized projection of the somatomotor system in the cerbral cortex yields the somatotopic arrangement known as the sensory homunculus, depicted in Figure 9.2.

Sensory information reaching the cerebral cortex along the extralemniscal ascending system crosses in the spinal cord before reaching the brainstem. From the brainstem topographically distinct collateral projections are sent to the reticular formation; collaterals are also sent to the limbic system (the "visceral brain"), which includes the cingulate gyrus, hippocampus, and amygdaloid nucleus and is thought to influence the affective quality of sensations. Second-order neurons relay sensory signals to nonspecific thalamic nuclei, and third-order neurons relay sensory signals to the cerebral cortex, mostly to area S2.

9.2.3   Cerebral cortex

The impact of cortical processing of afferent interoceptive information on consciousness, and on behavior, remains to be elucidated. For example, in comparison to our extensive knowledge about the implications of somatosensory projections (e.g., see Figure 9.2), the viscerosensory areas of the cortex have been surprisingly neglected (Newman, 1974). Exactly what regions of the cortex participate in the resolution of visceral sensibility remains unclear (Chernigovskiy, 1960/1967). For example, the recent volume on the neurophysiology of visceral afferents (Cervero & Morrison, 1986) does not discuss CNS processing of afferent signals beyond what occurs in the brainstem (Jordan & Spyer, 1986).

Three lines of evidence, however, indicate that interoceptive afferents project to distinct cortical regions and can affect both consciousness and behavior. This evidence results from experiments employing Pavlovian conditioning procedures, gross recording of electroencephalogram (EEG) desynchronization, and specific recording of sensory evoked potentials (EPs). With respect to conditional reflexes, the paradigms described earlier in some detail have established that higher nervous centers not only receive afferent impulses originating from various internal sites but also analyze and differentiate them (Adám, 1967; Bykov, 1954/1957). For instance, in man, stimulation of stomach electrodes placed 8 cm apart and stimulated separately with a delay of 105 ms results in distinct sensations at two discriminable loci (Razran, 1961).

Cortical desynchronization elicited by interoceptive stimulation can provide an objective index of the physiological threshold of higher nervous system processing (Adám, 1967 1978). Study of EEG desynchronization – a shift in brain wave activity from slow- and large-amplitude potentials to fast and small-amplitude potentials – provides the basis for an "objective psychophysics" (Adám, 1967, 1978). Studies in man indicate that some processing of interoceptive information in higher centers fails to reach consciousness. For example, EEG desynchronization elicited by the inflation of balloons in the stomach is not associated with subjective experience (Adám, 1967). Similarly, inflations of balloons in the intestine elicit arousal patterns, but on most trials these arousal patterns are not accompanied by any sensations of discomfort (Adám, 1967).

The organization of terminations of visceral processes in the brain and the implications of these findings for behavior have also been examined with evoked potentials measured either directly from the cortex in animals or from the scalp in humans. For example, evoked potentials have been recorded in animals from the thalamus, the posterior hypothalamus, and the reticular formation following stimulation of vagal, splanchnic, and pelvic nerves (Andrews, 1986; Adám, 1967; Chernigovskiy, 1960/1967; Newman, 1974). Information from practically every organ reaches the cortex (Chernigovskiy, 1960/1967). Various visceral receptor fields are projected to topographically distinct areas in the reticular formation

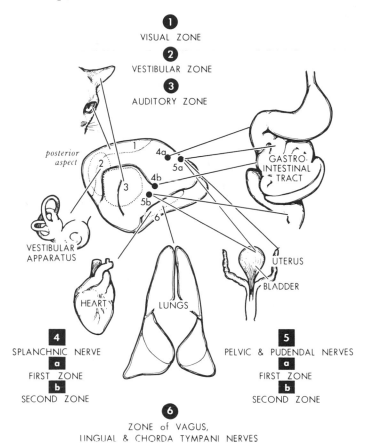

Figure 9.3. Termination of visceral afferents in cat cerebral cortex. (Adapted from Chernigovskiy, 1967/1960.)

(Adám, 1967), and all modalities of visceral sensation are represented in the ventrobasal complex of the thalamus. Afferent impulses from the abdominal viscera are distributed by the thalamus to somatosensory areas 1 and 2 precisely in the position to be expected on anatomical grounds (Newman, 1974).

There is a close connection between the zones of visceral organs and the zones of somatosensibility in the brain. Splanchnic projections in the thalamus, for example, overlap the arm and leg areas in the posterolateral nucleus (Newman, 1974). Projection of visceral afferents in cat cerebral cortex, determined largely through evoked potential analyses, are shown in Figure 9.3. As is shown, the classic and vestibular senses are distributed over a much larger area than are the visceral projections. However, there is discrete visceral representation in the cortex, including a large vagal zone.

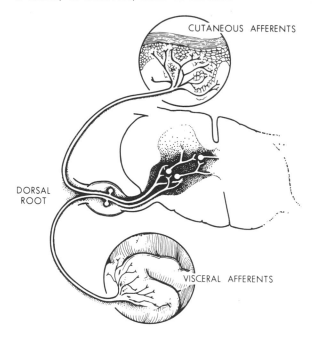

Figure 9.4. Viscero-somatic convergence in the spinal cord. (Adapted from Guyton, 1981.)

9.2.4   *Referred pain*

If we are aware normally of any visceral sensation, it is the sensation of pain. Most pain that arises from nociceptors in internal organs is carried in C-fibers along visceral sympathetic afferents into the spinal cord and along the spinothalamic tract with other pain signals. Pain sensations from the colon, rectum, and bladder are relayed through sacral segments, and those from the pharynx and trachea are relayed through cranial nerves. In addition to these direct communications of pain, there is also the phenomenon of referred pain. This phenomenon highlights visceral-somatic interactions that might actually result in the overshadowing of visceral sensations by somatosensory ones.

Disease in internal organs is often accompanied by pain localized at some characteristic place on the surface of the body. Many afferents from the skin and the internal organs that enter the CNS at a given spinal segment are connected with the same dorsal horn neurons, and branches from visceral afferents synapse in the spinal cord with some of the same second-order neurons that receive sensory information from the skin (Figure 9.4). Accordingly, when visceral fibers are stimulated, pain signals from the viscera are conducted through at least some of the same neurons that conduct pain signals from the skin. These interactions result in the interpretation that pain arising from the viscera originates in a particular segment of the body surface. Such a hypothesis – the "convergence-projection" theory of Ruch – has received experimental support (Cervero & Tattersall, 1986).

9.2.5 *Functions of visceral afferents*

We cannot change voluntarily the activity of the intestines, the liver, the kidneys, the spleen, metabolism, or cell permeability (Bykov, 1954/1957). Moreover, sensations from interoceptors are characteristically vague, poorly localized, and yield only "faint" (Adám, 1967) or "obscure" (Chernigovskiy, 1960/1967) sensations. Despite a highly organized afferent interoceptive system, therefore, it is unclear what functions the visceral afferents serve given the fact that these interoceptors contribute little to ordinary consciousness (Sherrington, 1948).

Visceral afferents serve at least three functions. The primary function of visceral afferents is homeostasis, the maintenance of the normal functioning of organs and systems (Adám, 1967; Chernigovskiy, 1960/1967). Visceral government is highly complex and operates during wakefulness and sleep. A second function is to inform higher centers about conditions that necessitate active voluntary responses, such as hunger, thirst, and excretion (Adám, 1967), as well as provide warning signals in emergency conditions (Whitehead & Drescher, 1980). Finally, visceral afferents serve an intermediate function: They may influence behaviors without giving rise to specific subjective sensations (Adám, 1967). Such intermediate functions would include contributions to emotional states (e.g., Sherrington, 1948) and unconscious control of states of awareness and operant behavior (Adám, 1967).

In summary, we can envision a continuum of signals arising from visceral events, ranging from glucose activation in the liver and gastric secretions to synthetic sensations like hunger and thirst to emergency states like vomiting and angina. Along this continuum, a psychophysiology of visceral sensation must contend with many serious obstacles, including the strong homeostatic mechanisms that keep all functions in check, the relatively small cortical space devoted to visceral afferents, and the overshadowing of visceral senses by cutaneous ones, as in referred pain.

9.3 PSYCHOPHYSICS OF INTEROCEPTION

9.3.1 *Sensory psychophysics*

Excellent discussions of sensory psychophysics, including its history, detection, recognition, discrimination, and scaling techniques, may be found in the edited volume by Carterette and Friedman (1974) and in texts by Baird and Noma (1978), Coren, Porac, and Ward (1984), D'Amato (1970), Gescheider (1976), and Stevens (1975). Considering the availability of these volumes, only a brief review will be presented here.

The goal of sensory psychophysics involves seeking answers to two primary questions: (1) what is the ability of humans to detect changes in stimulus intensity and (2) what is the ability of humans to judge changes in stimulus intensity?

9.3:1.1 *Detection*

Detection tasks are designed to reveal absolute sensory (or stimulus) thresholds, difference thresholds, and terminal thresholds. The absolute sensory threshold (*reiz limen*) is the smallest amount of stimulus energy necessary to produce a sensation. The difference threshold (*difference limen*) is the amount of change in a stimulus intensity required to produce a "just noticeable difference," or JND, in sensation

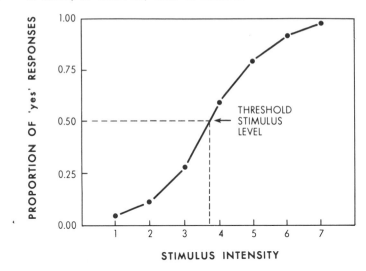

Figure 9.5. Psychometric function obtained with method of constant stimuli.

intensity. The terminal threshold is the stimulus level beyond which further increases in intensity no longer produce alterations in sensory magnitude.

Three tasks have been used to determine absolute and difference thresholds. Each consists of an experimental procedure and a mathematical treatment of the data. In the *method of constant stimuli*, experimenters present a constant set of stimuli to subjects for a fixed number of presentations. A wide range of stimulus intensities is chosen, varying from an undetectable stimulus to one that is always detected. These stimuli are presented repeatedly, and a psychometric function plotting the percentage of correct detections as a function of stimulus intensity is determined. Such a plot is displayed in Figure 9.5, which shows that the absolute threshold value is the stimulus intensity detected on 50 percent of the trials.

In the *method of limits*, stimulus intensities are changed progressively by only a small amount until the boundary of sensation is reached. The transition point is determined using both ascending and descending sequences of stimulus presentations that control for errors of habituation or perseverance (tendency to say yes in descending series) and errors of expectation or anticipation (tendency to say yes on ascending series; Coren et al., 1984). Variations of this technique include the staircase method, wherein stimulus intensity is controlled by the observer, and the forced-choice method, wherein the subject is forced to choose among several carefully specified observations only one of which contains the stimulus (Gescheider, 1976).

The third procedure, the *method of adjustment*, requires the subject to adjust a comparator stimulus to match a standard stimulus presented by the experimenter.

Sensory thresholds derived from these procedures do not take into account false alarms, that is, the rate at which subjects indicate the presence of a stimulus when in fact none was presented. To address this problem, as well as other problems introduced by response biases, signal detection theory (SDT) was developed. In signal detection tasks, the subject is presented a series of trials in which the stimulus signal is either present or absent. The subject may correctly identify the presence or absence of a signal (a hit/correct rejection) or incorrectly identify a signal when in fact it was absent (false alarm) or miss the presence of a signal (a miss).

Mathematical treatment of hits, misses, and false alarm proportions produces two estimates of the stimulus discrimination capabilities of a subject: (1) detection ability and (2) the criterion used to judge the presence or absence of a stimulus. The first of these, d', represents the observer's capability for making a discrimination. The second, *beta*, provides an index of the subject's criterion for acting on information arising from the discrimination. β is thus an index of response bias, or riskiness of the observer in acting on the perceived discrimination. More details about complex mathematical and theoretical issues in SDT may be obtained in Baird and Noma (1978), Gescheider (1976), and Swets (1973).

9.3.1.2 *Magnitude scaling*

When one desires to assess the perceived *magnitude* of stimulus intensities, one turns to the construction of psychological magnitude functions, which plot the subject's attribution of the magnitude of the sensory experience against the corresponding objectively measured physical magnitude of the stimulus.

Principles for direct magnitude scaling have been derived primarily from the seminal contributions of Stevens (1956, 1975). In direct scaling, observers make judgments of sensations that are then transformed into measurements of sensory magnitude. Stevens showed that physical intensity ratios yield corresponding sensation ratios according to a power function, $\Psi = k\varnothing^n$, where Ψ is the sensory judgment of the stimulus, k is a scaling constant, $\varnothing$ is the physical magnitude of the stimulus, and n is the relative sensitivity. This formulation (Stevens's Power Law) states that magnitude estimations for various sensory dimensions increase in proportion to stimulus intensity raised to a power.

There are two types of sensory scaling tasks: category scaling and ratio scaling. In category scaling, the goal is to construct "equal sensation intervals" between stimuli of various intensities; in ratio scaling tasks, the goal is to construct "equal sensation ratios" between stimuli of various intensities (Baird & Noma, 1978). The former tasks differ from the latter tasks in the following manner. In the construction of category scales, the subject works with a limited range and type of numbers to describe stimulus attributes; the extreme values of the scale are anchored by numerals supplied by the experimenter. In ratio tasks, there is no limit to either the range or type of the numbers an individual may use to estimate sensory attributes of the stimulus. Exponents derived from category tasks are smaller compared to those derived from ratio tasks (Baird & Noma, 1978).

Three types of ratio tasks have been used to quantify sensations. In the first type, magnitude estimation, the observer supplies a number to match the subjective magnitude of each of several stimulus levels. For example, an individual might rate the perceived magnitude of a series of auditory tones. In one version of the task, the experimenter provides a standard value (a modulus) for the stimulus of intermediate intensity; subsequent estimations by the observer are referred to that standard. In the other version, free, or "open," ratio estimation, the *subject* provides an estimate of the stimulus level of intermediate intensity, and subsequent estimations are referred to this standard estimate. To minimize response bias, the latter version is generally preferred to the former (Stevens, 1975). When the estimations of several observers obtained with free ratio estimation are combined, the method of modulus

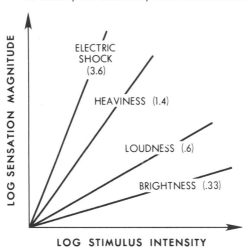

Figure 9.6. Psychological magnitude functions for various sensory stimuli.

equalization adjusts all the individual estimates to a common standard (Stevens, 1975).

The second ratio scaling task, magnitude production, requires the observer to manipulate the intensity of a stimulus to match the subjective magnitude of a numerical value supplied by the experimenter. In the third type of ratio task, cross-modality matching, individuals manipulate the intensity of a stimulus in one modality (e.g., hand grip strength) to match the perceived intensity of the magnitude of the stimulus of a different modality (e.g., light intensity).

Regardless of the technique employed, the measure of correspondence between sensation intensity and stimulus magnitude is the slope of the regression line fitted between pairs of scores obtained from two scales: numerical attributes of the sensation and the corresponding initiating stimulus. The slope of the regression line between these corresponding units, when plotted on logarithmic coordinates, *is* the measured exponent n in Stevens's power function. Theoretically, the exponent provides information about the sensory processing of stimulus energies. When $n = 1$, changes in psychological magnitude correspond directly to changes in stimulus intensity. When $n > 1$, small ranges of physical stimuli are expanded into a wide range of psychological magnitudes; when $n < 1$, wide ranges of physical stimuli are judged with little corresponding change in psychological magnitude. Psychometric functions for various stimuli according to Stevens (1975) are shown in Figure 9.6. Exponents for shock (3.6), heaviness (1.4), loudness (0.6), and brightness (0.33) are shown.

9.3.2   Sensory psychophysics and perception of visceral afferents

As with any other sensory scaling task, when assessing visceral perception, we need to consider the parameters or dimensions subjects attend to when they participate in sensory scaling tasks. For example, in the case of hearing it is generally accepted that the attributes of loudness and pitch are closely linked with the physical properties of sound intensity and frequency. Such information is generally lacking for visceral sensations. Nonetheless, an increasing number of studies have investigated sensations arising from various physiological systems using standard psychophysical techniques.

The most frequent standard psychophysical technique applied to the quantification of visceral sensations is signal detection. For example, the ability of individuals to detect spontaneous electrodermal responses (EDRs) was examined by Stern (1972). Subjects received 15 signal trials (a decrease in skin resistance of 100 Ω or greater) and 15 nonsignal trials. Half the subjects received training with 15 min of feedback about spontaneous fluctuations prior to the detection task. On average, trained subjects detected both large and small EDRs at better than chance levels and detected larger EDRs more readily than small ones.

Signal detection theory also has been applied to the perception of gastric (stomach) contractions. In one study, Griggs and Stunkard (1964) examined the abilities of both an obese and a nonobese subject to detect stomach contractions. Both subjects received 30 signal and 30 nonsignal trials. Both subjects detected strong contractions more readily than weak contractions. In a related experiment, the ability of 20 subjects to detect small stomach contractions was examined (Whitehead & Drescher, 1980). Subjects received approximately 200 trials. Signal trials were delivered following peak contraction, and nonsignal trials were delivered 12–15 s following peak contraction. Only 10 subjects detected stomach contractions significantly better than chance. This difference in detectability, compared to the earlier study, may relate to a stricter criterion employed by Whitehead and Drescher. Also, it was found that d' obtained on a heartbeat discrimination task correlated 0.51 with d' obtained on the gastric discrimination task. This is apparently the only study to explicitly compare visceral perceptual ability across response systems.

The (descending) method of limits has been employed to determine the threshold for sensations induced by rectal distension (Wald & Tunuguntla, 1984; Whitehead et al., 1980; Whitehead, Orr, Engel, & Schuster, 1981). In each of these experiments, a rubber balloon positioned in the rectum was inflated with air in successively smaller increments, from 50 to 5 ml, and the smallest volume of rectal distension sensed by subjects was determined. Despite using only descending sequences of stimulus presentations, the findings among these studies are quite robust: The subjective threshold response to rectal distension was between 10 and 20 ml in continent young adults (average stimulus levels of 12.5, 10.7, and 10.0 ml) and was reliably higher among incontinent patients (Wald & Tunuguntla, 1984; Whitehead et al., 1980). The subjective threshold response to rectal distension is absent during sleep (Whitehead et al., 1981). Magnitude scaling techniques have also been applied to visceral sensations. For example, in two related studies the ability of humans to scale pulsatile sensations elicited by a blood pressure cuff inflated over a range of pressures was examined with the technique of cross-modality matching (Papillo, Tursky, & Friedman, 1981; Tursky et al., 1982). In both studies, subjects judged the average intensity of pulsations beneath the cuff over a fixed number of heart cycles and adjusted either the loudness of tones or the length of lines to indicate sensation intensity. The distribution of these judgments, as well as the magnitude of cuff pressure oscillations, were symmetrical about a maximum value when the applied cuff pressure approximated mean arterial pressure.

Finally, many aspects of breathing including sensations of airflow, breathing frequency, and lung volume displacement have been evaluated with threshold detection, magnitude scaling, and cross-modality matching procedures. Since 1970 (Bakers & Tenney, 1970), various breathing maneuvers have been examined with Stevens's magnitude scaling techniques. The most widely studied sensations are those associated with resistive and elastic loads (for review, see Zechman & Wiley, 1986). Experimentally induced resistive loads mimic the type of flow limitation experienced by patients with obstructive lung disease (e.g., chronic bronchitis), and experimentally induced elastic loads mimic the type of volume restriction experienced by patients with interstitial lung disease (e.g., pulmonary fibrosis). The first investigations of the ability of human subjects to detect graded increases in either the resistive or elastic components to breathing were conducted by Campbell and his colleagues (Bennett, Jayson, Rubenstein, & Campbell, 1962; Campbell, Freedman, Smith, & Taylor, 1961). Magnitude scaling techniques were first applied to the perception of resistive and elastic loads fairly recently (Gottfried, Altose, Kelsen, Fogarty, & Cherniack, 1978).

Nearly 100 published reports on the ability of humans to detect and scale inspiratory volumes, static forces, and added loads have now appeared. Agreement on the receptor mechanisms giving rise to human judgments on respiratory scaling tasks has not emerged, but accumulating evidence suggests that sensory feedback from the upper airways, lungs, chest wall, and diaphragm could underlie the perception of respiratory stimuli.

9.4   ASSESSMENT STRATEGIES IN CARDIAC SELF-PERCEPTION

Virtually all of the current behavioral research on visceral self-perception has arisen from an interest in either biofeedback theory or Jamesian theories of emotion. Although these theories refer to and talk about *visceral* perception, much of the research derived from them has focused on *cardiac* perception. In addition, although SDT has been used to assess cardiac perception, the measurement of heart rate perceptual sensitivity generally has not involved traditional psychophysical scaling techniques. Accordingly, much of the remainder of this chapter is devoted to a detailed review of the methods and techniques used to assess cardiac perception.

The cardiac signal (a discrete occurrence) is a simple signal to define and is easily measured and quantified. However, it is yet unclear which component of the signal individuals attend to when they participate in a cardiac perception task. There are several discrete occurrences during a cardiac cycle, any of which might be perceived, including the opening and closing of valves and the contraction of atrial and ventricular muscle fibers. On the other hand, a discrete myocardial event may not be perceived; rather, subjects may perceive a pulse at a peripheral artery (either as pressure, movement, or sound) or they may perceive somatosensory stimulation from the pressure of the heart against the chest wall (e.g., Jones, Jones, Rouse, Scott, & Caldwell, 1987).

Alternatively, subjects may perceive heart *rate* and not individual beats. Although heart rate is a derivative measure of beats over time, it is possible that a subject may be sensitive *not* to individual beats but to the pattern or rhythm of beats over time. If heart rate is perceived, then it may be confounded with other physiological and cognitive activities such as respiration rate, physical exertion, and emotional state. Awareness of these conditions and their effects on heart rate, as well as self-awareness of one's averge heart rate, may allow a subject to guess, quite accurately, her or his heart rate without any awareness or perception of ongoing physiological activity. Such knowledge, however, is less likely to influence a subject's estimate of the occurrence or nonoccurrence of a heart *beat* when heartbeat discrimination tasks are employed (see what follows). As noted previously, it could be argued that techniques that assess heartbeat perception also do not necessarily assess perception of actual myocardial activity (i.e., ventricular contraction) but assess the perception of correlated events that result from cardiac activity (i.e., movement of or pressure against the chest cavity as a result of ventricular contraction).

The procedures that have been employed to assess cardiac perception can be divided into three basic categories; questionnaires, tracking techniques, and discrimination tasks.

The best known and most widely used questionnaire designed to assess a subject's awareness of visceral activity is Mandler, Mandler, and Uviller's (1958) Autonomic Perception Questionnaire (APQ). The APQ consists of 21 items that are designed to measure the perception of bodily sensations during states of anxiety, including five items that deal specifically with heart activity (e.g., "When you feel anxious, how often are you aware of any change in your heart action?" [Mandler et al., 1958)]). However, a number of studies have found no relationship between the APQ and other more objective measures of cardiac perception such as tracking tasks or heartbeat discrimination procedures (McFarland, 1975; Whitehead, Drescher, & Blackwell, 1976).

The subjective nature of the APQ is often criticized, primarily because a subject's self-report on the APQ is frequently unrelated to cardiac perception determined objectively. By the same token, other self-report measures that are not validated against external criteria may similarly be invalid. For instance, recent data from our laboratory (Reed, 1986) suggest that there is *no* relationship between a subject's actual ability to perceive cardiac activity as assessed by a discrimination procedure and self-reported awareness of cardiac activity as assessed by the question "How aware of your heart were you while performing this task?"

9.4.1 *Tracking techniques*

Tracking techniques can be divided into two basic categories; self-report and behavioral. Self-report tasks require subjects to focus on their internal experience and report verbally on the number of heartbeats perceived over a fixed time period. Behavioral tasks require the subjects to act (usually tap a finger or press a button) on the perception of each individual heartbeat.

9.4.1.1 *Self-report tasks*

The simplest tracking technique, used by Schandry and his associates (Schandry, 1980, 1981; Schandry & Specht, 1981) and by Dale and Anderson (1978), requires subjects to count the number of heartbeats that they perceive in a fixed time interval. Other techniques (Carroll & Wheelock, 1980; Donelson, 1966) require subjects to adjust the rate of a pulsing external signal until it equals their heart rate in a modification of the method of adjustments. As a result of either the scoring procedure used (the number of estimated heartbeats compared to the number of actual heartbeats) or the instructional set provided subjects (adjusting an externally generated *pulsing signal rate* to their *heart rate*), these studies assessed heart *rate* perception; no external criteria were used against which to evaluate the accuracy of a subject's perception of beats in these experiments.

Such studies are susceptible to the criticism that the obtained judgments of rate may reflect prior belief more than they characterize actual perception of changes in heart rate. Schandry (Schandry, 1980, 1981; Schandry & Specht, 1981), however, has argued that because subjects were unaware of the length of time per trial and because the duration of each trial varied, subjects could not use knowledge of average heart rate to perform the task. Varying the trial length would, in fact, make random guessing futile.

Schandry and Specht (1981) have provided additional data to support these assumptions. They asked subjects to estimate their heart rates under varying conditions of arousal (rest, knee bends, and preparing to give a speech), and the results indicated that increases in heart rates were associated with better perception scores. Furthermore, although heart rate was identical during both physical (knee bends) and psychological (preparing to give a speech) stress, better perception scores were associated with the *physical* stress. Schandry and Specht (1981) argued that the increase in the estimated number of beats could not be associated correctly with an actual increase in number of beats unless subjects, in fact, perceived the increase in cardiac rate.

Although Schandry's data suggest that some subjects can estimate the number of heartbeats that occur over a fixed time interval and that their estimates are affected differentially by arousal levels, it is also possible that the estimates were based on knowledge of average heart rate, on knowledge of the effects of stress on heart rate, or on temporal coincidences. Schandry and Specht's data would be more convincing if their subjects reported a *decrease* in their estimated number of heartbeats when exposed to disgust-eliciting stimuli, which are, counterintuitively, known to elicit heart rate decreases. To summarize, experiments on self-report of heartbeat counting show promise of providing a plausible index of accurate visceral perception. However, these findings are neither conclusive nor definitive.

9.4.1.2   *Behavioral tasks*

Behavioral tracking of heartbeats is a simple and straightforward procedure that has a great deal of face validity. When subjects perceive heartbeats, they tap their fingers (or push a button, etc.) in time with the perceived beats. These procedures may require subjects to track their heartbeats at a rate equivalent either to heart rate or to individual heartbeats.

McFarland (1975) asked subjects to press a button in rhythm with their heartbeats, and he defined a heart activity perception (HAP) score, $HAP = 1 - [(|A - E|)/A]$, where A is the actual number of heartbeats and E is the estimated number of heartbeats. McFarland's (1975) instructions focused subjects' attention on their heart *rates*, not on individual beats, and his scoring procedure was identical to that of the nonbehavioral tracking procedures. Therefore, his procedure is subject to the same criticisms as those applied to the self-report techniques: There is no way to determine whether a subject's estimate is based on actual perception or on knowledge of heart rate and educated guessing.

Although perception scores on these tasks are determined by the relationship of the estimated number of heartbeats to the actual number of heartbeats, different laboratories have used different mathematical transformations to define perceptual accuracy. Perception scores vary from simple absolute-difference scores $|A - E|$ (Donelson, 1966) to ratio transformations such as McFarland's HAP to more complex transformations (Schandry & Specht, 1981).

Aside from the difficulty of comparing studies that use different scoring procedures, it is difficult to determine which scoring procedure reflects accurately the ability to perceive cardiac activity and if the Law of Initial Values should be considered in this context. For example, if simple-difference scores are used, a 3-beat-per-minute (BPM) difference between estimated heart rate and actual heart rate might be treated equivalently regardless of the actual heart rate (HR) level (e.g., $43HR_{estimate} - 40HR_{actual} = 83HR_{estimate} - 80HR_{actual}$), whereas if a ratio score is used, the error data are intimately connected with the actual heart rate level [e.g., $(43HR_{estimate} - 40HR_{actual})/40HR_{actual} = 2(83HR_{estimate} - 80HR_{actual})/80HR_{actual}]$.

Studies that have used absolute-difference scores between actual and estimated values have failed also to consider whether subjects underestimate or overestimate the actual number of heartbeats. This presents additional difficulties. For example, in the case of *under*estimation, if subjects are, in fact, truly accurate perceivers, then it must be assumed that they did not perceive some beats. On the other hand, in the case of *over*estimation, subjects are apparently perceiving beats that are not there. In the absence of the use of SDT to analyze various hit and false alarm proportions, it is impossible to determine if these different error types represent differences in response bias or whether they are representative of different levels of perceptual sensitivity.

An additional problem with these scoring techniques is that the concept of expected values is not addressed. That is, what score would be expected by chance in those tasks, and what evidence would be needed to determine that the obtained perception scores were significantly different from chance? Furthermore, none of the studies employing behavioral tracking addressed either the criterion or the construct validity of heartbeat detection. That is, what is the evidence that the derived perception scores are a valid reflection of actual heartbeat detection, and what set of related behaviors can be demonstrated to be predictable from individual differences in heartbeat detection ability?

Despite these difficulties, behavioral tracking procedures have one major advantage over nonbehavioral procedures. With the self-report techniques, the experimenter knows only the number of beats the subject reported perceiving. The relationship between the counted beats and the actual heartbeats is unknown. With finger-tapping procedures, the relationship between each beat and each tap can be examined. Kleinman and Brener (1970) were the first experimenters to examine the beat-by-beat relationship between heartbeats and corresponding finger taps. Rather than using the number of taps as the dependent measure, Kleinman and Brener (1970) used the *latencies* from heartbeat to tap. We shall discuss Kleinman and Brener's approach in greater detail. First, however, we consider in detail scoring procedures using tap latencies as well as consider the problems inherent in them.

When using heartbeat-to-tap latencies as the dependent measure, the simplest and most obvious scoring procedure would be to calculate the mean of the tap latencies for each subject. However, mean tap latency provides no information about heartbeat detection. Different subjects could have different reaction times regardless of heartbeat perception accuracy. For example, one subject might have a very quick reaction time and tap 150 ms after the *R*-wave and therefore have consistently short tap latencies; another subject might have a slower reaction time and tap 350 ms after the *R*-wave and therefore have consistently long tap latencies. In addition, a subject tapping randomly would have a mean tap latency equal to approximately half the mean interbeat interval (IBI). There would be no way to differentiate between a mean tap latency obtained by perception of cardiac activity and a mean tap latency obtained by chance.

What *is* of interest is the consistency or *variability* of the tap latencies. The use of variability measures assumes that each subject has a stable reaction time and that the point in the cardiac cycle at which the heartbeat is perceived is constant. Therefore, a subject who perceives heartbeats accurately would be expected to have a tap latency with a small variance. Chance responding, however, should result in a relatively large variance.

Reed and Katkin (1987) have discussed in detail the implications of tap latency variability as an appropriate measure of cardiac discriminability. They asked subjects to press a key each time they perceived a heartbeat. Perception scores were defined as the standard deviations of the heartbeat-to-tap latencies. The data yielded a normal distribution of standard deviation scores, suggesting that some subjects were much more consistent than others in their tap latencies. However, post hoc analysis revealed that the standard deviation scores were an *artifact of heart rate*. There was a significant positive correlation between the mean IBI and heartbeat-to-tap latency variability such that the subjects with the smaller tap latency standard deviations had shorter IBIs. Reed and Katkin (1987) noted that random tapping by a subject with a slow heart rate would allow the possibility of taps with longer latencies than would random tapping by a subject with a fast heart rate. Consequently, the definition of "good heartbeat perception" cannot be derived from the observation of small standard deviations alone.

In order to remove the influence of heart rate on tap latencies, Reed and Katkin (1987) examined the standard deviations of the heartbeat-to-tap latencies both as a proportion of the IBI within which it fell (each tap latency divided by the IBI within which it occurred) and as a proportion of the average IBI (each tap latency divided by the mean IBI). However, Reed and Katkin demonstrated, via the simulation of idealized perfect perceivers compared to random responders, that these two statistics were affected also by the heart rate and the heart rate variability of subjects.

Another scoring approach tested by Reed and Katkin (1987) to minimize the effect of heart rate and heart rate variability on the heartbeat-to-tap latency employed the concept of *maximum expected variance* (MEV). The logic for this was that if a subject tapped randomly, there would be a MEV that could be calculated and that this MEV would be determined by the subject's heart rate and heart rate variability. A subject's perceptual accuracy, therefore, was defined as the observed heartbeat-to-tap latency variance divided by the MEV. It was expected that this procedure would compensate for individual differences both in heart rate and heart rate variability. The MEV was determined by calculating the variance of a set of points rectangularly distributed from zero to the upper limit of a distribution similar to that expected by random tapping. Employing a simulation model, however, different heart rates and heart rate variabilities affected the scores obtained by both the idealized perceivers and the random tappers.

The final approach developed by Reed and Katkin (1987) was the calculation of a randomness index. Theoretically, if a subject is tapping accurately to each perceived heartbeat, then the variance of the intertap intervals (ITIs) should be similar to the variance of the IBIs (as an IBI increases, the corresponding ITI should also increase, resulting in similar variances). Randomness was defined as the quotient of the standard deviation of the IBIs and the standard deviation of the ITIs. The closer the value was to 1, the less random the tapping. The randomness index was then multiplied by the tap variance. A smaller score should have indicated better cardiac perception, but this mathematical transformation also was not immune to the influences of heart rate and heart rate variability.

Thus it appears that the dependent measure of choice should not be the variance of the heartbeat-to-tap latencies. To summarize, Reed and Katkin (1987) have demonstrated that these latency variances are an artifact partially of subjects' heart rates and partially of heart rate variabilities. This artifact results from constraints placed on the variance by the length of the cardiac cycle. If subjects tap randomly, with no relationship to their heartbeats, then the frequency distribution of their tap latencies should be rectangular. That is, a tap is as likely to occur immediately after a heartbeat as it is likely to occur during the middle of the cardiac cycle or at the end of the cardiac cycle. Therefore, the maximum possible latency for any one tap is equal to the length of the IBI within which it falls. If two subjects tap randomly with the same rhythm, the subject with the shorter IBIs (faster heart rate) must necessarily have a smaller heartbeat-to-tap latency variance. Similarly, Reed and Katkin (1987) demonstrated that individual differences in heart rate variability place artifactual constraints on the limits of obtainable heartbeat-to-tap latency scores. Each of the statistical manipulations reduced the influence of one of the artifacts (e.g., heart rate or heart rate variability), but none of the approaches eliminated the influence of both heart rate and heart rate variability.

An alternative approach to scoring tap latency data was taken by Kleinman and Brener (1970). Rather than evaluating the central tendencies of the tap latencies, they evaluated their frequency distribution. Kleinman and Brener (1970) assigned each tap latency to one of five 180-ms categories such that a tap which occurred 200 ms after an *R*-wave would be included in category 2 (181–360 ms), whereas a tap that occurred 850 ms after an *R*-wave would be included in category 5 (721–900 ms). If subjects are aware of their heartbeats and respond with a consistent reaction time, then a majority of their tap latencies might be expected to fall within one specified category. However, if subjects are unaware of their heartbeats and tap randomly, then tap latencies should be expected to fall with equal frequency (rectangular distribution) in each of the five categories. Kleinman and Brener (1970) evaluated each subject's data to determine if there was a modal heartbeat-to-tap latency and then used the percentage of tap latencies above chance in the *modal* category as the perception score.

One of the problems associated with this procedure concerns the definition of the number and size of the categories. Data from Reed and Katkin (1987) suggest that the duration and number of categories contained in the frequency distribution will severely alter the results. If there are too many categories (e.g., 20 bins of 50 ms each), the data may be spread so thin as to reveal no pattern; if there are too few categories (e.g., 2 bins of 500 ms each), it would be difficult to say anything about cardiac perception. On the assumption that one would want to have at least 20 observations per category, we have determined that for frequency distributions using fewer than 200 cardiac cycles, five categories of equal duration represents a minimum acceptable number. Distributions composed of a larger number of observations might require using more categories.

Another fundamental problem concerns the definition of the range to be divided into five equal categories. Two possibilities exist: (1) using the longest heartbeat-to-tap latency as the range or (2) using the longest IBI value as the range. In either procedure there is the possibility that not all tap latencies have an *equal probability* of falling into each of the five categories. For example, if the range was 750 ms (yielding five categories, 1–150, 151–300, 301–450, 451–600, and 601–750) there might be some cardiac cycles shorter than the lower limit of the last category (in this example 601). In this case, the tap latency in that cycle could not possibly fall within the last category. Furthermore, it is virtually impossible for subjects to show a reaction time faster than 100 ms; therefore, it is expected that a category of 0–150 would be unlikely to have a high frequency of occurrence of finger taps even if a subject were a perfect detector. If the data are to be analyzed using any procedure employing expected frequencies, then the expected frequencies must be determined from the population (i.e., the percentages of all tap latencies for all subjects that fall into each of the categories). Simple probabilities (e.g., five categories yielding 20 percent probability for each category) are not adequate.

If the longest IBI is used to set the range and if the longest tap latency is shorter than the longest IBI, then no tap latencies will fall into one or more of the categories. For example, if the longest IBI was 1250 ms and the longest tap latency was 495 ms, then there could not be tap latencies in the last three categories (500–750, 751–1000, and 1001–1250). This would yield an inaccurate representation of the frequency distribution of tap latencies.

Once the categories have been defined, a scoring procedure must be determined. Kleinman and Brener (1970) defined their measure as the percentage of button presses (i.e., tap latencies) above chance in the *modal* category. As previously mentioned, calculating chance for each category must be determined from the population. In addition, simply using the modal category is questionable. Reed and Katkin (1987) showed that tap latency frequency distributions from subjects often show no single mode. In many cases two categories may have equally high frequencies, and in other cases the modal category may contain no more than one or two frequencies more than another category. Thus it is essential to determine whether any of the categories contain frequencies that are significantly different from chance. The Chi-square statistic provides the most useful technique for making this determination. If the frequency distribution is not different from chance expectation, it is not appropriate to infer that the subject is a good perceiver. However, this procedure and all of the scoring procedures using tap latencies have hidden traps that render them less than ideal. For instance, how do these scoring techniques handle missed taps and double taps? If a subject taps precisely 203 msec after a heartbeat on each tap but only taps to 10 out of 50 heartbeats, is that subject as good a perceiver as one who taps less consistently but taps to each heartbeat?

The problem of missed and extra taps leads to an additional conceptual difficulty. How can one be sure which tap belongs with which heartbeat? As experimenters, we *assume* that a tap was a response to the beat immediately preceding it, and in fact, we have little alternative if we want to analyze the data. However, a subject with an IBI of 600 ms cannot, by definition, have a tap latency greater than 600 ms. Now imagine two heartbeats (i.e., R-waves of the EKG) that occur 600 ms apart. Imagine further that a subject shows no finger tap between the two R-waves but taps at 50 ms after the second one. Is it possible, then, that the observed

50-ms heartbeat-to-tap latency is actually a latency of 650 ms after the first of the two *R*-waves?

In order to avoid these myriad methodological problems, an alternative technique was developed by Yates, Jones, Marie, and Hogben (1985). They focused their subjects' attention on specific individual heartbeats so that they could be more confident (although never completely certain) that a specific tap was a response to a specific heartbeat:

> The subject's attention was unambiguously focused onto a single cardiac cycle. . . . To warn the subject of an impending trial the trial light of the display panel was illuminated for 50 ms. The first *R*-wave following extinction of the trial light resulted in presentation of the tone which continued for a duration of three IBIs plus a delay determined by the stimulus position for that trial. Stimulus position was varied relative to the fifth *R*-wave. If, for example, the stimulus flash was to be presented coincidental with the *R*-wave the tone terminated 20 ms following the fourth *R*-wave; but if the stimulus flash was to be presented 100 ms after the *R*-wave the tone terminated 120 ms after the fourth *R*-wave. This procedure was adopted not only to focus the subject's attention onto a single heart cycle but also to prevent subjects from using the time delay between tone termination and stimulus presentation as a cue to discriminate between stimuli. (Yates et al., 1985, p. 562)

Subjects often respond mechanically to tracking tasks whether they believe they are perceiving their heartbeats or not. Also, numerous subjects have reported that the very act of tapping one's finger interferes with the ability to concentrate on the heartbeats (e.g., Flynn & Clemens, 1988). Focusing a subject's attention on a specific beat eliminates the necessity for the subjects to be constantly vigilant. Therefore, the response to each focused beat might be less contaminated by other distracting factors.

In summary, it appears that although tracking tasks provide a great deal of face validity, they contain enough ambiguity and lack of precision to render them dissatisfying as scientifically sound measures of cardiac self-perception. The behavioral tracking tasks, however, are certainly more satisfactory than the self-report tasks; further, the use of frequency analysis and the calculation of Chi-square statistics to evaluate the significance of a distribution's departure from chance ensures some modicum of certainty. Statistical analysis alone, however, does not overcome some of the fundamental conceptual confusion inherent in the analysis of tracking data. For that reason, a number of approaches using response discrimination techniques have been developed.

9.4.2 *Discrimination techniques*

The logic underlying discrimination techniques is quite simple. Subjects are presented with external stimuli such as lights, tones, or vibrations that bear differing relationships to heartbeats. For instance, one set of stimuli (S^+) may be contingent on heartbeats and a second set of stimuli (S^-) may be noncontingent. Subjects are asked to discriminate between the S^+ and S^- stimuli. Presumably, discrimination ability is an index of the ability to perceive the heartbeats. As with the tracking techniques, some discrimination tasks ask subjects to make discriminations based on heart rate perception and other discrimination tasks ask subjects to make discriminations based on heartbeat perception. We discuss these tasks separately.

9.4.2.1 *Heart rate discrimination*

Heart rate discrimination paradigms ask subjects to compare their heart rates, during separate time periods. For instance, some studies ask subjects to report whether their heart rates during a "task" period are faster or slower than during a baseline period (Epstein & Stein, 1974; Mandler & Kahn, 1960; Ross, 1982), whereas other studies ask subjects to indicate during which of two distinctly defined time periods their heart rates had "reached a peak" (Ashton, White, & Hodgson, 1979; Grigg and Ashton, 1982, 1984).

These studies are susceptible to certain methodological contaminants. Using respiratory and muscular manipulations, subjects can easily influence their heart rates so that they can determine when the heart rate is fastest or slowest. It would be simple for subjects to experiment until they find a particular manipulation that gives them the desired results. In fact, Mandler and Kahn (1960) concluded that "the apparent heart rate discrimination was spurious. What had actually controlled... behavior was well-developed change in...the respiratory cycle" Therefore, for our purposes, these techniques cannot be considered valid measures of cardiac perception.

9.4.2.2 *Heartbeat discrimination*

The development of a reliable and valid heartbeat discrimination task has progressed in a series of steps, with each new step building on the concepts of the previously developed technique. First in this series was the paradigm reported by Brener and Jones (1974). They presented subjects with 10-s trains of vibratory stimuli. On half of the trials (S^+ trials) these stimuli were triggered by the subject's own heartbeats, and on the other half (S^- trials) the stimuli were triggered by a clock pulse generator set at a frequency equal to the subject's heart rate. The subject's task was to discriminate which trains of vibratory stimuli were heartbeat driven and which were clock driven. Unfortunately, it is possible to discriminate between the two sets of vibratory stimuli without any awareness of the heartbeat, even if the noncontingent stimuli are presented in a simulated heartbeat rhythm. Subjects easily can use respiratory or muscular responses to affect the stimuli triggered by their heart rates but not the stimuli triggered by the pulse generator. It would be a simple task to determine which trains of stimuli were affected by such maneuvers and which were not, making the discrimination task possible without any awareness of actual cardiac activity.

Whitehead, Drescher, Heiman, and Blackwell (1977) preserved the essential features of the Brener and Jones (1974) technique but modified the stimuli so that *both* sets of stimuli (S^+ and S^-) were contingent on the subject's heartbeat. In their paradigm, one set of stimuli were presented 128 ms after each EKG R-wave for 10 consecutive R-waves and the other set of stimuli were presented 384 ms after each R-wave. Since both trains of stimuli are generated by the subject's own heartbeats, any form of physiological manipulation will affect both trains equally. Therefore, subjects cannot use respiratory or muscular manipulations to distinguish between the two sets of stimuli. In addition, the interstimulus interval for both sets of stimuli is equal to the IBI. Therefore, there are no discriminable temporal or rhythmic differences between the two trains of stimuli. Subjects *must* use their heartbeats as a reference point in order to discriminate between the two trains of

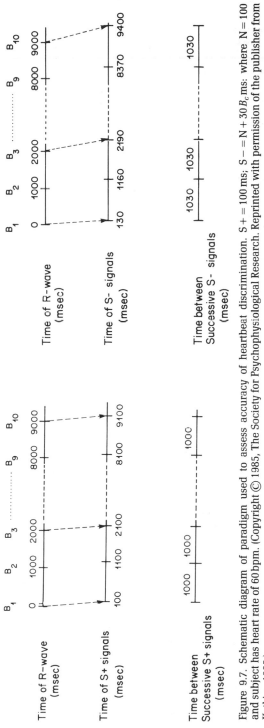

Figure 9.7. Schematic diagram of paradigm used to assess accuracy of heartbeat discrimination. $S+ = 100$ ms; $S- = N + 30\,B_c$ ms; where $N = 100$ and subject has heart rate of 60bpm. (Copyright © 1985, The Society for Psychophysiological Research. Reprinted with permission of the publisher from Katkin, 1985.)

stimuli. If they do not perceive their heartbeats, then the S^+ and S^- signals, in and of themselves, will appear to be identical.

Whitehead et al. (1977) found that only a small proportion of their subjects were able to perform well on the task. Now that they had an apparently valid measure of cardiac perception, there was nothing to measure; few people actually were able to perceive their heartbeats. Katkin, Morell, Goldband, Bernstein, and Wise (1982) believed that Whitehead et al.'s (1977) procedure underestimated a subject's ability to discriminate heartbeats. Whitehead's procedure requires subjects to discriminate a 256-ms time difference. Even if subjects are able to perceive their heartbeats, it is possible that they are unable to discriminate between a 128-ms delay and a 384-ms delay. Therefore, Katkin, Morell, et al. (1982) developed a modification of the Whitehead procedure. Essentially they modified Whitehead's paradigm so that S^+ stimuli were presented 100 ms after each consecutive R-wave but the S^- stimuli were presented at a continuously increasing delay after each R-wave (Figure 9.7). Thus subjects were asked to discriminate between one train of tones with a consistent fixed relationship to the heartbeat and a second train of tones with an increasing delay from the heartbeat. This procedure preserves the contributions of the Whitehead technique: Both trains of stimuli are generated by a subject's actual heartbeat, and there are no discriminable temporal differences between the two trains of tones. If subjects can perceive their heartbeats, the increasing delay from the R-wave should make the discrimination easier.

Recent studies have examined the parameters of both the Whitehead and the Katkin tasks. Both the Katkin and the Whitehead paradigms present S^+ stimuli at about 100 ms after the R-wave. However, recent evidence suggests that subjects, in fact, most often perceive their heartbeats between 200 and 300 ms after the R-wave, with a range of 100–400 ms (Brener & Kluvitse, 1988; Clemens, 1984; Davis, Langer, Sutterer, Gelling, & Marlin, 1986; Yates et al., 1985).

In Brener and Kluvitse's (1988) paradigm subjects are no longer forced to choose between a "right" and "wrong" response. Instead, subjects listen to trains of tones presented at intervals of 0, 100, 200, 300, 400, or 500 ms after each R-wave. The subjects are allowed to switch between the intervals as often as they like and to listen to any interval for as long as they like. When they are satisfied that the tones of a specific interval coincide with their heartbeats, they signal the judgment. Over a series of 60 trials, a frequency distribution of their interval choices is developed. Since all six time intervals are generated by the subject's heartbeats, it is impossible for them to distinguish among the intervals without using their heartbeats as reference points. Therefore, if subjects choose one interval significantly more often than the other five intervals, the only apparent reason must be that they have at least some tacit awareness of the occurrence of their heartbeats or some correlate of their heartbeats. Brener and Kluvitse interpreted their results as providing "unambiguous evidence that individuals are capable of detecting cardiac activity," but they did not attempt to assess these individual differences. For instance, a significant Chi-square statistic would indicate that one interval (or possibly more than one interval) was chosen significantly more often than the other intervals. Nevertheless, the data presented by Brener and Kluvitse (1988) suggest that their procedure appears to be the current procedure of choice for reliable and valid assessment of individual differences in the accuracy of self-perception of cardiac activity.

As Brener and Kluvitse (1988) point out, their paradigm "does not involve *a priori* judgments of which events the individual will employ in detecting cardiac activity" and "since there are no 'right' or 'wrong' answers the task...does not arbitrarily favor good performance in some subjects more than in others and is therefore likely to provide a less biased test of cardiac detection." In other words, this procedure allows one to assess heartbeat perception ability without addressing the question of whether myocardial activity itself is perceived or some correlated hemodynamic event that occurs consistently at a positive onset synchrony. In addition, this procedure avoids major problems inherent in tracking techniques, such as how to handle missed or extra taps. Finally, this procedure has as much face validity as the tracking techniques and is easier to both understand and employ compared to other discrimination techniques.

Now that we have discussed the methodological and theoretical problems involved in assessing visceral perception generally and cardiac perception ability specifically, we turn our focus to some of the possible applications of these techniques.

9.5 APPLICATIONS

9.5.1 *Social behavior*

Among the many areas to which visceral perception methodology may potentially be applied, perhaps none may be more relevant than arousal-based theories of social behavior. *Arousal* has been postulated to be an intervening variable for many social behaviors, including emotional labeling (Schachter & Singer, 1962) and attitude formation and attitude change (Cacioppo & Petty, 1979). Moreover, theories of cognitive consistency (Brehm & Cohen, 1962), of antisocial (Zillmann, 1978) and prosocial (helping) behavior (Piliavin, Piliavin, & Rodin, 1975), and of interpersonal behaviors such as social facilitation (Zajonc, 1968) and interpersonal attraction (Berscheid & Walster, 1974) contain elements that include components of arousal and perceived arousal.

Although arousal is an important, if not central, construct for these theories, most of them postulate some level of *awareness* of arousal as the key ingredient. Yet these theories have generated little empirical research on the relationship between visceral perceptual accuracy and arousal-based social behaviors. If the perception of visceral arousal is an important component of social behaviors, then the assessment of individual differences in ability to perceive that arousal must be addressed (Blascovich & Katkin, 1983): "To the extent that various forms of social behaviors are dependent on the experience of visceral arousal, visceral perceptual ability is crucial. Therefore, individual differences in the ability to perceive arousal responses should affect the experience and expression of arousal-based social behaviors" (Blascovich and Katkin, 1982, p. 90).

With the assessment techniques now available, these relationships can be and have been tested empirically. Jones and Hollandsworth (1981) have reported that under *exercise*-induced arousal, subjects, demonstrate improved hearbeat detection ability. In addition, Katkin, Blascovich, Reed, Adamec, Jones, and Taublieb (1982) have reported that under conditions of increased *psychological* arousal (viewing affectively toned slides) subjects demonstrate increased heartbeat detection ability. These studies support the hypothesis that there is a relationship between level of physiological arousal and visceral perceptual ability. Furthermore, these data imply a causal relationship between arousal and visceral perception; the ability to detect heartbeats increases as a function of increasing levels of arousal.

To the extent that there are individual differences in the degree to which increased arousal is perceived, it now seems possible that many theories of arousal-based social behavior can be examined more closely to see if the observed behavior is truly arousal based or based on the self-perception of arousal. In a direct test of the relationship between visceral perception and the experience of emotions, Hantas, Katkin, and Blascovich (1982) asked subjects who were either good heartbeat detectors or poor heartbeat detectors to rate their degree of subjective distress while viewing slides of mutilated accident victims. The results indicated that those subjects who were better able to perceive their heartbeats rated themselves as experiencing greater distress, irrespective of their actual level of arousal, as reflected in their heart rates. In other words, the intensity of emotional experience for the good perceivers was related to their ability to perceive visceral activity and not to their actual level of activity alone. In fact, both the good and poor heartbeat detectors showed similar degrees of cardiac rate reactivity to the negative stimuli. This represents an experimental test of the Jamesian and the neo-Jamesian (Schachter & Singer, 1962) view, which asserts that emotional experience depends upon both the induction of arousal *and its perception*. It is possible that the ability to perceive heartbeats and the intensity of emotional experience are, in fact, both correlates of a third trait factor, but there is as yet no evidence of what that might be. Extensive batteries of common tests of anxiety, hostility, emotionality, Type A behavior, and even androgyny have been administered to subjects in our laboratories without unearthing any significant relationship to heartbeat detection ability.

9.5.2   *Neuropsychology: lateralization of cardiac afferents*

Recent evidence supports the view that afferent feedback from the myocardium is represented in the cortex and that it may be lateralized. Schandry, Sparrer, and Weitkunat (1986) have found evidence that there is an evoked potential (N100) contingent on the occurrence of the R-wave and that subjects trained to be good heartbeat detectors demonstrate enhanced evoked potentials. Furthermore, in two separate studies using visual-evoked potentials, Walker and Sandman (1979, 1982) have shown evidence of a link between cardiac events and right-hemisphere cortical responses to stimulation but not left-hemisphere responses. Hugdahl, Franzon, Andersson, and Walldebo (1983) also have demonstrated that information presented exclusively to one cerebral hemisphere or the other results in discriminatively different cardiovascular responses.

Taken together, these studies suggest that afferentation from the cardiovascular system is represented cortically and that the right hemisphere may be more involved than the left hemisphere in its processing. Additional support for the idea that cerebral lateralization may play an important role in the processing of cardiovascular afferentation may be derived from the results of an experiment by Davidson, Horowitz, Schwartz, and Goodman (1981). Using a finger-tapping paradigm, they found that subjects tracked their heartbeats more accurately when tapping with their left hands (right hemisphere) than their right hands. In addition, both Hantas, Katkin, and Reed (1984) and Montgomery and Jones (1984) have demonstrated that right-hemisphere-preferent subjects, as defined by assessment of conjugate lateral eye movement responses to verbal and spatial questions (see Gur & Gur, 1977), perform significantly better on heartbeat detection tasks than left-hemisphere-preferent subjects. Reed (1986) found that under conditions of arousal, right-hemisphere-preferent subjects showed an increase in visceral perceptual ability, whereas left-hemisphere-preferent subjects showed a *decrement* in visceral perceptual ability. In order to test for the possibility that these results were an artifact of superior temporal perception ability for right-hemisphere-preferent subjects in general, Reed (1986) also tested subjects for time perception on an analogous task that mimicked the heartbeat task but consisted solely of externally presented signals. No differences were observed between right- and left-hemisphere-preferent subjects.

9.5.3 *Behavioral medicine*

An area in which the assessment of visceral perceptual ability has profound implications is in behavioral medicine. For example, sensations arising from the body are characteristically vague, hard to localize, and hard to quantify. Development of an appropriate vocabulary for such sensations through extended study may be useful because patients find it difficult generally to merely describe sensations (Guz, 1977; Mason, 1961).

In addition, there are a number of serious disorders, such as essential hypertension, asthma, and diabetes, that are characterized by a patient's inability to perceive symptoms. For instance, hypertension is often described as a "silent killer" because patients are unable to detect severe elevations in their blood pressure. If hypertensive patients could be taught to become aware of their visceral activity, then perhaps they could learn to attend to those stiuations that are associated with hypertensive episodes and perhaps take steps to modify their behaviors. At the least, enhanced awareness of hypertensive symptomatology would allow patients to monitor their medication usage more appropriately and perhaps allow them to regulate their dosage more appropriately. A related area of application analogous to hypertension is symptom discrimination in asthma. The ability of individuals to attend to bronchoconstriction varies widely, and asthmatic patients unable to detect acute fluctuations in airway caliber could be at an increased risk for both more frequent and severe attacks of asthma.

An alternative approach to the problem of symptom perception has been proposed by Pennebaker and colleagues (Pennebaker, 1982; Pennebaker & Hoover, 1984; Skelton & Pennebaker, chapter 19). They have argued that, in fact, the specific visceral response related to a particular disorder need not be perceived if a consistent correlate of the visceral response is perceptible. This argument suggests that it is not important to train a patient to become more sensitive to, say, blood pressure elevations or blood glucose elevations. Rather, a careful evaluation of the subject's symptom reporting, in conjunction with physiological assessment, should be carried out in order to determine if the patient is aware of a specific phenomenological symptom that is reliably related to the target symptom. Pennebaker suggests further that the correlated perceived symptom is likely to be idiosyncratic and that each patient may report a different, consistently reliable correlate of the target symptom. The advantage of this approach, according to Pennebaker, is that it may be easier to train patients to attend to their "naturally occurring" symptoms than to train them to make what appear to be extremely difficult discriminations. The disadvantages of this approach are the high probability of false alarms and the fact that when patients are trained to focus on their target symptoms, a change in the naturally occurring relationship between the underlying disorder and the correlated symptomatology may result.

9.6   CONCLUSION

In this chapter we have reviewed historical and contemporary developments in both experimental psychology and neurophysiology that provide the foundation for a psychophysiology of interoception. We have demonstrated that a psychophysiology of visceral sensation must contend with many serious obstacles including the strong homeostatic mechanisms that keep all functions in check, the relatively small cortical space devoted to visceral afferents, and the overshadowing of visceral sensations by cutaneous ones, as in referred pain. On the other hand, we have reviewed evidence demonstrating that a large number of visceral sensations reach consciousness and that standard psychophysical techniques can be used to quantify and describe such sensations. The delineation of the parameters or dimensions that subjects attend to when they participate in visceral scaling tasks remains a formidable empirical challenge.

A variety of psychological theories either stipulate or imply that the self-perception of internal visceral events has important consequences for behavior. Until recently such assertions have been impossible to test scientifically because of limitations associated with objective and valid techniques available for the assessment of visceral self-perception. In this chapter we have reviewed the development of such techniques and have focused on the methodological pitfalls associated with a number of techniques that possess reasonably high face validity. It now seems clear that at least for heart rate, we can be confident in the validity of assessment of self-perception using response discrimination techniques, particularly the technique recently developed by Brener and Kluvitse. Furthermore, it is also evident that experiments employing these techniques can be used to test hypotheses about diverse areas of psychological interest including arousal-based social behavior, the cortical representation of visceral events, and the alleviation of symptoms of psychophysiological disorders.

NOTE

Preparation of this chapter was supported, in part, by Research Grant MH-38629 from the National Institute of Mental Health awarded to ESK; by National Institutes of Health Biomedical Research Support Grant 2507RR0706722 awarded to AH; and by Research Fellowship MH08976 from the National Institute of Mental Health awarded to SDR.

REFERENCES

Adám, G. (1967). *Interoception and behavior.* Budapest: Akadémiai Kiadó.
Adám, G. (1978). Visceroception, awareness, and behavior. In G. E. Schwartz & D. Shapiro (Eds.), *Consciousness and self-regulation: Advances in research and theory* (Vol. 2, pp. 199–213). New York: Plenum Press.
Andrews, P. L. R. (1986). Vagal afferent innervation of the gastrointestinal tract. In F. Cervero & J. F. B. Morrison (Eds.), *Progress in brain research: Vol. 67. Visceral sensation* (pp. 207–225). Amsterdam: Elsevier.
Ashton, R., White, K. D., & Hodgson, G. (1979). Sensitivity to heart rate: A psychophysical study. *Psychophysiology, 16,* 463–466.

Baird, J. C., & Noma, E. (1978). *Fundamentals of scaling and psychophysics.* New York: Wiley.

Bakers, J. H. C. M., & Tenney, S. M. (1970). The perception of some sensations associated with breathing. *Respiration Physiology, 10,* 85–92.

Bennett, E. D., Jayson, M. I. V., Rubenstein, D., & Campbell, E. J. M. (1962). The ability of man to detect non-elastic loads to breathing. *Clinical Science, 23,* 155–162.

Bergman, J. S., & Johnson, H. J. (1971). The effects of instructional set and autonomic perception on cardiac control. *Psychophysiology, 8,* 180–190.

Berscheid, E., & Walster, E. (1974). Physical attractiveness. In L. Berkowitz (Ed.), *Advances in experimental social psychology* (Vol. 7, pp. 157–215). New York: Academic Press.

Blanchard, E. B., Young, L. D., & McLeod, P. (1972). Awareness of heart activity and self-control of heart rate. *Psychophysiology, 9,* 63–68.

Blascovich, J., & Katkin, E. S. (1982). Arousal-based social behaviors: Do they reflect differences in visceral perception? In L. Wheeler (Ed.), *Review of personality and social psychology* (pp. 73–95). Beverly Hills, CA: Sage.

Blascovich, J., & Katkin, E. S. (1983). Visceral perception and social behavior. In J. Cacioppo and R. Petty (Eds.), *Social psychophysiology: A source book* (pp. 493–509). New York: Guilford Press.

Boring, E. G. (1915a). The sensation of the alimentary canal. *American Journal of Psychology, 26,* 1–57.

Boring, E. G. (1915b). The thermal sensitivity of the stomach. *American Journal of Psychology, 26,* 485–494.

Boring, E. G. (1942). *Sensation and perception in the history of experimental psychology.* New York: Appleton-Century-Crofts.

Brehm, J. W., & Cohen, A. R. (1962). *Explorations in cognitive dissonance.* New York: Wiley.

Brener, J. (1974a). A general model of voluntary control applied to the phenomena of learned cardiovascular change. In P. A. Obrist, A. H. Black, J. Brener, & L. V. DiCara (Eds.), *Cardiovascular psychophysiology – Current issues in response mechanisms, biofeedback and methodology* (pp. 365–391). Chicago: Aldine.

Brener, J. (1974b). Factors influencing the specificity of voluntary cardiovascular control. In L. V. DiCara (Ed.), *Limbic and autonomic nervous systems research* (pp. 335–368). New York: Plenum Press.

Brener, J. (1977). Sensory and perceptual determinants of voluntary visceral control. In G. E. Schwartz & J. Beatty (Eds.), *Biofeedback: Theory and research* (pp. 29–66). New York: Academic Press.

Brener, J., & Jones, J. M. (1974). Interoceptive discrimination in intact humans: Detection of cardiac activity. *Physiology and Behavior, 13,* 763–767.

Brener, J., & Kluvitse, C. (1988). Heart beat detection: Judgments of the simultaneity of external stimuli and heart beats. *Psychophysiology, 25,* 554–561.

Brener, J., Ross, A., Baker, J., & Clemens, W. J. (1979). On the relationship between cardiac discrimination and control. In N. Birbaumer & H. D. Kimmel (Eds.), *Biofeedback and self-regulation* (pp. 51–70). Hillsdale, NJ: Erlbaum.

Bykov, K. M. (1957). *The cerebral cortex and the internal organs.* New York: Chemical Publishing. (Original work published 1954.)

Cacioppo, J. T., & Petty, R. E. (1979). Attitudes and cognitive response: An electrophysiological approach. *Journal of Personality and Social Psychology, 37,* 2181–2199.

Campbell, E. J. M., Freedman, S., Smith, P. S., & Taylor, M. E. (1961). The ability of man to detect added elastic loads to breathing. *Clinical Science, 20,* 223–231.

Carroll, D. (1977). Cardiac perception and cardiac control: A review. *Biofeedback & Self-Regulation, 2,* 349–369.

Carroll, D., & Wheelock, J. (1980). Heart rate perception and the voluntary control of heart rate. *Biological Psychology, 11,* 169–180.

Carterette, E. C., & Friedman, M. P. (Eds.). (1974). *Handbook of perception: Vol. 2. Psychophysical judgment and measurement.* New York: Academic Press.

Cervero, F., & Morrison, J. F. B. (Eds.) (1986). *Progress in brain research: Vol. 67. Visceral senation.* Amsterdam: Elsevier.

Cervero, F., & Tattersall, J. E. H. (1986). Somatic and visceral sensory integration in the thoracic spinal column. In F. Cervero & J. F. B. Morrison (Eds.), *Progress in brain research: Vol. 67. Visceral sensation* (pp. 189–205). Amsterdam: Elsevier.

Chernigovskiy, V. N. (1967). *Interoceptors* (G. Onischenko, Trans.). Washington, DC: American Psychological Association. (Original work published 1960.)

Clemens, W. J. (1984). Temporal arrangement of signals in heartbeat discrimination procedures. *Psychophysiology, 21,* 187–190.

Coren, S., Porac, C., & Ward, L. M. (1984). *Sensation and perception* (2nd ed). Orlando, FL: Academic Press.

Dale, A., & Anderson, D. (1978). Information variables in voluntary control and classical conditioning of heart rate: Field dependence and heart-rate perception. *Perceptual and Motor Skills, 47,* 79–85.

D'Amato, M. R. (1970). *Experimental psychology: Methodology, psychophysics, and learning.* New York: McGraw-Hill.

Davidson, R. J., Horowitz, M. E., Schwartz, G. E., & Goodman, D. M. (1981). Lateral differences in the latency between finger tapping and the heart beat. *Psychophysiology, 18,* 36–41.

Davis, M. R., Langer, A. W., Sutterer, J. R., Gelling, P. D., & Marlin, M. (1986). Relative discriminability of heartbeat-contingent stimuli under three procedures for assessing cardiac perception. *Psychophysiology, 23,* 76–81.

Donelson, F. E. (1966). *Discrimination and control of human heart rate.* Unpublished doctoral dissertation, Cornell University.

Dworkin, B. R., & Miller, N. E. (1986). Failure to replicate visceral learning in the acute curarized rat preparation. *Behavioral Neuroscience, 100,* 299–314.

Epstein, L. H., & Stein, D. B. (1974). Feedback-influenced heart rate discrimination. *Journal of Abnormal Psychology, 83,* 585–588.

Fillenz, M., & Widdicombe, J. G. (1972). Receptors of the lungs and airways. In E. Neil (Ed.), *Handbook of sensory physiology: Vol. 3. Enteroceptors* (pp. 81–112). Berlin: Springer-Verlag.

Flynn, D. M., & Clemens, W. J. (1988). On the validity of heartbeat tracking tasks. *Psychophysiology, 25,* 92–96.

Fudge, R., & Adams, H. E. (1985). The effects of discrimination training on voluntary control of cephalic vasomotor activity. *Psychophysiology, 22,* 300–306.

Gannon, L. (1977). The role of interoception in learned visceral control. *Biofeedback & Self-Regulation, 2,* 337–347.

Geldard, F. A. (1972). *The human senses* (2nd ed.). New York: Wiley.

Gescheider, G. A. (1976). *Psychophysics: Method and theory.* Hillsdale, NJ: Erlbaum.

Gottfried, S. B., Altose, M. D., Kelsen, S. G., Fogarty, C. M., & Cherniack, N. S. (1978). The perception of changes in airflow resistance in normal subjects and patients with chronic airways obstruction. *Chest, 73* (Suppl.), 286–288.

Grigg, L., & Ashton, R. (1982). Heart rate discrimination viewed as a perceptual process: A replication and extension. *Psychophysiology, 19,* 13–20.

Grigg, L., & Ashton, R. (1984). Heart rate discrimination and heart rate control: A test of Brener's theory. *International Journal of Psychophysiology, 2,* 185–201.

Griggs, R. C., & Stunkard, A. (1964). The interpretation of gastric motility. II. Sensitivity and bias in the perception of gastric motility. *Archives of General Psychiatry, 11,* 82–89.

Gur, R. C., & Gur, R. E. (1977). Correlates of conjugate lateral eye movements in man. In S. Harnad (Ed.), *Lateralization in the nervous system* (pp. 261–281). New York: Academic Press.

Guyton, A. C. (1981). *Textbook of medical physiology* (6th ed.). Philadelphia: Saunders.

Guz, A. (1977). Respiratory sensations in man. *British Medical Bulletin, 33,* 175–177.

Hantas, M., Katkin, E. S., & Blascovich, J. (1982). Relationship between heartbeat discrimination and subjective experience of affective state. *Psychophysiology, 19,* 563. (Abstract).

Hantas, M., Katkin, E. S., & Reed, S. D. (1984). Cerebral lateralization and heartbeat discrimination. *Psychophysioloy, 21,* 274–278.

Harris, V. A., & Katkin, E. S. (1975). Primary and secondary emotional behavior: An analysis of the role of autonomic feedback on affect, arousal, and attribution. *Psychological Bulletin, 82,* 904–916.

Harver, A., Baird, J. C., McGovern, J. F., & Daubenspeck, J. A. (1988). Grouping and multidimensional organization of respiratory sensations. *Perception & Psychophysics, 44,* 285–292.

Hugdahl, K., Franzon, M., Andersson, B., & Walldebo, G. (1983). Heart-rate responses (HRR) to lateralized visual stimuli. *The Pavlovian Journal of Biological Science, 18,* 186–198.

Iggo, A. (1986). Afferent C-fibers and visceral sensation. In F. Cervero & J. F. B. Morrison (Eds.), *Progress in brain research: Vol. 67. Visceral sensation* (pp. 29–36). Amsterdam: Elsevier.

Iggo, A., & Ilyinsky, O. B. (Eds.) (1976). *Progress in brain research: Vol. 43. Somatosensory and visceral receptor mechanisms.* Amsterdam: Elsevier.

James, W. (1884). What is an emotion? *Mind, 9,* 188–205.

Jones, G. E., & Hollandsworth, J. G. (1981). Heart rate discrimination before and after exercise-induced augmented cardiac activity. *Psychophysiology, 18,* 252–257.

Jones, G. E., Jones, K. R., Rouse, C. H., Scott, D. M., & Caldwell, J. A. (1987). The effect of body position on the perception of cardiac sensations: An experiment and theoretical implications. *Psychophysiology, 24,* 300–311.

Jordan, D., & Spyer, K. M. (1986). Brainstem integration of cardiovascular and pulmonary afferent activity. In F. Cervero & J. F. B. Morrison (Eds.), *Progress in brain research: Vol. 67. Visceral sensation* (pp. 295–314). Amsterdam: Elsevier.

Katkin, E. S. (1985). Blood, sweat and tears: Individual differences in autonomic self-perception. *Psychophysiology, 22,* 125–137.

Katkin, E. S., Blascovich, J., Reed, S. D., Adamec, J., Jones, J., & Taublieb, A. B. (1982). The effect of psychologically induced arousal on accuracy of heartbeat self-perception. *Psychophysiology, 19,* 568. (Abstract).

Katkin, E. S., Morell, M. A., Goldband, A., Bernstein, G. L., & Wise, J. A. (1982). Individual differences in heartbeat discrimination. *Psychophysiology, 19,* 160–166.

Katkin, E. S., & Murray, E. N. (1968). Instrumental conditioning of autonomically mediated behavior: Theoretical and methodological issues. *Psychological Bulletin, 70,* 52–68.

Kimble, G. A. (1961). *Hilgard and Marquis' conditioning and learning* (2nd ed.). New York: Appleton-Century.

Kimmel, H. D. (1967). Instrumental conditioning of autonomically mediated behavior. *Psychological Bulletin, 67,* 337–345.

Kleinman, R. A., & Brener, J. (1970). *The effects of training in heartbeat discrimination upon the subsequent development of learned heart rate control.* Unpublished manuscript, University of Tennessee.

Malliani, A., Lombardi, F., & Pagani, M. (1986). Sensory innervation of the heart. In F. Cervero & J. F. B. Morrison (Eds.), *Progress in brain research: Vol. 67. Visceral sensation* (pp. 39–48). Amsterdam: Elsevier.

Mandler, G., & Kahn, M. (1960). Discrimination of changes in heart rates: Two unsuccessful attempts. *Journal of the Experimental Analysis of Behavior, 3,* 21–25.

Mandler, G., Mandler, J. M., & Uviller, E. T. (1958). Autonomic feedback: The perception of autonomic activity. *Journal of Abnormal and Social Psychology, 56,* 367–373.

Mason, R. E. (1961). *Internal perception and bodily functioning.* New York: International Universities Press.

McFarland, R. A. (1975). Heart rate perception and heart rate control. *Psychophysiology, 12,* 402–405.

Miller, N. E. (1969). Learning of visceral and glandular responses. *Science, 163,* 434–445.

Montgomery, W. A., & Jones, G. E. (1984). Laterality, emotionality, and heartbeat perception. *Psychophysiology, 21,* 459–465.

Newman, P. P. (1974). *Visceral afferent functions of the nervous system.* London: Edward Arnold.

Paintal, A. S. (1977). Thoracic receptors connected with sensation. *British Medical Bulletin, 33,* 169–174.

Paintal, A. S. (1986). The visceral sensations – some basic mechanisms. In F. Cervero & J. F. B. Morrison (Eds.), *Progress in brain research: Vol. 67. Visceral sensation* (pp. 3–19). Amsterdam: Elsevier.

Papillo, J. F., Tursky, B., & Friedman, R. (1981). Perceived changes in the intensity of arterial pulsations as a function of applied cuff pressure. *Psychophysiology, 18,* 283–287.

Pennebaker, J. W. (1982). *The psychology of physical symptoms.* New York: Springer-Verlag.

Pennebaker, J. W., & Hoover, C. W. (1984). Visceral perception versus visceral detection: Disentangling methods and assumptions. *Biofeedback & Self-Regulation, 9,* 339–352.

Piliavin, I., Piliavin, J. A., & Rodin, J. (1975). Costs, diffusion, and the stigmatized victim. *Journal of Personality and Social Psychology, 32,* 429–438.

Razran, G. (1961). The observable unconscious and the inferable conscious in current Soviet psychophysiology: Interoceptive conditioning, semantic conditioning, and the orienting reflex. *Psychological Review, 68,* 81–147.

Reed, S. D. (1986). *Relationship among hemispheric preference, visceral self-perception, autonomic arousal and emotions.* Unpublished doctoral dissertation, State University of New York at Buffalo.

Reed, S. D., & Katkin, E. S. (1987). *Finger tapping methodology for assessment of cardiac perception.* Unpublished manuscript.

Ross, A. (1982). Concurrent assessment of heart rate discrimination and control. *Biological Psychology, 14,* 231–244.

Schachter, S., & Singer, J. E. (1962). Cognitive, social, and physiological determinants of emotional state. *Psychological Review, 69,* 379–399.

Schandry, R. (1980). Perception of heart activity and personality. *Psychophysiology, 17,* 298. (Abstract).

Schandry, R. (1981). Heart beat perception and emotional experience. *Psychophysiology, 18,* 483–488.

Schandry, R., Sparrer, B., & Weitkunat, R. (1986). From the heart to the brain: A study of heartbeat contingent scalp potentials. *International Journal of Neuroscience, 30,* 261–275.

Schandry, R., & Specht, G. (1981). The influence of psychological and physical stress on the perception of heart beats. *Psychophysiology, 18,* 154. (Abstract).

Schmidt, R. E. (Ed.) (1986). *Fundamentals of sensory physiology* (3rd ed.). Berlin: Springer-Verlag.

Sherrington, C. (1948). *The integrative action of the nervous system* (2nd ed.). New Haven: Yale University Press.

Skinner, B. F. (1938). *The behavior of organisms: An experimental analysis.* New York: Appleton-Century.

Stern, R. M. (1972). Detection of one's own spontaneous GSRs. *Psychonomic Science, 29,* 354–356.

Stevens, S. S. (1956). The direct estimation of sensory magnitude – loudness. *American Journal of Psychology, 69,* 1–25.

Stevens, S. S. (1970). Neural events and the psychophysical law. *Science, 170,* 1043–1050.

Stevens, S. S. (1975). *Psychophysics: Introduction to its perceptual, neural, and social prospects.* New York: Wiley.

Swets, J. A. (1973). The relative operating characteristic in psychology. *Science, 182,* 990–1000.

Tursky, B., Papillo, J. F., & Friedman, R. (1982). The perception and discrimination of arterial pulsations: Implications for the behavioral treatment of hypertension. *Journal of Psychosomatic Research, 26,* 485–493.

Wald, A., & Tunuguntla, A. K. (1984). Anorectal sensorimotor dysfunction in fecal incontinence and diabetes mellitus. *New England Journal of Medicine, 310,* 1282–1287.

Walker, B. B., & Sandman, C. A. (1979). Human visual evoked responses are related to heart rate. *Journal of Comparative and Physiological Psychology, 93,* 717–729.

Walker, B. B., & Sandman, C. A. (1982). Visual evoked potentials change as heart rate and carotid pressure change. *Psychophysiology, 19,* 520–527.

Whitehead, W. E., & Drescher, V. M. (1980). Perception of gastric contractions and self-control of gastric motility. *Psychophysiology, 17,* 552–558.

Whitehead, W. E., Drescher, V. M., & Blackwell, B. (1976). Lack of relationship between Autonomic Perception Questionnaire scores and actual sensitivity for perceiving one's heart beat. *Psychophysiology, 13,* 177. (Abstract).

Whitehead, W. E., Drescher, V. M., Heiman, P., & Blackwell, B. (1977). Relation of heart rate control to heartbeat perception. *Biofeedback & Self-Regulation, 2,* 371–392.

Whitehead, W. E., Engel, B. T., & Schuster, M. M. (1980). Perception of rectal distension is necessary to prevent fecal incontinence. In G. Adám, I. Meszaros, & E. I. Banyai (Eds.), *Advances in physiological science: Vol. 17. Brain and behavior* (pp. 203–209). Budapest: Akadémiai Kiádo.

Whitehead, W. E., Orr, W. C., Engel, B. T., & Schuster, M. M. (1981). External anal sphincter response to rectal distension: Learned response or reflex. *Psychophysiology, 19,* 57–62.

Widdicombe, J. G. (1986). Sensory innervation of the lungs and airways. In F. Cervero & J. F. B. Morrison (Eds.), *Progress in brain research: Vol. 67. Visceral sensation* (pp. 49–64). Amsterdam: Elsevier.

Willis, W. D., Jr. (1986). Visceral inputs to sensory pathways in the spinal cord. In F. Cervero & J. F. B. Morrison (Eds.), *Progress in brain research Vol. 67. Visceral sensation* (pp. 207–225). Amsterdam: Elsevier.

Yates, A. J., Jones, K. E., Marie, G. V., & Hogben, J. H. (1985). Detection of the heartbeat and events in the cardiac cycle. *Psychophysiology, 22,* 561–567.

Zajonc, R. (1968). Attitudinal effects of mere exposure. *Journal of Personality and Social Psychology, 9,* 1–27.

Zechman, F. W., Jr., & Wiley, R. L. (1986). Afferent inputs to breathing: Respiratory sensation. In A. P. Fishman (Ed.), *Handbook of physiology: Sec. 3. The respiratory system* (Vol. 2, Part 1, pp. 449–474). Bethesda, MD: American Physiological Society.

Zillmann, D. (1978). *Hostility and aggression.* Hillsdale, NJ: Erlbaum.

PART   III

Systemic psychophysiology

10 *The electrodermal system*

MICHAEL E. DAWSON, ANNE M. SCHELL, AND
DIANE L. FILION

Electrodermal activity (EDA) has been one of the most widely used – some might add "abused" – response systems in the history of psychophysiology. The purpose of this chapter is to provide a tutorial overview of EDA for the interested student, researcher, and practitioner who are not specialists in this particular system. As with other chapters in this volume, we begin with a historical orientation and then discuss the physical, inferential, and psychological–social aspects of EDA.

10.1 HISTORICAL BACKGROUND

10.1.1 *The discovery of electrodermal activity*

The empirical study of the electrical changes in human skin began approximately 100 years ago when Vigouroux (1879, 1888) measured tonic skin resistance levels from various patient groups as a clinical diagnostic sign. In the same laboratory, Féré (1888) found that by passing a small electrical current across two electrodes placed on the surface of the skin, one could measure momentary decreases in skin resistance in response to a variety of stimuli (visual, auditory, gustatory, olfactory, etc). The basic phenomenon discovered by Féré is that the skin momentarily becomes a better conductor of electricity when external stimuli are presented. Shortly thereafter, Tarchanoff (1890) reported that one could measure similar changes in electrical potential between two electrodes placed on the skin without applying an external current. Hence, Féré and Tarchanoff are said to have discovered the two basic methods of recording electrodermal activity in use today. Recording the skin resistance (or its reciprocal, skin conductance) response relies on the passage of an external current across the skin and hence is referred to as the *exosomatic method*, whereas recording the skin potential response does not involve an external current and hence is referred to as the *endosomatic method*. The present chapter will focus on the exosomatic method of recording skin resistance and conductance because this clearly is the method of choice among contemporary researchers (Fowles et al., 1981).

It is interesting and somewhat humbling to find that the very early investigators identified many of the important aspects of EDA that remain of interest today. For example, the tonic–phasic distinction was implied in the earliest of these publications. The tonic level of skin resistance or conductance is the absolute level of resistance or conductance at a given moment in the absence of a measurable phasic response and is referred to as SRL (skin resistance level) or SCL (skin conductance level). Superimposed on the tonic level are phasic decreases in resistance (increases in conductance) referred to as SRRs (skin resistance responses)

295

or SCRs (skin conductance responses). Similar distinctions are made with skin potential and are referred to as SPLs and SPRs. (It should be noted that other terms have been used to refer to EDA phenomena in the history of this response system, particularly psychogalvanic reflex, PGR, and galvanic skin response, GSR.)

Even more humbling is the fact that many of the variables and phenomena intensively studied today were already being investigated in this early research. For example, the ability of various types of sensory stimuli to elicit phasic EDA changes was clearly in evidence. The fact that stronger stimulation would elicit larger responses as well as the fact that repetitions of the same stimulus would lead to habituation were noted. Moreover, the effectiveness of mental images, mental effort (e.g., solving arithmetic problems), emotions, and uncertainties in eliciting EDA also was demonstrated. Individual differences in EDA were observed and questions regarding the utility of this new measure in distinguishing normal from pathological groups were being raised. Clearly, these early investigators recognized the psychophysiological significance of this newly discovered phenomenon and laid the foundation for more than a century of subsequent research. A detailed historical review of these early articles is provided by Neumann and Blanton (1970), and English translations of some of the classic early reports on electrodermal phenomena can be found in Porges and Coles (1976).

10.1.2 Issues in EDA research

Several issues identified in this early research have continued to be a source of considerable speculation and investigation in the history of this response system. One set of such issues concerns the mechanisms and functions of EDA. In terms of peripheral mechanisms, Vigouroux proposed what became known as the "vascular theory" of EDA (Neumann & Blanton, 1970). The vascular theory associated changes in skin resistance with changes in blood flow. Tarchanoff (1890) favored a "secretory theory," which related EDA to sweat gland activity. This theory was supported later by Darrow (1927) when he measured EDA and sweat secretion simultaneously from a group of graduate students at the University of Chicago. He found that the two measures were closely related, although the phasic EDA would begin about 1 s before moisture would appear on the surface of the skin. Thus, it was concluded that activity of the sweat glands, not sweat on the skin per se, was critical for EDA. (Other lines of evidence indicating that sweat glands are the major contributors to EDA have been reviewed by Fowles, 1986, pp. 74–75.) Since it was generally known at the time that palmar sweat glands are innervated by the sympathetic chain of the autonomic nervous system, EDA was said to reflect sympathetic activation. In terms of more central physiological mechanisms, work by early investigators such as Wang and Richter indicated that EDA was complexly determined by both subcortical and cortical areas (for a review of this early research, see Darrow, 1937). In the same review article, Darrow proposed that "the function of the secretory activity of the palms is primarily to provide a pliable adhesive surface facilitating tactual acuity and grip on objects" (1937, p. 641).

Issues surrounding the proper methods of recording and quantifying EDA also have been important in the history of this response system. Lykken and Venables (1971) noted that EDA has continued to provide useful data "in spite of being frequently abused by measurement techniques which range from the arbitrary to the positively weird" (p. 656). In fact, we would date the beginning of the modern era of EDA research to the early 1970s when Lykken and Venables (1971) proposed standardized techniques of recording skin conductance and standardized units of measurement. This was followed shortly by an edited book on EDA that contains several useful review chapters (Prokasy & Raskin, 1973), including a particularly outstanding chapter by Venables and Christie (1973). Published around the same time were several other excellent reviews (Edelberg, 1972a; Fowles, 1974; Grings, 1974).

Another issue of central importance concerns the psychological significance of EDA. From the beginning, this response system has been closely linked with the psychological concepts of emotion, arousal, and attention. Early in this century, Carl Jung added EDA measurements to his word association experiments in order to objectively measure the emotional aspects of "hidden complexes." An American friend joined Jung in these experiments and enthusiastically reported that "every stimulus accompanied by an emotion produced a deviation of the galvanometer to a degree in direct proportion to the liveliness and actuality of the emotion aroused" Peterson, 1907, cited in Neumann & Blanton, 1970, p. 470). About half a century later, when the concept of emotion was less in favor, Woodworth and Schlosberg (1954) devoted most of one entire chapter of their classic textbook in experimental psychology to EDA, which they described as "perhaps the most widely used index of activation" (p. 137). They supported this indexing relationship by noting that tonic SCL is generally low during sleep and high in activated states such as rage or mental work. The authors also related phasic SCRs to attention, noting that such responses are sensitive to stimulus novelty, intensity, and significance.

Many of the issues identified in the preceding discussion have remained important for contemporary psychophysiologists and are discussed in the remainder of this chapter. In the next section we first present a summary of the basic physiological mechanisms and proper recording techniques of EDA, followed by a presentation of the methods of measuring and quantifying various EDA components. We then discuss the relative advantages and disadvantages of EDA as a response system of choice for the researcher and finally end with a section devoted to a discussion of the psychological significance of EDA.

10.2   PHYSICAL CONTEXT

10.2.1   *Anatomical–physiological basis*

The skin is a selective barrier that serves the function of preventing entry of foreign matter into the body and selectively facilitating passage of materials from the bloodstream to the exterior of the body. It is an adaptive organ that aides in the maintenance of water balance and of constant core body temperature, functions accomplished primarily through vasoconstriction–dilation and through variation in the production of sweat. As Edelberg (1972a) points out, it is not surprising that an organ with such vital and dynamic functions constantly receives signals from control centers in the brain, and he suggests that "we can listen in on such signals by taking advantage of the fact that their arrival at the skin is heralded by measurable electrical changes that we call electrodermal activity" (Edelberg, 1972a, p. 368).

There are two forms of sweat glands in the human body: the eccrine, which have been of primary interest to psychophysiologists, and the apocrine, which have been relatively unstudied. The distinction between these two is usually made on the basis of location and function (Robertshaw, 1983). Whereas apocrine sweat glands typically open into hair follicles and are found primarily in the armpits and the genital areas, eccrine glands cover most of the body and are most dense on the palms and soles of the feet. The function of the apocrine glands is not yet well understood, and this may account for the subordinate status they currently hold within the field of psychophysiology. However, there have been some recent suggestions in the literature that apocrine glands may be more interesting than was once believed. For example, in mammals such as dogs and monkeys, apocrine glands are believed to produce a secretion that when modified by bacteria on the surface of the skin, serves as an identifying or sexual scent hormone (pheromone). Some authors have suggested that apocrine glands in humans may serve a similar function (e.g., Jakubovic & Ackerman, 1985). It has also been noted that there is some evidence that suggests that apocrine gland secretion is induced by any emotional stress that causes sympathetic nervous system discharge (Jakubovic & Ackerman, 1985). To date, the evidence still appears to be inconclusive, and a recent review of the literature concluded that the responsivity of the apocrine glands to emotional, stressful, or sexually arousing stimuli is still under debate (Shields, MacDowell, Fairchild, & Campbell, 1987).

In contrast to the apocrine gland, a great deal is known about the function of the eccrine sweat gland. For example, it is known that the primary function of most eccrine sweat glands is thermoregulation. However, those located on the palmar and plantar surfaces have been thought of as being more concerned with grasping behavior than with evaporative cooling (Edelberg, 1972a) and have been suggested to be more responsive to significant or emotional stimuli than to thermal stimuli. Although all eccrine glands are believed to be involved in emotion-evoked sweating, such sweating is usually most evident in these areas primarily because of their high density (Shields et al., 1987). The measurement of EDA by psychophysiologists is primarily concerned with this psychologically induced sweating.

Figure 10.1 shows the basic peripheral mechanisms involved in the production of EDA. The extreme outer layer of the skin, the stratum corneum or horny layer, consists of a layer of dead cells that serves to protect the internal organs. Below the stratum corneum lies the stratum lucidum, and just below that is the stratum Malpighii. The stratum Malpighii actually consists of three cell layers, the granular layer, the spinous layer, and the deepest layer, the stratum germinativum, which consists of cells that are continually reproducing and replacing the dead cells on the skin's surface. The eccrine sweat gland itself consists of a coiled compact body, which is the secretory portion of the gland, and the sweat duct, the long tube that is the excretory portion of the gland. The sweat duct remains relatively straight in its path through the stratum Malpighii and stratum lucidum and then it spirals through the stratum corneum and opens to the surface of the skin as a small pore (Edelberg, 1972a).

Many models have been suggested for explaining how these peripheral mechanisms relate to the electrical activity of the skin and to the transient increases in skin conductance elicited by stimuli, but probably still the most widely accepted is Edelberg's (1972a) sweat circuit model. According to this model, there are two peripheral mechanisms that contribute to EDA: the filling of the sweat duct and the activity of a selective membrane that lies somewhere in the epidermis. It is suggested that the duct-filling component is involved in the production of SCRs and that both the duct-filling and membrane components are involved in the

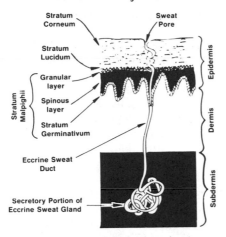

Figure 10.1. Eccrine sweat gland. (Adapted from Hassett, 1978.)

response recovery. According to Edelberg (1972a), the sweat ducts are ordinarily filled to the Malpighian layer, and the amount of standing sweat in the glands is a major determinant of tonic level measures of EDA. The phasic increases in skin conductance are a result of increases in the standing level of sweat in the ducts. Response recovery represents either the gradual diffusion of sweat through the duct wall into the stratum corneum or the action of the selective membranes through the active reabsorption of the sweat. A more complete description of this electrical model of the skin can be found in Edelberg (1972a). Although little doubt exists about the importance of duct filling in SCR production, the role of the selective membrane is not as well understood, and alternatives to the membrane model have been suggested (Fowles, 1986, pp. 87–88).

To understand how these electrical properties of the skin are measured, it is useful to first think of the sweat ducts (the long tubular portion of the gland that opens onto the skin surface) as a set of variable resistors wired in parallel. As just described in the Edelberg sweat circuit model, columns of sweat rise in the ducts in varying amounts and in varying numbers of sweat glands, depending on the degree of sympathetic activation. The higher the sweat rises in a given gland, the lower the resistance in that variable resistor. Any change in the level of sweat in the ducts changes the values of the variable resistors and yields observable changes in EDA.

Historically both the sympathetic and parasympathetic divisions of the autonomic nervous system (ANS) were considered as possible mediators of EDA. This is partially due to the fact that the neurotransmitter involved in the mediation of eccrine sweat gland activity is acetylcholine, generally a parasympathetic neurotransmitter, rather than norepinephrine, the neurotransmitter typically associated with sympathetic activation (Venables & Christie, 1980). Now, however, it is generally conceded that human sweat glands receive predominantly sympathetic cholinergic innervation but that some adrenergic fibers also exist in close proximity (Shields et al., 1987). Evidence for the predominant sympathetic control of EDA has been provided by studies that have measured sympathetic action potentials in peripheral nerves while simultaneously recording EDA. The results of such research have shown that within normal ranges of ambient room temperature and subject thermoregulatory states, there is a high correlation between bursts of sympathetic nerve activity and SCRs (Wallin, 1981).

The neuroanatomical mechanisms involved in the central nervous system control of EDA have been reviewed in detail by Edelberg (1972a) and by Venables and Christie (1973) and are discussed only briefly here. Edelberg (1972a) described three basically independent pathways that lead to the production of SCRs. One pathway involves control by the premotor cortex descending through the pyramidal tract, a second pathway involves activation of hypothalamic and limbic centers, and the third pathway involves activation of the reticular formation. Edelberg (1973) suggests that thermoregulatory sweating is primarily controlled by the hypothalamus, that SCRs elicited in situations requiring fine motor control are controlled primarily by the premotor cortex, and that SCRs elicited in situations requiring gross motor activity are controlled primarily through the reticular formation. In addition, Edelberg (1972a, 1973) suggests that SCRs elicited by startling or threatening stimuli may be thermoregulatory responses that would be adaptive for situations requiring fighting, escape, and so on. In these situations, extensive motor activity would be required that would result in increased body temperature. The activation of the sweat glands would thus aid in heat loss and maintenance of body temperature. Edelberg suggests that the SCRs elicited by startling or threatening stimuli are controlled by activation of the hypothalamic and limbic centers. Venables and Christie (1973) offer a description of the central control pathways similar to Edelberg's but suggest that the cortex will be the dominant influence unless otherwise prevented.

10.2.2   *Physical recording basis*

As briefly described earlier, EDA is measured by passing a small current through a pair of electrodes placed on the surface of the skin. The principle invoked in the measurement of skin resistance or conductance is that of Ohm's Law, which states that skin resistance (R) is equal to the voltage applied between two electrodes placed on the skin surface (V) divided by the current being passed through the skin (I). This law can be expressed as $R = V/I$. If the current is held constant, then one can measure the voltage between the electrodes, which will vary directly with skin resistance. Alternatively, if the voltage is held constant, one can measure the current flow, which will vary directly with the reciprocal of skin resistance, skin conductance.

Lykken and Venables (1971) developed a strong case for the direct measurement of skin conductance over measurement of skin resistance based in part on the earlier work and recommendations of Darrow (1934, 1964). Skin conductance has been shown to be more linearly related to the number of active sweat glands and their rate of secretion because the individual sweat glands function as resistors in parallel, and the conductance of a parallel circuit is simply the sum of all of the conductances in parallel. On the other hand, the overall resistance of a parallel circuit is a complex function of each of the individual resistances. Thus, unlike the relationship of SRR and SRL, the SCR is potentially independent of SCL since a given increment in the number of active sweat glands will produce the same increment in the total conductance of the pathway regardless of the level of basal activity. A description of constant-voltage circuits that allow the direct measurement of skin conductance can be found in Lykken and Venables (1971) as well as in Fowles et al. (1981).

Although there are several substantial advantages of recording skin conductance directly with a constant-voltage circuit, it nevertheless is possible to measure skin resistance initially and then subsequently transform the data to conductance if one has access only to a constant-current system. Conductance is simply the reciprocal of resistance, but it is important to remember that this is a nonlinear transformation. Thus, the conclusion one reaches can be quite different depending on whether one uses resistance or conductance units (e.g., see Hassett, 1978, pp. 166–167, or Woodworth & Schlosberg, 1954, p. 141). Given the typical values of skin conductance, Edelberg (1967) provides the following equation for converting SRL to SCL:

$$\text{SCL } (\mu \text{Siemens}) = 1000/\text{SRL } (\Omega)$$

Thus, an SRL of $100,000\,\Omega$ is equivalent to an SCL of $10\,\mu\text{S}$. However, as Edelberg notes, one cannot use this equation to convert phasic changes in resistance (SRR) to phasic changes in conductance (SCR). Instead, one must convert the pre-SRR level and the peak SRR level each to conductance and then compute the difference between the two conductances. As emphasized by Lykken and Venables (1971), these extra computational steps involve considerable labor as well as increased likelihood of errors. Both of these difficulties can be avoided rather easily by simply measuring skin conductance directly with a constant-voltage system in the first place.

In addition to a constant-voltage circuit for the direct recording of skin conductance, special consideration must be given to the choice of recording electrodes, electrode paste, and electrode placement. Silver-silver chloride electrodes are the type most typically used in skin conductance recording because they minimize the development of bias potentials and polarization. These electrodes can be easily attached through the use of double-sided adhesive collars that also serve the purpose of helping to control the size of the skin area that comes in contact with the electrode paste, an important function since it is the contact area, not the size of the electrode, that affects the conductance values. The electrode paste is the conductive medium between the electrodes and the skin. Probably the most important concern in choosing an electrode paste is that it preserve the electrical properties of the bioelectrical signals of the response system of interest. Since in the measurement of EDA a small current is passed through the skin, the electrode paste interacts with the tissue over which it is placed. For this reason, the use of a paste that closely resembles sweat in its salinity is recommended (Venables & Christie, 1980). Instructions for making such paste are given in Fowles et al. (1981, p. 235). Commercial EKG or EEG gels should not be used because they usually contain near saturation levels of NaCl and therefore may introduce measurement errors.

Skin conductance is recorded with both electrodes on active sites (bipolar recording); hence it does not matter in which direction the current flows between the two electrodes. Skin conductance recordings are typically taken from the locations on the palms, with several acceptable placements. The most common electrode placements are the thenar eminences of the palms and the volar surface of the medial or distal phalanges of the fingers (see Figure 10.2 for a diagram of these placements). Since it is critical in EDA recording that the electrical properties of the response system be preserved, the electrode sites for bipolar recording should not receive any special preparation such as cleaning with alcohol and abrading the skin, which might severely reduce the natural resistive/conductive properties of the skin.

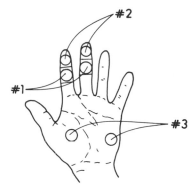

Figure 10.2. Illustration of three recommended electrode placements for recording electrodermal activity. Placement 1 involves volar surfaces of medial phalanges, placement 2 involves volar surfaces of distal phalanges, and placement 3 involves thenar and hypothenar eminences of palms. Note that each pair of electrodes represents a separate electrode configuration and that only one of the three configurations would be used at a time.

However, since a fall in conductance has been noted following the use of soap and water (Venables & Christie, 1973) and since the length of time since the last wash will be variable across subjects when they arrive at the laboratory, it is recommended that they be asked to wash their hands with a nonabrasive soap prior to having the electrodes attached. It is recommended that the electrodes be kept on the same hand to avoid ECG artifact and that the placement sites be clean and dry (Venables & Christie, 1973).

10.3   INFERENTIAL CONTEXT

10.3.1   Quantification procedures

Figure 10.3 shows tracings of two hypothetical skin conductance recordings during a 20-s rest period and then during three repetitions of a simple discrete stimulus (e.g., tone). Several important aspects of EDA can be seen in Figure 10.3. First, it can be seen that tonic SCL begins at 10 μS in the upper tracing and at 5 μS in the lower tracing. Although tonic SCL can vary widely between different subjects and within the same subject in different psychological states, the typical range is between 2 and 20 μS with the types of apparatus and procedures described here. Computing the logarithm of SCL can significantly reduce skew and kurtosis in the SCL data and is recommended by Venables and Christie (1980).

It can also be seen in the lower tracing of Figure 10.3 that the SCL drifts downward from 5 to nearly 4 μS during the rest period. It is common for SCL to gradually decrease while subjects are at rest, then rapidly increase when novel stimulation is introduced, and finally gradually decrease again when the stimulus is repeated (e.g., Montagu, 1963). These large "tidal" shifts in tonic SCL probably deserve more attention than they receive in the current literature.

Phasic SCRs are only a small fraction of the SCL and have been likened to small waves superimposed on the tidal drifts in SCL (Lykken & Venables, 1971). If the SCR occurs in the absence of an identifiable stimulus, as shown in the rest phase of Figure

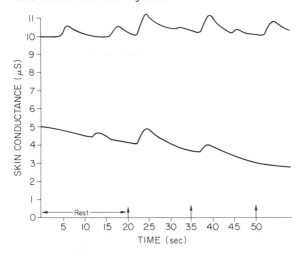

Figure 10.3. Tracing of two hypothetical skin conductance recordings during 20-s rest period and then during three repetitions of a simple discrete stimulus. Arrows represent the presentation of a stimulus. (From Dawson & Nuechterlein, 1984).

10.3., it is referred to as a "spontaneous" or "nonspecific" SCR (NS-SCR). The most widely used measure of NS-SCR activity is its rate per minute, which typically is between 1 and 3 per min while the subject is at rest. However, responses can be elicited by sighs, deep breaths, and bodily movements, so unless these also are monitored it is impossible to say which responses truly are NS-SCRs.

Presentation of a novel, unexpected, significant, or aversive stimulus will likely elicit an SCR called a "specific" or "event-related" SCR (ER-SCR). In this chapter we employ the abbreviation ER-SCR although it is customary in psychophysiological literature to simply use the term SCR to refer to an event-related skin conductance response. We believe that the term ER-SCR is generally useful because it reduces ambiguity and serves as a reminder that the response in question is assumed to have been elicited by a specific stimulus.

As is also the case with NS-SCRs, one must decide upon a minimum amplitude change in conductance to count as an ER-SCR. A common minimum response amplitude is 0.05 μS, which is a largely arbitrary value that happens to be the minimum change that can be reliably detected through visual inspection of most polygraph recordings. This arbitrary minimum will probably decrease as computer scoring becomes more popular because the computer can reliably detect much smaller changes. Another decision regarding ER-SCRs concerns the latency window during which time a response will be assumed to be elicited by the stimulus. Based on frequency distributions of response latencies to simple stimuli, it is common to use a 1–3s latency window. Hence, any SCR that begins between 1 and 3s following stimulus onset is considered to be elicited by that stimulus. It is important to select reasonably short latency windows, perhaps even shorter than 1–3s, so as not to have the NS-SCR rate contaminate the measurement of ER-SCRs (e.g., Levinson, Edelberg, & Bridger, 1984).

Having decided on a minimum response amplitude and a latency window in which a response will be considered an ER-SCR, one can measure several aspects of

Table 10.1. *Electrodermal measures, definitions, and typical values*

Measure	Definition	Typical Values
Skin conductance level (SCL)	tonic level of electrical conductivity of skin	2–20 μS
Change in SCL	gradual changes in SCL measured at two or more points in time	1–3 μS
Frequency of NS-SCRs	number of SCRs in absence of identifiable eliciting stimulus	1–3 per min
ER-SCR amplitude	phasic increase in conductance shortly following stimulus onset	0.2–1.0 μS
ER-SCR latency	temporal interval between stimulus onset and SCR initiation	1–3 s
ER-SCR rise time	temporal interval between SCR initiation and SCR peak	1–3 s
ER-SCR half recovery time	temporal interval between SCR peak and point of 50% recovery of SCR amplitude	2–10 s
ER-SCR habituation (trials to habituation)	number of stimulus presentations before two or three trials with no response	2–8 stimulus presentations
ER-SCR habituation (slope)	rate of change of ER-SCR amplitude	0.01–0.5 μS per trial

the ER-SCR besides its mere occurrence and frequency. Definitions and typical values of the major EDA component measures are given in Table 10.1 and shown graphically in Figure 10.4. For example, the size of the ER-SCR is quantified as the amount of increase in conductance measured from the onset of the response to its peak. The size of an ER-SCR typically ranges between 0.2 and 1.0 μS.

When a stimulus is repeated several times and an average size of the ER-SCR is to be calculated, one may choose to compute mean SCR amplitude or magnitude. Magnitude refers to the mean value computed across all stimulus presentations including those without a measurable response, whereas amplitude is the mean value computed across only those trials on which a measurable (nonzero) response occurred (Humphreys, 1943). Prokasy and Kumpfer (1973) argue strongly against use of the magnitude measure in large part because it confounds frequency and amplitude, which do not always covary. A magnitude measure can create the impression that the response size is changing when, in fact, response frequency is changing. Hence, these authors recommend separate assessments of frequency and amplitude rather than magnitude. However, it is important to note that a complication with the amplitude measure is that the N used in computing average response size can vary depending on how many measurable responses a subject gives, and the data of subjects without any measurable response must be eliminated. Thus, a subject who responds on each of 10 stimulus presentations with a response of 0.50 μS will have the same mean SCR amplitude as a subject who responds on only the first stimulus presentation with a response of 0.50 μS and does not respond thereafter. We concur with Venables and Christie (1980) that there are arguments for and against both amplitude and magnitude and that although no absolute resolution is possible, it is important to keep the difference between the two measures clearly in mind. In fact, we recommend that in most situations it is

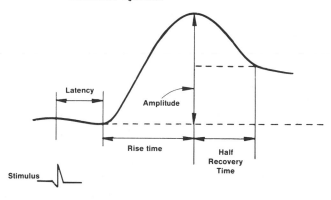

Figure 10.4. Graphical representation of major EDA components.

reasonable to compute and compare results obtained with SCR frequency, amplitude, and magnitude.

Like SCL, ER-SCR amplitude and magnitude are frequently found to be positively skewed and also leptokurtotic, and a logarithmic transformation is often used to remedy these problems. If measurements are being made of ER-SCR magnitude, so that zero responses are included, log(SCR + 1.0) may be calculated since the logarithm of zero is not defined (Venables & Christie, 1980). Another common practice is to use a square-root transformation, $\sqrt{SCR}$, to normalize ER-SCR data, which does not require the addition of a constant (Edelberg, 1972a). In some cases the choice of the square-root or logarithmic transformation should be guided by considerations of achieving or maintaining the homogeneity of variance across several groups, if variances tend to increase as means or squares of means increase across groups (Ferguson, 1976). If skew, kurtosis, or homogeneity of variance problems do not exist in a particular set of data, transformations need not be performed.

In addition to response size, one can also measure temporal characteristics of the ER-SCR including latency, rise time, and half recovery time. These temporal characteristics of the SCR waveform are not quantified as commonly as amplitude, and their relationship to psychophysiological processes is not as well understood at this time. Edelberg (1970, 1972b), for example, intensively studied half recovery time and suggested that rapidly recovering responses are related to "mobilization for goal directed behavior" (1970, p. 538), whereas Venables (1974) proposed that short recovery times are indicative of "openness to the environment" (p. 131). However, subsequent research has raised many questions about the peripheral mechanisms affecting this EDA component (e.g., Bundy & Fitzgerald, 1975); hence the unique informational utility of half recovery time is questionable at the present time (see Fowles, 1986, pp. 84–87). This is not to say that SCR half recovery time is without discriminating power but rather only that its qualitatively different informational properties relative to other EDA components is questioned.

The usual pattern of electrodermal responding is that high SCL, large SCR amplitude, short latency, short rise time, and short recovery time tend to cluster together. However, the correlations among the EDA components generally are not very high, usually less than 0.50 (Lockhart & Lieberman, 1979; Martin & Rust, 1976; Venables & Christie, 1980). The size and consistency of these relationships is compatible with the hypothesis that many of the EDA components may represent partially independent sources of information, although as indicated in the preceding discussion of half recovery time, this is a controversial hypothesis. The one exception to the weak relationships among EDA components is the rather consistently high correlation between SCR rise time and half recovery time. Based on the latter relationship, Venables and Christie (1980) suggest that SCR rise time and half recovery time may be essentially redundant measures, and since recovery time is not always as available as rise time (due to subsequent NS-SCRs), rise time may be the preferred measure.

A problem with quantifying the SCR components occurs when a response is elicited before an immediately preceding response has had time to recover. It is customary to measure the amplitude of each response from its own individual deflection point (Edelberg, 1967; Grings & Lockhart, 1965). However, the amplitude as well as the temporal characteristics of the second response are distorted by being superimposed on the recovery of the first response. For example, the measurable amplitude of the second response will be smaller given its occurrence following the first response. The amount of distortion of the second response is a function of the size of the first response and the time since the first response (Grings & Schell, 1969). Although there is no good solution to the response interference effect, it can be pointed out that response frequency may be the least distorted aspect of the response in this situation.

Another problem with quantifying the EDA components concerns the existence of large variability due to extraneous individual differences. Thus, whether an SCL of 8 μS is considered high, moderate, or low will depend upon that specific subject's range of SCLs. For example, one can see in Figure 10.3 that an SCL of 8 μS would be relatively low for the subject depicted in the upper tracing but would be relatively high for the subject depicted in the lower tracing. Similarly, an ER-SCR of 0.5 μS may be relatively large for one person but relatively small for another. Lykken, Rose, Luther, and Maley (1966) have proposed an interesting method to correct for this individual difference factor. The correction procedure involves computing a range for each individual subject and then expressing the subject's momentary value as a proportion of this range. For example, one may compute a subject's minimum SCL during a rest period and a maximum SCL while the subject blows a balloon to bursting and then express the subject's present SCL as a proportion of her or his individualized range according to the following formula:

$$(SCL - SCL_{min})/(SCL_{max} - SCL_{min})$$

For SCR data, the minimum SCR can be assumed to be zero and the maximum can be estimated by the presentation of some strong or startling stimulus. Each SCR can then be corrected for individual differences in range simply by dividing each SCR by that subject's maximum SCR. The rationale underlying these procedures is that an individual's maximum and minimum SCL and SCR are due mainly to physiological differences unrelated to psychological processes (e.g., thickness of the corneum). It is the variation within these physiological limits that is normally of psychological interest (Lykken & Venables, 1971).

Although the range correction procedure can reduce error variance and increase the power of statistical tests in some data sets, it also can be problematic in others.

For example, range correction would be inappropriate in a situation where two groups being compared had different ranges (Lykken & Venables, 1971). Also, the range correction procedure relies upon adequate and reliable estimates of maximum and minimum values, and estimates of these individual extreme values can be unreliable. For this reason, Ben-Shakhar (1985) has recommended using within-subject standardized scores to adjust for individual differences because this transformation relies upon the mean, a more stable and reliable statistic than the maximum response. As with any transformation procedure, the presently discussed procedures should be used thoughtfully and cautiously.

Another important aspect of ER-SCRs is their decline in amplitude and eventual disappearance with repetition of the eliciting stimulus (ER-SCR habituation). Habituation is a ubiquitous and adaptive phenomenon whereby subjects become less responsive to familiar and nonsignificant stimuli. There are several methods of quantifying habituation of the ER-SCR (Siddle, Stephenson, & Spinks, 1983). One simple method involves counting the number of stimulus repetitions required to reach some predetermined level of habituation (e.g., two or three consecutive trials without measurable ER-SCRs). This "trials-to-habituation" measure is useful and has been widely employed since its use by Sokolov (1963), but it is subject to considerable distortion by the occurrence of a single response. For example, whether an isolated ER-SCR occurs on trial 3 can make the difference between a trials-to-habituation score of 0 (indicative of an atypical nonresponder) and one of 3 (indicative of a typical rate of habituation). To reduce the chances of having a single isolated response contaminate the trials-to-habituation measure, Levinson and Edelberg (1985) argue for a two-trial rather than a three-trial criterion.

Another common measure of habituation is based on the rate of decline of ER-SCR magnitude across trials as assessed by a "trials" main effect or interaction effect within an analysis of variance. This measure, however, does not provide information about habituation in individual subjects and moreover can be distorted by differences in initial levels of responding.

A third measure of habituation is based on the regression of ER-SCR magnitude on the logarithm of trial number (Lader & Wing, 1966; Montagu, 1963). The regression approach provides a slope and an intercept score (the latter reflecting initial response amplitude), which usually are highly correlated with each other. Covariance procedures have been used to remove the dependency of slope on intercept, providing what Montagu (1963) has called an "absolute rate of habituation." However, this technique rests on the assumptions that slope and intercept reflect different underlying processes and that the treatment effects under investigation do not significantly affect the intercepts (Siddle et al., 1983). Use of the slope measure also assumes that subjects respond on a sufficient number of trials to compute a meaningful slope measure, which may not be the case with some types of subjects with mild innocuous stimuli. Nevertheless, to the extent that these assumptions can be justified, the slope measure is often preferable because (1) unlike the analysis-of-variance approach, individual habituation scores can be derived; (2) unlike the trials-to-habituation measure, isolated SCRs have less of a contaminating effect; (3) unlike the trials-to-habituation measure, the slope measure makes fuller use of the magnitude data; and (4) unlike the trials-to-habituation measure, the slope measure can discriminate between subjects who show varying degrees of habituation but who fail to completely stop responding for two or three consecutive trials.

10.3.2   *Paradigms to study EDA components*

Now that the principal EDA components have been identified and defined, we can describe basic experimental paradigms used to study the relationships of these components to psychological states and processes. In this section we identify three general types of paradigms: (1) those that involve the presentation of discrete stimuli, (2) those that involve the presentation of chronic stimuli, (3) those that involve the measurement of individual differences in EDA. In the final section of this chapter we discuss some of the applications and theoretical issues involved in these paradigmatic studies of EDA.

The ER-SCR is elicited by almost any novel, potentially important, discrete stimulus in the environment. One of the most widely used paradigms in psychophysiology involves measuring the elicitation and habituation of various indices of the orienting response, of which the ER-SCR is a reliable and easily measurable component. This paradigm typically consists of the repetitive presentation of a simple discrete innocuous stimulus (commonly a tone) with interstimulus intervals varying between 20 and 60 s. The initial elicitation and then subsequent habituation of the ER-SCR can be measured in this paradigm as a component of the orienting response. The typical finding with this paradigm is that the ER-SCR rapidly declines in amplitude with stimulus repetition and eventually disappears completely. The rate of the decline and disappearance of the ER-SCR varies with such factors as stimulus significance, stimulus intensity, and the length of the interval between stimuli (see review by Siddle et al., 1983). The shape of the response also changes with stimulus repetition as the latency, rise time, and half recovery time become longer (Lockhart & Lieberman, 1979; Martin & Rust, 1976). Moreover, the background tonic SCL generally declines and the frequency of NS-SCRs becomes less. All in all, the picture that emerges is one of a less active and less reactive response system with stimulus repetition.

We turn next to a paradigm that involves the presentation of some type of continuous, chronic stimulus or situation such as that involved in performing an ongoing task. Bohlin (1976), for example, required one group of subjects to perform arithmetic problems and a second group of subjects was threatened with delivery of electric shock for poor performance on the arithmetic task. Both groups then were presented a series of discrete innocuous tones during the task so that the elicitation and habituation of ER-SCRs could be measured. It was found that the ongoing task (and threat) (1) increased SCL, (2) reversed the usual decline over time in SCL, (3) increased the overall frequency of NS-SCRs, (4) increased the frequency and magnitude of ER-SCRs, and (5) retarded the rate of ER-SCR habituation (at least with the trials-to-habituation measure). These results demonstrated the sensitivity of these EDA components to simple but powerful manipulations in the ongoing stimulus situation.

The EDA individual difference paradigm is fundamentally different from the preceding two paradigms. Whereas the other paradigms treat EDA as a dependent variable under stimulus control, the individual difference paradigm treats EDA as an independent variable. That is, EDA is considered to be a relatively stable subject trait related to behavioral and psychological individual differences. Consistent with this view is the fact that EDA components exhibit moderate test–retest stability. The test–retest reliability coefficients generally range between .50 and .70 when measured over a range of a few days to a few months (Bull & Gale, 1973; Lacey &

Lacey, 1958a; Schell, Dawson, & Filion, 1988; Siddle & Heron, 1976). Another line of evidence consistent with the assumptions of the individual difference paradigm is that many of the EDA components appear to have a partial genetic influence (Lykken, Iacono, Haroian, McGue, & Bouchard, 1988).

Individual differences in the rate of NS-SCRs and the rate of ER-SCR habituation have been used to define a trait called electrodermal lability (e.g., Crider & Lunn, 1971; Katkin, 1975; Lacey & Lacey, 1958a). Electrodermal "labiles" are those subjects who show high rates of NS-SCRs and/or slow ER-SCR habituation, whereas electrodermal "stabiles" are those who show few NS-SCRs and/or fast ER-SCR habituation. The behavioral and psychological differences associated with this individual difference are presented in the last section of the chapter.

10.3.3   *Advantages and disadvantages of the use of EDA*

When one is considering use of EDA as an indicator of some psychological state or process of interest, it is well to remember that in the great majority of situations, changes in electrodermal activity do not occur in isolation. Rather, they occur as part of a complex of responses mediated by the ANS.

Experimental operations such as those already described designed to increase the arousal level of the subject (Bohlin, 1976), which have the effect of increasing SCL and/or NS-SCR rate, also would be expected generally to act to increase heart rate level and blood pressure and to decrease finger pulse volume, to mention a few of the more commonly measured ANS responses. (See, e.g., Eason & Dudley, 1970; Engel, 1960; Kahneman, Tursky, Shapiro, & Crider, 1969.) Stimuli that elicit an ER-SCR would also be expected to elicit certain components of heart rate response (e.g., Bohlin & Kjellberg, 1979; Graham & Clifton, 1966) and a peripheral vasoconstriction (Uno & Grings, 1965), and these response components would ordinarily be increased in magnitude by the same operations that would increase ER-SCR magnitude. The response or responses chosen for monitoring by a particular investigator will reflect considerations such as those discussed in the following.

Although it is true that operations that alter EDA also typically alter other ANS response measures, so that the electrodermal response occurs as part of a response complex, it is also true that different components of that response complex may correlate poorly with each other across individuals. Suppose, for instance, that one instructs subjects to pay close attention to a series of tones delivered to one ear and to ignore a second series of tones presented to the other ear. One would expect to find larger ER-SCRs, greater heart rate deceleration, and greater peripheral blood pulse volume responses elicited by the attended than the nonattended tones. However, across subjects the magnitude of the SCR, the heart rate response, and the blood pulse volume response would probably correlate poorly if at all.

The poor intercorrelation across subjects of the different components of the global ANS response pattern reflects in large part what is termed *individual response stereotypy* (Engel, 1960; Lacey & Lacey, 1958b; Wenger, Clemens, Coleman, Cullen, & Engel, 1961; see Stern & Sison, chapter 7). This is, individuals tend (some more strongly than others) to produce the same pattern to relative change across physiological systems, and that pattern differs across individuals. One person, for instance, may tend to show large EDA changes with increased arousal (large relative to other individuals) while showing only moderate heart rate changes and small blood volume changes. Another individual may show the reverse pattern, with large blood volume responses and small EDA changes. Thus, the decision about which particular physiological response one wishes to monitor is an important one, and the investigator may wish to record more than one. We now briefly examine the advantages and disadvantages of EDA as a response system of choice, particularly vis-à-vis the other most often used autonomic response measure, heart rate.

For some researchers, EDA may be the response system of choice because, unlike most ANS responses, it provides a direct and undiluted representation of sympathetic activity. As has been pointed out, the eccrine sweat glands are entirely under the neural control of the sympathetic nervous system. If heart rate is observed to slow, on the other hand, this could be due to decreased sympathetic activation of the heart via the cardiac nerves, increased parasympathetic input via the vagus nerve, or some combination of the two. With heart rate as with most ANS functions (pupil diameter, gastric motility, blood pressure), a change in activity in response to stimuli or situations of psychological significance cannot be unambiguously laid to either sympathetic or parasympathetic activity but may be due to either one or to a combination of both. Thus, the researcher who wishes an unalloyed measure of sympathetic activity may prefer to monitor EDA, whereas the experimenter who wishes a broader picture of both sympathetic and parasympathetic activity may prefer heart rate if constraints of instrumentation will allow only one to be recorded. The advantages to the experimenter of the potential bidirectionality of the heart rate response are discussed elsewhere in this volume (Papillo & Shapiro, chapter 14). Similarly, if for some reason (perhaps the use of medication with side effects on cholinergic or adrenergic systems) one wishes to monitor a response that is predominantly cholinergically mediated below the cerebral level but is also influenced by sympathetic activity, EDA would be the choice.

In addition to the preceding considerations arising from the neuroanatomy of the electrodermal system, EDA has what many researchers view as the advantage of being relatively free compared to heart rate from somatic influences. If the subject is sitting fairly quietly and if marked changes in respiration rate and depth are avoided, there is little moment-to-moment change in EDA due to the respiration cycle or to general muscle tonus. Heart rate, on the other hand, is strongly influenced by both respiration and by striate muscle tension, both tonically and phasically, as heart rate follows the respiration cycle (respiratory sinus arrhythmia) and also phasic changes in muscle tension and activity (e.g., Obrist, 1981, pp. 47–118; Porges, McCabe, & Yongue, 1982). Thus, compared to heart rate, EDA is relatively free of somatic influence. After surveying the data for conditioned emotional response learning in several animal species, Roberts (1974, p. 187) concluded: "The electrodermal and cardiac control systems are organized very differently with respect to neural mechanisms that determine striate muscular activity and motivational or attentional arousal. Unlike heart rate, which appears to be regulated primarily by movement control mechanisms, electrodermal activity appears to be determined mainly by motivational or attentional arousal, or by some other nonsomatic process."

Another advantage of the use of the ER-SCR is that its occurrence is generally quite discriminable. Thus, on a single presentation of a stimulus, one can determine by quick inspection whether or not an SCR has occurred. On the other hand, on an individual stimulus presentation, the presence of a heart rate response may be difficult to distinguish from ongoing changes in heart rate, reflecting changes in muscle tonus or respiratory sinus arrhythmia. For instance, the triphasic deceleratory–acceleratory–deceleratory heart rate response that appears in long interstimulus interval classical conditioning or during a long (8.0-s) reaction time foreperiod (Bohlin & Kjellberg, 1979) is often discriminable only when one averages second-by-second heart rate changes following stimulus presentation over a number of trials, just as in order to discriminate the cortical evoked potential recorded from the scalp from background EEG activity, one must average over a number of stimulus presentations. This may be disadvantageous for the researcher who has a strong interest in activity occurring on a few individual trials, such as those that immediately precede and follow discrete events, such as the delivery of an instruction to the subject or the attainment of a verbalizable insight or formulation of a new hypothesis by the subject.

In addition to being more discriminable on the individual trial, the ER-SCR also has the advantage of being more sensitive than is the heart rate response to paired stimulus paradigms with short interestimulus intervals. For instance, in the electrodermal system, discrimination classical conditioning occurs with very short intervals between the reinforced conditioned stimulus (CS+) and unconditioned stimulus (UCS), although nonreinforced test trials are required to measure the conditioned response uncontaminated by the unconditioned response. A CS+ test trial of 0.5 s duration will elicit a reliably larger ER-SCR than will a nonreinforced CS– of the same duration. The discrimination between the significant CS+ and the nonsignificant CS– by the ER-SCR that follows immediately after CS onset is as great with CS–UCS intervals of 0.5s duration as with intervals of 5.0s duration (Lockhart & Grings, 1964). The very short duration stimulus is sufficient to elicit a fully developed ER-SCR that is responsive to the information content of the stimulus. Heart rate responses, on the other hand, are generally viewed as being anticipatory in nature (anticipating the cognitive or motor demands of present or upcoming stimuli), and the most reliable signs of conditioning occur during the late portions of long CS–UCS intervals.

In addition to decisions made on the basis of neuroanatomical control and basic response characteristics, an investigator may prefer EDA to other response systems because of the nature of the situation in which he or she is assessing subjects. Fowles (1980, 1988) has argued convincingly that heart rate is influenced primarily by activation of a neurophysiological behavioral activation system involved in responding during appetitive reward seeking, to conditioned stimuli associated with reward, and during active avoidance. On the other hand, EDA is influenced primarily by activation of a neurophysiological behavioral inhibition system involved in responding to punishment, passive avoidance, or frustrative nonreward. This latter system is viewed as an anxiety system. Thus, if an investigator is studying the reaction of subjects to a situation or to discrete stimuli that elicit anxiety but in which or to which no active avoidance response can be made, the electrodermal system would be predicted to be the physiological system that would be most responsive.

A final advantage of the use of EDA relative to other response systems lies in the fact that of all forms of ANS activity, individual differences in EDA are most reliably associated with behavioral differences and psychopathological states. The correlates of some of these stable EDA differences between individuals will be discussed in some detail in what follows.

Thus, like any single response system, EDA has distinct advantages and disadvantages as a response system to monitor. The ideal situation, of course, is one in which the researcher can record more than one response measure. When ANS activity is of primary interest, EDA and heart rate are probably the two most common choices, EDA for its neuroanatomical simplicity, trial-by-trial visibility, and utility as a general arousal/attention indicator and heart rate for its potential differentiation of more subtle psychological states of interest to the researcher.

10.4   PSYCHOLOGICAL–SOCIAL CONTEXT

In this section, we review in more detail the EDA results that occur in the three types of paradigms identified earlier: (1) that which involves the presentation of discrete stimuli, (2) that which involves the presentation of chronic stimuli, and (3) that which involves measuring the correlates of EDA individual differences.

10.4.1   *Effects of discrete stimuli*

Ever since the discovery of EDA in the late nineteenth century, attempts have been made to specify the nature of the stimuli that elicit SCRs. As a result of this attempt, we now know that the stimuli to which the SCR is sensitive are wide and varied, that it is sensitive to stimulus novelty, intensity, emotional content, and significance (e.g., Raskin, 1973). It might be argued that because EDA is sensitive to such a wide variety of stimuli, it is not a clearly interpretable measure of any particular psychological process (e.g., Landis, 1930). This view is certainly correct in the sense that it is impossible to identify an isolated SCR as an "anxiety" response, or an "anger" response, or an "attentional" response. However, the psychological meaning of an SCR becomes interpretable by taking into account the stimulus condition or experimental paradigm in which the SCR occurred. The better controlled the experimental paradigm, the more conclusive the interpretation. That is, by having only one aspect of the stimulus change across conditions (e.g., task significance) while eliminating other differences (e.g., stimulus novelty, intensity, etc.), then one can more accurately infer the psychological process mediating the resultant SCR. Thus, the inference of a psychophysiological process requires knowledge of both a well-controlled stimulus situation as well as a carefully measured response. We now turn to some of the experimental paradigms in which EDA is most often measured and has proven to be the most useful.

One such paradigm, which relies on the SCR's sensitivity to stimulus significance, is the physiological detection of deception ("lie detection"). For example, one detection of deception technique, the Guilty Knowledge Test (GKT), involves recording SCRs while presenting subjects with a series of multiple-choice-type questions (Lykken, 1959). For example, a suspect in a burglary case might be asked to answer "no" to each of the alternatives given for a question concerning details about the burglary. For each question, the correct alternative would be intermixed among other plausible alternatives. The theory behind the technique is that the correct answer to each question will be more significant to a guilty subject than will the other alternatives, whereas for the innocent subject all of the alternatives would be of equal significance. Therefore, the guilty subject is expected to respond consistently more to the correct alternatives, whereas the innocent subject is expected to respond randomly (Lykken, 1959). Evidence indicates that in fact guilty subjects can be detected nearly 90 percent of the time and innocent subjects can be correctly classified nearly 100 percent of the time with a properly constructed GKT (Grings & Dawson, 1978, pp. 162–163).

Tranel, Fowles, and Damasio (1985) developed another type of paradigm with which to study the effects of significant facial stimuli on SCRs. In their initial investigations SCRs were recorded from normal college students while being presented a set of slides depicting familiar faces of famous people (e.g., Ronald Reagan, Bob Hope, etc.) and faces of unfamiliar people. A total of 55 slides were presented including 5 initial buffer items, 42 presentations of the nonsignificant stimuli (unfamiliar faces), and 8 intermixed presentations of the significant stimuli (famous faces). Subjects were instructed simply to sit quietly and look at each slide. The results revealed that the average SCR was much larger to slides of significant faces ($\bar{X} = 1.26$ μS) than to the nonsignificant faces ($\bar{X} = 0.19$ μS).

Tranel and Damasio (1985) later employed this paradigm with two prosopagnosic patients. Patients with prosopagnosia lose the ability to recognize faces. One patient had a pervasive syndrome and showed a complete failure to recognize any of the faces of famous people (as well as faces of family members, close friends, or even herself). Despite this syndrome, this patient exhibited more frequent as well as larger SCRs to the significant faces than the nonsignificant faces. Bauer (1984) used a paradigm patterned more closely after the GKT with another prosopagnosic patient and also observed SCR discrimination without verbal discrimination.

Whereas the GKT of Lykken (1959) appears to be quite adequate to detect concealed information (and hence the guilty person) and the paradigm of Tranel et al. (1985) appears adequate to test for recognition of famous faces, one may question whether either paradigm is sufficient to demonstrate the effect of stimulus significance on SCR. It may be argued that both paradigms confounded relative novelty with relative stimulus significance. If guilty subjects dichotomize items into relevant and irrelevant categories in the GKT (Ben-Shakhar, 1977), then the relevant category is presented less often than the irrelevant category, and this relative novelty may contribute to the differential SCRs. With the slides of famous faces, the significant category of stimuli is presented less often than the nonsignificant category, and this difference in relative novelty may have contributed to the differential SCRs. The number of presentations of relevant/significant stimuli should be equal to that of irrelevant/nonsignificant stimuli in order to unambiguously demonstrate the effect of stimulus significance on SCRs. As mentioned earlier in this section, close control over stimulus properties (i.e., novelty, significance) is necessary in order to infer the psychological processes eliciting the SCR.

Another paradigm that highlights the importance of stimulus significance and in which relative stimulus novelty is controlled involves discrimination classical conditioning of SCRs. For example, Dawson and Biferno (1973) employed a discrimination classical conditioning paradigm in which subjects were asked to rate their expectancy of the UCS (a brief electric shock) after each presentation of CS+ and CS−. Tones of 800 and 1,200 Hz were presented equally often and served as the reinforced CS+ and the nonreinforced CS−, counterbalanced across subjects. Thus, for each conditioning trial, the subject's expectancy of shock as well as the SCR was recorded. The results showed that subjects tended to respond equally to the reinforced CS+ and to the nonreinforced CS− until they became aware of the contingency between the conditioned stimuli and the shock. There was no evidence of SCR discrimination conditioning prior to the development of awareness, but once the subject became aware, the CS + became more significant than the CS −, and there was an abrupt increase in the magnitude of the SCRs elicited by the CS +.

The SCR discrimination conditioning data suggest that subjects must be consciously aware of the differential stimulus significance before differential SCRs are elicited, whereas the earlier reviewed findings with prosopagnosic patients suggest that conscious awareness is not necessary for SCR discrimination. This apparent contradiction may possibly be resolved by the hypothesis that conscious awareness is necessary for the initial learning of stimulus significance but not for the later evocation of SCRs to previously learned significant stimuli (Dawson & Schell, 1985). However, we should note that the results obtained from one of the prosopagnosic patients studied by Tranel and Damasio (1985) do not appear consistent with this hypothesis. This patient suffered only from anterograde prosopagnosia in that she failed to recognize only new faces experienced since the onset of her prosopagnosia. When this patient was exposed to slides of faces of persons with whom she had contact only since the onset of her illness (physicians, psychologists, etc.), she was not able to recognize these faces, but she still gave more frequent and larger SCRs to these significant faces compared to nonsignificant faces. Thus, the SCR data of this patient suggest that learning of facial cues may have occurred at some level without apparent conscious awareness. These provocative data call into question the generality of the necessity of awareness, but the results should be replicated with more than one patient and with sensitive measures of awareness.

As mentioned earlier, ER-SCRs elicited by discrete nonaversive stimuli are generally considered to be part of the orienting response (OR) to novel or significant stimuli. We believe that the data reviewed in this section can be interpreted within this theoretical setting. The task of subjects exposed to the GKT is to deceive or conceal knowledge and the correct item is more relevant to this task than are incorrect alternative items. Thus, subjects orient more to the task-significant items than the task-nonsignificant items. Likewise, faces of famous people may be perceived as more significant and attention demanding than the faces of unfamiliar people, and the signal (CS +) of an impending shock is more significant than the signal (CS −) of no shock. Thus, the results observed here are consistent with the notion that the SCR is highly sensitive to stimulus significance, although the reader is reminded of the caveat regarding the confounding of stimulus frequency with stimulus significance in some of these paradigms. Other research that indicates the importance of stimulus significance has been presented by Bernstein and Taylor (1979), who support the hypothesis that the skin conductance OR is due to the interaction of the informativeness of the eliciting stimuli and the potential significance of that information.

There have been several models proposed to account for the elicitation of autonomic ORs such as the SCR (see Siddle et al., 1983, for a review). For example, an interesting information–processing model has been proposed by Öhman (1979). This model distinguishes between automatic preattentive processing and controlled capacity-limited processing. Autonomic orienting is elicited when the preattentive mechanisms call for additional controlled processing. According to this model, there are two conditions under which this call is made. First, the call is made and the OR is elicited when the preattentive mechanisms fail to identify the incoming stimulus because there is no matching representation in short-term memory. Thus, the OR is sensitive to stimulus novelty. Second, the call is made and the OR is elicited when the preattentive mechanisms recognize the stimulus as significant. Thus, the OR represents a switch from automatic to controlled processing based on preliminary preattentive analysis of stimulus novelty and stimulus significance.

In conclusion, in this section we have described some of the experimental paradigms in which EDA is most often measured and has proven to be most useful. Within this description we have emphasized that because EDA is sensitive to a wide variety of stimuli, determining the psychological meaning of any particular SCR is dependent on a well-controlled stimulus situation. In addition we have suggested a theoretical model that can be used to account for the ER-SCRs elicited in the paradigms described.

10.4.2 *Effects of chronic stimuli*

We turn now to an examination of the effects of more chronic, long-lasting stimuli or situations as opposed to the brief, discrete stimuli already reviewed. Chronic stimuli might best be thought of as modulating increases and decreases in tonic arousal. Hence, the most useful electrodermal measures in the context of chronic stimuli are SCL and frequency of NS-SCRs because they can be measured on an ongoing basis over relatively long periods of time.

One type of chronic stimulus situation that will reliably produce increases in electrodermal activity involves the necessity of performing a task. The anticipation and performance of practically any task will increase both SCL and the frequency of NS-SCRs, at least initially. For example, Lacey, Kagan, Lacey, and Moss (1963) recorded palmar SCL and heart rate during rest and during the anticipation and performance of eight different tasks. The tasks ranged from those that required close attention to external stimuli, such as listening to an irregularly fluctuating loud white noise, to those that required close attention to internal information processing and rejection of external stimuli, such as solving mental arithmetic problems. The striking finding emphasized by Lacey et al. (1963) was that heart rate increased in "stimulus rejection" tasks and decreased in "stimulus intake" tasks. However, the impressive finding for present purposes was that SCL increased in each and every one of the task situations. Typically, SCL increased about 1 μS above resting level during anticipation and then increased another 1 or 2 μS during performance of the task. The largest increase in SCL occurred during the white-noise task, which, interestingly, was one of the tasks that produced heart rate slowing.

More recently, Munro, Dawson, Schell, and Sakai (1987) observed that large increases in SCL and NS-SCR frequency were induced by a different task-significant situation. In this case, college student subjects were tested during a 5-min rest period and then during performance of a continuous-performance vigilance task. The task stimuli consisted of a series of digits presented visually at a rapid rate of 1 per s with an exposure duration of 48 ms; the subject's task was to press a button whenever the digit 0 was presented. Both the number of NS-SCRs and SCL increased sharply from the resting levels during this demanding task and then gradually declined as the task continued.

The finding that electrodermal activity is reliably elevated by task stimuli suggests that tonic EDA can be a useful index of a process related to "energy regulation" or "energy mobilization." An attentional/information processing inter-pretation of this finding might be that tasks require an effortful allocation of attentional resources and that this is associated with heightened autonomic activation (Jennings, 1986). A different but not necessarily mutually exclusive explanation would invoke the concepts of stress and affect rather than attention and effortful allocation of resources. According to this view, laboratory tasks are stressors and a reliable physiological response to stressors is increased sympathetic activation, particularly EDA arousal.

Social stimulation constitutes another class of chronic stimuli that generally produce increases in EDA arousal. Social situations are ones in which the concepts of stress and affect are most often invoked. For example, early research related EDA recorded during psychotherapeutic interviews to concepts such as "tension" and "anxiety" on the part of both the patient and therapist (e.g., Boyd & DiMascio, 1954; Dittes, 1957). In one such study, Dittes (1957) measured the frequency of NS-SCRs of a 36-year-old patient during 42 hours of psychotherapy. The results of this study indicated that the frequency of NS-SCRs was inversely related to the judged permissiveness of the therapist, and Dittes concluded that EDA reflects "the anxiety of the patient, or his 'mobilization' against any cue threatening punishment by the therapist" (pp. 157, 303).

Schwartz and Shapiro (1973) reviewed electrodermal findings in several areas of social psychophysiology up to 1970. The areas included (1) attitudes (e.g., statements with which a subject disagrees elicit larger SCRs than ones with which the subject agrees), (2) empathy (e.g., observing another individual experience pain elicits large SCRs, particularly if the observer imagines how he or she would feel in the situation), (3) small groups and social interaction (e.g., the electrodermally activitating effects of failure are reduced in group situations with freedom to initiate attempts at problem solving with other individuals), and (4) cross-cultural and ethnic differences (e.g., electrodermal responses to electric shocks differ among different ethnic groups, presumably because of different attitudes toward pain). Schwartz and Shapiro (1973) point out that understanding the physiological effects of social variables is important not only to social psychophysiologists but to all psychophysiologists. The authors' overall conclusion most relevant to the present chapter was that "electrodermal activity, given its high sensitivity to psychological stimuli and its ease of measurement, appears to be an excellent dependent variable in social psychophysiological research" (p. 410).

A more recent series of studies has related the effects of threatening social stimuli on EDA to the study of relapse among schizophrenic patients. It has been well documented that the emotional attitudes expressed by a family member toward a schizophrenic patient can be a powerful predictor of later relapse of the patient. That is, patients are at increased risk for relapse if their relatives are critical, hostile, or emotionally overinvolved with them at the time of their illness (Brown, Birley, & Wing, 1972; Vaughn & Leff, 1976; Vaughn, Snyder, Jones, Freeman, & Falloon, 1984). The term *expressed emotion* (EE) is used to designate this continuum of affective attitudes ranging from low EE (less critical) to high EE (more critical) on the part of the relative.

It has been hypothesized that heightened autonomic arousal may be a mediating factor between the continued exposure to a high-EE relative and the increased risk of relapse (Turpin, 1983). According to this notion, living with a high-EE family member produces excessive stress and autonomic hyperarousal. Autonomic hyperarousal has been characterized as one of several transient intermediate states that can produce deterioration in the patient's behavior, which then can negatively affect people around the patient. Hence, a vicious cycle can be created whereby the increased arousal causes changes in the patient's behavior, which have an aggravating effect on the social environment, which in turn serves to further increase autonomic arousal. Unless such a cycle is broken (e.g., by removal from that social environment), it can lead to the return of schizophrenic symptoms and a clinical relapse (Dawson, Nuechterlein, & Liberman, 1983; Nuechterlein & Dawson, 1984).

One prediction derived from this model is that patients exposed to high–EE relatives should show heightened sympathetic arousal compared to patients exposed to low–EE relatives. The first study to test this prediction obtained rather clear confirmatory results (Tarrier, Vaughan, Lader, & Leff, 1979). These investigators measured the EDA of remitted patients living in the community whose relatives' level of EE had already been determined by Vaughan and Leff (1976). Patients were tested in their homes for 15 min without the key relative and for 15 min with the key relative present. The frequency of NS-SCR activity of the patients with high-EE relatives and low-EE relatives did not differ when the relative was absent from the testing room, but after the key relative was present, the patients with high-EE relatives exhibited higher rates of NS-SCRs than did patients with low-EE relatives. These results indicate that the presence of high-EE and low-EE relatives have differential effects on EDA, which is consistent with the hypothesis that differential autonomic arousal plays a mediating role in the differential relapse rates of the two patient groups.

In a subsequent investigation, Sturgeon Turpin, Kuipers, Berkowitz, and Leff (1984) employed very similar testing procedures with acutely ill hospitalized patients. In this case, it was found that patients with high-EE relatives exhibited more NS-SCRs than patients with low-EE relatives whether or not the key relative was present in the testing room. Sturgeon et al. speculated that this pattern of results may indicate that patients from high-EE homes undergo a more sustained elevation of sympathetic arousal than patients from low-EE homes when they experience an exacerbation of schizophrenic symptoms. Another possibility is that the patients knew that the high-EE relatives were at the hospital and they were anticipating the relatives joining them. In either event, these studies demonstrate the powerful effects of social stimulation on EDA and the potential importance and applicability of these effects in the area of psychopathology. More complete reviews of these studies and their implications can be found in Dawson, Liberman, and Mintz (in press) and Turpin, Tarrier, and Sturgeon (1988).

10.4.3   *Correlates of EDA individual differences*

In the immediately preceding sections of this chapter we discussed the utility of EDA as a dependent variable reflecting situational levels of arousal/activation or attentiveness/responsiveness to individual stimuli. In this section we consider the correlates of EDA viewed as a stable trait of the individual, as an individual difference variable. Individual differences in EDA are reliably associated with behavioral differences and psychopathological states of some importance, and we examine some of these.

As mentioned earlier, individuals who demonstrate a high frequency of NS-SCR production while at rest or who habituate slowly to repeated presentations of simple stimuli are termed *electrodermal labiles*, whereas individuals who produce few NS-SCRs or who habituate rapidly are termed *electrodermal stabiles* (Lacey & Lacey,

1958a; Mundy-Castle & McKiever, 1953). Also mentioned in the preceding, electrodermal lability is an individual trait that has been found to be relatively reliable over time, and labiles differ from stabiles with respect to a number of psychophysiological variables, including measures of both electrodermal and heart rate responsiveness (e.g. Schell et al., 1988).

Electrodermal lability is a trait that has been of interest in psychological research in part because many investigators have reported that labiles outperform stabiles on tasks that require sustained vigilance. When individuals perform a signal detection task that is sustained over time, deterioration across time in the accurate detection of targets is frequently observed, a phenomenon referred to as vigilance decrement (e.g., Davies & Parasuraman, 1982). Numerous experimenters have reported that when vigilance decrement occurs, it is more pronounced among electrodermal stabiles than among labiles. As time on the task goes by, labiles are apparently better able to keep attention focused on the task and to avoid a decline in performance (Coles & Gale, 1971; Crider & Augenbraun, 1975; Hastrup, 1979; Munro, et al. 1987; Vossel & Rossman, 1984). Munro et al., for instance, reported that with a difficult attentional capacity-demanding detection task, stabiles showed a significant decrement over time in the signal detection measure d', which reflects perceptual sensitivity, whereas labiles did not. Furthermore, the degree of task-induced sympathetic arousal as measured by increases in NS-SCR rate was negatively correlated across subjects with d' decrement.

Researchers investigating these sorts of behavioral differences between electrodermal stabiles and labiles have concluded that lability reflects the ability to allocate information-processing capacity to stimuli that are to be attended (Katkin, 1975; Lacey & Lacey, 1958a; Schell et al., 1988). As Katkin (1975, p. 172) concluded, "electrodermal activity is a personality variable that reflects individual differences in higher central processes involved in attending to and processing information." Viewing electrodermal lability in this way suggests that future research would show that labiles differ from stabiles in a variety of situations that involve information-processing tasks.

In addition to the differences between electrodermal stabiles and labiles within the normal population, reliable abnormalities in lability are associated with psychopathology. Most often reported in severe psychopathology is extreme electrodermal stability in the form of very rapid habituation of the OR or failure to show an OR at all, perhaps because of an association between extreme stability and impaired information processing. The finding of abnormalities in EDA has been most often reported for schizophrenia, and although abnormalities of orienting in other response systems have also been reported in that disorder, EDA is the system most often found to be abnormal (e.g. Bernstein et al., 1982; Dawson & Nuechterlein, 1984; Öhman, 1981).

In a well-known study, Gruzelier and Venables (1972) presented a series of nonsignal tones to a large group of schizophrenic patients and to normal controls. Although all of the normal controls initially responded to the stimuli and then showed habituation of the SCR, the schizophrenic group showed a bimodal distribution at both extremes of habituation. Fifty-four percent of the schizophrenics failed to give even one SCR-OR, whereas 42 percent not only responded but failed to meet the habituation criterion. The former group is referred to as "nonresponders" and the latter group as "responders."

Bernstein et al. (1982) examined a series of 14 related studies in which samples of

American, British, and German schizophrenics and normal controls were studied using a common methodology and response scoring criteria. Their consistent finding was that approximately 50 percent of schizophrenics were nonresponders, compared to only 5–10 percent of controls. A minority of the studies also reported the existence of a responder subgroup of schizophrenics showing slower than normal habituation. The responder–nonresponder distinction is a potentially important one because, like other electrodermal stabiles, nonresponders are more likely to show impaired performance on tasks involving selective attention and vigilance. Furthermore, nonresponders and responders have been reported to show different symptomatology, with responders generally displaying symptoms such as excitement, anxiety, manic behavior, belligerence, and inappropriate mannerisms, whereas nonresponders tend to show symptoms such as emotional withdrawal and conceptual disorganization. Research has indicated that the EDA abnormalities associated with schizophrenia may be trait-like (present during remission) as well as state-like (aggravated during the active stages of the disorder), may be found in those at high risk for schizophrenia as well as those who actually have the disorder, and may have prognostic utility (see Dawson & Nuechterlein, 1984, for a review of these issues).

Abnormalities in EDA have also been associated with depression. Mirkin and Coppen (1980) reported a higher than normal incidence of very rapid habituation, or complete failure to orient, in unmedicated depressives, and numerous investigators have reported abnormalities among depressive inpatients and outpatients in the form of low levels of SCL and/or small ER-SCRs to different classes of stimuli (Dawson, Schell, & Catania, 1977; Iacono et al., 1983; Lader & Noble, 1975; Ward, Doerr, & Storrie, 1983). These EDA abnormalities have both state-like and trait-like characteristics. (It should pointed out that heart rate abnormalities, usually in the form of high heart rate levels, are also generally reported in depression.) Dawson et al. (1977), for instance, reported lower tonic SCL and smaller ER-SCRs to neutral and task-related tones and unpleasant loud noises among unipolar depressed patients than among controls and found that these differences to a large extent continued to exist even after the patients had received a series of electroconvulsive therapy treatments that produced a marked degree of clinical improvement.

Electrodermal activity has also been found to be abnormal in other forms of psychopathology such as psychopathy (Hare, 1975) and severe anxiety disorders (Zahn, 1986). For all these disorders, investigation of the EDA abnormalities that appear as stable individual differences between patients and controls and the relationship of these differences to symptomatology and prognosis may help to shed light on the nature of the disorders themselves.

10.5 SUMMARY AND CONCLUSIONS

Social and behavioral scientists employ EDA widely to investigate a host of situational variables that may affect arousal and/or anxiety, stimulus variables that affect the multifaceted attentional process and stimulus significance, and individual differences that may be related to behavioral differences or psychopathological states. Thus EDA, among the first psychophysiological response systems to be investigated, remains of considerable interest and application today.

The physical and physiological processes that mediate EDA are fairly well understood, and there is general agreement on the optimal recording methods to be used and on quantification procedures. Electrodermal activity can be accurately recorded relatively inexpensively, it is not seriously affected by artifact due to small movements of skeletal musculature, and the SCR can be readily discerned on single trials. All in all, it is a response system that has much to recommend it and will remain an important tool in a wide variety of areas of psychological research.

REFERENCES

Bauer, R. M. (1984). Autonomic recognition of names and faces in prosopagnosia: A neuropsychological application of the guilty knowledge test. *Neuropsychologia, 22,* 457–469.

Ben-Shakhar, G. (1977). A further study of the dichotomization theory of detection of information. *Psychophysiology, 14,* 408–413.

Ben-Shakhar, G. (1985). Standardization within individuals: A simple method to neutralize individual differences in skin conductance. *Psychophysiology, 22,* 292–299.

Bernstein, A., Frith, C., Gruzelier, J., Patterson, T., Straube, E., Venables, P., & Zahn, T. (1982). An analysis of the skin conductance orienting response in samples of American, British, and German schizophrenics. *Biological Psychology, 14,* 155–211.

Bernstein, A. S., & Taylor, K. W. (1979). The interaction of stimulus information with potential stimulus significance in eliciting the skin conductance orienting response. In H. D. Kimmel, E. H. van Olst, & J. F. Orlebeke (Eds.), *The orienting reflex in humans* (pp. 499–519). Hillsdale, NJ: Erlbaum.

Bohlin, G. (1976). Delayed habituation of the electrodermal orienting response as a function of increased level of arousal. *Psychophysiology, 13,* 345–351.

Bohlin, G., & Kjellberg, A. (1979). Orienting activity in two-stimulus paradigms as reflected in heart rate. In H. D. Kimmel, E. H. van Olst, & J. F. Orlebeke (Eds.), *The orienting reflex in humans* (pp. 169–198). Hillsdale, NJ: Erlbaum.

Boyd, R. W., & DiMascio, A. (1954). Social behavior and autonomic physiology (a sociophysiologic study). *Journal of Nervous and Mental Disease, 120,* 207–212.

Brown, G., Birley, J. L. T., & Wing, J. K. (1972). Influence of family life on the course of schizophrenia. *British Journal of Psychiatry, 121,* 241–248.

Bull, R. H. C., & Gale, M. A. (1973). The reliability of and interrelationships between various measures of electrodermal activity. *Journal of Experimental Research in Personality, 6,* 300–306.

Bundy, R. S., & Fitzgerald, H. E. (1975). Stimulus specificity of electrodermal recovery time: An examination and reinterpretation of the evidence. *Psychophysiology, 12,* 406–411.

Coles, M. G. H., & Gale, M. A. (1971). Physiological reactivity as a predictor of performance in a vigilance task. *Psychophysiology, 8,* 594–599.

Crider, A., & Augenbraun, C. (1975). Auditory vigilance correlates of electrodermal response habituation speed. *Psychophysiology, 12,* 36–40.

Crider, A., & Lunn, R. (1971). Electrodermal lability as a personality dimension. *Journal of Experimental Research in Personality,* 145–150.

Darrow, C. W. (1927). Sensory, secretory, and electrical changes in the skin following bodily excitation. *Journal of Experimental Psychology, 10,* 197–226.

Darrow, C. W. (1934). Quantitative records of cutaneous secretory reactions. The significance of skin resistance in the light of its relation to the amount of perspiration. *Journal of General Psychology, 11,* 445–448.

Darrow, C. W. (1937). Neural mechanisms controlling the palmar galvanic skin reflex and palmar sweating. *Archives of Neurology and Psychiatry, 37,* 641–663.

Darrow, C. W. (1964). The rationale for treating the change in galvanic skin response as a change in conductance. *Psychophysiology, 1,* 31–38.

Davies, D. R., & Parasuraman, R. (1982). *The psychology of vigilance.* London: Academic Press.

Dawson, M. E., & Biferno, M. A. (1973). Concurrent measurement of awareness and electrodermal classical conditioning. *Journal of Experimental Psychology, 101,* 55–62.

Dawson, M. E., Liberman, R. P., & Mintz, L. I. (in press). Sociophysiology of expressed emotion in the course of schizophrenia. In P. R. Barachas (Ed.), *Sociophysiology of social relationships.* New York: Oxford Press.

Dawson, M. E., & Nuechterlein, K. H. (1984). Psychophysiological dysfunctions in the developmental course of schizophrenic disorders. *Schizophrenia Bulletin, 10,* 204–232.

Dawson, M. E., Nuechterlein, K. H., & Liberman, R. P. (1983). Relapse in schizophrenic disorders: Possible contributing factors and implications for behavior therapy. In M. Rosenbaum, C. M. Franks, & Y. Jaffe (Eds.), *Perspectives on behavior therapy in the eighties* (pp. 265–286). New York: Springer.

Dawson, M. E., & Schell, A. M. (1985). Information processing and human autonomic classical conditioning. In P. K. Ackles, J. R. Jennings, & M. G. H. Coles (Eds.), *Advances in psychophysiology* (Vol. 1, pp. 89–165). Greenwich, CT: JAI Press.

Dawson, M. E., Schell, A. M. & Catania, J. J. (1977). Autonomic correlates of depression and clinical improvement following electroconvulsive shock therapy. *Psychophysiology, 14,* 569–578.

Dittes, J. E. (1957). Galvanic skin response as a measure of patient's reaction to therapist's permissiveness. *Journal of Abnormal and Social Psychology, 55,* 295–303.

Eason, R., & Dudley, L. (1970). Physiological and behavioral indicants of activation. *Psychophysiology, 7,* 223–232.

Edelberg, R. (1967). Electrical properties of the skin. In C. C. Brown (Ed.), *Methods in psychophysiology* (pp. 1–53). Baltimore: Williams & Wilkins.

Edelberg, R. (1970). The information content of the recovery limb of the electrodermal response. *Psychophysiology, 6,* 527–529.

Edelberg, R. (1972a). Electrical activity of the skin: Its measurement and uses in psychophysiology. In N. S. Greenfield & R. A. Sternbach (Eds.), *Handbook of psychophysiology* (pp. 367–418). New York: Holt.

Edelberg, R. (1972b). Electrodermal recovery rate, goal-orientation, and aversion. *Psychophysiology, 9,* 512–520.

Edelberg, R. (1973). Mechanisms of electrodermal adaptations for locomotion, manipulation, or defense. *Progress in Physiological Psychology, 5,* 155–209.

Engel, B. T. (1960). Stimulus-response and individual-response specificity. *Archives of General Psychiatry, 2,* 305–313.

Féré, C. (1888). Note on changes in electrical resistance under the effect of sensory stimulation and emotion. *Comptes Rendus des Seances de la Societe de Biologie (Series 9), 5,* 217–219.

Ferguson, G. A. (1976). *Statistical analysis in psychology and education.* New York: McGraw-Hill.

Fowles, D. C. (1974). Mechanisms of electrodermal activity. In R. F. Thompson & M. M. Patterson (Eds.), *Methods in physiological psychology. Part C. Receptor and effector processes,* (pp. 231–271). New York: Academic Press.

Fowles, D. C. (1980). The three arousal model: Implications for Gray's two-factor theory for heart rate, electrodermal activity, and psychopathology. *Psychophysiology, 17,* 87–104.

Fowles, D. C. (1986). The eccrine system and electrodermal activity. In M. G. H. Coles, E. Donchin, & S. W. Porges (Eds.), *Psychophysiology: Systems, processes, and applications* (pp. 51–96). New York: Guilford Press.

Fowles, D. C. (1988). Psychophysiology and psychopathology: A motivational approach. *Psychophysiology, 25,* 373–391.

Fowles, D., Christie, M. J., Edelberg, R., Grings, W. W., Lykken, D. T., & Venables, P. H. (1981). Publication recommendations for electrodermal measurements. *Psychophysiology, 18,* 232–239.

Graham, F. K., & Clifton, R. K. (1966). Heart rate change as a component of the orienting response. *Psychological Bulletin, 65,* 305–320.

Grings, W. W. (1974). Recording of electrodermal phenomena. In R. F. Thompson & M. M. Patterson (Eds.), *Bioelectric recording technique. Part C: Receptor and effector processes* (pp. 273–296). New York: Academic Press.

Grings, W. W., & Dawson, M. E. (1978). *Emotions and bodily responses: A psychophysiological approach.* New York: Academic Press.

Grings, W. W., & Lockhart, R. A. (1965). Problems of magnitude measurement with multiple GSRs. *Psychological Reports, 17,* 979–982.

Grings, W. W., & Schell, A. M. (1969). Magnitude of electrodermal response to a standard stimulus as a function of intensity and proximity of a prior stimulus. *Journal of Comparative and Physiological Psychology, 67,* 77–82.

Gruzelier, J. H., & Venables, P. H. (1972). Skin conductance orienting activity in a heterogeneous sample of schizophrenics: Possible evidence of limbic dysfunction. *Journal of Nervous and Mental Disease, 155,* 277–287.

Hare, R. D. (1975). Psychophysiological studies of psychopathy. In D. C. Fowles (Eds.), *Clinical applications of psychophysiology* (pp. 77–105). New York: Columbia University Press.

Hassett, J. (1978). *A primer of psychophysiology.* San Francisco: Freeman.

Hastrup, J. L. (1979). Effects of electrodermal lability and introversion on vigilance decrement. *Psychophysiology, 16,* 302–310.

Humphreys, L. G. (1943). Measures of strength of conditioned eyelid responses. *Journal of General Psychology, 29,* 101–111.

Iacono, W. G., Lykken, D. T., Peloquin, L. T., Lumry, A. E., Valentine, R. H., & Tuoson, V. B. (1983). Electrodermal activity in euthymic unipolar and bipolar affective disorders. *Archives of General Psychiatry, 40,* 557–565.

Jakubovic, H. R., & Ackerman, A. B. (1985). Structure and function of the skin, Section I: Development, morphology, and physiology. In S. L. Moschella & H. J. Hurley (Eds.), *Dermatology* (Vol. 1, pp. 1–74). Philadelphia: Saunders.

Jennings, J. R. (1986). Bodily changes during attending. In M. G. H. Coles, E. Donchin, & S. W. Porges (Eds.), *Psychophysiology: Systems, processes, and applications* (pp. 268–289). New York: Guilford Press.

Kahneman, D., Tursky, B., Shapiro, D., & Crider, A. (1969). Pupillary, heart rate, and skin resistance changes during a mental task. *Journal of Experimental Psychology, 79,* 164–167.

Katkin, E. S. (1975). Electrodermal lability: A psychophysiological analysis of individual differences in response to stress. In I. G. Sarason & C. D. Spielberger (Eds.), *Stress and anxiety* (Vol. 2, pp. 141–176). Washington, DC: Aldine.

Lacey, J. I., & Lacey, B. C. (1958a). The relationship of resting autonomic activity to motor impulsivity. *Research Publications of the Association for Nervous and Mental Diseases, 36,* 144–209.

Lacey, J. I., & Lacey, B. C. (1958b). Verification and extension of the principle of autonomic response-stereotypy. *American Journal of Psychology, 71,* 50–73.

Lacey, J. I., Kagan, J., Lacey, B. C., & Moss, H. A. (1963). The visceral level: Situational determinants and behavioral correlates of autonomic response patterns. In P. H. Knapp (Ed.), *Expression of the emotions in man* (pp. 161–196). New York: International Universities Press.

Lader, M., & Noble, P. (1975). The affective disorders. In P. H. Venables & M. J. Christie (Eds.), *Research in psychophysiology* (pp. 258–281). New York: Wiley.

Lader, M. H., & Wing, L. (1966). *Psychological measures, sedative drugs, and morbid anxiety.* London: Oxford University Press.

Landis, C. (1930). Psychology of the psychogalvanic reflex. *Psychological Review, 37,* 381–398.

Levinson, D. F., & Edelberg, R. (1985). Scoring criteria for response latency and habituation in electrodermal research: A critique. *Psychophysiology, 22,* 417–426.

Levinson, D. F., Edelberg, R., & Bridger, W. H. (1984). The orienting response in schizophrenia: Proposed resolution of a controversy. *Biological Psychiatry, 19,* 489–507.

Lockhart, R. A., & Grings, W. W. (1964). Interstimulus interval effects in GSR discrimination conditioning. *Journal of Experimental Psychology, 67,* 209–214.

Lockhart, R. A., & Lieberman, W. (1979). Information content of the electrodermal orienting response. In H. D. Kimmel, E. H. van Olst, & J. F. Orlebeke (Eds.), *The orienting reflex in humans* (pp. 685–700). Hillsdale, NJ: Erlbaum.

Lykken, D. T. (1959). The GSR in the detection of guilt. *Journal of Applied Psychology, 43,* 383–388.

Lykken, D. T., Iacono, W. G., Haroian, K., McGue, M., & Bouchard, T. J. (1988). Habituation of the skin conductance response to strong stimuli: A twin study. *Psychophysiology, 25,* 4–15.

Lykken, D. T., Rose, R. J., Luther, B., & Maley, M. (1966). Correcting psychophysiological measures for individual differences in range. *Psychological Bulletin, 66,* 481–484.

Lykken, D. T., & Venables, P. H. (1971). Direct measurement of skin conductance: A proposal for standardization. *Psychophysiology, 8,* 656–672.

Martin, I., & Rust, J. (1976). Habituation and structure of the electrodermal system. *Psychophysiology, 13,* 554–562.

Mirkin, A. M., & Coppen, A. (1980). Electrodermal activity in depression: Clinical and biochemical correlates. *British Journal of Psychiatry, 137,* 93–97.

Montagu, J. D. (1963). Habituation of the psycho-galvanic reflex during serial tests. *Journal of Psychosomatic Research, 7,* 199–214.

Mundy-Castle, A. C., & McKiever, B. L. (1953). The psychophysiological significance of the galvanic skin response. *Journal of Experimental Psychology, 46,* 15–24.

Munro, L. L. Dawson, M. E., Schell, A. M., & Sakai, L. M. (1987). Electrodermal lability and rapid performance decrement in a degraded stimulus continuous performance task. *Journal of Psychophysiology, 1,* 249–257.

Neumann, E., & Blanton, R. (1970). The early history of electrodermal research. *Psychophysiology, 6,* 453–475.

Nuechterlein, K. H., & Dawson, M. E. (1984). A heuristic vulnerability/stress model of schizophrenic episodes. *Schizophrenia Bulletin, 10,* 300–312.

Obrist, P. A. (1981). *Cardiovascular psychophysiology: A perspective* (pp. 47–118). New York: Plenum Press.

Öhman, A. (1979). The orienting response, attention and learning: An information processing perspective. In H. D. Kimmel, E. H. van Olst, & J. F. Orlebeke (Eds.), *The orienting reflex in humans* (pp. 443–471). Hillsdale, NJ: Erlbaum.

Öhman, A. (1981). Electrodermal activity and vulnerability to schizophrenia: A review. *Biological Psychology, 12,* 87–145.

Porges, S. W., & Coles, M. G. H. (Eds.). (1976). *Psychophysiology.* Stroudsberg, PA: Dowden, Hutchinson & Ross.

Porges, S. W., McCabe, P. M., Yongue, B. G. (1982). Respiratory–heart rate interactions: Psychophysiological implications for pathophysiology and behavior. In J. T. Cacioppo & R. E. Petty (Eds.), *Perspectives in cardiovascular psychophysiology* (pp. 223–264). New York: Guilford Press.

Prokasy, W. F., & Kumpfer, K. L. (1973). Classical conditioning. In W. F. Prokasy & D. C. Raskin (Eds.), *Electrodermal activity in psychological research* (pp. 157–202). New York: Academic Press.

Prokasy, W. F., & Raskin, D. C. (Eds.). (1973). *Electrodermal activity in psychological research.* New York: Academic Press.

Raskin, D. C. (1973). Attention and arousal. In W. F. Prokasy & D. C. Raskin (Eds.), *Electrodermal activity in psychological research* (pp. 125–155). New York: Academic Press.

Roberts, L. E. (1974). Comparative psychophysiology of the electrodermal and cardiac control systems. In P. A. Obrist, A. H. Black, J. Brener, L. V. Dicara (Eds.), *Cardiovascular psychophysiology: Current issues in response mechanisms, biofeedback, and methodology* (pp. 163–189). Chicago: Aldine.

Robertshaw, D. (1983). Apocrine sweat glands. In L. A. Goldsmith (Ed.), *Biochemistry and physiology of the skin* (pp. 642–653). New York: Oxford University Press.

Schell, A. M., Dawson, M. E., & Filion, D. L. (1988). Psychophysiological correlates of electrodermal lability. *Psychophysiology, 25,* 619–632.

Schwartz, G. E., & Shapiro, D. (1973). Social psychophysiology. In W. F. Prokasy & D. C. Raskin (Eds.), *Electrodermal activity in psychological research* (pp. 377–416). New York: Academic Press.

Shields, S. A., MacDowell, K. A., Fairchild, S. B., & Campbell, M. L. (1987). Is mediation of sweating cholernergic, adrenergic, or both? A comment on the literature. *Psychophysiology, 24,* 312–319.

Siddle, D. A. T., & Heron, P. A. (1976). Reliability of electrodermal habituation measures under two conditions of stimulus intensity. *Journal of Research in Personality, 10,* 195–200.

Siddle, D. A. T., Stephenson, D., & Spinks, J. A. (1983). Elicitation and habituation of the orienting response. In D. Siddle (Ed.), *Orienting and habituation: Perspectives in human research* (pp. 109–182). Chichester: Wiley.

Sokolov, E. N. (1963). *Perception and the conditioned reflex.* New York: Macmillan.

Sturgeon, D., Turpin, G., Kuipers, L., Berkowitz, R., & Leff, J. (1984). Psychophysiological responses of schizophrenic patients to high and low expressed emotion relatives: A follow-up study. *British Journal of Psychiatry, 145,* 62–69.

Tarchanoff, J. (1890). Galvanic phenomena in the human skin during stimulation of the sensory organs and during various forms of mental activity. *Pflugers Archive für die Gesamte Physiologie des Menschen und der Tiere, 46,* 46–55.

Tarrier, N., Vaughn, C., Lader, M. H., & Leff, J. P. (1979). Bodily reactions to people and events in schizophrenics. *Archives of General Psychiatry, 36,* 311–315.

Tranel, D., & Damasio, A. R. (1985). Knowledge without awareness: An autonomic index of facial recognition by prosopagnosics. *Science, 228,* 1453–1454.

Tranel, D., Fowles, D. C., & Damasio, A. R. (1985). Electrodermal discrimination of familiar and unfamiliar faces: A methodology. *Psychophysiology, 22*, 403–408.

Turpin, G. (1983). Psychophysiology, psychopathology, and the social environment. In A. Gale & J. A. Edwards (Eds.), *Physiological correlates of human behavior* (pp. 265–280). New York: Academic Press.

Turpin, G., Tarrier, N., & Sturgeon, D. (1988). Social psychophysiology and the study of biopsychosocial models of schizophrenia. In H. Wagner (Ed.), *Social psychophysiology* (pp. 251–272). Chichester: Wiley.

Uno, T., & Grings, W. W. (1965). Autonomic components of orienting behavior. *Psychophysiology, 1*, 311–329.

Vaughn, C., & Leff, J. P. (1976). The influence of family and social factors on the course of psychiatric illness. *British Journal of Psychiatry, 129*, 125–137.

Vaughn, C. E., Synder, K. S., Jones, S., Freeman, W. B., & Falloon, I. R. H. (1984). Family factors in schizophrenic relapse: A California replication of the British research on expressed emotion. *Archives of General Psychiatry, 41*, 1169–1177.

Venables, P. H. (1974). The recovery limb of the skin conductance response in "high risk" research. In S. A. Mednick, F. Schulsinger, J. Higgins, & B. Bell (Eds.), *Genetics, environment and psychopathology* (pp. 117–133). Amsterdam: North-Holland.

Venables, P. H., & Christie, M. J. (1973). Mechanisms, instrumentation, recording techniques, and quantification of responses. In W. F. Prokasy & D. C. Raskin (Eds.), *Electrodermal activity in psychological research* (pp. 1–124). New York: Academic Press.

Venables, P. H., & Christie, M. J. (1980). Electrodermal activity. In I. Martin and P. H. Venables (Eds.), *Techniques in psychophysiology* (pp. 3–67). Chichester: Wiley.

Vigouroux, R. (1879). Sur le rôle de la résistance électrique des tissues dans l'électro-diagnostic. *Comptes Rendus Société de Biologie (Series 6), 31*, 336–339.

Vigouroux, R. (1888). The electrical resistance considered as a clinical sign. *Progrès Médicale, 3*, 87–89.

Vossel, G., & Rossman, R. (1984). Electrodermal habituation speed and visual monitoring performance. *Psychophysiology, 21*, 97–100.

Wallin, B. G. (1981). Sympathetic nerve activity underlying electrodermal and cardiovascular reactions in man. *Psychophysiology, 18*, 470–476.

Ward, N. G., Doerr, H. O., & Storrie, M. C. (1983). Skin conductance: A potentially sensitive test for depression. *Psychiatry Research, 10*, 295–302.

Wenger, M. A., Clemens, T. L., Coleman, M. A., Cullen, T. D., & Engel, B. T. (1961). Autonomic response specificity. *Psychosomatic Medicine, 23*, 185–193.

Woodworth, R. S., & Schlosberg, H. (1954). *Experimental psychology* (rev ed.). New York: Holt.

Zahn, T. P. (1986). Psychophysiological approaches to psychopathology. In M. G. H. Coles, E. Donchin, & S. W. Porges (Eds.), *Psychophysiology: Systems, processes, and applications* (pp. 508–610). New York: Guilford Press.

11 *The skeletomotor system*

JOHN T. CACIOPPO, LOUIS G. TASSINARY, AND
ALAN J. FRIDLUND

> The principal function of the nervous system is the coordinated innervation of the musculature. Its fundamental anatomical plan and working principles are understandable only on these terms.   (Sperry, 1952, p. 298)

> Certain complex actions are of direct or indirect service under certain states of the mind, in order to relieve or gratify certain sensations, desires, etc.; and *whenever the same state of mind is induced, however feebly, there is a tendency through the force of habit and association for the same movements to be performed*, though they may not be of the least use.   (Darwin, 1873/1872, p. 28, italics added)

> There has been a marked hesitation in thinking of the motor system as having anything significant to contribute to higher mental processes....The violinist Itzhak Perlman, in trying to play a difficult note raises his eyebrows (if it is a high note) and keeps them raised until the note has been played. His face and body perform a rich program of varied movements. Why, again? With few exceptions (Piaget, 1954), it is generally believed that these motions are secondary and ancillary. But suppose that a good part of musical memory is in fact lodged in these peculiar movements. Suppose that they are significant.   (Zajonc & Markus, 1984, pp. 81–84)

11.1 INTRODUCTION

The skeletomotor system is the final common pathway through which humans interact with and modify their environment. The specificity and sophistication of the skeletomuscular system enable the vast repertoires of adaptive reflexes and skilled behaviors associated with living organisms (cf. Smith and Kier, 1989). The electrophysiological signals emanating from the muscular system have been of interest for over four centuries due to the complexity of their organization and dynamics; their clinical applications; and their value as indices of and possible contributors to processes such as cognition, motivation, and emotion.

In this chapter, we provide an introduction to psychophysiological research on the skeletomotor system. We begin by reviewing the history of this research and by articulating some of the major issues, limitations, and advantages of surface electromyography (EMG). We then review briefly the physiological basis of the EMG, and we summarize and update the recent guidelines for surface EMG recording in humans by Fridlund and Cacioppo (1986). We continue with a discussion of the social context for EMG recording and of psychophysiological principles, paradigms, and applications that have emerged from research on the skeletomotor system. Due to the anatomy and electrophysiology of the skeletomotor system, many of the topics and issues addressed in this chapter are of general importance in psychophysiology.

325

Finally, a major theme in this chapter is that technical competence in recording EMG activity is necessary but not sufficient for securing scientifically meaningful data. This is because analyzing what underlies any muscular act is complex. Physiologically, similar limb displacements or feature distortions are often achieved by distinctly different muscular actions (e.g., Gans & Gorniak, 1980); control over these actions can be achieved peripherally through reflex arcs or centrally through the extrapyramidal or pyramidal mediation (e.g., Henneman, 1980a–c). At the behavioral level, muscular acts do not always occur as intended (e.g., as when one performs clumsily), are sometimes nonobvious (e.g., as when one "hides feelings" or inhibits an action), are often misleading as to goals (e.g., as when one deceives), and may not always be in the service of a single psychological endpoint (e.g., as when one lowers the brows in sadness vs. to communicate a point). For EMG signals to be of theoretical significance, therefore, one must consider the physiological, social, and inferential contexts in which these signals are acquired. Hence, in this chapter we address all three of these aspects of surface electromyography. Additional information on electromyography can be found in Basmajian and DeLuca (1985), Loeb and Gans (1986), Fridlund and Cacioppo (1986), Goldstein (1972), Strong (1970), and Lippold (1967).

11.2   HISTORICAL BACKGROUND

At least two distinct themes in the development of electromyography in psychophysiology can be identified. The first is the history of the physiology of the muscles, which derives from the writings of the early Greek philosophers and physicians, and of the field of neurophysiology, which can be traced to Francesco Redi's (1925/1671) deduction that the shock of the electric ray fish (the *Torpedo torpedo*) emanated from specialized muscle tissue (Wu, 1984). Redi's work provided early evidence that the muscles were a source of electricity (Basmajian & DeLuca, 1985). Within four decades, William Croone (1633–1684), through a bequest in his will, founded the revered Croonian lecture of the Royal Society on the physiology of "muscular motion." These annual lectures have been delivered each year for over 250 years; no other field of physiology has an older lectureship devoted to its advancement (Fulton, 1926).

The second theme relates to the theory guiding much of the psychophysiological research using EMG, which owes a debt to the work of such figures as Duchenne (1959/1867), Spencer (1855), Darwin (1873/1872), and James (1884, 1890), all of whom emphasized relatively subtle patterns of muscular actions as a way of characterizing and understanding organismic–environmental transactions more generally.

11.2.1   *The history of muscle physiology*

The history of muscle physiology can be broken into four partially overlapping phases (Fulton, 1926): (1) early history, fourth century B.C. to late 1700s; (2) electrophysiology, late 1700s to present; (3) thermodynamics and chemistry of contraction, mid-1800s to present; and (4) neural control of contraction, late 1800s to present.[1]

11.2.1.1   *Early history*

The first period was characterized by both experimental and theoretical investigations into the causes of animal movement. In his books *De Motu Animalium* and *De*

Incessu Animalium, Aristotle (384–322 B.C.) provided clear descriptions of coordinated motor acts (e.g., locomotion and the importance of the mechanism of flexion). Claudius Galen (131–201 A.D.), along with his many other discoveries in experimental physiology (see Cacioppo & Tassinary, chapter 1), may have been the first to observe that a muscle is still capable of contracting even after surgical removal from the body. Galen also was the first to note correctly that muscles can only contract or relax.

11.2.1.2 *Electrophysiology*

Francesco Redi (1925/1671) and his pupil Stephano Lorenzini (1678) were the first to dissect the torpedo ray and to conclude that the electric organ was a specialized muscle tissue (Wu, 1984). Giovanni Borelli (1680) proposed that the current emanating from this specialized muscle resulted from rapid contractions that produced numerous sharp blows and a numbing of anything touching it. It was not until 1762 that Pieter van Musschenbroek, the inventor of the Leyden jar (an early device used for storing electrostatic charge), noted that the pain incurred upon touching a charged Leyden jar and an electric eel were similar and suggested that the pain from the muscle contractions of the eel was also electrical. Contrary to the then prevalent theory that the torpedo's shock was mechanical in nature, Edward Bancroft (1769, as cited in Wu, 1984) and John Walsh (1773) conducted studies demonstrating that the eel and torpedo's shock could be transmitted through liquids. The notion that muscle contraction was electrical in nature continued to be doubted, however, because muscle contraction was not associated with the sparks that were commonly observed in studies of airborne electrostatic charge. Walsh, in 1776, was finally able to demonstrate that the current from an electric eel could produce a spark:

The strongest shocks of the gymnotus will pass a very short interruption in the circuit…. When the interruption is formed by the incision made by a pen-knife on a slip of tin-foil that is pasted on glass, and that slip is put into the circuit, the shock in passing through the interruption, will shew a small but vivid spark, plainly distinguishable in a dark room. (Cavallo, 1786, pp. 309–311)

Direct evidence for a relationship between muscle contraction and electricity was not obtained until the late eighteenth century when Luigi and Lucia Galvani (and, later, their nephew, Aldini) conducted a series of studies on muscular contractions evoked by the discharge of static electricity (Galvani, 1953/1791). The Galvanis also reported that the muscles of a frog's legs were depolarized merely by touching them with metals rods, and he noted that the intensity of the contraction depended on the type of metal used (Foley, 1954). Galvani interpreted these observations as meaning electricity was stored in the muscles. Alessandro Volta initially endorsed Galvani's hypothesis. However, upon replication and careful observations using a sensitive condensing electroscope he had invented earlier, Volta (1792/1816) argued that the muscle contractions did not result from current arising within the organism but rather from electrical current generated because dissimilar metals touched the muscle preparation. Although Volta was correct in asserting that electric current can arise from the contact of dissimilar metals, so too was Galvani's hypothesis that living cells produce electricity. Galvani (1952/1794) repeated his experiments, but to stimulate the muscles he used nerves from a severed spinal cord rather than a metal arc. He again found that the muscles contracted when brought into contact with the severed nerve.[2] Alexander von Humboldt (1797) subsequently replicated Galvani's findings using a large variety of animals, but according to Fulton (1926, p. 38), the notoriety accorded Volta for his many inventions minimized the impact of these observations for almost 40 years.[3]

It was not until the early-nineteenth century that the galvanometer, a sensitive instrument for measuring electric currents, was invented. In 1833, Carlo Matteucci used a galvanometer to demonstrate an electrical potential between an excised frog's nerve and its damaged muscle. In 1841, the renowned physiologist Johannes Müller (1801–1858) handed Matteucci's recent publication to one of his students, and seven years later the student published the results of an extensive series of investigations on the electrical basis of muscular contraction (Du Bois-Reymond, 1849). Du Bois-Reymond provided the first evidence of electrical activity in human muscles during voluntary contraction. Du Bois-Reymond's classic experiment involved placing a blotting cloth on each of the hands or forearms and immersing them in separate vats of saline solution. Each of these "electrodes" was attached to a galvanometer. Du Bois-Reymond observed minute deflections of the galvanometer when the muscles in the arms and hands were flexed. He further reasoned that the impedance (nonconductive nature) of the skin made the small voltage changes emanating from the muscles especially difficult to detect. To reduce this impedance, he created a blister on each forearm, removed the blistered skin, and placed the electrodes over these raw regions. Du Bois-Reymond found that contracting the arms and hands now resulted in much larger deflections in the galvanometer.

11.2.1.3 Thermodynamics and chemistry

The study of the thermodynamics of muscle contraction owes a debt to another of Müller's students, Hermann Ludwig Ferdinand von Helmholtz (1821–1894). Fueled by the desire to abolish the notion of vital forces underlying muscular actions, von Helmholtz began an investigation into the chemical transformations occurring in frog muscle during contraction. Based on the recently proposed Law of Conservation of Energy (i.e., the First Law of Thermodynamics), von Helmholtz reasoned that the heat of combustion combined with the transformation of food material should produce a quantity of heat measurable at the muscle surface during contraction. By stimulating an isolated muscle through its nerve and employing a sensitive thermocouple, von Helmholtz was able to demonstrate a rise in temperature during contraction.

Von Helmholtz's demonstration not only provided the experimental basis for his classic paper on the conservation of energy, but also it proved instrumental in focusing subsequent investigations on the central problem of understanding the physiochemical processes involved in converting neural energy to mechanical work. A historical account of our understanding of the physical processes involved in muscle contraction can be found in Needham (1971).

11.2.1.4 Neural control

Based on experimental observations using electrical stimulation, muscle physiologists since the time of Galvani attributed graded muscular responses to graded variations in the intensity of the stimulation. Until late in the nineteenth century, many erroneously inferred from this high correlation between the intensity of exogenous electrical stimulation and the intensity of contraction that the *actual size* of the neural impulses was proportional to the stimulus intensity.

Experimental work at the turn of the century by Bowditch (1871), Gotch (1902), Lucas (1909), and others challenged this belief, strongly suggesting that graded muscular responses resulted from the firing of individual contractile units rather than from variation in the size of the nerve impulse. Direct evidence for the "all-or-none" character of the response of muscle fibers was not obtained, however, until the work of Pratt and his colleagues in the early 1900s (Pratt, 1917; Pratt & Eisenberger, 1919). They provided graded electrical stimulation to individual muscle fibers either individually or in small groups while simultaneously photographing the spatial displacement of mercury droplets sprinkled over the muscle surface. They directly observed through a microscope that additional fibers contracted coincident with each quantal step in the displacement of a mercury droplet.

11.2.2 Skeletomotor activation and patterning

Detecting myoelectric signals using surface electrodes remained difficult throughout the nineteenth and early twentieth centuries. Electrically stimulating a muscle cutaneously was considerably simpler, however, and gained wide attention. Perhaps best known for this work was Guillaume Duchenne, who used this technique to investigate the dynamics and function of intact skeletal muscles (Duchenne, 1959/1867). At this point, the two lines of history mentioned at the outset of this section dovetail, as Darwin (1873/1872) corresponded with Duchenne in an effort to test his observations about facial expressions and bodily gestures.

Darwin's (1873/1872) interest in muscular action grew from his belief that phylogenesis was continuous and that behaviors as well as biological structures were in part inherited. He focused on the expression of emotions in man and animals to illustrate the latter. Darwin suggested that expressive movements stemmed primarily from the inheritance of acquired habit, secondarily through what he termed antithesis, and thirdly through the adventitious wiring of the nervous system. Darwin's (1873/1872) mechanism of inheritance was primarily Lamarckian:

That some physical change is produced in the nerve-cells or nerves which are habitually used can hardly be doubted, for otherwise it is impossible to understand how the tendency to certain acquired movements is inherited. (p. 29)

This was not the only mechanism of origin of expressions and behaviors, however, as the processes of variation and natural selection were also embraced:

Nor must we overlook the part which variation and natural selection may have played; for the males which succeeded in making themselves appear the most terrible to their rivals, or to their other enemies, if not of overwhelming power, will on an average have left more offspring to inherit their characteristic qualities, whatever these may be and however first acquired, than have other males. (p. 104)

Although Darwin's (1873/1872) observations were limited to overt actions, he suggested that "whenever the same state of mind is induced, however feebly, there is a tendency through the force of habit and association for the same movements to be performed, though they may not be of the least use" (p. 28). This suggestion presaged contemporary studies of the patterns of muscle contractions and facial actions that are undetectable to the naked eye (see Cacioppo, Martzke, Petty, & Tassinary, 1988).

The somatic components of William James's (1884, 1890) theory of emotions, James's (1890) ideomotor theory, and the various motor theories of thinking prevalent at the turn of the century (cf. McGuigan, 1978) further fueled interest in objective measures of subtle or fleeting muscle contractions. Among the more creative procedures used to magnify tiny muscular contractions was the placement of a flattened wine glass on the tongue to serve as a sensor during thought and of mechanical extensions from the wine glass to amplify the movements of the tongue (see McGuigan, 1979). However, accurate, reliable, and sensitive noninvasive recordings awaited the development of metal surface electrodes, vacuum tube amplifiers, and the cathode-ray oscilloscope early this century and the subsequent pioneering work of Edmund Jacobson (1925, 1927, 1930a–d, 1931a–c, 1932) on electrical measurements of muscle unit action potentials during imagery.

Jacobson's general approach has much to offer contemporary investigators. Briefly, he trained subjects in progressive relaxation, thereby obtaining very low basal levels of muscle tonus, and then ran subjects through a series of mental tasks. Clicks of a telegraph key were presented to mark the onset and offset of each task. Subjects were instructed to engage in a particular "mental activity" following the first click and to relax any muscular tensions present following the second. Tasks included "imagine throwing a ball," "imagine counting," "recall a poem," and "imagine the Eiffel Tower in Paris." Jacobson also employed a control procedure of instructing his subjects on some trials that "upon hearing the first signal do not bother to think." The results of these studies indicated that (1) EMG responses were evoked by these tasks, (2) these responses were minute and highly localized, and (3) these localized responses often occurred in the part of the body that one would use had the task called for an overt response (e.g., see Jacobson, 1932). This work was criticized primarily for not definitively achieving mentally quiescent comparison periods (e.g., Humphrey, 1951; Max, 1937), but successful replications of some of Jacobson's early work using different comparison tasks have been reported (McGuigan, 1978, chapters 6 and 7).

11.2.3   Issues in EMG research

Subsequent research using surface EMG has extended these early observations, documenting patterns of covert skeletomotor activity that differentiate both within and between emotional and cognitive processes (e.g., see reviews by Cacioppo & Petty, 1981a; Cacioppo, Losch, Tassinary, & Petty, 1986; Fridlund, 1988; Fridlund & Izard, 1983; McGuigan, 1978) as well as between normal and clinical populations (e.g., van Boxtel, Goudswaard, & Janssen, 1983; Malmo, 1975; Schwartz, Fair, Salt, Mandel, & Klerman, 1976; Whatmore & Ellis, 1959). The more important issues in Jacobson's early work and in subsequent psychophysiological research include the extent to which the EMG responses reflect: (1) specific or global activation; (2) phasic activation, tonic activation, or modulated thresholds for activation; and (3) characteristics of the stimulus (situation) or the individual (disposition). To address these issues, it has been necessary to monitor multiple measures of EMG activity. Furthermore, it has often been advantageous to monitor EMG responses across time using within-subjects designs; to use appropriate controls for assessing practice, sensitization, and carryover effects; to employ time-locked recording procedures; and to perform idiographic analyses at least when individual differences are of concern.

In addition, understanding the relative advantages and disadvantages of EMG in studies of psychology is important for its correct application and interpretation. Most of the striated muscles in the human body are bilaterally symmetrical in pairs (i.e., one on each side of the body), with estimates of the number of distinct muscles in the body ranging from 450 (Anson, 1966) to 639 (Khan, 1943) to 792 (Tomovic & Bellman, 1970). The general distribution of muscles across the body, as depicted in Anson (1966), is as follows: 37 bilaterally symmetrical muscle pairs in the head and face; 29 pairs in the neck and shoulder girth; 54 pairs in the shoulders, arms, and hands; 21 pairs in the spinal region; 15 pairs in the thoracoabdominal region; 9 pairs in the pelvic outlet; and 62 pairs in the hip, thighs, legs, and feet (Figure 11.1).

From a functional perspective, each striated muscle can be characterized as a linear actuator, with the potential states being limited to onset of contraction, offset of contraction, and relaxation (Tomovic & Bellman, 1970), wherein maximal muscle contraction results in a reduction in length to approximately 57 percent of that observed at rest (cf. Willis & Grossman, 1977). However, the structural arrangements of the striated muscles (e.g., as agonist–antagonist pairs, or through their interdigitation) expand dramatically the number of outcomes that can be achieved by this fairly simple system. The relatively small number of muscles in the head and neck, for instance, have been estimated to enable the encoding of some 6,000 to 7,000 appearance changes (Izard, 1971; see Figure 11.1 left panel). With this flexibility comes adaptability:

Speaking of muscles as linear actuators, it must always be kept in mind how inadequate the engineering performance criteria are when extended in any routine fashion to the biological world. For instance, we are so used to wheeled vehicles that we forget that there is a very close relation between their efficiency and road conditions. Animal locomotion, however, is practically independent of environmental constraints. This optimization criterion is therefore much more essential for the survival goal. (Tomovic & Bellman, 1970, p. 273)

This skeletomuscular architecture and its flexibility of action are also the source of the major limitations in EMG studies of psychology or behavior. First, it is feasible to obtain measurements over only a small number of muscles in the human body in any given experiment. Yet because the action of the striated muscles is multiply determined, monitoring activity from a single site may only provide global or ambiguous information about the associated psychological or behavioral process. Ekman (1982) observed, for instance, that emotions, with the possible exception of happiness, cannot be identified by the activity of a single muscle: "Disgust might be measured by the activity of two muscles, and surprise by the activity of three. To measure anger, fear, or sadness, many muscles need to be measured" (Ekman, 1982, p. 79).

Second, many limb displacements and feature distortions can be achieved by the actions of different or differently activated striated muscles. Electromyographic responses may therefore *appear* unreliable if the focus is on the motor/behavioral output rather than the mechanisms by which these outcomes were achieved (Gans & Gorniak, 1980). Third, the imperfect selectivity of surface electrodes and the close proximity of the various striated muscles make it difficult to pinpoint exactly which muscles are contracting. Hence, when using surface electrodes, it is appropriate

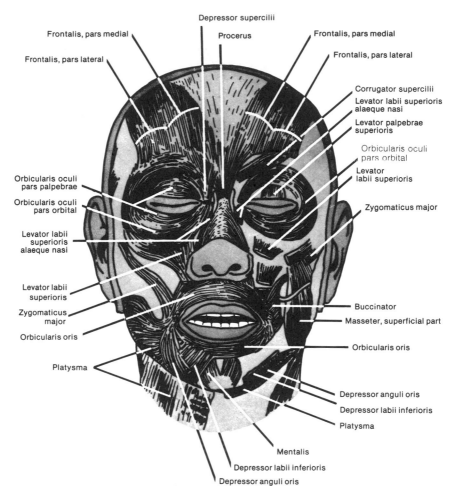

Depressor supercilii

Frontalis, pars medial

Procerus

Frontalis, pars medial

Frontalis, pars lateral

Frontalis, pars lateral

Corrugator supercilii

Levator labii superioris alaeque nasi

Levator palpebrae superioris

Orbicularis oculi pars orbital

Levator labii superioris

Orbicularis oculi pars palpebrae

Orbicularis oculi pars orbital

Zygomaticus major

Levator labii superioris alaeque nasi

Levator labii superioris

Zygomaticus major

Orbicularis oris

Buccinator

Masseter, superficial part

Orbicularis oris

Platysma

Depressor anguli oris

Depressor labii inferioris

Platysma

Mentalis

Depressor labii inferioris

Depressor anguli oris

Figure 11.1. *a*: Schematic representation of selected facial muscles. Overt facial expressions of emotion are based on contractions of underlying musculature that are sufficiently intense to result in visibly perceptible dislocations of skin and landmarks. More common visible effects of strong contractions of depicted facial muscles include the following. Muscles of lower face: *depressor anguli oris,* pulls lip corners downward; *depressor labii inferioris,* depresses lower lip; *orbicularis oris,* tightens, compresses, protrudes, and/or inverts lips; *mentalis,* elevates chin boss and protrudes lower lip; *platysma,* wrinkles skin of neck and may draw down both lower lip and lip corners. Muscles of midface: *buccinator,* compresses and tightens cheek, forming a "dimple"; *levator labii superioris alaeque nasi,* raises center of upper lip and flares nostrils; *levator labii superioris,* raises upper lip and flares nostrils, exposing canine teeth; *masseter,* raises lower jaw; *zygomaticus major,* pulls lip corners up and back. Muscles of upper face: *corrugator supercilii,* draws brows together and downward, producing vertical furrows between brows; *depressor supercilii/procerus,* pulls medial part of brows downward and may wrinkle skin over bridge of nose; *frontalis, pars lateral,* raises outer brows, producing horizontal furrows in lateral regions of forehead; *frontalis, pars medial,* raises inner brows, producing horizontal furrows in medial region of forehead; *levator palpebrae superioris,* raises upper eyelid; *orbicularis oculi pars orbital,* tightens skin surrounding eye, causing "crows-feet" wrinkles; *orbicularis oculi, pars palpebrae,* tightens skin surrounding eye causing lower eyelid to rise. Descriptions are consistent with those in Daniels and Worthingham (1986). Ekman and Friesen (1978), Kendall and McCreary (1980), Izard (1971), and Weaver (1977). (From J. T. Cacioppo, J. S. Martzke, R. E. Petty, & L. G. Tassinary, 1988. Reproduced with permission.)

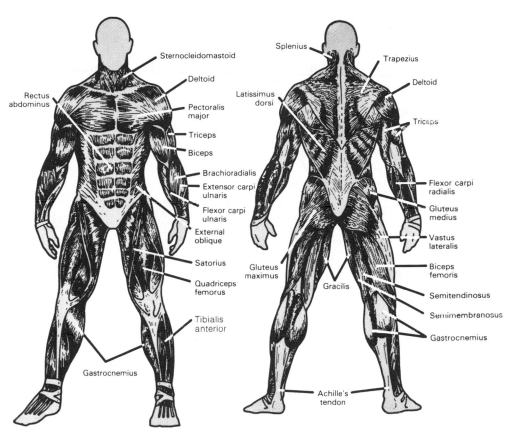

b: Schematic representation of major muscle groups of human body. Overt skeletomotor actions based on contractions of underlying musculature that are sufficiently intense to result in movements of skeletostructure. Front (ventral) view: *Sternocleidomastoid*, rotates face toward side opposite contracting muscle and, when paired muscles are contracted, flexes vertebral column to move neck and face toward chest: *deltoid*, abducts arm; *pectoralis major*, flexes, adducts, and medially rotates arm; *biceps brachii*, flexes and supinates arm; *triceps brachii*, extends forearm; *external oblique*, bends vertebral column laterally toward contracting muscle and, when paired muscles are contracted, compresses abdomen; *brachioradialis*, flexes forearm; *flexor carpi ulnaris*, flexes and adducts wrist; *extensor carpi ulnaris*, extends and abducts wrist; *sartorius*, flexes leg and flexes and rotates thigh laterally; *quadriceps femoris*, composite of four muscles (*rectus femoris*, *vastus lateralis*, *vastus medialis*, and *vastus intermedius*), which extend leg, and *rectus fermoris*, which flexes thigh; *tibialis anterior*, dorsiflexes and inverts foot; *gastrocnemius*, plantar flexes foot; *rectus abdominis*, flexes vertebral column. Back (dorsal) view: *splenius*, rotates head toward side same size as contracting muscle and, when paired muscles are contracted, extends head; *trapezius*, adducts, rotates, and elevates scapula (back part of shoulder) and extends head; latissimus *dorsi*, extends, adducts, and rotates arm medially; *gluteus medius*, abducts and rotates thigh medially; *gluteus maximus*, extends and rotates thigh laterally; *deltoid*, abducts arm; *flexor carpi radialis*, flexes and abducts wrist; *hamstrings*, composite of three muscles (*biceps femoris*, *semitendinosus*, and *semimembranosus*), which flex leg and extend thigh: *gracilis*, flexes leg and adducts thigh; *vastus lateralis*, extends leg. Descriptions are consistent with those in Daniels and Worthingham (1986), Langley, Telford, and Christensen (1974), Schmidt and Thews (1983), and Tortora (1983). *Note on terminology: Abductor* moves bone away from midline of body; *adductor* moves bone closer to midline; *levator* produces upward movement; *depressor* produces downward movement; *sphincter* decreases size of opening; *flexor* usually

(*contd. on next page*)

only to refer to EMG signals as reflecting activity from sites or muscle regions (e.g., *"corrugator supercilii* muscle region"). Fourth, surface EMG recording, although noninvasive, can be obtrusive and potentially reactive. Electrodes attached to the surface of the skin and leads traveling to preamplifiers, for instance, can restrict an individual's movement or make the individual tense or self-conscious. Finally, until recently there was no theoretically derived or empirically verified standard for the placement of surface electrodes to detect activity in a particular region of the face or, to some extent, the body. The absence of such a standard weakened comparisons across laboratories or across individuals and sessions within laboratories.

Progress has been made in overcoming many of these limitations (e.g., Fridlund & Cacioppo, 1986; Tassinary, Cacioppo, & Geen, 1989; Tassinary, Cacioppo, Geen, & Vanman, 1987), and this progress is reviewed in the sections that follows. In addition, surface EMG recording offers several unique advantages that complement the study of overt behavior through traditional means (see, also, Cacioppo & Petty, 1983; Fridlund, 1987). First, EMG responses, in contrast to measures such as response latencies or verbal reports, can be collected continuously without the individual's attention or labor. Second, the detection and quantification of EMG signals over a muscle region can be performed with the assistance of computers more sensitively, reliably, and quickly than can fine-grain analyses of overt behavior. Third, analyses of subtle somatic patterns and their time course may provide a means of differentiating underlying mechanisms of control over overt behaviors that are visibly identical.

Fourth, many subtle psychological (e.g., emotional) processes or events are not accompanied by visually perceptible actions or significant visceral changes, and these facts have hindered theory and research of psychological processes (e.g., Graham, 1980; Rajecki, 1983; cf. Cacioppo, Petty, et al., 1986). Darwin (1873/1872) recognized this limitation in the study of emotional expressions, stating that "the study of expression is difficult, owing to the movements being often extremely slight, and of a fleeting nature" (p. 12). It is now clear, however, that fast or low-level changes in EMG activity can occur without leading to any visible limb displacement or feature distortions on the surface of the skin. Facial expressions, for instance, result from movements of facial skin and connective tissue due to the contraction of facial muscles that create folds, lines, and wrinkles in the skin and the movement of facial landmarks such as the brows and corners of the mouth (e.g., Ekman & Friesen, 1978; Izard, 1971; Rinn, 1984). Although muscle activation must occur if these facial distortions are to be achieved (see Figure 11.1), it is possible for muscle activation to occur in the absence of any overt facial action if the activation is weak or transient or if the overt response is aborted. This holds for nonfacial striated muscles as well (e.g., see Coles, Gratton, Bashore, Eriksen, & Donchin, 1985).

In the face, this is due to the structure and elasticity of the facial skin, facial sheath, adipose tissue, and facial muscles. The muscles of expression are attached to

---

decreases anterior (or, in a few cases, posterior) angle at joint; *extensor* usually increases anterior (or, in a few cases, posterior) angle at joint; *supinator* turns palm upward or anteriorly; *pronator* turns palm downward or posteriorly; *dorsiflexor* flexes foot at ankle joint; *plantar flexor* extends foot at ankle joint.

other muscles, bones, or a facial sheath below the surface of the facial skin and adipose tissue; not unlike a loose chain, the facial muscles can be pulled a small distance (i.e., contracted slightly) before exerting a significant force on the object to which they are anchored (cf. Tassinary et al., 1989). In addition, the elasticity of the facial sheath, facial skin, and adipose tissue forms a low-pass mechanical filter, attenuating the visible effects of very rapid contractions (Fridlund, 1987; cf. Fridlund & Cacioppo, 1986).

In summary, measures of EMG and of observable muscular actions each have unique advantages and disadvantages. Neither is necessarily better or more capable of capturing completely the information provided by the other. A general congruence between the results based on EMG recordings and those obtained through fine-grain analyses of overt behavior is to be expected given the physiological basis of the surface EMG (see what follows). Therefore, the wealth of information that exists regarding nonverbal behavior and displays during such processes as thinking, communication, deception, and emotion (e.g., see Scherer & Ekman, 1982) provides a rich theoretical resource for research on subtler, more fleeting responses or on underlying mechanisms.

Yet EMG recordings and fine-grain behavioral observations do not coincide completely. As noted, EMG recordings can reveal muscular activity or patterns of activity too small or fleeting to evoke detectable movements or whose corresponding muscle contractions are counteracted by contraction of an antagonist. Ekman (1982) reported an interesting, illustrative study conducted by Ekman, Schwartz, and Friesen. Surface EMG recordings and high-quality videorecordings were secured simultaneously as individuals deliberately intensified the contraction of specific facial muscles (the *corrugator supercilii* and *medial frontalis*). Results revealed that measurements of facial feature distortions using Ekman and Friesen's (1978) Facial Action Coding System (FACS) and measurements from surface EMG over these muscle regions were highly correlated ($r = +.85$). Nevertheless, reliable EMG signals emerged at levels lower than could reliably be detected visually. These results speak well both for the validity of facial EMG measurement and for the possibility of tracking at least limited features of moment-by-moment psychological processes even in the absence of a visually detectable motor response (see, also, Cacioppo & Petty, 1979a; Cacioppo et al., 1988; Fridlund, Schwartz, & Fowler, 1984; Schwartz, 1975). Moreover, because individuals may be less likely to control momentary or minute muscular contractions that do not result in observable actions, discrepancies between EMG responses underlying covert versus overt responses may be of special interest (cf. Cacioppo, Petty, et al., 1986). We return to these issues following a discussion of the technical aspects of the surface EMG.

11.3 PHYSICAL CONTEXT

Almost three quarters of a century ago, Baines (1918, cited in Basmajian & DeLuca, 1985) argued that appropriate technical considerations should precede the collection or interpretation of data related to electrophysiological phenomena. In their survey of the EMG literature, Basmajian and DeLuca (1985) strongly concurred, observing that "this call still echoes among the numerous abuses that have been promulgated throughout the past seven decades" (p. 6).

Although fascination or concern with technical issues and "state-of-the-art" equipment can be overdone, an understanding of the physiological system one is studying and the bioelectrical principles underlying its responses serve several important purposes. These include the (1) intimation or stimulation of theory and development of operational definitions and procedures; (2) discrimination of signal from artifact; (3) safety of the individuals involved; (4) digital data acquisition and analysis and derivation of descriptive parameters that are reliable and valid representations of the physiological events of interest; and (5) guidance of inferences based on physiological data (see, also, Cacioppo & Tassinary, chapter 1; Cacioppo & Tassinary, 1989). In this section, therefore, we review the physiological basis of the surface EMG, and we outline principles and technical issues involved in obtaining valid measures of EMG activity.

11.3.1   *Anatomical and physiological basis of the surface electromyogram*

The striated muscles in the human body are capable of different types of muscular activity. They have tone, maintain postures, make reflexive movements in response to sensory stimuli, actuate spontaneous rhythmic contractions, and produce both spontaneous and voluntary contractions that can occur independent of immediate external stimuli (Willis & Grossman, 1977). A schematic of the central organization and control of the several hundred skeletomuscles in the human body is presented in Figure 11.2. A detailed description of the central organization and control of the motor system, although important, is beyond the scope of the present chapter. Interested readers can consult Henneman (1980a–c), Kandel and Schwartz (1985), and Willis and Grossman (1977).

At the peripheral level, one finds that each striated muscle is innervated by a single motor nerve whose cell bodies are primarily located in the ventral horn of the spinal cord or, in the case of the muscles of the head, in the cranial nerves of the brain stem. All behavior – that is, all actions of the striated muscles, regardless of the source of the neural signal (e.g., reflex arcs, pyramidal neurons emanating from the motor cortex) – result from neural signals traveling along these motor nerves. For this reason, the set of lower motor nerves has been designated the final common pathway (Sherrington, 1923/1906).

Closer inspection of these neuromuscular units reveals that the typical striated muscle consists of hundreds or thousands of separate, elongated muscle fibers bound together by a sheet of connective tissue. The motor nerve traveling to the muscle consists of numerous individual motoneurons, which as a collective are referred to as a motoneuron pool. Each motoneuron axon divides into a number of small branches, termed *axon fibrils*, just before reaching the muscle; each axon fibril, in turn, forms a junction, called a motor end plate, on an individual muscle fiber (Figure 11.3). Each motoneuron innervates a number of interspersed muscle fibers within a muscle, and each muscle fiber is usually innervated by only one motoneuron. An important functional consequence of this structure is that muscle fibers do not contract individually but rather there is a concerted action by each set of muscle fibers innervated by a single motoneuron. Therefore, the most elementary functional unit within the "final common pathway" is the motoneuron cell body, its axon, its axon fibrils, and the individual muscle fibers innervated by these axon fibrils. This functional, physiological entity is called a motor unit (see Figure 11.3).

The axons of the motoneurons within a motoneuron pool vary in diameter, and this structural feature also has important functional consequences. Generally, the

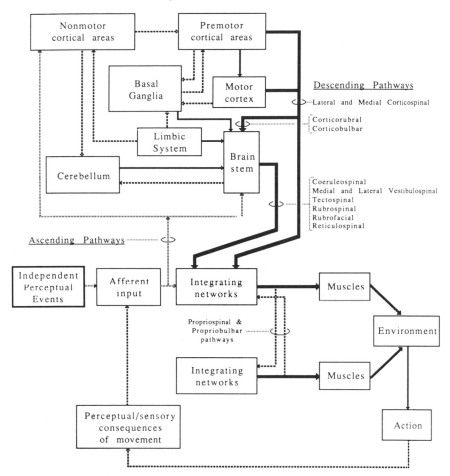

Figure 11.2. Major components of motor system. Solid lines represent efferent pathways, heavy dashed lines represent feedback pathways, and light dashed lines represent afferent pathways. Converging arrows do not necessarily imply convergence on same individual neurons. Crossing of pathways as well as details of specific connections within brain areas are not indicated. Note that arrows denote strong influences; they do not imply direct (monosynaptic) connections. Note also that list of descending pathways is representative; it is not meant to be exhaustive. The thalamus and hypothalamus have been omitted for clarity. (Modified and redrawn from Figure 33.3 of Ghez, 1985, based on Hinsey, 1940, and Kuypers, 1982.)

smaller the diameter of a motoneuron, the smaller the number of axon fibrils and consequently the smaller the number of muscle fibers it innervates. Hence, activation of muscle via small motoneurons produces smaller and more precise actions than activation of the same muscle by the depolarization of large motoneurons. In addition, the smaller the diameter of the motoneuron, the lower tends to be the critical firing threshold of its cell body and the more fatigue resistant (i.e., the greater the glycolytic capacity) the muscle fibers innervated by the

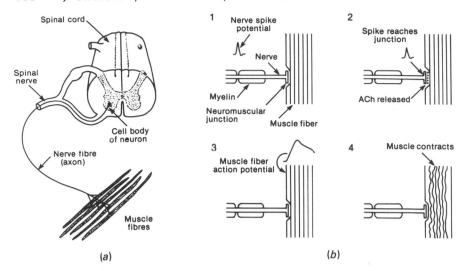

Figure 11.3. *Left panel (a):* Schematic of motor unit. (From Basmajian & DeLuca, 1985. Reproduced with permission.) *Right panel (b):* Sequence of events involved in transmission across neuromuscular junction: 1, nerve action (spike) potential approaches junction; 2, spike reaches junction and triggers release of ACh; 3, ACh acts on muscle fiber to produce muscle action potential; 4, muscle contracts. (From Thompson, 1967. Reproduced with permission.)

motoneuron. These relationships constitute the size principle (Henneman, 1980b), and it contributes to the graded contraction and coordinated actions of muscles. More specifically, the force of contraction produced by a muscle is attributable to small motoneurons initially discharging intermittently and then discharging more frequently. Stronger muscle contractions are attributable to the depolarization of increasingly large motoneurons within the motoneuron pool. As muscle contraction approaches maximal levels, further increases in contraction are again attributable to the individual motoneurons firing more quickly (Petrofsky & Phillips, 1982). If maximal contraction is required for an extended period, the physiochemical mechanisms underlying muscle contraction are unable to sustain brief refractory periods, and muscular quivering (tetany) develops.

The ratio of muscle fibers to motoneurons (innervation ratio) varies even more dramatically across than within muscles and is related to the precision of the movement of the particular muscles involved. Consistent with the principles outlined in the preceding, muscles with low innervation ratios (i.e., few muscles fibers per motoneuron and, hence, small motor units) are capable of producing actions more rapidly and with greater precision than are muscles with high innervation ratios. For example, the extrinsic muscles of the eye, which are capable of very fast and fine movements, have innervation ratios around 10:1, whereas the more slowly and grossly acting postural muscles have innervation ratios of around 3,000:1 (Basmajian & DeLuca, 1985).

The depolarization of a motoneuron results in the quantal release of acetylcholine at motor end plates (see Figure 11.3). The activating neurotransmitter acetylcholine is quickly metabolized by the enzyme cholinesterase so that continued efferent discharges are required for continued propagation of muscle action potentials (MAPs) and fiber contraction. Nonetheless, the transient excitatory potential within a motor end plate can lead to a brief (e.g., 1-ms) depolarization of the resting membrane potential of the muscle cell and an MAP that is propagated bidirectionally across the muscle fiber with constant velocity and undiminished amplitude. In the process, the physiochemical mechanism responsible for muscle contraction is activated (cf. Loeb & Gans, 1986). As the MAP travels along the muscle fiber, a small portion of this electrical activity passes through the extracellular fluids to the skin. It is these voltage changes that constitute the major portion of the surface EMG signal. Thus, the EMG does not provide a direct measure of tension or muscular contraction (mechanical events) but rather the electrical activity that accompanies these mechanical events.

Of course, the voltage changes that are detected in surface EMG recording do not emanate from a single MAP but from MAPs traveling across many muscle fibers within a motor unit (i.e., motor unit action potential, or MUAP) and even from MAPs traveling across several to hundreds of thousands of motor fibers due to the activation of multiple motor units. The surface EMG represents the aggregated electrical signals that reach the skin at a given moment in time. Not only are the details of the individual MAPs lost, but so too are the precise muscular origins. Reliable and sensitive information about the aggregate actions (or inactions) of motoneuron pools across time can nonetheless be obtained by careful attention to the elements of EMG recording and analysis (e.g., see Cacioppo, Marshall-Goodell, & Dorfman, 1983; Lippold, 1967; Petrofsky & Phillips, 1982). It is to these topics that we turn next.

11.3.2 *Physical recording basis*

The physical components for EMG recording are depicted schematically in Figure 11.4. These components include detection of the bioelectrical signals emanating from the subject; preamplification and preliminary signal conditioning; signal amplification, display, digitization, and storage; EMG signal representation; and inferential statistical analysis. In this section, we survey common problems of and standard methods for dealing with each of these physical components of EMG recording.

11.3.2.1 *Detecting the bioelectrical signals*

As outlined in the preceding section, the EMG signal emanating from the muscle is a quasi-random train of motor unit action potentials discharged by the contraction of striate muscle tissue. The signal train is characterized by a frequency range of several hertz to over 1 kHz and by amplitudes ranging at the surface of the skin from fractions of a microvolt to a few thousand microvolts. These frequency and amplitude characteristics are broader than most bioelectrical events of interest to psychophysiologists, and they overlap both a variety of nonmuscular physiological responses (e.g., electroencephalographic, cardiodynamic) and the ubiquitous external AC signals that power most laboratory lights, electrical transformers, and equipment (see Marshall-Goodell, Tassinary, & Cacioppo, chapter 4). Consequently, detection of high-quality EMG signals from a localized muscle region requires careful attention to noise reduction and grounding practices (to eliminate extraneous

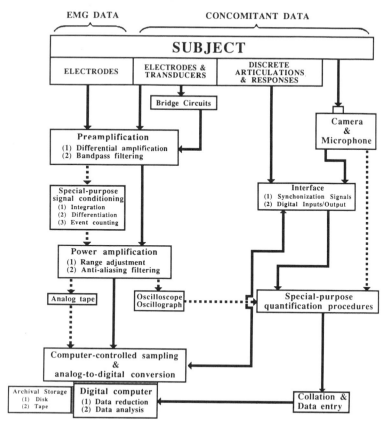

Figure 11.4. Major components of laboratory system for detection of EMG signals; preamplification and preliminary signal conditioning; power amplification, digitization, display, and data storage; and data processing (signal representation, statistical analyses). (Adapted from Cacioppo, Marshall-Goodell, & Gormezano, 1983, Loeb & Gans, 1986, and Shapiro & Crider, 1969.)

electrical noise), electrode site preparation and placement (to minimize the detection of irrelevant bioelectrical signals), and appropriate differential preamplification and preliminary signal conditioning (to further enhance signal-to-noise ratio).

Noise reduction and grounding procedures. Loeb and Gans (1986) define *noise* as any unwanted signal. The specific bioelectrical signal of interest can be obscured by noise from: (1) external electrical sources (e.g., through capacitive or inductive coupling from AC lines, movement of electrode interface or leads, electrical cross-talk in the recording componentry); (2) physiological responses whose frequency/amplitude characteristics overlap those for EMG recording (e.g., EKG, EEG); (3) EMG signals emanating from muscles whose actions are not of immediate interest at the target-recording site (i.e., cross-talk from somatic actions within the organism); and (4) EMG signals from target sites that result from "irrelevant" actions one tried to minimize or eliminate by the design of the experiment (e.g., movement artifacts). It is little wonder that noise is the "bane of the electrophysiologist's existence" (Loeb & Gans, 1986, p. 21).

The most problematic extraneous electrical noise in the laboratory is narrow-band noise because it arises from several common sources, it radiates through walls and air, and its frequency range overlaps that of the EMG signal. Sixty-hertz noise emanates from AC power lines, lights, relays, and transformers. Although many EMG preamplifiers include a notch filter to attenuate 60-Hz noise, the filter is neither completely effective nor selective. That is, notch filters attenuate frequencies to a varying degree on both sizes of 60 Hz – a bandwidth that can represent a significant portion of the total power in an EMG signal. It is therefore preferable to minimize electrical noise prior to amplification. This can be done through appropriate placement and shielding of equipment and careful grounding of the subject and equipment (Bramsley, Bruun, Buchthal, Guld, & Petersen, 1967; Strong, 1970).

Televisions, video monitors, and computer terminals all use cathode-ray tubes (CRTs), and they generate high-frequency electrical noise (ranging from 15 kHz to several hundred kilohertz) from the transformers used for CRT beam deflection These electrical signals can be eliminated by placing the devices (and any unshielded AC power cords) at least 2 ft away from EMG electrodes, electrode leads, data lines, and equipment. In addition, the use of coaxial cable with shielded connectors is recommended to minimize the leakage of radio-frequency (RF) noise. Fridlund and Cacioppo (1986) and McGuigan (1979) describe procedures for measuring laboratory electrical noise sources.

Wide-band, or white-noise, is usually attributable to Brownian motion (i.e., atoms and molecules randomly colliding with each other) in electronic devices. This noise is minimized by keeping electrode impedances low and amplifier filters set tightly to the proper bandwidth (Loeb & Gans, 1986; Strong, 1970).

Biological noise includes all endogenous signals that are not part of the bioelectrical signal of interest. The placement of a ground electrode does *not* prevent artifacts from cross-talk. This is because the impedance into the ground electrode tends to exceed the access impedance of the volume-conductive tissues between the spurious current source and the recording electrode (Loeb & Gans, 1986; see Marshall-Goodell et al., chapter 4). In the sections that follow, we outline several procedures for minimizing biological noise. Additional details and discussions are provided by Loeb and Gans (1986), Strong (1970), and Basmajian and DeLuca (1985).

The subject affixed with electrodes should also be grounded at one and only one point on her or his body. If multichannel recordings are being made, then the ground planes for the recording channels should be strapped together rather than using separate grounds for each. Similarly, all equipment in the laboratory should be grounded at exactly one point, and any equipment touched by the subject should be nonconductive. These procedures further minimize 60-Hz noise in the recordings and enhance the safety of the subject by eliminating the possibility of ground loops (i.e., unintended current flow due to imperfect grounding).

Electrode selection and placement. Psychophysiologists typically use surface rather than needle electrodes for EMG recording. This is due to the noninvasive nature of surface recording and to the research questions asked thus far by psychophysiologists (i.e., the usual interest is in muscles rather than motor units within muscles). Surface EMG electrodes are less sensitive to exact anatomical placement since they detect the MAPs from a cluster of motor units rather than a single unit. As previously noted, the discrete electrical discharges from individual MAPs summate spatially and temporally during motor unit recruitment to yield an aggregate that reflects the action of motoneuron pools. This aggregate response develops in an orderly manner from the individual MAPs – at least in a probabilistic sense – such that, generally, progressively larger motoneurons are added to or progressively smaller units subtracted from the total output from a motoneuron pool (Henneman, 1980a). Consequently, surface EMG recordings correlate well with the overall level of contraction of muscle groups underlying and near the electrodes, especially when limb movement is constrained and contractions are neither minimal nor maximal (Lawrence & DeLuca, 1983; Lippold, 1967).

Because most EMG amplifiers are AC coupled (see what follows), the electrical stability of the electrodes is not as important as, for instance, when recording skin conductance (e.g., see Dawson, Schell, & Filion, chapter 10). Nonpolarizing electrodes such as silver–silver chloride (Ag/AgCl) electrodes are nevertheless preferable to stainless steel or other alloys due to variations in amplifier design, minimization of electrode artifact, and special problems inherent in detecting low-level signals (Fridlund, Tassinary, & Cacioppo, 1988).

Surface electrodes are available in a variety of sizes. Electrodes with small detection surfaces and housings allow closer interelectrode spacing and consequently higher selectively.[4] Factors such as the electrode size, electrode positioning, and interelectrode distance over a particular site can affect the detected EMG signals and, hence, should be held constant across experimental conditions. Fridlund and Cacioppo (1986) found that electrodes with 0.5 cm diameter Ag/AgCl detection surfaces and 1.5 cm diameter housings are used commonly for limb and trunk EMG sites, and miniature electrodes with 0.25 cm diameter Ag/AgCl detection surfaces and 0.5 or 1.0 cm diameter housings are used when greater recording selectivity is required, such as for facial EMG sites. Ad hoc recommendations were also offered for the use of a 1.0 cm interelectrode spacing for 0.25 cm electrodes and 1.5 cm spacing for the 0.5 cm electrode in bipolar EMG recording unless an explicit rationale exists for employing a different interelectrode spacing. Only closely spaced electrodes and differential amplification can yield spatially selective EMG recordings. Using widely spaced electrodes or electrodes that are not aligned with respect to the underlying striate muscle makes sense only if one is not interested in spatially selective EMG recording.

Specification of surface electrode placements over target muscle groups is important to ensure that findings are comparable across individuals, sessions, or laboratories. Several studies offer empirically and anatomically derived recommendations for EMG recording for facial, masticatory, and articulatory muscle activity using subdermal electrodes (e.g., Compton, 1973; Fridlund & Cacioppo, 1986; Isley & Basmajian, 1973; O'Dwyer, Quinn, Guitar, Andrews, & Neilson, 1981; Seiler, 1973; Vitti et al., 1975), and additional studies have examined the reliability of EMG measurements in relatively large, well-defined muscles (Gans & Gorniak, 1980; Komi & Buskirk, 1970). This research supports two principles of electrode orientation for differential recording over a given muscle region: (1) electrodes should be arranged to span maximally the gradient desired (e.g., in line with the underlying muscle whose activity is of interest) to maximize the recording of its activity and

(2) electrodes should be arranged distal and/or perpendicular to gradients of extraneous signal sources (e.g., proximal muscles) to attenuate the recording of their activity. At the present time, only a handful of studies have established optimal electrode sites for bipolar surface EMG recording. Factors that must be balanced in implementing these principles in specifying electrode sites include (1) proximity of a proposed site to underlying muscle mass with minimal intervening tissue or interfering signals (such as from the electrocardiogram); (2) position of electrodes relative to muscle tissue fiber size, location, and orientation (e.g., electrodes generally should be aligned parallel to the course of the muscle fibers to maximize sensitivity and selectivity to the muscle of interest); (3) avoidance of straddling the motor end plate region; (4) ease of location of sites via anatomical landmarks that show relative uniformity across individuals; (5) ease of electrode attachments to these sites without undue obstruction of vision or movement or problems from skin folds, bony obstructions, and so on; and (6) minimizing cross-talk from proximal deep and superficial muscles (Fridlund & Cacioppo, 1986; Tassinary et al., 1989).

Davis (1952) was the first to offer recommendations for recording the muscle activity involved in movements of the limbs, neck, jaw, lower lip, and eyebrows. Davis, however, presented no evidence for the choice of particular sites over others and on occasion based placements on incorrect anatomical assumptions (cf. Fridlund & Cacioppo, 1986); consequently, only those regarding limb and neck placements are currently recommended (cf. Zipp, 1982).

Tassinary et al. (1989) provided relevant data for the *corrugator supercilii, depressor supercilii,* and *zygomaticus major* muscle regions, regions that have proven informative in studies of emotion. Based on anatomical data regarding the location of these muscles (see Figure 11.1a), several experiments were conducted to isolate the sites for surface EMG recording that met the six criteria outlined in the preceding. Subjects posed a series of facial actions and expressions twice while facial EMG activity was sampled. The activity of a specific muscle or set of muscles was verified with visible coding using the FACS (Ekman & Friesen, 1978). The surface recording sites identified as providing both sensitive and relatively selective measures of activation of specific muscle regions are illustrated in Figure 11.5.

Tassinary et al. (1987) provided relevant data for recording over the perioral muscle region and, in particular, for detecting silent language processing. Five sites in the perioral region were compared for their ability to differentiate facial actions due to the activation of discrete facial muscles in the perioral region. In addition to four electrode sites place over the *mentalis, orbicularis oris superior, orbicularis oris inferior,* and *depressor anguli inferioris* (see Figure 11.1), a standard electrode placement (i.e., "chin") recommended by Davis (1952) to measure general perioral EMG activity was included. Activation of specific muscles or sets of muscles was again achieved by poses and was verified using the FACS. Following their correct performance of the poses on two separate occasions, subjects were asked to read affectively neutral passages silently, subvocally, and aloud. Only EMG responses recorded over the *mentalis, orbicularis oris inferior,* and chin muscle regions differentiated quiescent baseline activity from silent reading. Of these three sites, only the site depicted in Figure 11.5 for the *orbicularis oris inferior* muscle region demonstrated high discriminant validity when poses activating this versus proximal superficial muscles were contrasted.

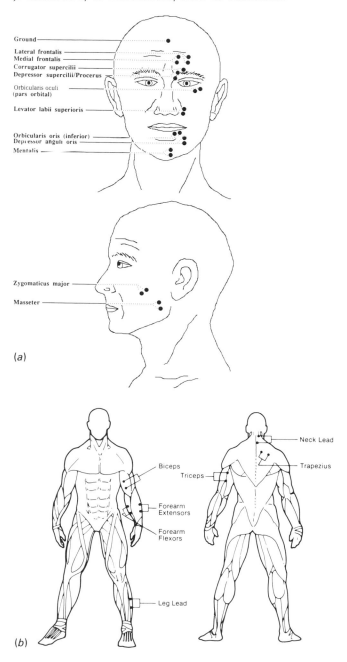

Figure 11.5. Atlas of EMG electrode placements for surface differential recording over selected facial muscle regions (a) and limb, body, and neck muscle regions (b). Detailed descriptions of electrode placements relative to physical landmarks are provided by Tassinary, Cacioppo, and Geen (1989), Fridlund and Cacioppo (1986), and Zipp (1982).

Site preparation. Surface EMG electrodes can be attached to the skin using double-stick adhesive collars. A conductive medium (paste or gel) is used between the electrode surface and skin. This medium serves several functions: (1) stabilizing the interface between the skin and each electrode surface to minimize movement artifacts or alterations in recording area; (2) reducing interelectrode impedances by forming a conductive pathway across the hornified layers of the skin; and (3) stabilizing the hydration and conductivity of the underlying skin.

Prior to the application of the conductive medium and electrodes, the electrode site on the surface of the skin is usually cleaned to remove dirt and oil, and the site is typically abraded to lower interelectrode impedances to 5 or 10 kΩ. The electrodes are then commonly affixed in a bipolar configuration, as illustrated in Figure 11.5. The placement of the ground electrode close but not directly adjacent to the EMG sites being monitored can also help minimize extraneous electrical noise in EMG recording. As already noted, however, only one ground electrode should be used, and all inputs should be configured to share this ground. Finally, to avoid obstructing movement due to the attachment of surface electrodes, thought should be given to the orientation of electrode collars and wires. Electrode wires, for instance, can be draped and secured using surgical adhesive tape to minimize distraction, annoyance, or obstruction of movement or vision.

11.3.2.2 *Preamplification and preliminary signal conditioning*

Electromyographic signals are "small" in two ways: They have low voltage and low current. As Loeb and Gans (1986) note, low-current signals coming from relatively high source impedances such as electrodes are particularly sensitive to noise picked up from external, extraneous signals (i.e., narrow-band noise), irrelevant, internally generated signals (i.e., biological noise) and the random motion of atoms and molecules within the amplification circuitry (i.e., wide-band noise). An amplifier supplies both voltage gain (turning low into high voltages), which can be controlled by the investigator, and current gain, a function of the ratio of the input and output impedances of the amplifier. The current gain of EMG preamplification is intentionally approximately zero to minimize source drain at the electrode site.

Electromyographic signals are amplified using differential amplifiers wherein the difference signal between two electrodes (with respect to a third, ground electrode) is amplified and carried through the signal-processing chain (Faulkenberry, 1977). Any bioelectrical or extraneous electrical signal that is common to both electrodes (the "common-mode" signal) is therefore attenuated (see Marshall-Goodell et al., chapter 4).

The most commonly used method of recording EMG signals is bipolar, in which electrode pairs are aligned parallel to the course of the muscle fibers. This alignment, coupled with the *common-mode rejection* of differential amplification, produces relatively sensitive and selective recording of the activity of the underlying muscle groups (Basmajian & DeLuca, 1985; see also Cooper, Osselton, & Shaw, 1980, chapter 3). Functional descriptions and circuit diagrams for differential EMG recording apparatus can be found in Fridlund and Fowler (1978) and Fridlund, Price, and Fowler (1982).

The second method of recording is monopolar, single ended, or common reference, which involves the placement of one EMG electrode over each target site (i.e., muscle group) of interest. The difference signal between the activity at each target site and a common reference electrode (which, in theory, is in contact with an isoelectric site on the subject's body) is differentially amplified and carried through the signal-processing chain. Common reference recording is characterized by (1) a much more general pickup region than bipolar recording and (2) sensitivity to variations in the absolute *level* of electrical activity (assuming the ground electrode reflects an isoelectric state). Bipolar recording, in contrast, is sensitive to variations in the *gradient* of electrical activity between the two active electrodes. Due to these distinctions, the selection of the common reference or the bipolar method depends entirely on the question posed by the investigator (e.g., see Tassinary et al., 1989; Marshall-Goodell et al., chapter 4).

Regardless of the approach adopted, the signals recorded across time can be conceptualized as constituting a waveform. Any waveform can be represented in terms of the linear addition of pure sinusoidal waveforms of various frequencies, and this is the basis of Fourier analysis. A spectral analysis of a time series of raw EMG amplitudes, for instance, describes the time series by the weighting factors needed to synthesize it from a series of sinusoids that are harmonically related (see Porges & Bohrer, chapter 21). This is an important analytic procedure in surface EMG recording because by identifying the range of frequencies containing most of the energy of the signal, an investigator can better know the amplifiers, electrodes, and passband to employ.

A schematized representation of a train of raw EMG signals is presented in the upper panel of Figure 11.6. As noted in the preceding, some filtering of the raw EMG signal is performed to increase the signal-to-noise ratio, decrease 60-Hz or EKG/EEG artifact, and reduce intersite cross-talk. The primary energy in the surface EMG signal lies between approximately 10 and 200 Hz (Hayes, 1960; van Boxtel, Goudswaard, & Shomaker, 1984). Between 10 and 30 Hz, this power is due primarily to the firing rates of motor units; and beyond 30 Hz this is due to the shapes of the aggregated motor unit action potentials (Lindstrom, 1970; Petrofsky & Phillips, 1982). Attenuating the high frequencies in the EMG signal (e.g., using 500-Hz low-pass filters) reduces amplifier noise but rounds peaks of the detected motor unit action potentials. Retaining sharp signal peaks may be important for waveform or spectral analysis of signal motor units or motor units action potential trains but is less critical for obtaining overall estimates of muscle tension. Attenuating the low frequencies (e.g., using 70-Hz high-pass filters) reduces 60-Hz noise from AC power lines, EEG and EKG artifacts, and to some extent, intersite cross-talk (due to the intervening tissue's preferential transmission of low frequencies) but also eliminates a significant portion of the EMG signal. Use of an overly restricted EMG signal passband may result in inaccurate appraisal of the level and form of EMG activity. Hence, selection of an EMG detection passband must proceed based on susceptibility to artifact, presence of extraneous electrical noise at the source and high-frequency noise internal to the amplifier, consideration of the amplitude of the EMG signals to be detected, need to minimize cross-talk, and variations across conditions in muscular fatigue. A passband from 10 to 500 or 1000 Hz is satisfactory for wide-band monitoring; if low-frequency artifact and intersite cross-talk are problematic, then a 90- or 100-Hz high-pass filter may be used, but the investigator should realize one consequence of this selection is that weak signals from the target region will be attenuated as well.[5]

Frequency (e.g., Fast Fourier Transform, or FFT) analyses have occasionally been performed on surface EMG recordings to determine whether there are shifts in the

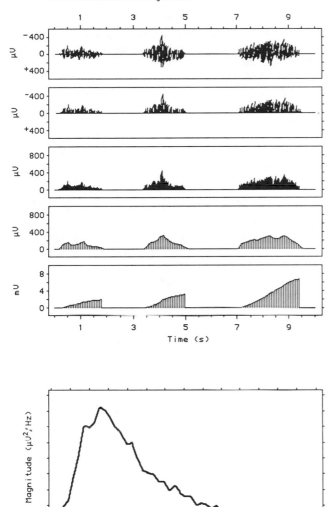

Figure 11.6. Schematic representations of EMG signals. From top to bottom: Raw EMG signal, full-wave rectified EMG signal, full-wave rectified and smoothed EMG signal, full-wave rectified and integrated EMG signal, and EMG power spectrum.

EMG spectra (i.e., magnitude or power at different frequencies) as a function of some psychological or behavioral variable. One robust finding is that shifts in EMG spectra are observed with fatigue (e.g., Mulder & Hulstijn, 1984). Part of the lack of attention to spectral analyses of the surface EMG in psychophysiology is attributable to the following factors: (1) to perform spectral analyses requires that the raw EMG signal be recorded at high rates (see what follows), making the application of FFTs costly; (2) unlike respiration or heart rate, the EMG is not an inherently periodic physiological event but rather is semistochastic; and (3) thus far, spectral analysis has proven no more sensitive to the few psychological manipulations that have been examined than the relatively inexpensive process of rectification and smoothing (e.g., see McGuigan, Dollins, Pierce, Lusebrink, & Corus, 1982).

The terms *integration* and *smoothing* are often confused. Integration is the temporal summation or accumulation of EMG activity, whereas smoothing refers to integration with a built-in signal decay and is accomplished by low-pass filtering, envelope detection, or averaging of the signal (see Figure 11.6). The total energy in an EMG spectra at any moment in time is equivalent to the rectified and smoothed EMG response; hence, when frequency components of the raw signal are not of interest, considerable economy in terms of data acquisition and signal processing can be achieved by rectification and smoothing prior to digitization and data storage.

The most frequently used on-line "smoother" in psychophysiological research is the contour follower, which is a precision rectifier connected to a low-pass filter (Fridlund, 1979). It acts as a running averager of ongoing EMG activity by providing a varying voltage proportional to the envelope of the EMG signal. Precision contour followers usually have selectable time constants. Short, in contrast to long, time constants produce sensitivity to momentary fluctuations in EMG signals. When measuring a rapidly changing EMG signal, a long time constant blurs rapid changes and signal peaks, and the output can therefore underestimate or overestimate EMG signal strength at any point in time. Conversely, if EMG signals that vary slowly are of primary interest, short time constants will be too sensitive to momentary EMG fluctuations, and the economic advantages of smoothing will be sacrificed.

11.3.2.3 *Signal recording, digitization, and storage*

Output from preamplification and preliminary signal processing may then be passed to power amplifiers to drive such devices as pen-writing galvanometers, FM tape recorders, and analog-to-digital (A/D) converters (see Figure 11.4). Characteristics of the signal passed from preamplification to this stage determine decisions made at the amplification stage. For instance, the gain required in amplification is dependent on the amplitude characteristics of the signal passed from the preamplifiers.

The rate at which the analog output of the amplification stage is digitized (i.e., the sampling rate for A/D conversion) is a function of the highest frequency present in the signal passed through the amplification stage. The Nyquist relation specifies that signals be sampled at a rate at least twice that of the fastest EMG frequency component of interest. The Nyquist relation, however, assumes both perfect filtering and continuous sampling. A good rule of thumb in laboratory practice, therefore, is to sample at four to eight times the highest frequency of interest to avoid aliasing and allow reconstruction of the original waveform with minimal smoothing. For instance, sampling rates of several kilohertz per channel might be required when digitizing the raw EMG signal, whereas sampling rates of 10–200 Hz per channel can yield satisfactory outputs if precision contour followers with moderate to long time constants are applied prior to digitization.

The process of digitization is accomplished by devices known as A/D converters, and their precision and noise characteristics are important to consider as well. For example, surface EMG recording over the *corrugator supercilii* muscle region can yield signals from fractions of a microvolt to several hundred microvolts. The standard 8-bit A/D converter, although widely available and inexpensive, offers insufficient resolution (1 part in 256) for detecting weak changes in EMG activity across a range in excess of about 100 μV. Twelve and 16-bit A/D converters offer a resolution of 1 part in 4,096 and 65,536, respectively; they consequently allow both very weak and very strong muscular contractions to be digitized precisely. One drawback to more precise A/D converters is that they require longer conversion times, placing a ceiling on sampling rates. Fast and precise 12–16-bit A/D converters are now widely available with conversion rates in excess of 100 kHz.

Most A/D converters offer input multiplexers that can be configured for single-ended or differential input. One might assume that passing each EMG channel from the differential amplifier to a single input on the A/D converter would be adequate since the output of the amplifier is the signal of interest. There is a potentially serious problem with this procedure, however. Any variations between the local ground at the amplifier and the local ground for the A/D converter, no matter how minute, can confound detection of the EMG signals being digitized. To avoid this possible source of noise, the input to the A/D converters can be configured for differential recording, and each output from an EMG amplifier can be 'differenced' from the ground at the amplifier.

Data storage can be accomplished in analog or digital form. Chart and pen recordings offer a simple visual aid in identifying likely artifacts, but high-frequency signals (e.g., EMG > 75 Hz) are truncated, and digitization of these chart and pen recordings is inefficient and potentially unreliable. Oscilloscopes allow on-line visual inspection of the full range of EMG frequencies, but they are not mass storage devices. Frequency-modulated or pulse-code-modulated tape decks are often useful because they can store the original signal indefinitely with minimal distortion of its amplitudes or frequency components, but decks with a wide recording bandwidth are expensive. Assuming the raw EMG signal was recorded, EMG activity can be replayed either through contour followers with varying time constants and various filters or directly to the A/D converters for purposes of comparison or analysis. Alternatively, the EMG signal can be digitized on-line and stored in digital form. This alternative can be satisfactory if forethought is given to matters such as on-line signal conditioning (e.g., filtering) and A/D conversion rate.

Finally, to ensure that the digitized signals are, in fact, in reasonable correspondence with the input signals emanating from the subject, a precision signal generator can be used to simulate low-level biological signals. These known signals should be varied from zero to several hundred microvolts and from 10–1,000 Hz to mimic the range of EMG signals. Problems such as extraneous electrical interference; amplifier or computer bus noise; improper preamplifier, amplifier, or A/D converter calibration; and undersampling (and consequent aliasing) manifest as discrepancies between the (known) input and digitized signals. This procedure should be repeated for each channel periodically and each time an addition or modification is made to the signal processing sequence. Illustrative designs for signal generators are available in Sheatz (1972) and Helmer (1986).

11.3.2.4 *EMG signal representation*

Electromyographic activity unfolds over time, and like most other psychophysiological responses, the raw signal is too complex to analyze without considerable data reduction. Whether features of the EMG signal are to be represented in the time domain, amplitude domain, or frequency domain, the first step involves the conversion of the digitized signal to a descriptive (e.g., physiological) unit of measurement. The numbers assigned to EMG signals of different amplitudes depend on: (1) the electrical unit chosen for description of the signal, (2) the accuracy of the calibration procedure and amplifier's gain setting, and (3) the type of integration method and length of time constant or reset criterion used. We focus on the former factors here. Interested readers can consult Fridlund and Cacioppo (1986) and Basmajian and DeLuca (1985) for additional details.

EMG activity as a voltage–time function. Reference is often made to digitizing analog bioelectrical signals at each peak (e.g., see Cooper, Osselton, & Shaw, 1980, p. 237). In laboratory practice, however, analog signals more commonly are digitized at equal time intervals of duration 1/(sampling rate) (e.g., once every A/D conversion). Hence, EMG signals can be viewed as a voltage–time function, where: (1) the ordinate represents bounded signal amplitudes scaled typically in terms of microvolts (μV) and (2) the abscissa represents discrete intervals of time of width 1/(sampling rate). The quantification of the amplitudes at each recording/conversion cycle is determined by the direction and magnitude of the measured voltage and is expressed in units of microvolts (μV) or microvolts peak-to-peak (μV_{p-p}). (The latter terminology is reserved for measurements of amplitudes made from negative to positive peaks). The EMG voltage–time envelope, like the motor unit action potential, is bipolar and asymmetrical about electrical zero.

Most psychophysiological research using EMG has focused on some variation of EMG signal amplitude as the dependent variable (cf. Cacioppo, Marshall-Goodell, & Dorfman, 1983). Recording EMG signals with AC-coupled amplifiers (or DC amplifiers with zero offsets) ensures that the average value will be zero. Hence, simple averaging of the raw EMG amplitudes is uninformative.

Counting or averaging the EMG signal's peaks, or tallying its directional changes or zero crossings, are relatively easy methods to implement and are useful for gauging gross differences in EMG activity provided a sufficiently high sampling rate is used (Grieve & Cavanaugh, 1973; Willison, 1963). These parameters are further limited in that they do not vary linearly with contraction and are unreliable at the extremes of muscular contraction.

Lippold (1967) maintained that the total energy in an EMG signal at a given moment in time, or what Lippold referred to as the integrated EMG (IEMG) signal, represents overall muscular contraction more accurately than the number or average amplitude of peaks in the EMG signal. Subsequent research has largely corroborated Lippold's assertion given limb movements are constrained and contractions are not extreme (Basmajian & DeLuca, 1985; Goldstein, 1972; Winter, Rau, Kadefors, Broman, & DeLuca, 1980). However, the term IEMG has been used in this research to refer to several different processing techniques. Two of the most common processing techniques in contemporary research are (1) the rectified EMG signal, smoothed using a contour follower, expressed as average voltage (μV or μV avg), and (2) the root-mean-square (rms) EMG, which is expressed as an rms voltage (μV or μV rms).[6] Both processing techniques transform the EMG voltage–time function into a contoured waveform that is nonnegative and bounded in time and amplitude. The moment-by-moment amplitude of this function respresents an estimate of the total energy of the signal at the time; the mean amplitude of this voltage–time function represents the average level of electrical energy emanating from the underlying muscle region(s) during a given recording epoch; and the integral of this function (e.g., the sum of the amplitudes) represents the total electrical activity (i.e., the size of the response) emanating from the underlying muscle region(s) during the recording epoch. Mean amplitude and total electrical energy are redundant when the sampling rate and length of the recording epochs are constant across conditions.

Cacioppo, Marshall-Goodell, and Dorfman (1983) demonstrated that although traditional measures of smoothed or integrated EMG amplitudes are generally representative of the level of isometric muscular contraction, they are insensitive to the distribution of amplitudes and to the manner in which the EMG signals emerge across time. Thus, one consequence of the traditional focus on the amplitude domain of the EMG signal is that the form of the response across time has been largely ignored. A notable exception is Malmo's (Davis & Malmo, 1951; Malmo, 1965, 1975) use of *EMG gradients*, which he defined as a "progressively rising level of voltage reflecting gradually rising tension in the specific muscle group on which the electrodes are placed" (Malmo, 1975, p. 34). Electromyographic gradients have been used to assess variations across time in tonic muscle tension and are depicted by plotting the mean (or rms) EMG amplitude for two or more consecutive recording epochs.

Cacioppo and Dorfman (1987) (see also Dorfman & Cacioppo, chapter 20) have recently extended work on representing EMG waveforms in the time, amplitude, and frequency domains to derive a systematic and comprehensive representation of nonnegative bounded waveforms predicated on the moments of the waveform in a given domain. Nonnegative bounded waveforms are an important class in psychophysiology, ranging from IEMG activity in the time domain, EMG or IEMG activity in the amplitude domain, and the power spectrum of the EMG signals. The waveform of EMG signals can be distorted in numerous ways, including threshold settings, rectification, and filtering (Loeb & Gans, 1986). Although an important goal in EMG recording is to preserve the original signals with as little distortion as possible, a more serious problem for waveform analyses is when distortion in a signal (e.g., due to filter settings) varies across comparison conditions.

Baselines. As in psychophysiology generally, it is often desirable to obtain both basal measures of activity and response measures that are uncontaminated by the basal (e.g., prestimulus) level of activity. The notion of "basal" activity can be ambiguous when applied to EMG signals, however. This is because the true "physiological baseline" for EMG activity is zero; hence, the lowest empirical baseline for EMG recording is the system noise floor. On these grounds, Fridlund and Izard (1983) questioned the pro forma baseline correction of EMG scores.

In laboratory practice, EMG recording levels seldom show zero activity because the alert experimental subject is rarely completely relaxed. Therefore, it is important to consider the EMG activity that exists in the absence of experimental stimuli both to assess individual differences and to help achieve a measure of the experimental treatments free from prestimulus EMG activity. In assessing basal EMG activity, care is required to avoid any confounding of measurements with task-irrelevant activity (e.g., adaptation, fatigue, apprehension). The procedures commonly used include recording during prestimulus periods and recordings during pseudotrials (Johnson & Lubin, 1972). The use of pseudotrials has the advantage that assessments are obtained under conditions identical to the experimental trials except that there are no experimental stimuli to which to respond.

Obtaining measures of the response free from the influence of prestimulus levels can be more complicated. Perhaps the oldest procedure is to subtract the prestimulus period mean from that observed during the stimulus period. This procedure is satisfactory if mean amplitude is the only parameter of interest and the prestimulus state will not confound the stimulus period state (cf. Caltoppo, Marshall-Goodell, & Dorfman, 1983, pp. 276–277). On the other hand, significant differences across conditions in prestimulus period EMG activity contraindicates the use of this procedure.

A closed-loop baseline procedure offers an alternative to the use of simple change or residualized scores (McHugo & Lanzetta, 1983). Briefly, the presentation of experimental stimuli or treatments is programmed to be contingent on acceptably low levels of somatic activity across the recording sites. In this way, task-specific EMG responses are quantified while minimizing the confounding effects of extraneous muscular activity or basal differences in somatic activity across treatments, a procedure that is reminiscent of Jacobson's (1932) use of progressive relaxation in studies of EMG and imagery. Using a closed-loop baseline has the advantage over simple change scores, too, in that time series (see Gottman, chapter 22) and waveform moment analyses (see Dorfman & Cacioppo, chapter 20) can be performed with fewer restrictions. A potential liability of the closed-loop procedure is that achieving low levels of EMG activity may be one outcome of a subject's idiosyncratic strategies, and experimenters using the closed-loop baseline may be shaping subjects inadvertently for these strategies.

In summary, because the physiological baseline for EMG signals is zero, the rationale for baseline corrections of EMG signals (e.g., covariance analyses, change scores, range corrections) is weak at best. Fridlund, Schwartz, and Fowler (1984) compared baseline-corrected and range-corrected with uncorrected EMG signals and found that corrected EMG scores did not improve the ability to discriminate facial displays within subjects. It is simply unknown at this time whether these corrections would prove useful empirically in discriminating among treatments between subjects.

Standard scores. Standard scores, range-corrected scores, and change scores have been used in an attempt to achieve a metric common to all sites or subjects. For example, standardizing EMG scores within sites and subjects has been used in an attempt to reduce individual and site variability. Although this procedure can provide a powerful means of attenuating individual variability in EMG research, it has limitations that are often unrecognized. Dorfman (cited in Fridlund & Cacioppo, 1986) offered the following numeric illustration (see Table 11.1).

Briefly, let T_i represent a within-subjects treatment and S_j represent a particular subject. Mean EMG measures are presented in the left columns of Table 11.1, and the corresponding standardized EMG measures are in the other two sections. Even though standardization was within subjects, the order of the treatment means $T_1, \ldots T_3$, and the intervals between individual data points within subjects were altered by standardization. If one had used only T_1 and T_2 in this study, both untransformed and z-scores would have indicated that $T_2 > T_1$ (see middle columns of Table 11.1). Such a result might obtain, for instance, if EMG activity over the *corrugator supercilii*

Table 11.1. *Hypothetical data showing hazards of EMG score standardization*

Subjects	Raw scores in hypothetical study 1 $(T_1 - T_2)$ and study 2 $(T_1 - T_3)$					Standard scores in hypothetical study 1				Standard scores in hypothetical study 2				
	T_1	T_2	T_3	X	SD	T_1	T_2	X	SD	T_1	T_2	T_3	X	SD
S_1	3	2	1	2.00	1.00	0.707	−0.707	0.0	1.00	1	0	−1	0.00	1.00
S_2	1	2	10	4.33	4.93	−0.707	0.707	0.0	1.00	−0.675	−0.473	1.15	0.00	1.00
S_3	1	2	10	4.33	4.93	−0.707	0.707	0.0	1.00	−0.675	−0.473	1.15	0.00	1.00
X	1.67	2.00	7.00			−0.236	0.236			−0.120	−0.320	0.43		

muscle region were being recorded and T_1 and T_2 represented imagery conditions that generally evoked mild happiness and anger, respectively.

If this within-subjects study were then perfectly replicated (i.e., the same raw data were obtained in response to T_1 and T_2), but treatment T_3 was added (where, e.g., T_3 represented imagery conditions that generally evoked sadness), then the untransformed scores for T_1 and T_2 would, by definition, remain unchanged. Such a result would, of course, be interpreted as being consistent with the previous study showing that the induction of sadness or anger is associated with increased EMG activity over the *corrugator supercilii* muscle region. Inspection of the raw data reveals there is considerable individual variability in EMG activity, however, and one might reason that these data should be standardized within subjects, purportedly to obtain a measure of the effects of treatments free from individual differences.

Inspection of the z-scores in the right columns of Table 11.1 reveals the potential flaw in this reasoning; the standardized EMG measures now make it *appear* that $T_1 > T_2$. If the raw data were not first inspected, such a result would be interpreted as a failure to replicate the previous study even though the actual outcomes of hypothetical studies 1 and 2 were *identical*. This apparent failure to replicate is attributable entirely to an erroneously applied nonlinear transformation. The point is not that EMG data should never be standardized or transformed, but rather that for the sake of replicability, the application of any nonlinear transformation of EMG signals (or psychophysiological data) should be accompanied both by an explicit justification (cf. Levey, 1980) and an acknowledgment of any differences in the ordering of the untransformed versus transformed means.[7]

11.3.2.5 *Statistical analysis*

Perhaps due to the large number of muscles and to the fact that their coordination is required to communicate, anticipate, adapt, and react, it is analyses of the form or pattern of somatic activity – across sites and across time – that are potentially most informative in psychophysiological research. Before proceeding to a review of some of this research, we discuss briefly selected issues involved in statistical analyses of these data. A more detailed discussion of multivariate analyses of psychophysiological data is provided by Russell (chapter 23; see also Fridlund & Izard, 1983).

Multivariate procedures have several advantages over univariate analyses in EMG research. They provide a quantitative index of whether or not the obtained measures (or subsets of measures) varied as a function of conditions. Second, they can provide information about the configuration of responding across time (e.g., Cacioppo, Petty, & Marshall-Goodell, 1984) or sites (e.g., Fridlund et al., 1984).

There are problems in relying entirely on multivariate procedures, however. First, research in which multiple psychophysiological measures are obtained tends to be expensive to conduct and can yield huge quantities of data even though the number of cases (e.g., subjects) is relatively small. Most multivariate procedures, however, require 8–10 cases per variable per treatment group. An insufficient number of cases in the sample threatens the reliability of the configurations (factor weightings) identified in multivariate analyses of these data.

Second, the results of the analyses can depend heavily on the particular set of variables (in particular, their variance–covariance structure) included in the analysis (Harris, 1975). This is because the inclusion or deletion of another psychophysiological measure or set of measures can affect the variance–covariance structure of the data and lead to dramatic changes in the weighting (i.e., apparent patterning) of one or more measures obtained in the original multivariate analysis. Instability in weights in a multivariate analysis is less of a problem when (1) the psychophysiological measures are not highly correlated, a situation which lessens the chances of variables serving a suppressor or moderator influence on the solutions; (2) obtaining a multivariate effect is sufficient without regard for the dependent variable weights that accounted for it, as when using MANOVA to assess whether or not there is an overall difference across treatments; (3) cross-validation on new data establishes the robustness of the multivariate solution; and (4) the directions of the univariate effects corroborate the multivariate solutions (Fridlund & Cacioppo, 1986). Multivariate data analyses, which appear to reveal order not discernible in univariate or graphical analyses, should be interpreted cautiously, however.

11.3.3   *Social recording basis*

Social factors and processes are of increasing interest to psychophysiologists for several reasons. First, psychophysiological research was once thought to be exempt from the laboratory artifacts that have led others to consider the physical and social context in which the research was conducted (e.g., Rosenthal & Rosnow, 1969). The vulnerability of physiological responses to instructional sets (Sternbach, 1966), intentional distortions (e.g., Ekman, 1985; Honts & Hodes, 1982), and social biases (Ekman & Friesen, 1975; Tognacci & Cook, 1975) vitiates this notion. Nowhere is this vulnerability more apparent in psychophysiology than in studies of the skeletomotor system (Cacioppo, Petty, & Tassinary, 1989; Fridlund & Izard, 1983). A serious consideration of these factors can contribute to the construction of more sensitive, artifact-free psychophysiological experimentation and, hence, to stronger inferences. We begin this section by briefly discussing two major ways in which social factors can contribute to artifactual results in EMG research. Interested readers may also wish to consult Cacioppo, Petty, and Marshall-Goodell (1984, 1985), Christie and Todd (1975), Gale and Baker (1981), Fridlund and Izard (1983), Gale and Christie (1987), and Fridlund and Cacioppo (1986).

A second reason for situational and social factors gaining wider attention in psychophysiology is that these factors have been found to moderate the influence of nonsocial factors on physiological responding. This point, too, is perhaps clearest in studies of skeletomotor response. The expression of a person's joy following successful completion of a task, for instance, can be magnified, attenuated, or masked because of the presence of others. Comprehensive psychophysiological theories must accommodate such moderating influences. We therefore end this section with a brief survey of social moderators of EMG responses to nonsocial stimuli or states. Interested readers may wish to consult Cacioppo, Losch, et al. (1986) and Fridlund (in press) for additional discussions of these and related issues.

11.3.3.1 *Social factors as laboratory artifacts*

As Gale and Baker (1981) noted: "In psychophysiological studies, experimenter–subject interactions are particularly important since the procedures may involve bodily contact, partial removal of clothing, skin abrasion, touching, and application and removal of electrodes" (p. 373). This somewhat unique and extended interaction between subjects and experimenters may result in subjects becoming anxious, distracted, or aware of the experimenter's expectations. In any case, significant laboratory artifacts may be introduced.

Demand characteristics. Orne (1962) suggested that many subjects try to discern the true purpose of an experiment and behave accordingly. To the extent that subjects can discern the experimental hypotheses and manipulate their actions accordingly, EMG studies are vulnerable to experimental demand confounds. Fridlund and Izard (1983) argued that many facial EMG studies of emotion and emotional imagery could be interpreted in terms of demand characteristics. Specifically, they reasoned that placing multiple electrodes on a person's face can make the person acutely aware of her or his facial expressions. Subjects who desired to please the experimenter or contribute to "science" might make faces in accordance with what they believed were the experimental hypotheses. Particularly susceptible, Fridlund and Izard (1983) suggested, were studies in which the experimental hypothesis was obvious, such as the early studies of facial EMG activity during emotional imagery (cf. Schwartz, 1975). Not all previous research using facial EMG to study emotion was susceptible to this interpretation (cf. Cacioppo & Petty, 1979a), and recent studies whose designs minimized experimental demands have still found that subtle emotions could be discriminated using facial EMG (Cacioppo et al., 1984; Cacioppo, Petty, et al., 1986; Fridlund et al., 1984; McHugo, Lanzetta, Sullivan, Masters, & Englis, 1985). Hence, experimental demands do not appear to be necessary for facial EMG patterning during emotions, but they nevertheless remain a potential source of bias in many EMG studies.

A variety of procedures can be used to minimize or assess the effects of experimental demands in EMG research. These include: (1) designing the laboratory setting to minimize subjects' perceptions of being scrutinized; (2) giving subjects peripheral experimental hypotheses; (3) using dummy electrode placements over bodily areas that lower subjects' awareness that voluntary bodily responses are being monitored; (4) employing cover stories that divert subjects' awareness from the fact that physiological actions over which they could exert voluntary control are being recorded[8]; (5) challenging subjects to guess the hypothesis at the end of the study and analyzing suspicious subjects separately; and (6) conducting "simulation" studies in which the EMG study is described to a naive group of subjects, who are then asked to predict how subjects would respond in the setting or how they should respond to confirm the experimenter's hypothesis.

Evaluation apprehension. Naive subjects may be apprehensive about participating in research involving the use of electrodes and electrical recording equipment. Such apprehension, although possibly of interest in its own right (Fridlund, Hatfield, Cottam, & Fowler, 1986), can create a level of tension or hypervigilance in the subject that is unrepresentative and that can obscure the effects of the experimental treatments. This apprehension is in addition to the potential apprehension that subjects may feel about being evaluated by experimenters who are presumably experts in human behavior. Rosenthal (1966) suggested that this "evaluation apprehension" may also lead subjects to distort their actions in a socially desirable fashion. If an experimenter's behavior or experimental treatment makes subjects especially anxious or aware that they are being evaluated, then the data may be significantly biased.

Procedures for minimizing evaluation apprehension have been suggested and, in addition to those outlined in the preceding section, include: (1) providing a tour of portions of the laboratory to prospective subjects while explaining the principles underlying bioelectrical recording, briefly demonstrating hook-up procedures, and briefing them on the tasks and procedures involved in the study prior to seeking informed consent or scheduling them for participation; (2) allowing time before the beginning of the experimental procedures for subjects to adapt to the laboratory; (3) using buffer trials or stimuli to allow adaptation to the experimental procedure; (4) employing a closed-loop baseline to ensure subjects are not tense or aroused before initiating the next trial; and (5) minimizing the sense subjects have that they are being "observed" or evaluated, for instance, by automating procedures, assuring subjects that their responses are anonymous, and using hidden cameras when visually monitoring subjects.

Subject variables as potential independent variables. Finally, various attributes of the subjects can affect EMG measures and, therefore, are important to assess or control by means of the experimental design. These attributes include age; intramuscular temperature, which can be affected by muscle activity as well as ambient temperature; and muscle strength, which is correlated with sex (cf. Goldstein, 1972).

11.3.3.2 *Social determinants of somatic actions*

In the previous section, we saw that the nature of the interaction between the experimenter and subject is a source of both bias in psychophysiological research and a means for its solution. In this section, we briefly review illustrative research demonstrating how social factors can also moderate the influence of nonsocial factors on EMG responses.

Display rules. The classic observations of Charles Darwin (1873/1872) suggested that facial expressions of emotion were universal. The study of emotions was advanced yet further when, building on the pioneering observations of Darwin, it was found that (1) individuals perform at better than chance levels when matching emotion terms to photographs of faces held to represent happiness, sadness, surprise, anger, disgust, and fear; (2) the inductions of states in which individuals report positive and negative emotions are associated with distinctive facial actions; (3) cultural influences can alter significantly these outcomes; (4) displays similar to those of the adult can be found in neonates and the blind as well as sighted adults; (5) specific patterns of activity in the autonomic nervous system are observed when facial prototypes connoting emotion are constructed muscle by muscle and by reliving past experiences reported as emotional; and (6) variability in emotional expressions observed across individuals and cultures could be attributed to factors such as differences in which emotion was evoked or the sequence or blend of emotions evoked and to cultural prescriptions regarding facial display of emotions (e.g., see Ekman, 1973, 1982; Ekman & Friesen, 1978; Ekman, Levenson, & Friesen, 1983; Ekman et al., 1987; Izard, 1971, 1977; Steiner, 1979; Tomkins, 1962).

According to Ekman's notion of display rules, a given emotion will not always be displayed in the same fashion due to the influence of personal habits, situational pressures, and cultural norms. In an early study on display rules, Japanese or American students were exposed to a disgusting film while being videotaped unobtrusively or with an authoritarian experimenter present (Ekman, 1972; Friesen, 1972). Results revealed that both the Japanese and American students displayed revulsions while viewing the film in solitude, but the Japanese students masked their feelings of revulsion by smiling during the film when the experimenter was present (cf. Fridlund, in press).

The influence of an observer on people's facial expressions of emotion emphasizes the dual role played by muscular responses. Because the skeletomotor system is the only means individuals have of approaching, avoiding, or modifying physical elements in their environment, one might expect that somatic responses in part reflect or serve to gratify certain goals or desires. An individual who accidentally touches a hot platter is likely to exhibit a rapid withdrawal, just as an individual who begins to ingest wretched food is likely to express disgust and rapidly expel the offending food (Darwin, 1873/1872).

The skeletomotor system is also the primary means individuals have of communication and effecting change in the social environment. Not surprisingly, therefore, somatic responses such as facial expressions can be affected strongly by the perceived presence of observers. Kraut and Johnson (1979), for instance, related the observed frequency of smiling to simultaneously occurring events in a wide range of naturalistic settings (e.g., bowling alleys, public walkways, hockey arenas). Their results indicated that people were most likely to smile while speaking with other people; they were significantly less likely to smile perceptibly when an event caused them to experience positive emotions (e.g., bowling a strike) when their faces were unobserved than observed (see, also, Fridlund, in press).

Social facilitation and social loafing. Facial expressions of emotion are not the only somatic responses that are affected by the presence of observers. Chapman (1974), for instance, monitored EMG activity over the forehead region as subjects listened to a story while unobserved, watched by a concealed observer, or watched by an unconcealed observer. Chapman found that EMG activity over the forehead region was higher during the story when the subject was observed than when unobserved and slightly though not significantly higher when the observer was present than when concealed. Groff, Baron, and Moore (1983) further demonstrated that the presence of observers led to more vigorous motor responses. These data fit well with observations dating as far back as 1898 demonstrating that an individual's performance on a task can be altered dramatically simply by moving the task from a nonsocial to a social context. Triplett (1898) is credited with being the first to notice that individuals perform well-practiced actions (e.g., bicycle riding) more quickly or vigorously when others were engaged in the same task rather than when alone, and Meumann (1904; cited in Cottrell, 1972) several years later reported the same effect occurred as a result of simple observation. Zajonc (1965) organized much of this research with his proposal that the presence of conspecifics lowered the threshold for the single most likely response to a task. Hence, according to Zajonc's theory of social facilitation, coactors or audiences facilitate the performance of easy tasks and impair the performance of difficult tasks (see review by Geen & Gange, 1977). The important point here is that not only performance but also physiological responses such as EMG activity over the forehead region and the vigor of a forearm flexion have been found to vary as a function of the presence of observers (cf. Cacioppo & Petty, 1986, pp. 658–664).

The presence of others has also been shown to lessen rather than heighten effort and the vigor of somatic responses when by their presence an individual is rendered anonymous or unaccountable for her or his performance. Latane, Williams, and Harkins (1979) have dubbed this effect "social loafing." In an illustrative series of studies, Latane et al. (1979) instructed subjects to clap or shout as loudly as possible. On some trials, subjects were led to believe their individual performance was being monitored, whereas on other trials they were led to believe their performance was being pooled with those of varying numbers of other subjects. On all trials, subjects heard a masking noise through headphones as they clapped or shouted, so they could not tell how loudly they or others were performing. Results revealed that subjects expended more physical effort (i.e., clapped or shouted more loudly) when they believed they were personally accountable for their performance than when they were able to diffuse their responsibility for performing the task. Hence, the presence of others can enhance or reduce muscular responses depending on whether the presence of others increases or decreases the threat of social sanctions or embarrassment based on one's performance.

Mimicry. Mimicry here refers to the elicitation of a localized motor response through witnessing the same response being performed by another. Evidence for motor mimicry includes such demonstrations as wincing at another's pain (Vaughan & Lanzetta, 1980), straining at another's effort (Markovsky & Berger, 1983), and smiling at another's evident delight (Dimberg, 1982). Motor mimicry in psychology has traditionally been conceptualized as primarily intrapersonal, representing either primitive empathy, a conditioned emotional response based on one's direct experience, or an expression of vicarious emotion (Allport, 1968). Consistent with this emphasis, Dimberg (1982) reported that subtle decreases in EMG activity over the *corrugator supercilii* muscle region and increases in EMG activity over the *zygomaticus major* muscle region were observed when subjects viewed pictures of smiling faces, whereas the opposite pattern of facial EMG activity was observed when subjects viewed pictures of angry faces. Englis, Vaughan, and Lanzetta (1982) provided evidence that counterempathic as well as empathic responses could manifest in subtle changes in facial EMG activity.

A recent pair of studies by Bavelas, Black, Lemery, and Mullett (1986) suggests the intensity of *visible* motor mimicry is influenced strongly by the communicative significance of the mimesis as well. For instance, in one study the victim of what appeared to be a painful injury was either increasingly or decreasingly visible to the observing subject. Results revealed that the subject's motor mimicry was signi-

RESPONSE ORIGIN

		Endogenous	Exogenous
RESPONSE PARAMETER	Dependent variable	Double dissociation	Reflex probe
	Independent variable	Conditional probability	Manipulated response

Figure 11.7. Illustrative paradigms in psychophysiological research involving skeletomotor system.

ficantly affected by the visibility of the victim. Thus, the research on mimicry is consistent with the preceding suggestion that social factors can influence somatic responding in the service of interpersonal (i.e., communicative) goals as well as personal feelings and emotions.

11.4 INFERENTIAL CONTEXT

Understanding the physiological basis of EMG and the electrical principles underlying its measurement is important in conducting meaningful research, but it is not sufficient. As Shapiro and Crider (1969, p. 3) noted:

In the most concrete sense, physiological variables are measures of nothing but themselves, and cannot be taken as ready-made indicators of...psychological constructs. A response measure, whether of overt or covert functioning, has meaning only in the context of observation.

General discussions of the issues involved in moving from physiological data to psychological or behavioral inferences have been provided by Cacioppo and Tassinary (chapter 1) and Strube (chapter 2). In this section, we review several general and promising paradigms in psychophysiological studies of EMG activity. In so doing, we also highlight some of the information about cognitive, emotional, and behavioral processes that has come from EMG studies.

11.4.1 *Psychophysiological paradigms*

One of the challenges in psychophysiological research is to create paradigms that allow strong inferences about psychological constructs based on physiological responses. Much of the variety and complexity in the experimental paradigms in this area can be characterized in terms of a 2 (Somatic Response as the Dependent vs. Independent/Blocking Variable) × 2 (Endogenous vs. Exogenous Origin of Somatic Response) multidimensional space (Figure 11.7). Within these general paradigms, answers have been sought to questions regarding the psychological, behavioral, and health significance of somatic activity and the extent to which skeletomotor activity reflects specific or global activation, phasic activation, tonic activation, or modulated thresholds for activation; and characteristics of the stimulus situation or the individual's disposition.

11.4.1.1 *Outcome paradigms*

Outcome paradigms are the simplest and most prevalent in psychophysiology. Although variations include the double-dissociation paradigm and the double-dissociation with constant stimuli paradigm (see subsequent discussion), the essence of the outcome paradigm, as illustrated in Figure 11.7, is that a psychological or behavioral process is manipulated while one or more physiological (e.g., EMG) responses are monitored. Edmund Jacobson's (e.g., 1932) original EMG studies summarized at the beginning of this chapter are cases in point as are studies based on the logic of the subtractive and additive factors methods (see Cacioppo & Tassinary, chapter 1).

Studies conducted within this general paradigm on phasic EMG responses since Jacobson have found that, despite large variations within and across individuals in skeletomotor response, reliable and oftentimes minute patterns of EMG activity accompany thought, emotion, and imagery. Cacioppo and Petty (1981a) summarized this research as follows: (1) there are foci of somatic activity in which changes mark particular psychological processes (e.g., emotion and the mimetic muscles, language processes, and the musculature employed in speech); (2) inhibitory as well as excitatory changes in somatic activity can mark a psychological process; (3) changes in somatic activity are patterned temporally as well as spatially; (4) changes in somatic activity become less evident as the distance of measurement from the focal point increases; and (5) foci can be identified a priori by (a) analyzing the overt reactions that initially characterized the particular psychological process of interest but appeared to drop out with practice and (b) observing the somatic sites that are involved during the "acting out" of the particular psychological process of interest.

In an illustrative study, Shaw (1940) instructed subjects to lift or imagine lifting weights. He found that the amplitude of EMG activity over the preferred arm increased as subjects lifted heavier and heavier weights; this same trend held when subjects imagined lifting the weights. Similarly, Schwartz and his colleagues (e.g., Schwartz et al., 1976; cf. Schwartz, 1975) found that clinically (dysphorically) depressed subjects displayed higher levels of EMG activity over the brow (*corrugator supercilii*) muscle region and lower levels of EMG activity over the cheek (*zygomaticus major*) muscle region when they imagined unpleasant experiences than when they imagined pleasant ones. Nondepressed subjects displayed patterns similar to those produced by the depressed subjects, but the pattern accompanying pleasant imagery was accentuated and the pattern accompanying unpleasant imagery was attenuated in the normal subjects. Furthermore, when the subjects were asked to imagine their typical day, normal subjects displayed a pattern similar to that evinced when they imagined a pleasant experience, whereas depressed subjects displayed a pattern similar to that exhibited while they imagined an unpleasant experience.

Although the early and contemporary EMG research in psychophysiology focused primarily on specific phasic changes in EMG activity, much of the research from 1940 to 1975 focused on general or tonic changes in tension, activation, or arousal (e.g., see reviews by Duffy, 1962; Goldstein, 1972; Malmo, 1959, 1975). Germana (1974), for instance, suggested that although skilled or habitual actions are characterized by a well-orchestrated patterning of skeletomotor activity, response uncertainty leads to a general activation of the musculature. Germana further suggested that the basic significance of this general activation across functionally disparate muscle regions is extensive preparation for overt behavior. Finally, the two conditions identified by Germana as being likely to produce response uncertainty, and consequent somatic activation, were novel stimuli and conditioned stimuli during the initial stages of conditioning. Interestingly, recent research provides some support for Germana's suggestion that the pattern of activation of the musculature during response uncertainty contributes to "a greater equalization within the distribution of behaviorally selective probabilities" (e.g., see Coles et al., 1985; see, also, Coles, Gratton, & Fabiani, chapter 13).

Malmo (e.g., Davis & Malmo, 1951; Malmo, 1965, 1975; Wallerstein, 1954), in contrast, used EMG gradients to depict variations across time in tonic muscle tension. Malmo (1965) summarized his findings as follows: (1) EMG gradients are observed in certain muscles, namely, those that are chronically the most reactive within an individual or those whose actions (or whose paired muscles' actions) are specifically required by the situation, and (2) the steepness of the EMG gradient throughout the entire course of the sequence reflects the stress or effort involved in the entire sequence from beginning to end.

In an illustrative study, subjects played a video game that required they stop a "ball" from passing across the screen by maneuvering a video "bat" to intercept the ball (Svebak, Dalen, & Storfjell, 1981). Subjects rotated a knob held between the thumb and index finger to control the location of the bat. Two versions of the game were employed. In the *easy* version, an unimpeded ball bounced across the screen in approximately 3 s, whereas in the *difficult* version the ball traveled at approximately twice this rate. Both versions required the subject to engage in continuous performance for 150 s, and EMG activity was recorded over the forearm flexor of the passive arm during baseline and task periods. Results revealed the EMG gradient associated with the difficult game was steeper than that associated with the easy game.

In a similar vein but on a shorter time scale, Davis (1940) recorded EMG activity over several muscle regions (e.g., forearm extensors) as subjects performed a choice reaction time task under unwarned, fixed-foreperiod or variable-foreperiod conditions. Davis observed that EMG activity was higher in the foreperiod when the subject was warned than unwarned; EMG activity began to rise approximately 200–400 ms following the warning signal and continued to rise until the overt response was completed; and EMG activity was higher (and reaction time shorter) with a fixed than variable foreperiod. Davis concluded that the EMG responses during the foreperiod reflected a set for motoric response.

Despite these encouraging findings, there is no more consensus within the EMG field than within other fields of psychophysiology regarding which measure best reflects general motivation, tension, or activation. Meyer (1953) suggested eyeblink rate provided the best overall measure of generalized tension. Consistent with the notion that sympathetico-tonia resulted in scleral dryness and increased blinking, Meyer, Bahrick, and Fitts (1953) reported that individuals who score high on anxiety inventories also have high blink rates. However, Rossi (1959) found a similar relationship between manifest anxiety scores and EMG activity over forearm extensors. Similarly, Davis, Malmo, and Shagass (1954) administered white-noise blasts at 1-min intervals to two groups of subjects: individuals with anxiety disorders and normals. Results revealed that although the noise blast evoked a slightly larger EMG response over the forearm extensor region in the anxious than normal individuals, the more significant difference occurred immediately following the stressor. The elevation in EMG activity in normals was sharply delimited, returning to basal levels within seconds of the termination of the noise burst, whereas the elevation in EMG in the anxious subjects lingered.

Fridlund et al. (1986) recently replicated and extended these molar findings using EMG measures over the head, neck, and limbs. Subjects first rested quietly for 15 min and then were exposed to 5 min of 105 dB binaural white-noise stimulation. High-, in contrast to low-, anxious subjects exhibited higher levels of EMG activity primarily over the head and neck preceding the stimulus and more generally during the stimulus. Within-subjects principal components analyses of EMG activity during these periods failed to reveal evidence for a general, intercorrelated tensional factor; instead, the EMG elevations in the highly anxious subjects consisted largely of uncorrelated response bursts. They believed the EMG responses indicated anxious hypervigilance.

Woodworth and Schlosberg (1954, pp. 173–179) made the interesting suggestion that EMG activity, particularly in the neck (e.g., splenius), may be an indicator of the level of activation due to the possibility that a disproportionate share of proprioceptive impulses to the central nervous system originated in this muscle region. This suggestion is interesting in light of the sparse evidence for the notion of a coherent tensional factor (e.g., see Fridlund, Fowler, & Pritchard, 1980). Consistent with Woodworth and Schlosberg's suggestion, Eason and White (1961) had subjects perform a variety of vigilance tasks (e.g., rotary tracking) while recording EMG activity over the *splenius* and *trapezius* of the neck, *trapezius* of the shoulder, and the *deltoid* and *biceps* of the right arm. The major finding in these studies was that the general level of EMG activity (most consistently that recorded over the neck muscles) varied as a function of the effort subjects expended on tasks.

In summary, substantial increases in task difficulty, the subjective effort expended on tasks, or stressors have been found to lead to elevated EMG activity over the neck in seated subjects during vigilance tasks and in task-relevant musculature in general. In addition, an inhibition of EMG activity over irrelevant musculature is sometimes observed during such tasks, particularly when the response to the task is well practiced (e.g., see Germana, 1974; Goldstein, 1972). Although these findings contradict the simple-minded view of general tension or arousal, this research clearly indicates that muscle tonus can be an informative outcome measure:

> The literature of muscle tonus has been burdened in the past and is still being burdened by observations which have not taken into account the functional significance of tonic activity. Tonic manifestations have been sought for indiscriminately in all muscles, at all times, and not infrequently the operative procedure of the investigator has caused the very tonicity he has sought for to vanish. (Fulton, 1926, p. 384)

11.4.1.2 *Double-dissociation paradigm*

Whether EMG changes reflect specific actions and patterns or general somatic changes often has important theoretical implications. The *double-dissociation paradigm* from physiological psychology (Teuber, 1955) can therefore be particularly powerful in EMG research. This paradigm is so named because: (1) one or more treatments that should evoke a specific somatic action or pattern is contrasted with one or more treatments that should not evoke the target action or pattern and (2) one or more measures of the target somatic response are included as well as one more measures of nontarget somatic response. The former establishes discriminant validity of the treatments, whereas the latter demonstrates the discriminant validity of the responses.

To illustrate, there has long been a hypothesis that silent-language processing is associated with increased activation of the speech (e.g., perioral) musculature (see McGuigan, 1978). As McGuigan (1970) noted, there are a number of studies demonstrating that EMG activity over the perioral musculature increased from basal levels when individuals engaged in silent-language processing. These results alone are not particularly informative because such a psychophysiological outcome could be attributed to aspects of the task that had nothing to do with language processing (e.g., orthographic or auditory analyses may be associated with a tensing of the lips) or to general increases in tension or arousal (e.g., due to the motivation or apprehension that stemmed from the presentation of the task). The inclusion of nonlanguage as well as language tasks speaks to the first of these interpretational problems, and the measurement of EMG activity over nontarget as well as target sites speaks to the second.

In most applications of the double-dissociation paradigm, different subjects or stimuli are used to achieve treatments that theoretically should and should not evoke a specific somatic action or pattern. In a particularly comprehensive series of studies, for instance, McGuigan and Bailey (1969) recorded EMG activity over the chin, tongue, and forearm muscle regions while subjects silently read, memorized prose, listened to prose, listened to music, and attentively listened to "nothing." Results revealed that EMG activity over the perioral musculature increased dramatically while subjects performed silent-language tasks.

Double dissociation with constant stimuli. Although the outcome observed by McGuigan and Bailey (1969) is consistent with the hypothesis that silent-language processing leads to increased perioral EMG activity, Cacioppo and Petty (1979b, 1981b) noted that the grounds for such an inference would be strengthened further if the subjects and the physical characteristics of the target stimuli were held constant within the double-dissociation paradigm. In an illustrative study, EMG activity was monitored over the *inferior orbicularis oris* and the *superficial forearm flexor* muscle regions while subjects responded to questions about visual presentations of trait adjectives (Cacioppo & Petty, 1979b). The treatment condition was varied by what subjects were asked about a set of stimuli rather than by varying subjects or stimuli. Specifically, half the questions required that subjects perform a semantic analysis of the stimulus word (e.g., "Is the following descriptive of you?"), whereas half did not (e.g., "Is the following printed in uppercase letters?"). In addition, half of the trait adjectives within each treatment condition were self-descriptive, and half were not; half were printed in uppercase letters and half in lowercase letters; and half of the questions for each type of task called for a button press signifying yes, whereas half called for a button press signifying no. Results revealed EMG activity over the perioral region was greater during the language than nonlanguage task, whereas EMG activity over the nonpreferred forearm did not differ as a function of task. Because the type of stimulus presented or type of subject tested did not vary along with the extent of silent-language processing presumed to be manipulated in this double-dissociation design, one can be somewhat more confident that silent-language processing involving short-term memory leads to increased EMG activity over the perioral region.

11.4.1.3 *Conditional probability paradigm*

Most psychologists, like many psychophysiologists, have sought to use physiological data to infer psychological or behavioral constructs such as anxiety, emotion, and depression. In this effort, the target physiological events have been identified as those that have been shown to vary as a function of the theoretical construct of interest. Electromyographic activity over the forehead region has been of interest, for instance, because anxiety and tension are often accompanied by increased EMG activity over this site. However, knowing that the manipulation of a psychological or behavioral factor leads to a particular somatic response does not logically imply that this somatic response indexes the psychological or behavioral factor (see Cacioppo & Tassinary, 1989). Chapter 1 outlined how probability theory can be used to guide the construction of comparison conditions. Briefly, let Ψ represent the abstract construct of interest and Φ represent skeletomotor activity. It should be clear from probability theory that $P(\Psi/\Phi)$ cannot be assumed to equal $P(\Phi/\Psi)$, as they can differ dramatically. In fact, however, $P(\Psi/\Phi) = P(\Psi, \Phi)/[P(\Psi, \Phi) + P(\text{Not} - \Psi, \Phi)]$. Hence, it can be seen that the utility of the target skeletomotor response to serve as an index of an abstract construct is weakened by the occurrence of the skeletomotor response in the absence of the construct of interest (see chapter 1).

Although one cannot logically identify all possible factors that might influence the target skeletomotor response/pattern, the preceding formula makes it clear that information about the value of a target physiological response/pattern as an index of a construct can be gained by quantifying the extent to which the construct of interest is present given the presence of the target physiological response. That is, one can block on the presence or absence of the target skeletomotor response (or on variations of the target physiological response) and analyze the extent to which the construct of interest is evident. In so doing, an endogenous skeletomotor response pattern is used as a blocking variable (see Figure 11.7).

Cacioppo et al. (1988) utilized a conditional probability paradigm to examine the extent to which specific forms of EMG response over the brow region indexed variations in emotions evoked during an interview. As noted in the preceding, previous research has demonstrated that mild negative emotional imagery and unpleasant sensory stimuli tends to lead to more EMG activity over the brow (*corrugator supercilii*) and less EMG activity over the cheek (*zygomaticus major*) and ocular (*orbicularis oculi*) muscle regions than mild positive imagery and stimuli. This previous research did *not* address whether facial EMG responses provided a sensitive and specific index of emotions, however, since there is a multiplicity of events that can change facial EMG activity. To address this question, Cacioppo et al. (1988) obtained facial EMG and audiovisual recordings while individuals were interviewed about themselves. Afterward, individuals were asked to describe what they had been thinking during specific segments of the interview marked by distinctive EMG responses over the brow region in the context of ongoing but stable levels of activity elsewhere in the face. Consistent with the notion that expressive/behavioral components of emotion are "*sometimes brought unconsciously into momentary action by ludicrously slight causes*" (Darwin, 1873/1872, p. 184), minute EMG responses over the *corrugator supercilii* muscle region were observed to covary with subtle variations in emotion during the interview even though the overt facial expressions evinced by subjects were rated similarly across conditions by observers. Furthermore, it was reasoned that certain forms of EMG response, such as jagged bursts rather than graded increases and decreases in EMG activity, would be especially predictive of variations in emotion due to theoretical differences in $P(\text{Not-}\Psi, \Phi)$.[9] Support for this reasoning was also found. These results illustrate the power of the conditional probability paradigm and provide evidence that specific patterns of facial EMG response can actually *index* variations in emotion, at least within this limited context (see, also, Fridlund et al., 1984).

Interestingly, a classic study by Max (1935) can be viewed within this paradigm as well. Max hypothesized that EMG activity would increase during problem solving and that this activity would be evident not only in the speech musculature of normal speaking individuals, but also in the hands of deaf mutes (since their speech originated in their fingers). In a test of this reasoning, EMG activity was recorded over the arm and finger muscles as normal and deaf subjects slept. Max observed a general decrease in EMG activity as subjects fell asleep, and occasional bursts of EMG activity were observed over the finger muscles during their sleep. When the latter occurred, subjects were awakened and were asked to report if and what they had been dreaming. Max (1935) found that EMG activity over the finger muscles was associated with dreaming in the deaf subjects but not in the normals.

Shimizu and Inoue (1986) recently completed a study of sleep and dreams that bears on the utility of perioral EMG activity as a marker of silent-language processing in normals as well. Electroencephalographic (EEG), electrooculographic (EOG), perioral EMG, and nonoral EMG activity were recorded as subjects slept. Subjects were awakened during either rapid eye movement (REM) or Stage 2 sleep, as determined by inspection of the EEG and EOG recordings. When subjects reported dreaming, subjects were asked whether or not they had been speaking in their dreams. Dream recall during REM sleep occurred in approximately 80% of the awakenings, and it occurred during Stage 2 sleep in approximately 28% of the awakenings. Awakenings without dream recall were excluded from further analyses, as were awakenings preceded by phasic discharges in the perioral musculature that were accompanied by any whispering or vocalization. Results revealed that when phasic discharges over the perioral musculature were observed within the 30 s preceding the awakening, subjects reported having been speaking in their dreams in 88% of the awakenings from REM sleep and 71% of the awakenings during State 2 sleep. Moreover, when phasic discharges over the perioral musculature were not observed within the 30 s preceding the awakening, subjects reported having been speaking in their dreams in only 19% of the awakenings from REM sleep and in none of the awakenings during Stage 2 sleep.

In summary, previous research has indicated that situations in which subjects report negative emotional reactions are accompanied by EMG activity over regions of the mimetic muscles (e.g., the brow) and that silent-language and numeric tasks that load working memory influence the EMG activity over the speech muscle region. The research reviewed in this section further suggests that EMG discharges over the brow and over the muscle regions involved in speech can be used in at least some situations (see chapter 1) to mark episodes of affect and silent-language processing, respectively.

11.4.1.4 *Reflex paradigms*

We have made the case throughout the chapter that the skeletomotor system is a primary means through which the organism interacts with its environment. A detailed discussion of how environmental information is transformed into observable skeletomotor activity is beyond the scope of this chapter, although the interested reader is referred to the excellent tutorial by Gallistel (1980). Other theoretical discussions of traditional and recent approaches to this problem can be found in Asby (1960) and Kugler and Turvey (1987), respectively. However, in order to convey some of the issues involved, we first describe what is arguably the simplest internal mechanism for mediating organismic–environmental transactions (i.e., the monosynaptic reflex) and then briefly describe how this mechanism can be used to probe ongoing psychophysiological processes. The reader further interested in the history of the reflex is encouraged to consult the monographs by Fearing (1930) and Liddell (1960).

Definition. Reflexes generally refer to any automatic reaction of the nervous system to stimuli impinging upon the body or arising within it (Merton, 1987). Although there have been clear analytical attempts to define the concept of the reflex in precise logical and empirical terms from within both physiology (Sherrington, 1923/1906) and psychology (Skinner, 1931), the definition of the reflex and the functional significance of reflexes in the intact organism remain active topics of research (e.g., Berkinblit, Feldman, & Fukson, 1986).

From a physiological perspective, reflexes can be defined as a discrete type of behavior mediated by a reflex arc, thus providing both functional and structural constraints on the definition (Gallistel, 1980). Structurally, a reflex arc is an anatomical entity consisting of (1) receptors, tuned to transduce to specifiable classes of environmental stimuli into neural signals; (2) sensory neurons, which conduct the output signals from the receptors to the central nervous system (CNS); (3) mediators, either a single synapse or a small set of interneurons, that relay the sensory output to an appropriate subset of motoneurons or neurohumoral cells; (4) motoneurons/neurohumoral cells, which conduct the signal from the CNS to particular effectors; and (5) the effectors themselves, which impact on the environment as a function of neural and/or hormonal input.

Functionally, four conditions must be met in order for a particular behavior to be classified as reflexive. First, the effector response to any single sensory stimulus of sufficient intensity to actually elicit a response must rise to a single peak and then decline rapidly. Second, response duration and amplitude must be determined strictly by the intensity of the elicitor and current states of the intervening synapses and effector organs. Third, signal conduction can proceed in only one direction ("the irreversibility of conduction"). And finally, the actual result of the activation of the effectors cannot directly modify subsequent effector output (i.e., there should be no feedback from the effectors to any part of the reflex arc).

From a psychological perspective, Skinner (1931) argued that the concept of the reflex is fundamentally both behavioral and statistical and that it reduces simply to "the observed correlation of the activity of an effector (i.e., a response) with the observed forces affecting a receptor (i.e., a stimulus)" (p. 438). He argued that the functional attributes of unlearned, unconscious, and involuntary as well as any physiological attributes so often claimed to define a reflex were actually incidental properties of the class of reflexes that were first discovered and investigated by neurophysiologists. Generalizing the concept beyond its historical beginnings, he partitioned the experimental study of the reflex into two parts. First, there is the investigation of the correlation between a specifiable stimulus class (*S*) and response class (*R*), that is, the latency, threshold, and range of variation in *S* and *R* over which the correlation holds. Second, there is the investigation of variations in these characteristics as a function of third variables. This latter investigation would include assessing changes in reflex strength (i.e., the magnitude of the correlation) as a function of variables such as motivation, drive, response preparation, and so on.

Reflex probe technique. Since the turn of the century, the scientific study of the reflex has proceeded in two directions. Disciplines concerned with the control of movement (e.g., neurophysiology, physiological psychology, psychology) have generally followed the tradition of Sherrington (1923/1906) and examined reflexes as integral to the regulation of behavior. Predicated on this view of the reflex as a relatively invariant unit of behavior, the accompanying research and theory focuses on specifying the rules by which reflexes combine to generate coordinated, goal-directed movements.

In neurology and psychophysiology, however, the reflex is viewed in a manner more consistent with the behaviorist generalization of the concept articulated by Skinner. In the field of neurology this conceptualization led initially to widespread confusion, with the early part of the century referred to as an open season for the "hunting of the reflex" (Wartenberg, 1946). During this time, any stimulus–response correlation was "fair game" to be named and reified. An unfortunate result was that many reflexes were "discovered" by one author after another, each time renamed and claimed to be unique.

However, it is now possible to use parameters of reflex responses as markers of CNS function (Kimura, 1973) because of increasingly detailed information about the neural circuits mediating specific reflexes (Ongerboer de Visser, 1983) and the development of standardized testing conditions (Bickerstaff, 1975; Desmedt, 1973; Hugon, 1973). For example, Kimura, Giron, and Young (1976) divided 81 Bell's palsy patients into two groups based on temporal changes in the electrically elicited direct and reflex blink responses. Direct blinks were those evoked by the stimulation of the motoneuron axons, whereas reflex blinks were those evoked by sensory nerves. The results were striking: All of the 56 patients who maintained direct motor responses until the recovery of the blink reflex experienced at least a 50 percent recovery of facial nerve function at the end of 2 months, whereas none of the 25 patients who had lost direct blink responses prior to reflex recovery demonstrated any indication of facial nerve function at the end of 2 months.

As a tool in the investigation of psychological processes, surface electromyography provides an ongoing record of muscular activity while minimally interfering with the behavior under study. The unique advantage of the reflex probe technique, however, is that it allows estimation of changes in the excitability of spinal and brainstem motor structures that may be manifest in neither overt behavior nor in peripheral EMG activity. The use of the reflex as a probe into ongoing psychological processes further exemplifies the examining of variations in reflex characteristics as a function of third variables. Although Skinner (1931) intended this experimental procedure to be used to quantify the influences of external variables on the reflex behavior of intact organisms, that logic of the situation allows one to use variations in reflex strength as an indicant of internal psychological processes as well. In the former case the focus is on the description of behavior, whereas in the latter case one infers the operation of either intervening variables or hypothetical constructs.

Early investigations of reflexes revealed that psychological factors (i.e., attention) could impact on aspects of reflex response. Clinical neurologists looked upon these influences as nuisance variables, factors that could increase the likelihood of both false positives and false negatives in their diagnosis of CNS function. However, the enormous potential to use such procedures in psychophysiological investigations was apparent from the turn of the century (Dodge, 1911; Sherrington, 1923/1906). Surprisingly, for reasons that remain somewhat unclear (see Ison & Hoffman, 1983), the use of this technique was sporadic until the mid-1960s and early 1970s.

The power of the reflex probe technique for psychophysiological inference can be most clearly seen in the work on attentional processes (e.g., Anthony, 1985; Graham, Stock, & Zeigler, 1981) and on response preparation (e.g., Boelhouwer, Bruggemans, & Brunia, 1987; Brunia, 1984). For example, Anthony (1985) reviews numerous experiments on the modulation of the blink reflex by manipulations affecting attention. The general conclusion from such studies is that the amplitude and/or latency of the blink can be used in specific situations to measure how attention is allocated to different sensory modalities. Specifically, in paradigms in which the subject is warned of an impending target stimulus, the amplitude of the blink is reliably enhanced or suppressed in the warning interval as a function of the match or mismatch, respectively, between the modalities of the two stimuli. In addition, reliable changes in the degree of facilitation or inhibition across the warning interval suggest that the selective allocation of attention may begin as early as the onset of the warning stimulus but that the rate of allocation speeds up dramatically approximately 2 s before the onset of the target stimulus (cf. Davis, 1940).

11.4.1.5 Manipulated response paradigms

Questions about the contributions of skeletomotor actions to psychological states or processes have typically been addressed by manipulating skeletomotor actions to achieve the desired configuration, verifying the configuration using some observational procedure such as Ekman and Friesen's (1978) facial action coding system and measuring the outcome variables of interest (e.g., subjective states, autonomic responses; see Figure 11.7). Although skeletomotor actions have occasionally been manipulated through operant conditioning procedures (e.g., Hefferline, Keenan, & Harford, 1959; McCanne & Anderson, 1987), the most common approaches have been to instruct subjects either to exaggerate/suppress general skeletomotor configurations or to achieve a particular pose by varying the actions of individual muscles (e.g., see reviews by Laird, 1984; Matsumoto, 1987).

Muscle-by-muscle induction paradigm. In an illustrative study utilizing the muscle-by-muscle induction variant of this general approach, Ekman et al. (1983) instructed individuals to contract individual muscles until prototypes of the expressions of happiness, sadness, fear, anger, disgust, or surprise were constructed. The construction of each emotional expression was preceded by the construction of an equally effortful nonemotional expression. Each expression was held for 10 s and was subsequently verified as having been achieved by the experimenter. Averaged data during emotional faces minus that during nonemotional ones revealed that the anger face was associated with elevated heart rate and palmar skin temperature, fear and sad faces were associated with elevated heart rate and relatively low levels of palmar skin temperature, and the remaining expressions were associated with relatively low levels of heart rate and skin temperature.

Research utilizing the muscle-by-muscle induction paradigm has sometimes yielded inconsistent results (e.g., Tourangeau & Ellsworth, 1979; cf. Tassinary et al., 1989). Methodological issues that could contribute to inconsistent results and flawed interpretations include improper controls for somatic tension or effort; floor and ceiling effects in emotional responding; and the specification and construction of the appropriate configuration of skeletomotor actions, at appropriate levels of intensity overall and relative to one another, with naturalistic durations and appropriate forms of response across time. Interested readers might wish to see relevant commentaries by Cacioppo and Petty (1986), Fridlund (1988), Hager and Ekman (1981), Laird (1984), and Matsumoto (1987).

Exaggeration–suppression paradigm. Vaughan and Lanzetta (1981) employed the exaggeration–suppression variant of this paradigm to assess the possible influence of facial expressions on vicarious emotional arousal. Subjects were exposed to a videotaped model displaying pain, ostensibly from receiving electric shocks. One group of subjects was instructed to *inhibit* any facial expressions when the model was shocked, a second group was instructed to *amplify* their facial expressions when the model was shocked, and a third (*control*) group received no instructions about modulating their facial expressions. Results revealed that the amplify group exhibited larger skin conductance responses, heart rate increases, and facial EMG activity in response to the model's display of pain than the other two groups, which did not differ from one another.

Based on the emerging research showing that manipulations of overt facial expressions can influence affective responses, Wells and Petty (1980) tested the hypothesis that affectively relevant bodily movements could also influence attitudinal responses toward a persuasive appeal. Specifically, head movements (nodding in agreement or disagreement) were chosen for study because of their strong association with agreeing and disagreeing responses in a wide variety of cultures (Eibl-Eibesfeldt, 1972). Darwin (1873/1872), in fact, suggested that head shaking has a universal negative meaning that originated from food refusal.

In their study, subjects were led to believe that they were participating in con-summer research on the sound quality of stereo headphones; in particular, how the headphones tested (e.g., in terms of sound quality, comfort) when listeners were engaged in movement (e.g., walking, dancing, jogging). One group of subjects was told that they should move their heads up and down once per second to test the headphones (vertical head movements condition), a second was told to move their heads from side to side once per second (horizontal head movements condition), and a third (control) group was told nothing about head movements. After subjects were given the instructions, a tape from a purported campus radio program was played. The tape began and ended with music, and a "station editorial" was introduced between the two musical selections. Subjects either heard an editorial in favor of raising tuition at their university or one in favor reducing tuition. The key dependent measure was what subjects indicated tuition at their university should be. Results revealed that although subjects believed the appropriate level of tuition was higher following the "increase tuition" than "decrease tuition" editorial, a significant interaction revealed that subjects in the vertical-head-movements condition advocated more tuition than subjects in the horizontal-head-movements condition following the "increase tuition" message, and the opposite occurred following the "decrease tuition" message; in both instances, judgments by subjects in the control condition fell between these two. That is, vertical head movements led to greater agreement with the message in both cases than did horizontal head movements. Whether these results reflect the effects of peripheral feedback per se or of memories and cognitive sets that might have been evoked by the head movements remains to be determined.

11.4.2   Range of applications

As we describe throughout this chapter, the surface EMG technique is valuable in studying a variety of psychological and behavioral processes. The technique also finds wide use in clinical practice, research, and forensics. We list a few general areas to illustrate the breadth of its application.

11.4.2.1   Headache and stress reduction

A popular use of surface EMG detection is in clinical biofeedback for tension headache and stress reduction. This use stemmed from a clinical report by Budzynski and Stoyva (1969), who used EMG activity from a bilateral forehead site over the *lateral frontalis*. In the typical clinical regimen, patients hear tones or clicks whose pitch or rate varies with the envelope of the smoothed, rectified electromyogram; patients learn to lower the tone or click rate by relaxing their muscles. Budzynski and Stoyva promulgated "frontalis EMG biofeedback" as a treatment for muscle contraction ("tension") headache, but this procedure was soon extended to general stress management (e.g., Stoyva & Budzynski, 1974).

Budzynski and Stoyva chose the *frontalis* site because they claimed that muscle tention there was uniquely indicative of whole-body tension. This rationale was eventually discredited, both in normals (Alexander, 1975; Fridlund, Cottam, & Fowler, 1982; Fridlund et al., 1980; Shedivy & Kleinman, 1977; Whatmore, Whatmore, & Fisher, 1981) and in anxious students (Fridlund et al., 1986).

The rash of frontalis EMG biofeedback studies published in biofeedback's halcyon days consisted mostly of case reports and uncontrolled clinical trials (see Alexander & Smith, 1979, for review), and the claimed incremental efficiacy over simple relaxation or meditation techniques is in doubt. The few studies that were done with adequate controls indicated the EMG biofeedback for stress control is equivalent in efficacy to the panoply of stress-reduction techniques. By 1980, an NIMH report on claims for EMG biofeedback's unique efficacy in headache and stress management was skeptical (NIMH, 1980). Moreover, the last ten years have seen a devaluation of the role of muscle tension in "tension" headache (Chun, 1985), and an emphasis on vascular dysfunction, secondary ischemia, and nocigenic metabolites in the etiology (Pikoff, 1984). Clinicians now tend to use "frontalis EMG biofeedback" as a variant of relaxation training.

Psychosomatic medicine researchers in the 1940s and 1950s were interested in painful, idiopathic muscular contractions occurring in stress or conflict (Malmo, 1965; Malmo & Shagass, 1949a, b; Malmo, Shagass, Belanger, & Smith, 1951; Malmo, Shagass, & Davis, 1951; Malmo & Smith, 1955). These examples of "symptom specificity" have occasionally been treated with EMG biofeedback to relax the muscles. However, these idiopathic contractions are today regarded most often as secondary to any number of disorders, including joint disturbance (e.g., temporomandibular joint disorder), major depression, Briquet's syndrome, anxiety disorders, or infectious illness. Treatment of the primary disorder is the preferred intervention.

11.4.2.2 *Physical medicine and rehabilitation*

Basmajian (1963) confirmed early the supposition that given sufficiently precise feedback, individuals could learn to control single motor units. His finding, and his pioneering application of EMG biofeedback methods in physical medicine, soon led to the widespread use of surface EMG to enhance recovery of function in muscles that were rendered nonfunctional by stroke, illness, and accidents (Basmajian & DeLuca, 1985). In the rehabilitation setting, feedback derived from the surface EMG signal is used, depending upon the disorder, either to relax or tense spastic muscles (e.g., chronic unilateral neck spasms; spastic cerebral palsy; see DeBacher, 1979) or to activate atrophied or functionally denervated muscles (e.g., hemiplegia from stroke; Basmajian, Kukulka, Narayan, & Takebe, 1975). Following facial anastomosis surgery (graft of a facial nerve branch from the functional side of the lower face to the nonfunctional side, often after a stroke has induced hemiparesis), biofeedback is often used to restore bilateral symmetry to the hemiparetic face.

Electromyographic biofeedback in rehabilitation is now standard procedure, and there were early reports of incremental efficacy over standard physical therapy (see Fernando & Basmajian, 1978). Despite this early enthusiasm, it is still not clear that the mechanism of the EMG biofeedback is the source of its putative efficacy. Most individuals with neuromuscular disability are chronically depressed, and their hopes for success of the biofeedback often ameliorate the depression and rejuvenate their efforts in physical therapy.

11.4.2.3 *Forensic polygraphy*

Canny criminal suspects who undergo a polygraph test often use a variety of countermeasures to foil the test. By pressing their toes hard against the floor or biting their tongues, they can generate autonomic responses that confuse the polygraph examiner (Honts, Hodes, & Raskin, 1985; Reid & Inbau, 1977). Recently, Honts, Raskin, and Kircher (1983) found that surface EMG detected from the examinee's gastrocnemius (anterior thigh) and temporalis (temple) muscles permitted detection of 90 percent of experimental subjects who used tongue biting or toe pressing to defeat the test. Using surface EMG is not routine in polygraphy because of both its novelty and the added expense of the EMG equipment. We expect that it will become used more widely.

11.4.2.4 *Polysomnography*

In studies of sleep, the onset of paradoxical or rapid eye movement (REM) sleep is reliably accompanied by a loss of normal muscle activity in the face and limbs. This loss of tension is thought to block the acting out of dreams. In both clinical and research polysomnography (i.e., measurement during sleep of physiological responses like heart rate, sweat gland response, respiration, eye movement, etc.; see Rechtschaffen & Kales, 1968), surface EMG is typically recorded from the chin, over the *mentalis* muscle (whose action elevates the chin boss). Changes in activity over this site corroborate transitions to and from paradoxical sleep (Kupfer & Reynolds, 1983). Surface EMG has also been used to study: (1) leg spasms in nocturnal myclonus ("restless legs syndrome"); (2) abdominal actions in airway apneas (breathing difficulties due to paradoxical sleep-related epiglottal collapse); and (3) nocturnal bruxism, or tooth grinding (see Association of Sleep Disorders Centers, 1979; Guilleminault, 1982; Hauri, 1977).

11.4.2.5 *Miscellaneous*

Surface EMG is a viable, precise way of measuring muscular contraction in an ongoing fashion in many situations wherein observation is too imprecise or awkward. In addition to those uses we detailed, we just mention a few more: (1) measuring eyeblink rates and amplitudes in conditioning and vigilance studies; (2) determining muscle tension in ergonomic design and man–machine interface studies; (3) timing and quantifying precisely the onset of responses in reaction time tasks, including incipient responses that precede the overt response; (4) corroborating timing or force irregularities in neurological finger-tapping tasks; and (5) discerning the specific muscles that maintain posture, coordinate gait, and participate in skilled acts.

With the decreasing expense of the instrumentation required for sensitive and precise EMG measurement, the availability of guidelines and standards, and the emergence of conceptual frameworks and paradigms to aid in the interpretation of EMG responses, the surface EMG technique should find even wider application.

11.5   CONCLUSION

The skeletomotor system has been central to the field of neurophysiology since Francesco Redi's indirect observation in 1666 that living muscles generate electrical current. The centrality of the skeletomotor system within the field of psychology is illustrated by William James's (1890) early suggestion that the "Will" (i.e., an idea or image) triggers the waiting musculature:

> We may then lay it down for certain that every representation of a movement awakens in some degree the actual movement which is its object; and awakens it in a maximum degree whenever it is not kept from doing so by an antagonistic representation present simultaneously to the mind....We do not have a sensation or a thought and then have to *add* something dynamic to get a movement. (pp. 526–527)

Moreover, the concepts of muscle activation, muscle tension, and skeletomotor patterning have long been related to thinking (e.g., Jacobson, 1932; James, 1890; McGuigan, 1978), feeling (e.g., Darwin, 1873/1872; James, 1884), behaving, imagined or real (e.g., Jacobson, 1932; Shaw, 1940), sleeping (e.g., Larson & Foulkes, 1969; Max, 1935), and learning (e.g., Bills, 1927; Courts, 1942) and to the constructs of motivation (e.g., Bartoshuk, 1955; Malmo, 1965), arousal or activation (e.g., Kennedy & Travis, 1948; Woodworth & Schlosberg, 1954), attention (e.g., Lynn, 1966; Pavlov, 1927), personality (e.g., Goldstein, 1964), psychosomatic disease (e.g., Malmo, Shagass, & Davis, 1950; Malmo, 1975), and psychopathology and psychotherapy (e.g., Jacobson, 1938).

Early theories attempted to explain many psychological processes entirely in terms of peripheral skeletomotor actions. This resulted in an exciting and active period for psychophysiology, but the disconfirmation of categorical predictions made by these motor theories was inevitable, resulting in a brief downturn in interest in transient or weak skeletomotor actions. Nonetheless, many interesting results from this early period have been replicated, however, and coupled with advances in signal acquisition and analysis, these data are being incorporated within theoretical frameworks highlighting the integrated actions of the central and peripheral nervous systems. As illustrated in this chapter, contemporary EMG studies are diverse. Among the key directions are: (1) the spatial and temporal patterning that characterizes specific organismic–environmental transactions; (2) incipient actions of the skeletomotor system and their relation to ongoing psychological processes; (3) surface EMG in studies of the potential influence of striated muscle actions and patterns on supraphysiological constructs such as thought, emotion, and motivation; (4) the diagnosis and therapeutic use of EMG in psychopathology and psychosomatic disorders; and (5) interactions between the skeletomotor and other physiological systems (see, also, Papillo & Shapiro, chapter 14; Coles et al., chapter 13). These directions, we believe, bode well for EMG research in psychology.

NOTES

Preparation of his chapter was supported by National Science Foundation Grant Nos. BNS-8414853, BNS-8706156, and BNS-8940915.

1 Interested readers may wish to consult Fulton (1926), Wu (1984), and Brazier (1959) for additional details about the history of muscle physiology and electromyography. Readers interested in additional details about the physical basis and neural control of muscle contraction are encouraged to consult the recent works of Hoyle (1983) and Loeb and Gans (1986), and those interested in more information about related clinical applications are encouraged to consult Monnier (1970).

2 This was also the first evidence of the injury current in muscles, which is the current flow resulting from the potential difference between injured and intact tissue (Wu, 1984). Extensive study of this phenomenon during the nineteenth century resulted in the discovery of the action potential.

3 Volta's study of muscle actions contributed significantly to his inventing the first electric battery. Volta's battery was constructed by interposing layers of two different metals and pasteboards and soaking them in salt water. Volta asserted that this "artificial electric organ" was essentially the same as the natural electric organ of the torpedo or electric eel (Wu, 1984).

4 It is the closer spacing that can be achieved with small electrodes, not their higher electrode impedances, which enables greater recording selectivity: "Only closely spaced bipolar electrodes with differential amplification can make such recordings spatially selective" (Loeb & Gans, 1986, p. 24).

5 One important implication is that a failure to find significant treatment differences in EMG activity could be due to the selection of an inappropriate recording bandpass rather than to an actual absence in EMG activity across treatments. It is often advisable, therefore, to use a wide bandpass (e.g., 10–500 or 1,000 Hz) when recording EMG activity and subsequently apply filters to copies of the stored data.

6 The rms of the EMG signal can be calculated by summing the squares of each EMG amplitude within a recording bin, and performing the square root (see Marshall-Goodell et al., chapter 4). The rms is superior to mean amplitude as a measure of sinusoidal alternating current, and Basmajian and DeLuca (1985) have extended this argument to motor unit action potentials as well. It is of interest to note that the measures of mean amplitude, rms amplitude, and total electrical energy are closely related mathematically, with each emphasizing a different aspect of the amplitude distribution of a waveform. Interested

readers may wish to consult Cacioppo and Dorfman (1987). For alternative forms of averaging, see Basmajian and DeLuca (1985), Fridlund and Cacioppo (1986), or Dorfman and Cacioppo (chapter 20).

7 One common practice is to conduct analyses on standardized scores but present means of the raw data. It should be clear, however, that this practice can also be misleading in instances such as that depicted in Table 11.1. Finally, although the example discussed in the text focused on the use of standard scores to achieve a "comparable" metric across subjects, it is simple to demonstrate that the same limitations can arise when using standard scores to obtain comparability across recording sites.

8 For instance, Cacioppo, Petty, et al. (1986) placed electrodes on the side and back of the head and neck as well as on subjects' face and body; and subjects were told that the electrodes were placed around their brain to help isolate and identify the neural processes involved in processing pictorial stimuli through a process of triangulation. To the extent that the electrodes on the body and the dummy electrodes on the neck and head diverted subjects' attention from their voluntary facial actions, which debriefing suggested they did, then this explanation was factually accurate.

9 For instance, gradual rises and falls in EMG activity over the brow region were suggested to reflect paralinguistic signals as well as emotions, whereas more ballistic EMG responses over the brow region were depicted as less likely to serve as paralinguistic signals during an interview.

REFERENCES

Alexander, A. B. (1975). An experimental test of assumptions relating to the use of electromyographic biofeedback as a general relaxation technique. *Psychophysiology, 12,* 656–662.
Alexander, A. B., & Smith, D. D. (1979). Clinical applications of EMG biofeedback. In R. J. Gatchel & K. P. Price (Eds.), *Clinical applications of biofeedback: Appraisal and status* (pp. 112–133). New York: Pergamon.
Allport, G. W. (1968). The historical background of modern social psychology. In G. Lindzey & E. Aronson (Eds.), *The handbook of social psychology* (2nd ed.). Menlo Park, CA: Addison-Wesley.
Anson, B. J. (1966). *Morris' human anatomy* (12th ed.). New York: McGraw-Hill.
Anthony, B. J. (1985). In the blink of an eye: Implications of reflex modification for information processing. *Advances in Psychophysiology: A Research Annual, 1,* 167–218.
Ashby, W. R. (1960). *Design for a brain: The origin of adaptive behavior.* New York: Wiley.
Association of Sleep Disorders Centers. (1979). Diagnostic classification of sleep and arousal disorders (1st ed.). *Sleep, 2,* 1–137.
Bartoshuk, A. (1955). Electromyographic gradients as indicants of motivation. *Canadian Journal of Psychology, 9,* 215–230.
Basmajian, J. V. (1963). Control and training of individual motor units, *Science, 141,* 440–441.
Basmajian, J. V., & DeLuca, C. J. (1985). *Muscles alive: Their functions revealed by electromyography* (5th ed.). Baltimore: Williams & Wilkins.
Basmajian, J. V., Kukulka, C. G., Narayan, M. G., & Takebe, K. (1975). Biofeedback treatment of foot-drop after stroke compared with standard rehabilitation technique: Effects on voluntary control and strength. *Archives of Physical Medicine and Rehabilitation, 56,* 231–236.
Bavelas, J. B., Black, A., Lemery, C. R., & Mullett, J. (1986). "I *show* how you feel": Motor mimicry as a communicative act. *Journal of Personality and Social Psychology, 50,* 322–329.
Berkinblit, M. B., Feldman, A. G., & Fukson, O. I. (1986). Adaptability of innate motor patterns and motor control mechanisms. *Behavioral and Brain Sciences, 9,* 585–638.
Bickerstaff, E. R. (1975). *Neurological examination in clinical practice.* Oxford: Blackwell Scientific Publications.
Bills, A. G. (1927). Facilitation and inhibition in mental work. *Psychological Bulletin, 34,* 386–309.
Boelhouwer, A. J. W., Bruggemans, E., & Brunia, C. H. M. (1987). Blink reflex magnitude during the foreperiod of a warned reaction time task: Effects of precueing. *Psychophysiology, 24,* 625–631.

Bowditch, H. P. (1871). Uber die Eigenthumlichkeiten der Reizbarkeit welche die Muskelfasern des Herzens zeigen. *Ber, d. Konigl. Sachs. d. Ges. D. Wissen., 23*, 652–689. Cited in Fulton (1926).

Borelli, G. A. (1680). *De motu animalium* (pp. 276–277). Leiden: P. Vander Aa, 1710.

Bramsley, G. R., Bruun, G., Buchthal, F., Guld, C., & Petersen, H. S. (1967). Reduction of electrical interference in measurements of bioelectrical potentials in a hospital. *Acta Polytechnica Scandanavia, Electrical Engineering Series, 15*, 1–37.

Brazier, M. A. (1959). The historical development of neurophysiology. In J. Field (Ed.), *Handbook of physiology: Vol. 1, Section I. Neurophysiology* (pp. 1–58). Washington, DC: American Physiological Society.

Brunia, C. H. M. (1984). Selective and aselective control of spinal motor structures during preparation for a movement. In S. Kornblum & J. Requin (Eds.), *Preparatory states and processes*. Hillsdale, NJ: Erlbaum.

Budzynski, T. H., & Stoyva, J. M. (1969). An instrument for producing deep muscle relaxation by means of analog information feedback. *Journal of Applied Behavior Analysis, 2*, 231–237.

Cacioppo, J. T., & Dorfman, D. D. (1987). Moments in psychophysiological research: Topographical analysis of non-negative bounded waveforms. *Psychological Bulletin, 102*, 421–438.

Cacioppo, J. T., Losch, M. L., Tassinary, L. G., & Petty, R. E. (1986). Properties of affect and affect-laden information processing as viewed through the facial response system. In R. A. Peterson, W. D. Hoyer, & W. R. Wilson (Eds.), *The role of affect in consumer behavior: Emerging theories and applications* (pp. 87–118). Lexington, MA: Heath.

Cacioppo, J. T., Marshall-Goodell, B. S., & Dorfman, D. D. (1983). Skeletal muscular patterning: Topographical analysis of the integrated electromyogram. *Psychophysiology, 20*, 269–283.

Cacioppo, J. T., Marshall-Goodell, B. S., & Gormezano, I. (1983). Social psychophysiology: Bioelectrical measurement, experimental control, and analog-to-digital data acquisition. In J. T. Cacioppo & R. E. Petty (Eds.), *Social psychophysiology: A sourcebook* (pp. 666–692). New York: Guilford Press.

Cacioppo, J .T., Martzke, J. S., Petty, R. E., & Tassinary, L. G. (1988). Specific forms of facial EMG response index emotions during an interview: From Darwin to the continuous flow hypothesis of affect-laden information processing. *Journal of Personality and Social Psychology, 54*, 592–604.

Cacioppo, J. T., & Petty, R. E. (1979a). Attitudes and cognitive response: An electrophysiological approach. *Journal of Personality and Social Psychology, 37*, 2181–2199.

Cacioppo, J. T., & Petty, R. E. (1979b). Lip and nonpreferred forearm EMG activity as a function of orienting task. *Biological Psychology, 9*, 103–113.

Cacioppo, J. T., & Petty, R. E. (1981a). Electromyograms as measures of extent and affectivity of information processing. *American Psychologist, 36*, 441–456.

Cacioppo, J. T., & Petty, R. E. (1981b). Electromyographic specificity during covert information processing. *Psychophysiology, 18*, 518–523.

Cacioppo, J. T., & Petty, R. E. (1983). *Social psychophysiology: A sourcebook*. New York: Guilford Press.

Cacioppo, J. T., & Petty, R. E. (1986). Social processes. In M. G. H. Coles, E. Donchin, & S. Porges (Eds.), *Psychophysiology: Systems, processes, and applications* (pp. 646–679). New York: Guilford Press.

Cacioppo, J. T., Petty, R. E., Losch, M. E., & Kim, H. S. (1986). Electromyographic activity over facial muscle regions can differentiate the valence and intensity of affective reactions. *Journal of Personality and Social Psychology, 50*, 260–268.

Cacioppo, J. T., Petty, R. E., & Marshall-Goodell, B. (1984). Electromyographic specificity during simple physical and attitudinal tasks: Location and topographical features of integrated EMG responses. *Biological Psychology, 18*, 85–121.

Cacioppo, J. T., Petty, R. E., & Marshall-Goodell, B. (1985). Physical, social, and inferential elements of psychophysiological measurement. In P. Karoly (Ed.), *Measurement strategies in health psychology* (Vol. 1, pp. 263–300). New York: Wiley.

Cacioppo, J. T., Petty, R. E., & Morris, K. J. (1985). Semantic, evaluative, and self-referent processing: Memory, cognitive effort, and somatovisceral activity. *Psychophysiology, 22*, 371–384.

Cacioppo, J. T., Petty, R. E., & Tassinary, L. G. (1989). Social psychophysiology: A new look. *Advances in Experimental Social Psychology, 22*, 39–91.

Cacioppo, J. T., & Tassinary, L. G. (1989). The concept of attitude: A psychophysiological analysis. In H. L. Wagner & A. S. R. Manstead (Eds.), *Handbook of psychophysiology: Emotion and social behaviour.* Chichester: Wiley.

Cavallo, T. (1786). *A complete treatise on electricity, in theory and practice* (3rd ed., Vol. 2). London: C. Dilly. Cited in Wu (1984).

Chapman, A. J. (1974). An electromyographic study of social facilitation: A test of the "mere presence" hypothesis. *British Journal of Psychology, 65,* 123–128.

Christie, M. J., & Todd, J. L. (1975). Experimenter-subject-situational interactions. In P. H. Venables & M. J. Christie (Eds.), *Research in psychophysiology.* London: Wiley.

Chun, W. X. (1985). An approach to the nature of tension headache. *Headache, 25,* 188–189.

Coles, M. G. H., Gratton, G., Bashore, T. R., Eriksen, C. W., & Donchin, E. (1985). A psychophysiological investigation of the continuous flow model of human information processing. *Journal of Experimental Psychology: Human Perception and Performance, 11,* 529–553.

Compton, R. W. (1973). Morphological, physiological, and behavioral studies of the facial musculature of the Coati (Nasua). *Brain, Behavior, and Evolution, 7,* 85–126.

Cooper, R., Osselton, J. W., & Shaw, J. C. (1980). *EEG technology* (3rd ed.). London: Butterworth.

Cottrell, N. B. (1972). Social facilitation. In C. G. McClintock (Ed.), *Experimental social psychology.* New York: Holt, Rinehart & Winston.

Courts, F. A. (1942). Relations between muscular tension and performance. *Psychological Bulletin, 39,* 347–367.

Daniels, L., & Worthingham, C. (1986). *Muscle testing: Techniques of manual examination* (5th ed.). Philadelphia: Saunders.

Darwin, C. (1873). *The expression of the emotions in man and animals.* New York: Appleton. (Original work published 1872.)

Davis, J. F., & Malmo, R. B. (1951). Electromyographic recording during interview. *American Journal of Psychiatry, 107,* 908–916.

Davis, J. F. (1952). *Manual of surface electromyography.* Montreal: Laboratory for Psychological Studies, Allan Memorial Institute of Psychiatry.

Davis, J. F., Malmo, R. B., & Shagass, C. (1954). Electromyographic reaction to strong auditory stimulation in psychiatric patients. *Canadian Journal of Psychology, 8,* 177–186.

Davis, R. C. (1940). Set and muscular tension. *Indiana University Publications, Science Series,* No. 10.

DeBacher, G. (1979). Biofeedback in spasticity control. In J. V. Basmajian (Ed.), *Biofeedback – Principles and practice for clinicians.* Baltimore: Williams & Wilkins.

Desmedt, J. E. (1973). A discussion of the methodology of the Triceps Surae T- and H-reflexes. In J. E. Desmedt (Ed.), *New developments in electromyography and clinical neurophysiology* (Vol. 3). Basel: Karger.

Dimberg, U. (1982). Facial reactions to facial expressions. *Psychophysiology, 19,* 643–647.

Dodge, R. B. (1911). A systematic exploration of a normal knee jerk, its technique, the form of muscle contraction, its amplitude, its latent time and its theory. *Zeitschrift für Allgemeine Physiologie, 12,* 1–58.

Du Bois-Reymond, E. (1849). *Untersuchungen ueber thiersiche elektricitaet* (Vol. II, 2nd part). Berlin: Reimer-Verlag. Cited in Basmajian & DeLuca (1985).

Duchenne, G. B. (1959). *Physiology of motion: Demonstrated by means of electrical stimulation and clinical observations and applied to the study of paralysis and deformities* (E. Kaplan, Trans. & Ed.). Philadelphia: Lippincott. (Original work published 1867.)

Duffy, E. (1962). *Activation and behavior.* New York: Wiley.

Eason, R. G., & White, C. T. (1961). Muscular tension, effort, and tracking difficulty: Studies of parameters which affect tension levels and performance efficiency. *Perceptual and Motor Skills, 12,* 331–372.

Eibl-Eibesfeldt, I. (1972). Similarities and differences between cultures in expressive movement. In R. A. Hinde (Ed.), *Nonverbal communication.* Cambridge: Cambridge University Press.

Ekman, P. (1972). Universal and cultural differences in facial expressions of emotion. In J. Cole (Ed.), *Nebraska symposium on motivation,* (Vol. 19, pp. 207–218). Lincoln: University of Nebraska Press.

Ekman, P. (1973). *Darwin and facial expression: A century of research in review.* New York: Academic Press.

Ekman, P. (1982). Methods for measuring facial action. In K. R. Scherer & P. Ekman (Eds.),

Handbook of methods in nonverbal behavior research (pp. 45–90). Cambridge: Cambridge University Press.

Ekman, P. (1985). *Telling lies: Clues to deceit in the marketplace, politics, and marriage.* New York: Norton.

Ekman, P., & Friesen, W. V. (1975). *Unmasking the face.* Englewood Cliffs, NJ: Prentice-Hall.

Ekman, P., & Friesen, W. V. (1978). *Facial action coding system (FACS): A technique for the measurement of facial actions.* Palo Alto, CA: Consulting Psychologists Press.

Ekman, P., Friesen, W. V., O'Sullivan, M., Chan, A., Diacoyanni-Tarlatzis, I., Heider, K., Krause, R., LeCompte, W. A., Pitcairn, T., Ricci-Bitti, P. E., Scherer, K., Tomita, M., & Tzavaras, A. (1987). Universals and cultural differences in the judgments of facial expressions of emotion. *Journal of Personality and Social Psychology, 53,* 712–717.

Ekman, P., Levenson, R. W., & Friesen, W. V. (1983). Autonomic nervous system activity distinguishes among emotions. *Science, 221,* 1208–1210.

Englis, B. G., Vaughan, K. B., & Lanzetta, J. T. (1982). Conditioning of counter-empathic emotional responses. *Journal of Experimental Social Psychology, 18,* 375–391.

Faulkenberry, L. M. (1977). *An introduction to operational amplifiers.* New York: Wiley.

Fearing, F. (1930). *Reflex action: A study in the history of physiological psychology.* Baltimore: Williams & Wilkins.

Fernando, C. K., & Basmajian, J. V. (1978). Biofeedback in physical medicine and rehabilitation. *Biofeedback and Self-Regulation, 3,* 435–455.

Foley, M. G. (1954). *Galvani: Effects of electricity on muscular motion.* Norwalk, CT: Bundy Library.

Fridlund, A. J. (1979). Contour-following integrator for dynamic tracking of electromyographic data. *Psychophysiology, 16,* 491–493.

Fridlund, A. J. (1987). Advances in analyzing the facial electromyogram. *Face Value, 1,* 4–5.

Fridlund, A. J. (in press). Evolution and facial action in reflex, emotion, and paralanguage. In P. K. Ackles, J. R. Jennings, & M. G. H. Coles (Eds.), *Advances in psychophysiology* (Vol. 4). Greenwich, CT: JAI Press.

Fridlund, A. J., & Cacioppo, J. T. (1986). Guidelines for human electromyographic research. *Psychophysiology, 23,* 567–589.

Fridlund, A. J., Cottam, G. L., & Fowler, S. C. (1982). In search of the general tension factor: Tensional patterning during auditory stimulation. *Psychophysiology, 19,* 136–145.

Fridlund, A. J., & Fowler, S. C. (1978). An eight-channel computer-controlled scanning electromyograph. *Behavior Research Methods & Instrumentation, 10,* 652–662.

Fridlund, A. J., Fowler, S. C., & Pritchard, D. A. (1980). Striate muscle tensional patterning in frontalis EMG biofeedback. *Psychophysiology, 17,* 47–55.

Fridlund, A. J., Hatfield, M. E., Cottam, G. L., & Fowler, S. C. (1986). Anxiety and striate-muscle activation: Evidence from electromyographic pattern analysis. *Journal of Abnormal Psychology, 95,* 228–236.

Fridlund, A. J., & Izard, C. E. (1983). Electromyographic studies of facial expressions of emotions and patterns of emotions. In J. T. Cacioppo & R. E. Petty (Eds.), *Social psychophysiology: A sourcebook* (pp. 243–286). New York: Guilford Press.

Fridlund, A. J., Price, A. W., & Fowler, S. C. (1982). Low-noise, optically isolated electromyographic preamplifier. *Psychophysiology, 19,* 701–705.

Fridlund, A. J., Schwartz, G. E., & Fowler, S. C. (1984). Pattern recognition of self-reported emotional state from multiple-site facial EMG activity during affective imagery. *Psychophysiology, 21,* 622–637.

Fridlund, A. J., Tassinary, L. G., & Cacioppo, J. T. (1988). On the utility of non-polarizing electrodes in human surface electromyographic recording. *Psychophysiology, 25,* 488.

Friesen, W. V. (1972). *Cultural differences in facial expression in a social situation: An experimental text of the concept of display rules.* Unpublished doctoral dissertation, University of California, San Francisco.

Fulton, J. F. (1926). *Muscular contraction and the reflex control of movement.* Baltimore: Williams & Wilkins.

Gale, A., & Baker, S. (1981). In vivo or in vitro? Some effects of laboratory environments, with particular reference to the psychophysiological experiment. In M. J. Christie & P. G. Mellet (Eds.), *Foundations of psychosomatics.* Chichester: Wiley.

Gale, A., & Christie, B. (1987). *Psychophysiology and the electronic workplace* (pp. 3–15). Chichester: Wiley.

Gallistel, C. R. (1980). *The organization of action: The new synthesis.* Hillsdale, NJ: Erlbaum.

Galton, F. (1884). Measurement of character. *Fortnightly Review, 42*, 179–185.

Galvani, L. (1952). *Dell'uso e dell'attivita dell'arco conduttore nelle contrazione dei muscoli, Supplemento al trattato.* Bologna: A. S. Tomaso d'Aquino. *Galvani-Volta* (B. Dibner, Trans.). Norwalk, CT.: Burndy Library. (Original work published in 1794.)

Galvani, L. (1953). *De viribus electricitatis in motu musculari.* Bologna: Typographia Instituti Scientiarum. (R. M. Green, Trans.) *Commentary on the effect of electricity on muscular motion.* Cambridge, MA: Elizabeth Licht. (Original work published in 1791.)

Gans, C., & Gorniak, G. C. (1980). Electromyograms are repeatable: Precautions and limitations. *Science, 210*, 795–797.

Geen, R. G., & Gange, J. J. (1977). Drive theory of social facilitation: Twelve years of theory and research. *Psychological Bulletin, 84*, 1267–1288.

Germana, J. (1974). Electromyography: Human and general. In R. F. Thompson & M. M. Patterson (Eds.), *Bioelectric recording techniques: Part C: Receptor and effector processes* (pp. 155–163). New York: Academic Press.

Ghez, C. (1985). Introduction to the motor systems. In E. R. Kandel & J. H. Schwartz (Eds.), *Principles of neural science* (2nd ed., pp. 429–442). New York: Elsevier.

Goldstein, I. B. (1964). Role of muscle tension in personality theory. *Psychological Bulletin, 601*, 413–425.

Goldstein, I. B. (1972). Electromyography: A measure of skeletal muscle response. In N. S. Greenfield & R. A. Sternbach (Eds.), *Handbook of psychophysiology* (pp. 329–366). New York: Holt, Rinehart & Winston.

Gotch, F. (1902). The submaximal electrical response of nerve to a single stimulus. *Journal of Physiology, 28*, 395–416.

Graham, F. K., Strock, B. D., & Zeigler, B. L. (1981). Excitatory and inhibitory influences on reflex responsiveness. In W. A. Collins (Ed.), *Aspects of the development of competence: The Minnesota symposia on child psychology* (Vol. 14, pp. 1–38). Hillsdale, NJ: Erlbaum.

Graham J. L. (1980). A new system for measuring nonverbal responses to marketing appeals. *1980 AMA Educator's Conference Proceedings, 46*, 340–343.

Grieve, D. W., & Cavanaugh, P. R. (1973). The quantitative analysis of phasic electromyograms. In J. E. Desmedt (Ed.), *New developments in electromyography and clinical neurophysiology* (Vol. 2, pp. 487–496). Basel: Karger.

Groff, B. D., Baron, R. S., & Moore, D. L. (1983). Distraction, attentional conflict, and drivelike behavior. *Journal of Experimental Social Psychology, 19*, 359–380.

Guilleminault, C. (Ed.) (1982). *Sleeping and waking disorders: Indication and techniques.* Menlo Park, CA: Addison-Wesley.

Hager, J. C., & Ekman, P. (1981). Methodological problems in Tourangeau and Ellsworth's study of facial expression and experience of emotion. *Journal of Personality and Social Psychology, 40*, 358–362.

Harris, R. (1975). *A primer of multivariate statistics.* New York: Academic.

Hauri, P. (1977). *The sleep disorders.* Kalamazoo, MI: Upjohn Pharmaceuticals.

Hayes, K. J. (1960). Wave analyses of tissue noise and muscle action potential. *Journal of Applied Physiology, 15*, 749–752.

Hefferline, R. F., Keenan, B., & Harford, R. A. (1959). Escape and avoidance conditioning in human subjects without their observation of the response. *Science, 1*, 1338–1339.

Helmer, R. J. (1986) A test-signal generator for low-frequency instrumentation. *Behavior Research Methods, Instruments, and Computers, 18*, 372–376.

Henneman, E. (1980a). Organization of the motoneuron pool: The size principle. In V. E. Mountcastle (Ed.), *Medical physiology* (14th ed., Vol. 1, pp. 718–741). St. Louis: Mosby.

Henneman, E. (1980b). Organization of the motor systems: A preview. In V. E. Mountcastle (Ed.), *Medical physiology* (14th ed., Vol. 1, pp. 669–673). St. Louis: Mosby.

Henneman, E. (1980c). Skeletal muscle: The servant of the nervous system. In V. E. Mountcastle (Ed.), *Medical physiology* (14th ed., Vol. 1, pp. 674–702). St. Louis: Mosby.

Hinsey, J. C. (1940). The hypothalamus and somatic responses. In J. F. Fulton, S. Walter, & A. M. Frantz (Eds.), *Research publications of the Association for Research in Nervous and Mental Disease* (Vol. 20, pp. 657–685). Baltimore: Williams & Wilkins.

Honts, C. R., & Hodes, R. L. (1982). The effects of multiple physical countermeasures on the detection of deception. *Psychophysiology, 19*, 564–565.

Honts, C. R., Hodes, R. L., & Raskin, D. C. (1985). Effects of physical countermeasures on the physiological detection of deception. *Journal of Applied Psychology, 79*, 177–187.

Honts, C. R., Raskin, D. C., & Kircher, J. C. (1983). Detection of deception: Effectiveness of physical countermeasures under high motivation conditions. *Psychophysiology*, *20*, 446–447.

Hoyle, G. (1983). *Muscles and their neural control*. New York: Wiley.

Hugon, M. (1973). Methodology of the Hoffman reflex in man. In J. E. Desmedt (Ed.), *New developments in electromyography and clinical neurophysiology* (Vol. 3, pp. 277–293). Basel: Karger.

Humboldt, F. H. A. von (1797). *Versuche uber die gereizte Muskel- und Nervenfaser nebst Vermuthungen uber chemischen Processes des Lebens in der Thier und Pflanzwelt* (Vol. 1). Poznan: Decker. Cited in Fulton (1926).

Humphrey, G. (1951). *Thinking*. New York: Wiley.

Isley, C. L., & Basmajian, J. V. (1973). Electromyography of the human cheeks and lips. *Anatomical Record*, *176*, 143–148.

Ison, J. R., & Hoffman, H. S. (1983). Reflex modification in the domain of startle: II. The anomalous history of a robust and ubiquitous phenomenon. *Psychological Bulletin*, *94*, 3–17.

Izard, C. E. (1971). *The face of emotion*. New York: Appleton-Century–Crofts.

Izard, C. E. (1977). *Human emotions*. New York: Plenum Press.

Jacobson, E. (1925). Voluntary relaxation of the esophagus. *American Journal of Physiology*, *72*, 387–394.

Jacobson, E. (1927). Action currents from muscular contractions during conscious processes. *Science*, *66*, 403.

Jacobson, E. (1930a). Electrical measurements of neuromuscular states during mental activities: I. Imagination of movement involving skeletal muscle. *American Journal of Physiology*, *91*, 567–608.

Jacobson, E. (1930b). Electrical measurements of neuromuscular states during mental activities: II. Imagination and recollection of various muscular acts. *American Journal of Physiology*, *94*, 22–34.

Jacobson, E. (1930c). Electrical measurements of neuromuscular states during mental activities: III. Visual imagination and recollection. *American Journal of Physiology*, *95*, 694–702.

Jacobson, E. (1930d). Electrical measurements of neuromuscular states during mental activities: IV. Evidence of contraction of specific muscles during imagination. *American Journal of Physiology*, *95*, 703–712.

Jacobson, E. (1931a). Electrical measurements of neuromuscular states during mental activities: V. Variation of specific muscles contracting during imagination. *American Journal of Physiology*, *96*, 115–121.

Jacobson, E. (1931b). Electrical measurements of neuromuscular states during mental activities: VI. A note on mental activities concerning an amputated limb. *American Journal of Physiology*, *96*, 122–125.

Jacobson, E. (1931c). Electrical measurements of neuromuscular states during mental activities: VII. Imagination, recollection and abstract thinking involving the speech musculature. *American Journal of Physiology*, *97*, 200–209.

Jacobson, E. (1932). Electrophysiology of mental activities. *American Journal of Psychology*, *44*, 677–694.

James, W. (1884). What is an emotion? *Mind*, *9*, 188–205.

James, W. (1890). *The principles of psychology*. New York: Holt.

Johnson, L. C., & Lubin, A. (1972). On planning psychophysiological experiments: Design, measurement, and analysis. In N. S. Greenfield & R. A. Sternbach (Eds.), *Handbook of psychophysiology* (pp. 125–158). New York: Holt, Rinehart & Winston.

Kahn, F. (1943). *Man in structure and function* (George Rosen, Trans.) (Vol. 1). New York: Knopf.

Kandel, E. R., & Schwartz, J. H. (1985). *Principles of neural science* (2nd ed.). New York: Elsevier.

Kendall, P. T., & McCreary, E. K. (1980). *Muscles: Testing and function* (3rd ed.). Baltimore: Williams & Wilkins.

Kennedy, J. L., & Travis, R. C. (1948). Prediction and control of alertness: II. Continuous tracking. *Journal of Comparative and Physiological Psychology*, *41*, 203–210.

Kimura, J. (1973). The blink reflex as a test for brainstem and higher central nervous system function. In J. E. Desmedt (Ed.), *New developments in electromyography and clinical neurophysiology* (Vol. 3). Basel: Karger.

Kimura, J., Giron L. T., & Young, S. M. (1975). Electrophysiological study of Bell's palsy: Electrically elicited blink reflex in assessment of prognosis. *Archives of Otolaryngology*, *102*, 140–143.

Komi, P. V., & Buskirk, E. R. (1970). Reproducibility of electromyographic measurements with inserted wire electrodes and surface electrodes. *Electromyography*, *10*, 357–367.

Kraut, R. E., & Johnson, R. E. (1979). Social and emotional messages of smiling: An ethological approach. *Journal of Personality and Social Psychology*, *37*, 1539–1553.

Kugler, P. N., & Turvey, M. T. (1987). *Information, natural law, and the self-assembly of rhythmic movement*. Hillsdale, NJ: Erlbaum.

Kupfer, D. J., & Reynolds, C. F. (1983). Sleep disorders. *Hospital Practice*, February, 101–109.

Kuypers, H. G. J. M. (1982). A new look at the organization of the motor system. In H. G. J. M. Kuypers & G. F. Martin (Eds.), *Progress in brain research: Anatomy of descending pathways to the spinal cord* (Vol. 57, pp. 381–403). Amsterdam: Elsevier.

Laird, J. D. (1984). The real role of facial response in the experience of emotion: A reply to Tourangeau and Ellsworth, and others. *Journal of Personality and Social Psychology*, *47*, 909–917.

Langley, L. L., Telford, I. R., & Christensen, J. B. (1974). *Dynamic anatomy and physiology* (4th ed.). New York: McGraw-Hill.

Larson, J. D., & Foulkes, D. (1969). Electromyogram suppression during sleep, dream recall and orientation time. *Psychophysiology*, *5*, 548–555.

Latane, B., Williams, K. D., & Harkins, S. G. (1979). Many hands make light the work: The causes and consequences of social loafing. *Journal of Personality and Social Psychology*, *37*, 822–832.

Lawrence, J. H., & DeLuca, C. J. (1983). Myoelectrical signal vs. force relationship in different muscles. *Journal of Applied Physiology*, *54*, 1653–1659.

Levey, A. B. (1980). Measurement units in psychophysiology. In I. Martin & P. H. Venables (Eds.), *Techniques in psychophysiology*. Chichester: Wiley.

Liddell, F. O. T. (1960). *The discovery of the reflexes*. Oxford: Clarendon.

Lindstrom, L. R. (1970). *On the frequency spectrum of EMG signals*. Technical Report, Research Laboratory of Medical Electronics, Chalmers Institute of Technology, Goteborg, Sweden.

Lippold, O. C. J. (1967). Electromyography. In P. H. Venables & I. Martin (Eds.), *Manual of psychophysiological methods* (pp. 245–298). New York: Wiley.

Loeb, G. E., & Gans, C. (1986). *Electromyography for experimentalists*. Chicago: University of Chicago Press.

Lorenzini, S. (1678). *Osservazioni intorno alle Torpedini* (J. Davis, Trans.). Florence: 1'Onofri. [*The curious and accurate observations of Mr. Stephen Lorenzini of Florence*, pp. 66–72. London: Jeffery Wale, 1705.]

Lucas, K. (1909). The "all-or-none" contraction of amphibian skeletal muscle. *Journal of Physiology*, *38*, 113–133.

Lynn, R. (1966). *Attention, arousal and the orientation reaction*. Oxford: Pergamon.

Malmo, R. B. (1959). Activation: A neuropsychological dimension. *Psychological Review*, *66*, 367–386.

Malmo, R. B. (1965). Physiological gradients and behavior. *Psychological Bulletin*, *64*, 225–234.

Malmo, R. B. (1975). *On emotions, needs, and our archaic brain*. New York: Holt, Rinehart & Winston.

Malmo, R. B., & Shagass, C. (1949a). Physiologic studies of reaction to stress in anxiety and early schizophrenia. *Psychosomatic Medicine*, *11*, 9–24.

Malmo, R. B., & Shagass, C. (1949b). Physiologic study of symptom mechanisms in psychiatric patients under stress. *Psychosomatic Medicine*, *11*, 25–29.

Malmo, R. B., Shagass, C., & Davis, F. H. (1950). Symptom specificity and bodily reactions during psychiatric interview. *Psychosomatic Medicine*, *12*, 362–376.

Malmo, R. B., Shagass, C., & Davis, J. F. (1951). Electromyographic studies of muscular tension in psychiatric patients under stress. *Journal of Clinical & Experimental Psychopathology*, *12*, 45–66.

Malmo, R. B., & Smith, A. A. (1955). Forehead tension and motor irregularities in psychoneurotic patients under stress. *Journal of Personality*, *23*, 391–406.

Markovsky, B., & Berger, S. M. (1983). Crowd noise and mimicry. *Personality and Social Psychology Bulletin*, *9*, 90–96.

Matsumoto, D. (1987). The role of facial response in the experience of emotion: More methodological problems and a meta-analysis. *Journal of Personality and Social Psychology,* 52, 769–774.

Max, L. W. (1935). An experimental study of the motor theory of consciousness: III. Action-current responses in deaf mutes during sleep, sensory stimulation and dreams. *Journal of Comparative Psychology,* 19, 469–486.

Max, L. W. (1937). An experimental study of the motor theory of consciousness: IV. Action-current responses in the deaf during awakening, kinaesthetic imagery and abstract thinking. *Journal of Comparative Psychology,* 24, 301–344.

McCanne, T. R., & Anderson, J. A. (1987). Emotional responding following experimental manipulation of facial electromyographic activity. *Journal of Personality and Social Psychology,* 52, 759–768.

McGuigan, F. J. (1970). Covert oral behavior during the silent performance of language. *Psychological Bulletin,* 74, 309–326.

McGuigan, F. J. (1978). *Cognitive psychophysiology: Principles of covert behavior.* Englewood Cliffs, NJ: Prentice-Hall.

McGuigan, F. J. (1979) *Psychophysiological measurement of covert behavior: A guide for the laboratory.* Hillsdale, NJ: Erlbaum.

McGuigan, F. J., & Bailey, S. C. (1969). Logitudinal study of covert oral behavior during silent reading, *Perceptual and motor skills,* 28, 170.

McGuigan, F. J., Dollins, A., Pierce, W., Lusebrink, V., & Corus, C. (1982). Fourier analysis of covert speech behavior. *Pavlovian Journal of Biological Science,* 17, 49–52.

McHugo, G., & Lanzetta, J. T. (1983). Methodological decisions in social psychophysiology. In J. T. Cacioppo & R. E. Petty (Eds.), *Social psychophysiology: A sourcebook* (pp. 630–665). New York: Guilford Press.

McHugo, G., Lanzetta, J. T., Sullivan, D. G., Masters, R. D., & Englis, B. G. (1985). Emotional reactions to a political leader's expressive displays. *Journal of Personality and Social Psychology,* 49, 1513–1529.

Merton, P. A. (1987). Reflexes. In R. L. Gregory (Ed.), *The Oxford companion to the mind.* New York: Oxford University Press.

Meyer, D. R. (1953). On the interaction of simultaneous responses. *Psychological Bulletin,* 20, 204–220.

Meyer, D. R., Bahrick, H. P., & Fitts, P. M. (1953). Incentive, anxiety, and the human blink rate. *Journal of Experimental Psychology,* 45, 183–287.

Monnier, M. (1970). *Functions of the nervous system: Vol. 2. Motor and psychomotor functions.* New York: Elsevier.

Mulder, T., & Hulstijn, W. (1984). The effect of fatigue and repetition of the task on the surface electromyographic signal. *Psychophysiology,* 21, 528–534.

National Institutes of Mental Health. (1980). *Biofeedback: Issues in treatment assessment.* NIMH Science Reports, Washington, DC: Author.

Needham, D. M. (1971). *Machina carnis. The biochemistry of muscular contraction in its historical development.* London: Cambridge University Press.

Ongerboer de Visser, B. W. (1983). Anatomical and functional organization of reflexes involving the trigeminal system in man: Jaw reflex, blink reflex, corneal reflex, and exteroceptive suppression. In J. E. Desmedt (Ed.), *Motor control mechanisms in health and disease* (pp. 727–738). New York: Raven Press.

Orne, M. T. (1962). On the social psychology of the psychological experiment: With particular reference to demand characteristics and their implications. *American Psychologist,* 17, 776–783.

O'Dwyer, N. J., Quinn, P. T., Guitar, B. E., Andrews, G., & Neilson, P. D. (1981). Procedures for verification of electrode placement in EMG studies of orofacial and mandibular muscles. *Journal of Speech and Hearing Research,* 241, 273–288.

Pavlov, I. P. (1927). *Conditioned reflexes.* New York: Oxford University Press.

Petrofsky, J. S., & Phillips, C. A. (1982). The electromyogram: A potentially attractive tool for the noninvasive assessment of muscle function. In J. A. Herd, A. M. Gotto, P. G. Kaufman, & S. M. Weiss (Eds.), *Cardiovascular instrumentation: Proceedings of the working conference on applicability of new technology to biobehavioral research.* Washington, DC: National Heart, Lung, and Blood Institute.

Piaget, J. (1954). *The construction of reality in the child.* New York: Basic Books.

Pikoff, H. (1984). Is the muscular model of headache still viable? *Headache,* 24, 186–198.

Pratt, F. H. (1917). The all-or-none principle in graded response of skeletal muscle. *American Journal of Physiology, 44,* 517–542.

Pratt, F. H., & Eisenberger, J. P. (1919). The quantal phenomena in muscle: Methods with further evidence of the all-or-none principle in graded response for the skeletal fibre. *American Journal of Physiology, 49,* 1–54.

Rajecki, D. W. (1983). Animal aggression: Implications for human aggression. In R. G. Geen & E. J. Donnerstein (Eds.), *Aggression: Theoretical and empirical reviews* (Vol. 1, pp. 189–211). New York: Academic Press.

Rechtschaffen, A., & Kales, A. (Eds.). (1968). *A manual of standardized terminology, techniques and scoring system for sleep stages of human subjects.* Washington DC: U.S. Government Printing Office (National Institute of Health Publication No. 204).

Redi, F. (1925). *Esperienze intorno a diverse cose naturali e particolarmente a quelle che ci sono portate dalle Indie* (pp. 47–51). Florence. (Original work published1617.) Reprinted in *Le Piu Belle Pagine di Francesco Redi,* P. Giacosa (Ed.), pp. 105–109. Milan: Fratelli Treves, Editori. Cited in Wu (1984).

Reid, J. E., & Inbau, F. E. (1977). *Truth and deception: The polygraph ("lie detector") technique.* Baltimore: Williams & Wilkins.

Rinn, W. E. (1984). The neuropsychology of facial expression: A review of the neurological and psychological mechanisms for producing facial expressions. *Psychological Bulletin, 95,* 52–77.

Rosenthal, R. (1966). *Experimenter effects in behavior research.* New York: Appleton-Century-Crofts.

Rosenthal, R., & Rosnow, R. (Eds.) (1969). *Artifact in behavioral research.* New York: Academic Press.

Rossi, A. M. (1959). An evaluation of the manifest anxiety scale by the use of electromyography. *Journal of Experimental Psychology, 58,* 64–69.

Scherer, K. R., & Ekman, P. (1982). *Handbook of methods in nonverbal behavior research* (pp. 45–90). Cambridge: Cambridge University Press.

Schmidt, R. F., & Thews, G. (1983). *Human physiology.* Berlin: Springer-Verlag.

Schwartz, G. E. (1975). Biofeedback, self-regulation, and the patterning of physiological processes. *American Scientist, 63,* 314–324.

Schwartz, G. E., Fair, P. L., Salt, P., Mandel, M. R., & Klerman, G. L. (1976). Facial muscle patterning to affective imagery in depressed and nondepressed subjects. *Science, 192,* 489–491.

Seiler, R. (1973). On the function of facial muscles in different behavioral situations: A study based on the muscle morphology and electromyography. *American Journal of Physical Anthropology, 38,* 567–572.

Shapiro, D., & Crider, A. (1969). Psychophysiological approaches to social psychology. In G. Lindzey & E. Aronson (Eds.), *The handbook of social psychology* (Znd ed., Vol. 3). Reading, MA: Aldison-Wesley.

Shaw, W. A. (1940). The relation of muscular action potentials to imaginal weight lifting. *Archives of Psychology,* No. 247.

Sheatz, G. C. (1972). A differential microvolt test signal adjustable to given laboratory requirements. *Psychophysiology, 9,* 658–659.

Shedivy, D. I., & Kleinman, K. M. (1977). Lack of correlation between frontalis EMG and either neck EMG or verbal ratings of tension. *Psychophysiology, 14,* 182–186.

Sherrington, C. S. (1923). *The integrative actions of the nervous system.* New Haven: Yale University Press. (Original work published 1906.)

Shimizu, A, & Inoue, T. (1986). Dreamed speech and speech muscle activity. *Psychophysiology, 23,* 210–215.

Skinner, B. F. (1931). The concept of the reflex in the description of behavior. *The Journal of General Psychology: Experimental, Theoretical, Clinicial, and Historical Psychology, 5,* 427–457.

Smith, R. R., Kier, W. M. (1989). Trunks, tongues, and tentacles: Moving with skeletons of muscle. *American Scientist, 77,* 28–35.

Spencer, H. (1855). *Principles of Psychology* (1st ed.). New York: Appleton.

Sperry, R. (1952). Neurology and the mind–brain problem. *American Scientist, 40,* 291–312.

Steiner, J. E. (1979). Human facial expression in response to taste and smell stimulation. *Advances in Child Development and Behavior, 13,* 257–295.

Sternbach, R. A. (1966). *Principles of psychophysiology.* New York: Academic.

Stoyva, J., & Budzynski, T. (1974). Cultivated low arousal: An anti-stress response? In L. V. DiCara (Ed.). *Recent advances in limbic and autonomic nervous system research* (pp. 370–394). New York: Plenum Press.

Strong, P. (1970). *Biophysical measurements.* Beaverton, OR: Textronix.

Svebak, S., Dalen, K., & Storfjell, O. (1981). The psychological significance of task–induced tonic changes in somatic and autonomic activity. *Psychophysiology, 18,* 403–409.

Tassinary, L. G., Cacioppo, J. T., & Geen, T. R. (1989). A psychometric study of surface electrode placements for facial electromyographic recording: I. The brow and cheek muscle regions. *Psychophysiology, 26,* 1–16.

Tassinary, L. G., Cacioppo, J. T., Geen, T. R., & Vanman, E. (1987). Optimizing surface electrode placements for facial EMG recordings: Guidelines for recording from the perioral muscle region. *Psychophysiology, 24,* 615–616.

Teuber, H. L. (1955). Physiological psychology. *Annual Review of Psychology, 6,* 267–294.

Thompson, R. F. (1967). *Foundations of physiological psychology.* New York: Harper & Row.

Tognacci, L. N., & Cook, S. W. (1975). Conditioned autonomic responses as bidirectional indicators of racial attitude. *Journal of Personality and Social Psychology, 31,* 137–144.

Tomkins, S. S. (1962). *Affect, imagery, and consciousness.* New York: Springer.

Tomovic, R., & Bellman, R. (1970). A systems approach to muscle control. *Mathematical Biosciences, 8,* 265–277.

Tortora, G. J. (1983). *Principles of human anatomy* (3rd ed.). New York: Harper & Row.

Tourangeau, R., & Ellsworth, P. C. (1979). The role of facial response in the experience of emotion. *Journal of Personality and Social Psychology, 37,* 1519–1531.

Triplett, N. (1898). The dynamogenic factors in pacemaking and competition. *American Journal of Psychology, 9,* 507–533.

van Boxtel, A., Goudswaard, P., & Janssen, K. (1983). Absolute and proportional resting EMG levels in muscle contraction and migraine headache patients. *Headache, 23,* 215–222.

van Boxtel, A., Goudswaard, P., & Shomaker, L. R. B. (1984). Amplitude and bandwidth of the frontalis surface EMG: Effects of electrode parameters. *Psychophysiology, 21,* 699–707.

Vaughan, K. B., & Lanzetta, J. T. (1980). Vicarious instigation and conditioning of facial expressive and autonomic responses to a model's expressive display of pain. *Journal of Personality and Social Psychology, 13,* 909–923.

Vaughan, K. B., & Lanzetta, J. T. (1981). The effects of modification of expressive displays on vicarious emotional arousal. *Journal of Experimental Social Psychology, 17,* 16–30.

Vitti, M., Basmajian, J. V., Ouclette, P. L., Mitchell, D. L., Eastman, W. P., & Seaborn, R.D. (1975). Electromyographic investigations of the tongue and circumoral muscular sling with fine-wire electrodes. *Journal of Dental Research, 54,* 844–849.

Volta, A. (1816). Memoria prima sull' elettricita animale. In *Collezione dell'Opere* (Vol. 2). Florence: G. Piatti. (Original work published 1792.) Cited in Wu (1984).

Wallerstein, H. (1954). An electromyographic study of attentive listening. *Canadian Journal of Psychology, 8,* 228–238.

Walsh, J. (1773). Of the electric property of the torpedo. *Philosophical Transactions of the Royal Society, 63,* 461–480.

Wartenberg, R. (1946). *The examination of reflexes: A simplification.* Chicago: Year Book Publishers.

Weaver, C. V. (1977). Descriptive anatomical and quantitative variation in human facial musculature and the analysis of bilateral asymmetry. *Dissertation Abstracts International* (University Microfilms, No. 77–24, 305).

Wells, G. L., & Petty, R. E. (1980). The effects of overt head-movements on persuasion: Compatibility and incompatibility of responses. *Basic and Applied Social Psychology, 1,* 219–230.

Whatmore, G., & Ellis, R. M. (1959). Some neurophysiological aspects of depressed states: An electromyographic study. *Archives of General Psychiatry, 1,* 70–80.

Whatmore, G., Whatmore, N. J., & Fisher, L. D. (1981). Is frontalis activity a reliable indicator of the activity in other muscles? *Biofeedback and Self-Regulation, 6,* 305–314.

Willison, R. G. (1963). A method for measuring motor unit activity in human muscles. *Journal of Physiology, 168,* 35–36.

Willis, W., & Grossman, R. (1977). *Medical neurobiology* (2nd ed.). St. Louis: Mosby.

Winter, D. A., Rau, G., Kadefors, R., Broman, H., & DeLuca, C. J. (1980). *Units, terms, and*

384   J. CACIOPPO, L. TASSINARY, AND A. FRIDLUND

standards in the reporting of EMG research. Report by the Ad Hoc Committee of the International Society of Electrophysiological Kinesiology.

Woodworth, R. S., & Schlosberg, H. (1954). *Experimental psychology.* New York: Holt.

Wu, C. H. (1984). Electric fish and the discovery of animal electricity. *American Scientist, 72,* 598–607.

Zajonc, R. B. (1965). Social facilitation. *Science, 149,* 269–274.

Zajonc, R. B., & Markus, H. (1984). Affect and cognition: The hard interface. In C. E. Izard, J. Kagan, & R. B. Zajonc (Eds.), *Emotions, cognition, and behavior* (pp. 73–102). Cambridge: Cambridge University Press.

Zipp, P. (1982). Recommendations for the standardization of lead positions in surface electromyography. *European Journal of Applied Physiology, 50,* 41–54.

12 *The electrocortical system*

WILLIAM J. RAY

The recording of electrical activity from the scalp has intrigued scientists and lay people alike. Inherent in the idea of recording electrical activity from the scalp was the possibility of having an objective marker that reflected underlying psychological processes. Hans Berger (1929), the discoverer of the human electroencephalogram (EEG), reflected upon this possibility in one of his first papers on EEG:

Naturally, in the course of the investigations various questions quite spontaneously forced themselves upon my mind, e.g. whether in the human electroencephalogram too, as has been found in the animal experiment, changes occur under the influence of peripheral stimuli; furthermore, the question whether one would be able to demonstrate a difference of the electroencephalogram in wakefulness from that of sleep, how it would behave in narcosis and others of this kind. Above all, however, what about the question which already preoccupied Fleischl von Marxow when he wrote that under certain circumstances one would perhaps be able to go so far as to observe the electrical concomitants of the events in one's own brain? (Berger, 1929, p. 72)

As one will see in this chapter, Berger's speculation has been answered in the affirmative and EEG has offered useful insights into psychological processing. However, as one will also see, with the introduction of new techniques and theoretical approaches, there are new questions on both a basic and a more theoretical level yet to be resolved. In this chapter, we discuss classical and contemporary approaches to the study of psychological phenomena through the use of EEG. Related phenomena such as event-related potentials will be discussed in chapter 13. Alternative technologies such as neuromagnetometry are briefly introduced and referenced in the final section of this chapter.

12.1 HISTORICAL AND THEORETICAL INTRODUCTION

In 1791, Galvani published the idea that nerves contain an intrinsic form of electricity and marked a turning point in the history of electrophysiology (see Brazier, 1961, for a discussion of the early history of electrophysiology before the discovery of EEG). Less than 60 years later, Du Bois-Reymond (1848) discovered that activity in a peripheral nerve was accompanied by recordable changes in electrical potential. This discovery encouraged the scientific community to look for changes in the electrical activity emanating from the nervous system that could be used as an indicant of its function. One person who built upon this research was the English physician Richard Caton. Caton worked in a period of history in which localization of function in the cortex was of great interest. During this period, researchers demonstrated that if particular parts of the cortex were electrically stimulated, then activation followed in specific muscle groups related to that cortical site (cf. Ferrier, 1875; Fritsch & Hitzig, 1870). What was not known was whether there existed a connection between the electrical activity of the brain and external sensory stimuli such as light. Caton was able to demonstrate such connections existed in the brains of both rabbits and monkeys (Caton, 1875). He further reported in this and a later publication (Caton, 1877) that it was also possible to record "feeble currents" from electrodes on the surface of the skull. Thus, the EEG was born.

It was some 54 years later before there existed evidence that human beings also display potential differences across the surface of the scalp. Hans Berger (1929) reported in great detail on the appearance of electrical activity recorded from the scalp, although his first recordings had been made some five years earlier (Berger, 1929). Berger named the electrical activity recorded from the scalp *Elektrenkephalogramm* as well as named two distinctive rhythmic components of the EEG, alpha and beta waves. Because Berger, a German psychiatrist at the University of Jena, was not recognized for physiological research, his first reports on the EEG were received skeptically. Instead, it was not until 1934 that a scientific demonstration by Adrian and Mathews at the meeting of the British Physiological Society in Cambridge that EEG received widespread acceptance. However, a present-day reading of Berger's published reports displays sophistication as to the nature and basis of EEG as well as providing interesting reading. Fourteen of these papers published between 1929 and 1938 carried the common title "On the Electroencephalogram of Man" and are available as a translated collection (Gloor, 1969) from which the Berger quotations in this chapter are taken.

In the first papers of the series, Berger (1929) sought to discover what physiological activities were related to EEG activity. He reported that EEG cannot be attributed to cerebral pulsations, cerebral blood flow, blood flow through scalp vessels, EKG, skeletal or smooth muscle artifact, eye movement, or electrical properties of the skin. He reached these conclusions by such procedures as measuring the time between the presentation of a stimulus, one of which was the firing of a cap pistol, and the resultant EEG changes, showing that EEG changes preceded blood flow changes. Likewise, Berger showed that manipulations of respiration, known to influence cerebral blood flow, did not affect EEG. Berger's discussion of the EEG can be seen as reflecting the classic psychophysical tradition in which changes in physical stimuli (e.g., changes in intensity of light or sound) are mapped on changes in psychological processes (e.g., the subjective experience of brightness or loudness). For example, a function could be determined that related an external stimuli to the internal experience. From this perspective, Berger (1929) reported surprise to find that stimulation did not increase electrical activity as might be expected given a model that assumed that an increase in stimulation would be related to an increase in electrical activity. Rather, Berger found that with stimulation alpha waves (8–12 cycles per second activity) were no longer present in the record. Berger also found that alpha decreased with voluntary movement or intention to move and mental work (e.g., mental arithmetic). Based on these findings, Berger discussed alpha in two different although similar ways.

Berger first viewed alpha as a correlate of attention. In this way he drew upon the interest of his historical period in the attempt to time fluctuations in attention. Berger (1929) described this idea as follows:

It is evident that the durations of these periodic fluctuations of the E.E.G. correspond very well with those of the fluctuations of attention reported by various investigators, for which Wundt assumed a central origin and which therefore he named waves of apperception.... [Mosso] thought it likely that fatigue of a nerve cell of the brain already sets in after 3–4 seconds of activity. We know of numerous phenomena exhibiting such a short periodicity, e.g. the oscillating fluctuations of memory images and other psychological processes to which I merely wish to allude here. (Berger, 1929, p. 80)

In his early reports, Berger described alpha as a "concomitant phenomena of those nervous processes which have been termed psychophysical, i.e. of those material cortical processes which under certain circumstances can also be associated with phenomena of consciousness" (Berger, 1929, p. 91).

For Berger, alpha was also seen as a generalized reaction of the brain. This more global interpretation of changes in alpha activity was based on the assumption that any sensory stimulus would produce a localized increased potential at a particular sensory center. This center in turn exerted a generalized inhibitory effect on the rest of the cortex. This inhibition manifested itself by a disappearance of alpha. In essence, Berger hypothesized that alpha activity represented the concomitants of psychophysiological processes taking place in the brain and that under certain circumstances these could be associated with conscious mental processes. The model suggests that alpha is associated with passive psychological processes (e.g., stream of consciousness). With stimulation, consciousness is narrowed and mental activity ceases to be passive. At this point, alpha activity is reduced and the person has an active EEG. In passive EEG, the brain is assumed to work as a whole that is undifferentiated and unstructured, whereas in active EEG (attention to sensory stimulus), a topographic pattern develops. This pattern may move as mental activity progresses. Further, contained in this speculation is the idea that electrical activity in the brain could influence the structure of the nervous system. As one can observe in the following quote, the general model suggests a decrease in potential during mental work that is an expression of inhibition:

During sensory perception vigorous activity occurs in the area of the involved sensory center by which other processes taking place simultaneously in the cerebrum are influenced. This manifests itself in an alteration of the E.E.G.... From the focus of activity which is formed in the sensory center, inhibitory influences spread to all other parts of the cerebrum. This general inhibition arising from the local excitation causes a cessation of those nervous processes whose concomitant phenomena appear in the E.E.G. as alpha waves. The alpha waves disappear and only the beta waves remain. One could also imagine that the energy required for the genesis of the nervous processes which are associated with alpha-waves issued up elsewhere, i.e. precisely in the active sensory center, and that therefore this would cause the energy to flow off to this area. (Berger, 1929, p. 88)

Berger further suggests that this inhibition of the EEG in those cortical areas not directly affected by the stimulus would function to increase the efficiency of the active center itself, "or that of creating the conditions which are required for the occurrence of a conscious sensation" (Berger, 1929, p. 178).

Concerning the frequency components of the EEG, Berger was the first to name and describe the characteristics of alpha and beta activity to be discussed later in this chapter. He believed that alpha reflected specific neural functioning of the brain, whereas beta (higher frequency activity) reflected only metabolic and nutritional processes. Berger (1929) later modified this view and suggested it was beta that "must be regarded as the material concomitant phenomena of mental

Table 12.1. *Levels of consciousness in terms of psychological states and EEG*

Behavioral state	EEG
Excited emotion	Fast, mixed frequencies with low to moderate amplitude
Alert	Mainly fast, low-amplitude waves
Relaxed wakefulness	Optimal alpha rhythm
Drowsiness	Reduced alpha and occasional low-amplitude slow waves
Light sleep	Sleep spindles and slow waves; loss of alphas
Deep sleep	Large and very slow waves; random, irregular patterns

Source: After Lindsley, 1952.

processes!" (Berger, 1929, p. 297, thirteenth report). Concerning their origin, alpha was seen to be related to large pyramidal cells of deeper layers of the cortex, and beta activity was related to small superficial cortical neurons. Overall, Berger accepted the idea that cortical activity was regulated from the thalamic center in such a manner that when thalamic regulation was lessened, cortical activity would become disorganized and loss of consciousness resulted.

In summary, the initial work of Hans Berger generated a number of hypotheses and theoretical speculations that continue to influence EEG research to this day. It is impressive that within a 10-year period Berger not only named the EEG and its major frequency components alpha and beta, but also investigated the timing of EEG and external stimuli, evoked responses, the merits of bipolar and unipolar recordings, as well as the application of Fourier analysis for describing the frequency components of the EEG. For more information on the history of the EEG, there exist a number of interesting and informative sources in addition to the writing of Berger himself (cf. Brazier, 1961; Lindsley & Wicke, 1974; Walter, 1953).

Historically, the most consistent view of EEG functioning in relation to psychological research has been in terms of arousal or activation. The traditional arousal model has assumed a unitary continuum ranging from sleep to high activity, which were thought to be indexed by any one of a number of psychophysiological measures (cf. Duffy, 1957, 1962). With the discovery of the role of the reticular activating system in desynchronization of EEG (cf. Moruzzi & Magoun, 1949), arousal seemed to have a firm theoretical basis on which to stand and a physiological mechanism by which to explain emotionality and arousal. Electroencephalography offered a convenient measure reflecting the activity of the reticular activating system (Lindsley, 1951). In this model, Lindsley (1952) describes a continuum in which lower levels of consciousness such as deep sleep are associated with large-amplitude low-frequency activity, whereas more alert activity and strong excitement are associated with high-frequency low-amplitude waves. Middle levels of alertness such as drowsiness and relaxed wakefulness are indexed by middle-range frequencies of EEG activity. This information is summarized in Table 12.1.

Daniel (1966) tested the basic arousal model by asking subjects to engage in periods ranging from relaxation to arousal. He reported overall mixed results with no single EEG parameter (i.e., amplitude distribution, frequency spectrum, power

spectrum, wavelength distribution, autocorrelation, and cross-correlation) supporting the arousal model in a convincing manner. Further, there was no support for the
idea that low-voltage high-frequency EEG activity is a unique property of arousal. In
summary, the arousal interpretation of EEG has played a major role in the history of
EEG research, but its historically simple presentation offers only a limited view of a
complex picture.

12.2   PHYSIOLOGICAL BASIS

Presently, there does not exist a definitive understanding of the origin of the EEG.
However, there do exist a number of suggestive theories that offer alternative
explanations of how elementary neural generators are synchronized and result in
the topological and frequency distribution understood as EEG. One of the first
theories of EEG genesis suggested that EEG reflected the summation of rapid
"all-or-none" depolarizations (i.e., action potentials) both from neighboring cells and
across time (Adrian & Matthews, 1934). However, this model has not been supported.
For example, in an overview of EEG, Cooper, Osselton, and Shaw (1980) point out
that although EEG must represent the summated activity of thousands of cells, it is
not possible to explain the slow potential changes of the EEG as the resultant of the
summation of nerve action potentials. This reasoning is supported by the work of
such researchers as Li and Jasper (1953), who demonstrated that the EEG of cats
could be recorded even after neural action potentials were abolished under deep
anaesthesia. Thus, the EEG is thought to result primarily from the subthreshold
synaptic and dendritic potentials that may summate and reflect the strength of the
stimulus rather than those that fire in an all-or-nothing manner (Bishop & Clare, 1953;
Purpura, 1959). Elul (1972) reviewed evidence from animal studies to suggest that
nerve cells in the cerebral cortex produce wave activity that reflects membrane
conductance in these neurons. His evidence was based on the demonstration that if
the activity of these neurons was blocked by drugs, then surface EEG disappeared.
Further, Elul suggested that the generator of the EEG is probably a group of
synapses, rather than the entire neuron, that are activated together. Elul referred to
this group of synapses as a "synaptic functional unit," which he described as
analogous to a motor unit in a skeletal muscle. The implication of this is that there
need not exist a special class of EEG generators but that all neurons may be
potentially involved in the generation of EEG. Further, it was suggested that only a
small proportion of the total possible number of cell groups need to be synchronized
at any one time. The particular set of neurons in synchrony could change from
moment to moment. Although there exists no direct evidence, Elul suggested that
the functional significance of the changing groups of sychronized cortical neurons
may reflect a subcortical "scanning" mechanism that would facilitate the identification and processing of cortical output by subcortical centers. Although the EEG
potentially could be generated by all neurons, the control in terms of a "pacemaker"
function of this cortical activity would come from subcortical sources (e.g., the
thalamus). In summary, Elul (1972) has suggested that there exist synaptic
functional units that would be analogous to a motor unit and that these synaptic
functional units generate the EEG. These synaptic functional units are composed of
a group of literally thousands of synapses sharing the same presynaptic input, which
would allow for depolarization or hyperpolarization as a unit. Within this model, the
EEG would result from a shifting of these functional units such that different

Table 12.2. *Major EEG frequencies and amplitudes*

Name	Frequency (Hz)	Amplitude (μV)
Delta	0.5–3.5	up to 100–200
Theta	4–7.5	<30
Alpha	8–12	30–50
Slow beta	13–19	<20
Fast beta	20–30	<20
Gamma	30–50	<10
Sleep spindles	12–14	5–100

generators at different times would be involved in the EEG recorded from surface electrodes. The control of such processes would be located in the subcortical areas and functionally represent a means to identify which particular cortical areas were active at any one time.

Presently, some researchers (e.g., Lutzenberger, Elbert, & Rockstroh, 1987) assume that we know enough to state clearly that EEG originates in the depolarizations of the dendritic trees of a pyramidal cell in the cerebral cortex. They base their argument on the fact that no subcortical structure would be large enough to generate 30–50 μV of potential difference on the scalp. These researchers also suggested that both the quantity of pyramidal neurons (some 70–80 percent of cortical neurons) and the restrictive geometry of the dendritic tree in the basket and stellate cells for producing scalp potentials further supported their position for the origin of EEG.

12.3   DESCRIPTION OF THE EEG

The resultant EEG recorded from the surface of the head can be represented by various types of periodic activity. Before the use of computers in EEG analysis, components of the record were identified by sight. Thus, by tradition, classification of EEG activity has been related largely to specific waveforms, frequency components, amplitude components, and amount of time that a particular frequency occurred in the EEG (see Cooper et al. 1980, for an extended discussion of each of these types of analysis). The major types of EEG activity are presented in Table 12.2.

It should be noted that these frequency divisions are approximate, although some factor analytic studies have suggested that these represent more than just arbitrary divisions. As better frequency analysis techniques have been applied, researchers have also made finer discriminations within a particular band. For example, beta is often divided into an upper beta band that begins around 20 Hz and ends above 30 Hz and a lower beta band composed of frequencies ranging from around 13 to 20 Hz. Finally, it should also be noted that high test–retest EEG frequency component reliability has been reported suggesting the normal EEG may be treated as a stable intra-individual trait (Gasser, Bacher, & Steinberg, 1985).

In the following sections, the major frequency bands will be discussed beginning with alpha since the majority of EEG work has been performed using this band. Beta activity is then discussed. Finally, theta and delta are discussed. These lower frequencies pose some interesting questions since the visual presence of low frequencies in the waking EEG record has been associated with pathology, whereas the presence of low-frequency activity as identified through mathematical signal analysis techniques may have important psychological implications for normal cognition.

12.3.1   *Alpha activity*

Alpha can be seen in about three-fourths of all individuals when they are awake and relaxed. Asking these individuals to close their eyes and relax will produce an immediate increase in alpha activity. In the spontaneous record alpha can be seen under a variety of conditions generally coming in bursts of several seconds each. Alpha activity is characterized by high-amplitude low-frequency (8–12 Hz) waveforms in the EEG. From its inception, alpha activity has been associated with particular levels of consciousness and awareness. Conversely, the reduction of alpha activity (alpha blocking) has been associated with sensory stimulation or mental activity.

Historically, alpha activity was first named by Hans Berger (1929). Since alpha could be recorded from any location on the cortex, Berger believed alpha activity to have a general function (Gloor, 1969). Darrow (1947) further investigated alpha and suggested that alpha waves were associated with vasoconstriction whereas alpha blocking and the enhancement of beta was associated with vasodilation and in turn related to vagal mechanisms (see Gullickson, 1973, for a collection and discussion of Darrow's work). Further, alpha was shown to be sensitive to hyperventilation, which suggested to Darrow (1947) that alpha might have a homeostatic function of maintaining and controlling internal cerebral functioning. Grey Walter (1953) speculated that the alpha rhythm reflected a mechanism that scanned the environment for information that was input once each alpha cycle. Thus, Walter (1953) pointed out that if someone was asked to scan 100 words, this would require about 10 s, or one word for each alpha cycle. He also suggested this is the basis for the illusion of movement when one light is turned off just before another is turned on in the same field of vision. Walter further considered visual imagination and alpha rhythms to be mutually exclusive. Lindsley (1952) suggested a distinction should be made between alpha activity and the alpha rhythm. Alpha activity was to be seen as the basic metabolic rhythm of brain cells that is always present even when a large number of cortical cells were not synchronized such that the alpha rhythm could not be recorded from the surface of the scalp with EEG electrodes. Since sensory input or mental activity was known to produce an EEG record of lower amplitude and higher frequency activity (referred to as alpha blocking), the presence of alpha was hypothesized to be related to a lack of activity in a particular area of the brain and in this manner used to infer information processing in particular locations. Alpha blocking as originally reported in the early EEG work has been recently confirmed by Grillon and Buchsbaum (1986), who presented 10 lights and tones of different intensities, which resulted in decreased amplitude of alpha. These researchers reported a differential reactivity with tones and lights in terms of frequency of alpha in various cortical areas. Their work also suggested that breaking the alpha band down into smaller frequency components may prove valuable as well as supporting the view that alpha activity is disrupted by a mechanism that involves the activation of specific sensory systems.

Another line of research has suggested that stimuli are processed at discrete temporal intervals and that the concurrent alpha rhythm can be a marker for maximal stimulus processing (see Surwillo, 1986, for an expanded discussion of the central timing hypothesis). The origin of this model has been attributed to Bishop (1933, 1936) and his speculation regarding the existence of a cortical excitability cycle. Since that time a number of researchers have considered several related possibilities including the possibility that alpha provides a means of pulsing and coding sensory impulses (Lindsley, 1952), that alpha is a scanning function that serves as a central regulating mechanism for coordinating afferent and efferent signals (Walter, 1953), and that alpha serves the function of a clock (Gooddy, 1958; Wiener, 1958). This type of thinking has been tested by presenting stimuli at various points in a single alpha cycle while the subject responds to the onset of the stimulus (Kristofferson, 1967). Surwillo, in a number of studies (e.g., Surwillo, 1963), reported that a positive association exists between alpha frequency and reaction time. Specifically, it is assumed that maximal stimulus processing can occur only at a particular part of a single alpha wave. Thus, with the lower alpha frequency reported in older populations there would be less opportunity for processing compared to the faster alpha rhythm seen earlier in life. Surwillo's general position is that the EEG frequency reflects a "biological clock" that determines information processing (cf. Surwillo, 1968; see also Marsh & Thompson, 1977, and Woodruff, 1978, 1983, for reviews of this work in relation to aging).

12.3.1.1 Generation of alpha

Although the early work of Lindsley and Wicke (1974) led to an accepted position that the gross anatomical locus for the generation of alpha activity was in the thalamus, there were numerous variations as well as alternative theories for the anatomical locus, the physiological substrate, and the functional significance of alpha activity. Andersen and Andersson (1968) have suggested that alpha results from activity generated by pyramidal cells in the cortex that are kept in synchrony by pacemaker neurons located in the thalamus. Although the Andersen and Andersson model of a thalamic pacemaker is widely accepted, it is not without its critics (cf. Nunez, 1981). The objection of Nunez is based on his view of EEG as composed of standing and traveling waves whose frequency is dependent on global properties of the brain rather than a fixed spatial pattern of input to the cortex from subcortical structures. In relation to this, Nunez points out that anatomically most of the input to a given area comes not from the thalamus but from other cortical regions via association fibers. Thus, he concludes that corticocortical interactions may be more important in determining EEG properties than thalamocortical interactions. Further, Nunez suggests that the ratio of corticocortical connections to thalamocortical connections, which differs across species, may be a major factor in determining the spatial and temporal properties of the EEG in different species.

In a different view, alpha also has been seen to be related to electromechanical properties exterior to the cortex. One such theory of alpha was presented by Lippold (1973) in which he suggested that alpha activity could be totally explained as an artifact of the mechanisms of the eye. To be specific, Lippold suggested that alpha is derived from a translational eye tremor that elicits oscillatory corneo-retinal potentials transmitted through the cerebral ventricles to a maximum at the occipital recording sites. This proposal was evaluated experimentally by Cavonius and

Estevez-Uscaryn (1974), who presented visual stimulation to either the left or right visual half-fields. They reasoned that if Lippold was correct, visual stimulation to either half-field should modify alpha activity across both hemispheres. What was found was that alpha blocking occurred only in the hemisphere anatomically connected with the particular half-field given stimulation.

Yet another electromechanical explanation of alpha speculated that cardiac activity was the basis of EEG alpha. This theory suggested that the applied force of arterial pulsations induce alpha by modulating standing intracranial DC potentials at a resonant frequency approximating 10 Hz (Castillo, 1983; Kennedy, 1959). A study by Hogan and Fitzpatrick (1987) sought to rule out both the cardiac and the eye muscle hypotheses using an isolated canine brain preparation. These authors reasoned that if alpha was present when the canine brain was isolated and presented blood in a continuous manner, then mechanical explanations would not be viable. This indeed was the case, and the study makes electromechanical explanations of EEG difficult to support.

Although a number of studies have sought to identify the origin of alpha, at this time two will be briefly reviewed along with the logic they present. Both studies utilized dogs since dogs have an alpha rhythm similar to humans in its localization frequency band, and reactivity to eye closure. Lopes da Silva and Storm van Leeuwen (1978) conducted an intriguing study designed to show the origin of alpha to be within the cortex. These researchers began with the simple assumption that the area of the brain generating alpha activity should form a dipole field oriented perpendicularly to the surface of the brain. It this were the case, then one would expect to find the opposite polarity as one moved from one end of the dipole to the other. Mathematically, this should be seen in the measure of phase between two signals that share a common component (see section 12.4.5 as well as Porges and Bohrer, chapter 21). In order to test this idea, Lopes da Silva and Storm van Leeuwen (1978) recorded telemetric EEG over a period of time in free-running dogs with implanted electrodes in the visual cortex. Alpha was recorded when the dog closed its eyes in a dimly lit room. The results demonstrated an opposite phase relationship (180°) between alpha rhythms recorded at the surface and that recorded from depth electrodes within the cortex. The authors conclude that these results are proof of the cortical origin of EEG alpha. Further, these results suggest that alpha does not sweep over the entire cortex but that there exist epicenters of alpha activity from which this activity spreads in several directions "just like water springing from small fountains" (Lopes da Silva & Storm van Leeuwen, 1978, p. 331). These authors interpret their work to suggest that one of the neuronal generators of alpha is located at the level of the large pyramidal cells in the visual cortex.

12.3.2 Beta activity

Beta activity has been defined as low-amplitude (2–30 μV) high-frequency (13–50 Hz) rhythms. Jasper and Andrews (1938) divided this band into an 18–30 Hz component they called beta waves and a 30–50 Hz component they referred to as gamma waves, although the term is infrequently seen in the literature today. In psychophysiological research beta generally includes the 20–30 Hz band, although various researchers may also include lower or higher frequency components. Historically, beta activity has been reported to be affected by tactile, auditory, and emotional stimulation (Lindsley & Wicke, 1974) as well as blocked by voluntary effort (Jasper & Penfield, 1949). Walter (1953) associated beta activity with tension as would be seen in states of anxiety. Both Darrow (1957) and Sokolov (1963) suggested that beta represents a process of cortical activation. Sokolov, for instance, associated beta with the orienting response such that beta should appear when stimuli are perceived as novel and disappear with habituation or problem solving. Vogel, Broverman, and Klaiber (1968) followed this line of reasoning and present evidence that individuals who did better on automatized tasks (e.g., reading color names, naming familiar objects) as compared to more spatial tasks (e.g., embedded figures, object assembly, and block design) showed less beta on more difficult math tasks than individuals who perform better on the more spatial tasks. Vogel et al. interpret these results to suggest that the former individuals who also attempted more difficult tasks were better able to habituate to their method of dealing with the task. This interpretation is also consistent with the hemispheric nature of the tasks in that one would expect individuals who perform best on naming and reading tasks (primarily left hemispheric for many individuals) would also find math problems (also primarily left hemispheric) easier than those individuals who do best on spatial tasks (primarily right hemispheric tasks). Ray and Cole (1985) suggested the involvement of beta in the processing of positive and negative emotional stimuli with more beta being present in the right temporal area during positively as opposed to negatively valenced emotional tasks.

12.3.3   Theta activity

Theta activity refers to EEG activity in the 4–8 Hz range. The term *theta waves* or *theta rhythm* was introduced by Grey Walter (1953) in the 1940s. He suggested that whereas alpha waves scan for information, theta waves scan for pleasure. Although not an easy statement to understand, Walter meant by this that in the same way that visual imagination and alpha are mutually exclusive, theta and the experience of pleasure are mutually exclusive. Thus, the cessation of a pleasurable activity is associated with theta activity. Although the scanning hypothesis is one possibility, it is a speculative possibility in an area in which alternatives abound including the simple suggestion that alpha and theta activity reflect content, quiescent organismic states. Developmentally, EEG activity in the theta range is seen in children between 1 and 6 years of age with the amount of theta activity decreasing with age. Other areas of research have suggested an involvement of theta with learning disabilities (e.g., Sklar, Hanley, & Simmons, 1972).

   Although theta activity has been associated with a variety of psychological processes including hypnagogic imagery, REM (rapid eye movement) sleep, problem solving, hypnosis, and meditation, there is little understanding concerning its nature (see Schacter, 1977, for a review). Schacter (1977) concluded his comprehensive review of the theta literature by suggesting that one cannot articulate in exact terms the relationship between theta and psychological processes. In fact, the literature suggests two very different relationships of theta and cognitive processes. On the one hand, theta has been associated with conditions of low levels of alertness (e.g., hypnagogic states, REM sleep, and sleep deprivation) and as such has been associated with decreased information processing. One interpretation of this association is that of inhibition of attention. On the other hand, theta has been associated with active and efficient processing of various types of problem solving and perceptual tasks. Vogel et al. (1968) suggested that these differences represent the existence of two different types of behavioral inhibition. Class I inhibition referred to a gross inactivation of an entire excitatory process that results in the induction of a relaxed, less active behavioral state. Class II inhibition, on the other hand, referred to a selective inactivation of particular responses such that particular patterns of activity are possible as illustrated by overlearned behavior. According to Vogel et al. (1968), the occurrence of low-frequency activity (including both theta and delta) during periods of performance in which old responses are being practiced would be an example of Class II inhibition. Further, it is suggested that there is a positive correlation between slow wave activity and efficiency of performance. However, it is unclear whether this correlation is direct or indirect.

It should also be noted that there exists a research area in animal EEG work that refers to theta. However, this area uses different conventions in that theta is broadly defined in terms of frequency and measured from electrodes located within the midbrain, particularly the hippocampus. In general, the animal work suggests two types of theta: type 1, which is related to movement and has a frequency range of 7–12 Hz in rats and rabbits, and type 2, which is related to immobility and has a frequency range of 4–9 Hz in rats and rabbits (see Bland, 1986, and Vanderwolf & Robinson, 1981, for a more detailed discussion of this area).

12.3.4 Delta activity

Delta activity refers to low-frequency EEG activity (0.5–4 Hz). It was named delta by Walter (1937) since the names alpha, beta, and gamma had been previously used. Delta is most commonly associated with sleep in the normal human and is a predominant frequency of the human newborn during the first two years of life. Pathological conditions such as brain tumors and vascular lesions are also associated with delta activity, although these will not be discussed in this chapter. One of the earliest studies with frequencies including delta was work by Hoagland, Cameron, and Rubin (1938). In this research, a delta index composed of all EEG frequencies below alpha was constructed and reported to increase in responses to "emotional stimulation in the form of probing remarks and questions of an intimate personal nature" (p. 247). Later research has examined the presence of both general and focal slow wave activity in terms of aging, with this work being reviewed by Marsh and Thompson (1977).

Although visually detected delta in the awake adult is considered abnormal, more sensitive signal-processing techniques (e.g., Fourier analysis) often show delta activity in the normal EEG record. For example, in a study by Grillon and Buchsbaum (1986), delta was reported to be responsive to intensities of light but not tones in the frontal areas. Tucker, Dawson, Roth, and Penland (1985), who also used signal-processing techniques for delta recognition, reported increases in delta power over left anterior regions during a word fluency task. Further, Tucker et al. reported delta power to be present across several adjacent frequency intervals in the delta band and not a clear peak, as would be expected if the delta were visible in the EEG. Thus, it may be important to distinguish delta activity that can be visually observed from that reported through signal–processing techniques (e.g., Fourier analysis) representing power across the frequencies of the delta band. Likewise, the interpretation of these two different types of delta would suggest different psychophysiological processes.

12.4   RECORDING OF THE EEG

12.4.1   *Introduction*

To record and quantify the EEG, electrical signals of only a few microvolts must be detected on the scalp and then amplified by a factor of 10^4–10^6. With such an amplification factor, care must be taken such that the final signal is indeed representative of the EEG and not artifact. To accomplish this end, EEG electrodes must be chosen and appropriately placed on the scalp along with a conductive gel such that unwanted noise is not introduced into the signal. The important electromechanical processes at this point are appropriate electrodes and amplification techniques. Historically, much attention was directed toward making electrodes, creating an electrode paste, and designing an appropriate amplifier with many of the initial psychophysiology texts largely directed toward this end (e.g., Brown, 1967; Strong, 1970; Venables & Martin, 1967). Today excellent electrodes and amplifiers can be purchased for the purpose of recording EEG, with some systems offering over 20 channels. However, such equipment presents both problems and promises, and thus it is imperative to understand the major questions in terms of EEG recording techniques. The interested reader should consult a source such as Cooper et al. (1980) for a thorough discussion of these issues. This understanding is particularly important as newer computerized devices (e.g., BEAM) are developed in which the EEG is presented only in a graphic representation following numerous amplification and analysis stages (see section 12.6). Numerous possibilities exist for artifacts to influence the final EEG record in such devices.

12.4.2   *Electrode location and recording*

The standard method for electrode placement is the International 10–20 system (Jasper, 1958). This system is so named since it represents 10 and 20 percent deviations from four anatomical landmarks. These four landmarks are the nasion (the bridge of the nose), the inion (the bump at the back of the head just above the neck), and the left and right preauricular points (depression in front of the ears above the cheekbone). The electrode locations are denoted by reference to both a frontal–posterior location (F = frontal, P = parietal, C = central, T = temporal, O = occipital) and a left–right location (odd numbers = left hemisphere, z = midline, even numbers = right hemisphere). Thus, the designation P_3 refers to an electrode placed above the parietal lobe on the left side of the cortex. This framework is presented in Figure 12.1.

When a researcher records electrical activity from the brain, it should be noted that one is, in actuality, comparing the signals from two recording electrodes. What is recorded is the signal or rhythm that is not common to both sites. Any shared or common signal is canceled out electrically. Thus, with EEG one is always measuring the electrical or potential difference between two electrode sites. Hence, a theoretical distinction is made between "active" sites and "inactive" sites. When EEG is recorded by comparing the signal between two active sites, this is referred to as bipolar recording. For example, one could record EEG activity from the left frontal (F_3) and the left parietal (P_3) areas. Since there are assumed to be EEG generators under both of these electrodes, both sites would be considered active. Bipolar recordings from some 15–30 electrodes are the common procedure of clinical EEG

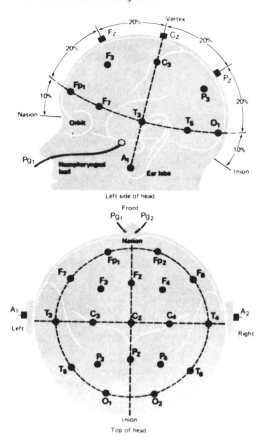

Figure 12.1. International 10–20 electrode system. (Reprinted from Stern, Ray, & Davis, 1980.)

examinations. This procedure allows for the visual detection of unusual waveforms not common to normal brain activity, such as epileptic discharges. However, most psychophysiological research is directed toward a description of normal EEG activity and somewhat by tradition has been performed in relation to an inactive reference site. Recordings in which one electrode is seen to be inactive are referred to as monopolar, or common, reference recording. The most common inactive reference sites are the ear lobes, which may be electrically connected and referred to as linked ears (AA), the nasion, the vertex, or the neck ring configuration (see Stephenson & Gibbs, 1951, and Nunez, 1981, for a discussion of noncephalic references). The term *inactive* suggests that such sites may be viewed as not reflecting a source of the EEG itself and thus allows a neutral site for reference. A procedure for electrically connecting the two ears (referred to as linked ears) has been the choice of clinical EEG procedures and is also widely used in research. Recently, Katznelson (1981) has discussed the idea of an inactive reference in some detail. Among his theoretical points is the idea that a linked-ears reference will display a reduced hemispheric difference and suggested a neck ring procedure for studies of hemispheric lateralization. Various researchers have informally suggested the actual empirical magnitude of this reduction is small and continue to recommend linked ears. Other researchers have suggested that a more appropriate reference to use in EEG research is that of a network of leads spaced across the scalp and mathematically averaged together. This average value then is used as the reference. The reference electrode question is an important one, and the interested reader should consult additional sources (e.g., Katznelson, 1981) for a discussion of these as well as newer approaches. One newer approach at this time is the Laplacian current source density derivation, which seeks to mathematically identify those areas of high cortical activity (sources) versus those of less cortical activity (sinks). Gevins et al. (1987) utilize this procedure in order to distinguish the electrical activity of the brain preceding accurate and inaccurate motor responses. At the present time, there is no general consensus among researchers as to the best electrode reference to use for monopolar recordings, although an average reference composed of a number of equally spaced electrodes has merit. However, the linked-ears reference remains in common use by tradition and has the ability to reduce heart rate artifacts in the EEG.

12.4.3   *Artifacts in the EEG record*

In order to simplify the process of electrode placement, a number of EEG researchers use specially designed helmets fitted with electrode sockets or the electrodes themselves at the 10–20 electrode locations. However, when using such devices, care still must be taken not only to ensure accurate location but also to ensure the absence of major artifacts. A variety of potential artifacts can be introduced into the EEG signal from both the normal physiology of the subject and the experimental environment. Such noncortical activity as the beating of the heart, the movement of the eyeballs and eyelids, and muscular activity from the face and neck may all enter into the EEG signal. Paradoxically, one of the best means of learning to cope with artifacts is to learn how to produce them on command. In this way it becomes easier to recognize artifacts and develop procedures for removing them. One procedure for minimizing artifacts is to set up the experimental situation such that movement is reduced or controlled for. Another procedure is to visually monitor the data and then discard those trials with artifact. Additionally, a computer program can be written to detect and correct such artifacts as eye movements (cf. Jervis, Nichols, Allen, Hudson, & Johnson 1985). External artifacts can come from such sources as elevator motors and electric lights as well as the polygraph and computer connections themselves. Most of these problems can be dealt with through either appropriate filtering of the signal (e.g., to remove 60 Hz activity) or careful shielding and grounding of the connections. Newer electrodes and amplifier circuits have greatly reduced external sources of artifacts in EEG recordings.

12.4.4   *Amplification*

In terms of amplification, the two factors of sensitivity and frequency response are important. Sensitivity refers to the magnitude of the incoming signal required for detection by the amplifier and to both the amplification factor (ratio of output to input voltage) of the amplifier and the writing device (e.g., a pen recorder). Sensitivity is often described in terms of voltage required for a particular pen deflection (e.g., $5\,\mu$V/mm). Frequency response refers to the frequency range that the amplifier is able to reproduce accurately (i.e., with minimal distortion and with equal sensitivity). Most EEG amplifiers have a frequency response from DC (0 Hz) to 100 Hz or more. Additionally, there are filters in almost all EEG machines for restricting this range. For example, the typical EEG recording involves frequencies between 0.5 and 30 Hz. For such a recording a low-pass filter would be set such that all frequencies above 30 Hz would be attenuated. Likewise, the high-pass filter would be set at 0.5 Hz. On some equipment the high-pass filter is labeled in terms of either frequency at which the sensitivity is 70.7 percent (-3 dB), referred to as turnover frequency, or in terms of time constants (e.g., 0.03, 0.1, 0.3, 1, 5, 10). There is a relationship between these measures [turnover frequency $= \frac{1}{2}\pi$ (time constant)] such that a 0.03 time constant would attenuate all frequencies below 5.3 Hz, a 0.1 time constant would attenuate below 1.6 Hz, and a 0.3 time constant below 0.53 Hz. Time constants on the order of 10s would be used for recording very slow signals such as the readiness potential (RP) or the contingent negative variation (CNV).

Once the EEG signal is detected and amplified, it can then be displayed visually with a strip-chart recorder. Whereas signal parameters historically have been extracted directly from this physical record, many laboratories today use this record primarily as a convenient check on signal fidelity. In most research laboratories, the amplified analog EEG signal is both written on a strip-chart recorder and sent to an analog-to-digital converter and then stored and analyzed by a digital computer. All quantification and analysis is thus actually performed on a digitized representation of the original EEG signal.

12.4.5 EEG analysis

As one can imagine, the spontaneous EEG produces a large amount of ongoing data that is multiplied in terms of the number of channels to be examined. Historically, EEG data were analyzed visually. Using such a procedure, a researcher would visually identify the frequency band under study. Quantification would be composed of the amount of time that a particular frequency was present in the record in relation to the total time of the record. There were also historical attempts to develop signal analyzers. However, with the availability of computers, sophisticated signal analysis procedures became available to EEG researchers (e.g., Bendat & Piersol, 1986; Roberts & Mullis, 1987). For a historical overview of signal-processing techniques that have been applied to the EEG, see Brazier (1980).

The analog EEG signal is first converted to a digital form using an analog-to-digital converter that can be manipulated mathematically by means of a digital computer. One question that must be determined is the rate at which the EEG signal is sampled so that an accurate record can be obtained by the computer. One can look toward engineering studies in signal processing for important guidelines. However, it should be noted that most engineering models assume that the signal under consideration (e.g., the EEG) can be viewed as being composed of a number of sines and cosines. Further, it is assumed that the signal either goes on infinitely or was transformed with filters that have an infinite roll-off (i.e., the beginning and end of the signal is not abrupt) and that there is a random relationship in terms of phase between the sampling frequency and the highest frequency in the signal as well as conditions to ensure that the signal under consideration does not contain excessive noise. Given these and other restrictive considerations, engineering studies have shown that a sampling rate of twice the highest frequency of a given signal to be sampled will contain all the basic information in that signal. Thus, if one were interested in accurately describing a signal with the highest frequencies below 30 Hz, then one must sample at a rate of at least twice 30 Hz. This sampling rate is referred to as the Nyquist frequency. However, EEG cannot be assumed to meet all the conditions required for accurate representation in engineering terms. Thus, in practice, most EEG researchers use a more conservative sampling rate of at least three to five times the highest frequency under consideration such that EEG researchers sample at 100 Hz or higher for describing frequencies in the 0.5–30 Hz range.

Before a sampled EEG epoch can be analyzed through a signal analysis technique such as Fourier, windowing may be necessary. Windowing is required since one does not analyze infinite EEG records but selects a particular time epoch or window for examination. For signal-processing purposes it is important that the beginning and end of a particular window be treated in a special way in order to attenuate the frequency characteristics that are mistakenly introduced into the power spectrum by the abrupt onset and offset of the epoch. Thus, windowing is designed to reflect more accurately the EEG signal. One of the more common windows is the Hanning window (also referred to as the cosine-bell window). There are additional windows that are described in detail in signal-processing texts (cf. Harris, 1978; Nuttall, 1981). Once the signal is converted to an appropriate digital form and shaped through the use of a windowing technique, the data are prepared for signal processing. The most common signal-processing procedure for EEG data is that of Fourier analysis.

Fourier analysis is a time series technique designed to decompose a signal into its frequency components (see Porges & Borher, chapter 21; Gottman, chapter 22). The technique is named after the French mathematician Fourier, who suggested that any given time series can be described as a corresponding sum of sine and cosine functions. Using this information, he described how to determine, in the frequency domain, the amplitude and phase information of a known temporal signal. What Fourier analysis allows one to do is to move from the EEG signal as expressed in terms of time into basic parameters that describe the frequency components of the signal. Basically, the Fourier transform creates a graph that plots the frequency of a signal against the amplitude of that frequency (referred to as "power" if squared). This procedure is also referred to as spectral analysis or power spectral analysis. Specific forms of the Fourier transform, generally referred to as the Fast Fourier Transform (FFT), have been developed especially for computer applications (see Cohen, 1986, for further discussion including the required programming).

A related signal analysis technique that is increasingly being used with the EEG is coherence analysis, including measurements of phase. Whereas Fourier gives the power spectral density for each channel, coherence gives the covariance of spectral energies between any given pair of channels at a particular frequency. Coherence is equivalent to the absolute value of the cross-correlation function in the frequency domain and may be considered to reflect the number and strength of connections between spatially distant cortical generators. In simple terms, coherence reflects the manner in which two signals covary at a particular frequency. The related measurement of phase reflects the extent to which these EEG measures are also in synchrony. That is, do two signals of the same frequency have peaks at the same time? Such an analysis has been used with both normal and abnormal populations (e.g., Koles & Flor-Henry, 1987; O'Connor, Shaw, & Ongley, 1979; Shaw et al., 1979; Thatcher, Walker, & Gudice, 1987; Tucker et al., 1985). Good discussions of coherence may be found in Cooper et al. (1980), recent EEG articles (e.g., Ford, Goether, & Dekker, 1986; Thatcher, Krause, & Hrybyk, 1986; Tucker & Roth, 1984), traditional signal-processing references (cf. Bendat & Piersol, 1986), as well as Gottman (chapter 22) and Porges and Bohrer (chapter 21). Further, Thatcher et al. (1987) discuss the use of measures of phase relation between EEG signals as estimates of cortical connection in terms of lead and lag times between separate generators of EEG as a means to describe neurophysiological network properties.

12.5 RESEARCH APPLICATIONS

Since the discovery of the EEG, individuals have sought to understand its relationship to various psychological and physiological processes as well as how individual differences ranging from sex to anxiety to intelligence are reflected in the EEG. Some processes – sleep, for example – are more ongoing and use EEG to define the change from one particular stage of sleep to another (Rechtschaffen & Kales, 1968). Likewise, EEG has been used to index the effects of pharmacological agents (cf. Fink, 1984). Although beyond the scope of this chapter, sleep and drug research present excellent examples of how EEG measures led to advances in understanding sleep, brain processes, and drug actions not available through other conventional methods such as self-report (Dement, 1974). Another use of the EEG is to describe the processing of particular types of tasks as with the hemispheric work comparing verbal versus spatial tasks or the processing of positive versus negative emotional tasks. A third use of EEG measures is to describe individual differences examining how various types of individuals compare with one another using the EEG to reflect underlying brain processes. Electroencephalographic studies offer particular promise in the study of nonconscious processes or in work with special populations such as infants, stroke victims, or individuals with psychiatric disorders. In this section of the chapter a number of these research areas and the manner in which EEG has been utilized are considered as well as assumptions made concerning the meaning of the EEG.

12.5.1 *Developmental aspects of EEG*

There are two ways in which EEG has been used in developmental research. The first way is as a descriptive tool in which EEG changes are mapped across the life span. The second is as an indicator of processing such as emotional or cognitive involvement in various tasks as well as indexing underlying physiological mechanisms. In terms of the first, some of the earliest work in this area was performed by Lindsley (1936, 1939) and continued by Henry (1944). Henry examined the EEG of 95 children across a 5-year period. In this monograph he reported on the developmental aspects of alpha, the absence of an association between alpha and skeletal maturity, and the relationship of alpha to IQ. More recently, EEG activity across the complete life span has been considered (e.g., Marsh & Thompson, 1977; Woodruff, 1978, 1983). The general view from these reports suggests that neuroanatomical development in the first years of life is reflected in the rhythmic EEG activity. Until 3–4 months of life, the infant EEG is of low voltage (less than 50 μV) and not well organized. Around 3 months of age, some dramatic changes take place in which an occipital rhythm of 3–4 Hz of more than 50 μV amplitude appears. Since this is also the time that the Babinski, Moro, and grasp reflexes disappear, these EEG changes have been interpreted as reflecting central nervous system development. By the end of the first year, the occipital EEG rhythm is in the 6–7 Hz range. Further, EEG changes parallel dendritic and myelinization changes that appear first in the sensory and then in the motor areas. Electroencephalographic changes during the next 12 years are less rapid. By age 12, the modal occipital EEG frequency is between 10 and 11 Hz, mirroring that of the adult. Traditionally, it has been assumed that alpha activity decreased with age. However, recently it has been suggested that this finding may be related to types of medication and other such factors and is not an aspect of human development.

More recently, Thatcher et al. (1987) used coherence and phase relations measurements from 577 children ranging in age from 2 months to 26 years to map underlying hemispheric changes. They concluded that the left hemisphere develops at a faster rate than the right in terms of the EEG phase relationship between frontal and occipital areas. They also found evidence of growth spurts at particular ages. Overall, these researchers suggest five dominant growth periods in terms of intrahemispheric cortical coupling across the life span. The first, from birth to 3 years of age, can be described as a decrease in coherence and phase. The second, from age 4 to 6 years, involved more synchronized patterns, mainly in terms of left hemispheric coupling. The third period, from ages 8 to 10, involved right hemispheric connections between the temporal and frontal areas. The final two periods, from ages 11 to 14 and 15 to adulthood, mainly involved bilateral connections within the frontal areas. Thatcher et al. point out that these periods are consistent with the Piagetian stages of cognitive development. Thus, this research suggests the possibility of a genetically programmed unfolding of specific cortical connections at specific ages, which are reflected in the EEG. Additionally, a valuable aspect of EEG research may be to help clarify the underlying mechanisms of more macrotheoretical presentations such as that of Piaget.

12.5.2   EEG measures of hemispheric lateralization

One basic conceptualization of the role of the central nervous system has been derived from the work of Roger Sperry and his colleagues with split-brain patients (see Sperry, 1982, for an overview). This research has led to the conclusion that the left hemisphere is more involved in the processing of verbal/analytic material, whereas the right hemisphere is more involved in the processing of visuospatial/ synthetic material. Although initially based on research with epileptic patients, other research using a variety of techniques including dichotic listening, tachisto-scopic presentation, lateral eye movements, blood flow measures, evoked potentials, as well as EEG has given support to the original formulation (see Bryden, 1982, Corballis, 1983, and Springer & Deutsch, 1985, for general reviews of these areas).

In one of the first studies using EEG as an index of hemispheric processing, Morgan, McDonald, and Macdonald (1971) reported proportionally less alpha activity over the right occipital areas (as compared to the left) during spatial tasks (imagining scenes) as compared to analytic ones (mental arithmetic and word construction). Using an undifferentiated EEG frequency band width ranging between 1 and 35 Hz, Galin and Ornstein (1972) reported EEG hemispheric differences in the parietal and temporal areas between spatial right hemispheric tasks (solving Kohs blocks and Minnesota Form Board) and verbal left hemispheric tasks (writing a letter and mentally composing a letter). A later study (Doyle, Ornstein, & Galin, 1974) reported that the task-dependent asymmetries were strongest in the alpha band, and numerous researchers have limited their research to this band. In general, researchers have reported EEG results consistent with the hemispheric lateralization hypothesis (see Davidson & Ehrlichman, 1980; Donchin, Kutas, & McCarthy, 1977; and Yingling, 1980, for a presentation of these studies).

There are a number of methodological issues ranging from the site of the reference electrode to the mode of analysis to the meaning of the EEG itself that remain open issues at this time. Donchin et al. (1977), in their review of electrocortical measures of hemispheric lateralization, suggested that a number of logical and methodological issues exist making interpretation of existing studies difficult. Gevins et al. (1979) proposed that previous lateralized differences in electrocortical measures did not relate to cognitive processing but rather reflected inconsistencies in stimulus properties, limb movements during tasks, and/or performance factors such as subject ability or engagement in a given task. Ray and Cole (1985) have demonstrated that the attentional demands of the task also influence EEG hemispheric alpha ratios. This type of methodological criticism suggests that simple EEG ratio measures of alpha activity along a single verbal–spatial continuum might not be presenting the entire story in terms of hemispheric lateralization. The positive side of the picture is that in spite of a lack of exact meaning of the EEG in hemispheric studies, it is stable over time both in terms of task-related EEG asymmetries over sessions (Amochaev & Salamy, 1979; Ehrlichman & Wiener, 1979) and in terms of a stable intra-individual trait (Gasser et al., 1985).

12.5.3 *Hemispheric laterality and emotion*

Cognitive processes have been associated not only with differential hemispheric involvement, but also with emotionality. Support has accumulated from a variety of sources for the idea that lateralized central nervous system activity and emotionality are functionally related (see Tucker, 1981, for a review). In addition, recent evidence suggests that an anterior–posterior dimension must also be considered. For example, Robinson, Kubos, Starr, Rao, and Price (1984) have reported differential anterior–posterior as well as hemispheric involvement with mood disorders. In an examination of stroke patient groups, Robinson et al. found that patients with left frontal lesions reported significantly more severe depression, whereas less depression was noted in patients with lesions in the posterior left hemisphere. A different pattern was seen in the right hemisphere, with depression being more pronounced in patients with lesions in the right posterior areas, whereas patients with anterior lesions were more cheerful.

Electrocortical research has also suggested differential hemispheric activation related to emotionality with both psychiatric populations (Flor-Henry, 1979) and normal populations (Davidson, Schwartz, Saron, Bennett, & Goldman, 1979; Erlichman & Weiner, 1980; Harman & Ray, 1977; Tucker, Stenislie, Roth, & Shearer, 1981) using a variety of emotionally valenced tasks. The particular emotional valence associated with each hemisphere has varied. For example, in one of the first studies to examine EEG correlates of emotional functioning, Harman and Ray (1977) reported differential hemispheric changes over time with the recall of positive and negative past events. Left hemispheric temporal power (3–30 Hz) increased during recall of positive events and decreased during recall of negative events. Using similar tasks and recording sites, Ehrlichman and Wiener (1980) also reported greater right hemispheric activation (relatively more alpha activity in the left hemisphere than right hemisphere) during positive emotional tasks.

Other research requiring subjects to evaluate emotional stimuli has also reported hemispheric differences. Davidson et al. (1979) required subjects to subjectively rate how well they liked or disliked various parts of a television show using a pressure-sensitive device. Bilateral frontal and parietal EEG activity in the alpha range was compared during liked and disliked segments. The results indicated relatively greater right frontal alpha activity during the favored segments and relatively greater left frontal alpha activity during disliked segments. No significant differences were reported for parietal activity. Tucker et al. (1981) used a mood induction procedure and then presented subjects with cognitive tasks. Tucker found negative mood to be associated with greater left frontal EEG alpha activity. Using a three-mode factor analytic technique (PARAFAC), Ray and Cole (1985) reported greater beta in the right temporal area during positively as opposed to negatively valenced emotional tasks. Davidson and his colleagues have also reported finding temporal differences in EEG processing using emotional films with a depressed population (Henriques, Davidson, Straus, Senulis, & Saron, 1987).

12.5.3.1 *EEG methodological and theoretical questions in relation to emotionality*

Since the EEG studies examining emotion, mood, and preference have used a variety of tasks and procedures involving different frequency bands and areas of the cortex, it remains unclear whether different EEG results may be attributed to variations in EEG measures being recorded (e.g., different frequency bands and/or data transformations), the manner in which different areas of the cortex (e.g. frontal, parietal, and temporal) are involved in the processing of emotional material, or the task requirements themselves (e.g., the validity of the emotions produced). Part of the problem is also a definitional one since emotionality and arousal have been linked for years in the experimental literature. In fact, emotionality as defined in many of the experimental studies dating back to the 1930s meant nothing more than activity on the part of an organism. Today, there is often little distinction between constructs such as emotionality, feelings, and moods, and thus specificity is missing in terms of precise EEG mappings.

In EEG research with awake subjects the common assumption was that alpha activity was inversely related to levels of arousal and beta activity was directly related to levels of arousal. One common assumption dating back to the early days of EEG research, for instance, was that alpha blocking involves the replacement of alpha waves by beta waves (e.g., Adrian & Matthews, 1934). However, informal as well as published reports have shown this not to be the case (e.g., Elliott, 1964). In our own laboratory, as well as in others, there is common skepticism toward the inverse alpha–beta assumption. For example, for various tasks we have found beta activity to increase or decrease with increases in alpha as well as to have no relationship (McCarthy & Ray, 1988). In one study, alpha was found to be sensitive to attentional factors, whereas beta reflected the type of task (Ray & Cole, 1985). In particular, the arousal assumption places a much too important role on EEG alpha and assumes less specificity in the cortex than is usually assumed to be the case. Indeed, although cognitive psychology has moved beyond a simple arousal model, this transition has not been clearly reflected in EEG research. In sum, the power in one frequency band can be used to infer neither the relative nor the absolute power in other frequency bands.

12.5.4 *Individual differences*

The study of EEG and individual differences has existed since the beginning studies of Berger and Adrian and Matthews (cf. Lemere, 1936). One of the most experimentally investigated conceptualizations of individual differences has been the introversion–extraversion dimension. The study of introversion–extraversion as developed by Hans Eysenck (1967) had a neuropsychological basis that has often been tested through EEG approaches (Gale, 1981, 1983; Gale and Edwards, 1986). The general theory suggested that one difference between introverts and extraverts is the threshold of arousal of the brainstem reticular formation and its relation to an optimum arousal level. Specifically, extraverts have been conceptualized as having a high threshold for arousal, leading to a state of underarousal, whereas introverts have been conceptualized as having a lower threshold for arousal, leading to overarousal. According to the theory, this results in the extravert seeking to increase arousal through contact with new and varied stimulation, whereas the introvert attempts to reduce arousal levels through avoiding stimulation or engaging in familiar and unchanging activities.

Given that extraverts are seen to be underaroused, the EEG prediction by researchers was that extraverts would show greater relative power in the lower EEG frequencies (e.g., alpha) interpreted by these researchers to be indicative of relative underarousal, whereas introverts would display greater relative power in the high-frequency bands (e.g., beta), suggestive of more active processing and greater arousal. A number of studies report such findings for extraverts and introverts at baseline rest conditions. However, other studies have also found either no differences or the opposite relationship. Numerous studies related to the Eysenck arousal question are reviewed in great detail by Gale (1983) and Gale and Edwards (1983, 1986). As they point out in their review, there are a variety of questions related to personality measurement as well as the appropriate task and EEG parameters yet to be answered.

Another interesting individual difference measure is the relationship between sex and spatial ability. It is well known that males score higher on spatial ability tests than females. There has been some speculation that this is related to neurological organization and thus hemispheric differentiation (cf., McGlone, 1980). Based on some initial work by Furst (1976) with EEG and Gur and Revich (1980) with blood flow, Ray, Newcombe, Semon, and Cole (1981) sought to determine if different EEG activity in high and low spatial ability males and females was associated with successful solving of spatial problems. Results revealed evidence for the hypothesized relationship, but only for males. In addition, high and low spatial ability males showed equal but opposite correlations with performance. EEG ratios (right − left/ right + left) with performance were negative (-0.77 during baseline and -0.53 during tasks) for high spatial ability males but positive (0.77 and 0.56, respectively) for low spatial ability males. This was interpreted as suggesting that different areas of the brain were associated with successful performance in each group. Further it was suggested that high and low spatial ability males adopted opposite approaches to solving spatial tasks, one a more right hemispheric (spatial/synthetic) and the other a more left hemispheric (verbal/analytic). In addition, the higher baseline correlations suggest that EEG may be useful as a measure to examine the set or preparation that an individual brings to a task. In future work, it would be interesting to determine if these baseline differences in ongoing EEG are related to the slow wave potentials seen as a subject prepares for a task presentation (cf. Birbaumer, Elbert, Rockstroh, Lutzenberger, & Schwartz, 1981).

12.6   NEW DEVELOPMENTS AND EEG RESEARCH

Although human EEG research has been in development for over 50 years, new instrumentation and techniques suggest that we are entering a stage in which important new developments are possible. One of the most important recent developments is the personal computer, making sophisticated EEG analysis possible with limited resources. Likewise, laboratory computers are reaching speeds in terms of operations per second that allow for a large variety of parameters to be calculated almost simultaneously. One new technique involves a method of graphically representing EEG activity across the surface of the cortex through color coding of EEG parameters. Referred to as BEAM (brain electrical activity mapping), this technique maps EEG information on a color computer screen in relation to the amplitude and frequency of the EEG at each of a number of brain sites simultaneously (cf. Duffy, 1982; Duffy, McAnulty, & Schachter, 1984). This technique offers a visual representation of EEG data that is useful for the graphic presentation of abnormal patterns of activity, as found in epilepsy, for example. However, technology is not enough, as Freeman and Skarda (1985) point out: It is also important for an appropriate nomenclature and set of conventions to be developed if graphic presentations of the EEG are to progress in a meaningful manner. This should also aid in the development of a guiding theory to help interpret these large-scale graphic displays.

A strictly empirical computer-based approach was developed by John and his colleagues (Harmony, 1984; John, 1977; Thatcher & John, 1977). These researchers proposed a statistical approach to EEG interpretation, referred to as Neurometrics, for the differential diagnosis of a variety of clinical disorders. The basic procedure involved the development of a normative EEG data base collected cross-culturally from healthy individuals that served as a basis of comparison. When statistical features of certain EEG parameters (e.g., absolute power, relative power, mean frequency, coherence, and asymmetry) in this data base were compared with EEGs of patients showing a variety of cognitive, psychiatric, and neurological dysfunctions, a high incidence of abnormal values in the clinical groups was found (cf. John, Prichep, Fridman, & Easton, 1988). Specific statistical patterns of EEG activity were associated with particular disorders such that a computerized differential classification was possible for some disorders. Further, the magnitude of these statistical deviations was found to increase with severity of the disorder. The promise of this research is the ability to objectively diagnose a variety of clinical and neurological disorders.

A recent development is the application of nonlinear dynamics to the study of EEG (e.g., Skarda & Freeman, 1987). The basic idea is that seemingly irregular or quasi-random patterns of EEG activity could have been generated from relatively simple deterministic systems. The use of nonlinear dynamics or "chaos" theory as it is often called is an attempt to describe the nature of the EEG signal in mathematical and topological terms, especially that of a phase space. A simple way to understand the question is to ask how many differential equations are required to model a particular segment of EEG activity. If a few equations are required, the EEG activity could be said to be low dimensional. If, however, EEG activity was totally random, then an infinite number of equations would be required. Destexhe, Sepulchre, and Babloyantz (1988) use such an approach and report that processes such as deep sleep and epileptic EEG are of a lower dimension than normal alpha activity. Such information has important implications for modeling EEG activity in a variety of pathological and normal conditions and should lead to a better understanding of EEG processes. However, this research is in its early stages in a variety of laboratories around the world including our own, and it will be some time before the usefulness of the approach can be assessed.

In the last 10 years a number of new technologies have emerged that promise to offer new ways to noninvasively probe the regional activity of the brain during psychological processing. These include regional cerebral blood flow (RCBF) studies (cf. Larsen, Skinhoj, & Lassen, 1978), computerized axial tomography (CAT scan), positron emission tomography (PET scan) (cf. Phelps & Mazziotta, 1985), nuclear magnetic resonance (NMR imaging), and magnetoencephalography (MEG, cf. Rose Smith, & Sato, 1987). Andreasen (1988) has compared these approaches in relation to psychiatric applications. Holder (1987) has reviewed these and newer techniques in terms of future possibilities including the suitability for imaging neuronal discharge. Holder suggested that at present two techniques, that of impedance imaging and that of electron spin resonance, offer the greatest potential for imaging neuronal discharges in the human brain. Impedance imaging, which is similar in principle to currently used impedance techniques for studying cardiovascular activity, and electron spin resonance, which is similar to NMR techniques, are both in the development phase. In general, these techniques offer a structural, more microlevel approach, which complements the more macrolevel information contained in the EEG. At this point the long-term potential and applications for various methods of representing brain activity, including the EEG, have yet to be fully evaluated but appear substantial.

NOTE

I would like to thank Thomas Elbert, Paul McCarthy, Judy Ray, Jules Thayer, and Don Tucker as well as the editors of this volume for thoughtful suggestions concerning this chapter.

REFERENCES

Adrian, E. D., & Matthews, B. H. C. (1934). Berger rhythm: Potential changes from the occipital lobes of man. *Brain, 57,* 355–385.
Amochaev, A., & Salamy, A. (1979). Stability of EEG laterality effects. *Psychophysiology, 16,* 242–246.
Andersen, P., & Andersson, S. (1968). *Physiological basis of the alpha rhythm.* New York: Appleton-Century-Crofts.
Andreasen, N. (1988). Brain imaging: Applications in psychiatry. *Science, 239,* 1381–1388.
Bendat, J. S., & Piersol, A. G. (1986). *Random data, analysis and measurement* (2nd ed.). New York: Wiley.
Berger, H. (1929). Uber das Elektrenkephalogramm des Menschen. Translated and reprinted in Pierre Gloor, Hans Berger on the electroencephalogram of man. *Electroencephalography and clinical neurophysiology (Supp. 28,)* 1969, Amsterdam: Elsevier.
Birbaumer, N., Elbert, T., Rockstroh, B., Lutzenberger, W., & Schwartz, J. (1981). EEG and slow

cortical potentials in anticipation of mental tasks with different hemispheric involvement. *Biological Psychology, 13,* 251–260.

Bishop, G. H. (1933). Cyclic changes in excitability of the optic pathway of the rabbit. *American Journal of Physiology, 103,* 213–224.

Bishop, G. H. (1936). The interpretation of cortical potentials. *Cold Spring Harbor Symposium on Quantitative Biology, 15,* 305–317.

Bishop, G. H., & Clare, M. H. (1953). Response of cortex to direct electrical stimuli applied at different depths. *Journal of Neurophysiology, 16,* 1–19.

Bland, B. (1986). The physiology and pharmacology of hippocampal formation theta rhythms. *Progress in Neurobiology, 26,* 1–54.

Brazier, M. A. B. (1961). *A history of the electrical activity of the brain, the first half century.* New York: Macmillan.

Brazier, M. A. B. (1980). The early developments of quantitative EEG analysis: The roots of modern methods. In R. Sinz & M. Rosenzweig (Eds.), *Psychophysiology 1980.* Amsterdam: Elsevier.

Brown, C. (1967). *Methods in psychophysiology.* Baltimore: Williams & Wilkins.

Bryden, M. P. (1982). *Laterality.* New York: Academic Press.

Castillo, H. T. (1983). A cardiac hypothesis for the origin of EEG alpha. *IEEE Transactions in Biomedical Engineering, BME-30,* 793–796.

Caton, R. (1875). The electric currents of the brain. *British Medical Journal, 2,* 278.

Caton, R. (1877). Interim report on investigation of the electric currents of the brain. *British Medical Journal, 1(Supp.),* 62–65.

Cavonius, C. R., & Estevez-Uscaryn, D. (1974). Local suppression of alpha activity by pattern in half visual field. *Nature, 251,* 412–413.

Cohen, A. (1986). *Biomedical signal processing.* Boca Raton, FL: CRC Press.

Cooper, R., Osselton, J., & Shaw, J. (1980). *EEG technology* (3rd ed.) London: Butterworths.

Corballis, M. C. (1983). *Human laterality.* New York: Academic Press.

Daniel, R. S. (1966). Electroencephalographic pattern quantification and the arousal continuum. *Psychophysiology, 2,* 146–160.

Darrow, C. W. (1947). Psychological and psychophysiological significance of the electroencephalogram. *Psychological Review, 54,* 157–168.

Darrow, C. W. (1957). Electroencephalographic "blocking" and "adaptation." *Science, 126,* 74–75.

Davidson, R., Schwartz, G., Saron, C., Bennett, J., & Goldman, D. (1979). Frontal versus parietal EEG asymmetry during positive and negative affect. *Psychophysiology, 16,* 202–203.

Davidson, R. J., & Ehrlichman, H. (1980). Lateralized cognitive processes and the electroencephalogram. *Science, 207,* 1005–1006.

Dement, W. (1974). *Some must watch while others must sleep.* San Francisco: Freeman.

Destexhe, A., Sepulchre, J., & Babloyantz, A. (1988). A comparative study of the experimental quantification of deterministic chaos. *Physics Letters A, 132,* 101–106.

Donchin, E., Kutas, M., & McCarthy, G. (1977). Electrocortical indices of hemisperic utilization. In S. Harnad, S. Doty, L. Goldstein, J. Jaynes, & G. Kravthamer (Eds.), *Lateralization in the nervous system.* New York: Academic Press.

Doyle, J. Ornstein, R., & Galin, D. (1974). Lateral specialization of cognitive mode: II. EEG frequency analysis. *Psychophysiology, 11,* 567–578.

Du Bois-Reymond, E. (1848). *Untersuchungen uber thierische Elektricitat.* Berlin: Reimer.

Duffy, E. (1957). The psychological significance of the concept of "arousal" or "activation." *Psychological Review, 64,* 265–275.

Duffy, E. (1962). *Activation and behavior.* New York: Wiley.

Duffy, F. (1982). Topographic display of evoked potentials: Clinical applications of brain electrical mapping (BEAM). *Annuals of the New York Academy of Sciences, 388,* 183–196.

Duffy, F., McAnulty, G., & Schachter, S. (1984). Brain electrical activity mapping, In N. Geschwind & A. Galaburda (Eds.), *Cerebral dominance.* Cambridge, MA: Harvard University Press.

Ehrlichman, H., & Wiener, M. (1979). Consistency of task related EEG asymmetries. *Psychophysiology, 16,* 247–252.

Ehrlichman, H., & Wiener, M. (1980). EEG asymmetry during covert mental activity. *Psychophysiology, 17,* 228–235.

Elliott, R. (1964). Physiological activity and performance: A comparison of kindergarten children with young adults. *Psychological Monographs, 78* (No. 10, Whole # 587).

Elul, M. R. (1972). The genesis of the EEG. *International Review of Neurobiology, 15,* 227–272.

Eysenck, H. (1967). *The biological bases of personality.* Springfield. IL: Thomas.

Ferrier, D. (1875). Experiments on the brains of monkeys. *Proceedings of the Royal Society (London), 23,* 409–505.

Fink, M. (1984). Pharmacoelectroencephalography: A note on its history. *Neuropsychobiology, 12,* 173–178.

Flor-Henry, P. (1979). On certain aspects of the localization of the cerebral systems regulating and determining emotion. *Biological Psychiatry, 14,* 677–698.

Ford, M., Goethe, J., & Dekker, D. (1986). EEG coherence and power in the discrimination of psychiatric disorders and medication effects. *Biological Psychiatry, 21,* 1175–1188.

Freeman, W., & Skarda, C. (1985). Spatial EEG patterns, nonlinear dynamics and perception: The neo-Sherringtonian view. *Brain Research Reviews, 10,* 147–175.

Fritsch, G., & Hitzig, E. (1870). Uber did elektrische Erregbzarkeit des Grosshirns. *Archiv für Anatomie Physiologic und Wissenschaftlichi Medium, 37,* 300–332. [Translated by G. Von, Bonin, *The cerebral cotex,* Springfield, IL: Thomas.

Furst, C. (1976). EEG alpha asymmetry and visuospatial performance. *Nature, 260,* 254–255.

Gale, A. (1981). EEG studies of extraversion-introversion: What's the next step? In R. Lynn (Ed.), *Dimensions of personality: Essays in honour of H. J. Eysenck.* Oxford: Pergamon Press.

Gale, A. (1983). Electroencephalographic correlates of extraversion and introversion. In R. Simz & M. R. Rosenweig (Eds.), *Psychophysiology 1980.* Amsterdam: Elsevier Biomedical Press.

Gale, A., & Edwards, J. (1983). EEG and human behavior. In A. Gale & J. Edwards (Eds.), *Physiological correlates of human behavior* (Vol. 2). London: Wiley.

Gale, A., & Edwards, J. (1986). Individual differences. In M. Coles, E. Donchin, & S. Porges (Eds.), *Psychophysiology, systems, processes, and applications.* New York: Guilford Press.

Galin, D., & Ornstein, R. (1972). Lateral specialization of cognitive mode: An EEG study. *Psychophysiology, 9,* 412–418.

Gasser, T., Bacher, P., & Steinberg, H. (1985). Test–retest reliability of spectral parameters of the EEG. *EEG and Clinical Neurophysiology, 60,* 312–319.

Gevins, A., Morgan, N., Bressler, S., Cutillo, B., White, R., Illes, J., Greer, D., Doyle, J., & Zeitlin, G. (1987). Human neuroelectric patterns predict performance accuracy. *Science, 235,* 580–585.

Gevins, A., Zeitlin, G., Doyle, J., Yingling, C. D., Schaffer, R. E., Callaway, E., & Yeager, C. L. (1979). Electroencephalogram correlates of higher cortical functions. *Science, 203,* 665–668.

Gloor, P. (1969). Hans Berger on the electroencephalogram of man. *Electroencephalography and clinical neurophysiology (Supp. # 28).* Amsterdam: Elsevier.

Gooddy, W. (1958). Time and the nervous system. The brain as a clock. *Lancet, 7031,* 1139–1144.

Grillon, C., & Buchsbaum, M. (1986). Computed EEG topography of response to visual and auditory stimuli. *EEG and Clinical Neurophysiology, 63,* 42–53.

Gullickson, G. (1973). *The psychophysiology of Darrow.* New York: Academic Press.

Gur, R. C., & Reivich, M. (1980). Cognitive effects on hemispheric blood flow in humans: Evidence for individual differences in hemispheric activation. *Brain and Language, 9,* 78–92.

Harman, D., & Ray, W. J. (1977). Hemispheric activity during affective verbal stimuli: An EEG study. *Neuropsychologia, 15,* 457–460.

Harmony, T. (1984). *Neurometric assessment of brain dysfunction in neurological patients.* Hillsdale, NJ: Lawrence Erlbaum.

Harris, F. (1978). On the use of windows for harmonic analysis with the discrete Fourier transform. *Proceedings of the IEEE, 66,* 51–83.

Henriques, J., Davidson, R., Straus, A., Senulis, J., & Saron, C. (1987). Emotion-elicited EEG asymmetries differ in depressed and control subjects. *Psychophysiology, 24,* 591–592.

Henry, C. (1944). Electroencephalograms of normal children. *Monographs of the Society for Research in Child Development, IX, 3* (Serial No. 39).

Hoagland, H., Cameron, D., & Rubin, M. (1938) Emotion in man as tested by the delta index of the electroencephalogram: I. *The Journal of General Psychology, 19,* 227–245.

Hogan, K., & Fitzpatrick (1987). The cerebral origin of the alpha rhythm. *Electroencephalography and Clinical Neurophysiology, 69,* 79–81.

Holder, D. S. (1987). Feasibility of developing a method of imaging neuronal activity in the human brain: A theoretical review. *Medical and Biological Engineering and Computing, 25,* 2–11.

Jasper, H. (1958). Report on the committee on methods of clinical examination in electroencephalography. *Electroencephalography and Clinical Neurophysiology, 10,* 370–375.

Jasper, H., & Andrews, H. (1938). Electroencephalography. III. Normal differentiation of occipital and precentral regions in man. *Archives of Psychiatry, 39,* 96–115.

Jasper, H., & Penfield, W. (1949). Electrocorticograms in man: Effect of voluntary movement upon the electrical activity of the precentral gyrus. *Archives of Psychiatry, 183,* 183–174.

Jervis, B., Nichols, M., Allen, E., Hudson, N., & Johnson, T. (1985). The assessment of two methods for removing eye movement artefact from the EEG. *Electroencephalography and Clinical Neurophysiology, 61,* 444–452.

John, E. (1977). *Functional neuroscience: Vol. 2. Neurometrics: Clinical applications of quantitative electrophysiology.* Hillsdale, NJ: Erlbaum.

John, E., Prichep, L., Fridman, J., & Easton, P. (1988). Neurometrics: Computer-assisted differential diagnosis of brain dysfunctions. *Science, 239,* 162–169.

Katznelson, R. (1981). EEG recording, electrode placement, and aspects of generator localization. In P. L. Nunez (Ed.), *Electrical fields of the brain.* New York: Oxford University Press.

Kennedy, J. (1959). A possible artifact in electroencephalography. *Psychological Review, 66,* 347–352.

Koles, Z., & Flor-Henry, P. (1987). The effects of brain function on coherence patterns in the bipolar EEG. *International Journal of Psychophysiology, 5,* 63–71.

Kristofferson, A. B. (1967). Successiveness discrimination as a two-state, quantal process. *Science, 158,* 1337–1339.

Larsen B., Skinhoj, E., & Lassen, N. (1978). Variations in regional cortical blood flow in the right and left hemispheres during automatic speech. *Brain, 101,* 193–209.

Lemere, F. (1936). The significance of individual differences in the Berger rhythm. *Brain, 59,* 366–375.

Li, C., & Jasper, H. (1953). Microelectrode studies of the electrical activity of the cerebral cortex in the cat. *Journal of Physiology, 121,* 117–140.

Lindsley, D. (1936). Brain potentials in children and adults. *Science, 84,* 354.

Lindsley, D. (1939). A longitudinal study of the occipital rhythm in normal children: Frequency and amplitude standards. *Journal of Genetic Psychology, 55,* 197–213.

Lindsley, D. (1951). Emotion. In S. S. Stevens (Ed.), *Handbook of experimental psychology.* New York: Wiley.

Lindsley, D. (1952). Psychological phenomena and the electroencephalogram. *Electroencephalography and Clinical Neurophysiology, 4,* 443–456.

Lindsley, D., & Wicke, J. (1974). The electroencephalogram: Autonomous electrical activity in man and animals. In R. Thompson & M. Patterson (Eds.), *Bioelectric recording techniques: Part B. Electroencephalography and human brain potentials.* New York: Academic Press.

Lippold, O. (1973). *The origin of the alpha rhythm.* London: Churchill Livingstone.

Lopes da Silva, F., & Storm van Leeuwen, W. (1978). The cortical alpha rhythm in dogs: The depth and surface profile of phase. In M. Brazier & H. Petsche (Eds.), *Architectonics of the cerebral cortex.* New York: Raven Press.

Lutzenberger, W., Elbert, T., & Rockstroh, B. (1987). A brief tutorial on the implications of volume conduction for the interpretation of the EEG. *Journal of Psychophysiology, 1,* 81–89.

Marsh, G., & Thompson, L. (1977). Psychophysiology of aging. In J. Birren & W. Schaie (Eds.), *Handbook of the psychology of aging.* New York: Van Nostrand Reinhold.

McCarthy, P., & Ray, W. (1988). Interactions between alpha and beta EEG frequencies. *Psychophysiology, 25,* 434.

McGlone, J. (1980). Sex differences in human brain asymmetry: A critical survey. *Behavioral and Brain Sciences, 3,* 215–263.

Morgan, A., McDonald, P., & Macdonald, H. (1971). Differences in bilateral alpha activity as a function of experimental task, with a note on lateral eye movements and hypnotizability. *Neuropsychologia, 9,* 459–469.

Moruzzi, G., & Magoun, H. W., (1949). Brain stem reticular formation and activation of the EEG. *EEG and Clinical Neurophysiology, 1,* 455–473.

Nunez, P. (1981). *Electrical fields of the brain.* New York: Oxford University Press.

Nuttal, A. (1981). Some windows with very good sidelobe behavior. *IEEE Transactions on Acoustics, Speech and Signal Processing, 29,* 84–91.

O'Connor, K., Shaw, J., & Ongley, C. (1979). The EEG and differential diagnosis in psychogeriatrics. *British Journal of Psychiatry, 135,* 156–162.

Phelps, M., & Mazziotta, J. (1985). Positron emission tomography: Human brain function and biochemistry. *Science, 228,* 799–809.

Purpura, D. (1959). Nature of electrocortical potentials and synaptic organizations in cerebral and cerebellar cortex. *International Review of Neurobiology, 1,* 42–163.

Ray, W. J., & Cole, H. C. (1985). EEG alpha activity reflects attentional demands, and beta activity reflects emotional and cognitive processes. *Science, 228,* 750–752.

Ray, W. J., Newcombe, N., Semon, J., & Cole, P. (1981). Spatial abilities, sex differences, and EEG functioning. *Neuropsychologia, 19,* 719–722.

Rechtschaffen, A., & Kales, A. (Eds.) (1968). *A manual of standardized terminology, techniques and scoring system for sleep stages of human subjects.* Public Health Service, Washington, DC: U.S. Government Printing Office.

Roberts, R., & Mullis, C. (1987). *Digital signal processing.* Reading, MA: Addison Wesley.

Robinson, R., Kubos, K., Starr, L., Rao, K., & Price, T. (1984). Mood disorders in stroke patients. *Brain, 107,* 81–93.

Rose, D., Smith, P., & Sato, S. (1987). Magnetoencephalography and epilepsy research. *Science, 238,* 329–355.

Schacter, D. (1977). EEG theta waves and psychological phenomena: A review and analysis. *Biological Psychology, 5,* 47–82.

Shaw, J., Brooks, S., Colter, N., O'Connor, K. (1979). A comparison of schizophrenic and neurotic patients using EEG power and coherence spectra. In J. Gruzelier & P. Flor-Henry (Eds.), *Hemispheric asymmetries of function in psychopathology.* Amsterdam: Elsevier/North-Holland.

Skarda, C., & Freeman, W. (1987). How brains make chaos in order to make sense of the world. *Behavioral and Brain Sciences, 10,* 161–195.

Sklar, B., Hanley, J., and Simmons, W. (1972). An EEG experiment aimed toward identifying dyslexic children. *Nature, 240,* 414–416.

Sokolov, E. N. (1963). Higher nervous functions: The orienting reflex. *Annual Review of Physiology, 25,* 545–580.

Sokolov, E. N. (1965). The orienting reflex, its structure and mechanism. In L. G. Veronin, A. N. Leotrev, A. R. Luria, E. N. Sokolov, & O. S. Vinogradov (Eds.), *Orienting reflex and exploratory behavior.* Washington, DC: American Institute of Biological Sciences.

Sperry, R. (1982). Some effects of disconnecting the cerebral hemispheres. *Science, 217,* 1223–1226.

Springer, S. P., & Deutsch, G. (1985). *Left brain, right brain.* San Francisco: W. H. Freeman.

Stephenson, W., & Gibbs, F. (1951). A balanced non-cephalic reference electrode. *Electroencephalography and Clinical Neurophysiology, 3,* 237–240.

Stern, R., Ray, W., & Davis, C. (1980). *Psychophysiological Recording.* New York: Oxford University Press.

Strong, P. (1970). *Biophysical measurements.* Beaverton: Tektronix, Inc.

Surwillo, W. W. (1963). The relation of simple response time to brain-wave frequency and the effects of age. *Electroencephalography and Clinical Neurophysiology, 15,* 105–114.

Surwillo, W. W. (1968). Timing of behavior in senescence and the role of the central nervous system. In G. Talland (Ed.), *Human aging and behavior.* New York: Academic Press.

Surwillo, W. W. (1986). *Psychophysiology.* Springfield IL: Thomas.

Thatcher, R., & John, E. (1977). *Foundations of cognitive processes.* Hillsdale, NJ: Erlbaum.

Thatcher, R., Krause, P., & Hrybyk, M. (1986). Cortico-cortical associations and EEG coherence: A two-compartmental model. *EEG and Clinical Neurophysiology, 64,* 123–143.

Thatcher, R. W., Walker, R. A., & Giudice, S. (1987). Human cerebral hemispheres develop at different rates and ages. *Science, 236,* 1110–1113.

Tucker, D., & Roth, D. (1984). Factoring the coherence matrix: Patterning of the frequency specific covariance in a multi-channel EEG. *Psychophysiology, 21,* 228–236.

Tucker, D. M. (1981). Lateral brain function, emotion, and conceptualization. *Psychological Bulletin, 89,* 19–46.

Tucker, D. M., Dawson, S., Roth, D., & Penland, J. (1985). Regional changes in EEG power and coherence during cognition: Intensive study of two individuals. *Behavioral Neuroscience, 99,* 564–577.

Tucker, D. M., Stenisle, C., Roth, R., & Shearer, S. (1981). Right frontal lobe activation and right hemisphere performance decrement during a depressed mood. *Archives of General Psychiatry, 38,* 169–174.

Vanderwolf, C., & Robinson, T. (1981). Reticulo-cortical activity and behavior: A critique of the arousal theory and a new synthesis. *Behavioral and Brain Sciences, 4,* 459–514.

Venables, P., & Martin, I. (Eds.). (1967). *A manual of psychophysiological methods.* Amsterdam: North-Holland.

Vogel, W., Broverman, D., & Klaiber, E. (1968). EEG and mental abilities. *Electroencephalography and Clinical Neurophysiology, 24,* 166–175.

Walter, W. (1937). Electroencephalogram in cases of cerebral tumour. *Proceedings of the Royal Society of Medicine. 30,* 579–598.

Walter, W. G. (1953). *The living brain.* New York: Norton.

Wiener, N. (1958). Time and the science of organization (first part). *Scientia (Milano), 93,* 199–205.

Woodruff, D. (1978). Brain electrical activity and behavior relationships over the life span. In P. Baltes (Ed.), *Life span development and behavior* (Vol. 1). New York: Academic Press.

Woodruff, D. (1983). Arousal, Sleep and aging. In J. Birren and W. Schaie (Eds.), *Handbook of the psychology of aging* (Vol. 2). New York: Van Nostrand Reinhold.

Yingling, C. D. (1980). Cognition, action, and mechanisms of EEG asymmetry. In G. Pfurtscheller, P. Buser, F. Lopes da Silva, & H. H. Petsche (Eds.), *Rhythmic EEG activities and cortical functioning.* Amsterdam: Elsevier/North-Holland Biomedical Press.

13 *Event-related brain potentials*

MICHAEL G. H. COLES, GABRIELE GRATTON,
AND MONICA FABIANI

13.1 INTRODUCTION

Ever since Berger (1929) demonstrated that it is possible to record the electrical activity of the brain by placing electrodes on the surface of the scalp, there has been considerable interest in the relationship between these recordings and psychological processes. Whereas Berger and his followers focused their attention on spontaneous rhythmic oscillations in voltage, that is, on the electroencephalogram, or EEG (see chapter 12), more recent research has concentrated on those aspects of the electrical potential that are specifically time locked to events, that is, on event-related potentials, or ERPs. The ERPs are regarded as manifestations of brain activities that occur in preparation for or in response to discrete events, be they internal or external to the subject. Conceptually, the ERPs are regarded as manifestations of specific psychological processes. Later in this chapter, we shall review what is known about their underlying sources and their relationship to physiological function (section 13.2). However, we shall focus for the most part on the relationship between the potentials and psychological function (sections 13.3–5).

13.1.1 *Deriving event-related potentials*

The procedures used to derive ERPs begin with the same amplifiers and filters used to obtain EEG (Figure 13.1). Electrodes are attached to the scalp at various locations and connected to amplifiers. The locations are usually chosen according to the International 10–20 system (Jasper, 1958) such that between-laboratory and between-experiment comparisons are possible. The outputs of the amplifiers are converted to numbers by a device for measuring electrical potentials, an analog-to-digital converter. The potentials are sampled at a frequency ranging from 100 to 10,000 Hz (cycles per second) and may be stored for subsequent analysis.

The ERP is small (a few microvolts) in comparison to the EEG (about 50 μV). Thus, the analysis generally begins with a procedure to increase the discrimination of the *signal* (the ERP) from the *noise* (background EEG). The most common procedure involves *averaging* samples of the EEG that are time locked to repeated occurrences of a particular event. The number of samples used in the average will depend on the signal-to-noise ratio. However, in all cases the samples are selected so as to bear a constant temporal relationship to an event. Since all those aspects of the EEG that are not time locked to the event are assumed to vary randomly from sample to sample, the averaging procedure should result in a reduction of these potentials leaving the event-related potentials visible.[1] The resulting voltage $\times$ time function

413

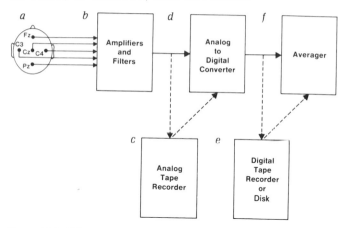

Figure 13.1. Schematic representation of operations involved in recording event-related brain potentials. (a) Top view of head, indicating placements of five electrodes (Fz, C3, Cz, C4, and Pz) from which EEG is recorded: Note that other locations are also frequently used. (b) EEG signal is then transferred to amplifying and filtering system. (c) Amplified and filtered signal may be stored temporarily on analog magnetic tape. (d) Analog signal is then converted into a digital signal by sampling potential at high frequency (usually at least 100 Hz) by analog-to-digital converter. (e) Digitally transformed signal may be stored on digital store device (magnetic tape or disk). (f) Finally, ERPs are extracted from digitized EEG signal by averaging point by point across large sample of trials (more than 20).

(Figure 13.2) contains a number of positive and negative peaks that are then subjected to a variety of measurement operations (see section 13.3.2). These peaks are generally described in terms of their characteristic polarity and latency. Thus, P300 refers to a positive peak with a modal latency of 300 ms. Other descriptors can include reference to the psychological or experimental conditions that control the potential (e.g., readiness potential, mismatch negativity) and to the scalp location at which the potential is maximal (e.g., frontal P300). Note that each peak in the ERP waveform is usually associated with a particular distribution across the scalp. Thus, spatial (topographic) distribution is regarded as an important discriminative characteristic of the ERP (Donchin, 1978; Sutton & Ruchkin, 1984). The relationship between spatial distribution and underlying brain activity will be discussed in section 13.2, whereas section 13.3 provides a more thorough description of the methods used to extract and measure ERPs. Section 13.4 reviews some of the more commonly measured components.

13.1.2   *The endogenous versus exogenous distinction*

From a psychological point of view, it is convenient to distinguish between different types of ERPs. First we can identify those ERPs whose characteristics are mostly controlled by the physical properties of an external eliciting event. Such potentials are considered to be obligatory and are referred to as *sensory* or *exogenous*. Second, we can identify ERPs whose characteristics are determined more by the nature of the interaction between the subject and the event. For example, some ERPs vary as a function of the information-processing activities required of the subject; others can

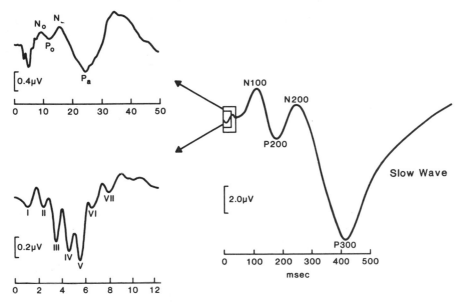

Figure 13.2. Schematic representation of ERP components elicited by auditory, infrequent target stimuli. Three panels represent three different voltage × time functions: Left bottom panel shows very early sensory components (with latency of less than 10 ms); left top panel shows middle latency sensory components with latency of between 10 and 50 ms. Note different voltage and time scales uses in three panels as well as different nomenclatures used to label peaks (components). (Copyright 1979, Plenum Publishing Corporation. Adapted with permission of author and publisher from Donchin, 1979).

be elicited in the absence of an external eliciting event. These potentials are referred to as *endogenous*. Naturally, it is the endogenous potentials that are the focus of those researchers interested in cognitive function. (For a discussion of the distinction between exogenous and endogenous potentials, see Donchin, Ritter, & McCallum, 1978.)

13.2 PHYSIOLOGICAL BASIS OF ERPs

In this section, we review evidence that relates the scalp-recorded electrical activity to its underlying anatomical and physiological basis. For a detailed review of this relationship, see Nunez (1981) or Allison, Wood, and McCarthy (1986).

13.2.1 *From the brain to the scalp: the generation of ERPs*

It is generally assumed that ERPs are distant manifestations of the activity of populations of neurons within the brain. This activity can be recorded on the surface of the scalp because the tissue that lies between the source and the scalp acts as a volume conductor. Since the electrical activity associated with any particular neuron is small, it is only possible to record at the scalp the integrated activity of a large number of neurons. Two requirements must be met for this integration to occur: (1) the neurons must be active synchronously and (2) the electric fields

Open Field   Closed Field

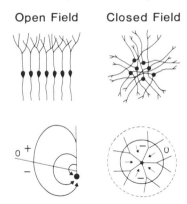

Figure 13.3. Schematic representation of configuration of neurons whose simultaneous polarization does or does not result in potential detectable by distant electrode. Electric fields generated by polarization of neurons organized in layers (such as those shown in the left panel) add together to form powerful fields that can be detected from distant (e.g., scalp) electrodes ("open field"). Fields generated by neurons organized concentrically (such as those shown in right panel) cancel each other to produce very small fields that cannot be detected by scalp electrodes ("closed field"). (Copyright 1947, Alan R. Liss, Inc. Reprinted with permission of author and publisher from Lorente de No, 1947.)

generated by each particular neuron must be oriented in such a way that their effects at the scalp cumulate. As a consequence, only a subset of the entire brain electrical activity can be recorded from scalp electrodes.

Two considerations further restrict the likely sources of the ERP. First, since the ERP represents the synchronous activity of a large number of neurons, it is probably not due to the summation of presynaptic potentials (spikes) because these potentials have a very high frequency and short duration. On the other hand, postsynaptic potentials, having a relatively slower time course, are more likely to be synchronous and therefore to summate to produce scalp potentials. Thus, it is commonly believed that most scalp ERPs are the summation of the postsynaptic potentials of a large number of neurons that are activated (or inhibited) synchronously (see Allison et al., 1986).

A second consideration concerns the orientation of neuronal fields. Since the electric fields associated with the activity of each individual neuron involved must be oriented in such a way as to cumulate at the scalp, only neural structures with a specific spatial organization may generate scalp ERPs. Lorente de No (1947) specified the spatial organizations that are required for the distant recording of the electrical activity of a neural structure. He distinguished between two types, "open fields" and "closed fields" (Figure 13.3).

A structure having an open-field organization is characterized by neurons that are ordered so that their dendritic trees are all oriented on one side of the structure, whereas their axons all depart from the other side. In this case, the electric fields generated by the activity of each neuron will all be oriented in the same direction and summate. Only structures with some degree of open-field organization generate potentials that can be recorded at the scalp. Open fields are obtained whenever neurons are organized in layers, as in most of the cortex, parts of the thalamus, the cerebellum, and other structures.

A structure with a closed-field organization is characterized by neurons that are concentrically or randomly organized. In both cases, the electric fields generated by each neuron will be oriented in very different, sometimes opposite, directions and therefore will cancel each other. Examples of closed-field organization are given by some midbrain nuclei.

From this analysis it is clear that ERPs represent just a sample of the brain electrical activity associated with a certain event. Thus, it is entirely possible that a sizeable portion of the information-processing transactions that occur after (or before) the anchor event are silent as far as ERPs are concerned. For this reason, some caution should be used in the interpretation of ERP data. For instance, if an experimental manipulation has no effect on the ERP, we cannot conclude that it does not influence brain processes.

13.2.2   *From the scalp to the brain: inferring the sources of ERPs*

So far we have examined how particular properties of neuronal phenomena may determine whether they will be recorded at the scalp. We have approached the problem of ERP generation in a direct fashion, from properties of the generators to predictable scalp observations. In most cases, however, we have only limited information about the neural structure(s) responsible for a specific aspect of the ERP. Our data base consists of observations of voltage differences between scalp electrodes or between scalp electrodes and a reference electrode. To determine which neural structures are responsible for the scalp potential, that is, to identify the neural generators of ERPs, we must solve the inverse problem. We have to infer the unique combination of neural generators whose activity results in the potential observed at the scalp.

In solving this problem, we are confronted with an indefinite number of unknown parameters. In fact, an indefinite number of neural generators may be active simultaneously, and each of them may vary in amplitude, orientation of the electric field, and location inside the head. Since a limited number of observations (the voltage values recorded at different scalp electrodes) is used to estimate an indefinite number of parameters, it is clear that the inverse problem does not have a unique solution. A further complication is that the head is not a homogeneous medium. Therefore, the electric field generated by the activity of particular structures is difficult to compute. A particularly important distortion of the electric fields is caused by the skull, a very low conductance medium that reduces and smears electric fields. For all these reasons, we cannot determine unequivocally which structures are responsible for the ERP observed at any point in time when the only information available is given by the potentials recorded at scalp electrodes.

In spite of these problems, investigators have tried to identify the neural sources of the scalp ERP using a variety of approaches involving both noninvasive and invasive techniques. Noninvasive techniques are based on scalp recordings. They involve complex mathematical procedures and depend on a number of restrictive assumptions. Invasive techniques are based on recordings from indwelling electrodes (in humans or in animals) or on lesion data.

A noninvasive approach to the inverse problem is to generate several alternative hypotheses about neural structures that may be active at a particular point in time and that may be responsible for an observed scalp ERP. The distribution of potentials across the scalp that would be generated by each of these structures can then be computed using a direct approach. Finally, the structure whose activity best accounts for the observed scalp distribution can be identified. This approach requires that specific neurophysiological knowledge exists about candidate underlying structures. First, we must have some reason to restrict the number of candidate neural generators to a manageable number. Second, we must have sufficient knowledge of the anatomy and physiology of each of these candidate neural generators to be able to compute the distributions of the scalp potentials associated with their activity. At present, such knowledge exists only in a very limited number of cases (see, e.g., Scherg & von Cramon, 1985).

A more sophisticated and promising noninvasive procedure involves the use of magnetic field recordings. Magnetic fields generated by brain activity are extremely small in relation to magnetic fields generated by environmental and other bodily sources. Therefore, their measurement is both difficult and expensive. The advantage of measuring the magnetic field is that it is practically insensitive to variations of the conductive media (such as those due to the presence of the skull). It is therefore much easier to compute the source of a particular field. An in-depth discussion of the problems and peculiarities of the magnetic technique is beyond the scope of this chapter and can be found elsewhere (Beatty, Barth, Richer, & Johnson, 1986). We only note here that using the magnetic technique to determine the source of neural components still requires assumptions about the number of neural structures active at a particular moment in time.

Invasive techniques for the identification of the sources of ERP components are based on the implantation of electrodes within the brain of humans or animals. Research on humans has been made possible by the need for recording EEG activity in deep regions of the brain for diagnostic purposes (Halgren et al., 1980; Wood et al., 1984). A problem with the human research is that the indwelling electrodes are located according to clinical rather than scientific criteria and therefore may fail to map the regions involved in the generation of scalp ERPs. This may be solved by research on animals (Buchwald & Squires, 1983; Csepe, Karmos, & Molnar, 1987; Starr & Farley, 1983). However, animal research is problematic because it is difficult to determine whether the ERP observed in animals corresponds to that observed in humans. This is because of fundamental differences in the anatomy of animal and human brains. Finally, a general problem with depth recording is that it is difficult to know the extent to which the scalp-recorded ERP is due to the activity of the structures that have been identified by the indwelling electrodes. This problem can be resolved in animal research if lesions in the structure identified as the candidate generator result in elimination of the scalp potential.

In summary, although several techniques have been used for identifying the source of ERP components, none of them appears to be likely to give definitive answers in all cases. However, the convergence of several techniques may provide useful information about the neural structures whose activity is manifested at the scalp by the ERP.

13.3   THE INFERENTIAL CONTEXT

In this section, we review the process through which we come to make inferences about psychological processes and states from the measurement of ERPs. To begin with, however, we need to address a number of assumptions about the "meaning" of the ERP and a variety of measurement issues.

13.3.1 *The concept of components*

As we noted, the ERP can be described as a voltage × time function. We assume that the various voltage fluctuations represented by this function reflect the activities of neuronal populations and that, in turn, these neuronal populations are responsible for the execution of some psychological process. In practice, the tendency in cognitive psychophysiology has been to focus on processes identified by cognitive psychologists as candidate psychological processes.

The total ERP is assumed to be a manifestation of the aggregate of a number of ERP "components." The components can be defined in three different ways (Fabiani, Gratton, Karis, & Donchin, 1987; Näätanen & Picton, 1987). First, components can be defined in terms of the peaks and troughs (maxima and minima) that are observed in the ERP trace. Second, components can be defined as aspects of the ERP waveforms that are functionally associated; that is, they covary across subjects or conditions or location on the scalp. Third, components can be defined in terms of those neural structures that generate them. These definitions may converge in some circumstances. However, as Näätanen and Picton (1987) have indicated, a peak in the ERP waveform (e.g., the N1) may represent the summation of several functionally and structurally distinct components. Thus, the adoption of one or another of these definitions will have important consequences for the interpretation of the component structure of the ERP waveform. A corollary of this is that different measurement procedures will be required depending on the type of component definition that is adopted. These procedures will be reviewed in subsequent sections after a brief discussion of general measurement issues.

13.3.2 *General measurement issues*

13.3.2.1 *Artifacts*

The potential recorded at the scalp can be influenced by sources of electrical activity that do not arise from the brain. Examples of these sources of artifacts include the movement of eyeballs and eyelids, tension of the muscles in the head and neck, and the electrical activity generated by the heart. These artifacts can be dealt with in the following ways. First, one can set up the recording situation so that artifacts are minimized. This can be accomplished by suitable choice of electrode locations and of the subject's task and environment. Second, one can simply discard records that contain artifacts. Unfortunately, this procedure may lead to a bias in the selection of the observations and/or subjects. Third, one can use filters (see section 13.3.2.2) to attenuate artifactual activity. This procedure is useful when the frequency of the artifactual activity is outside the frequency range of the ERP signal of interest. For example, the frequency of electromyographic activity is higher than that of most endogenous ERP components. Fourth, one can attempt to measure the extent of the artifact and then remove it from the data. This procedure has been used most frequently in the case of ocular artifacts (e.g., Gratton, Coles, & Donchin, 1983).

13.3.2.2 *Signal-to-noise-ratio*

The ERP consists of a series of fluctuations in voltage that are time locked to an event. These voltage changes are typically small (a few microvolts) in relation to the

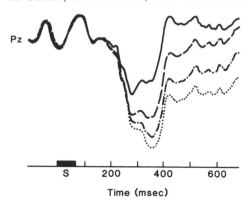

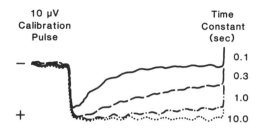

Figure 13.4. ERPs elicited by counted, rare tones (*upper panel*). Data recorded with four different high-pass filter settings (time constant) are superimposed. Stimulus occurrence is indicated by *S* on the time scale. Calibration pulses (*lower panel*) are plotted on same voltage × time scale as ERPs. Note reduction in amplitude and deformation of ERP waveshape produced by progressively shorter time constants, which reduce low-frequency activity. (Copyright 1979, The Society for Psychophysiological Research. Reprinted with permission of author and publisher, from Duncan-Johnson & Donchin, 1979).

background EEG (about $50\mu V$) in which they are imbedded. Thus, a major measurement problem concerns the extraction of the ERP signal from the background noise.

Several procedures have been advocated to increase the signal-to-noise ratio, including filtering, averaging, and pattern recognition (see Coles, Gratton, Kramer, & Miller, 1986, for a more detailed discussion).

Filtering involves the attenuation of noise, whose frequency is different from that of the signal. For example, most endogenous components have frequencies of between 0.5 and 20 Hz. Thus, at the time of recording or later at the time of analysis, analog or digital filters can be used to attenuate activity outside this frequency range. Great care should be taken in the selection of filters. The amplitude and latency of an ERP component (as well as the general ERP waveform) will be distorted if the bandpass of the filter excludes frequencies of interest (Figure 13.4).

Averaging involves the summation of a series of EEG epochs (or trials) each of which is time locked to the event of interest. These EEG epochs are assumed to be given by two sources: first, the ERP, and second, other voltage fluctuations that are not time locked to the event. Since, by definition, these other fluctuations are random with respect to the event, they should average to zero, leaving the time-locked ERP both visible and measurable. If it is the case that (1) the ERP "signals" are constant over trials, (2) the noise is random across trials, and (3) the ERP signals are independent of the background noise, then the signal-to-noise ratio will be increased by the square root of the number of trials included in the average. Note that the utility of the averaging procedure also depends on the fact there are no correlated signals (such as the EOG; see section 13.3.2.1) that are also time locked to the event.

One of the problems with the averaging procedure is that the three assumptions described in the previous paragraph may not always be satisfied in the typical experiment. In particular, if the latency of the ERP varies from trial to trial (latency jitter), the average ERP waveform will not be representative of the actual ERP of any individual trial. A related problem is that the investigator may be interested in measures of the ERP on individual trials. Thus, a major thrust in ERP methodology has been to derive procedures for single-trial analysis.

Pattern recognition techniques allow the investigator to identify segments of the EEG epoch that contain specific features, such as a particular pattern of peaks and troughs characteristic of an ERP component. The advantage of these techniques is that they allow the investigator to identify and measure components on individual trials. Examples of pattern recognition techniques are cross-correlation, the Woody filter (Woody, 1967), and stepwise discriminant analysis (Donchin & Herning, 1975; Horst & Donchin, 1980; Squires & Donchin, 1976). In the case of cross-correlation and the Woody filter, the individual trial epoch is scanned to determine the segment that best resembles an "ideal" template corresponding to the component of interest. In the case of a discriminant function, the procedure begins with the selection of two sets of waveforms that are presumed to differ in terms of a specific component. Then features are identified (in the form of numerical weights) that best discriminate between the two sets of waveforms. These features are considered to represent the defining characteristic of the component, and individual trials can be examined to determine the extent to which the features are present. Note that the cross-correlation and Woody filter procedures can yield both amplitude and latency estimates for individual trials, whereas discriminant function procedures yield only amplitude estimates. (For a general discussion of pattern recognition techniques, see Glaser & Ruchkin, 1976.)

13.3.3 *Component quantification*

In this section, we describe procedures that have been used to quantify ERP components. As mentioned earlier, these measurement operations will depend on the way in which ERP components are defined.

13.3.3.1 *Peak measurement*

As indicated in section 13.1, components can be defined in terms of peaks or troughs having characteristic polarities and latency ranges. Thus, the measurement operation involves the assessment of either amplitude of the peak in microvolts or its latency in milliseconds (Figure 13.5). Amplitude is usually referred either to the baseline, preevent, voltage level (base-to-peak amplitude), or to some other peak in

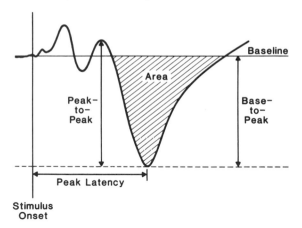

Figure 13.5. Schematic representation of ERP waveform, indicating different procedures for component quantification. Three types of peak measures are indicated.
Peak latency is obtained by measuring interval (in ms) between external triggering
event and positive or negative peak in waveform. Base-to-peak amplitude measure
is obtained by computing voltage difference (in μV) between voltage at peak point
and baseline level (usually average prestimulus level). Peak-to-peak amplitude
measure is obtained by computing voltage difference (in μV) between voltage at
peak point and voltage at a previous peak of opposite polarity. Area measure is
obtained by integrating voltage between two timepoints.

the ERP waveform (peak-to-peak amplitude). Latency is referred to the time of
occurrence of the event.

When the component under analysis does not have a definite peak, it is customary
to measure the integrated activity across a particular latency range (area measure).

13.3.3.2 *Covariation measures*

As already mentioned, components can also be defined in terms of segments of the
ERP waveform that exhibit covariation across subjects, conditions, or scalp
locations. As a consequence, procedures are needed to identify and measure these
segments.

One of the most commonly used procedures in Principal Component Analysis
(PCA). This procedure can be applied to describe the structure of the variance associated with a set of ERP waveforms. This structure is inferred from the pattern of
covariance between the voltage values for each timepoint in the waveform. The
outcome of PCA is a set of components each characterized by a particular pattern of
weights (loadings, or eigenvectors) for each timepoint (Figure 13.6). Then, the
weights for each component can be used as a linear filter to derive measures of
amplitude of each component in a particular waveform. Each point in the waveform
is multiplied by the weight for that point. The resulting values are summed to yield
factor scores (or measures of component amplitude). A more detailed description of
the application of PCA to ERPs can be found in Donchin and Heffley (1978).

GRAND MEAN WAVEFORM

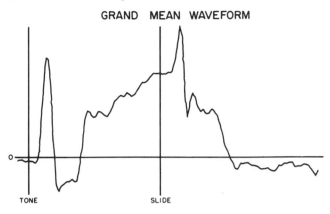

COMPONENT LOADINGS

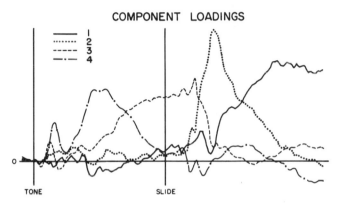

Figure 13.6. Example of application of principal component analysis (PCA) to the study of ERPs. Series of ERP waveforms (whose grand average is plotted in upper panel) is decomposed in several constituent components, whose time courses (component loadings) are shown in lower panel. The component loadings are then used to determine degree to which particular component is present in each ERP waveform. (Copyright 1982, Elsevier Science Publishers. Reprinted with permission of author and publisher from Duncan-Johnson & Donchin, 1982).

13.3.3.3 *Source activity measures*

A third way of defining components is in terms of underlying sources. According to this definition, we should quantify the activity of these sources to provide latency and amplitude measures of the different components. As we noted earlier (section 13.2), the relationship between scalp electrical activity and source activity is difficult, if not impossible, to describe. Thus, for the time being, this type of component measurement, although theoretically important, is practically unfeasible.

13.3.3.4 *Problems in component measurement*

In this section we discuss two specific problems that arise during component measurement.

The first problem concerns the commensurability of the measurements of different waveforms. Is a particular component recorded under a particular set of circumstances the same as that recorded in another situation? This is a particular problem when we define components as a peak observed at a particular latency. For example, if the latency of the peak differs between two experimental conditions, we would be led to conclude that different components are present in the two sets of data. How can we be sure that the same component varies in latency between the two conditions rather than that two different components are present in the two different conditions? The problem is not resolved by using PCA. In this case, how can we know whether two components extracted by separate PCAs conducted on different sets of data reflect the same activity? A solution to this problem can only be derived from a careful examination of the pattern of results obtained and from a comparison of these results with what we already know about different ERP components. Of course, this means that we are including a large number of empirical and theoretical arguments in the definition of each ERP component, which, of course, may differ from one component to another and from time to time. Thus, the definition of a component may include not only polarity and latency, but also distribution across the scalp and sensitivity to experimental manipulations (see, e.g., Fabiani et al., 1987). Thus, it is clear that a correct interpretation of ERP component structure requires some background information about the components themselves (see section 13.4).

A second problem in component measurement is that of component overlap. Usually, ERP components do not appear in isolation, but several of them may be active at the same moment in time. This reflects the parallel nature of brain processes. When this occurs, it is difficult to attribute a particular portion of scalp activity to a particular component. Peak and area measures are particularly susceptible to this problem, but even PCA can, in some cases, misallocate variance across different components (see Wood & McCarthy, 1984). As a result, we may attribute a difference obtained between two particular experimental conditions to the wrong component.

Several procedures have been proposed to solve the problem of component overlap, but none of them seems to have universal validity. In some cases, it can be assumed that only one component varies between two experimental conditions. In this case, the variation of this component can be isolated by subtracting two sets of waveforms. Unfortunately, very rarely can we assume that the effect of an experimental variable is so selective. Furthermore, the subtraction procedure implies that only amplitude, and not latency, varies across experimental conditions.

A procedure that may help solve both these problems is vector filtering (Gratton, Coles, & Donchin, 1989). This procedure begins with the assumption that components can be defined in terms of scalp distribution. Any component can be represented by a specific profile of amplitude values at different electrode locations. This profile is then used as a *distributional filter* to determine the extent to which the component is present in a particular epoch (Figure 13.7). This procedure can be applied to several components simultaneously, and thus, it is possible to separate the contribution of several overlapping components to an observed waveform. Note

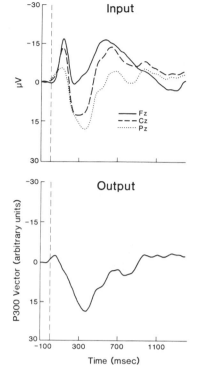

Figure 13.7. Example of application of vector filtering to the study of ERPs. Waveforms from three electrode locations, shown in upper panel, are used to determine contribution of a particular component (e.g., P300), which is characterized by the specific profile of amplitudes at different electrode locations. The result of this operation is shown in lower panel.

that, in contrast to PCA, neither the latency nor the time course of the component (but only the scalp distribution) need be constant over trials. The assumption of constancy of distribution may be more valid than assumptions of constancy of latency and time course.

Note that distributional filters perform the same kind of operations in the spatial domain that frequency filters perform in the frequency domain. Whereas frequency filters apply different weights to activity in different frequency bands, distributional filters apply different weights to activity from different spatial locations.

13.3.4 *Experimental logic*

In this section, we review the experimental procedures that lead to a specification of the functional significance of the components. Some theory about the functional significance of a component is essential to the understanding of the changes that this component will exhibit as a function of specific contexts. The development of a theory about the functional significance of a component is a complex process that involves studies of the component's antecedents and consequences as well as speculations about the psychological function it manifests.

To illustrate this process, we shall focus on the approach adopted in our laboratory (see Coles, Gratton, & Gehring, 1987; Donchin, 1981; Donchin & Coles, 1988a, b; Donchin, Karis, Bashore, Coles, & Gratton, 1986). Although this approach is oriented toward cognitive ERP research and to the P300 component in particular, there is no reason, in principle, why it could not be applied to other approaches to ERPs and to other components.

13.3.4.1 *Antecedent conditions*

In the case of all ERP components, the initial phase in the process begins with the "discovery" of a component. For most endogenous ERP components, this discovery occurred during the 1960s and 1970s; for the P300, this occurred in 1965 (Sutton, Braren, Zubin, & John, 1965). After this report, there followed a period in which attempts were made to map out the antecedent conditions that influence the amplitude and latency of the component.

For amplitude, a large series of studies focused on the "oddball" paradigm in which subjects are presented with two stimuli or classes of stimuli that occur in a Bernouilli sequence. The probability of one stimulus is generally less than that for the other, and the subject's task is to count the rarer of the two stimuli. The basic conclusion of these kinds of studies is that the amplitude of the P300 is sensitive to the probability of task-relevant events (see, e.g., Duncan-Johnson & Donchin, 1977, and Figure 13.8; see also Donchin, Karis, et al., 1986). Further research indicated that it is subjective, rather than objective, probability that controls the amplitude of P300 (Squires, Wickens, Squires, & Donchin, 1976). In addition, the stimuli or stimulus classes can be as diverse as male versus female names (Kutas, McCarthy, & Donchin, 1977) or pictures of politicians versus pictures of others (Towle, Heuer, & Donchin, 1980) or even the absence of the stimulus (Sutton, Tueting, Zubin, & John, 1967). Furthermore, the scalp distribution is independent of the modality of the stimulus (Simson, Vaughan, & Ritter, 1976).

A second factor controlling the amplitude of P300 is the task relevance of the eliciting event. Thus, P300s are only elicited if the subject must use the stimuli to perform the assigned task. If the events occur while the subject is performing another task (such as a word puzzle), then even rare events do not elicit the P300 (see Figure 13.8; Duncan-Johnson & Donchin, 1977). Furthermore, the P300 to an event is directly related to the event's utility in terms of the subject's task (Bosco et al., 1986; Johnson & Donchin, 1978).

A final series of studies (see Donchin, Kramer, & Wickens, 1986) has demonstrated that the P300 is related to the processing resources demanded by a particular task. In a dual-task situation, P300 amplitude to primary-task events increases with the perceptual/cognitive resource demands, whereas the P300 response to the concurrent secondary task decreases (Sirevaag, Kramer, Coles, & Donchin, 1984).

As far as P300 latency is concerned, the research has focused on the identification of those processes that have elapsed prior to the elicitation of P300. As an initial observation, it can be noted that if P300 amplitude is sensitive to probability, then, at the very least, processes required to establish the rareness of an event must occur prior to the P300 process. On the basis of this observation, Donchin (1979) proposed that P300 latency may reflect stimulus evaluation or categorization time. This idea was supported by the observation that the correlation between P300 latency and reaction time is higher when subjects are given accuracy rather than speed

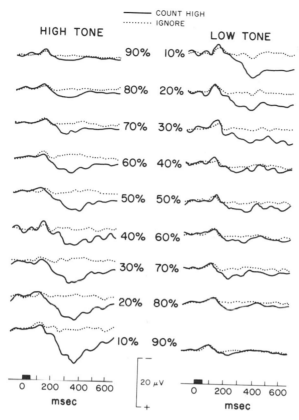

Figure 13.8. Grand-average ERP waveforms at Pz from 10 subjects for counted (high, left column) and uncounted (low, right column) stimuli (tones) with different a priori probabilities. Probability level is indicated by percentage value beside each waveform. Waveforms from condition in which subjects were instructed to ignore stimuli are also presented for comparison. Occurrence of stimulus is indicated by black bar on time scale. Positive voltages are indicated by downward deflections of waveforms. Note that P300 amplitude is inversely proportional to probability of eliciting stimulus ("probability effect"), and at same probability level, P300 is larger for counted than uncounted stimuli ("target effect"). (Copyright 1977, The Society for Psychophysiological Research. Reprinted with permission of author and publisher from Duncan-Johnson & Donchin, 1977.)

instructions. Furthermore, as categorization becomes more difficult, P300 latency becomes longer (Figure 13.9; Kutas et al., 1977).

If P300 latency reflects stimulus evaluation time, then it should not be affected by factors that influence response-related processes. Several studies (Magliero, Bashore, Coles, & Donchin, 1984; McCarthy & Donchin, 1981; Ragot, 1984) demonstrate that manipulations that should affect the duration of response-related processes (i.e., stimulus–response compatibility) have little or no effect on P300 latency, whereas manipulations of stimulus complexity have a large effect. (Both these manipulations have a substantial efffect on reaction time.) Thus, it appears

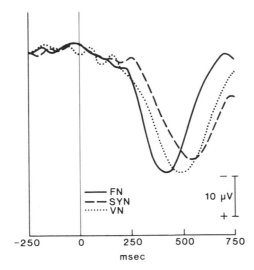

Figure 13.9. ERP waveforms at Pz averaged across subjects for three different semantic categorization tasks. Solid line indicates ERPs obtained during task in which subjects had to distinguish between word *David* and word *Nancy* (FN condition). Dotted line indicates ERPs obtained during task in which subjects had to decide whether word presented was male or female name (VN condition). Dashed line indicates ERPs obtained during task in which subjects had to decide whether word was or was not synonym of word *Prod* (SYN condition). These three tasks were considered to involve progressively more difficult discriminations. Note latency of P300 peak is progressively longer as discrimination is made more difficult. (Copyright 1977, The AAAS. Adapted with permission of author and publisher from Kutas, McCarthy, & Donchin, 1977.)

that the P300 is more dependent on the completion of processes of stimulus evaluation and categorization than on those related to the current overt response.

13.3.4.2 *Formation of theory*

Taken together, these data suggest that the P300 is dependent on (1) the subjective probability of task-relevant effects, (2) the value or meaning of the event in the context of the task, and (3) the psychological resources allocated to the processing of the event. Furthermore, the P300 is not emitted until the event has been categorized. If responses are based on incomplete stimulus evaluation, the P300 will occur after the overt response. (See also Johnson, 1986, for a discussion of the determinants of P300, and Donchin et al., 1984, for a discussion of the relationship between P300 and the orienting reflex.)

With these observations in mind, one can proceed to speculate about the functional significance of the P300. Thus, Donchin (1981; Donchin & Coles, 1988a, b) argued that it is a manifestation of a process related to the updating of models of the environment or context in working memory. Such an updating will depend on the processing of the current event (hence, the P300 latency – stimulus evaluation time relationship) but will have implications for the processing of and response to future events.[2]

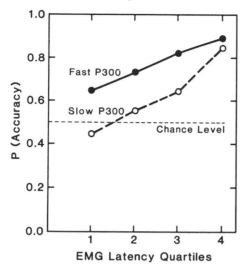

Figure 13.10. Accuracy of reaction-time responses given at different latencies ("speed–accuracy functions") for trials with "fast" and "slow" P300. Response latency (defined in terms of onset of EMG response) is plotted on abscissa. Probability that response would be correct is plotted on ordinate. Note that the probability of giving a correct response increases as response latency increases. At very short response latencies, responses are at chance level of accuracy (.5). At long response latencies, responses are usually accurate. Speed–accuracy function for those trials with P300 latency shorter than median latency (fast P300 trials) are indicated by solid lines. Speed–accuracy function for those trials with P300 latency longer than median latency (slow P300 trials) are indicated by dashed lines. Note that, for each response latency, the probability of giving a correct response is higher when P300 on that trial (reflecting speed of stimulus at processing on that trial) is fast than when it is slow. (Copyright 1985, The American Psychological Association. Reprinted with permission of publisher from Coles, Gratton, Bashore, Eriksen, & Donchin, 1985).

13.3.4.3 *Consequences*

These kinds of statements relating to functional significance can be tested by an examination of the predicted consequences of variation in the latency or amplitude of the P300 for the outcome of the interaction between the subject and the environment.

For example, as far as P300 latency is concerned, if the P300 occurs after the stimulus has been evaluated, then the quality of the subject's response to that event should depend on the timing of that response relative to the occurrence of the P300. Thus, Coles, Gratton, Bashore, Eriksen, and Donchin (1985) showed that, for a given response latency, response accuracy was higher the shorter the P300 latency. This is illustrated in Figure 13.10.

For P300 amplitude, we expect that to the extent the subject's future behavior depends on the degree to which an event leads to a change in their model of the environment, that behavior will be related to P300 amplitude. Thus, there have been several studies that have demonstrated a relationship between the memorability of an event, assessed at some future time, and the amplitude of the P300 response to the event at the time of initial presentation (see action 13.4.4.1, for a detailed discussion).

As another example, we have demonstrated that the subject's future strategy as revealed in overt behavior can be predicted from the P300 response to current events (Donchin, Gratton, Dupree, & Coles, 1988). In particular, in a speeded choice reaction time task, the amplitude of the P300 following an error was related to the latency and accuracy of overt responses on subsequent trials.

These kinds of experiments that investigate the predicted consequences of variation in the P300 response for overt behavior provide tests of the theories of the functional significance of the P300. As a result, the theories are refined or revised, until, eventually, we are confident enough to proceed to use the ERP measure to monitor information-processing activities (see, e.g., Coles et al., 1985; Kramer, Sirevaag, & Braune, 1987).

13.3.5   *The role of neurophysiology*

As we noted earlier, there are serious problems in trying to infer the source of a given ERP component from its distribution on the scalp. Thus, the identification of a particular ERP component with a particular intracranial source must depend on a variety of converging methodologies including magnetic and intracranial recordings in humans and animals, neuropsychological research, and lesion studies in animals.

What are the consequences of knowing the intracranial source for theorizing about the functional significance of an ERP component? We should emphasize that by *functional significance* we mean a specification of the information-processing transactions that are manifested by the component, not its neurophysiological significance.

In the case of the P300, there has been considerable speculation that at least one source lies in the hippocampus (Halgren et al., 1980; Okada, Kaufman, & Williamson, 1983). If, in fact, this speculation is supported by future research, we could incorporate what is known about the psychologically relevant functions of the hippocampus into our theory of the P300 (and vice versa). In this regard, it is interesting to note the similarity between theories of hippocampal function that emphasize its role in memory (O'Keefe & Nadel, 1978) and the theory of P300 outlined in the previous sections that emphasizes its relationship to *context updating*.

Note that we can articulate a theory of the functional significance of P300 without any knowledge of its neural origin. However, when its neural origin is known, then the theory can be refined and developed on the basis of what is known about the underlying neural structures. In this sense, then, neurophysiological knowledge may be useful, but not necessarily critical, to the psychophysiological enterprise. Of course, such knowledge is critical for those who wish to use ERPs as a sign of neurophysiological function.

13.3.6   *Using the measure: psychophysiological inference*

In the preceding sections, we have considered the ways in which ERP researchers establish the functional significance of the ERP components. In a sense, this research can be considered as establishing the validity of ERP components as measures of particular psychological activities. In this section, we consider the ways in which the measures are used to make inferences about psychological processes. We shall review a series of inferential steps, from the crudest to the most sophisticated, that depend to a greater and greater extent on assumptions about the functional significance of the ERP. For the purposes of elucidating the inferential process, we shall consider an experiment in which subjects are run in two different conditions.

13.3.6.1 *Inference 1: Conditions are different*

At the most fundamental level, we can ask whether or not the two conditions are associated with different responses. The analytic procedure necessary to answer this question would involve a univariate or multivariate analysis of variance (with condition and timepoint as factors). Given that such an analysis yields a significant condition by timepoint interaction, we can infer that the conditions are different. If we assume that the ERP is a sign of brain activity and/or that it reflects some psychological process, then we can infer that the brain activity and associated psychological processing are different in the two conditions.

13.3.6.2 *Inference 2: Conditions differ at a particular time*

The second level of inference concerns the time at which the two conditions differ. This inference could be made on the basis of post hoc tests of the significant condition by time interaction. It would take the form of "by at least X milliseconds, processing of stimuli in condition A is different than processing of stimulus in condition B." This kind of inference is frequently made in studies of selective attention where an important theoretical issue concerns the relative time at which an attended event receives preferential processing. As with the most primitive form of inference, we need only assume that the ERP is a reflection of some aspect of psychological processing.

13.3.6.3 *Inference 3: Conditions differ with respect to the latency of some process*

For this level of inference, additional assumptions and measurement operations must be made. First, we must assume that the latency of a particular ERP component is related to the latency of a particular psychological process. For example, we argued previously that P300 does not occur until the evaluation process is complete. Second, we must adopt a procedure to identify the component in question and to measure its latency (see section 13.3). Then, we use an analytic procedure (analysis of variance, t-test, etc.) to evaluate the difference between the conditions with respect to the component latency. As a result of this procedure, we make the inference that the conditions differ with respect to the timing of process X.

13.3.6.4 *Inference 4: Conditions differ with respect to the degree to which some process occurs*

At the most complex level, we can use ERPs to infer that a particular process occurs to a greater degree under one condition than under another. In this case, we must assume that a particular ERP component is a manifestation of process X. We must further assume that changes in the magnitude of the component correspond directly

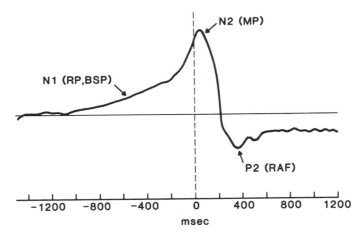

Figure 13.11. Typical movement-related potential (recorded from a central electrode, Cz) preceding voluntary hand movement. Note that potential begins about 1
sec before movement (indicated by dashed vertical line). Potential can be
subdivided into different components as follows: N1 (RP, readiness potential, BSP,
Bereitschaftspotential); N2 (MP, motor potential); and P2 (RAF, reafferent potential).
(Copyright 1980, Elsevier Science Publisher. Adapted with permission of author and
publisher from Kutas & Donchin, 1980.)

to changes in the degree to which the process is invoked. Then, we must devise a
suitable measurement procedure to identify and assess the magnitude of the
component. Finally, we can proceed with the usual inferential test and determine
whether or not the conditions differ with respect to the degree of process X.

13.4   A SELECTIVE REVIEW OF ERPs

In this section, we consider some of the research on the functional significance of a
variety of different ERP components. We begin with a discussion of ERPs that occur
prior to a marker event. This is followed by a brief overview of sensory and cognitive
ERP components that occur after the marker event.

13.4.1   *Event-preceding potentials*

13.4.1.1 *Movement-related potentials*

One class of event-preceding potentials includes those that are apparently related to
the preparation for movement. These potentials were first described by Kornhuber
and Deecke (1965), who found that prior to voluntary movements a negative
potential develops slowly, beginning some 800 ms before the initiation of the
movement (Figure 13.11). These *readiness potentials* (or *Bereitschaftspotentials*) were
distinguished from those that followed the movement, the *reafferent potentials*. In a
condition in which a similar but passive movement was involved, only postmove-
ment potentials were observed. Both readiness and reafferent potentials tend to be
maximal at electrodes located over motor areas of the cortex. Furthermore, some
components of the potentials are larger at electrode locations contralateral to the

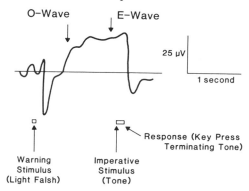

Figure 13.12. Schematic representation of typical contingent negative variation (CNV) recorded from Cz. The CNV is negative portion of wave between presentation of warning and imperative stimuli. Early portion of CNV is labeled O-wave (orienting wave), late portion is labelled E-wave (expectancy wave). (Copyright 1983, Elsevier Science Publisher. Adapted with permission of author and publisher from Rohrbaugh & Gaillard, 1983.)

responding limb (at least for hand and finger movements). Indeed, this kind of lateralization has become an important criterion for movement-related potentials.

The investigation of movement-related potentials has developed along several different paths, including (1) the discovery and classification of different components of the movement-related potential (for reviews, see Brunia, Haagh, & Scheirs, 1985, and Deecke et al., 1984), (2) analysis of the neural origin using the scalp topography of ERPs (e.g., Vaughan, Costa, & Ritter, 1972) or magnetic field recordings (e.g., Deecke, Weinberg, & Brickett, 1982; Okada, Williamson, & Kaufman, 1982), (3) analysis of the functional significance of different components (see Brunia et al., 1985, and Deecke et al., 1984, for reviews), and (4) recording of movement-related potentials in special populations (e.g., in mentally retarded children, Karrer & Ivins, 1976, and in Parkinson's patients, Deecke, Englitz, Kornhuber, & Schmitt, 1977). In general, these studies confirm that the potential described by Kornhuber and Deecke is generated, at least in part, by neuronal activity in motor areas of the cortex and is a reflection of processes related to the preparation and execution of movements.

Recently, movement-related potentials have been applied to the investigation of human information processing. In particular, we have used the measure to index the commitment to a specific motor response in choice reaction-time paradigms (see Bosco et al., 1986; De Jong, Wierda, Mulder, & Mulder, 1988; Gehring, Gratton, Coles, & Donchin, 1986; Gratton, Coles, Sirevaag, Eriksen, & Donchin, 1988; Kutas & Donchin, 1980). We have demonstrated that the speed and accuracy of a subject's reaction time response is, in part, related to the degree of prior preparation manifested by the movement-related potential.

13.4.1.2 *The contingent-negative variation (CNV)*

The CNV was first described by Walter, Cooper, Aldridge, McCallum, and Winter (1964) as a slow negative wave that occurs during the foreperiod of a reaction-time task (Figure 13.12). The wave tends to be largest over central (vertex) and frontal areas. Researchers investigating the functional significance of CNV have manipulated several aspects of the S1–S2 paradigm, including the subject's task, the discriminability of the imperative stimulus, foreperiod duration, stimulus probability, presence of distractors, and so on. The component has been variously described as related to expectancy, mental priming, association, and attention (for a review, see Donchin et al., 1978; Rohrbaugh & Gaillard, 1983).

A central controversy in research in this area over the past decade concerns whether the CNV consists of one or several functionally distinct components. A further but related question is whether the late portion of the CNV (just prior to the imperative stimulus) reflects more than the process of motor preparation as the subject anticipates making a response to the imperative stimulus. This controversy was raised by Loveless and his co-workers (e.g., Loveless & Sanford, 1974; see also Connor & Lang, 1969), who argued that the CNV consists of two components, an early orienting wave (the O-wave) and a later expectancy wave (the E-wave). Subsequent research by these investigators led them to argue that the E-wave is a readiness potential and reflects nothing more than motor preparation. Research by Rohrbaugh, Syndulko, and Lindsley (1976) and by Gaillard (1978; see also Rohrbaugh & Gaillard, 1983) also supports this interpretation. However, the question of the functional significance of the latter component (the E-wave) remains controversial. Some investigators have claimed that because a late E-wave is evident even in situations in which no overt motor response is required, the E-wave has a significance over and above that of motor preparation. However, it is clear that even though the overt motor response requirement may be removed from these situations, attention to a stimulus necessarily involves some motor activity associated with adjustment of the sensory apparatus. Perhaps the most persuasive arguments for a nonmotor role for the late CNV comes from a recent study of Damen and Brunia (1987). These authors found evidence for a motor-independent wave that precedes the delivery of feedback information in a time estimation task.

13.4.2   Sensory components

The presentation of stimuli in the visual, auditory, or somatosensory modality elicits a series of voltage oscillations that can be recorded from scalp electrodes. In practice, sensory potentials can be elicited either by a train of relatively high frequency stimuli or by transient stimuli. In the former case, the ERP responses to different stimuli overlap in time. The waveforms have quite fixed periodic characteristics that are driven by the periodic stimulation and are therefore referred to as *steady state* (see Regan, 1972). In the case of transient stimuli, the responses from different stimuli are separated in time.

For both steady-state and transient potentials the potentials appear to be obligatory responses of the nervous system to external stimulation. In fact, the earlier components of all sensory potentials (within, say, 100 ms) are invariably elicited whenever the sensory system of interest is intact. In this sense, they are described as exogenous potentials. They are thought to represent the activity of the sensory pathways that transmit the signal generated at peripheral receptors to central processing systems. Therefore, these components are *modality specific*, that is, they differ both in wave shape and scalp distribution as a function of the sensory modality in which the eliciting stimulus is presented. As would be expected of manifestations of primitive sensory processes, the sensory components are influenced primarily by stimulus parameters such as intensity, frequency, and so on. For a review of these components, see Hillyard, Picton, and Regan (1978).

For clinical purposes, sensory-evoked potentials are used in the diagnosis of neurological diseases (i.e., demyelinating diseases, cerebral tumors and infarctions, etc.). Of particular diagnostic importance are the auditory potentials (diseases involving the posterior fossa) and the steady-state visual potential (multiple sclerosis). Auditory potentials can also be used to diagnose hearing defects in uncooperative subjects.

Since most sensory potentials appear to be insensitive to psychological factors, they have not been used extensively in the study of psychological processes. We should note, however, that there have been reports that some of the middle-latency components (between 10 and 100 ms after stimulus) may reflect selective attention (McCallum, Curry, Cooper, Pocock, & Papakostopoulos, 1983; Michie, Bearpark, Crawford, & Glue, 1987). The relationship between the N100 component (in the visual, auditory, and somatosensory modality) and attention will be reviewed later in this section.

13.4.3   The early negativities

Several negative components have been described in the period between 100 and 300 ms after the presentation of an external stimulus. In this section, we examine two families of negative components that have been associated with selective attention and elementary feature analysis. Although these components have been grouped because of functional similarities and latency into a few large subgroups (N100s, N200s, etc.), their scalp distribution and morphology vary as a function of the modality of the eliciting stimulus. Therefore, these potentials may be considered to lie at the interface between "purely" exogenous (described in section 13.4.2) and purely endogenous components (described later in this section).

13.4.3.1   The N100s

First indications that ERPs could be used to investigate attentional processes came from studies in which the ERP response to attended stimuli was compared to that to unattended stimuli (e.g., Eason, Aiken, White, & Lichtenstein, 1964; Hillyard, Hink, Schwent, & Picton, 1973). These kinds of studies suggested that attended stimuli are associated with a more negative ERP between 100 and 200 ms. Subsequent research has been concerned with two issues: (1) the use of ERPs to test theories of selective attention and (2) the nature of the attentional effect on ERPs.

Selective attention refers to the ability of the human information-processing system to selectively analyze some stimuli and ignore others. Two metaphors have been associated with selective attention, that of filtering (see Broadbent, 1957) and that of resources (see Kahneman, 1973; Norman & Bobrow, 1975). Filtering theories have focused on the debate about the locus of the filter: Does filtering occur at an early, perceptual level (early selection theories, Broadbent, 1957) or at later stages of processing (late selection theories, Deutsch & Deutsch, 1963)? According to the resource metaphor, selective attention is a mechanism by which the system allocates more resources to process information coming through a particular attended channel than through other unattended channels.

In a typical paradigm (Hillyard et al., 1973), four types of stimuli are presented.

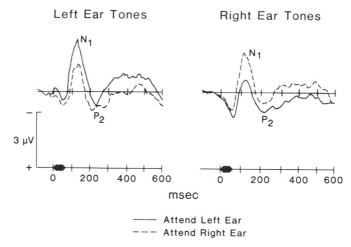

Figure 13.13. Effects of attention on early components of auditory event-related potential recorded at central electrode (Cz). Left panel shows ERPs for tones presented in left ear. Note that difference between ERPs to attended tones (solid line) versus those for unattended tones (dashed line) consists of a sustained negative potential. Similar difference can be seen for tones presented to right ear (see right panel). (Copyright 1981, Elsevier Science Publishers. Adapted with permission of author and publisher from Knight et al., 1981.)

The stimuli (tones) differ along two dimensions (location and pitch), each having two levels (left vs. right ear and standard vs. deviant pitch). The subject is instructed to attend to stimuli at a particular location and to detect target tones of a deviant pitch (e.g., left ear tones of high pitch). To investigate attention effects, ERPs to standard tones occurring in the attended location (channel) are compared to those to standard tones in the unattended channel.

Using this paradigm, Hillyard and his colleagues have observed a larger negativity with a peak latency of about 100–150 ms for stimuli presented in the attended channel (Figure 13.13 shows data from a similar experiment by Knight, Hillyard, Woods, & Neville, 1981). The moment in time at which the waveforms for attended and unattended stimuli diverge is considered as the time at which filtering starts playing a role. Hillyard and his colleagues originally interpreted their data in terms of a modulation of the sensory N100 response (Hillyard et al., 1973). Thus, they considered these data as evidence for early selection.

Later research has shown that the difference between the ERP waveforms for the attended and unattended channels cannot be considered only in terms of the amplitude variation of peak with a latency between 100 and 150 ms (N100). Rather, it can be characterized by the superimposition of a negative component lasting several hundred milliseconds (Naatanen, 1982). This component has been labeled "Processing Negativity." The onset latency of the Processing Negativity is related to the difficulty of the discrimination between the attended and the unattended channel (Hansen & Hillyard, 1983). The Processing Negativity interpretation of the selective attention effect is consistent with the resource metaphor. Rather than indicating a filtering process in the information-processing flow, the Processing Negativity might reflect a selective allocation of processing resources to the attended channel.

Similar variations in the amplitude of ERP components with a latency of 100–200 ms have been observed for visual (Harter & Aine, 1984) and somatosensory (Desmedt & Robertson, 1977) stimuli. In these modalities, however, the difference between the attended and unattended channels is characterized more by an amplification of the ERP peaks than by the superimposition of a sustained negativity (Harter & Aine, 1984; Michie et al., 1987). Again, this may be viewed either in terms of early filtering that reduces the processing of irrelevant information or in terms of extra resources devoted to processing the critical information.

This review is necessarily an oversimplification of the complexity of ERP we have loosely referred to as N100. For example, in a recent review Naatanen and Picton (1987) identified no less than six different components that are active around the time of N100!

13.4.3.2 *The N200s*

Although the amplitude of the N100 (or of the Processing Negativity) appears to reflect the selection of information from a particular perceptual channel, the amplitude of the N200 component reflects the detection of deviant features. As with N100, N200 is used to refer to a family of components, one for each modality, that are similar in function and latency. Thus, different N200s can be observed for the visual modality (with maximum at the occipital electrode) and for the auditory modality (with maximum at the central or at the frontal electrode).

Squires, Squires, and Hillyard (1975) manipulated stimulus frequency and task relevance independently and found that the N200 was larger for rare stimuli, regardless of their task relevance. A similar observation has been made by Naatanen (1982) in the kind of paradigm used by Hillyard and his colleagues that we described in the previous section. Note that to isolate N200 effects, the comparison of interest is between the rare targets and the frequent non-targets rather than between the attended and the unattended channels (as is the case with N100 effects). The N200s will be observed to rare stimuli presented on either channel; therefore, the N200 does not require selective attention for its appearance (Squires et al., 1975).[3] Not only does the amplitude of the N200 depend on stimulus probability, the latency of the N200 component is dependent on the difficulty of the discrimination between target and nontarget stimuli (Naatanen, 1982). Furthermore, the amplitude of the N200 is also proportional to the difference between frequent and rare stimuli (Figure 13.14). Therefore, Naatanen proposed that the N200 reflects the operation of an automatic "mismatch detector," and he labeled this component "mismatch negativity." Since the N200 appears to be related to the automatic detection of surprising (rare) events, this component has been related to the *orienting reflex* (see Naatanen & Gaillard, 1983). Furthermore, since the N200 is related to the automatic processing of rare features, it may be a reflection of the automatic stage of feature analysis proposed by some recent theories of perception (see Treisman & Gelade, 1980).

The N200 has been used in the investigation of mental chronometry. In particular, Ritter, Simson, Vaughan, and Macht (1982) and Renault (1983) have observed that the latency of this component covaries with reaction time. The high correlation between N200 latency and reaction time may reflect the importance of automatic feature discrimination processes (signaled by the N200) in determining the latency of the overt response. However, the subtraction technique used by Ritter et al. (1982)

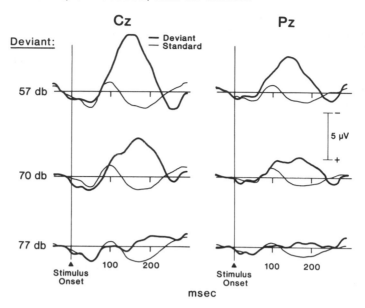

Figure 13.14. Effects of deviance on "mismatch negativity." Standard (80-dB) tone was presented on 90% of trials and deviant tone (57, 70, or 77 dB, in different blocks) was presented on 10% of trials. The ERP to a standard tone is indicated by thin line in each panel; ERP to deviant tone is indicated by thick line. As degree of mismatch between stimuli increases, mismatch negativity also increases (magnitude of difference between standard and deviant ERPs increases). (Copyright 1987, The Society for Psychophysiological Research. Adapted with permission of author and publisher from Naatanen & Picton, 1987.)

to derive their measures of N200 must be interpreted with caution since the latencies of the components in the original waveforms differ. Furthermore, motor potentials, which are characterized by a large negativity, will also covary quite strictly with reaction times. Thus, it is important to disambiguate the N200 component from motor potentials when the former component is used in the study of mental chronometry.

13.4.4   The late cognitive components

In this section, we review a sample of the research dealing with two major endogenous components, the P300 and the N400. For reasons of space we do not discuss in detail other late components, particularly a group of "slow waves." At the present time, the functional significance of the slow waves is largely unknown. However, see Sutton and Ruchkin (1984) and the research on the O-wave (section 13.4.1.2) for further information.

13.4.4.1 The P300

In section 13.3.4, we reviewed research on the antecedents of P300 and briefly alluded to attempts to evaluate a theory of P300 by studying its consequences. In this section, we focus on a series of studies that have sought to investigate the relationship between P300 and the memorability of events that elicit it.

As we noted earlier (section 13.3.4), unexpected events that are relevant to the subject's task elicit large P300s. This led Donchin (1981; Donchin & Coles, 1988a,b) to formulate the *context-updating* hypothesis of the functional significance of P300. This hypothesis allows one to generate predictions about the consequences of the elicitation of large P300 component. The context-updating hypothesis assumes that the elicitation of a P300 reflects a process involved in the updating of representations in working memory. Rare or unexpected events should lead to an updating of the current memory schemas because only by so doing can an accurate representation of the environment be maintained. The updating process may involve the "marking" of some attribute of the event that made it "distinctive" with respect to other events. This updating of the memory representation of an event is assumed to facilitate the subsequent recall of the event by providing valuable retrieval cues so that the greater the updating that follows an individual event, the higher the probability of later recalling that event. The P300 amplitude is assumed to be proportional to the degree of updating of the memory representation of the event. Therefore, as the updating process is supposed to be beneficial to recall, P300 amplitude should also predict the subsequent recall of the eliciting event.

The relationship between P300 and memory has been tested in various paradigms. For example, Karis, Fabiani, and Donchin (1984) recorded ERPs to words presented in a series that contained a distinctive word (an *isolate*) (cf. von Restorff, 1933). The isolation was achieved by changing the size of the characters in which the word was displayed. As is well documented (Cimbalo, 1978; von Restorff, 1933; Wallace, 1965), isolated items are better recalled than are comparable nondeviant items (the von Restorff effect). The isolated items, being rare and task relevant, can be expected to elicit large P300s. Thus, we could predict that the recall variance would be related to the very factors that are known to elicit and control P300 amplitude. Karis et al. (1984) found that the magnitude of the von Restorff effect depends on the mnemonic strategy employed by the subjects. Rote memorizers (i.e., subjects who rehearse the words by repeating them over and over) showed a large von Restorff effect and poor recall performance relative to elaborators (i.e., subjects who combine words into complex stories or images in order to improve their recall). For all subjects, isolates elicited larger P300s than nonisolates. For rote memorizers, isolates subsequently recalled elicited larger P300s on their initial presentation than did isolates that were not recalled. This relationship between recall and P300 amplitude was not observed in elaborators (Figure 13.15). It is noteworthy that the amplitude of a frontal-positive slow wave was correlated with subsequent recall in the elaborators, suggesting that this component may be related to the degree of elaborative processing.

Karis et al., (1984) interpreted these data as evidence that all subjects "noticed" the isolated words and reacted by updating their memory representations and producing large P300s. The differences among the subjects emerged when subjects tried to memorize the stimuli by using different types of rehearsal strategies. These strategies interacted with the retrieval processes: When subjects used rote strategies, changes in the stimulus representation induced by the isolation and manifested by P300 made it easier to recall the word. For the elaborators, whose recall depended on the networks of associations formed as the series were presented, the effects of the initial memory activation and updating manifested by

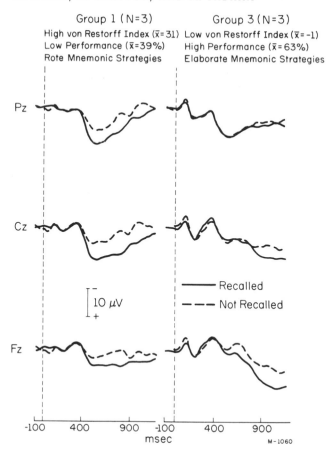

Figure 13.15. ERPs elicited by "isolated" words that were later recalled (solid line) or not recalled (dashed line). Left column shows ERPs for subjects who used rote mnemonic strategies; right column shows ERPs for subjects who used elaborative strategies. Note that amplitude of P300 is related to subsequent recall for rote memorizers but not for elaborators. (Copyright 1986, Elsevier Science Publishers. Reprinted with permission of publisher from Fabiani, Karis, Donchin, 1986b.)

P300 were not noticeable because they were overshadowed by the more powerful elaborative processing that occurred after the time frame of P300.

The interpretation of the data of the Karis et al. (1984) study capitalized on different strategies used by different subjects. The hypothesis that the relationship between P300 amplitude and subsequent recall indeed depends on the mnemonic strategy used by the subject was tested in a subsequent study in which strategy was manipulated by instruction on a within-subject basis (Fabiani, Karis, & Donchin, 1985; see also Fox & Michie, 1987). Strategy instructions were effective in manipulating the performance of the subjects. When instructed to use rote strategies, subjects recalled fewer words and displayed a larger von Restorff effect than when they used elaborative strategies. Analyses of ERPs also supported our predictions. When subjects were instructed to use rote strategies, the P300s elicited by words subsequently recalled were significantly larger than those elicited by words subsequently not recalled. Such a relationship was not observed when subjects used elaborative strategies. In addition, when rote strategies were used, subjects recalled the size of the words better than in the elaborative condition. This suggests that *size* is a *distinctive* attribute of the memory representation of the word, such as to help recall in the case of rote instructions.

In another experiment, Fabiani, Karis, and Donchin (1986a) employed an incidental memory paradigm (an "oddball" task) to reduce the use of elaborative strategies. The results confirmed the prediction that stimuli that were subsequently recalled had larger P300s at the time of initial presentation than those for stimuli that were not recalled.

All the studies described in the preceding paragraphs use either the von Restorff paradigm or the oddball paradigm. However, the memory effect is not limited to isolated or rare items. It is also present for the nonisolates and for the frequent items in the oddball experiment.

In several recent studies, memory paradigms have been used that do not capitalize on stimuli for which the P300 is expected to be enhanced, that is, paradigms in which neither the distinctiveness nor the probability of occurrence of the stimuli to be memorized are manipulated. A seminal study in this respect is that by Sanquist, Rohrbaugh, Syndulko, and Lindsley (1980), who found that larger amplitude P300s (or late positive components) were elicited, in a same–different judgment task, by stimuli that were correctly recognized in a subsequent recognition test. Johnson, Pfefferbaum, and Kopell (1985) recorded ERPs in a study–test memory paradigm. They reported that the P300 associated with subsequently recognized words was slightly but not significantly larger than that elicited by nonrecognized words. Paller, Kutas, and Mayes (1985) recorded ERPs in an incidental memory paradigm in which the subjects were asked to make either a semantic or a nonsemantic decision and were subsequently and unexpectedly tested for their recognition or recall of the stimuli. They found that ERPs elicited during the decision task were predictive of subsequent memory performance in that the P300 (late positive complex) was larger for words subsequently recalled or recognized than for words not recalled or recognized. Similarly, Paller, McCarthy, and Wood (1987) recorded ERPs in two semantic judgment tasks that were followed by a free recall and by a recognition test. The ERPs to words later remembered were more positive than those to words later not remembered even though the memory effect was smaller for recognition than for recall. Neville, Kutas, Chesney, and Schmidt (1986) recorded ERPs to words that were either congruous or incongruous with a preceding sentence in a task in which subjects were asked to judge whether or not the word was congruent with the sentence. They found that the amplitude of a late positive component (P650) predicted subsequent recognition.

Taken together, the experiments described in this section suggest that the P300, as well as other late components of the ERP, can have an important role in illuminating some of the cognitive processes that accompany stimulus encoding and that are usually opaque to traditional techniques. Although the first group of studies conducted in our laboratory has focused on the interaction between distinctiveness and rehearsal strategies in determining the ERP–memory relationship, the other studies have shown that such a relationship is widespread over a variety of different memory paradigms. It is important to emphasize that memory is a complex phenomenon that can be influenced by a multitude of variables and that can be probed with a number of different tests. Thus, it is unlikely that a single component of the ERP can be identified as the "memory component." It is much more likely, and indeed more interesting, that a series of ERP components will prove to be significant in different memory tasks.

13.4.4.2 *The N400*

The N400 component of the ERP was first described by Kutas and Hillyard (1980a), who recorded ERPs in a sentence-reading task. In this paradigm, words are presented serially, and the subject is asked to read them silently in order to answer questions about the content of the sentence at the end of the experiment. In two studies reported by Kutas and Hillyard (1980a), 25 percent of the sentences ended with a semantically incongruous (but syntactically correct) word. These incongruous words elicited an N400 component that was larger than that elicited by words that were congruous with respect to the meaning of the sentence. Furthermore, the amplitude of the N400 appeared to be proportional to the degree of incongruity: Moderately incongruous words ("he took a sip from the waterfall") had a smaller N400 than strongly incongruous words ("he took a sip from the transmitter"). Kutas and Hillyard (1982) reported that the N400 to incongruous endings was slightly larger and more prolonged over the right than the left hemisphere.

These results have been replicated and extended repeatedly using variations of the sentence-reading paradigm described. The aim of these studies has been to determine whether the N400 is a manifestation of a distinctively semantic process or whether it is elicited by other kinds of deviance. Kutas and Hillyard (1984) found that the amplitude of the N400 was inversely related to the subject's expectancy of the terminal word (cloze probability), whereas it was insensitive to sentence constraints (i.e., to the number of possible alternative endings). Kutas and Hillyard (1980b) recorded ERPs to the terminal word in a sentence. This word could be semantically or physically deviant or not deviant. They interpreted their data as indicating that an N400 followed semantic deviation, whereas late positive complex (P300) followed physical deviation.[4] In addition, Kutas and Hillyard (1983) inserted a number of semantic and grammatical anomalies in prose passages. They found that large N400s were associated with the semantic anomalies embedded in the text, whereas the negativities recorded to grammatical errors were inconsistent and had a scalp distribution different from that of the N400. Kutas, Lindamood, and Hillyard (1984) found that anomalous words that were semantically related to the sentence's "best completion" ("the pizza was too hot to drink") elicited smaller N400s than anomalous words unrelated to the best completion ("the pizza was too hot to cry"). This suggests that the degree of semantic relatedness is an important determinant of the N400 (Figure 13.16).

A large N400 component is also evoked by semantic anomalies presented in the auditory modality (McCallum, Farmer, & Pocock, 1984) or in anomalies embedded in American Sign Language (ASL) gestures (Neville, 1985). However, Macar and Besson (1987) did not find N400 responses to anomalous endings of musical tunes.

N400-like components have also been recorded in paradigms other than sentence reading. For example, Fischler, Bloom, Childers, Roucos, and Perry (1983) recorded ERPs in a sentence verification paradigm. In this paradigm, sentences are presented in segments ("a robin / is / a bird"), and two dimensions are orthogonally manipulated: whether the sentences are positive or negative ("is," "is not") and

THE PIZZA WAS TOO HOT TO...

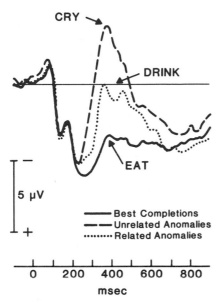

Figure 13.16. Effects of anomalous sentence endings on N400. The ERPs (from Pz) depicted were recorded following visual presentation of words that varied in their relationship to previous words in sentence. For example, for sentences such as "The pizza was too hot to...," three endings were possible. *Best completion:* "eat"; *Related anomaly:* "drink"; *Unrelated anomaly:* "cry." Note that N400 component is only present for anomalies and is larger for unrelated than for related anomalies. (Copyright 1984, Lawrence Erlbaum Publishers. Adapted with permission of author and publisher from Kutas, Lindamood, & Hillyard, 1984.)

whether they are true or false. The subject is required to indicate whether the sentence is true or false. A large negativity was elicited by false affirmative ("a robin/is/a tree") and true negative ("a robin/is not/a tree") sentences, that is, by sentences in which the first and last element were semantically unrelated. In a similar study (Fischler, Childers, Achariyapaopan, & Perry, 1985) subjects were required to learn the occupation of fictitious people. They were then asked to indicate whether sentences of the type "John / is / a dentist" were true or false. They found that false statements were associated with larger negativities than true statements.

Rugg recorded N400-like components in a semantic priming paradigm (Rugg, 1985) and in a rhyme judgment task (Rugg & Barrett, 1988), although there are some differences between the scalp distribution of the negativity recorded in these paradigms and that recorded in the sentence-reading task.

In general, research reviewed in this section suggests that there is a brain response (the N400) that is specifically sensitive to the violation of semantic expectancies. Measures of this component, then, should prove useful in testing theories and models relating to semantic priming (e.g., Van Petten & Kutas, 1987).

13.5   POTENTIAL APPLICATIONS OF ERP RESEARCH

In this section we consider the possible contribution of ERP research to problems that arise in various branches of psychology, with a particular emphasis on social psychology. Before we review some specific research examples, we need to consider two general issues related to the application of ERP research.

First, as we noted earlier, for some ERP components there is sufficient knowledge about the *physiological* significance for them to be used us markers of physiological functioning. This knowledge has led to the use of ERPs in neurological diagnosis (see, e.g., Halliday, Butler, & Paul, 1987, for a review). Second, we have devoted much of this chapter to a discussion of the *psychological* significance of ERP components; that is, we have attempted to show that the components are manifestations of particular cognitive activities. One implication of this is that to the extent that questions that arise in any branch of psychology can be recast in terms of questions about cognitive activities, there is at least the possibility that the measurement of ERPs will be useful.

In the following sections, we review several examples of how such research has proceeded or might proceed. For reviews of other applications of ERP research to cognitive and engineering psychology, see Donchin, Karis, et al. (1986) and Donchin, Kramer, and Wickens (1986).

13.5.1   *ERPS and emotion*

13.5.1.1   *Emotion and cognition*

In previous sections of this chapter, we have emphasized the view that ERPs can be regarded as manifestations of cognitive processes. For the most part, the ERP literature contains few studies of ERP–emotion relationships. This tendency to emphasize the cognitive rather than the emotional is probably due to the belief that the psychophysiological analysis of emotions is more the province of students of the autonomic nervous system. However, recent attempts to reevaluate the distinction between cognition and emotion call into question the justification for their psychophysiological separation. For example, if the experience of emotion is attributed, at least in part, to the process of cognitive appraisal (e.g., Arnold, 1960), then the so-called cognitive ERPs have the potential to be useful in the analysis of appraisal processes. Similarly, if emotions are believed to influence cognitive processes (e.g., Bower, 1981), it may be that ERPs will be useful in describing such an influence.

These kinds of ideas are behind the recent analysis of ERPs in situations in which subjects anticipate and receive emotional stimuli (Johnston, Miller, & Burleson, 1986; Klorman & Ryan, 1980; Simons, MacMillan, & Ireland, 1982) and in studies of subjects suffering from emotional dysfunction (Miller, 1986; Yee & Miller, 1988). In the following sections, we review two other kinds of studies in which there is evidence of concern with cognitive–emotion issues.

13.5.1.2   *Lie detection*

In preceding sections, we have emphasized that ERPs can be used to explore situations involving emotion if these situations can be viewed in terms of the information-processing activities. In the case of lie detection, studies using autonomic measures have similarly emphasized the importance of cognitive factors. Thus, rather than propose a specific emotional "lie-response," these studies have sought to use the measures to determine whether an individual has specific knowledge (cf. the guilty-knowledge test, Lykken, 1974; Podlesny & Raskin, 1977).

In the case of studies of lie detection using ERPs, researchers have used a paradigm in which stimulus words or phrases relating to a crime would be categorized in one way if the information they represented was unknown to the individual and in another way if the information was known (see Farwell& Donchin, 1986). The role of the ERPs, then, is to identify the categorization rule being used by the subject. This is accomplished by using a variant of the oddball task. Three classes of stimuli are presented: (1) words or phrases related to the crime (the probe stimuli); (2) words of phrases unrelated to the crime and unknown to the subject (irrelevant stimuli); and (3) words or phrases unrelated to the crime but known to the subject (target stimuli). The subject is instructed to count the target stimuli.

Thus, the critical question is whether the subject will categorize the probe stimuli as irrelevant (indicating no knowledge) or as target stimuli (indicating knowledge). This question is answered by setting up the probabilities of the different stimuli such that the probe stimuli would elicit a large response (P300) if they are categorized as targets. Farwell and Donchin (1986) have shown that if the probabilities of irrelevant, probe, and target stimuli are .67, .17, and .16, respectively, the procedure is effective in determining the categorization rule used by the individual. In this way, the presence of guilty knowledge can be determined.

In this example, the role of the ERP is to determine whether a particular set of stimuli is classified by the subject as belonging to one of two other categories. In principle, then, it could be used in any situation in which the experimenter is interested in identifying classification rules.

13.5.1.3 *Bargaining*

Bargaining, like most forms of social interaction, involves both cognitive and emotional processes. Thus, bargaining presents an interesting topic of study for the analysis of cognitive–emotional relationships.

In the study to be described in this section (Karis, Druckman, Lissak, & Donchin, 1984), the focus was on the cognitive ERP responses to events believed to have emotional consequences. The subject was engaged in a "bargaining" session with the computer. The object of bargaining was the purchase of a used car. The subject and the computer alternated in making their concessions until they agreed on a price. The subject's objective was to buy the car at the lowest possible price. The ERPs were recorded while the subject viewed the computer's concession.

An interesting aspect of this study was that the computer adopted either one of two strategies in making its concessions: It could be either "generous" or "stingy." When the computer was in the generous mode, it would concede 80 percent of the subject concession, whereas when it was in the stingy mode, it would concede only 20 percent of the subject concession. Thus, it was important to the subject to guess the computer's strategy in order to take advantage of it.

Switches in the computer's strategy (which occurred randomly) reliably elicited P300s that were larger than those recorded to trials in which the strategy remained the same. This can be viewed in terms of cognitive processes: To the extent that

P300 represents a process of context updating, it seems reasonable that the subject would need to update her or his mental schema at the moment in which a task-relevant event changes. Another interesting aspect of this study is that a photograph of the subject's face was taken every time the subject saw the computer's concession. The facial expression of the subject was then analyzed in terms of the emotions displayed. It is interesting to note that, on some occasions, the subject smiled when the concession was generous. Thus, the appraisal of a concession (as manifested by the ERP) was, in some cases, associated with the facial expression of emotion.

13.5.2   ERPs and "payoff" manipulations

The social interaction between experimenter and subject can have an influence on the strategy adopted by the subject in performing her or his assigned task. Subjects approach experimental situations with hypotheses about the goals of the experiment and, most importantly, the payoffs associated with different goals. Information about these payoffs can be derived from explicit instructions as well as more implicit forms of communication between subject and experimenter.

In most ERP studies, we try to constrain the subject's task so as to reduce the options available to the subject. In this way, assumptions can be made about the processes used by the subject to perform the task.

In several studies, instructions or payoff schedules have been deliberately manipulated in order to alter the subject's strategy in performing the task. In this case, the ERP focus is on understanding how strategic changes are implemented. An example of this approach has been described in section 13.4.4, The P300, where we saw that mnemonic strategies manipulated by instruction were important determinants of the P300–recall relationship and, by implication, of the role of the rehearsal of distinctiveness cues in memory.

In the following two sections, we review other examples of this kind of approach.

13.5.2.1 Decision making

The way in which humans reach decisions is an important problem for social psychologists. Most theories of decision making agree that subjective probability and payoff structure are fundamental determinants of human choices (Fishbein & Ajzen, 1975).

Karis, Chesney, and Donchin (1983) investigated the role of these two dimensions in determining the amplitude of P300. In this study, subjects had to predict which of three stimuli (the numbers 1, 2, or 3) would next occur. The probabilities of the three stimuli were .45, .10, and .45, respectively. The subjects were rewarded for correct predictions following one of two schedules run in different blocks. In one schedule ("all-or-none"), subjects were only rewarded for correct predictions. In another payoff schedule ("linear"), subjects not only were rewarded for correct choices, but also received half bonuses when their predictions were off by 1 (i.e., a 1 occurred when a 2 was predicted). Thus, in the linear schedule, the optimal strategy was to predict 2 (objectively the rare event).

Karis et al. found that although subjects did indeed vary their overt predictions following the payoff schedules, their P300s were always larger for the rare stimuli (the 2s). That the subjects were aware of the probability structure in each of the two conditions was confirmed by subjective reports. These results indicate that P300 reflects subjective probability rather than a conscious decision about which stimulus was most rewarding.

Karis et al. also studied variations in subject's strategy. In particular, they were able to quantify the "riskiness" of a particular choice by estimating the expected loss with respect to the optimal behavior. They observed that P300 amplitude was proportional to the riskiness of the prediction. They interpreted this result in terms of differences in the relevance of the information conveyed by the stimulus in cases of high- and low-risk choices.

13.5.2.2 *Speed–accuracy instructions*

Kutas, McCarthy, and Donchin (1977) analyzed the relationship between P300 and reaction time when subjects were given speed or accuracy instructions. Whereas the timing of the reaction time response in relation to the P300 changed with instruction, the latency of the P300 itself was only slightly affected. Thus, in this case, the effect of instructions was to change the coupling between the processes associated with P300 and those associated with overt behavior. In terms of information processing, it appears that speed instructions lead the subject to generate an overt response before information has been fully processed.

A similar modulation of the relationship between the processing of stimulus information and the timing of the overt response has been described by Gratton et al. (1988; see also Gehring et al., 1986). In this case, measures of the readiness potential (see section 13.4.1.1) were diagnostic of the strategic mode of the subject (accurate vs. fast).

13.5.3   *ERPs and communication*

In this chapter, we have considered ERPs as a tool for investigating cognitive processing. In particular, we have emphasized how ERPs can be used to obtain information about cognitive functions that would not be available in other ways. In somewhat more extreme terms, we may consider ERPs as a communication device.

An interesting example of this approach is given by a recent study by Farwell, Donchin, and Kramer (1986). These investigators have devised a technique that allows people to communicate by exploiting the relationship between ERPs and attention. Subjects in this study were presented with a matrix of letters that were illuminated in rapid succession. By examining the ERP responses to each of the flashes, they were able to determine the letters to which the subjects were attending. Thus, letter by letter, the subjects were able to communicate entire words by means of their ERPs. This type of communication device may be particularly useful for cases in which people cannot communicate in other ways, such as in cases of patients that have lost any motor ability as a consequence of trauma and disease.

13.5.4   *Summary*

In the examples reviewed in this section, we have seen how ERPs can be used to study or, in one case, enhance social behavior, broadly defined. The underlying theme of these examples has been that if the question of interest can be considered in terms of the information-processing transactions that occur, ERPs may be a useful tool. This is because ERPs can be regarded as manifestations of information-processing activities.

Upon analysis, there appear to be several other instances in which such a conception is quite feasible, such as when the interest of the investigator is on the cognitive processing of social information. For example, the recent development of *social cognition* as a subdiscipline within social psychology has led to the treatment of a subset of *social processes* as involving the operation of the cognitive apparatus on social information (see, e.g., Wyer & Srull, 1984). The only restriction in the application of ERPs to this domain is that the information be presented discretely so that segments of the EEG can be identified that are time locked to the events of interest.

In other cases, considerable efforts may be needed in order to apply the model of cognitive psychophysiology. For example, evaluations of social interactions would require not only that the interactions be structured so as to permit discrete events to be identified. One would also need to incorporate repetitions of the "same" event into the interaction (if averaging is necessary to extract stable ERPs) and, most importantly, to identify the putative cognitive processes associated with the events. The imposition of this kind of structure may result in a distortion of the essence of the interaction process.

On the basis of the foregoing examples and discussion, there appears to be good reason to expect considerable benefit from an application of a cognitive psychophysiology based on ERPs in various areas within psychology, particularly social psychology. Just as problems in cognitive psychology are proving more tractable when psychophysiological measures are added to those measures traditionally available, problems in social psychology may prove to be similarly more tractable. However, the benefits of such an application will only accrue if the psychophysiological measures are derived under appropriate circumstances and if such circumstances can be created without distortion of the phenomenon of interest.

NOTES

Preparation of this chapter was supported in part by grants MH41445 and NS24986. Bill Gehring, and Greg Miller made helpful comments on preliminary drafts.

1 Note that this assumption may not always be valid, as, for example, in the case of variability in the latency and other characteristics of the ERP from sample to sample (see section 13.3.2.2). Furthermore, the ERP derived by averaging may include potentials that do not originate in the brain but are time locked to the event (see section 13.3.2.1).
2 Note that other theories of P300 have been offered by, e.g., Desmedt (1980), Rosler (1983), and Verleger (1988). Both Desmedt and Verleger propose that the P300 is related to the termination, or *closure*, of processing periods, whereas Rosler proposed that P300 reflects controlled processing. As we have argued elsewhere (Donchin & Coles, 1988a,b), these theories do not account for the richness of the results concerning the consequences of the P300 that have accrued in the last decade.
3 Note that in this paradigm the P300 is only elicited by rare targets presented on the attended channel. Thus, the P300 is only elicited by task-relevant stimuli, while the N200 appears to be "automatically" elicited by rare stimuli regardless of their task relevance.
4 We should note that there is some controversy concerning whether or not a P300 *follows* the

occurrence of an N400 in the case of semantic deviation. For present purposes, it is sufficient to note that the physical deviation was *not* followed by an N400.

REFERENCES

Allison, T., Wood, C. C., & McCarthy, G. (1986). The central nervous system. In M. G. H. Coles, S. W. Porges, & E. Donchin (Eds.), *Psychophysiology: System, processes, and applications* (pp. 5–25). New York: Guilford Press.

Arnold, M. B. (1960). *Emotion and personality.* New York: Columbia University Press.

Beatty, J., Barth, D. S., Richer, F., & Johnson, R. A. (1986). Neuromagnetometry. In M. G. H. Coles, S. W. Porges, & E. Donchin (Eds.), *Psychophysiology: Systems, processes, and applications* (pp. 26–40). New York: Guilford Press.

Berger, H. (1929). Uber das Elektrenkephalogramm das menchen. *Archiv für Psychiatrie, 87,* 527–570.

Bosco, C. M., Gratton, G., Kramer, A. F., Wickens, C. D., Coles, M. G. H., & Donchin, E. (1986). Information extraction and components of the event-related potential. *Psychophysiology, 23,* 426. (Abstract)

Bower, G. H. (1981). Mood and memory. *American Psychologist, 36,* 129–148.

Broadbent, D. E. (1957). A mathematical model for human attention and immediate memory. *Psychological Review, 64,* 205–215.

Brunia, C. H. M., Haagh, S. A. V. M., & Scheirs, J. G. M. (1985). Waiting to respond: Electrophysiological measurements in man during preparation for a voluntary movement. In H. Heuer, U. Kleinbeck, & K. H. Schmidt (Eds.) *Motor behavior. Programming, control and acquisition* (pp. 35–78). Berlin: Springer-Verlag.

Buchwald, J., & Squires, N. (1983). Endogenous auditory potentials in the cat: A P300 model. In C. Woody (Ed.), *Conditioning* (pp. 503–515). New York: Plenum Press.

Cimbalo, R. S. (1978). Making something stand out: The isolation effect in memory performance. In M. M. Grunneberg, P. E. Morris, & R. N. Sykes (Eds.), *Practical aspects of memory* (pp. 101–110). New York: Academic Press.

Coles, M. G. H., Gratton, G., Bashore, T. R., Eriksen, C. W., & Donchin, E. (1985). A psychophysiological investigation of the continuous flow model of human information processing. *Journal of Experimental Psychology: Human Perception and Performance, 11,* 529–553.

Coles, M. G. H., Gratton, G., & Gehring, W. J. (1987). Theory in cognitive psychophysiology. *Journal of Psychophysiology, 1,* 13–16.

Coles, M. G. H., Gratton, G., Kramer, A. F., & Miller, G. A. (1986). Principles of signal acquisition and analysis. In M. G. H. Coles, E. Donchin, & S. W. Porges (Eds.), *Psychophysiology: Systems, processes, and applications* (pp. 183–221). New York: Guilford Press.

Connor, W. H., & Lang, P. J. (1969). Cortical slow-wave and cardiac rate responses in stimulus orientation and reaction time conditions. *Journal of Experimental Psychology, 82,* 310–320.

Csepe, V., Karmos, G., & Molnar, M. (1987). Effects of signal probability on sensory evoked potentials in cats. *International Journal of Neuroscience, 33,* 61–71.

Damen, E. J. P., & Brunia, C. H. M. (1987). Changes in heart rate and slow brain potentials related to motor preparation and stimulus anticipation in a time estimation task. *Psychophysiology, 24,* 700–713.

Deecke, L., Bashore, T., Brunia, C. H. M., Grunewald-Zuberbier, E., Grunewald, G., & Kristeva, R. (1984). Movement-associated potentials and motor control. In Karrer, R., Cohen, J., & Tueting, P. (Eds.), *Brain and information: Event-related potentials* (pp. 398–428). New York: New York Academy of Science.

Deecke, L., Englitz, H. G., Kornhuber, H. H., & Schmitt, G. (1977). Cerebral potentials preceding voluntary movement in patients with bilateral or unilateral Parkinson akinesia. In J. E. Desmedt (Ed.), *Attention, voluntary contraction, and event-related cerebral potentials. Progress in clinical neurophysiology* (Vol. 1, pp. 151–163). Basel: Karger.

Deecke, L., Weinberg, H., & Brickett, P. (1982). Magnetic fields of the human brain accompanying voluntary movements. Bereitschaftsmagnetfeld. *Experimental Brain Research, 48,* 144–148.

De Jong, R., Wierda, M., Mulder, G., & Mulder, L. J. W. (1988). The timing of response preparation. *Journal of Experimental Psychology: Human Perception and Performance, 14,* 682–692.

Desmedt, J.E. (1980). P300 in serial tasks: An essential post-decision closure mechansim. In H.H. Kornhuber & L. Deecke (Eds.), *Motivation, motor, and sensory processes of the brain. Progress in brain research* (Vol. 54, pp. 682–686). Amsterdam: Elsevier North-Holland.

Desmedt, J. E., & Robertson, D. (1977). Differential enhancement of early and late components of the cerebral somatosensory evoked potentials during forced-paced cognitive tasks in man. *Journal of Physiology, 271,* 761–782.

Deutsch, J. A., & Deutsch, D. (1963). Attention: Some theoretical considerations. *Psychological Review, 70,* 80–90.

Donchin, E. (1978). Use of scalp distribution as a dependent variable in event-related potential studies: Excerpts of preconference correspondence. In D. Otto (Ed.), *Multidisciplinary perspectives in event-related brain potentials research* (EPA-600/9-77-043, pp. 501–510). Washington, DC: U.S. Government Printing Office.

Donchin, E. (1979). Event-related brain potentials: A tool in the study of human information processing. In H. Begleiter (Ed.), *Evoked potentials and behavior* (pp. 13–75). New York: Plenum Press.

Donchin, E. (1981). Surprise!...Surprise? *Psychophysiology, 18,* 493–513.

Donchin, E., & Coles, M. G. H. (1988a). Is the P300 component a manifestation of context updating? *Behavioral and Brain Sciences, 11,* 343–356.

Donchin, E., & Coles, M. G. H. (1988b). On the conceptual foundations of cognitive psychophysiology: A reply to comments. *Behavioral and Brain Sciences, 11,* 408–427.

Donchin, E., Gratton, G., Dupree, D., & Coles, M. G. H. (1988). After a rash action: Latency and amplitude of the P300 following fast guesses. In G. Galbraith, M. Klietzman, & E. Donchin (Eds.), *Neurophysiology and psychophysiology: Experimental and clinical application* (pp. 173–188). Hillsdale, NJ: Erlbaum.

Donchin, E., Heffley, E. (1978). Multivariate analysis of event-related potential data: A tutorial review. In D. Otto (Ed.), *Multidisciplinary perspectives in event-related brain potential research* (EPA-600/9-77-043, pp. 555–572). Washington, DC: U.S. Government Printing Office.

Donchin, E., Heffley, E., Hillyard, S. A., Loveless, N., Maltzman, I., Ohman, A., Rosler, F., Ruchkin, D., & Siddle, D. (1984). Cognition and event-related potentials: II. In R. Karrer, J. Cohen, & P. Tueting (Eds.), *Brain and information: Event-related potentials. Annals of the New York Academy of Sciences, 25,* 39–57.

Donchin, E., & Herning, R. I. (1975). A simulation study of the efficacy of step-wise discriminant analysis in the detection and comparison of event-related potentials. *Electroencephalography and Clinical Neurophysiology, 38,* 51–68.

Donchin, E., Karis, D., Bashore, T. R., Coles, M. G. H., & Gratton, G. (1986). Cognitive psychophysiology and human information processing. In M. G. H. Coles, E. Donchin, & S. W. Porges (Eds.), *Psychophysiology: Systems, processes, and applications* (pp. 244–267). New York: Guilford Press.

Donchin, E., Kramer, A. F., & Wickens, C. D. (1986). Applications of event-related brain potentials to problems in engineering psychology. In M. G. H. Coles, E. Donchin, & S. W. Porges (Eds.), *Psychophysiology: Systems, processes, and applications* (pp. 702–718). New York: Guilford Press.

Donchin, E., Ritter, W., & McCallum C. (1978). Cognitive psychophysiology: The endogenous components of the ERP. In E. Callaway, P. Tueting, & S. H. Koslow (Eds.), *Event-related brain potentials in man* (pp. 349–411). New York: Academic Press.

Duncan-Johnson, C. C., & Donchin, E. (1977). On quantifying surprise: The variation of event-related potentials with subjective probability. *Psychophysiology, 14,* 456–467.

Duncan-Johnson, C. C., & Donchin, E. (1979). The time constant in P300 recording. *Psychophysiology, 16,* 53–55.

Duncan-Johnson, C.C., & Donchin, E. (1982). The P300 component of the event-related brain potential as an index of information processing. *Biological Psychology, 14,* 1–52.

Eason, R. G., Aiken, L. R., Jr., White, C. T., & Lichtenstein, M. (1964). Activation and behavior: II. Visually evoked cortical potentials in man as indicants of activation level. *Perceptual and Motor Skills, 19,* 875–895.

Fabiani, M., Gratton, G., Karis, D., & Donchin, E. (1987). The definition, identification, and reliability of measurement of the P300 component of the event-related brain potential. In P. K. Ackles, J. R. Jennings, & M. G. H. Coles (Eds.), *Advances in psychophysiology* (Vol. 1, pp. 1–78), Greenwich, CT: JAI Press.

Fabiani, M., Karis, D., & Donchin, E. (1985). Effects of strategy manipulation on P300 amplitude in a von Restorff paradigm. *Psychophysiology, 22,* 588–589. (Abstract).

Fabiani, M., Karis, D., & Donchin, E. (1986a). P300 and recall in an incidental memory paradigm. *Psychophysiology, 23,* 298–308.

Fabiani, M., Karis, D., & Donchin, E. (1986b). P300 and memory. In W. C. McCallum, R. Zappoli, & F. Denoth (Eds.), *Cerebral psychophysiology: Studies in event-related potentials* (pp. 63–69). Amsterdam: Elsevier. (Supplement 38 to *Electroencephalography and Clinical Neurophysiology.*)

Farwell, L. A., & Donchin, E. (1986). The "brain detector": P300 in the detection of deception. *Psychophysiology, 23,* 435. (Abstract.)

Farwell, L. A., Donchin, E., & Kramer, A. F. (1986). Talking heads: A mental prosthesis for communicating with event-related potentials of the EEG. *Psychophysiology, 23,* 435. (Abstract)

Fischler, I., Bloom, P. A., Childers, D. G., Roucos, S. E., & Perry, N. W., Jr. (1983). Brain potentials related to stages of sentence verification. *Psychophysiology, 20,* 400–409.

Fischler, I., Childers, D. G., Achariyapaopan, T., & Perry, N. W., Jr. (1985). Brain potentials during sentence verification: Automatic aspects of comprehension. *Biological Psychology, 21,* 83–105.

Fishbein, M., & Ajzen, I. (1975). *Belief, attitude, intention and behavior.* Reading, MA: Addison-Wesley.

Fox, A. M., & Michie, P. T. (1987). *P3 and memory relationship under instructed learning strategy conditions.* Paper presented at the 4th International Conference on Cognitive Neurosciences, June, Paris-Dourdan, France.

Gaillard, A. (1978). *Slow brain potentials preceding task performance.* Unpublished doctoral dissertation, Soesterberg, The Netherlands: Institute for Perception (TNO).

Gehring, W., Gratton, G., Coles, M. G. H., & Donchin, E. (1986). Response priming and components of the event-related brain potential. *Psychophysiology, 23,* 437–438. (Abstract)

Glaser, E. M., & Ruchkin, D. S. (1976). *Principles of neurobiological signal analysis.* New York: Academic Press.

Gratton, G., Coles, M. G. H., & Donchin, E. (1983). A new method for off-line removal of ocular artifact. *Electroencephalography and Clinical Neurophysiology, 55,* 468–484.

Gratton, G., Coles, M. G. H., Donchin, E. (1989). A procedure for using multielectrode information in the analysis of components of the event-related potentials: Vector filter. *Psychophysiology, 26,* 222–232.

Gratton, G., Coles, M. G. H., Sirevaag, E., Eriksen, C. W., & Donchin, E. (1988). Pre- and post-stimulus activation of response channels: A psychophysiological analysis. *Journal of Experimental Psychology: Human Perception and Performance, 14,* 331–344.

Halgren, E., Squires, N. K., Wilson, C. L., Rohrbaugh, J. W., Babb, T. L., & Randall, P. H. (1980). Endogenous potentials generated in the human hippocampal formation and amygdala by infrequent events. *Science, 210,* 803–805.

Halliday, A. M., Butler, S. R., & Paul, R. (Eds.) (1987). *A textbook of clinical neurophysiology.* Chichester: Wiley.

Hansen, J. C., & Hillyard, S. A. (1983). Selective attention to multidimensional auditory stimuli in man. *Journal of Experimental Psychology: Human Perception and Performance, 9,* 1–19.

Harter, M. R., & Aine, C. J. (1984). Brain mechanisms of visual selective attention. In R. Parasuraman & D. R. Davies (Eds.), *Varieties of attention* (pp. 293–321). London: Academic Press.

Hillyard S. A., Hink, R. F., Schwent, V. L., & Picton, T. W. (1973). Electrical signs of selective attention in the human brain. *Science, 182,* 177–180.

Hillyard, S. A., Picton, T. W., & Regan, D. (1978). Sensation, perception, and attention: Analysis using ERPs. In E. Callaway, P. Tueting, & S. H. Koslow (Eds.), *Event-related brain potentials in man* (pp. 223–321). New York: Academic Press.

Horst, R. L., & Donchin, E. (1980). Beyond averaging II: Single trial classification of exogenous event-related potentials using step-wise discriminant analysis. *Electroencephalography and Clinical Neurophysiology, 48,* 113–126.

Jasper, H. H. (1958). The ten-twenty electrode system of the International Federation. *Electroencephalography and Clinical Neurophysiology, 10,* 371–375.

Johnson, R., Jr. (1986). A triarchic model of P300 amplitude. *Psychophysiology, 23,* 367–384.

Johnson, R., Jr., & Donchin, E. (1978). On how P300 amplitude varies with the utility of the eliciting stimuli. *Electroencephalography and Clinical Neurophysiology, 44*, 424–437.

Johnson, R., Jr., Pfefferbaum, A., & Kopell, B. S. (1985). P300 and long-term memory: Latency predicts recognition time. *Psychophysiology, 22*, 498–507.

Johnston, V. S., Miller, D. R., & Burleson, M. H. (1986). Multiple P3s to emotional stimuli and their theoretical significance. *Psychophysiology, 23*, 684–694.

Kahneman, D. (1973). *Attention and effort.* Englewood Cliffs, NJ: Prentice-Hall.

Karis, D., Chesney, G. L., & Donchin, E. (1983). "... 'Twas ten to one; And yet we ventured...": P300 and decision making. *Psychophysiology, 20*, 260–268.

Karis, D., Druckman, D., Lissak, R., & Donchin, E. (1984). A psychophysiological analysis of bargaining: ERPs and facial expressions. In R. Karrer, J. Cohen, & P. Tueting (Eds.), *Brain and information : Event-related potentials* (pp. 230–235). New York: New York Academy of Sciences.

Karis, D., Fabiani, M., & Donchin, E. (1984). P300 and memory: Individual differences in the von Restorff effect. *Cognitive Psychology, 16*, 177–216.

Karrer, R., & Ivins, J. (1976). Steady potentials accompanying perception and response in mentally retarded and normal children. In R. Karrer (Ed.), *Developmental psychophysiology of mental retardation* (pp. 361–417). Springfield, IL: Thomas.

Klorman, R., & Ryan, R. M. (1980). Heart rate, contingent negative variation, and evoked potentials during anticipation of affective stimulation. *Psychophysiology, 17*, 513–523.

Knight, R. T., Hillyard, S. A., Woods, D. L., & Neville, H. J. (1981). The effects of frontal cortex lesions on event-related potentials during auditory selective attention. *Electroencephalography and Clinical Neurophysiology, 52*, 571–582.

Kornhuber, H. H., & Deecke, L. (1965). Hirnpotentialanderungen bei Wilkurbewegungen und passiven Bewegungen des Menschen: Bereitschaftpotential und reafferente Potentiale. *Pflugers Archives für die gesammte Physiologie, 248*, 1–17.

Kramer, A. F., Sirevaag, E. J., & Braune, R. (1987). A psychophysiological assessment of operator workload during simulated flight missions. *Human Factors, 29*, 145–160.

Kutas, M., & Donchin, E. (1980). Preparation to respond as manifested by movement-related brain potentials. *Brain Research, 202*, 95–115.

Kutas, M., & Hillyard, S. A. (1980a). Reading senseless sentences: Brain potentials reflect semantic incongruity. *Science, 207*, 203–205.

Kutas, M., & Hillyard, S. A. (1980b). Event-related brain potentials to semantically inappropriate and surprisingly large words. *Biological Psychology, 11*, 99–116.

Kutas, M., & Hillyard, S. A. (1982). The lateral distribution of event-related potentials during sentence processing. *Neuropsychologia, 20*, 579–590.

Kutas, M., & Hillyard, S. A. (1983). Event-related brain potentials to grammatical errors and semantic anomalies. *Memory and Cognition, 11*, 539–550.

Kutas, M., & Hillyard, S. A. (1984). Brain potentials during reading reflect word expectancy and semantic association. *Nature, 307*, 161–163.

Kutas, M., Lindamood, T. E., & Hillyard, S. A. (1984). Word expectancy and event-related brain potentials during sentence processing. In S. Kornblum & J. Requin (Eds.), *Preparatory states and processes* (pp. 217–237). Hillsdale, NJ: Erlbaum.

Kutas, M., McCarthy, G., & Donchin, E. (1977). Augmenting mental chronometry: The P300 as a measure of stimulus evaluation time. *Science, 197*, 792–795.

Lorente de No, R. (1947). Action potential of the motoneurons of the hypoglossus nucleus. *Journal of Cellular and Comparative Physiology, 29*, 207–287.

Loveless, N. E., & Sanford, A. J., (1974). Slow potential correlates of preparatory set. *Biological Psychology, 1*, 303–314.

Lykken, D. T. (1974). Psychology and the lie detector industry. *American Psychologist, 29*, 725–739.

Macar, F., & Besson, M. (1987). An event-related potential analysis of incongruity in music and other non-linguistic contexts. *Psychophysiology, 24*, 14–25.

McCallum, W. C., Curry, S. H., Cooper, R., Pocock, P. V., & Papakostopoulos, D. (1983). Brain event-related potentials as indicators of early selective processes in auditory target localization. *Psychophysiology, 20*, 1–17.

McCallum, W. C., Farmer, S. F., & Pocock, P. V. (1984). The effects of physical and semantic incongruities on auditory event-related potentials. *Electroencephalography and Clinical Neurophysiology, 59*, 477–488.

McCarthy, G., & Donchin, E. (1981). A metric for thought: A comparison of P300 latency and reaction time. *Science, 211*, 77–80.

Magliero, A., Bashore, T. R., Coles, M. G. H., & Donchin, E. (1984). On the dependence of P300 latency on stimulus evaluation processes. *Psychophysiology, 21*, 171–186.

Michie, P. T., Bearpark, H. M., Crawford, J. M., & Glue, L. C. T. (1987). The effects of spatial selective attention on the somatosensory event-related potential. *Psychophysiology, 24*, 449–463.

Miller, G. A. (1986). Information processing deficits in anhedonia and perceptual aberration: A psychophysiological analysis. *Biological Psychiatry, 21*, 100–115.

Näätanen, R. (1982). Processing negativity: An evoked potential reflection of selective attention. *Psychological Bulletin, 92*, 605–640.

Näätanen, R., & Gaillard, A. W. K. (1983). The orienting reflex and the N2 deflection of the event-related potential (ERP). In A. W. K. Gaillard & W. Ritter (Eds.), *Tutorials in ERP research: Endogenous components* (pp. 119–141). Amsterdam: North-Holland.

Näätanen, R., & Picton, T. (1987). The N1 wave of the human electric and magnetic response to sound: A review and an analysis of the component structure. *Psychophysiology, 24*, 375–425.

Neville, H. J. (1985). Biological constraints on semantic processing: A comparison of spoken and signed languages. *Psychophysiology, 22*, 576. (Abstract)

Neville, H. J., Kutas, M., Chesney, G., & Schmidt, A. L. (1986). Event-related brain potentials during initial encoding and recognition memory of congruous and incongruous words. *Journal of Memory and Language, 25*, 75–92.

Norman, D. A., & Bobrow, D. G. (1975). On data-limited and resource-limited processes. *Cognitive Psychology, 7*, 44–64.

Nunez, P. L. (1981). *Electric fields of the brain: The neurophysics of EEG.* London: Oxford University Press.

Okada, Y. C., Kaufman, L., & Williamson, S. J. (1983). The hippocampal formation as a source of the slow endogenous potentials. *Electroencephalography and Clinical Neurophysiology, 55*, 416–426.

Okada, Y. C., Williamson, S. J., & Kaufman, L. (1982). Magnetic fields of the human sensory-motor cortex. *International Journal of Neurophysiology, 17*, 33–38.

O'Keefe, J., & Nadel, L. (1978). *The hippocampus as a cognitive map.* Oxford: Oxford University Press.

Paller, K. A., Kutas, M., & Mayes, A. R. (1985). An investigation of neural correlates of memory encoding in man. *Psychophysiology, 22*, 607. (Abstract)

Paller, K. A., McCarthy, G., & Wood, C. C. (1987). *ERPs predictive of later performance on recall and recognition tests.* Paper presented at the 4th International Conference on Cognitive Neurosciences, Paris-Dourdan, France.

Podlesny, J. A., & Raskin, D. C. (1977). Physiological measures and the detection of deception. *Psychological Bulletin, 84*, 782–799.

Ragot, R. (1984). Perceptual and motor space representation: An event-related potential study. *Psychophysiology, 21*, 159–170.

Regan, D. (1972). *Evoked potentials in psychology, sensory physiology, and clinical medicine.* New York: Wiley.

Renault, B. (1983). The visual emitted potentials: Clues for information processing. In A. W. K. Gaillard & W. Ritter (Eds.), *Tutorials in event-related potential research: Endogenous components* (pp. 159–176). Amsterdam: North-Holland.

Ritter, W., Simson, R., Vaughan, H. G., Jr., & Macht, M. (1982). Manipulation of event-related potential manifestations of information processing stages. *Science, 218*, 909–911.

Rohrbaugh, J. W., & Gaillard, A. W. K. (1983). Sensory and motor aspects of the contingent negative variation. In A. W. K. Gaillard & W. Ritter (Eds.), *Tutorials in event-related potential research: Endogeneous components* (pp. 269–310). Amsterdam: North-Halland.

Rohrbaugh, J. W., Syndulko, K., & Lindsley, D. B. (1976). Brain components of the contingent negative variation in humans. *Science, 191*, 1055–1057.

Rosler, F. (1983). Endogenous ERPs and cognition: Probes, prospects, and pitfalls in matching pieces of the mind-body problem. In A. W. K. Gaillard, & W. Ritter (Eds.), *Tutorials in event-related potential research: Endogenous components* (pp. 9–35). Amsterdam: North-Holland.

Rugg, M. D. (1985). The effects of semantic priming and word repetition on event-related potentials. *Psychophysiology, 22*, 642–647.

Rugg, M. D., & Barrett, S. E. (1988). *Event-related potentials and the interaction between orthographic and phonological information in a rhyme-judgment task.* Manuscript submitted for publication.

Sanquist, T. F., Rohrbaugh, J. W., Syndulko, K., & Lindsley, D. B. (1980). Electrocortical signs of levels of processing: Perceptual analysis and recognition memory. *Psychophysiology, 17,* 568–576.

Scherg, M., & von Cramon, D. (1985). Two bilateral sources of the late AEP as identified by a spatio-temporal dipole model. *Electroencephalography and Clinical Neurophysiology, 62,* 32–44.

Simons, R. F., MacMillan, F. W., & Ireland, F. B. (1982). Anticipatory pleasure deficit in subjects reporting physical anhedonia: Slow cortical evidence. *Biological Psychology, 14,* 297–310.

Simson, R., Vaughan, H. G., Jr., & Ritter, W. (1976). The scalp topography of potentials associated with missing visual and auditory stimuli. *Electroencephalography and Clinical Neurophysiology, 40,* 33–42.

Sirevaag, E. J., Kramer, A. F., Coles, M. G. H., & Donchin, E. (1984). P300 amplitude and resource allocation. *Psychophysiology, 21,* 598–599. (Abstract)

Squires, K. C., & Donchin, E. (1976). Beyond averaging: The use of discriminant functions to recognize event-related potentials elicited by single auditory stimuli. *Electroencephalography and Clinical Neurophysiology, 41,* 449–459.

Squires, K. C., Squires, N. K., & Hillyard, S. A. (1975). Decision-related cortical potentials during an auditory signal detection task with cued intervals. *Journal of Experimental Psychology: Human Perception and Performance, 1,* 268–279.

Squires, K. C., Wickens, C., Squires, N. K., & Donchin, E. (1976). The effect of stimulus sequence on the waveform of the cortical event-related potential. *Science, 193,* 1142–1146.

Starr, A., & Farley, G. R. (1983). Middle and long latency auditory evoked potentials in cats. II Component distribution and dependence on stimulus factors. *Hearing Research, 10,* 139–152.

Sutton, S., Braren, M., Zubin, J., & John, E. R. (1965). Evoked potential correlates of stimulus uncertainty. *Science, 150,* 1187–1188.

Sutton, S., & Ruchkin, D. S. (1984). The late positive complex. Advances and new problems. In R. Karrer, J. Cohen, & P. Tueting (Eds.), *Brain and information: Event-related potentials. Annals of the New York Academy of Sciences, 425,* 1–23.

Sutton, S., Tueting, P., Zubin, J., & John, E. R. (1967). Information delivery and the sensory evoked potentials. *Science, 155,* 1436–1439.

Towle, V. L., Heuer, D., & Donchin, E. (1980). On indexing attention and learning with event-related potentials. *Psychophysiology, 17,* 291. (Abstract)

Treisman, A., & Gelade, G. (1980). A feature integration theory of attention. *Cognitive Psychology, 12,* 97–136.

Van Petten, C., & Kutas, M. (1987). Ambiguous words in context: An event-related analysis of the time course of meaning activation. *Journal of Memory and Language, 26,* 188–208.

Vaughan, H. G., Costa, L. D., & Ritter, W. (1972). Topography of the human motor potential. *Electroencephalography and Clinical Neurophysiology, 25,* 1–10.

Verleger, R. (1988). Event-related potentials and memory: A critique of the context updating hypothesis and an alternative interpretation of P3. *Behavioral and Brain Sciences, 11,* 343–356.

Von Restorff, H. (1933). Uber die Wirkung von Bereichsbildungen im Spurenfeld. *Psychologische Forschung, 18,* 299–342.

Wallace, W. P. (1965). Review of the historical, empirical, and theoretical status of the von Restorff phenomenon. *Psychological Bulletin, 63,* 410–424.

Walter, W. G., Cooper, R., Aldridge, V. J., McCallum, W. C., & Winter, A. L. (1964). Contingent negative variation: An electrical sign of sensorimotor association and expectancy in the human brain. *Nature, 203,* 380–384.

Wood, C. C., & McCarthy, G. (1984). Principal component analysis of event-related potentials: Simulation studies demonstrate misallocation of variance across components. *Electroencephalography and Clinical Neurophysiology, 59,* 298–308.

Wood, C. C., McCarthy, G., Squires, N. K., Vaughan, H. G., Woods, D. L., & McCallum, W. C. (1984). Anatomical and physiological substrates of event-related potentials. In R. Karrer, J. Cohen, & P. Tueting (Eds.), *Brain and information: Event-related potentials* (pp. 681–721). New York: New York Academy of Sciences.

Woody, C. D. (1967). Characterization of an adaptive filter for the analysis of variable latency neuroelectrical signals. *Medical and Biological Engineering, 5,* 539–553.

Wyer, R. S., & Srull, T. K. (1984). *Handbook of social cognition.* Hillsdale, NJ: Erlbaum.

Yee, C. M., & Miller, G. A. (1988). Emotional information processing: Modulation of fear in normal and dysthymic subjects. *Journal of Abnormal Psychology, 97,* 54–63.

14   *The cardiovascular system*

JAMES F. PAPILLO AND DAVID SHAPIRO

14.1   INTRODUCTION

In the preface to the most recent handbook of psychophysiology, the editors (Coles, Donchin, & Porges, 1986) define the field as the study of behavior from a perspective that emphasizes the biological mechanisms that underlie behavior. Psychophysiologists "seek to understand psychological phenomena by studying the activity of various organ systems and to evaluate the functional significance of the physiological phenomena by exploring them in a psychological context" (p. 1). Furthermore, these goals require a detailed knowledge of physiological systems and of the psychological context in which the physiological processes are observed. Thus, the enterprise fosters a symbiotic relationship between physiology and psychology.

The cardiovascular system is a major focus of interest of psychophysiological research, an interest that has grown considerably in recent years, especially with the emergence of behavioral medicine as a research specialty and increasing awareness that family and social setting, daily life stress, and individual behavior patterns play a significant role in cardiovascular health and disease.

From the standpoint of traditional physiology, the cardiovascular system is generally viewed as an apparatus for moving the blood and thereby carrying and exchanging materials between various tissues and organs. That the system forms a loop was shown for the first time by Harvey some 350 years ago (see Willis, 1965/1847). The system comprises the heart and blood vessels and complex control mechanisms for regulating their functioning. The physiologist focuses attention on the integration of cardiovascular functions as they pertain to selected normal and diseased states.

The knowledge derived from traditional physiological research on the cardiovascular system has been applied mainly in medical investigations of such topics as hemorrhage and hypotension, upright posture, exercise, hypertension, congestive heart failure, heart attacks, and arteriosclerosis (Vander, Sherman, & Luciano, 1970). Cardiovascular control centers in the brain mediate the effects of other factors on the circulation, such as those involved with temperature regulation and hunger as well as behaviors related to pain, emotion, and other psychological processes. The latter have not been mainstream topics in physiology, although they are attracting greater attention now (Reis & LeDoux, 1987).

For the psychophysiologist, the focus of attention is generally on psychological effects on the circulation – hence the classification of the cardiovascular system by psychophysiologists as a part of the autonomic nervous system and of the peripheral division of the nervous system. In effect, the cardiovascular system is seen in psychophysiology primarily from the standpoint of behavior and psychological

456

processes. The behavior of the cardiovascular system itself, however, is also dependent on local control mechanisms (e.g., cellular, metabolic, hormonal, receptor/reflexive, etc.) that can operate independently of the nervous system. For example, the presence of ventricular premature beats may be a risk factor for sudden death, but such symptoms are not necessarily affected by perturbations of the autonomic nervous system (Lown, 1987).

To follow the strictures laid down by Coles et al. (1986), one must be both psychologist and physiologist, which is not simply achieved as judged by the history and traditions of research in this area. Generally, scientists in the two disciplines employ concepts and research strategies congenial to their formal education and experience. In typical papers on cardiovascular physiology and cardiovascular medical science, the core emphasis is on the cardiovascular processes themselves and underlying structures and functions of the heart, blood vessels, and kidneys. As the major causes of the phenomena of concern are assumed to lie in their associated structures and functions, one can more or less ignore the particular psychosocial characteristics of the subjects being studied, the setting in which the measurements are taken, experimenter–subject interactions, and so on. Such variables are seen as contributing little to the variance of the phenomena in question. The study of interactions between the central nervous system and the cardiovascular system does provide an entree for the physiologist into the consideration of environmental/ psychological factors, but no simple identities are possible between psychological variables and properties of the central nervous system.

In contrast, psychologists have focused their attention on such concepts as stress, emotion, anxiety, tension, and arousal, and the physiological data obtained serve as crude counterparts or indices of the phenomena. A single physiological index may suffice, for example, heart rate or peripheral blood flow or finger temperature, and one index can well substitute for another. Such research is usually prompted by psychological theories, and physiological mechanisms or complications are more or less ignored. As stated, the psychophysiological perspective falls between or incorporates both traditions.

Finally, the issue of reductionism deserves brief comment. In our view, the stance of cardiovascular psychophysiology should not imply that physiological processes are examined to "explain" behavior, cognitive processes, or emotional states, or responses to stimuli. Rather, they serve to provide additional information about bodily processes taking place in association with the psychological phenomenon. Nor do the psychological variables explain the physiological changes taking place. The consideration of different domains of data and causation will hopefully lead to a better understanding and prediction of the behavior and of the physiology. As Schwartz (1982) has pointed out, however, cardiovascular psychophysiology requires the enormous and almost impossible task of integrating diverse knowledge and data. He proposes use of *systems theory* as a means of fostering an effective integration of different *levels* of the phenomena of interest. Whether such a systems perspective can be effectively incorporated into the thinking of cardiovascular researchers remains uncertain.

Perhaps a more modest goal of integration is the bringing together of advanced knowledge from different disciplines employing productive methods of measurement and investigation. A recent example of effective integration of psychophysiology and cardiology was proposed by Lane and Schwartz (1987). It is based on two bodies of research: the role of hemispheric specialization in the mediation of emotional arousal and the role of lateralized imbalance in sympathetic input to the heart in cardiac arrhythmogenesis. The authors use these two bodies of research with their associated methods and findings to develop the hypothesis that individuals who manifest more lateralized frontal lobe activity during emotional arousal may concomitantly generate more lateralized sympathetic input to the heart and be at increased risk for cardiac arrhythmias. This small-scale integration involved the bringing together of two streams of research from two disciplines, cardiology and psychophysiology. Such more modest attempts will likely become the building blocks of further integrative research in cardiovascular psychophysiology in the future, and other examples are given in this chapter. It is this perspective that guides our presentation of the cardiovascular response system.

14.2   STRUCTURE AND FUNCTION OF THE CARDIOVASCULAR SYSTEM

14.2.1   *Overview*

The primary function of the cardiovascular system is to help maintain adequate blood flow through the various body tissues in the face of constantly changing metabolic requirements. Even slight alterations in the need of most body tissues for energy (i.e., oxygen, nutrients, and other vital substances) will trigger a highly complex pattern of cardiovascular adjustments involving neural, humoral, and mechanical factors. Collectively, these adjustments serve to modify the quantity and/or distribution of blood flow through the circulation in an attempt to maintain a state of *metabolic homeostasis.*

In view of the complex nature of the physiological mechanisms involved in regulating blood flow, serious study of behavioral, psychological, and cardiovascular interrelationships requires more than a rudimentary knowledge of cardiovascular system structure and function. Although a detailed discussion of the cardiovascular system is beyond the scope of the present chapter, we shall briefly overview several of its organizational features essential for a rational approach to issues concerning the quantification, analysis, and interpretation of those cardiovascular response system measures of most interest to psychophysiologists. The reader interested in a more comprehensive review of the cardiovascular system is encouraged to consult one of several excellent texts devoted to this topic (e.g., Berne & Levy, 1986; Guyton, 1979; Guyton, 1986; Rushmer, 1976).

Figure 14.1 shows the distribution of blood flow to various body tissues in the human at rest as well as during various levels of exercise. In response to the stress associated with strenuous physical exercise, the distribution of blood flow becomes substantially altered. For example, blood flow to several areas normally receiving a small percentage of the total blood flow under resting conditions, such as the skeletal muscles (21%), heart muscle (4%), and skin (9%), is dramatically increased during intense physical exercise. Conversely, blood flow to the kidney and splanchnic regions (i.e., stomach, spleen, liver, and pancreas), which together receive approximately 43% of total blood flow during rest, is markedly reduced during periods of heavy exercise. The absolute quantity of blood flow to the brain remains fairly constant over a wide range of exercise levels.

It is important to note that changes in blood flow to particular body tissues during exercise closely parallel alterations in the energy requirements of those tissues. Thus, during exercise, perfusion of the active skeletal muscles as well as heart

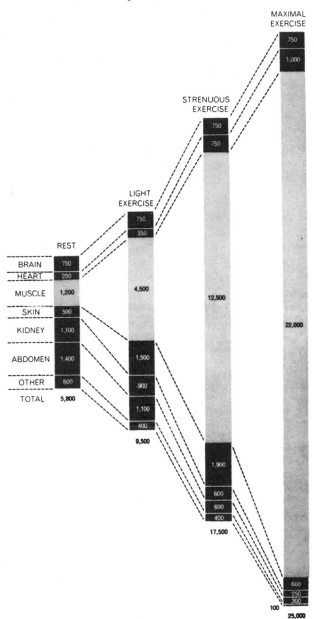

Figure 14.1. Distribution of blood flow to various body organs and tissues at rest as well as during periods of light, strenuous, and maximal exercise. Values represent blood flow in millimeters per minute. (From "The Physiology of Exercise," by C. B. Chapman & J. H. Mitchel, *Scientific American*, May 1965. Reprinted by permission.)

muscle increases in direct proportion to the increased energy needs of these tissues. However, in some organs (e.g., the kidneys), factors other than metabolic demand regulate the quantity of blood flowing through them during periods of rest. In the case of the kidneys, factors related to the clearance of substances from the blood and temperature regulation – major functions performed by these organs – cause a large quantity of blood to flow through them during resting conditions. From the point of view of metabolic requirements, the kidneys are overperfused during rest. During periods of physical exertion, the priorities attached to the various bodily functions become reorganized, and this reorganization is reflected in the altered pattern of blood flow distribution. As discussed in greater detail in what follows, shifts in blood flow distribution similar to those observed during exercise also occur in association with a variety of behavioral and psychological states, especially those associated with the *fight-or-flight* reaction.

14.2.2   Anatomy

Structurally, the cardiovascular system is comprised of the heart and vasculature (Figure 14.2). The primary function of the heart, a muscular pump, is to supply the energy required for the circulation of blood in the cardiovascular system. The vasculature serves as the distribution, exchange, and collection channels by which the blood, pumped by the heart, travels to and nurtures every living tissue in the body and is subsequently returned to the heart. The heart and vasculature each represents a complex and dynamic process controlled by autoregulatory, peripheral nervous system (i.e., autonomic) and central nervous system mechanisms. Further, interactions between heart and vascular actions provide an additional level of complexity for understanding the functioning of the cardiovascular system as a whole.

14.2.2.1 *The heart*

The heart is comprised of four chambers that function as two pumps in series. The right-side pump, composed of the right atrium and right ventricle, provides the energy necessary to move blood through the pulmonary circulation. The left-side pump, composed of the left atrium and left ventricle, provides the energy causing blood to flow through the systemic circulation. The atria receive, as input, blood returning from either the systemic (right atrium) or the pulmonary (left atrium) circulations. Blood entering the right atrium is oxygen deficient, whereas blood entering the left atrium is rich with oxygen. As a result of a common pacemaker (see what follows) and the *syncytial* nature of cardiac muscle fibers (Guyton, 1979), the two atria contract rhythmically and in synchrony, thereby causing these chambers to periodically empty their contents and to fill the ventricular chambers. A fraction of a second following atrial contraction, the blood-filled ventricles also contract in synchrony. Blood ejected from the ventricles travels, via the vasculature, either through the pulmonary (right ventricle) or systemic (left ventricle) portions of the circulatory system.

14.2.2.2 *The circulatory system*

An immense network of blood vessels comprises the vasculature. The major categories of blood vessels are arteries, arterioles, capillaries, venules, and veins.

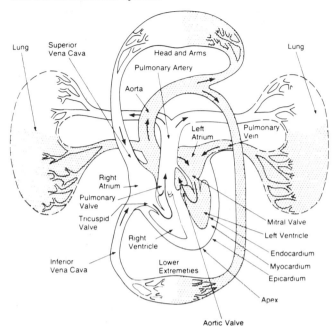

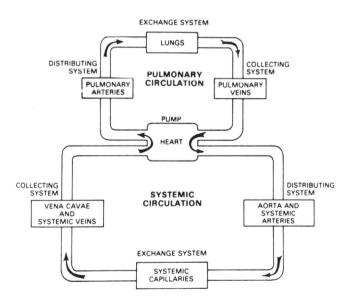

Figure 14.2. Human circulatory system. Top figure presents detailed schematic of circulation while bottom figure highlights functional divisions of circulatory system. See text for details. {*Top*}: From *Circulatory Physiology: The Essentials*, by J. J. Smith & J. P. Kampine. Copyright 1980 by Williams & Wilkins. Reprinted by permission. *Bottom:* From *A Primer of Psychophysiology*, by J. Hassett. Copyright 1978 by W. H. Freeman. Reprinted by permission.

These consecutive vascular segments differ from one another both in terms of structure and function.

Arteries and arterioles. The arteries (large vessels) and arterioles (small vessels) serve as the distributing channels carrying blood away from the heart and toward the body tissues. Arteries are thick-walled vessels that contain small amounts of smooth muscle and large amounts of collagen and elastin fibers. Because of the predominance of elastic elements in their walls, the major arteries are sometimes referred to as the "pressure-storing" blood vessels. Ejection of blood from the ventricles following each contraction of the heart causes passive expansion of the arteries due to their elastic nature. Subsequent recoil of the arteries causes the blood to be propelled toward adjacent vascular segments and thus progressively down the arterial tree. As distance from the heart increases, the size and inside diameter (i.e., *lumen*) of the arteries gradually decrease. In addition, the morphology of the small-diameter arteries in the periphery differs from the major arteries closer to the heart in that their walls contain a higher proportion of smooth muscle and a smaller amount of elastin fibers. As a result of their structure, the smallest arteries (arterioles) are often referred to as "resistance" vessels.

Unlike the major arteries, which passively expand and recoil in response to the output of the heart, the caliber of the arterioles is determined primarily by direct neural innervation from the sympathetic branch of the autonomic nervous system. Sympathetic innervations of the arterioles normally produce a continuous state of moderate *constriction* of these blood vessels commonly referred to as *vasomotor tone*. Variations in the degree of constriction/dilation of blood vessels is caused primarily by alterations in sympathetic nervous system activity. Thus, both *vasoconstriction* and *vasodilation* are controlled by the sympathetic branch of the autonomic nervous system. In addition to neurogenic influences, vasomotor tone may also be influenced by autoregulatory and hormonal mechanisms (cf. Rushmer, 1976).

An increase in sympathetic activation will produce either vasoconstriction or vasodilation depending on the type of adrenergic (sympathetic) receptors (alpha or beta) mediating the particular vascular bed under consideration. Stimulation of alpha-receptors located in the blood vessels serving the skin, skeletal muscles, abdominal viscera, and coronary arterioles produces vasoconstriction. Conversely, stimulation of beta-receptors that accompany alpha-receptors in the blood vessels of the heart (coronary arterioles) and skeletal muscles produces vasodilation.

Because the majority of vascular resistances throughout the body are in parallel, great precision and flexibility is permitted in controlling flow to individual organs. Thus, by controlling vascular resistance, blood flow to one area of the circulation may be either increased or decreased without substantially altering the flow to adjacent areas.

Capillaries. The actual transfer of oxygen and other nutrients from the blood to the tissues takes place across the walls of the capillaries, the smallest of the blood vessels. Composed of a single layer of endothelial cells, passive movement of gases across the capillary wall results primarily from both hydrostatic and osmotic pressure differences existing on the two sides of the capillary membrane. Capillaries receive no neural innervation and thus play no direct role in regulating blood flow.

Venules and veins. The venules (small vessels) and veins (large vessels) serve as the collecting channels carrying blood away from capillary beds and back toward the heart (i.e., *venous return*). Structurally, these blood vessels are characterized as having a large lumen, thin walls, and large capacity. Because of their thin walls, veins are highly susceptible to external compressional forces such as those produced by the contraction of skeletal muscles. The walls of venous blood vessels contain some smooth muscle and very small amounts of elastin fibers. Like the arterioles, the smooth muscle contained in veins is innervated by the sympathetic branch of the autonomic nervous system, which exerts considerable control over the state of constriction/dilation of these blood vessels.

As a result of their structure, veins are quite distensible and thus are often referred to as "volume-storing" blood vessels. In addition to its role in the transport of blood back toward the heart, the venous system also functions to provide a ready reservoir of blood for the heart to enhance cardiac filling and thereby increase the quantity of blood flowing through the circulation. At rest, approximately two-thirds of the total volume of blood in the human circulatory system remains in the venous system. During exercise, blood is displaced within the venous system in such a way as to augment the filling of the atria. For example, the quantity or volume of blood returning to the right atrium is determined primarily by the interplay between two distinct pools of blood contained within the venous system of the systemic circulation. A large, diffuse reservoir of blood, known as the *peripheral venous pool*, is comprised of blood stored in the multitude of veins serving the various organs throughout the body. A second, smaller pool of blood is concentrated in the great veins located in the thorax and is referred to as the *central venous pool*. During exercise or other behavioral states, constriction of veins (*venoconstriction*), resulting from both an increase in sympathetic nervous system activity and the mechanical compression of vessels associated with active muscles, causes blood to be shifted from peripheral to central venous pools. As a result of an increase in the central venous volume, the relative pressure difference between the great veins and the right atrium increases, thereby causing a greater volume of blood to be returned to the right heart.

14.2.2.3 *The movement of blood through the cardiovascular system*

Heart valves. As blood is forced through and is displaced within the cardio-vascular system, a series of one-way valves ensures unidirectional flow. In the heart, the tricuspid and mitral valves (also called the *atrioventricular*, or *AV*, *valves*) open toward the right and left ventricles, respectively, permitting blood to enter from the atria while simultaneously preventing blood from flowing back into the atria. Following contraction of the atria, the rapid buildup of pressure within the ventricles forces the AV valves to snap shut. The sudden closure of the AV valves produces the first of two heart-sounds ("*lub*-dub") that can be detected when the bell of a stethoscope, or other acoustical device, is positioned on the chest directly over the heart. A second set of valves, the aortic and pulmonary (also called *semilunar*), open and close in response to the relative pressure difference between the ventricles and either the aorta (*aortic valve*) or the main pulmonary artery (*pulmonary valve*). As the ventricles contract, the increase in pressure within these chambers forces the semilunar valves to open, thus allowing blood to be ejected into the circulatory system. As the ventricles subsequently relax, the greater pressures in the aorta and pulmonary artery, as compared to inside the ventricles, causes the semilunar valves to snap shut. The closure of these valves prevents blood from reentering the ventricles and, in the process, produces the second heart-sound ("dub").

Proper functioning of the heart valves is essential for the efficient pumping action of the heart. Current interest among psychophysiologists in assessing the status of the heart valves, particularly the mitral valve, has its basis in the putative association between certain valvular abnormalities and several psychological states including anxiety (Gorman et al., 1988) and stress (Combs, Shah, Shulman Klorman, & Sylvester, 1977). Recently, the timing of the heart sounds has been used as reference points in the measurement of several cardiodynamic parameters (see what follows).

Circulatory system. The lower portion of Figure 14.2 summarizes the major functional divisions of the circulatory system. Blood ejected by the right ventricle is propelled through the pulmonary circulation – first through the pulmonary arteries, followed, in turn, by the lungs and pulmonary veins. In the lungs, blood flows through the pulmonary capillaries where oxygen is absorbed into the blood and carbon dioxide is excreted from the blood into the alveoli. Following this exchange of gases at the pulmonary capillary sites, oxygen-enriched blood exits from the lungs and travels, via the pulmonary veins, into the left atrium. Blood ejected by the left ventricle is propelled through the systemic circulation – first through the systemic arteries, followed, in sequence, by the systemic capillaries and veins. With few exceptions (e.g., cartilage, epidermis, cornea, and lens), the systemic capillaries permeate every tissue of the body. At the systemic capillary sites, oxygen and carbon dioxide are exchanged in the direction reverse from that which takes place in the pulmonary circulation. Thus, in the systemic circulation, oxygen and other nutrients are removed from the blood and are replaced by carbon dioxide and other metabolic by-products formed by active tissues.

14.2.3   *Cardiodynamic and hemodynamic control mechanisms*

14.2.3.1   *The heart*

Electromechanical properties of the heart. The beating of the heart is an electromechanical event. Electrical impulses generated by specialized cells within the heart, referred to as pacemaker cells, initiate the mechanical contraction of heart muscle (*myocardium*). Pacemaker cells are "special" in the sense that they possess the inherent ability to spontaneously generate action potentials (i.e., depolarize) in a rhythmic fashion.

Numerous clusters of pacemaker cells are found in various regions of heart muscle (Figure 14.3). One such cluster of cells, known as the sinoatrial node (*SA node*), is located on the posterior wall of the right atrium. Because its rate of spontaneous depolarization is faster than other pacemaker cells, the SA node is responsible for initiating and timing the rhythmic contraction of the entire heart. Through a specialized conduction system (*Purkinje system*), electrical activity associated with the depolarization of cells in the SA node first spreads rapidly through the atria causing these chambers to contract in unison. This wave of

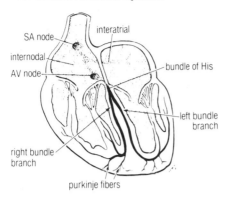

Figure 14.3. Conduction system of heart. (From *Pathophysiology: Clinical Concepts of Disease Processes*, by S. Anderson Price & L. McCarty Wilson. Copyright 1982 by McGraw-Hill. Reprinted by permission.)

electrical activity is then propagated through the internodal atrial tracts reaching the atrioventricular node (*AV node*). Following a brief delay in its passage through the AV node, thus allowing extra time for the ventricles to fill, transmission of this electrical activity then proceeds through the *bundle of His* followed by the right and left bundle branches, which terminate onto the ventricular muscle causing both ventricles to contract in synchrony.

The following four characteristics distinguish cardiac muscle from striated and smooth muscle fibers (Wilke, 1970):

1 repolarization of cardiac muscle fibers lasts approximately 100 ms;
2 the contraction phase is equal in duration to the duration of the cardiac action potentials;
3 the muscle tissue has an unstable resting potential that is the physiological basis for the intrinsic cardiac rhythm; and
4 the action potentials are freely conducted from one cell to another owing to the latticelike (i.e., syncytial) networking of cardiac muscle fibers.

The orderly transmission of electrical activity through the various portions of the heart gives rise to an electrical field that can easily be detected and measured with electrodes placed on the body's surface. The *electrocardiogram*, or ECG, is a graphical representation of the stereotypic pattern of electrical activity generated by the heart during each beat. Figure 14.4 presents a short segment of a schematized ECG recording. The major features of the ECG signal are the *P-wave*, the *QRS complex*, and the *T-wave*. The P-wave corresponds to the depolarization of the atria, the QRS complex to the depolarization of the ventricles, and the T-wave to the repolarization of the ventricles.

The intrinsic rate of firing of cells in the SA node is approximately 105–110 times per minute. However, in healthy adults at rest, the heart beats at an average rate of only 70 times per minute. This difference is due to the modulating effects of neural influences on the heart. The heart is innervated by both the sympathetic and parasympathetic branches of the autonomic nervous system. Fibers from both branches terminate on cells in the SA node and can modify the intrinsic rate of the heart. Parasympathetic fibers travel to the heart via the vagus nerve and release the

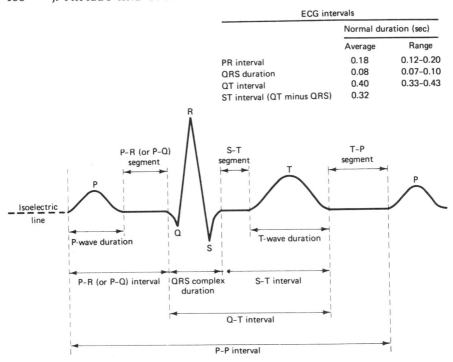

ECG intervals		
	Normal duration (sec)	
	Average	Range
PR interval	0.18	0.12-0.20
QRS duration	0.08	0.07-0.10
QT interval	0.40	0.33-0.43
ST interval (QT minus QRS)	0.32	

Figure 14.4. Normal ECG cycle recorded with bipolar limb lead II (Schematic). (From Hewlett-Packard Co., Palo Alto, California. Reprinted by permission.)

neurotransmitter acetylcholine on SA nodal cells. Acetylcholine acts to alter the course of the spontaneous depolarization of SA nodal cells to produce a decrease in their rate of firing. Thus, an increased parasympathetic outflow to the heart causes a reduction in heart rate (*negative chronotropic effect*). A continuous, tonic level of parasympathetic input to the heart is mainly responsible for the normal resting heart rate of approximately 70 beats per minute observed in healthy adult human subjects.

Sympathetic fibers innervating the heart release the neurotransmitter norepinephrine, which alters the course of spontaneous depolarization of SA nodal cells to produce an increase in heart rate (*positive chronotropic effect*). Phasic heart rate acceleration (*tachycardia*) can result from an increase in sympathetic activity, a decrease in parasympathetic activity, or some combination of the two. Similarly, phasic heart rate deceleration (*bradycardia*) can result from a decrease in sympathetic activity, an increase in parasympathetic activity, or both. Studies conducted on animals (cf. Randall, 1977) as well as on humans (cf. Obrist, 1981) have shown that, under varying conditions, the neural influences on the heart may operate either synergistically or antagonistically to produce alterations in heart rate. In view of these findings, it is important to emphasize that measures of heart rate alone provide ambiguous information concerning the neurogenic influences on the heart and, therefore, can lead to misleading conclusions regarding the effects of experimental variables on cardiovascular system functioning. Instead, measures of

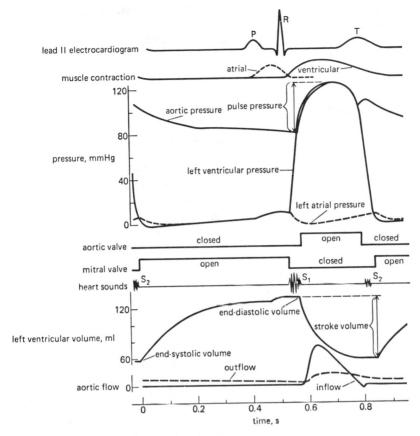

Figure 14.5. The cardiac cycle. See text for details. (From *Cardiovascular Physiology*, by L. J. Heller & D. E. Mohrman. Copyright 1981 by McGraw-Hill. Reprinted by permission.)

heart rate may only be interpreted as reflecting the net result of the interaction between both divisions of the autonomic nervous system. To more precisely assess the neurogenic mechanisms underlying an observed alteration in heart rate, additional measures of cardiac function must be obtained (see what follows).

The cardiac cycle. The *cardiac cycle* (Figure 14.5) encompasses the various electrical, mechanical, and valvular events associated with each heart beat and is comprised of two distinct phases: *systole* and *diastole*. For the sake of clarity, the following discussion of the cardiac cycle will be presented from the view of the left heart. It must be understood, however, that the mechanical and electrical events of the right heart mirror those in the left.

The *diastolic phase* of the cardiac cycle corresponds to the time period during which the left ventricle is in a state of relaxation. During this phase, which is initiated by the opening of the mitral valve, both the left atria and the left ventricle are being filled with blood returning from the pulmonary circulation. Near the end of ventricular diastole, the atria contract (ECG P-wave), causing an additional quantity of blood to be pumped into the ventricle.

The *systolic phase* corresponds to the period of time during which the left ventricle is contracting and blood is being ejected into the systemic circulation. As Figure 14.5 indicates, the systolic phase begins when electrical activity spreads through the left ventricle as represented by the QRS complex of the ECG waveform. Subsequent contraction of the ventricle causes intraventricular pressure to rise. When the pressure within the ventricle exceeds the pressure within the atria, the AV valve snaps shut, producing the first heart-sound. During the *isovolumic contraction period*, when the ventricle is a closed chamber with a fixed volume (*end diastolic volume*), intraventricular pressure continues to rise rapidly. Once the pressure within the ventricle exceeds the pressure in the aorta (the main trunk of the arterial system), the aortic valve suddenly opens and blood is ejected from the ventricle, first rapidly (*rapid ejection phase*) and then more slowly (*reduced rejection phase*) as the pressures within the ventricle and aorta begin to equalize. The peak pressure recorded in the aorta during ventricular ejection is known as the *systolic pressure*. As the strength of ventricular contraction continues to diminish (ECG T-wave), the point is reached whereby intraventricular pressure becomes lower than that in the aorta. It is this pressure difference that causes the aortic valve to snap shut, resulting in the second heart-sound and marking the end of the cardiac cycle. For a brief period of time following closure of the aortic valve, the ventricle once again becomes a closed chamber (*isovolumic relaxation period*) with a fixed volume (*end systolic volume*). It is important to note that, under resting conditions, not all of the end diastolic volume (EDV) is ejected from the heart during each heart cycle. The *ejection fraction*, the ratio of the quantity of blood ejected by the heart during each cycle (*stroke volume*) to EDV, provides a sensitive index of ventricular function. During the isovolumic relaxation period, intraventricular pressure decreases steadily and rapidly. When intraventricular pressure is reduced to a level lower than that in the left atrium, the mitral valve opens and the next cardiac cycle commences. During the diastolic phase, the lowest pressure recorded in the aorta is known as the *diastolic pressure*.

At the near normal resting heart rate of 75 beats per minute (bpm), the total duration of the cardiac cycle is approximately 800 ms. The diastolic phase comprises nearly three-fourths of this interval (600 ms), whereas the systolic phase comprises the remaining one-fourth (200 ms) of this interval. As heart rate increases, the duration of the diastolic phase is reduced disproportionately more than the systolic phase.

Cardiac output. At rest, the heart of a healthy human subject pumps approximately 5 l of blood each minute. This is known as the *cardiac output* and can be determined as the product of the number of heart beats per minute (*heart rate*) and the volume of blood ejected by the heart during each beat (*stroke volume*). Thus, cardiac output (CO) = heart rate (HR) × stroke volume (SV). During vigorous physical exercise, CO may exceed 25 l/min. As previously indicated, a major portion of this elevated CO is distributed to the vascular beds serving the exercising skeletal muscles.

Determinants of SV include *preload, afterload, contractility,* and HR. Preload refers to the volume of blood within the ventricles following atrial contraction but prior to ventricular contraction and is thus synonymous with end diastolic volume. On each beat of the heart, both end diastolic volume and SV vary as a direct function of the level of venous return. This fundamental cardiodynamic relationship is often referred to as *Starling's law of the heart.* The mechanism underlying this relationship is a simple one and is inherent in the structure of the heart muscle itself. Increased filling of the ventricle (i.e., end diastolic volume) causes a greater stretch of ventricular muscle fibers and thus an increase in the strength of the subsequent ventricular contraction (*positive inotropic effect*). As a result of this enhanced state of contractility, a greater proportion of the end diastolic volume is ejected from the ventricle into the circulation (i.e., both the ejection fraction and stroke volume are increased).

In addition to the purely mechanical control of contractility described in the preceding, a number of extrinsic factors, the most important of which involves the sympathetic branch of the autonomic nervous system, may also influence the force of ventricular contraction. Activation of sympathetic fibers innervating the heart causes norepinephrine to be released on cardiac muscle cells comprising the ventricles, which in turn causes these chambers to contract more forcefully. An increased sympathetic outflow to the heart produces both an increase in HR (as already discussed) and an increase in contractility. As will be discussed, several strategies and techniques have been proposed for obtaining noninvasive assessments of the sympathetic influences on the heart through measures of ventricular contractility.

Afterload refers to the resistance to the output of the heart during each cardiac cycle (i.e., SV) imposed by the pressure in the circulatory system. Changes in systemic arterial pressure can either facilitate (low pressure) or impede (high pressure) the ejection of blood from the left ventricle following the opening of the aortic valve. This effect, like Starling's law of the heart, exemplifies the interaction between cardiodynamic and hemodynamic factors in regulating cardiovascular system functioning.

Figure 14.6 summarizes the multiple determinants of CO. During exercise or other behavioral states, as HR increases, the duration of the cardiac cycle is substantially reduced, and as stated previously, there is a disproportionately greater reduction in the diastolic phase of the cycle as compared to the systolic phase. The reduction in the length of the diastolic phase serves to restrict ventricular filling time and might otherwise lead to a reduction in SV were it not for the fact that (1) most of the filling of the ventricle occurs during the initial period of diastole and (2) increased sympathetic outflow to the heart enhances ventricular contractility so that a greater proportion of the end diastolic volume is ejected. As a result, SV remains fairly constant over a wide range of exercise levels, whereas increases in CO are produced mainly by an increase in HR (Obrist, 1981).

14.2.3.2 *The circulatory system: pressure, flow, and resistance*

The major factors influencing the movement of blood through the circulatory system are pressure, flow, and resistance to flow. *Blood pressure* (BP) refers to the force exerted by the blood against the walls of blood vessels, and its primary function is to drive the output of the heart through the circulatory system. The absolute-pressure level within the circulatory system drops steadily as the distance from the heart increases. In the systemic circulation, it is the pressure gradient defined by the difference in pressure between the root of the aorta (high pressure)

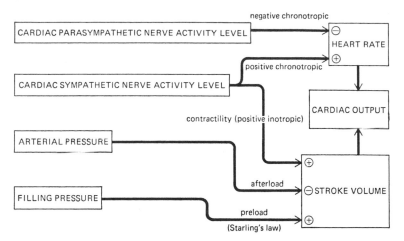

Figure 14.6. Multiple influences on cardiac output. See text for details. (From *Cardiovascular Physiology*, by L. J. Heller & D. E. Mohrman. Copyright 1981 by McGraw-Hill. Reprinted by permission.)

and the right atrium (low pressure), commonly known as the *systemic filling pressure* P_{sf}, which is the primary factor influencing venous return. When a subject becomes active behaviorally, either during exercise or in response to psychologically significant events, increased sympathetic activation leads to increases in HR and contractility and to greater constriction of the major arteries. Together, these changes serve to increase arterial BP, thereby elevating P_{sf}. The displacement of blood volume from the peripheral to the central venous pools resulting from increased sympathetic outflow and mechanical compression of the veins increases the quantity of blood available to be returned to the right heart. As a result, venous return increases and CO is enhanced during subsequent cardiac cycles (via Starling's law of the heart).

Systemic arterial BP plays a critical role in regulating blood flow to the various organs in the body and is determined as the product of CO and *total peripheral resistance* (TPR) (i.e., Arterial BP = CO × TPR). Thus, factors that determine CO (i.e., HR, contractility, SV, end diastolic volume, and venous return) also figure significantly in regulating arterial BP. An alteration in either CO or TPR, without a compensatory change in the other, will affect BP. Thus, any intervention (biological or psychological) that impacts BP must do so by altering CO, TPR, or both.

Total peripheral resistance refers to the level of resistance to blood flow caused by the relative state of constriction of all the blood vessels in the circulatory system. As previously indicated, the sympathetic branch of the autonomic nervous system plays a major role in regulating the caliber of blood vessels throughout the circulation and is thus a primary regulator of TPR. By mimicking the effects of sympathetic influences on blood vessels, various hormones circulating in the blood (e.g., antidiuretic hormone, angiotensin II, and histamine) also play a role, albeit a minor one, in determining TPR.

In view of the number of factors involved in its regulation, it would be erroneous to consider measures of BP as indexing a specific physiological process. Equivalent changes in BP at various points in time may be produced by completely different patterns of cardiodynamic and hemodynamic events. As a result. BP can provide only a general index of cardiovascular activity. To more precisely ascertain the mechanisms underlying an observed alteration in BP, additional measures of cardiovascular functioning must be obtained and evaluated.

Blood pressure is an important *controlled* and *controlling* variable with respect to cardiovascular functioning. The various cardiodynamic and hemodynamic factors that regulate BP are themselves partly regulated by BP. Through the operation of various negative-feedback mechanisms involving both the autonomic and central nervous systems, the BP level is normally maintained within a narrow range.

14.2.3.3 *Integrative control mechanisms*

Baroreceptor reflex. The *baroreceptor reflex* is the most important mechanism for regulating short-term alterations in BP. Pressure-sensitive receptors (baroreceptors) located in the arch of the aorta and carotid sinus are stimulated mainly by the rate of stretch of the walls of these vessels as blood is propelled through them. Afferent fibers from the baroreceptors travel via the aortic and carotid sinus nerves, join the vagus and glossopharyngeal nerves, respectively, and terminate at the cardiovascular regulatory centers of the medulla oblongata (Figure 14.7). In reponse to an increase in baroreceptor activity (resulting from an increase in BP), the medullary control centers initiate a series of events leading to immediate reductions in HR, myocardial contractility, SV, and vasomotor tone (*depressor response*) to rapidly return the BP to its original level. Conversely, a decrease in baroreceptor activity caused by a reduction in BP results in a series of cardiovascular adjustments designed to increase BP back toward its original level (*pressor response*). Thus, the baroreceptor reflex can be characterized as a negative-feedback mechanism that operates automatically (and quickly) to resist abrupt changes in BP.

As a direct result of the baroreceptor reflex, an inverse relationship between the direction of change in BP and the direction of change in both HR and vasomotor tone is typically observed. However, several higher cortical areas such as the thalamus, hypothalamus, and forebrain – areas implicated in the experience and expression of the emotions as well as other psychological processes – may override the operation of this reflex circuit, thus leading to profound, unbuffered alterations in BP (cf. Stephenson, 1984).

In addition to the baroreceptors, the cardiovascular control areas of the medulla oblongata receive information from a variety of other receptors (e.g., mechanoreceptors and chemoreceptors) located in both the peripheral and central nervous systems to form additional reflex circuits that help counteract temporary disturbances in cardiovascular system function (see Berne and Levy, 1986).

Respiratory effects on the cardiovascular system. Respiratory processes can have a profound influence on cardiovascular system functioning. In response to variations in the breathing pattern, a number of central and autonomic nervous system mechanisms as well as mechanical (heart) and hemodynamic adjustments are triggered, thereby causing both tonic and phasic changes in cardiovascular functioning. Respiratory and cardiovascular functions are coupled in the medulla oblongata. An important example of this coupling is a phenomenon known as

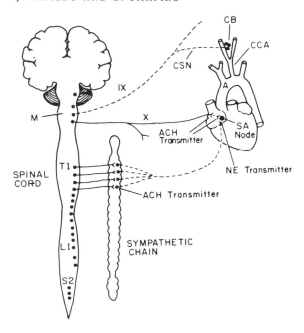

Figure 14.7. Schematic diagram of autonomic pathway serving carotid baroreceptor reflexes. The IX and X nerves are parasympathetic; outflow from upper thoracic region of spinal cord (T1 and three segments directly below, i.e., T2, T3, and T4) representing efferent sympathetic innervation. Long dotted line represents afferent neural connection from baroreceptor to medulla, solid line represents preganglionic autonomic nerves, and short dotted lines represent postganglionic autonomic nerves. Abbreviations: A, aorta; ACH, acetylcholine: CB, carotid baroreceptor; CCA, common carotid artery; CSN, carotid sinus nerve; L, lumbar; M, medulla; NE, norepinephrine; S, sacral; SA, sino atrial; T, thoracic; IX, glossopharyngeal; X, vagus nerve. (From "Mechanisms of the Cardiovascular Responses to Environmental Stressors," by R. P. Forsyth. In P. A. Obrist, A. H. Black, J. Brener, and L. V. Dicara (eds.), *Cardiovascular Psychophysiology: Current Issues in Response. Mechanisms, Biofeedback, and Methodology.* Copyright 1974 by Aldine. Reprinted by permission.)

respiratory sinus arrhythmia (RSA). This refers to the cyclical variations in HR that are linked, in time, to the inspiratory (HR acceleration) and expiratory (HR deceleration) phases of the respiratory cycle. The significance of RSA for improving our understanding of cardiovascular–behavioral interactions will be discussed in section 14.3.1 (see also, Lorig & Schwartz, chapter 17; Porges & Bohrer, chapter 21).

Kidney function and the cardiovascular system. Though not a part of the cardiovascular system per se, the kidneys play a major role in regulating cardiovascular system functioning. As the primary organs responsible for regulating total body fluid volume and maintaining electrolyte balance, the kidneys perform these functions mostly through control of arterial blood pressure. In response to a decrease in arterial BP, blood flow to the kidneys is reduced and the formation and excretion of urine by the kidneys is diminished. As a result of this sequence of events, the fluids and electrolytes consumed by mouth gradually accumulate, thereby increasing blood volume and, thus, reestablishing the normal blood volume and BP levels. Conversely, an increase in BP causes the kidneys to increase the formation and excretion of urine, which serves to lower blood volume. This lowered blood volume leads to a gradual decrease in systemic BP until it once again reaches a normal level.

An additional mechanism by which the kidneys can affect BP is initiated when the quantity of blood flow to the kidneys becomes insufficient. A reduced blood flow to the kidneys resulting from a decrease in arterial BP causes the kidneys to secrete the hormone *renin* directly into the bloodstream. Renin acts as an enzyme to convert one of the plasma proteins to a substance known as *angiotensin*. Angiotensin acts directly on the blood vessels to cause vasoconstriction, which serves to increase the arterial BP back toward normal.

Whereas the nervous system reflexes mentioned earlier serve to quickly counteract abrupt, short-term disturbances in BP, the kidneys are more important in the long-term control of cardiovascular functioning (i.e., over days, weeks, or longer).

14.3 MEASUREMENT OF CARDIOVASCULAR RESPONSES

14.3.1 *Cardiodynamics*

14.3.1.1 *Electrocardiography*

Electrocardiography refers to the recording of electrical potentials generated by the heart during each cardiac cycle. Because the human body is a good volume conductor, the relatively large bioelectric signal associated with myocardial activity can be reliably and continuously recorded by the placement of electrodes at the body surface. Comprehensive determinations of cardiac status are typically made by recording the ECG signal using a montage of 12 electrodes strategically positioned on the limbs and chest. Using 12-lead ECG techniques, a cardiologist may detect various irregularities in the electrical activity of the heart and may even identify specific regions of heart muscle involved in the genesis of many of these irregularities. In contrast, psychophysiologists have historically employed ECG techniques to simply assess the frequency or rate of cardiac activity. Recently, however, a number of investigators have become interested in more detailed analyses of the ECG waveform as the information obtained can potentially shed significant new light on cardiac–behavioral interactions.

For most applications where the frequency or rate of cardiac activity is the primary variable of interest, the exact positioning of ECG electrodes has relatively little significance due to the large size of the ECG signal. By convention, however, bipolar limb leads positioned in accordance with Einthoven's triangle (Figure 14.8) are most frequently used. A lead II configuration (e.g., one electrode placed above the right wrist and one placed above the left ankle) is often preferred because it produces the most pronounced QRS complex. Alternative electrode placements consistent with the lead II configuration but that are less susceptible to movement artifact can be employed (Thakor & Webster, 1985).

The morphologic characteristics of the normal ECG signal along with the intervals

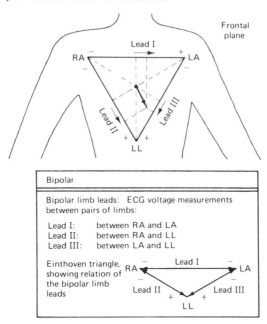

Figure 14.8. Einthoven's triangle. Abbreviations: RA, right arm; LA, left arm; LL, left leg. (From Hewlett-Packard Co., Palo Alto, California. Reprinted by permission.)

separating significant ECG events were presented in Figure 14.4. Briefly, the major components of the ECG signal can be described as follows.

1   The P-wave corresponds to the passage of electrical activity originating in the SA node through the atria (i.e., atrial depolarization). Enlargement of the atria may increase the amplitude or width of the P-wave. Certain cardiac arrhythmias may also alter the P-wave configuration.

2   The QRS complex corresponds to the passage of electrical activity originating in the SA node through the ventricles (i.e., ventricular depolarization). The normal QRS duration is a measure of ventricular depolarization time. The R-wave is the most prominent component in the electrocardiogram primarily because ventricular muscle cells are so numerous.

3   The T-wave represents the repolarization of the ventricles and is broader and smaller in amplitude in comparison to the R-wave because ventricular repolarization is less synchronous than depolarization.

4   The P–R interval is the time period from the beginning of the P-wave to the onset of the QRS complex and represents the time it takes for electrical activity to travel from the atria to the ventricles. Prolongation of this interval is usually indicative of a disturbance in impulse conduction through the AV node.

5   The S–T segment represents the interval between the end of ventricular depolarization and the beginning of ventricular repolarization. Abnormal depression or elevation of the S–T segment may be indicative of either injury or ischemia of the ventricular myocardium.

6   The Q–T interval encompasses both the QRS complex, the S–T segment, and the T-wave duration, and thus represents the elapsed time from the onset of ventricular depolarization to the end of ventricular repolarization.

7   The T–P segment represents the elapsed time from the end of ventricular repolarization to the onset of atrial depolarization in the next ECG cycle.

8 Heart period (HP), or interbeat interval (IBI), represents the elapsed time between two successive heart cycles and can be determined as the time (in milliseconds) between any point in the ECG cycle and the corresponding point in the succeeding cycle.

Because of its relatively large size, the R-wave is most often used in calculations of heart period (R−R interval). A related measure of cardiac activity, heart rate (HR), is defined as the reciprocal of heart period. The mathematical formula that follows is used to convert measures of heart period into heart rate expressed in beats per unit time:

$$HR = 1/HP \times K \tag{1}$$

where HR is heart rate (counts per unit time), HP is heart period (time), and K is scaling constant. For instance, if the time between two successive R-waves (i.e., heart period) is measured to be 1000 ms, and it is desired to convert this to beats per minute (i.e., 60,000 ms), then by formula (1):

$$HR = 1/1,000 \times 60,000$$
$$= 60 \text{ beats per minute}$$

Technical and methodological guidelines for recording the ECG have recently been published both for clinical applications (American Heart Association, 1967) and for basic psychophysiological research (Jennings et al., 1981).

Heart rate is expressed in terms of the raw number of heart beats per unit of time, typically 1 min, and can be obtained simply by counting the number of beats (e.g., R-waves) during the time period of interest. An alternative technique involves the use of an electronic device known as a cardiotachometer, which provides a continuous, beat-by-beat measure of heart rate. The electronic circuitry of the cardiotachometer calculates the reciprocal of the time between successive heart beats (i.e., heart period). The voltage output of this device is calibrated in terms of beats per minute and may be displayed on a polygraph and/or sampled by computer. It is important to point out that, at any moment, the cardiotachometer signal reflects the time period between the two previous cardiac cycles (R-waves). This lag must be considered when, during subsequent analyses of the data, determinations of heart rate are based on either real-time (e.g., 1-min) or cardiac time (e.g., 30 heart beats) units.

An alternative method of reporting heartbeat data, heart period, is based directly on the time interval (expressed in milliseconds) between successive heart cycles. Several special-purpose electronic devices for recording and processing heart period information have been developed (see Brener, 1980; Brown, 1972). Most often, however, measures of heart period are determined on-line by computer.

Several issues concerning the appropriate unit of measure for expressing cardiac activity data (i.e., rate vs. period) have received much attention in the literature. As discussed by Graham (1978b), whereas both rate and period measures share a common base (i.e., time), conversion of the data from one unit of measure to another could serve to exacerbate measurement errors and may cause statistical problems due to the nonlinear relationship between them. It is therefore possible, under certain conditions, to reach different conclusions depending on the unit of measure one chooses for expressing a particular set of cardiac activity data. Factors such as the magnitude of the effect under study as it compares to the size of measurement errors introduced in data collection (e.g., the computer sampling rate used for digitizing the data or, in the case of manual scoring, the speed at which the polygraph paper moves) and whether such measurement errors are found to be constant with one or the other measure must be considered in choosing between rate- or period-based measures of cardiac activity. For meeting the important assumptions of normality of distributions and homogeneity of variances underlying most parametric statistical techniques, the appropriate choice between rate- and period-based measures has been shown to depend on whether the analyses are to be performed on individual or group data, if adults or infants are used as subjects, and whether raw scores or change scores serve as the primary data (Graham, 1978a; Graham & Jackson, 1970; Jennings, Stringfellow, & Graham, 1974).

Another issue debated in the literature concerns whether successive changes in heart rate or heart period should be computed on the basis of real time (i.e., second by second) or so-called cardiac time (i.e., beat by beat). The choice of time units can be made on the basis of both practical and theoretical considerations. Theoretically, whether the process under investigation is believed to vary with real time or cardiac time should be the determining factor in deciding on the appropriateness of one unit over the other. When investigating short-term (phasic) changes in cardiac activity, if a fixed number of heart cycles serves as the basic unit of analysis, subjects with a fast heart rate will provide a smaller sample in terms of real time vis-à-vis those with a slow rate, whereas if a fixed real-time period is examined, the converse is true (see Graham, 1980, for a discussion of related considerations). On a practical note, converting beat-by-beat cardiac information into real-time units is somewhat costly in terms of computational effort. The algorithm for partitioning whole and fractional beats within real-time units can consume a significant amount of a computer's resources, particularly if the conversion is performed on-line. In constrast, the processing of heart activity data in cardiac time units (i.e., beat by beat) requires less computational effort. In terms of the statistical properties of the various combinations of time units and cardiac activity measures, Graham (1978b) has indicated that only heart rate expressed in real-time units and heart period expressed in cardiac time units provide unbiased estimates of the mean.

An additional consideration of extreme importance not only for the analysis of cardiac activity data but for most other physiological measures as well concerns the choice of adequate baseline procedures. Because the mere exposure to a laboratory setting or the wearing of an ambulatory monitor in the natural environment can profoundly affect baseline levels of autonomically mediated physiological activity, especially in highly anxious or reactive subjects, analysis of data collected without first obtaining adequate baseline measures could lead to incorrect interpretations of the data and the inability to make meaningful comparisons of data collected within and between laboratory settings.

The importance of properly assessing baseline levels of physiological activity is emphasized by the Law of Initial Values (LIV), which states that both the magnitude and, in extreme cases, the direction of elicited changes in physiological activity is partly determined by the prestimulus or baseline level of activity (see Stern & Sison, chapter 7). With respect to response magnitude, the LIV predicts an inverse relationship between the level of prestimulus activity and the degree of change elicited by the stimulus. Thus, if the baseline level of activity is low, relatively large responses are likely to be observed, whereas small-magnitude responses are likely when the prestimulus level is high. At extreme high or low prestimulus levels of activity, paradoxical changes may be elicited (i.e., a decrease in activity is observed when an increase is predicted and vice versa). A number of cardiovascular responses including heart rate (Hord, Johnson, & Lubin, 1964), vasomotor activity (Lovallo & Zeiner, 1975), and blood pressure (Lacey & Lacey, 1962) have been shown to be lawfully related to prestimulus levels as predicted by the LIV.

Hastrup (1986) recently surveyed a portion of the literature published in the journal *Psychophysiology* and found a high degree of variability as to the length of baseline assessment used by investigators. On the basis of the heart rate data reported in the studies examined, a significant negative correlation was obtained between length of baseline assessment and mean level of heart rate change. It was suggested that adaptation periods of at least 15 min be used to allow heart rate to stabilize prior to the start of experimental procedures. It was further suggested that the duration of adaptation periods be individualized by using a closed-loop baseline whenever feasible. For example, adaptation periods may be continued until some measure of heart rate activity (e.g., the coefficient of variation) does not exceed some value. Obrist (1981) has recently demonstrated that measurements of cardiovascular activity obtained during a period of relaxation on a day when no laboratory tasks are scheduled may provide a more appropriate assessment of baseline levels, especially in physiologically reactive subjects.

A variety of post hoc statistical techniques that can be applied to cardiac activity data to correct for variations in baseline levels observed among subjects and heterogeneity in covariance of repeated measures and to neutralize the effects of the LIV have been previously described in the literature (Benjamin, 1963; Cronbach & Furby, 1970; Jennings & Wood, 1976, 1977; Lacey & Lacey, 1962). Issues related to the assessment of heart rate variability (Heslegrave, Ogilvie, & Furedy, 1979; Varni, Clarke, & Giddon, 1971), the handling of individual differences in the range of heart rate response (Lykken, 1972), and the use of statistical techniques for analyzing heart rate data such as trend analysis (Wilson, 1974), time series analysis (Sayers, 1970), and spectral analysis (Sayers, 1980) have been previously discussed in the literature. Interested readers might also wish to consult Porges and Bohrer (chapter 21), Gottman (chapter 22), and Russell (chapter 23) for additional information.

14.3.1.2 *Phonocardiography*

Procedures and techniques associated with the recording of heart-sounds ("lub-dub") are referred to as *phonocardiography* (PCG). As the term implies, heart-sounds are acoustic phenomena. These sounds are caused by events associated with the sudden closing of the AV and semilunar heart valves during each cardiac cycle and are transmitted from the heart, through the body tissues, and directly to the thoracic surface. The instrument most commonly used by physicians to detect the heart-sounds is the stethoscope. By positioning the bell of the stethoscope on the chest surface directly above the heart, a physician can listen for subtle abnormalities in the intensity and quality of heart-sounds and can diagnose a variety of clinical disorders related to the mechanical malfunctioning of the heart based solely on these abnormal sounds. In the psychophysiology laboratory, heart-sounds are monitored using a piezoelectric transducer (i.e., crystal microphone) that is strapped to the chest surface in the same position as the bell of a. stethoscope. The phonocardiogram refers to the graphic representation of the voltage output recorded from the heart-sounds microphone (see Figure 14.5). The first heart sound (S1) is caused by the deceleration of blood associated with closure of the mitral and tricuspid valves (the AV valves). Since S1 corresponds to the onset of ventricular contraction, it may be used to indicate the beginning of the systolic phase of the cardiac cycle. The second heart-sound (S2) is produced by events associated with closure of the aortic and pulmonary valves (the semilunar valves). Since S2 corresponds to the onset of ventricular relaxation, it marks the beginning of the diastolic phase of the cardiac cycle. In comparison to S2, S1 can be characterized as lower in frequency and slightly longer in duration. Third and fourth heart-sounds, which are not present in all individuals, have thus far not received the attention of psychophysiologists (Burton, 1972).

14.3.1.3 *Measures of cardiac output*

Perhaps the greatest challenge presently confronting cardiovascular psychophys-iologists as well as others involved in the design and development of biomedical recording techniques concerns the search for reliable and valid noninvasive measurements of cardiac output, one of the most important cardiovascular parameters. Clinical assessments of cardiac output are routinely obtained using a variety of invasive techniques requiring either cardiac catheterization procedures involving arterial and venous punctures or surgical implantation of transducers to measure blood flow (see Guyton, Jones, & Coleman 1973). For example, dye dilution techniques involve the rapid injection of a known quantity of indicator (dye) into the bloodstream entering the right heart. Photosensitive detectors (densitometers) strategically placed to record the concentration of indicator substance as it exits the left heart make it possible to obtain precise estimates of cardiac output.

Echocardiography. Echocardiography represents a relatively new and highly so-phisticated technology that can safely provide valuable information concerning cardiovascular functioning. The basic technique involves attaching a specialized transducer (piezoelectric crystal) on the surface of the chest that both emits and receives an ultrasonic (2–3-MHz) sound beam that is directed at the heart. The transducer oscillates between a sending and receiving mode. As the emitted sound beam traverses the heart, ultrasonic waves are reflected back to the transducer whenever the beam crosses a boundary between various thoracic structures or substances (e.g., blood) having different acoustic impedance. These reflected ultrasonic waves, or "echos," are then converted to electrical voltages, amplified, and graphically recorded (as undulating lines) on paper along with a simultaneous ECG signal for reference to the cardiac cycle. The echocardiogram documents in detail the dimensions and motion of cardiac structures so that structural disorders of the heart can be evaluated. Information contained in the echocardiogram also enables one to obtain estimates of stroke volume, cardiac output, and intraventricu-lar volumes during the various phases of the cardiac cycle.

14.3.1.4 *Measures of ventricular contractility*

As discussed earlier, unlike the SA node and atria, which are innervated by both the sympathetic and parasympathetic branches of the autonomic nervous system, the ventricles receive direct innervations from the sympathetic branch only. Thus, a relatively pure measure of sympathetic influences on the myocardium may be obtained by assessing the strength of ventricular contraction (i.e., contractile force) during each heart cycle. Because contractile force directly influences SV and, therefore, CO, the development of noninvasive, beat-by-beat measures of ventricular contractility has received much attention from cardiovascular psychophysiologists.

dP/dt. One proposed technique for assessing contractility involves monitoring the pulse pressure at the site of the carotid artery and determining the first derivative (i.e., slope) of the recorded pulse pressure waveform (Obrist et al., 1972). Because the mechanical events of the heart cycle are faithfully encoded in pressure pulses recorded from arterial segments close to the heart, the rate of rise (*dP/dt*) of the pulse waveform recorded from the carotid artery can be used to index contractile force. The reliability of this technique has been shown to be limited, however, due primarily to the necessary use of a highly sensitive transducer for detecting the pressure pulse in the neck region. As a result of the transducer's sensitivity and location, the signal obtained is highly susceptible to movement artifact caused by head turning and swallowing. It must also be noted that measures of *dP/dt* can be markedly influenced by preload, afterload, and heart rate changes, which may limit the validity of this measure for assessing variations in cardiac contractility (Heslegrave & Furedy, 1980).

T-wave amplitude. A less obtrusive measure of myocardial contractility that has recently been proposed is based on the amplitude of the T-wave of the ECG signal (Heslegrave & Furedy, 1979; Matyas & King, 1976). As previously described, the ECG T-wave represents the repolarization of the ventricular myocardium and is a positive-going waveform when the ECG signal is recorded using a lead II configuration (see Figure 14.4). Several studies have demonstrated that T-wave amplitude becomes less positive and may actually become negative as the sympathetic influence on the ventricular myocardium increases (Furedy & Heslegrave, 1983). In addition, increases in T-wave amplitude have been reported to occur following the administration of the pharmacological agent propranolol, which blocks the beta-adrenergic receptors of the ventricles (Furberg, 1968; Stern & Eisenberg, 1969). Although the T-wave is fairly easy to record, changes in its amplitude are very small, measuring only 20–30 μV (Matyas & King, 1976). Important issues concerning both the reliability and validity of the T-wave amplitude measure for indexing beat-by-beat beta-adrenergic influences on the heart have been previously discussed in the literature (cf. Heslegrave & Furedy, 1979; Obrist, 1981; Schwartz & Weiss, 1983).

Systolic time intervals. Substantial evidence has accumulated indicating that the timing and duration of certain electrical and mechanical events associated with the systolic phase of the cardiac cycle may provide reliable information concerning the contractile state of the heart. Measurement of the *systolic time intervals* (STI) can be obtained from the simultaneous recordings of the ECG Q-wave, heart-sounds, and a peripherally detected arterial pulse (Figure 14.9). Three STIs are determined for assessing ventricular function: *preejection period* (PEP), *left ventricular ejection time* (LVET), and *electromechanical systole* (EMS). Electromechanical systole represents the period of time encompassing all electrical and mechanical events associated with the systolic phase of the cardiac cycle. As shown in Figure 14.9, EMS can be

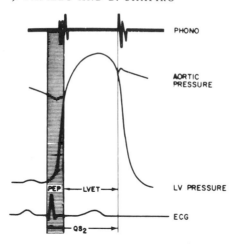

PHONO

AORTIC
PRESSURE

LV PRESSURE

ECG

Figure 14.9. Systolic time intervals. See text for details. (From "A Critical Review of the Systolic Time Intervals," by R. P. Lewis, S. E. Rittgers, W. F. Forester, & H. Boudoulas, *Circulation*, *56*, 146–158, 1977.)

calculated as the time period (in milliseconds) commencing with the ECG Q-wave (the beginning of ventricular depolarization) and ending with the detection of S2, that is, the second heart-sound (the closing of the semilunar valves). Electrome-chanical systole (Q–S2) is comprised of the subintervals PEP and LVET.

The LVET represents the period during which blood is being ejected from the ventricles into the circulatory system and is determined as the difference in time between the opening and closing of the semilunar valves. However, because the precise timing of the opening of the semilunar valves is difficult to assess, calculations of LVET are based on the timing of two aspects of the pulse waveform obtained from a peripheral site (e.g., carotid artery, finger, or pinna of the ear). The temporal relationship between the opening and closing of the semilunar valves is faithfully encoded in the pulse waveform and can be measured from the foot of the pulse upstroke (opening, onset of ejection) to the dicrotic notch (closing, end of ejection). Because both S2 and the dicrotic notch represent closure of the semilunar valves, the time difference between these two events provides a measure of arterial *transit time*, that is, the time required for the blood ejected from the left ventricle to reach a peripheral vascular site.

The PEP represents the period of time commencing with the onset of ventricular depolarization (ECG-Q-wave) and ending with the opening of the semilunar valves. In practice, PEP is derived from the measures of EMS and LVET (PEP = EMS − LVET).

There is substantial empirical evidence demonstrating that PEP, as measured using STI methodology, is highly correlated with more direct measures of myocardial contractility (Ahmed, Levinson, Schwartz, & Ettinger, 1972) and that PEP is specifically sensitive to beta-adrenergic influences on the heart (Harris, Schoenfeld, & Weissler, 1981).

Although manual scoring of the STIs directly from polygraph records is possible, the small magnitude (millisecond range) of even large changes in these intervals can produce significant errors in measurement. Recently, computer software for digitizing and processing the STIs has been developed (e.g., Divers, Katona, Dauchot, & Hung, 1977). Several excellent overviews covering STIs are currently available and should be consulted by the reader desiring greater detail (Larsen, Schneiderman, & Pasin, 1986; Lewis, Rittgers, Forester, & Boudoulas, 1977; Weissler, Stack, & Sohn, 1980).

Impedance cardiography. An alternative strategy for obtaining noninvasive assessments of cardiodynamic function is based on the measurement of changes in the electrical impedance of the thoracic region (Geddes & Baker, 1968). The technique known as *impedance cardiography* involves measuring pulsatile changes in the electrical impedance of the thorax to low-energy, high-frequency (20–200 kHz) alternating current. As shown in the upper portion of Figure 14.10, the technique employs four electrode bands positioned proximally and distally to the heart. Alternating current is presented through the outer electrode bands labeled 1 and 4. Electrode bands 2 and 3, positioned inside the current path, monitor the resulting changes in the impedance of the thoracic region to the applied current that are caused by mechanical events associated with the cardiac cycle.

Based on temporal and morphologic features of the differentiated waveform of the impedance signal (lower portion of Figure 14.10), a number of cardiodynamic indices can be easily obtained. The waveform labeled dz/dt represents the first derivative of the raw impedance signal (delta–Z) and, together with signals obtained from the ECG and PCG, is used in calculations of SV, CO, myocardial contractility, and the STIs (see Lamberts, Visser, & Zijlstra, 1984, for procedural and mathematical details). Several factors limiting the reliability of impedance cardiographic measures have been recognized (Miller & Horvath, 1978). First, changes in thoracic impedance may result from variations in the shape and volume of the lungs as well as the heart and can, therefore, contaminate measures of cardiac function. One strategy that has been used to minimize this problem involves obtaining impedance measurements during the same phase of each respiratory cycle (i.e., inspiration or expiration). Impedance measures are also susceptible to movement artifact so that assessments made during periods of physical activity are often difficult to interpret (Denniston et al., 1976). Studies directly comparing measures of SV obtained using impedance cardiography and invasive procedures have shown that impedance-based values generally overestimate the true SV (Lamberts, Visser, & Zijlstra, 1984). However, there is sufficient empirical evidence to justify the use of impedance cardiography for evaluating relative changes in SV and CO.

14.3.1.5 *Assessing parasympathetic influences on the cardiovascular system*

As previously described, the parasympathetic branch of the autonomic nervous system plays an important role in modulating heart function. Respiratory sinus arrhythmia (RSA) – the normal variation in heart rate occurring in synchrony with the inspiratory (HR acceleration) and expiratory (HR deceleration) phases of the respiratory cycle – depends almost entirely on an intact parasympathetic (vagal) innervation to the heart. Several biological mechanisms linking respiratory and heart activity have been proposed and include (1) central influences via a direct brainstem projection from respiratory to cardiac centers, (2) afferent feedback from stretch receptors in the lungs, and (3) volume receptor and baroreceptor reflexes elicited by alterations in blood flow from changing intrathoracic pressure (Porges,

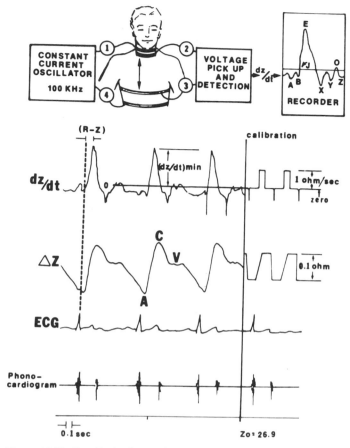

Figure 14.10. *Top:* Basic electronic circuits and electrode placements for recording impedance changes associated with cardiac activity. Delta-Z = impedance change during cardiac cycle. *Bottom:* Delta-Z = impedance change during cardiac cycle; dz/dt = first time derivative of delta-Z; $R-Z$ = time period beginning from R-wave of ECG and ending at point of peak ventricular ejection as represented by Z-spike of dz/dt waveform (dividing dz/dt by the $R-Z$ interval – the Heather index – provides highly sensitive measure of the ability of the heart to respond to stress). From "Impedance Cardiography and Photoplethysmography," by J. C. Buell. In *Cardiovascular Instrumentation: Applicability of New Technology to Biobehavioral Research,* J. A. Herd, A. M. Gotto, P. G. Kaufmann, & S. M. Weiss (Eds.). Copyright 1984 by the U.S. Department of Health and Human Services – NIH Publication No. 84–1954. Reprinted by permission.)

McCabe, & Yongue, 1982). Elimination of the vagal innervations to the heart through the use of either pharmacologic blockade or surgical ablation, has been shown to abolish RSA almost entirely, whereas elimination of the sympathetic innervations has no effect on RSA. This evidence strongly suggests that the major efferent limb of RSA is through the vagus nerve. On the basis of this evidence, it has been proposed that a noninvasive measure of the vagal influences on the heart may be obtained by quantifying RSA.

Several measurement strategies have been utilized for assessing the magnitude of RSA. The simplest strategy is based on relatively crude measures of heart rate variability such as the range or variance (e.g., Wheeler & Watkins, 1973). More recently, a peak-to-trough method for quantifying RSA has been proposed (Fouad Tarazi, Ferrario, Fighaly, & Alicandro, 1984; Katona & Jih, 1975). In the peak-to-trough method, the unfiltered R–R interval series is used to assess maximal heart period (or heart rate) differences corresponding to the inspiratory and expiratory phases associated with each respiratory cycle. For each respiratory cycle, the shortest R–R interval corresponding to inspiration is subtracted from the longest R–R interval corresponding to expiration. Thus, in using the peak-to-trough method, it is necessary to monitor both the ECG and respiration signals for quantifying RSA.

Assessments of RSA using the peak-to-trough method have been shown to produce precise estimates of variations in cardiac vagal tone resulting from both spontaneous and experimentally induced alterations in parasympathetic influences on the heart (e.g., Eckberg, 1983; Haddad, Jeng, Lee, & Lai, 1984; Raczkowska, Eckberg, & Ebert, 1983; Zemaityte, Varoneckas, & Sokolov, 1984). However, because respiratory activity represents just one of several sources contributing to heart rate variability (others sources include movement, blood pressure oscillations, and body temperature fluctuations), more sophisticated statistical techniques must be employed when the heart rate pattern is composed of numerous influences. Porges and his colleagues (Bohrer & Porges, 1982; Porges, 1986; Porges et al., 1982) have proposed the use of spectral analysis, a time-series technique, for partitioning the variance associated with RSA from the total heart rate (or heart period) variability. Spectral analysis is used to decompose the pattern of heart period variability into its constituent frequency components much as a prism decomposes sunlight into its constituent frequencies (i.e., colors). To calculate the component of heart period variability associated with respiratory activity, the spectral, or power, densities (proportional to variance) for each frequency within the range associated with normal spontaneous breathing are summed. At the normal, adult breathing rate of between 8 and 25 breaths per minute, the duration for each breath would range from 2.4 to 7.5 s and would have a frequency of between 0.13 and 0.42 Hz (respiratory frequency band). The sum of the spectral densities within the respiratory frequency band provides the measure of RSA amplitude, which is directly related to vagal tone to the heart. For additional information on the use of spectral analysis for assessing RSA, see chapter 21.

14.3.2 *Hemodynamics*

As previously discussed, an important component of the pattern of physiological responses associated with fight-or-flight reaction is the shifting of blood flow away from such areas as the skin, splanchnic bed, and kidney and toward the skeletal muscles. This redistribution of blood flow is controlled by two primary mechanisms: (1) alpha-adrenergic-mediated constriction of the blood vessels supplying the skin, gastrointestinal tract, kidneys, and liver and (2) beta-adrenergic-mediated dilation of the blood vessels supplying the skeletal muscles. With respect to the assessment of changes in the pattern of blood flow through the peripheral vasculature, the variables of most interest to psychophysiologists include rate of flow, resistance to flow, and pressure. It is important to note that each of these variables is *not* an independent measure of cardiovascular function. Rather, they should be considered as interrelated factors that together characterize blood flow. In accordance with

Poiseuille's Law, the following equation helps one to conceptualize the precise nature of the interrelationships among these and other factors regulating blood flow (Guyton, 1979):

$$\text{Blood flow (rate)} = \frac{\text{Pressure} \times (\text{diameter})^4}{\text{Length} \times \text{viscosity}} \qquad (2)$$

According to this equation, the rate of blood flow through a blood vessel is directly proportional to both the product of the pressure difference between the two ends of the vessel and the fourth power of vessel diameter and inversely proportional to the product of the length of the vessel and the viscosity of the fluid in the vessel. As previously indicated, blood vessel diameter is controlled to a large extent by the sympathetic (alpha-adrenergic) nervous system, and as a result of the fourth-power effect, small changes in vessel diameter (i.e., constriction or dilation) produce large changes in blood flow.

14.3.2.1 *Peripheral blood flow measurement*

Two strategies have been employed by psychophysiologists for obtaining noninvasive assessments of phasic and tonic alterations in peripheral blood flow. One strategy involves measuring blood flow through the skin capillary beds serving particular segments of the body such as the finger or ear. A second strategy involves measuring the quantity of blood flow through the skeletal muscles, particularly those in the forearm (i.e., forearm blood flow).

The most commonly used techniques for measuring peripheral blood flow are based on the method of *plethysmography* (derived from the Greek word meaning "enlargement" or "fullness"). Early plethysmographic techniques involved placing a limb or limb section (e.g., finger, hand, arm, leg) into an airtight, rigid chamber filled with either water (hydroplethysmography) or air (pneumoplethysmography). A tube extending from the chamber and containing the same medium as the chamber (i.e., water or air) is attached to a transducer, the output of which is displayed on a recording device. Because the chamber is sealed, alterations in the volume of blood flowing to the limb causes displacement of the medium inside the chamber. This displacement is converted to either an electrical or mechanical output, depending on the characteristics of the transducer attached to the tube. Several problems with this method were quickly noted (Lader, 1967). For instance, in the case of hydraulic plethysmography, it was necessary to maintain the water temperature as close as possible to normal body temperature (34°C) in order to minimize changes in vasomotor activity that might result from fluid temperature (ambient temperature and humidity changes can affect vasomotor activity in skin areas). Another problem concerns the lack of specificity of the blood flow measures obtained with respect to the particular segment under study. It became evident that measurements obtained using these techniques reflected not only changes in local flow but also changes in the flow through more distal portions of the extremities, such as the hand, as well (see Tursky & Jamner, 1982, for a more detailed discussion of historical developments in the field of plethysmography).

Photoplethysmography. A variety of sophisticated plethysmographic techniques is currently available to the psychophysiologist for measuring peripheral blood

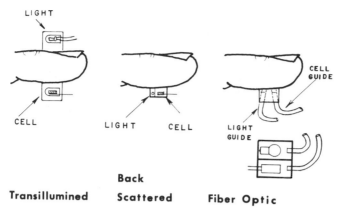

Figure 14.11. Three different methods for applying photoplethysmograph. (From "The Techniques of Plethysmography," by C. C. Brown. In *Methods in Psychophysiology*, C. C. Brown (Ed.). Copyright 1967 by Williams & Wilkins. Reprinted by permission.)

flow. These techniques differ primarily in terms of their operating principles and include those based on the measurement of changes in electrical impedance (impedance plethysmography), electrical resistance (strain gauge plethysmography), ultrasonic energy (Doppler flowometry), and the light absorption characteristics of blood (photoplethysmography). Several extensive overviews of these and other noninvasive techniques for measuring blood flow have previously been published (Brown, 1967; Jennings, Tahmoush, & Redmond, 1980; Tursky & Jamner, 1982). Cook (1974) provides a full discussion of the many factors that must be considered in obtaining and interpreting measures of peripheral vasomotor activity.

Photoplethysmography is the most widely used measurement technique for assessing peripheral blood flow in the psychophysiology laboratory. Because the technique measures changes in light rather than volume displacement, it has been suggested that the term *photometry* be used (Jennings et al., 1980). The technique is based on the differential light-absorbing characteristics of tissue and blood. Specifically, living tissue is relatively transparent to light in the infrared range (7,000–9,000 A), whereas blood is relatively opaque to light within this frequency range. Three different types of photoplethysmographs have evolved over the years, each one having both advantages and disadvantages in comparison to the others (Figure 14.11).

Using the transillumination method, the segment under study (e.g., a finger tip) is "sandwiched" between two elements (a light source and a photocell) attached to the skin surface. The light source (tungsten lamp or light-emitting diode) projects a beam of infrared light through the finger in the direction of the photocell positioned on the opposite side of the segment. Because blood scatters light within the infrared range, the quantity of light reaching the photocell is an inverse function of the amount of blood flowing through the finger. Thus, when the blood vessels supplying the finger constrict, the reduced blood flow allowed more light to reach the photocell, whereas dilation of blood vessels causes less light to reach the photocell.

The photocell is a special transducer that converts light energy into electrical

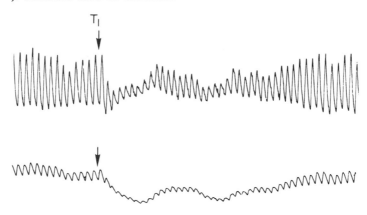

Figure 14.12. Pulse volume (*top*) and blood volume (*bottom*)₁ polygraph recordings obtained from output of finger photoplethysmograph. T_1 indicates onset of vasoconstriction. Pulse volume was recorded using 1 s time constant.

energy. The electrical output of the photocell can be either displayed on an analog recording device (e.g., polygraph) or digitized by computer. Figure 14.12 displays a sample of the analog signals typically recorded from a photoplethysmograph. In the upper trace, the pulsatile nature of blood flow can be seen where individual pulse waves reflect the pumping action of the heart during a single cardiac cycle. Thus, the ascending portion of the waveform represents the systolic phase and the descending portion the diastolic phase of the cardiac cycle. This measure of blood flow is referred to as *pulse volume* (PV) and provides information about beat-to-beat variations in blood flow. In the lower trace, a different view of blood flow is presented that is commonly referred to as *blood volume* (BV). Measures of BV reflect the overall engorgement of the area under study and is used to index more tonic changes in blood flow occurring over time. The effects of an acute period of vasoconstriction on both PV and BV measures can be seen in Figure 14.12 beginning at the point marked T_1. It is important to note that both components of blood flow (PV and BV) are obtained from the same output signal recorded from the photocell transducer. To measure BV, the output signal is recorded using a DC amplifier so that only slow changes in the overall engorgement of the body segment appear on the display. For the measurement of PV, the output signal from the photocell transducer is AC coupled to enable the pulsatile features of blood flow to be recorded.

Two other photoplethysmographic methods (back-scattered and fiber-optic) are simply variations on the transillumination method. In the back-scattered or reflectance method, the photosensitive transducer is positioned adjacent to the light source (see Figure 14.11). In this position, the photocell provides a measure of the quantity of infrared light that is reflected back as the result of the passage of blood underneath it. Although the analog signal produced by the reflectance transducer is identical in form to that obtained with the transillumination method, the former method is mainly sensitive to variations in blood flow through the superficial cutaneous vascular beds, whereas the latter can more easily detect vascular changes deep within the tissues. A problem shared by both of these methods concerns the use of light for measuring vasomotor activity. Over time, the small amount of heat generated by the light source can actually elicit changes in local vasomotor tonus (i.e., dilation). As pointed out by Webster (1978), this may or may not be desirable as the effect serves to enhance the amplitude of recorded pulses.

Several devices have recently been developed, such as fiber-optic photoplethysmographs, and those employing either a light-emitting diode (LED) or phototransistor as a source of low-intensity light, which effectively eliminate the problems associated with heat. Photoplethysmographs using LEDs and phototransducers have gained widespread use in psychophysiology laboratories in recent years (see Jennings et al., 1980).

Photoplethysmographic recordings are highly sensitive to movement artifact, limb position, respiratory actions, and environmental temperatures (Brown, 1967). Also, if during the course of an experiment the transducer must be removed and subsequently reattached, it is important to document this event as even slight changes in the positioning of the device can affect the recordings. Finally, it must be noted that blood flow measures obtained using photoplethysmographic techniques cannot be calibrated in terms of absolute blood flow units and thus can only provide an index of relative changes in blood flow.

Venous-occlusion plethysmography. A technique known as *venous-occlusion plethysmography* has been used extensively for measuring blood flow through the skeletal muscles of the limbs. This technique is similar in principle to the volume displacement technique described. For measuring *forearm blood flow* (FBF), two blood pressure cuffs are used: one positioned around the upper arm and the other around the wrist (labeled 8 and 9 in the upper portion of Figure 14.13). A mercury-in-silastic (or rubber) strain gauge is positioned lightly around that portion of the forearm having the largest circumference, that is, approximately midway between the blood pressure cuffs (labeled 10 in Figure 14.13). The strain gauge, a resistive device, changes in length as a function of changes in blood flow through the forearm. As the length of the strain gauge increases or decreases, the electrical resistance of the mercury column is altered in a predictable manner (i.e., length and resistance are inversely related). The change in strain gauge resistance can be recorded on a polygraph (lower portion of Figure 14.13) and/or sampled by computer.

To obtain a measure of FBF, the wrist cuff is first inflated to a level that effectively occludes the blood vessels carrying blood to the hand, thereby cutting off flow (i.e., above the systolic pressure level; see what follows). This is desirable because blood flow to the hand is controlled primarily by the vasculature serving skin rather than muscle and thus could contaminate the measurement of muscle blood flow. When a measure of FBF is desired, the upper-arm cuff is inflated to a level (e.g., 40–50 mm Hg) that effectively blocks blood from flowing out of the forearm via the veins, whereas blood flow into the segment is unaffected. Once the upper-arm cuff has been inflated, the circumference of the forearm begins to increase immediately as this segment becomes engorged with blood. This causes the mercury column of the strain gauge to be stretched and, therefore, its resistance to increase. The lower portion of Figure 14.13 demonstrates the *venous-occlusion slope* produced by the change in strain gauge resistance following inflation of the upper-arm cuff (i.e., venous occlusion). The rate of rise of this slope is directly proportional to the rate of

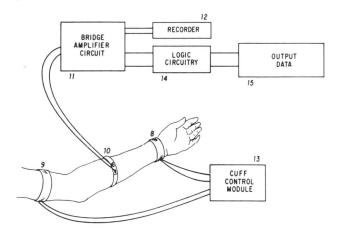

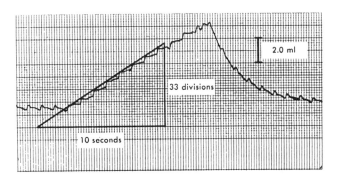

Figure 14.13. *Top:* Components used in venous-occlusion plethysmography (From "Measurement of Local Blood Flow during Behavioral Experiments: Principles and Practice," by R. B. Williams. In *Cardiovascular Instrumentation: Applicability of New Technology to Biobehavioral Research.* J. A. Herd, A. M. Gotto, P. G. Kaufmann, & S. M. Weiss (Eds.). Copyright 1984 by U.S. Department of Health and Human Services–NIH Publication No. 84–1654. Reprinted by permission). *Bottom,* Recording of venous-occlusion slope. (From "Volume Plethysmography in Vascular Disease: An Overview," by D. S. Sumner, 3d ed. In *Noninvasive Diagnostic Techniques in Vascular Disease,* E. F. Bernstein (Ed.). Copyright 1985 by C. V. Mosby Company. Reprinted by permission.]

change in forearm circumference, or blood volume. By properly calibrating the strain gauge prior to its placement, it is possible to express measures of forearm blood flow in absolute volume units (see Whitney, 1953, for details). This calibration, which corrects for individual differences in forearm volume, makes it possible to make valid comparisons of FBF measures obtained within as well as between individuals. By obtaining measures of *mean arterial blood pressure* (MAP) concomitantly with FBF, one can calculate *forearm vascular resistance* (FVR = MAP/FBF). The significance of this measure is that it provides information that allows the investigator to determine with some confidence whether an alteration in FBF is due to passive or active changes in vasoconstriction/vasodilation. For instance, if FBF increases as a result of passive withdrawal of sympathetic influences on the vasculature, the blood pressure would also fall and FVR would remain unchanged (Williams, 1984). Thus, measures of FBF and FVR, in combination with other cardiodynamic and hemodynamic indices, may enable the psychophysiologist to more precisely examine patterns of cardiovascular activity.

As with other techniques for measuring blood flow, venous-occlusion plethysmography is subject to a variety of problems that can limit its usefulness in certain applications. In particular, this technique is susceptible to movement artifact, and thus the subject must remain relatively still during assessment periods. In addition, the position of the limb during measurement is critical; the arm should be elevated to the heart level to nullify the potential effects on blood flow of hydrostatic pressure. Finally, the blood pressure cuffs can remain inflated for only brief periods of time (e.g., 60 s) to avoid ischemic pain, and so continuous measures of FBF are not possible.

14.3.2.2 *Blood pressure measurement*

The single factor having the greatest influence on the control of blood flow through the circulatory system is BP. Direct or invasive measurements of BP are obtained by inserting a cannula through the skin and directly into one of the major arteries, usually the brachial or radial arteries. A pressure-sensitive transducer attached to the external end of the cannula detects the phasic changes in arterial pressure following each heartbeat. The morphologic features observed in these pulsatile waveforms reflect the various phases of ventricular contraction during each cardiac cycle. The maximum pressure exerted in the artery following each heartbeat is called the systolic blood pressure (SBP), and the minimum pressure is called the diastolic blood pressure (DBP). Another measure often reported in the literature, pulse pressure, is simply the difference between the SBP and DBP. Mean arterial pressure represents the average pressure during the cardiac cycle and can also be estimated using the following formula:

$$MAP = 1/3 \, (SBP - DBP) + DBP \qquad (3)$$

In calculating MAP, the value 1/3 is used because during each pressure cycle the pressure remains at the systolic level for approximately one third of the total cycle duration. Thus, when averaged over the entire pressure cycle, the mean pressure is closer to the DBP than to the SBP level. It is important to note that the use of this weighted average will provide accurate measures of the true MAP for heart rates within the normal (i.e., resting) range. Since, as stated previously, the duration of the diastolic phase of the cardiac cycle is reduced disproportionately more than the systolic phase as the heart rate is increased, estimates of MAP using the preceding formula will be in error at high heart rate levels.

Mean arterial pressure is a particularly important BP measure as it reflects the average effective pressure that drives the blood through the circulatory system. At any instant, the MAP must be sufficient to cause the CO to flow through the resistance provided by the blood vessels.

Blood pressure values are expressed in millimeters of mercury (mm Hg) units. The "normal" systolic and diastolic values for adult individuals under resting conditions are approximately 120 and 80 mm Hg, respectively, and are typically reported in the format 120/80 mm Hg. As is the case for all physiological variables, there exists great variability in the BP values among individuals. Measures taken from the same individual at different times can also vary widely. Factors such as age, gender, weight, race, physical health, individual habits (e.g., caffeine, nicotine, alcohol, and sodium consumption as well as certain drugs) can all influence the normal BP range.

Both the pressure values and the pressure wave configurations are altered during transmission through the circulatory system. As compared to the pressures recorded in the ascending aorta, the systolic pressure values increase and the diastolic pressure values decrease (resulting in a higher pulse pressure) within the descending aorta and large arteries. However, the mean pressure within these vascular segments steadily decreases as distance from the heart increases. With further transmission of the pressure pulse, the changes in blood vessel size and structure causes the pulsatile waveform to become progressively smoother as it travels through the circulation. Thus, the intermittent, pulsatile output of the heart is transformed to a more steady and continuous flow that facilitates the exchange of nutrients and waste products between tissues and blood at the capillary sites. The BP values previously cited (120/80) represent measures obtained from the brachial artery. Steady pressures in the capillaries range from 20 to 30 mm Hg, whereas those in the systemic veins are in the range 0–20 mm Hg.

Standard auscultatory technique. Whereas intraarterial blood pressure recordings provide the most accurate measures of BP, ethical and safety considerations associated with the invasiveness of the procedure preclude its use in most studies involving human subjects. Several noninvasive BP-recording techniques have been developed that provide safe, intermittent assessments of BP and are widely used in the psychophysiology laboratory.

The most common technique used in clinical and laboratory assessments of BP is the *auscultatory technique.* Manual auscultatory technique involves the use of a blood pressure cuff (fit snugly around the upper arm) and a stethoscope. As illustrated in Figure 14.14, measures of BP are obtained by inflating the BP cuff first to a level that totally occludes the artery underneath the cuff and then gradually reducing the pressure at a fixed rate (i.e., 2–3 mm Hg/s). Prior to inflating the BP cuff, the bell of the stethoscope is placed over the brachial artery just distal to the lower edge of the cuff. The actual determinations of SBP and DBP are made by listening through the stethoscope for the characteristic *Korotkoff-sounds* (K-sounds) that are produced when the pressure pulse wave passes through the artery underneath the cuff. With the cuff pressure initially set to above the occluding level, no K-sounds are detected because transmission of the pressure pulses along the artery is interrupted at the point of occlusion. At this level, the cuff pressure exceeds the arterial systolic pressure. As the cuff pressure is slowly reduced from the occluding level, the difference between the pressure in the cuff and the pressure within the artery (i.e., BP) is reduced. Eventually, the cuff pressure level is reached, at which point arterial pressure just exceeds cuff pressure. At this point, the pressure pulse wave will penetrate the point of occlusion under the cuff, force open the artery, and pass to the other side. The bell of the stethoscope is positioned to detect the turbulence in the artery produced by the passing pressure pulse (i.e., a K-sound will be detected). Upon detection of the first K-sound, the level of applied cuff pressure can be read from a manometer (a pressure indicator calibrated in mm Hg

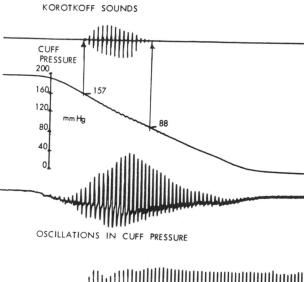

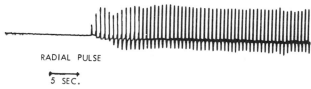

Figure 14.14. Comparison among auscultatory (*top*), oscillometric (*middle*), and palpatory (*bottom*) methods of measuring blood pressure. From *The Direct and Indirect Measurement of Blood Pressure*, by L. A. Geddes. (Copyright 1970 by Year Book Medical Publishers. Reprinted by permission.)

units) that is attached to the cuff. The pressure reading on the manometer when the first K-sound is detected represents the SBP. As cuff pressure continues to be slowly reduced, arterial pressure now exceeds the applied cuff pressure following each heart cycle and a series of K-sounds will be detected that first increase in loudness, then reach a maximum, and finally decrease as less counterpressure is applied to the arterial segment under the cuff. Depending on the particular criteria employed (American Heart Association, 1967), the pressure reading on the manometer when the K-sounds either become muffled in sound or disappear completely marks the arterial DBP level.

Although the auscultatory technique has become the standard method for measuring BP in both clinical and laboratory settings, it is not satisfactory for all psychophysiological studies. Specifically, since prolonged periods of cuff inflation cause ischemia and its associated discomfort, the bleed-down procedure described can be repeated, at most, approximately once every 1½ min or so (at least 30 s between cuff inflations is recommended to allow the return of normal blood flow to the arm). Thus, studies requiring more frequent measures of BP must employ a different technique. A further problem concerns the fact that the measures obtained with this technique consistently underestimate the true SBP and DBP. As indicated by Tursky (1974), at the points where the SBP and DBP are determined, the applied cuff pressure must be less than the true arterial pressure for either a K-sound to be detected (SBP) or for the K-sounds to disappear (DBP). The representativeness of single determinations obtained with this technique is affected by the inherent lability of BP. That is, BP normally varies from one heartbeat to the next, and this variability can be quite large in some individuals, reaching 30 mm Hg over a brief period of time (e.g., the time equal to 50 consecutive beats) (Tursky, Shapiro, & Schwartz, 1972). In view of the fact that determinations of SBP and DBP are each based on the pressure level associated with a single heart cycle, the values obtained during a single bleed-down may not truly represent the subject's average SBP or DBP levels during the period of measurement. For this reason, multiple readings should be obtained and averaged. Additional sources of errors in measurement associated with the auscultatory technique include bodily movement, defects in the hearing ability of the person taking the measurement, and a number of procedural errors such as improper positioning of the arm and improper deflation of the cuff pressure (Geddes, 1970; Steptoe, 1980). One of the most important factors influencing the accuracy of BP measurements is the size of the occluding cuff. Complete and even transmission of cuff pressure through the surrounding tissue is dependent on the relationship between the width of the cuff and the circumference of the limb to which it is applied. Inaccurate systolic and diastolic blood pressure determinations will result if the width of the cuff is either too large or too small with respect to limb diameter. The recommended cuff width is 20 percent wider than limb diameter or, alternatively, 40 percent of limb circumference (Geddes, 1970). For the average adult, this corresponds to a cuff width of approximately 12–14 cm wide. Pediatric cuffs of various sizes (2.5–9.0 cm) are commercially available and are recommended for use in measuring BP in children (Geddes, 1970). The inflatable bag should be long enough to completely encircle the limb. The standard length of the adult-size cuff is approximately 30 cm.

Constant-cuff technique. Tursky and colleagues (Shapiro, Tursky, Gershon, & Stern, 1969; Tursky, 1974; Tursky et al., 1972) have developed a method of recording BP that circumvents many of the problems associated with the auscultatory technique. The constant-cuff technique is an automated BP-recording technique that operates by tracking, over time, either the median systolic or diastolic BP. A significant feature of this technique is its use of a crystal microphone, in place of a stethoscope, for electronically detecting the presence and absence of K-sounds. The K-sound microphone is positioned under the distal edge of the cuff, and its output signal is fed either into solid-state logic circuits or a digital computer for processing. The measurement of SBP is initiated by first inflating the BP cuff to the pressure level at which roughly half the heartbeats (ECG R-wave) coincide with the detection of a K-sound. This marks the median SBP. Once the median SBP has been established, a series of cuff inflations is presented each lasting a period of time equaling 30–50 heart cycles (shorter or longer time periods can be used). During each cuff inflation period, the total number of K-sounds detected by the K-sound microphone indicates whether the current cuff pressure level is at, above, or below the median pressure. It has been empirically shown that when between 25 and 75 percent of the heart cycles during a cuff inflation trial coincide with a K-sound the cuff pressure equals the true arterial pressure with an accuracy of ± 2 mm Hg (Tursky et al., 1972). If fewer than 25 percent of the heart cycles coincide with a K-sound during a cuff inflation trial, cuff pressure exceeds the true arterial pressure and so the pressure applied to the cuff will be reduced by a fixed amount (e.g., 2–3 mm Hg) on the next trial. If greater that 75 percent of heart cycles are followed by a K-sound (i.e., cuff pressure is too low relative to arterial BP), the cuff pressure on the next trial will be increased by a fixed amount. In this way, the median SBP or DBP can be tracked from one cuff inflation trial to the next during a protracted period of time.

Beat-to-beat tracking technique. Shapiro, Greenstadt, Lane, and Rubinstein (1981) developed an alternative method that allows the tracking of BP (SBP or DBP) on a beat-to-beat basis. In this system, the cuff pressure is either increased or decreased by a fixed amount (2 or 3 mm Hg) following each heartbeat depending on whether or not a K-sound is detected. Within-subject comparisons of BP recorded intraarterially and using the beat-to-beat tracking procedure have shown good agreement between the two under both resting and moderately stressful conditons. The system makes it possible to follow changes in BP over relatively short periods of time (see Paller & Shapiro, 1983; Victor, Weipert, & Shapiro, 1984). However, dramatic and sudden shifts in BP may be difficult to track precisely with this system due to its inherent hysteresis. The multiplicity of pressure estimates (on each heartbeat) greatly improves the accuracy of measures of average values of pressure over periods of time (30 s, 1 min, etc.). Since only one pressure level can be tracked over time, two cuffs (one on each arm) are necessary to record beat-to-beat variations in SBP and DBP simultaneously. Use of the two-cuff system thereby provides assessments of SBP, DBP, calculated MAP, as well as pulse pressure on a beat-to-beat basis. Further work examining the relationship between changes in BP and characteristics of the K-sounds other than its mere presence or absence (amplitude, spectral composition, etc.) may improve the precision of the beat-to-beat tracking technique by permitting variable adjustments of pressure on each succeeding heartbeat.

Oscillometric technique. Posey, Geddes, Williams, and Moore (1969) have demonstrated that the gradual reducation in applied cuff pressure from the occluding level is accompanied by an orderly series of cuff pressure oscillations that are first detected at approximately the SBP, increase in amplitude until peaking at or near the MAP level, and then are gradually reduced in amplitude as cuff pressure nears the DBP level (see Figure 14.14). It was further shown that these cuff pressure oscillations result from the transmission of turbulence within the artery, produced when arterial blood flow is partially occluded, directly into the air in the BP cuff. By connecting a pressure transducer to the cuff, these slight oscillations in cuff pressure may be amplified and recorded on a polygraph or sampled and processed by computer. Attempts to validate measures of SBP and DBP obtained on the basis of changes in cuff pressure oscillation amplitude have generally proven unsuccessful (see Geddes, 1970). However, substantial evidence indicates that the point of maximum amplitude cuff oscillations is associated with MAP (Posey et al., 1969). Recent experiments have also demonstrated that when the level of applied cuff pressure is held constant within the range that produces cuff pressure oscillations (i.e., between SBP and DBP), beat-to-beat variations in the amplitude of the oscillations reflect changes in arterial BP (Geddes & Newberg, 1977). Thus, the *oscillometric technique* may provide useful information concerning relative changes in BP on a beat-by-beat basis (Papillo, Tursky, & Friedman, 1981; Tursky, Papillo, & Friedman, 1982).

Pulse transit time. A proposed alternative strategy for indirectly assessing beat-to-beat BP changes, one that does not require the use of an occluding cuff, is based on the time taken for a pressure pulse wave to travel along an arterial segment. The underlying assumption is that increases in BP are associated with decreases in the transit time. The *pulse transit time* (PTT) is designated as the time period (in milliseconds) required for a pulse wave to travel between two points along an artery (P–PTT) or, alternatively, the time duration commencing with the ECG R-wave and terminating with the arrival of the pulse wave at a peripheral site (R–PTT). For measuring PTT, a number of vascular sites have been chosen for recording the peripheral pressure pulse including the brachial, radial, temporal, and carotid arteries as well as the pinna of the ear. Techniques employed to detect the peripheral pulse have included piezoelectric strain gauges (Steptoe, 1976), photoplethysmographs (Martin, Epstein, & Cinciripini, 1980; Newlin & Levenson, 1979, 1980), and impedance plethysmographs (Williams & Williams, 1965).

Numerous studies have examined the extent to which measures of PTT correlate with measures of arterial BP obtained both directly and indirectly. Taken together, the results of these studies can best be characterized as ambiguous (Allen, Schneider, Davidson, Winchester, & Taylor, 1981; Gribbin, Steptoe, & Sleight, 1976; Lane, Greenstadt, Shapiro, & Rubinstein, 1983; Obrist, Light, McCubbin, Hutcheson, & Hoffer, 1979). It remains unclear as to whether measures of PTT are most closely associated with changes in SBP, MAP, or DBP. The strength of the correlation has been shown to vary widely depending on which aspect of the peripheral pulse (e.g., foot, peak, slope) is used in calculating PTT (Lane et al., 1983). One further point worth mentioning is that whereas P–PTT represents the actual transit time and is influenced primarily by vascular events, R–PTT includes, in addition, most of the PEP and is therefore influenced by cardiodynamic as well as hemodynamic factors. Thus, the relative contributions of the beta- and alpha-adrenergic influences operating on the cardiovascular system when measures are obtained can affect the strength of correlations observed between R–PTT and BP. In view of the inconsistencies reported in the literature concerning both the reliability and validity of PTT measures, it is suggested that extreme caution be used when interpreting the results of studies reporting BP data based solely on measures of PTT.

14.4   CONCEPTUAL ISSUES

14.4.1   *Social context*

It has long been recognized that the social and cultural environments exert profound influences on normal cardiovascular functioning and on cardiovascular pathophysiology (see Mesulam & Perry, 1972). In contemporary research, which heavily emphasizes the determinants of health and disease (in this context, cardiovascular disease), greater emphasis has been placed in developing an understanding of the health-damaging and health-protective factors occurring in the social milieu of any individual. The observations range from broad socioeconomic and social organization factors such as technological development, westernization, modernization, amount and rapidity of social change, and socioeconomic status to social factors in the family and extended social milieu of the individual (e.g., social support) to individual culturally based beliefs about the controllability of environmental threats and challenges. Hundreds of examples of such phenomena have been reviewed repeatedly, and no attempt will be made to detail them here (see Henry & Stephens, 1977; James, 1987; Kuller, Talbott, & Robinson, 1987; Lown, 1987). They derive from the thinking and research of anthropologists, sociologists, and epidemiologists that have led to hypotheses attempting to integrate the diverse phenomena. For example, James (1987) states that the "active pursuit of a Western lifestyle *under conditions that are not conducive to success* may represent one aspect of modernization that leads to higher blood pressures in third world populations undergoing rapid social and cultural changes" (p. 63). This rich literature stimulates many such hypotheses, and the observations are sometimes suggestive of ways of bringing social phenomena under experimental scrutiny in the laboratory. For example, this particular hypothesis may be translated into individual psychological mechanisms that can be defined and examined more precisely in the laboratory test situation. We can ask how success and failure experiences affect physiological functioning under task conditions varying in their difficulty or in their potential for resolution, or depending on the climate of cooperation or competition that prevails in the situation. Such translations have been effectively made in designs used in social psychophysiological studies, for example, see Glass (1977) and Van Egeren (1984).

In many respects, however, the field of social psychophysiology or sociophysiology has been built on other traditions of research specific to itself. In the simplest terms, as Stern and Ray (1984) put it, "all psychophysiology is sociophysiology," and thus all cardiovascular psychophysiology is by definition cardiovascular sociophysiology. The development of this endeavor has been traced out by Shapiro and Crider (1969), summarizing earlier studies, and brought up to date by Cacioppo and Petty (1983, 1986) and Waid (1984).

Contemporary topics in this field have been laid out by Cacioppo and Petty (1986) and include social facilitation of behavior and physiological responses; effects of other observers; attitude formation, maintenance, and change; affective reactions; message processing; and cognitive dissonance, to which we should add processes of social interaction and social communication in groups of individuals.

As in other sections of this chapter, we have emphasized the importance of combined biological–behavioral strategies of research. In the context of social psychophysiology, this same point has been discussed by Ohman and Dimberg (1984) in laying out some of the biological factors that constrain social behavior and, by extension, physiological responding in social situations. For example, emotional facial expressions and behavioral and physiological reactions to such expressions are greatly determined by response tendencies rooted in evolution and genetics. A greater appreciation of this perspective requires an incorporation of such knowledge into the research. We concur with the major conclusion drawn by Ohman and Dimberg (1984) (also following Brunswik, 1956) that we "make sure that the evolutionary and ecologically relevant dimensions are represented in the experiment" (p. 81). Although these authors wrote from a biological perspective, we can also add that a similar appreciation of the social or social–cultural context of behavior and physiological functioning is vital if not a necessity. This conclusion has important implications for the design of studies in cardiovascular psychophysiology, for example in the health area (see what follows), which has tended to rely on a few laboratory tests chosen because they are relatively simple, well studied, or easy to apply. One research strategy is to incorporate sociologists and social psychologists into our research groups so as to guide us toward the kind of experimentation most likely to advance our knowledge of these complex interactions. It is encouraging to see greater attention being paid to cardiovascular psychophysiological research focused on relevant social psychophysiological questions about sex differences in physiological responses to stress and in coronary heart disease (Stoney, Davis, & Matthews, 1987), effects of race on cardiovascular responses to stress (Anderson et al., 1986; Morell, Myers, Shapiro, Goldstein, & Armstrong, 1988), and interpersonal competition (Glass et al., 1980; Van Egeren, 1979).

14.4.2   Psychological–behavioral context

14.4.2.1 Attention, arousal, and directional fractionation of responses

In modern psychophysiology, the concept of arousal or activation has long been used to organize phenomena and guide experimental research. The concept derives in large measure from the early research of Walter Cannon (1979/1929) on the pattern of neuroendocrine responses associated with behavior variously labeled as the "emergency reaction" or "fight and flight" and is supported by extensive observations and theories on related brain and behavioral processes and mechanisms, as spelled out in the writings of Duffy (1957), Gellhorn (1964), Lindsley (1951), Malmo (1959), and Selye (1976). Of special relevance to an understanding of relations between psychological or emotional states and cardiovascular responses are other observations indicating that autonomic, electrocortical, skeletomotor, and other gross behavioral responses do not fall into a uniform response complex but rather are patterned according to the nature of the stimuli or situations confronting the individual and to the manner in which the individual interacts with external demands. Arguments that there are distinct forms of arousal were made decisively by Lacey in 1967, in which he presented evidence on dissociations of somatic and behavioral arousal, imperfectly correlated changes of different autonomic response systems, and differentiated patterns of response to different environmental emotional challenges. The seminal observations made by Lacey were instances of what he labeled "directional fractionation" in which "one or more physiological functions changes decisively in a direction opposite to the expectations inherent in Cannon-like views of the energizing and protective role of sympathetic activity" (Lacey, 1967, p. 33). Of major significance to cardiovascular functioning are the observations of the sensitivity of heart rate and blood pressure responses to the "directionality" of behavior and the demonstration that even these two closely related functions may show some dissociation. For example, during the 4-s preparatory interval of a reaction time task, Lacey (1967) noted a consistent pattern of heart rate deceleration and a corresponding small increase in blood pressure (see also Paller & Shapiro, 1983).

With respect to patterns of heart rate change and changes in other noncardiovascular autonomic measures, Lacey showed that the same degree of electrodermal responding could be coupled with heart rate acceleration in "environmental rejection" situations in which the task or stimulation is aversive or requires cognitive elaboration or could be coupled with heart rate deceleration in "environmental detection" or "environmental intake" situations in which the task requires the taking in of information – the "intent to note and detect external stimuli" (Lacey, 1967). Generally, these observations and distinctions have held up in contemporary research, although other interpretations have been offered of the significance of the directionality of heart rate change in relation to attention and performance of various motor and cognitive tasks (see Jennings, 1986). Coles (1984) argued that the various types of heart rate change – tonic shifts in level, decelerative and accelerative phasic changes, and short-latency variations in the duration of individual cardiac cycles – are manifestations of motor and perceptual preparatory responses and of fast and slower information-processing activities, which generally are under the control of the vagus (parasympathetic), and he concluded that measures of cardiac activity can be as useful as measures of cortical activity (such as event-related potentials) in the study of cognitive processes.

14.4.2.2 *Differentiation of emotional states*

The search for specific patterning of physiological responses has a long tradition in research on emotion. It is an area fraught with definitional problems given the multiple and varying patterns of subjective experience, verbal behavior, motor behavior, and physiological processes occurring during different emotional states. Contemporary research has given major attention to electrocortical and electromyographic indices, although the earlier classic studies by Ax (1953), Schachter (1957), and Funkenstein, King, and Drolette (1957) of anger and fear indicated that electrodermal and cardiovascular variables as well as indices of muscle tension could provide context-specific indices of these two emotional states. In recent research, localized electromyographic and specific self-report measures have been particularly sensitive to emotional states, demonstrating that different patterns of facial muscle activity and self-reports of emotional experiences accompany the generation of qualitatively different emotional imagery (see Cacioppo, Tassinary, & Fridlund, chapter 11; Fridlund & Izard, 1983; Schwartz, 1986). There are also observations indicating that relationships between blood pressure and heart rate vary as a function of emotion (Schwartz, Weinberger, & Singer, 1981). Another promising line of investigation has shown cardiovascular differentiation of emotional states based on the generation of specific patterns of facial features without the experience of emotion or reliving of specific emotions (Ekman, Levenson, & Friesen, 1983). Heart rate differentiated positive and negative emotions with further differentiation made possible using recordings of changes in finger temperature in the emotional conditions of the study. That posed facial expressions can elicit such differences is remarkable, given the apparent lack of affective experience or of associated differences in motor activity. These findings need to be repeated and their biological basis examined more thoroughly.

14.4.2.3 *Active–passive coping*

We have touched on attempts to classify the numerous response patterns occurring in transactions between the individual and the environment in dealing with various tasks or situations (e.g., fear/anger, environmental rejection/environmental intake). Such categorizations, although inevitably oversimplified and insufficient to account for the many different patterns of responses observed in groups let alone individual subjects, give the researcher a handle on how to select methods of testing subjects' reactions or a means of examining commonalities in response patterns. One of the most useful recent schemes derives from the work of Obrist and his colleagues (see Obrist, 1981, 1982, 1984) in which tasks were classified according to whether they required active or passive coping. Active coping tasks involve the exertion of sustained mental effort to deal with the demands of a task, and passive coping tasks are those in which the individual simply endures the experience, especially where there is no means of avoiding the task or its consequences, including the belief that coping is not possible. Active and passive coping tasks differ in the magnitude of physiological responses they elicit with mainly larger, more sustained cardiovascular and other physiological reactions in the active coping tasks. In addition, challenges requiring active coping tend to evoke greater beta-adrenergic stimulation of the heart, whereas passive coping tasks evoke greater vascular responses, presumably mediated by alpha-adrenergic receptors (see review of evidence in Light, 1987). The kind of reactivity associated with active coping is also deemed characteristic of certain individuals who are thereby predisposed to cardiovascular disease. Obrist (1982) finds the critical element in active coping to be the action that the cardiovascular system is concerned with, and he concludes that it is "easier conceptually to link cardiovascular activity with it than with behavioural processes such as motivation or emotion or attention, unless the latter can be viewed along an activity continuum" (p. 285). We have briefly discussed the frameworks of attention and emotion. For a discussion of the concepts of motivation and incentives as linked with responses of the cardiovascular system, see Fowles (1982, 1984).

14.5   CARDIOVASCULAR BEHAVIORAL MEDICINE

14.5.1   Hypertension

Through its role as a major risk factor for stroke and heart and kidney disease, hypertension, or high blood pressure, is the single most important cause of death in the United States (Surwit, Williams, & Shapiro, 1982). The World Health Organization has defined hypertension as abnormally elevated blood pressure greater than 160/95 mm Hg (World Health Organization, 1978). However, the significance of the elevation in blood pressure is relative, given that blood pressure is a continuous variable and the higher the blood pressure the greater the predictability of associated diseases (Kannel, 1977; Kannel & Sorlie, 1975). Of fundamental importance to psychophysiologists is primary (i.e., essential or idiopathic) hypertension in which the blood pressure is not secondary to kidney disease, tumors of the adrenal glands, narrowing of the aorta, or primary aldosteronism (Kaplan, 1980). This does not mean that primary hypertension is essentially a *psychosomatic*, or *stress-related*, disorder, but it is clear from various sources of evidence that psychological and social factors play a significant causative role in many inidividuals with this disorder.

Hypertension is the single most well-developed area of application of cardiovascular psychophysiology to a health problem. It is built on a basic literature of studies on the effects of various stimuli and tasks on heart rate, blood pressure, skin and muscle blood flow, and hormonal responses and on a technology of cardiovascular measurement, mainly noninvasive, that has been developed and refined, as presented in this chapter, and into which new methods are constantly being introduced. The application of psychophysiological principles to the study of hypertension represents an attempt to determine which patterns of behavioral, physiological, and neuroendocrine response occur reliably in association with particular kinds of interactions between the individual and the environment. In particular, the aim is to develop standard methods of assessing such response patterns in the individual so as to provide diagnostic indicators or psychophysiological markers of hypertension such as, for example, excessive heart rate, blood pressure, or other cardiovascular and neuroendocrine reactions to tasks requiring cognitive or behavioral adaptation (James, 1987; Light, 1987). Typically, comparative studies are carried out in hypertensive patients varying in severity of the disorder (e.g., borderline, fixed hypertension) or in risk for the disorder (e.g., positive vs. negative family history of hypertension, casual blood pressure level; see what follows). Major additional objectives are to develop methods of intervention and to evaluate their effectiveness in the behavioral management of hypertension (e.g., Benson, Shapiro, Schwartz, & Tursky, 1971; Chesney, Agras, et al., 1987; Chesney, Black, Swan, & Ward, 1987; Glasgow, Gaarder, & Engel, 1982; Goldstein, Shapiro, & Thananopavarn, 1984).

The framework and methods of cardiovascular psychophysiology provide models for testing the significance of emotional states, cognitive processes, and social behaviors for hypertension. The literature is rich in empirical studies and theoretical speculations on personality and behavioral styles, effects of anger, anxiety, and depression, and various kinds of social and occupational stress, urbanization and cultural change, prolonged illness, and so on (see Shapiro & Goldstein, 1982). A large body of knowledge has accumulated over the years about physical and structural/organic factors involved in the etiology and pathophysiology of hypertension, such as age, genetic disposition, dietary factors (e.g., sodium, potassium, calcium), exercise and physical conditioning, and obesity. Investigation into these factors has by and large dominated medical research on hypertension. The interaction of physical and psychological processes in this disorder needs closer scrutiny.

The multiplicity of causes of hypertension leads one to ask whether it is possible to determine the relative contributions of different behavioral and physiological factors and, more importantly, to consider how the different factors may interact with one another and the significance of such interactions. In recent research, attempts at the study of biological–behavioral interactions have become more prominent, one example being research on relations between behavioral stress and the renal control of body sodium and fluid volume. Decreased sodium and fluid excretion was shown to occur in saline-infused dogs during a shock-avoidance task along with a rise in blood pressure (Grignolo, Koepke, & Obrist, 1982). In parallel human studies, competitive mental tasks were shown to induce decreases in sodium and fluid excretion in those individuals with a family history of hypertension, with borderline hypertension, and more specifically only in those who showed above average heart rate reactivity to the task (Light, Koepke, Obrist, & Willis, 1983). These findings were interpreted by Light (1987) to suggest that a generalized increase in sympathetic activity was responsible for both the renal sodium retention and the cardiac responses but that the renal responses occurred only in those individuals who had a genetic disposition to retain sodium.

The reader is referred to various treatises that provide overviews of biomedical and psychophysiological research on hypertension (Cohen & Obrist, 1975; Folkow, 1982; Harris & Brady, 1974; Henry & Stephens, 1977; Obrist, 1981; Obrist, Light, Langer, & Koepke, 1986; Shapiro & Goldstein, 1982; Shepherd & Weiss, 1987; Steptoe, 1981; Weiner, 1979). Major strategies of investigation will be briefly summarized emphasizing what appear to be promising directions of current research.

14.5.1.1 *Psychological and psychophysiological differences between hypertensive and normotensive individuals*

This research is motivated by the following questions: Can one detect the influence of psychological or psychosocial factors in hypertension by comparing samples of known hypertensive and normotensive individuals? Do such samples differ in personality traits, emotional and behavioral characteristics in response to life stress, or in cardiovascular reactions to various psychological and physical stimuli differing in type and intensity of threat or challenge and performance requirement? The resulting literature was a major impetus for current developments in the behavioral medicine of hypertension (see reviews by Goldstein, 1981; Henry & Cassell, 1969; Krantz et al., 1987; Shapiro & Goldstein, 1982). Although the evidence does not support the existence of a unique "hypertensive personality" type, it is clear that anger-coping style and submissiveness are often associated with individuals who have hypertension (Cottington, Matthews, Talbott, & Kuller, 1986; Dimsdale et al., 1986; Gerardi, Blanchard, Andrasik, & McCoy, 1985; Perini, Muller, Rauchfleisch, Battegay, & Buhler, 1986; Schneider, Egan, Johnson, Drobny, & Julius, 1986).

Experimental studies provide supportive evidence, though not always consistent, that hypertensive individuals tend to be more reactive to experimentally induced mental and psychological stress, for example, during discussions of stressful topics (Schneider & Zangari, 1951; Williams, Kimball, & Williard, 1972), performance of mental arithmetic under time pressure (Brod, Fencl, Hejl, & Jurka, 1959), exercise (Groen et al., 1977), and exposure to various aversive and demanding stimuli (Jost, Ruilmann, Hill, & Gulo, 1952; Schachter, 1957). The stimuli used in such studies need not be emotionally provocative or demanding. Investigations of response to orthostatic stress (e.g., full-body tilt) also revealed differences between hypertensives and normals, reflecting differences in neural and cardiovascular control mechanisms involved in adaptation to postural change (Frohlich, Tarazi, Ulrych, Dustan, & Page, 1967; Hull, Wolthius, Cortese, Longo, & Triebwasser, 1977). For example, the responses to tilt of the patients with mild hypertension in the study by Frohlich et al. were categorized as either normal, hypotensive, or hypertensive. Those showing an orthostatic hypertensive pattern also showed marked increases in peripheral resistance during head-up tilt, and these patients also had a greater blood pressure response to the *Valsalva maneuver*. In a later study, correlated changes in plasma renin activity and cardiac output indicated that both functions were influenced by the sympathetic nervous system (Dustan, Tarazi, & Frohlich, 1970) (see discussion of these data in Dustan, 1987).

The most promising hypothesis to be advanced in this area of research derives from the work of Julius, Esler, and their colleagues indicating that in a subset of patients with mild hypertension the sympathetic nervous system plays a major role. These patients showed elevated levels of plasma renin activity, higher heart rate, and elevated plasma norepinephrine (Esler et al., 1977). Of special importance was the finding that this subgroup of patients differed from the low-renin group in scoring higher on personality tests measuring unexpressed anger. This research provides major support for the appropriateness of a combined biological–psychological characterization of individuals with hypertension.

The preceding research consists entirely of cross-sectional and clinical studies, making it difficult to establish whether psychological factors are primary or secondary to the disorder. For example, unexpressed anger or submissiveness may be a consequence rather than an antecedent of hypertension.

14.5.1.2 *Relationships between psychosocial variables and blood pressure*

This is a natural extension of the preceding research to the more general question of correlations between psychological or social factors and individual differences in blood pressure and other cardiovascular and hormonal variables. Also to be included are epidemiological studies comparing different populations in terms of blood pressure level. This research asks about the relations between blood pressure and personality traits and individual differences, cultural modernization and urbanization, socioeconomic status, race, social, industrial, and occupational stress, and crowding, among other things, finding generlly that blood pressure is affected by all of these (see James, 1987; Shapiro & Goldstein, 1982). It is difficult to establish causation in epidemiological studies. Moreover, the processes affecting normal variations in blood pressure may not be significant for hypertension itself. That is, pathophysiological development may only occur in conjunction with inherent neural or cardiovascular properties of the individual related to genetic factors, early development, obesity, diet, and so on. By the same token, as Shine (1987) has pointed out, reduction of risk factors through diet and exercise may reduce the discriminative value of personality factors. Moreover, although early elevations in blood pressure may predict subsequent elevations, mildly elevated blood pressure does not necessarily progress to established hypertension (Weder & Julius, 1985). Nonetheless, these studies provide evidence pointing to critical factors in the environment that affect blood pressure regulation and that could be significant for the development of hypertension in combination with other processes.

14.5.1.3 *Precursors of hypertension*

On the basis of the limitations of the preceding two strategies for providing definitive evidence about neural and psychological influences on the development of hypertension but exploiting the knowledge derived from this research, an alternate approach has emerged as a major strategy of contemporary research, that is, to select individuals at risk for hypertension and to examine their psychological, psychophysiological, and other relevant characteristics. Inasmuch as hypertension runs in families (Report of Task Force of Blood Pressure Control in Children, 1977), this risk factor has been targeted for investigation, along with other presumably inherited constitutional dispositions, such as heart rate or blood pressure level, variability, or reactivity. Children, adolescents, and young adults with and without a positive family history of hypertension have been investigated during exposure to various simple and challenging tasks of a psychological or physical nature. In general, those with a positive family history show greater reactivity than those with a negative family history (e.g., Falkner, Onesti, Angelakos, Fernandes, & Langman, 1979; Hastrup, Light, & Obrist, 1982; Manuck & Proietti, 1982). Stressors that encourage active coping appear to be more effective in uncovering such differences (see Light, 1981, 1987). However, there has been little attention given to the use of physical or other simple stimuli in this research. For example, in the study of cardiovascular adaptation to orthostatic stress, we have found differences in normotensives according to family history of hypertension (Weipert, Shapiro, & Suter, 1987).

Moreover, other biological processes may interact with this constitutional predis-position, as suggested in a study by Falkner, Onesti, and Angelakos (1981), who found that adding salt to the normal diet increased blood pressure and stress reactivity, but only in those individuals in the sample of normotensive adolescents who had a positive family history of hypertension, underscoring again the fruitful merging of biological and behavioral concepts and methods. Positive family history was associated with decreased sodium excretion in response to mental stressors (Light et al., 1983), a relationship that may also depend on individual differences in salt sensitivity (see Light, 1987).

Significant questions have been raised about the reliability and validity of classifying individuals according to family history (Hastrup, Hotchkiss, & Johnson, 1985; Watt, 1986). An alternate strategy is to use blood pressure level as the risk factor on which to select subjects, which by itself is highly predictive of subsequent blood pressure level and hypertension. Ewart, Harris, Zeger, and Russell (1986) used this approach and found that ninth and tenth graders selected with blood pressure between the 85th and 95th percentiles showed lower levels of pulse pressure and *reduced* systolic blood pressure response to mental stress. Contrary to expectations, when subjects were selected in this fashion, the data point to increased peripheral resistance and lower cardiac output associated with genetic risk in the normoten-sive adolescent. This study suggests that the critical evaluation of precursors of hypertension requires refining and distinguishing various methods of assessing risk of hypertension. Above all what is sorely needed in this research are longitudinal studies tracking individuals with defined characteristics over time such as in the work of Falkner, Kushner, Onesti, and Angelakos (1981). In this study, adolescents with borderline hypertension were followed over a 41-month period. Those with a strong family history of hypertension, a high resting heart rate, and an excessive cardiovascular response to mental stress progressed to fixed hypertension in this relatively short time period. A major issue is the design and selection of appropriate tests, whether of cognitive functions, performance under challenge or threat, physical demands, and/or tests or autonomic functions such as the cold pressor test, Valsalva maneuver, tilt and postural change, isometric exercise (handgrip), face immersion (diving reflex), drug and other tests of baroreceptor sensitivity, and aerobic or isotonic exercise (treadmill, bicycle, ergometer), and standard methods of quantifying and analyzing responses to these stimuli and tasks (see Shepherd et al., 1987).

14.5.2   *Other cardiovascular disorders*

The preceding section on hypertension was intended to provide an overview of research strategies in cardiovascular psychophysiology relevant to other areas of cardiovascular behavioral medicine. The limitations of space preclude comparable coverage of coronary heart disease, which is clearly a major interest of contempor-ary research, with growing involvement of psychophysiological investigators. Atherosclerosis, the underlying pathophysiological process akin to hypertension, through its association with coronary heart disease and cerebrovascular disease, accounts for more than half of the yearly mortality in the United States. In many respects, the environmental and psychological risk factors contributing to coronary heart disease parallel those occurring in hypertension, and many of the same generalizations about behavioral influences apply.

Given that the Type A behavior pattern has been demonstrated as an independent risk factor for heart disease (Rosenman et al., 1975), a major psychophysiological strategy has focused on examining how Type A individuals differ from others in their responses (physiological, biochemical) to laboratory stressors (see Krantz & Manuck, 1984). By and large, this literature indicates greater cardiovascular reactivity to various mental and performance challenges, harassment during social competition, and threats of self-esteem (see Schneiderman, 1987, for review). Williams (1987) hypothesized that the major critical component of Type A behavior is hostility/anger/cynicism, and supporting evidence is available for increased cardiovascular reactivity in relation to this factor. Of greatest importance to work out are the links between behavior or physiological reactivity and processes of atherogenesis (Herd, 1986). These links are doubly complicated by the operation of other risk factors, such as diet, smoking, physical conditioning, genetic disposition, and so on.

Schneiderman (1987) discusses the hypothesis that stress-induced increases in sympathetic nervous system activity and the release of plasma catecholamines are important links between emotional stress and atherogenesis. The release of catecholamines may lead to injury of the intimal endothelium of the coronary arteries, leading to excessive release of free fatty acids resulting in platelet aggregation, smooth muscle proliferation, and deposits of lipids at the lesion. Catecholamines may also affect buildup of cholesterol in the blood. In addition, other hormones such as cortisol and testosterone may contribute to the critical pathophysiology. Again, as in the case of hypertension, establishing the empirical evidence requires longitudinal studies of the course of atherosclerosis in relation to the kinds of data collected in the cardiovascular psychophysiology laboratory.

14.6 CONCLUSIONS

In recent years, cardiovascular psychophysiology has moved into a front-line position with increasing physiological sophistication on the part of behavioral and social scientists and increasing psychological–behavioral sophistication on the part of medical and biological scientists. This chapter could only offer some general outlines of the anatomy and physiology of the cardiovascular system and the measurement of cardiovascular responses with an introduction to topics of interest in contemporary research. We highlighted the application of cardiovascular psychophysiological methods in behavioral medicine as related to hypertension and coronary heart disease as this focus dominates the field. It forms an easy way to bridge the gap between biology and psychology and an area of obvious significance to public health. We have had to forgo discussion of several other major basic research topics and applications, such as the use of heart rate in studies of orienting and attention in children and adults (Coles, 1984; Graham, 1984; Jennings, 1986; Kagan, Reznick, Clarke, Snidman, & Coll, 1984), anxiety (Fowles, 1982; Schwartz, 1986), and attitude change (Cacioppo & Petty, 1982). Nor have we been able to cover in any detail the use of behavioral and psychological methods to modify cardiovascular responses to aversive and challenging stimuli or situations, including exercise (Perski, Engel, & McCroskery, 1982; Shapiro & Reeves, 1982). This last topic is of clinical potential for cardiovascular disorders in providing a means of reducing excessive cardiovascular reactivity to stressful stimuli, which may be a significant precursor of these disorders. Also of potential interest are related studies on the effects of behavioral influences on physical conditioning as well as the effects of physical conditioning on the ability to cope with environmental challenges and life stress.

The health of cardiovascular psychophysiology is predicated on the continued growth of fundamental knowledge gained from basic studies in humans and animals on the behavioral, neural, and humoral mechanisms that regulate cognitive, emotional, and physiological responding. It is our belief that this growth is now critically dependent on intensive collaborative efforts across disciplines such as cardiology, physiology, and psychology and that this represents the beginning of a problem-oriented approach to cardiovascular psychophysiology.

NOTE

Some of the material in this chapter has been adapted from a previous article (Shapiro & Goldstein, 1982). Preparation of this chapter was supported by NHLBI Research Grant HL-31184-03 and the MacArthur Foundation (Health Network: UCLA Node).

REFERENCES

Ahmed, S. S., Levinson, G. E., Schwartz, C. J., & Ettinger, P. D. (1972). Systolic time intervals as measures of the contractile state of the left ventricular myocardium in man. *Circulation, 46,* 559–571.

Allen, R. A., Schneider, J. A., Davidson, D. M., Winchester, M. A., & Taylor, C. B. (1981). The covariation of blood pressure and pulse transit time in hypertensive patients. *Psychopysiology, 18,* 301–306.

American Heart Association (AHA) (Kirkendall, W. M., Burton, A. C., Epstein, F. H., & Freis, E. D.) (1967). Recommendations for human blood pressure determinations by sphygmo-manometers. *Circulation, 36,* 503–509.

Anderson, N. B., Williams, R. B., Jr., Lane, J. D., Haney, T., Simpson, S., & Houseworth, S. J. (1986). Type A behavior, family history of hypertension and cardiovascular responses among Black women. *Health Psychology, 5,* 393–406.

Ax, A. F. (1953). The physiological differentiation between fear and anger in humans. *Psychosomatic Medicine, 15,* 433–442.

Benjamin, L. S. (1963). Statistical treatment of the law of initial values in autonomic research: A review and recommendation. *Psychosomatic Medicine, 25,* 556–566.

Benson, H., Shapiro, D., Tursky, B., & Schwartz, G. E. (1971). Decreased systolic blood pressure through operant conditioning techniques in patients with essential hypertension. *Science, 173,* 740–742.

Berne, R. M., & Levy, M. N. (1986). *Cardiovascular physiology.* St. Louis: Mosby.

Bohrer, R. E., & Porges, S. W. (1982). The application of time-series statistics to psychological research: An introduction. In G. Karen (Ed.), *Statistical and methodological issues in psychology and social science research.* Hillsdale, NJ: Erlbaum.

Brener, J. (1980). Measurement and quantification of heart rate. In I. Martin & P. H. Venables (Eds.), *Techniques in psychophysiology* (pp. 179–192). New York: Wiley.

Brod, J., Fencl, V., Hejl, Z., & Jurka, J. (1959). Circulatory changes underlying blood pressure elevation during acute emotional stress (mental arithmetic) in normotensive and hypertensive subjects. *Clinical Science, 18,* 269–279.

Brown, C. C. (1967). The techniques of plethysmography. In C. C. Brown (Ed.), *Methods in psychophysiology* (pp. 54–74). Baltimore: Williams & Wilkins.

Brown, C. C. (1972). Instruments in psychophysiology. In N. S. Greenfield & R. A. Sternbach (Eds.), *Handbook of psychophysiology* (pp. 154–196). New York: Holt, Rinehart, & Winston.

Brunswik, E. (1956). *Perception and the representative design of psychological experiments.* Berkeley: University of California Press.

Burton, A. C. (1972). *Physiology and biophysics of the circulation.* Chicago: Year Book Medical Publishers.

Cacioppo, J. T., & Petty, R. E. (1982). *Perspectives in cardiovascular psychophysiology.* New York: Guilford Press.

Cacioppo, J. T., & Petty, R. E. (Eds.). (1983). *Social psychophysiology: A sourcebook.* New York: Guilford Press.

Cacioppo, J. T., & Petty, R. E. (1986). Social processes. In M. E. Coles, E. Donchin, & S. W. Porges (Eds.), *Psychophysiology: Systems, processes, and applications* (pp. 646–680). New York: Guilford Press.

Cannon, W. B. (1979). *Bodily changes in pain, hunger, fear, and rage.* New York: Appleton. (Original work published in 1929.)

Chesney, M. A., Agras, W. S., Benson, H., Blumenthal, J. A., Engel, B. T., Foreyt, J. P., Kaufmann, P. B., Levenson, R. M., Pickering, T. G., Randall, W. C., & Schwartz, P. J. (1987). Task Force 5: Nonpharmacologic approaches to treatment of hypertension. *Circulation Supplement, 76,* 104–110.

Chesney, M. A., Black, G. W., Swan, G. E., & Ward, M. W. (1987). Relaxation training for essential hypertension at the worksite: I. The untreated mild hypertensive. *Psychosomatic Medicine, 49,* 250–264.

Cohen, D. H., & Obrist, P. A. (1975). Interactions between behavior and the cardiovascular system. *Circulation Research, 37,* 693–706.

Coles, M. G. H. (1984). Heart rate and attention: The intake-rejection hypothesis and beyond. In M. G. H. Coles, J. R. Jennings, & J. A. Stern (Eds.), *Psychophysiological perspectives* (pp. 276–295). New York: Van Nostrand Reinhold.

Coles, M. G. H., Donchin, E., & Porges, S. W. (Eds.). (1986). *Psychophysiology: Systems, processes, and applications.* New York: Guilford Press.

Cook, M. (1974). Psychophysiology of peripheral vascular changes. In P. A. Obrist, A. H. Black, J. Brener, & L. V. DiCara (Eds.), *Cardiovascular psychophysiology* (pp. 60–84). Chicago: Aldine Press.

Cottington, E. M., Matthews, K. A., Talbott, E., & Kuller, L. H. (1986). Occupational stress, suppressed anger, and hypertension. *Psychosomatic Medicine, 48,* 249–260.

Cronbach, L. J., & Furby, L. (1970). How should we measure change or should we? *Psychological Bulletin, 74,* 68–80.

Denniston, J. C., Maher, J. T., Reeves, J. T., Cruz, J. C., Cymerman, R., & Grover, R. F. (1976). Measurement of cardiac output by electrical impedance at rest and during exercise. *Journal of Applied Physiology, 40,* 91–95.

Dimsdale, J. E., Pierce, C., Schoenfeld, D., Brown, A., Zusman, R., & Graham, R. (1986). Suppressed anger and blood pressure: The effects of race, sex, social class, obesity, and age. *Psychosomatic Medicine, 48,* 430–436.

Divers, W. A., Katona, G., Dauchot, P. S., & Hung, J. C. (1977). Continuous real-time computation and display of systolic time intervals from surgical patients. *Computers in Biomedical Research, 10,* 45–59.

Duffy, E. (1957). The psychological significance of the concept of "arousal" or "activation." *Psychological Review, 64,* 265–275.

Dustan, H. P. (1987). Biobehavioral factors in hypertension: Overview. *Circulation Supplement, 76,* 57–60.

Dustan, H. P., Tarazi, R. C., & Frohlich, E. D. (1970). Functional correlates of plasma renin activity in hypertensive patients. *Circulation, 41,* 555–567.

Eckberg, D. L. (1983). Human sinus arrhythmia as an index of vagal cardiac outflow. *Journal of Applied Physiology, 54,* 961–966.

Ekman, P., Levenson, R., & Friesen, W. V. (1983). Autonomic nervous system activity distinguishes among emotions. *Science, 221,* 1208–1210.

Esler, M., Julius, S., Zweïfler, A., Randall, O., Harburg, E., Gardiner, H., & De Quattro, V. (1977). Mild high-renin essential hypertension: Neurogenic human hypertension? *New England Journal of Medicine, 296,* 405–411.

Ewart, C. G., Harris, W. L., Zeger, S., & Russell, G. A. (1986). Diminished pulse pressure under mental stress characterizes normotensive adolescents with parental high blood pressure. *Psychosomatic Medicine, 48,* 489–501.

Falkner, B., Kushner, H., Onesti, G., & Angelakos, E. T. (1981). Cardiovascular characteristics in adolescents who develop essential hypertension. *Hypertension, 3,* 521–527.

Falkner, B. Onesti, G., & Angelakos, E. (1981). Effect of salt loading on the cardiovascular response to stress in adolescents. *Hyptertension, 3,* 195–199.

Falkner, D., Onesti, G., Angelakos, E. T., Fernandes, M., & Langman, C. (1979). Cardiovascular response to mental stress in normal adolescents with hypertensive parents. *Hyptertension, 1,* 23–30.

Folkow, B. (1982). Physiological aspects of primary hypertension. *Physiological Review, 62,* 347–503.

Fouad, F. M., Tarazi, R. C., Ferrario, C. M., Fighaly, S., & Alicandro, C. (1984). Assessment of parasympathetic control of heart rate by a noninvasive method. *American Journal of Physiology, 246,* H838–H842.

Fowles, D. C. (1982). Heart rate as an index of anxiety: Failure of a hypothesis. In J. T. Cacioppo, & R. E. Petty (Eds.), *Perspectives in cardiovascular psychophysiology* (pp. 93–127). New York: Guilford Press.

Fowles, D. C. (1984). Arousal: An examination of its status as a concept. In M. G. H. Coles, J. R. Jennings, & J. A. Stern (Eds.), *Psychophysiological perspectives* (pp. 143–157). New York: Van Nostrand Reinhold.

Fridlund, A. J., & Izard, C. E. (1983). Electromyographic studies of facial expressions of emotions. In J. T. Cacioppo & R. E. Petty (Eds.), *Social psychophysiology* (pp. 243–286). New York: Guilford Press.

Frohlich, E. D., Tarazi, R. C., Ulrych, M., Dustan, H. P., & Page, I. H. (1967). Tilt test for investigating a neural component in hypertension: Its correlation with clinical characteristics. *Circulation, 36,* 387–393.

Funkenstein, D. H., King, S. H., & Drolette, M. E. (Eds.) (1957). *Mastery of stress.* Cambridge, MA: Harvard University Press.

Furberg, C. (1968). Effects of repeated work tests and adrenergic beta-blockade on electrocardiographic ST and T changes. *Acta Medica Scandinvica, 183,* 153–161.

Furedy, J. J., & Heslegrave, R. J. (1983). A consideration of recent criticisms of the T-wave amplitude index of myocardial sympathic activity. *Psychophysiology, 20,* 204–211.

Geddes, L. A. (1970). *The direct and indirect measurement of blood pressure.* Chicago: Year Book Publishers.

Geddes, L. A., & Baker, L. E. (1968). *Principles of applied biomedical instrumentation.* New York: Wiley

Geddes, L. A., & Newberg, D. C. (1977). Cuff pressure oscillations in the measurement of relative blood pressure. *Psychophysiology, 14,* 198–202.

Gellhorn, E. (1964). Motion and emotion. *Psychological Review, 71,* 457–472.

Gerardi, R. J., Blanchard, E. B., Andrasik, F., & McCoy, G. C. (1985). Psychological dimensions of office hypertenion. *Behavior Research and Therapy, 23,* 609–612.

Glasgow, M. S., Gaarder, K. R., & Engel, B. T. (1982). Behavioral treatment of high blood pressure II: Acute and sustained effects of relaxation and systolic blood pressure biofeedback. *Psychosomatic Medicine, 44,* 155–170.

Glass, D. (1977). *Behavior patterns, stress, and coronary disease.* New York: Wiley.

Glass, D. C., Krakoff, L. R., Contrada, R., Hilton, W. F., Kehoe, K., Mannucci, E. G., Collins, C., Snow, B., & Elting, E. (1980). Effect of harassment and competition upon cardiovascular and plasma catecholamine responses in Type A and Type B individuals. *Psychophysiology, 17,* 453–463.

Goldstein I. B. (1981). Assessment of hypertension. In L. A. Bradley & C. K. Prokop (Eds)., *Medical psychology: A new perspective* (pp. 37–54). New York: Academic Press.

Goldstein, I. B., Shapiro, D., & Thananopavarn, C. (1984). Home relaxation techniques for essential hyptertension. *Psychosomatic Medcine, 46,* 398–414.

Gorman, J. M., Goetz, R. R., Fyer, M., King, D. L., Fyer, A. J., Liebowitz, M. R., & Klein, D. F., (1980). The mitral valve proplapse–panic disorder connection. *Psychosomatic Medicine, 50,* 144–122.

Graham. F. K. (1978a). Normality of distributions and homogeneity of variance of heart rate and heart period samples. *Psychophysiology, 15,* 487–491.

Graham, F. K. (1978b). Constraints on measuring heart rate and period sequentially through real and cardiac time. *Psychophysiology, 15,* 492–495.

Graham, F. K. (1980). Representing cardiac activity in relation to time. In I. Martin & P. H. Venables (Eds.), *Techniques in psychophysiology* (pp. 192–197). New York: Wiley.

Graham, F. K. (1984). An affair of the heart. In M. G. H. Coles, J. R. Jennings, & J. A. Stern (Eds.), *Psychophysiological perspectives* (pp. 171–188). New York: Van Nostrand Reinhold.

Graham, F. K., & Jackson, J. C. (1970). Arousal systems and infant heart rate responses. In H. W. Reese & L. P. Lipsitt (Eds.), *Advances in child development and behavior* (Vol. 5, pp. 69–117). New York: Academic Press.

Gribbin, B., Steptoe, A., & Sleight, P. (1976). Pulse wave velocity as a measure of blood pressure change. *Psychophysiology, 13*, 86–90.

Grignolo, A., Koepke, J. P., & Obrist, P. A. (1982). Renal function, heart rate and blood pressure during exercise and shock avoidance in dogs. *American Journal of Physiology, 242*, R482–R490.

Groen, J. J., Hansen, B., Hermann, J. M., Shäfer, N., Schmidt, T. H., Selbmann, R. H., Uexkull, T. V., & Weckmann, P. (1977). Hemodynamic responses during experimental emotional stress and physical exercise in hypertensive and normotensive patients. In W. DeJong, A. P. Provoost, & A. P. Shapiro (Eds.), *Progress in brain research: Vol. 47. Hypertension and brain mechanisms*. Amsterdam: Elsevier.

Guyton, A. C. (1979). *Physiology of the human body*. Philadelphia: Saunders.

Guyton, A. C. (1986). *Textbook of medical physiology*. Philadelphia: Saunders.

Guyton, A. C., Jones, C. E., & Coleman, T. G. (1973). *Circulatory physiology: Cardiac output and its regulation*. Philadelphia: Saunders.

Haddad, G. G., Jeng, H. J., Lee, S. H., & Lai, T. L. (1984). Rhythmic variations in R-R interval during sleep and wakefulness in puppies and dogs. *American Journal of Physiology, 247*, H67–H73.

Harris, A. H., & Brady, J. B. (1974). Animal learning – visceral and autonomic conditioning. In M. R. Rosenzweig & L. W. Porter (Eds.), *Annual review of psychology* (pp. 107–133). Palo Alto: Annual Reviews.

Harris, W. S., Schoenfeld, C. D., & Weissler, A. M. (1981). Effects of adrenergic receptor activation and blockade on the systolic pre-ejection period, heart rate, and arterial pressure in man. *Journal of Clinical Investigation, 46*, 1704–1714.

Hastrup, J. L. (1986). Duration of initial heart rate assessment in Psychophysiology: Current practices and implications. *Psychophysiology, 23*, 15–17.

Hastrup, J. L., Hotchkiss, A. P., & Johnson, C. A. (1985). Accuracy of knowledge of family history of cardiovascular disorders. *Health Psychology, 4*, 291–306.

Hastrup, J. L., Light, K. C., & Obrist, P. A. (1982). Parental hypertension and cardiovascular response to stress in healthy young adults. *Psychophysiology, 19*, 615–622.

Henry, J. P., & Cassell, J. C. (1969). Psychosocial factors in essential hyptertension: Recent epidemiologic and animal experimental evidence. *American Journal of Epidemiology, 90*, 171–200.

Henry, J. P., & Stephens, P. M. (1977). *Stress, health, and the social environment: A sociobiologic approach to medicine*. New York: Springer-Verlag.

Herd, J. A. (1986). Behavioral influences on neuroendocrines and insulin sensitivity as precursors of coronary heart disease. In T.H. Schmidt, T. M. Dembroski, & G. Blumchen (Eds.), *Biological and psychological factors in cardiovascular disease* (pp. 389–405). Berlin: Springer-Verlag.

Heslegrave, R. J., Ogilvie, J. C., & Furedy, J. J. (1979). Measuring baseline-treatment differences in heart rate variability: Variance versus successive difference mean square and beats per minute versus interbeat interval. *Psychophysiology, 16*, 151–157.

Heslegrave, R. J., & Furedy, J. J. (1979). Sensitivities of HR and T-wave amplitude for detecting cognitive and anticipatory stress. *Psychophysiology, 22*, 17–23.

Heslegrave, R. J., & Furedy, J. J. (1980). Carotid *dP/dt* as a psychophysiological index of sympathetic myocardial effects: Some considerations. *Psychophysiology, 17*, 482–494.

Hord, D. J., Johnson, L. G., & Lubin, A. (1964). Differential effects of the law of initial values (LIV) on autonomic variables. *Psychophysiology, 1*, 79–87.

Hull, D. H., Wolthuis, R. A., Cortese, T., Longo, M. R., & Triebwasser, J. H. (1977). Borderline hypertension versus normotension: Differential response to orthostatic stress. *American Heart Journal, 94*, 414–420.

James, S. (1987). Psychosocial precursors of hyptertension: A review of the epidemiologic evidence. *Circulation Supplement, 76*, 60–67.

Jennings, J. R. (1986). Memory, thought, and bodily response. In M. G. H. Coles, E. Donchin, & S. W. Porges (Eds.), *Psychophysiology: Systems, processes, and applications* (pp. 290–308). New York: Guilford Press.

Jennings, J. R. (1986). Bodily changes during attending. In M. G. H. Coles, E. Donchin, & S. W. Porges (Eds.), *Psychophysiology: Systems, processes, and applications* (pp. 268–289). New York: Guilford Press.

Jennings, J. R., Berg, K. W., Hutcheson, J. S., Obrist, P., Porges, S., & Turpin, G. (1981). Publication guidelines for heart rate studies in man. *Psychophysiology, 3,* 226–231.

Jennings, J. R., Stringfellow, J. C., & Graham, M. (1974). A comparison of the statistical distributions of beat-by-beat heart rate and heart period. *Psychophysiology, 11,* 207–210.

Jennings, J. R., Tahmoush, A. J., & Redmond, D. P. (1980). Non-invasive measurement of peripheral vascular activity. In I. Martin & P. H. Venables (Eds.), *Techniques in psychophysiology* (pp. 69–137). New York: Wiley.

Jennings, J. R., & Wood, C. C. (1976). The ϵ-adjustment procedure for repeated measures analysis of variance. *Psychophysiology, 13,* 277–278.

Jennings, J. R., & Wood, C. C. (1977). Principal component separation of pre- and post-response effects on cardiac interbeat-intervals in a reaction time (RT) task. *Psychophysiology, 14,* 89–90.

Jost, H., Ruilmann, C. J., Hill, T. S., & Gulo, M. J. (1952). Studies in hypertension: II. Central and autonomic nervous system reactions of hypertensive individuals to simple physical and psychologic stress situations. *Journal of Nervous and Mental Diseases, 115,* 252–262.

Kagan, J., Reznick, J. S., Clarke, C., Snidman, N., & Coll, C. C. (1984). Cardiac correlates of behavioral inhibition in the young child. In M. G. H. Coles, J. R. Jennings, & J. A. Stern (Eds.), *Psychophysiological perspectives* (pp. 216–229). New York: Van Nostrand Reinhold.

Kannel, W. B. (1977). Importance of hyptertension as a major risk factor in cardiovascular disease. In J. Genest, E. Koiw, & O. Kuchel (Eds.), *Hyptertension* (pp. 888–910). New York: McGraw-Hill.

Kannel, W. B., & Sorlie, P. (1975). Hypertension in Framingham. In O. Paul (Ed.), *Epidemiology and control of hypertension.* Miami, FL: Symposia Specialists.

Kaplan, N. M. (1980). The control of hypertension: A therapeutic breakthrough. *American Scientist, 68,* 537–545.

Katona, P. G., & Jih, R. (1975). Respiratory sinus arrhythmia: A non-invasive assessment of parasympathetic cardiac control. *Journal of Applied Physiology, 39,* 801–805.

Krantz, D. S., DeQuattro, V., Blackburn, H. W., Eaker, E., Haynes, S., James, S. A., Manuck, S. B., Myers, H., Shekell, R. B., Syme, S. L., Tyroler, H. A., & Wolf, S. (1987). *Circulation Supplement, 76,* 84–89.

Krantz, D. S., & Manuck, S. B. (1984). Acute psychophysiologic reactivity and risk of cardiovascular disease. *Psychological Bulletin, 96,* 435–464.

Kuller, L. H., Talbott, E. O., & Robinson, C. (1987). Environmental and psychosocial determinants of sudden death. *Circulation Supplement, 76,* 177–186.

Lacey, J. I. (1967). Somatic response patterning and stress: Some revisions of activation theory. In M. H. Appley & R. Trumbull (Eds.), *Psychological stress: Issues in research* (pp. 4–44). New York: Appleton-Century-Crofts.

Lacey, J. I., & Lacey, B. C. (1962). The law of initial value in the longitudinal study of autonomic constitution: Reproducibility of autonomic responses and response patterns over a four year interval. *Annals of the New York Academy of Science, 38,* 1257–1290.

Lader, M. H. (1967). Pneumatic plethysmography. In P. H. Venables & I. Martin (Eds.), *A manual of psychophysiological methods* (pp. 159–184). Amsterdam: North-Holland.

Lamberts, R., Visser, K. R., & Zijlstra, W. G. (1984). *Impedance cardiography.* The Netherlands: Van Gorcum.

Lane, J. D., Greenstadt, L., Shapiro, D., & Rubinstein, E. (1983). Pulse transit time and blood pressure: An intensive analysis. *Psychophysiology, 20,* 45–49.

Lane, R. D., & Schwartz, G. E. (1987). Induction of lateralized sympathetic input to the heart by the CNS during emotional arousal: A possible neurophysiologic trigger of sudden cardiac death. *Psychosomatic Medicine, 49,* 274–285.

Larsen, P. B., Schneiderman, N., & Pasin, R. D. (1986). Physiological bases of cardiovascular psychophysiology. In M. G. H. Coles, E. Donchin, & S. W. Porges (Eds.), *Psychophysiology: Systems, processes, and applications* (pp. 122–165). New York: Guilford Press.

Lewis, R. P., Rittgers, S. E., Forester, W. F., & Boudoulas, H. A. (1977). A critical review of systolic time intervals. *Circulation, 56,* 146–158.

Light, K. C. (1981). Cardiovascular responses to effortful active coping: Implications for the role of stress in hypertension development. *Psychophysiology, 18,* 216–225.

Light, K. C. (1987). Psychosocial precursors of hypertension: Experimental evidence. *Circulation Supplement, 76,* 67–77.

Light, K. C., Koepke, J. P., Obrist, P. A., & Willis, P. W. (1983). Psychological stress induces sodium and fluid retention in men at high risk for hypertension *Science, 220,* 429–431.

Lindsley, D. B. (1951). Emotion. In S. S. Stevens (Ed.), *Handbook of experimental psychology* (pp. 473–516). New York: Wiley.

Lovallo, W., & Zeiner, A. R. (1975). Some factors influencing the vasomotor response to cold pressor stimulation. *Psychophysiology, 13*, 499–505.

Lown, B. (1987). Sudden cardiac death: Biobehavioral perspective. *Circulation Supplement, 76*, 186–196.

Lykken, D. T. (1972). Range correction applied to heart rate and GSR data. *Psychophysiology, 9*, 373–379.

Malmo, R. B. (1959). Activation: A neuropsychological dimension. *Psychological Review, 66*, 367–386.

Manuck, S., & Proietti, J. M. (1982). Parental hypertension and cardiovascular response to cognitive and isometric challenge. *Psychophysiology, 19*, 481–489.

Martin, J. E., Epstein, L. H., & Cinciripini, P. M. (1980). Effects of feedback and stimulus control of pulse transit time discrimination. *Psychophysiology, 17*, 431–436.

Matyas, T. A., & King, M. G. (1976). Stable T-wave effects during improvement of heart rate control with biofeedback. *Physiology and Behavior, 16*, 15–20.

Mesulam, M., & Perry, J. (1972). The diagnosis of lovesickness: Experimental psychophysiology without the polygraph. *Psychophysiology, 9*, 546–551.

Miller, J. C., & Horvath, S. M. (1978). Impedance cardiography. *Psychophysiology, 15*, 80–91.

Morell, M. A., Myers, H. F., Shapiro, D., Goldstein, I. B., & Armstrong, M. A. (1988). Psychophysiological reactivity to mental arithmetic stress in black and white normotensive men. *Health Psychology, 1*, 479–496.

Newlin, D. B., & Levenson, R. W. (1979). Measuring beta-adrenergic influences upon the heart: Pre-ejection period. *Psychophysiology, 16*, 546–553.

Newlin, D. B., & Levenson, R. W. (1980). Voluntary control of pulse transmission time to the ear. *Psychophysiology, 17*, 581–585.

Obrist, P. A. (1981). *Cardiovascular psychophysiology – A perspective.* New York: Plenum Press.

Obrist, P. A. (1982). Cardiac-behavioral interactions: A critical appraisal. In J. T. Cacioppo & R. E. Petty (Eds.), *Perspectives in cardiovascular psychophysiology* (pp. 265–296). New York: Guilford Press.

Obrist, P. A. (1984). Some thoughts on the "psychophysiological strategy." In M. G. H. Coles, J. R. Jennings, & J. A. Stern (Eds.), *Psychophysiological perspectives* (pp. 188–199). New York: Van Nostrand Reinhold.

Obrist, P. A., Howard, J. L., Lawler, J. E., Sutterer, J. R., Smithson, K. W., & Martin, P. L. (1972). Alterations in cardiac contractility during classical aversive conditioning in dogs: Methodological and theoretical implications. *Psychophysiology, 9*, 246–261.

Obrist, P. A., Light, K. C., Langer, A. W., & Koepke, J. P. (1986). Psychosomatics. In M. G. H. Coles, E. Donchin, & S. W. Porges (Eds.), *Psychophysiology: Systems, processes, and applications* (pp. 626–646). New York: Guilford Press.

Obrist, P. A., Light, K., McCubbin, J. A., Hutcheson, J. S., & Hoffer, J. L. (1979). Pulse transit time: Relationship to blood pressure and myocardial performance. *Psychophysiology, 16*, 292–301.

Ohman, A., & Dimberg, U. (1984). An evolutionary perspective on human social behavior. In W. M. Waid (Ed.), *Sociophysiology* (pp. 47–87). New York: Springer-Verlag.

Paller, K., & Shapiro, D. (1983). Systolic blood pressure and a simple reaction time task. *Psychophysiology, 20*, 585–589.

Papillo, J. F., Tursky, B., & Friedman, R. (1981). Perceived changes in the intensity of arterial pulsations as a function of applied cuff pressure. *Psychophysiology, 18*, 283–287.

Perini, C., Muller, F. B., Rauchfleisch, U., Battegay, R., & Buhler, F. R. (1986). Hyperadrenergic borderline hypertension is characterized by suppressed aggression. *Journal of Cardiovascular Pharmacology, 8*, s53–s56.

Perski, A., Engel, B. T., & McCroskery, J. H. (1982). The modification of elicited cardiovascular responses by operant conditioning of heart rate. In J. T. Cacioppo & R. E. Petty (Eds.), *Perspectives in cardiovascular psychophysiology* (pp. 296–315). New York: Guilford Press.

Porges, S. W. (1986). Respiratory sinus arrhythmia: Physiological basis, quantitative methods, and clinical implications. In P. Grossman, K. H. L. Jansen, & D. Vaitl (Eds.), *Cardiorespiratory and cardiosomatic psychophysiology* (pp. 101–115). New York: Plenum Press.

Porges, S. W., McCabe, P. M., & Yongue, B. G. (1982). Respiratory–heart rate interactions: Psychophysiological implications for pathophysiology and behavior. In J. T. Cacioppo & R.

E. Petty (Eds.), *Perspectives in cardiovascular psychophysiology* (pp. 223–264). New York: Guilford Press.

Posey, J. A., Geddes, L. A., Williams, H., & Moore, A. G. (1969). The meaning of the point of maximum oscillations in cuff pressure in the indirect measurement of blood pressure. Part 1. *Cardiovascular Research Bulletin, 8,* 15–25.

Raczkowska, M., Eckberg, D. L., & Ebert, T. J. (1983). Muscarinic cholinergic receptors modulate vagal cardiac responses in man. *Journal of the Autonomic Nervous System, 7,* 271–278.

Randall, W. C. (Ed.) (1977). *Neural regulation of the heart.* New York: Oxford University Press.

Reis, D. J., & Ledoux, J. E. (1987). Some central neural mechanisms governing resting and behaviorally coupled control of blood pressure. *Circulation Supplement, 76,* 2–10.

Report of Task Force on Blood Pressure Control in Children. (1977). *Pediatrics, 59,* 797–820.

Rosenman, R. H., Brand, R. J., Jenkins, C. D., Friedman, M., Straus, R., & Wurm, M. (1975). Coronary heart disease in the Western Collaborative Group Study: Final follow-up experience of $8\frac{1}{2}$ years. *JAMA, 233,* 872–877.

Rushmer, R. F. (1976). *Structure and function of the cardiovascular system.* Philadelphia: Saunders.

Sayers, B. M. (1970). Inferring significance from biological signals. In M. Clynes & J. H. Milsum (Eds.), *Biomedical engineering systems* (pp. 84–164). New York: McGraw-Hill.

Sayers, B. M. (1980). Pattern analysis of the heart rate signal. In I. Martin & P. H. Venables (Eds.), *Techniques in psychophysiology* (pp. 197–210). New York: Wiley.

Schachter, J. (1957). Pain, fear and anger in hypertensives and normotensives. *Psychosomatic Medicine, 19,* 17–29.

Schneider, R. A., & Zangari, V. M. (1951). Variations in clotting time, relative viscosity and other physiochemical properties of the blood accompanying physical and emotional stress in the normotensive and hypertensive subject. *Psychosomatic Medicine, 13,* 288–303.

Schneider, R. H., Egan, B. M., Johnson, E. H., Drobny, H., & Julius, S. (1986). Anger and anxiety in borderline hypertension. *Psychosomatic Medicine, 48,* 242–248.

Schneiderman, N. (1987). Psychophysiologic factors in atherogenesis and coronary artery disease. *Circulation Supplement, 76,* 41–48.

Schwartz, G. E. (1982). Cardiovascular psychophysiology: A systems perspective. In J. T. Cacioppo & R. E. Petty (Eds.), *Perspective in cardiovascular psychophysiology* (pp. 347–373). New York: Guilford Press.

Schwartz, G. E. (1986). Emotion and psychophysiological organization: A systems approach. In M. G. H. Coles, E. Donchin, & S. W. Porges (Eds.), *Psychophysiology: Systems, processes, and applications* (pp. 354–377). New York: Guilford Press.

Schwartz, G. E., Weinberger, D. A., & Singer, J. A. (1981). Cardiovascular differentiation of happiness, sadness, anger and fear following imagery and exercise. *Psychosomatic Medicine, 43,* 343–364.

Schwartz, P. J., & Weiss, T. (1983). T-wave amplitude as an index of cardiac sympathetic activity: A misleading concept. *Psychophysiology, 20,* 696–701.

Selye, H. (1976). *The stress of life.* New York: McGraw-Hill.

Shapiro, D., & Crider, A. (1969). Psychophysiological approaches in social psychology. In G. Lindzey & E. Aronson (Eds.), *Handbook of social psychology* (2nd ed., Vol. 3, pp. 1–49). Reading, MA: Addison-Wesley.

Shapiro, D., & Goldstein, I. B. (1982). Biobehavioral perspectives on hypertension. *Journal of Consulting and Clinical Psychology, 50,* 841–858.

Shapiro, D., Greenstadt, L., Lane, J. D., & Rubinstein, E. (1981). Tracking-cuff system for beat-to-beat recording of blood pressure. *Psychophysiology, 18,* 129–136.

Shapiro, D., & Reeves, J. L. (1982). Modification of physiological and subjective responses to stress through heart rate biofeedback. In J. T. Cacioppo & R. Petty (Eds.), *Perspectives in cardiovascular psychophysiology* (pp. 127–150). New York: Guilford Press.

Shapiro, D., Tursky, B., Gershon, E. E., & Stern, M. (1969). Effects of feedback and reinforcement on the control of human systolic blood pressure. *Science, 163,* 588–590.

Shepherd, J. T., & Weiss, S. M. (Eds.) (1987). *Circulation Supplement* (Vol. 76). American Heart Association: Conference on behavioral medicine and cardiovascular disease. Sea Island, GA, 1985.

Shepherd, J. T., Dembroski, T. M., Brody, M. J., Dimsdale, J. E., Eliot, E. S., Light, K .C., Miller, N. E., Myers, H. F., Obrist, P. A., Schneiderman, N., Skinner, J. E., & Williams, R. B., Jr. (1987). Task Force 3: Biobehavioral mechanisms in coronary artery disease. Acute stress. *Circulation Supplement, 76,* 150–158.

Shine, K. I. (1987). Conclusions. *Circulation Supplement, 76,* 225–227.

Stephenson, R. B. (1984). Modification of reflex regulation of blood pressure by behavior. *Annual Review of Physiology, 46,* 133–142.

Steptoe, A. (1976). Blood pressure control: A comparison of feedback and instructions using pulse wave velocity measurements. *Psycophysiology, 13,* 528–535.

Steptoe, A. (1980). Blood pressure. In I. Martin & P. H. Venables (Eds.), *Techniques in Psychophysiology* (pp. 247–273). New York: Wiley.

Steptoe, A. (1981). *Psychological factors in cardiovascular disorders.* London: Academic Press.

Stern, R. M., & Ray, W. J. (1984). Methods in sociophysiology. In W. M. Waid (Ed.), *Sociophysiology* (pp. 21–46). New York: Springer-Verlag.

Stern, S., & Eisenberg, S. (1969). The effect of propranolo (Inderol) on the electrocardiogram in normal subjects. *American Heart Journal, 77,* 192–195.

Stoney, C. M., Davis, M. C., & Matthews, K. A. (1987). Sex differences in physiological responses to stress and in coronary heart disease: A causal link? *Psychophysiology, 24,* 127–132.

Surwit, R. S., Williams, R. B., & Shapiro, D. (1982). *Behavioral approaches to cardiovascular disease.* New York: Academic Press.

Thakor, N. V., & Webster, J. G. (1985). Electrode studies for the long-term ambulatory ECG. *Medical and Biological Engineering and Computing, 23,* 1–7.

Tursky, B. (1974). The indirect recording of human blood pressure. In P. A. Obrist, A. H. Black, J. Brener, & L. V. DiCara (Eds.), *Cardiovascular psychophysiology* (pp. 93–105). Chicago: Aldine Press.

Tursky, B., & Jamner, L. D. (1982). Measurement of cardiovascular functioning. In J. T. Cacioppo & R. E. Petty (Eds.), *Perspectives in cardiovascular psychophysiology* (pp. 19–92). New York: Guilford Press.

Tursky, B., Papillo, J. F., & Friedman, R. (1982). The perception of arterial pulsations: Implications for the behavioral treatment of hypertension. *Journal of Psychosomatic Research, 26,* 485–493.

Tursky, B., Shapiro, D., & Schwartz, G. E. (1972). Automated constant cuff pressure system to measure average systolic and diastolic pressure in man. *IEEE Transactions in Biomedical Engineering, 19,* 271–276.

Van Egeren, L. (1979). Social interactions, communications, and the coronary-prone behavior pattern: A psychophysiological study. *Psychosomatic Medicine, 41,* 20–18.

Van Egeren, L. W. (1984). Social processes, biology, and disease. In W. M. Waid (Ed.), *Sociophysiology* (pp. 249–283). New York: Springer-Verlag.

Vander, A. J., Sherman, M. H., & Luciano, D. S. (Eds.). (1970). *Human physiology: The mechanisms of body function.* New York: McGraw-Hill.

Varni, J. G., Clarke, E., & Giddon, D. B. (1971). Analysis of cyclic heart rate variability. *Psychophysiology, 8,* 406–413.

Victor, R., Weipert, D., & Shapiro, D. (1984). Volutary control of systolic blood pressure during postural change. *Psychophysiology, 21,* 673–682.

Waid, W. M. (Ed.) (1984). *Sociophysiology.* New York: Springer-Verlag.

Watt, G. (1986). Design and interpretation of studies comparing individuals with and without a family history of high blood pressure. *Journal of Hypertension, 4,* 1–7.

Webster, J. G. (1978). Measurement of flow and volume of blood. In J. G. Webster (Ed.), *Medical instrumentation: Application and design* (pp. 385–433). Boston: Houghton Mifflin.

Weder, A. B., & Julius, S. (1985). Behavior, blood pressure variability, and hypertension. *Psychosomatic Medicine, 47,* 406–414.

Weiner, H. (1979). *Psychobiology of essential hypertension.* New York: Elsevier.

Weipert, D., Shapiro, D., & Suter, T. W. (1987). Family history of hypertension and orthostatic stress. *Psychophysiology, 24,* 251–257.

Weissler, A. M., Stack, R. S., & Sohn, Y. H. (1980). The accuracy of systolic time intervals as a measure of left ventricular function. In W. F. List, J. S. Gravenstein, & D. H. Spodick (Eds.), *Systolic time intervals.* New York: Springer-Verlag.

Wheeler, T., & Watkins, P. J. (1973). Cardiac denervation in diabetes. *British Medical Journal, 4,* 584–586.

Whitney, R. J. (1953). The measurement of volume changes in human limbs. *Journal of Physiology, 121,* 1–27.

Wilke, D. R. (1970). *Muscle.* London: Edward Arnold.

William, J. G. L., & Williams, B. (1965). Arterial pulse wave velocity as a psychophysiological measure. *Psychosomatic Medicine, 27,* 408–414.

Williams, R. B., Jr. (1984). Measurement of local blood flow during behavioral experiments: Principles and practice. In J. A. Herd, A. M. Gotto, P. G. Kaufmann, & S. M. Weiss (Eds.), *Proceedings of the working conference on applicability of new technology to biobehavioral research* (pp. 207–217). NIH Publication # 84–1654.

Williams, R. B., Jr. (1987). Psychological factors in coronary artery disease: Epidemiologic evidence. *Circulation Supplement, 76*, 117–124.

Williams, R. B., Jr., Kimball, C. P., & Williard, H. N. (1972). The influence of interpersonal interaction on diastolic blood pressure. *Psychosomatic Medicine, 34*, 194–198.

Willis, R. (1965). The works of William Harvey, M. D.: Translated from the Latin with a life of the author. New York: Johnson Reprint. (Originally published in London by Sydenhan Society, 1847.)

Wilson, R. S. (1974). CARDIVAR: The statistical analysis of heart rate data. *Psychophysiology, 11*, 76–85.

World Health Organization (1978). *Arterial hypertension: Report of WHO Expert Committee* (Technical Report Series, No. 628). Geneva: World Health Organization.

Zemaityte, D., Varoneckas, G., & Sokolov, E. (1984). Heart rhythm control during sleep. *Psychophysiology, 21*, 279–289.

15 *The ocular system*

JOHN A. STERN AND DOUGLAS N. DUNHAM

15.1 INTRODUCTION

That the eye is an important source of information *for* the observer can be readily documented. That it can serve as a channel of communication *with* others is well documented in our language. Who has not been the recipient of angry stares, a knowing wink, or if fortunate, a seductive glance? That it can serve as a source of information *about* the observer is less apparent. Our focus in this chapter will be on the eye, not as an instrument for sensing and perceiving the environment, not as a tool for conscious communication, but as an instrument for informing us about perceptual, cognitive, and affective activity. What aspects of the visual system provide such information to the observer? It will be our contention that all aspects of the visual system can provide us with clues about how the subject deals with information, whether that information comes in through the eyes or the other senses. In this chapter, we propose to look at three aspects of the visual system, namely, changes in pupil diameter, eye movements, and eyelid movements (i.e., eyeblinks).

Pupillary diameter changes can be readily observed by altering the amount of light impinging on the eye or through pharmacological manipulation. Those occasioned by more subtle psychological variables are not so readily observed and require special instrumentation for their recording and quantification (Beatty, 1982). Similarly, eye movements are readily observed and can be used to infer where a person is looking. They have been used since the late-nineteenth century to make inferences about the reading process (Huey, 1908) and have more recently been used as a tool to help in the diagnosis of psychiatric problems (Holzman, Kringlen, Levy, & Haberman, 1980), as an index of preferred modes of information processing (Bakan, 1971), and as an index of altered states of alertness (Stern, Goldstein, & Walrath, 1984). Eyelid activity, principally the eyeblink, has been used to judge the presence of symptoms of anxiety, whether situationally produced (Ponder & Kennedy, 1928) or as an organismic trait (Kanfer, 1960). There has been considerable debate in the literature on its utility as a measure of fatigue (Bitterman, 1945; Luckiesh & Moss, 1942). We (Stern, Walrath, & Goldstein 1984) have asked whether the nature or waveform of the eyeblink is affected by task demands and whether blinks are randomly occurring events or are more likely to occur at psychologically meaningful moments.

There are, thus, a variety of reasons why psychologists should pay more serious attention to this "window to the soul" than we have done in the past.

15.2   GROSS ANATOMY OF THE EYE

15.2.1   *Physical makeup of the pupil*

Beatty (1986) has stated that "the pupil provides psychophysiology with a window to the brain" (p. 43). Because of the link between pupillary activity and central nervous system (CNS) functioning (Loewenfeld, 1958; Lowenstein & Loewenfeld, 1962; Moruzzi, 1972), there is no doubt that the pupil can provide us with information regarding brain activation, cognitive processing, and attention (Beatty, 1982).

15.2.1.1   *The iris*

The iris is a disk-shaped, pigmented tissue with a central aperture (the pupil) that is elliptical in shape toward the nasal side. The amount of retinal stimulation is approximately proportional to pupil size; the main function of the iris, then, is to control the amount of light reaching the retina. It does this by adjusting the size of the pupil. The size of the pupil can range from 2 to 8 mm, with an average size of 4 mm. There are three main functions of the iridic musculature: (1) to adjust for ambient illumination; (2) to reduce the aperture of the lens, thus increasing depth of field; and (3) to regulate pupil diameter, improving visual acuity by reducing aberrations. Generally speaking, lens accommodation and the light reflex are the principal determinants of pupillary oscillation, with deviations due to CNS activity "superimposed" (Beatty, 1986). Iridic adjustment is controlled by two muscles: the sphincter pupillae and the dilator pupillae.

Sphincter pupillae. The sphincter pupillae is composed of smooth, ringlike muscle fibers 0.5–1.0 mm wide and 40–80 μm thick that serve to close the pupil by expanding the iris; it is controlled by *parasympathetic* postganglionic muscle fibers.

Dilator pupillae. The dilator pupillae serves to control the size of the pupil by contraction, which results in the retraction of the iris and the enlargement of the pupil. Because of the connection of their fibers, each muscle (sphincter and dilator) is able to act directly upon the other. The sphincter "stretches" the dilator, and the dilator "unfolds" the sphincter (Alexandridis, 1985). The dilator pupillae is innervated mostly by *sympathetic* nerve fibers.

15.2.1.2   *Efferent neuronal control of the pupil*

Parasympathetic innervation of the sphincter pupillae. This point of origin for control of the sphincter pupillae is at the Edinger–Westphal nucleus located in the central core of the midbrain. The neural pathway continues with efferent fibers exiting the brain through the third cranial nerve. The pathway to the eye is then interrupted by a synapse at the ciliary ganglion; at this point, excitatory projections are made to the sphincter pupillae via the ciliary ganglion (acetylcholine is the neurotransmitter substance) with some evidence of an inhibitory projection to the dilator pupillae.

Sympathetic innervation of the dilator pupillae. The sympathetic innervation of the dilator pupillae involves neural populations in three discrete areas. The origin of the first is at the hypothalamus projecting downward to the ciliospinal center of the lateral anterior horns (located in the upper thoracic and lower cervical regions of the spinal cord). Fibers for the second neuron arise from here, merge with the anterior roots, and continue to the cervical sympathetic trunk where they synapse with the superior cervical ganglion. Finally, sympathetic efferents join here and travel through the carotid plexus to the first division of the trigeminal nerve and directly to the dilator pupillae of the iris.

15.2.1.3 *Control of pupillae through more central brain regions*

Beatty (1986) contends that pupillary activity should be regarded as an indication of more complex central events rather than an insulated oculomotor response. The reticular activating system of the brainstem controls, in large part, pupillary movements. Why, then, should we expect that pupillary oscillations reflect cortical activity? Luria (1973) and Beatty (1982) suggest that there is an interaction between the reticular activating system and the cerebral cortex: The reticular activating system sends fibers to as well as receives fibers from the cerebral cortex; changes detected in the size of the pupil in response to a task requiring cognitive processing then most likely reflect cortical modulation of the reticular formation.

15.2.2 *Anatomical substrates responsible for eye movements*

15.2.2.1 *Afferent system*

In order to receive information, the eye must be focused "at the right place at the right time." Eye position is controlled by afferent as well as efferent limbs. Both limb systems are responsible for relaying sensory information regarding current eye position with the efferent system, in particular, controlling eye movements. Although visual input appears to be the primary determinant of eye position, proprioceptive inputs and "an internal 'memory' of eye position are likely to be present" (Feldon & Burde, 1987, p. 122).

15.2.2.2 *Efferent system*

The specific purpose of the efferent system is to coordinate the extraocular musculature to direct the eyes to a chosen target. These muscles are controlled by three pairs of cranial nerves whose nuclei "reside" in the brainstem, sending axons through the superior orbital fissure (by way of the sinus) and extending into the orbit to terminate on the individual ocular muscles.

15.2.2.3 *Eye movement system*

Obviously, one of the most important functions of the oculomotor system is to coordinate binocular movements of the eyes. Very complex anatomical and physiological relationships are responsible for these movements (called *version*), and the innervation of these muscles extends to different agonist muscles. The anatomical relationships responsible for coordinating horizontal and vertical eye movements have only recently been delineated.

Horizontal movements. It appears that conjugate eye movements are controlled by the paramedian pontine reticular formation. In primates, direct pathways have been identified, beginning at the paramedian pontine reticular formation, extending to the ipsilateral abducens motoneurons and interneurons, and projecting to the medial recticular subnuclei of the oculomotor nerve (Buettner-Ennever & Henn, 1976).

Vertical movements. Researchers have not been able to pinpoint, with much success, the subtrate responsible for vertical eye movements. Five areas have all been mentioned: the interstitial nucleus of Cajal, the nucleus of Darkschewitsch, the nucleus of the posterior commissure in the pretectum, the posterior commissure, and the rostral interstitial nucleus of the medial longitudinal fasciculus (Feldon & Burde, 1987). It is the latter that is considered the most likely candidate as the premotor nucleus for vertical eye movements (both upward and downward) (Buettner-Ennever, 1977). The "staging area," however, is thought to originate in the medial portion of the paramedian pontine reticular formation, which projects to the rostral interstitial nucleus of the medial longitudinal fasciculus from which extensions attach to the trochlear nucleus and the vertical subnuclei of the oculomotor nerve (Buettner-Ennever & Lang, 1978).

15.2.3   Eyelid musculature

15.2.3.1   Eyelid elevation

Voluntary and reflexive opening and closing of the eyelids are controlled by a motor system composed of the levator palpebrae superioris, the orbicularis oculi, and the smooth muscles of Mueller in the upper and lower eyelids. Contraction of the levator palpebrae superioris results in the elevation of the eyelid, raised approximately 10 mm against gravity. Elevation is further assisted by smooth muscle fibers, the muscles of Mueller, innervated by the sympathetic nervous system arising from the undersurface of the levator and inserting into the upper margin of the tarsus. The main muscle producing eyelid elevation is the levator muscle, but activity of the superior rectus muscle is also implicated. The activity of the former is normally associated with contraction of the superior rectus muscle (Fox, 1966); this relationship is supported by the connection of the two muscles to a common fascial sheath. This has been demonstrated in operations in which the superior rectus is recessed on the globe. In such operations, the levator is affected such that the upper eyelid will be raised, widening the palpebral fissure. On the other hand, resecting or advancing the superior rectus pulls the levator muscle forward, causing the eyelid to droop (called ptosis).

15.2.3.2   Eyelid closure

The seventh cranial nerve innervates the orbicularis oculi, the muscle responsible for eyelid closure. The orbicularis muscle can be broken down anatomically into two "portions": the palpebral portion and the orbital portion. The two portions work in conjunction with one another, with the orbital portion also working with the muscles of the eyebrow.

There are different functional groups in the orbicularis oculi: those responding in blinking and in the corneal reflex and those responding in blinking and in sustained activity, which lie mainly in the pretarsal region, the preseptal region, and the orbital region, respectively (Moses, 1987). These areas are not unique in their functioning. For example, when a blink is first initiated, the reciprocal innervation of the muscles determine the maintenance of the blink. That is, relaxation of the levator muscle, not contraction of the palpebral portion of the orbicularis, is the first physical stage of the blink. Moses (1987) notes that relaxation of the levator has particular importance "in that it allows the orbicularis to contract from the start against reduced resistance" (p. 8).

15.3 THE MEASUREMENT OF OCULOMOTOR VARIABLES: PUPIL, EYE MOVEMENTS, AND BLINKS

It has been said that Chinese jade merchants infer a potential customer's interest in a particular piece of jade by observing alterations in pupillary diameter. Similarly, an occasional poker player will claim to be able to judge an opponent's hand from looking at his pupils. Unfortunately, these observations are in need of experimental verification. The earliest and still most frequently used procedures involve *direct observations*. This, of course, is a tedious procedure and allows for only crude measures, such as making judgments about changes in pupil diameter of the order of "smaller" or "larger" from time 1 to time 2.

For eye position shifts, one can also use observational techniques to index alterations in gaze, eye movements associated with visual information abstraction, as well as involuntary eye movements associated with thinking. As a matter of interest, all of the *conjugate lateral eye movement* (CLEM) literature, as reviewed by Ehrlichman and Weinberger (1978), has used such observational procedures.

The counting of eyeblinks and relating eyeblinks to other bodily activity has been studied by such observational techniques (Ponder & Kennedy, 1928).

Of the various types of oculomotor activity that have been investigated, the dilation/constriction response of the pupil is perhaps the oldest. In fact, probably the earliest English reference to observation of the pupil is Travisa's 1495 translation of Batholomaeus (Janisse, 1977). Subsequent research has suggested that the pupil is used to acquire information *from* the environment, communicate information *to* the environment, and reflect "internal" processes, products *of the interaction between* the environment and the individual.

As an agent of acquisition, pupil diameter is known to fluctuate as a function of the amount of light entering the eye. Darwin (1872) found the pupil to be a valuable means of communication in animals, relating pupil size to "fear" and other emotions. Additionally, Bumke (1903), a German neurologist working with human subjects, noted that the pupil was continually dilated in anxious subjects. It was further demonstrated that the light reflex could be inhibited in subjects who were presented with emotional and painful stimuli (Bender, 1933; Gang, 1945).

More recent research has evaluated the utility of the pupillary response as a reflector of "internal" processes. Although Lowenstein and Loewenfeld (1951) deserve the title of "pioneer," studying the relationship between pupillary activity and internal processing, as early as 1896 Heinrich noted relationships between pupillary dilation and mental processing. Furthermore, Bumke (1911, translated in Hess, 1975) observed that "every active intellectual process, every psychical effort, every active mental image, regardless of content, particularly every affect, just as truly produces pupil enlargement, as does every sensory stimulus" (pp. 23–24).

15.3.1   *What can be recorded?*

15.3.1.1   *The pupil of the eye*

Whereas the actual recording of changes in pupil size is reasonably straightforward (given available technology), the experimenter is faced with the more complex issue of determining which aspect of the pupillary response to measure (e.g., pupil diameter, latency to peak size, area, variance, and minimum size). Janisse (1974) has suggested that the most appropriate measure depends on the question being asked; later in the chapter, we suggest that the task-evoked pupillary response (TEPR: changes in pupil diameter relative to baseline values) is a most appropriate index. Regardless of the index used, one must keep in mind variables that may confound measures of pupil size.

The light reflex. The light reflex is the primary determinant of pupil size. Therefore, it is important to keep the amount of light impinging on the retina as constant as possible. The luminance of a stimulus target upon which the subject's gaze falls must be uniform. Woodmansee (1966a) points out that as the subject alters her or his fixation point to different features of a stimulus, different levels of brightness exist, producing changes in pupil size (see also Goldwater, 1972; Janisse & Peavler, 1974; Loewenfeld, 1966; Woodmansee, 1966b; Zuckerman, 1971).

The near vision reflex, pupillary hippus, and fatigue. The effects due to the near vision reflex – the tendency for the pupil to constrict when focusing at a point near the subject – can be controlled with reasonable success by using viewing distances farther away from the subject; Hakerem and Sutton (1964) recommend 3–4 m.

Fatigued subjects are unreliable subjects since relatively lengthy trials will produce pupil size variation; for example, tired subjects may lose interest, fail to attend to the target, and lose or change focus (Janisse, 1977). In addition, fatigue enhances pupillary hippus, spontaneously occurring waves of dilation and constriction (Lowenstein and Loewenfeld, 1962; Woodmansee, 1966a,b).

Baseline values. Extreme values of pre- and post-trial pupillary diameter will largely determine the magnitude of the pupillary oscillations since the size of the pupil prior to experimental stimulus presentation will limit how much the pupil can constrict or dilate. If the pupil is large prior to experimental manipulation (e.g., 6–7 mm), then one should not expect a great deal of (absolute or percentage) dilation. In contrast, under the same conditions, the potential for constriction of a higher magnitude is present.

The Law of Initial Values (LIV; Wilder, 1958) states that an inverse relationship exists between subjects' baseline (or prestimulus) psychophysiological response and the magnitude of their subsequent response during stimulus presentation. The LIV only becomes a problem when pre- and poststimulus values are at their extremes. Fortunately, average pupil size is 4–6 mm, and Hansmann, Semmlow, and Stark (1974) reported that the relationship between prestimulus values and the magnitude of the response to stimuli is small if pupil diameter is within this range.

Response averaging. In view of all the variables that affect pupillary diameter, how might one enhance the signal-to-noise ratio? If the stimulus can be repeated a number of times, one may have recourse to response averaging. The assumption is that the signal of interest is elaborated by each presentation of the stimulus. Noise, on the other hand, is random with respect to stimulus presentation and should therefore sum to zero (or some minimal value), enhancing the signal-to-noise ratio. Since TEPRs are measured in fractions of a millimeter whereas the background noise may be of the order of a millimeter or more, response averaging is necessary to extract signal from noise.

15.3.1.2 *Eye movements*

A number of types of eye movements can be identified. The most common are *saccadic* movements, which involve rapid (usually conjugate) jumps of the eyes from one point to another. Saccades are initiated to place objects to be viewed on the fovea (the area of the retina that resolves images with high accuracy). What else need we know about saccades? The ability to take in visual information is markedly attenuated, not only during a saccade, but also for a brief period preceding and following saccade initiation and termination. This phenomenon is referred to as *saccade suppression* (Matin, 1974). Saccades occur in the horizontal and vertical planes as well as obliquely. The refractory period (or minimum delay between the termination of one saccade and the initiation of a new saccade) is on the order of 50 ms (Fischer & Ramsperger, 1984), although many authors claim this period to be of the order of 100–200 ms.

A second type of movement is *pursuit* (or slow tracking) movements. The eye can follow a slowly moving target if target motion does not exceed 20–30°/s. Pursuit movements allow for the stabilization of a moving image on the retina. During these eye movements, we have no difficulty perceiving the moving object. These eye movements can only be elicited by a moving object. Pursuitlike movements can also be produced by asking subjects to fixate on an object and requiring them to rotate their head slowly in the horizontal or vertical plane. These movements are referred to as compensatory eye movements since they compensate for head movements.

Vergence movements are focusing movements of the two eyes allowing us to foveate on near and far objects. These eye movements are even slower than pursuit movements, with maximum velocities of less than 10°/s. These various types of eye movements can thus be reasonably reliably discriminated on the basis of velocity characteristics.

15.3.1.3 *The eyelid*

Eyelid position is, in part, a function of gaze location. Looking low in the visual field produces not only a downward rotation of the eyeball to foveate an object, but also a downward movement of the upper eyelid as well. Similarly, looking upward produces a retraction of the upper eyelid and a lesser movement upward of the lower lid. The movements of the upper lid associated with gaze shifts can be readily identified by observation. Those of the lower lid are somewhat more difficult to detect.

Eyeblinks are periodic, symmetrical closures and reopenings of the eyelid. Three types of blinks can be identified, namely, the startle (or reflex), the voluntary, and the periodic blink. Such identification is based in part on a knowledge of eliciting conditions and in part on the waveform of the blink. The startle blink is a component of the startle reflex; it is one of the more sensitive measures of startle, one that habituates more slowly than most other components. The voluntary blink can be self-elicited or can occur in response to instruction. This blink can be readily discriminated from other types of blinks by its amplitude and waveform. Amplitudewise, it is generally larger than other blinks, that is, the eye closes further and the duration of the blink (from closure to reopening) is longer than most other blinks. The periodic, spontaneous, or endogenous blink occurs most frequently. As will be discussed, it is triggered, to a very limited extent, by environmental conditions such as humidity and the presence of air particulates such as dust and smoke. This blink may involve either full or partial closure of the eyelid, with closure duration between 150 and 300 ms. Unless made aware of a blink, the normal viewer does not perceive these interruptions in visual input.

How does one discriminate between a blink and an eye closure followed by reopening of the eyes some time later? One can a priori define a blink as involving a lid closure that does not exceed a given time period. However, our real concern is with the time period for which vision is obscured because the eyelid covers the pupil. This, of course, is more difficult to measure since both eye and eyelid position have to be taken into consideration. If gaze is directed low in the visual field, the point in time during the reopening of the lid for which gaze is obscured will be considerably less than if gaze is directed higher in the visual field.

Unfortunately, one cannot use gaze location at point of blink initiation to define gaze location at blink termination since eye movements in both the horizontal and vertical planes frequently occur during a blink. Because of these and other problems, we have "arbitrarily" (based on our observations) suggested that if blink closure duration, as defined in what follows, exceeds 300 ms, the closure should not be considered a blink. We have selected 300 ms, because we are reasonaly confident that if closure duration exceeds this period, we are most likely not looking at an "involuntary" or "spontaneous" blink. We suspect that blink closure durations between 200 and 300 ms are also "unusual" blinks and refer to these as *long closure duration blinks*.

How do we define closure duration? Since one cannot reliably measure, during the opening and closing phases of the blink, when the lid crosses the pupil (using extent technology), we operationally define closure duration as the difference between the point in time where the lid is closed half of the distance (of the blink) and the point in time during the reopening process where it passes that same (voltage) level. We can point to a number of problems with this procedure but believe it to be the most reasonable metric at the present time.

15.3.2   *Recording techniques*

15.3.2.1 *Pupillometry*

Early procedures involved the use of a still frame of a motion picture using infrared-sensitive film for recording pictures of the eye. Such pictures were then projected onto a screen and manually or semiautomatically measured by an operator.

Video procedures allow for the electronic identification of the sclera, iris, and pupil. The pupil, when illuminated with collimated light, reflects such light from the interior of the eye. This reflection is brighter than that for the iris. Video technology takes advantage of the differential reflectance of the sclera, iris, and pupil; when used to scan the eye in the horizontal plane, one can determine pupil size by identifying which scan line first crosses the pupil as well as which line last crosses the pupil. An alternative method is to use the vertical plane scan line as the index of pupil diameter; one selects the line that is midway between the top and bottom of the pupil by determining which intersected first with the pupil and which one is last to leave. If the pupil is partially obscured by the eyelid or eyelashes, using the horizontal plane, one can still measure the time of entrance of the scan line into the pupil and time to exit for the pupil, select the longest time, and identify pupillary diameter.

Other techniques for accomplishing these measures are available. Beatty (1986) provides a brief review of instrumentation used for the recording of pupillary diameter; another good reference is Young and Sheena (1975). This is an equally useful reference source for the evaluation of eye movements. A table comparing various procedures for recording oculomotor parameters is found at the end of their paper; it provides an excellent review of the relative advantages and disadvantages of the various techniques. This table is reproduced as Table 15.1.

15.3.2.2 Eye movements

A large variety of procedures for recording eye movements are available. These range from the use of special contact lenses to less invasive procedures such as photoelectric and other reflectance procedures, electrooculographic (EOG) procedures, as well as the video procedure already described. The technique used should depend on the purpose of the experiment. Thus, if exact knowledge of eye position with respect to the environment is necessary, EOG procedures should not be used. If, on the other hand, one desires high temporal resolution of an eye movement, then video techniques, where the resolution is not better than 16 ms for American and 20 ms for most European recording procedures, should not be used. If one wishes to record eye movements under conditions of nonrestraint, video procedures are contraindicated. If one is concerned with eye movement in the vertical plane, photoelectric techniques are to be avoided unless one is permitted to trim the eyelashes of the subject; eyelashes are excellent reflectors of infrared light. Let us briefly review these techniques.

Special contact lenses. Though relatively seldom used today, the use of contact lenses with mechanical lever systems were the earliest used procedures to measure eye movements (Huey, 1908). These were followed by contact lenses with mirrors mounted in them that reflected light that could be photographically tracked or with small iron pellets mounted in the lens that could be magnetically tracked. A tight-fitting contact lens, which has a small mark that can be tracked, is still the most accurate procedure for tracking the eye in both the horizontal and vertical plane; unfortunately, a snug fit of the contact lens makes removal difficult.

Video procedure. The procedure used for measuring pupil diameter is readily adapted for the measurement of eye position, especially in the horizontal plane. Using this method, one measures how much white of the eye has to be traversed before one shifts from the cornea to the iris or vice versa. This procedure is referred to as limbus tracking.

Table 15.1. *Comparison of eye-movement measuring techniques*

Method	Measurement range (degrees)		Accuracy		Speed or frequency response	Inference with normal vision
	Vertical	Horizontal	Vertical	Horizontal		
1. Corneal reflex (Mackworth camera)						
Polymetric lab V1164	± 9	± 9	0.5°	0.5°	photographic rate, 12–64 frames/s; television, 60 fields/s	medium
Polymetric mobile VO165	± 10	± 10	1°	1°	same as above	high: weight on head: optics near eye
NACREES	± 10–20	± 10–20	2°	2°	same as above	high: weight on head
2. Contact lens with						high
Lamp or radiant spot	Both ± 10–30	± 10–30	Precision 3′	3′	high	
Coil	*a*	*b*	15′	15′	high	
Mirror	± 10	± 10	2′	2′	high	
3. EOG	± 50	± 50–80	2°	1.5°	DC or 0.01–15 Hz limited by filtering	none
4. Limbus boundary						
Narco Eye Trac		± 10	4°	2°	2 ms 30 ms with recorder	medium
Narco Model 200	+ 10–20	± 20	2°	1°	4 ms; 26 ms with filtering	medium
5. Wide-angle Mackworth camera						
Polymetric V1166	40	40	2.5°	2.5°	same as method 1	medium: subject looks through apertures; special lighted stimuli are required
6. Pupil-center-corneal-reflection distance						
Honeywell oculometer	+ 30 − 10	± 30	1°	1°	0.1 s time constant	low
Whittaker eye view monitor	± 15°	± 22°	1°	1°	30–60 sample sec	low
U.S. Army Human Engineering Lab	30	40	2°	2°	60 sample sec filtered	low
7. Double Purkinje						
Image eye tracker	25°	25°	noise of 1 mm		300 Hz	low

a To make measurement, not to obtain fixation point.
b Larger than others.

522

Glasses acceptable	Contact lens acceptable	Subject variation problems eye color etc.	Subject cooperation required	Subject training required	Usable with young children	Calibration and setup time
?	possible source of error	none	high	low	?	low
no	possible source of error	none	high	low	no	high: biteboard
no	possible source of error	none	high	low	no	medium: fit headvabd, set light source
	no accept contact lens	eye must	high	high	no	
no yes no						high: lens must be filtered
yes	yes	medium: placement of cloctrodes and calibration is variable	medium	low	yes	high: requires electrode stablization and light adaptation
yes	yes	iris coloration a factor	high	low	yes	low
no	yes	iris coloration a factor	high	low	yes	low
?	possible source of error	none	high	low	yes	low
yes	possible source of error	low	low	low	yes	low: higher for maximum linearization
yes	same as above	low	low	low	yes	low
no	same as above	low	low	low	yes	low
	auto-correction possible	low	low	low	yes	low

Table 15.1. (*Cont.*)

Method	Head attachments required	Head stabilization requirement[a]	Subject discomfort	Subject awareness	Pupil diameter output also
1. Corneal reflex (Mackworth camera)					
	chinrest or biteboard	high head restraint or biteboard	medium	high	no
	biteboard	none	high	high	no
Polymetic lab V1164	head-mounted optics	none	medium	high	no
Polymetric mobile VO165 NACREES	contact lens	high low	high	high	no
2. Contact lens with Lamp or radiant spot Coil Mirror	yes, 2–6 electrodes	low low	low	high	no
3. EOG	head bracket and chinrest	high	low	high	no
4. Limbus boundary Narco	spectacles	none	low	high	no
Eye Trac	viewing through aperture	medium, head must be kept still	low	high	no
Narco Model 200	none	Mark II: head free. 1 in.'; Mark III: head free, 1 ft.'	low	low	yes
5. Wide-angle Mackworth camera Polymetric V1166	none	head free up to 1 ft.'	low	medium	yes
	none	1 ft'	low	low	yes
6. Pupil-centre-corneal-reflection distance					
Honeywell oculometer Whittaker eye view monitor U.S. Army Human Engineering Lab	chinrest or biteboard	none, head free 1 cm', biteboard for high precision	low	medium	no
7. Double Purkinje Image eye tracker					

Form of output	Status	Cost of operation	Remarks	Source of further information
photographic of videotape: low-resolution digital output	commercially available	high for film	—	Polymetric Co., P.O. Box D. Reseland, NJ 07068
same as above		high for film	higher resolution digital output is possible with other instruments	Instrumentation Marketing Corp., 820 South Mariposa, Burbank, CA 91506
same as above		high for film	headmounted TV camera	REES Inst. Ltd. Westminster House, Old Working, Surrey, United Kingdom
photographic or electrical	some commercial devices available	lens grindling may be costly	negative pressure application may be hazardous	
electrical record	commercially available	low	more suitable for eye motion than eye position	LT instruments, 4004 Osage, Houston, TX 770036; Grass Instruments, Quincy, MA 02169; ICS, 129 Laura Dr., Addison, IL 60101
analog and digital	commercially available	low	vertical position of eyelid is used to approximate vertical eye position	Narco Bio-Systems, Inc., Biometrics Division, 7651 Airport Blvd., Houston, TX 77017
analog and digital	commercially available	low	—	Narco (also see ICS)
photographic or videotape: low-resolution digitizer available	commercially available	high for film	point of regard output without motion artifact	Polymetric Co. (see above)
digital, analog, and fixation pointer on TV image of scene	commercially available	low	computer-based system; Mark III tracks head motion and has auto focus	Honeywell Radiation 2 Forbes Rd. Lexington, MA 02172
same as above	commercially available	low	tracks head motion and has autofocus available	Whittaker, Space Sci. Div., 335 Bear Hill Rd. Waltham, MA 02154
digital, analog, videotape, and graphic	Research laboratory	NA	—	U.S. Army/HEL Aberdeen Proving Ground, MD
analong output	small production	low	has auto focus: field and operation are dependent on pupil size suitable for image stabilization	Stanford Research Institute, Menlo Park, CA 94025

Photoelectric procedure. This procedure utilizes an infrared light source and two photocells sensitive to infrared light reflection. The pupil of the eye is a poorer reflector of light than the cornea. Thus, one can use differential reflectance of light from the pupil, cornea, and iris to track eye position. Such equipment is commercially available and has been used for many years to record eye movements during reading.

Electrooculographic procedure. This procedure involves the application of electrodes around the eyes. These electrodes do not record the muscle activity involved in moving the eyes; rather they record changes in the difference in electrical potential between the cornea and retina as the eye rotates. These potentials can be readily amplified and recorded on a strip chart or electromagnetically on analog tape. Care must be taken in both the preparation of the skin underlying the electrode and electrode placement. If the skin is not properly prepared, electrical potential changes associated, for example, with changes in skin resistance may generate slow potential changes that obviously have nothing to do with eye movements. If electrodes are not properly applied with respect to spatial location, one cannot discriminate between left–right and up–down eye movements. Silver–silver chloride pellet electrodes are recommended to minimize electrode artifacts.

Our recommendations (Oster & Stern, 1980) with respect to electrode placements are that for the recording of horizontal eye movements, the electrodes placed at the outer canthi be in line with the pupil; that is, with the subject looking straight ahead, these electrodes should be placed so that they are in a straight line drawn through the center (or top or bottom) of the pupil of the left and right eye. For vertical eye movements we recommend that the electrodes be placed on a line perpendicular to the horizontal line used for placing horizontal eye movement recording and that they be placed so that they bisect one of the two eyes. Young and Sheena (1975) recommend a number of other placements. Since these require a greater number of electrodes and, in our opinion, do not materially improve the resolution of horizontal and vertical eye movements, we have chosen not to describe them here.

We would like to warn the uninitiated that one should not attempt to discriminate between left and right eye movements (vergence movements) with EOG techniques. Some authors recommend that measuring the potential difference between the nasion and the left and right canthi allows one to measure eye movements of the two eyes independently. The problem is that the potential recorded from electrodes on the left and right inner margin of the eye or over the bridge of the nose is affected by movements of both eyes. If one could drive a lead wedge through the nasal bone and electrically isolate the left electrode from the right eye (and the right electrode from the left eye), one could then measure the horizontal displacement of one eye without that potential being affected by movements of the other eye. This, of course, is a procedure that is hypothetical but impractical as well as unethical. If one wishes to measure movements of the two eyes independently, we would recommend photoelectric reflectance procedures.

15.3.2.3 *Eyeblinks*

The eyeblink appears as an "artifact" in many eye movement recording procedures; that is, when the eye is closed, neither video nor reflectance techniques can record eye position. Electrooculographically, the movement of the eyelid across the cornea acts as a sliding resistor, one that significantly affects the recorded potential difference between the retina and cornea. This artifact is referred to as the *Rider artifact* and makes it impossible to record vertical eye movements concurrent with eyeblinks. However, the Rider artifact has little effect on the recording of horizontal eye movements.

The procedures for recording eye movements and their relative advantages are well described in a paper by Young and Sheena (1975). Oster and Stern (1980) provide an extended discussion of the procedure for recording EOG as well as reviewing the shortcomings and virtues of this technique.

15.3.3 Data reduction techniques: general comments

With the advent of digital computers, techniques for reducing signals that can be converted into voltage fluctuations are rapidly developing. We should be on the threshold of techniques that can automatically evaluate signals of interest. What needs to be measured is, in great part, a function of the questions asked. If we ask vague and general questions, such as what physiological measure best reflects attentional states, we cannot be very specific about the particular attributes to be abstracted from our biological measures. If, on the other hand, we ask questions such as "Is the waveform of the eyeblink (or saccade, or pupillary response) affected by alterations in attentional states?" we can specify the metric that needs to be applied to the biological signal in question.

Until the past 10–20 years, data reduction techniques involved the recording of data on strip charts or film and manually measuring the variable of interest. We have come a long way since those days; we now digitize and frequently analyze our biological signals at the time they are obtained. What determines the sampling rate for digitizing data? Should we sample as frequently as possible, or are there guidelines for determining sampling frequency? Sampling frequency should be dependent upon the spectral characteristics of the signal analyzed. If we are dealing with a slowly changing response, such as body temperature, we may reliably represent such changes by sampling infrequently (e.g., once per second). On the other hand, if we are concerned with an accurate representation of muscle activity, we have to sample more frequently, for example, once per millisecond (or a thousand times per second).

With respect to the signals of interest here, eye movement and eyelid movement sampling rates of 500 per second are adequate to capture the finer nuances of such movements. For pupillary diameter measurements, sampling data 20 times per second may be adequate.

15.3.3.1 Pupillometry

As previously mentioned, there are different aspects of pupillary change from which to choose (i.e., average diameter, average area, latency to peak dilation, peak size, etc.). When considering which aspect of the pupillary response to measure, one must keep in mind the variables (and their "solutions") previously mentioned. The original measure of pupillary activity used by Hess and Polt (1960) was expressed in terms of area. This index was superseded by changes in pupil *diameter* since changes in area due to constriction or dilation, relative to baseline measures, are not directly comparable; that is, given identical baseline values, a 1-mm *increase* in pupil diameter results in a greater change in area than a change in area due to a 1-mm *decrease* in pupil diameter. Additionally, pupil diameter is preferred over pupil area as an index since (1) diameter is easier to measure and (2) area is a derived measure based on diameter. When dealing with area as an index, one must assume that the pupil is spherical; however, we know that the pupil is not spherical but elliptical toward the nasal side. Thus, (vertically) measuring pupil diameter is the preferred measure.

Others have suggested (e.g., Beatty, 1982; Beatty & Wagoner, 1978; Kahneman, 1973) the TEPR as the most appropriate aspect of the pupillary response to record when relating such activity to the CNS. Beatty (1982) has eloquently summarized the reasoning behind the use of the TEPR as a reflector of processing load; a brief presentation of his arguments will be presented here.

Beatty (1982) states that "a task-evoked pupillary response bears the same relation to the pupillary record from which it is derived as does an event related brain potential to spontaneous electroencephalographic activity" (p. 276). During an information-processing task, systematic changes in CNS activity occur in response to critical events in the task; by performing time-locked averaging with respect to these critical events, phasic task-evoked dilations become evident, appearing between 100 and 200 ms after stimulus presentation and quickly terminating once the stimulus has been removed (and presumably after processing of the task has been completed). The TEPR is very small in comparison to pupillary changes induced by accommodation or by moderate changes in illumination so we must use time-locked averaging techniques to assure ourselves that changes in pupillary oscillations are indeed evoked by aspects of processing task.

15.3.3.2 *Eye movements*

Saccades. Outlined in what follows are aspects of saccadic eye movements measured by psychophysiologists interested in relating such eye movements to psychological constructs.

1. *Saccade latency:* The time between presenting a visual (or other) stimulus and the initiation of a saccade to foveate the stimulus.

2. *Saccade amplitude:* To determine how far the eye has moved between saccade initiation and termination.

3. *Direction of eye movement:* From a knowledge of eye position shifts in both the horizontal and vertical plane, one can reconstruct gaze location at the termination of an eye movement.

4. *Velocity:* Two velocity measures are found in the literature. The first is peak velocity (the fastest velocity attained during a saccade of a specified amplitude), and the second is average velocity (total time taken by the eye to saccade a specified distance). The relationship between saccade velocity and amplitude is linear over a reasonably wide angular range (0–50°); the larger the amplitude, the greater the peak velocity.

5. *Accuracy:* How does the eye shift from one position to the next? The idealized movement involves a single saccade. However, one frequently finds that the eye undershoots the target location and makes a "compensatory" saccade or glissade to slew the eye on target. Although overshoots occur less frequently, the usual eye movement that brings the eye back to the target is not saccadic in nature.

6. *Fixation pause.* Refers to the time between successive eye movements, usually saccades.

Slow eye movements (pursuit movements)

1. These movements are used to track a slowly moving target. If the eye falls behind (or gets ahead of) the target, saccadic eye movements are used to return the eyes to the target. These movements are sensitive not only to visual inputs, but also to inputs to the vestibular apparatus (vestibular nystagmus).

2. Slow eye movements (SEMs) are movements with a periodicity less than 0.8 Hz that occur as a subject becomes drowsy (Lehmann & Kuhlo, 1961). They occur most frequently after the eyes are closed but can occasionally be seen with the eyes partially open.

3. Although they have not received much attention in the literature, eye movements that are a combination of a saccade and a pursuit movement are readily identified in oculographic tracings. The common pattern is for saccades that shade into a pursuit movement. The amplitude of the slow component is usually less than 20 percent of the total distance moved, but the time necessary to make that movement is equal to the duration of the saccadic component. They are referred to as glissades in the literature (Bahill & Stark, 1975).

Vergence movements. These movements refer to coordinate movements, in opposite directions, for the two eyes to foveate an object. If the object is close to the eyes, the eyes will converge; if at a distance, they will diverge.

15.3.3.3 The eyelids

The eyelids serve a protective function, not only by shutting out visual input, but also by closing and reopening (blinking) to startling stimuli. They serve to spread lacriminal fluid over the eyeball and conjunctiva, and to rid the eye surface of foreign objects. We have both an upper and a lower eyelid. Both move during blinks. Both lids also move when gaze is shifted in the vertical plane. When gaze is shifted downward, the upper eyelid moves down. We usually measure blink amplitude, blink closure duration, and blink latency.

1. *Blink amplitude:* This is the distance the eyelid moves during a blink. As suggested, blink amplitude is, in part, determined by eye position. With the eye looking downward, blink amplitude will be smaller than when gaze is directed upward.

2. *Blink closure duration:* Since the reopening portion of a blink is considerably longer than the closing portion and since one can presume that once the pupil is no longer obscured by the eyelid, vision is again possible, a "convention" first described by Kennard and Glaser (1964) has been adopted to define closure duration. The measure is the time elapsing between the eyelid reaching half its closing amplitude and returning through that same level during reopening. It is assumed that this time is roughly equivalent to the duration for which the pupil is covered. As suggested earlier, this measure is, under other than the highly constrained conditions of the vision laboratory, only an approximation of the time that vision is obscured.

3. *Blink latency:* As we shall document later, blink latency is a psychologically meaningful measure. We have found it useful to evaluate it with respect to experimenter-controlled events but find it equally instructive to evaluate it with

respect to "internal," subject-controlled events such as eye movements and head movements.

15.4   INFERENTIAL CONTEXT: WHAT CAN WE LEARN ABOUT INTERNAL PROCESSES BY EVALUATING OCULOMOTOR PHENOMENA?

15.4.1   *What the pupil can tell us*

15.4.1.1 *Cognition and information processing*

Various manipulations of processing requirements imposed upon subjects have demonstrated that the TEPR is a reliable index of cognitive processing. Tasks used include short- and long-term memory tasks (Kahneman & Beatty, 1966), mental imagery (Paivio, 1973), mental arithmetic (Ahern & Beatty, 1979; Bradshaw, 1968), and language processing (Stanners, Headley, & Clark, 1972). Recently, Schluroff (1982) asked subjects to rate auditorily presented sentences of various lengths, construction, and content for comprehensibility while measuring mean pupil dilation. He was able to demonstrate that mean pupil dilation correlated more strongly with grammatical complexity than did subject ratings of sentence comprehensibilty, suggesting its usefulness as an "on-line" monitor of imposed cognitive load.

The TEPR appears to be a sensitive measure of within-task variations in processing load. For instance, Ahern (1978) examined the TEPR in the perception and comprehension of words where subjects were required to compare easy versus difficult words for similarity of meaning. Ahern demonstrated that the TEPR was responsive to word difficulty, the more difficult word leading to greater pupillary dilation that the simpler word.

Beatty (1982) has summarized the results of several studies that suggest that the TEPR also reflects between-task variations in processing load. In general, there is an orderly relationship between the amount of processing demand placed on the subject and the amplitude of the TEPR; that is, the more demanding the task – whether judged behaviorally, subjectively, or by an analysis of task requirements – the larger the TEPR. The results obtained by Dunham (1986), however, conflict with these conclusions; his data suggest that the TEPR reflects the actual amount of processing accomplished ("effort") rather than reflecting only the processing load imposed.

Finally, Ahern and Beatty (1979, 1981) demonstrated differences in TEPR between groups made up of individuals with varying levels of "psychometrically measured intelligence." Group 1 was made up of persons having SAT scores of 950 or less, with the other made up of those with SAT scores of 1,350 or greater. In three of the four tasks, the TEPR was consistently smaller in the group with the higher SAT scores than in the group with the lower SAT scores. They suggested that the between-group diferences were the result of the tasks being less demanding for those with higher "intelligence." However, concluding that the differences in the amplitude of the TEPRs between groups were due to differences in intelligence of the members of the respective groups is questionable since intelligence was evaluted on the basis of a static measure of scholastic aptitude (i.e., SAT scores); these scores bear a less than perfect relationship to intelligence, which in turn bears a less than perfect relationship to processing capacity.[1]

15.4.1.2 *Pharmacological and psychopathological effects*

The pupil can be useful for the study of pharmacological effects on the autonomic nervous system (ANS) given the reciprocal influences of the parasympathetic and sympathetic nervous systems. Additionally, aspects of physiologically based hypotheses of psychopathology may be tested, via the pupil, by inspecting the response itself and, by inference, determine the efficiency of the functioning of the brain centers known to be associated with the pupillary response.

Schizophrenia. Hakerem, Sutton, and Zubin (1964), using unmedicated, acutely ill schizophrenics, reported that these subjects had smaller dark-adapted pupils than chronic or normals as well as a shorter constriction time in response to a series of light flashes. Additionally, Lidsky, Hakerem, and Sutton (1971), using unmedicated, recent admissions to a mental hospital, reported a significantly *lower* construction to 36-s light pulses in patients when initial diameter was controlled. Further research has supported these findings (cf. Rubin & Barry, 1972). Zahn (1986) concludes that differences in the pupillometric activity between schizophrenics and normals appear to be due to higher sympathetic nervous system activity in the schizophrenics.

Hyperactivity. It was Satterfield and Dawson (1971) who stimulated interest in the use of autonomic measures to test the low-arousal hypothesis of hyperactivity. Research employing pupillometric techniques to assess ANS activity has demonstrated that hyperactive children required to sit upright and focus their gaze on a spot so that pupil size can be recorded have marginally greater pupil size than their controls (Zahn, Little, & Wender, 1978). These researchers also reported that the smaller pupillary dilation (to reaction-time stimuli) in hyperactive children disappeared after baseline pupil size was covaried out. Additionally, smaller anticipatory heart rate deceleration during reaction-time foreperiods in hyperactive children compared to controls was found. Zahn contends that these results "can be thought to be a fairly direct physiological manifestation of the attentional problems in hyperactive children...[but] can also be seen as another manifestation of a general lack of autonomic responsivity to the environment, which has also been amply documented" (Zahn, 1986, p. 565).

Stress and anxiety. The pupil has not been used extensively as a measure of ANS activity in stress-related studies; Plouffe and Stelmack (1979) reported that pupillometric data have not been effective in the differentiation of variable levels of "anxiety." Work by Stanners, Coulter, Sweet, and Murphy (1979) suggest that the pupil response to cognitive activity may overshadow the effects of affective variables such as anxiety. Cognitive demands appear to take priority over arousal factors. Two experiments were conducted in which pupillary response as well as other behavioral measures were recorded. In the first experiment, 24 female undergraduates who reported different degrees of fear of snakes listened to passages describing imagined interactions with a snake. The control passages were identical to the aversive passages except they made no mention of snakes. The arousal manipulations had no effect on the pupillary response, whereas behavioral data indicated that the arousal variables had been effective. The authors did demonstrate that the cognitive demands of the experiment were reflected by changes in pupil size.

The second experiment, using 30 male undergraduates, employed two types of tasks: one that exercised both arousal ("incentive") and cognitive factors and another that manipulated arousal only ("threat of shock"). Here, pupil response as well as heart rate, skin conductance, and EMG activty were recorded. This experiment also demonstrated that cognitive demands take priority over arousal factors in affecting the pupillary response.

Perhaps pupillary oscillations are not due to fear, anxiety, or stress per se but instead are a result of the attentive processes and/or the processing of the incoming stimuli. As Cacioppo and Petty (1986) point out:

Although, to date, no experiment has documented the course of the pupillary response during the presentation of persuasive communications or documented its utility in gauging the cognitive load on a recipient of a persuasive message, the pupillary response may prove to be a sensitive marker of this attitudinal processing component. (p. 670)

15.4.1.3 *Alertness and fatigue*

We now briefly survey literature regarding pupillary oscillations in fatigued subjects. Lowenstein and Loewenfeld (1951) demonstrated that changes in the ANS due to fatigue could be estimated using the pupillary light reflex. They were able to distinguish four types of fatigue in normal individuals by observing the shape of the pupillary response curve:

(1) syntonic reaction type of the well-balanced person; (2) reaction of central sympathetic irritability in the hyperactive normal subject; (3) reaction of central sympathetic weakness; and (4) reaction of central sympathetic irritative weakness. Using the pupillary response, they developed distinctions between two concepts: fatigue and fatigability. In the following passage, Lowenstein and Loewenfeld (1951) explain the distinction:

The shape of each individual reflex to light is an indicator of the degree to which the centers of control are disintegrated; it therefore is a measure of the actual condition of fatigue at the moment of reflex excitation. The length of the rhythmically appearing periods of decrement and increment of autonomic (pupillary) reflex activity and the rate of deterioration of the reflex to light within each period are a measure of fatigueability. (p. 581)

In a more recent study, Yoss, Moyer, and Hollenhorst (1970) were able to identify eight "pupillographic" stages of alertness and sleep. They found, in general, that pupil diameter is large and stable in an alert subject, medium and unstable in a drowsy subject, and small and stable when the subject is asleep, with pupil diameter and waveform in the intermediate stages following the same digressive patterns.

The point is that the pupillary response does indeed reflect ANS activity as well as CNS activity. It is important to be cognizant of this effect when designing studies (e.g., the recognition that it is possible to obtain an order effect due to fatigue).

15.4.1.4 *Affect and attitudes*

The work of E. H. Hess and collaborators was instrumental in a reawakening of interest in the use of pupillographic measures to index affective and attitudinal states. In what many consider a landmark study, Hess and Polt (1960) reported "discovery" of a "reliable" relationship between pupil response (measured in percentage difference in mean pupil *area*) and pictoral stimuli (photographic slides of a baby, of a mother holding a child, of a partially nude man, of a partially nude woman, and of a landscape). Using six subjects, Hess and Polt reported that pupil area of their female subjects was quantitatively larger than that of the males in response to the pictures of the baby, the mother and baby, and the partially nude male. In contrast, the area of the males' pupils increased more to the partially nude female and landscape pictures. The females' pupils actually decreased in *area* when shown the landscape pictures.

This study had major flaws. In subsequent research, Hess tried to deal with some of the procedural flaws of his initial work. In one such attempt, Hess (1965) argued that only after stimulus novelty is "habituated" can one evaluate the impact of attitudes on the pupillary response. Any pupillary response, then, can be said to covary with a person's attitude; that is, the greater the liking for a stimulus, the greater the pupil dilation, and the more dislike, the greater the constriction. Hess stated that this relationship appears only after the novelty, interest, and other effects of the stimuli have been reduced through multiple exposures.

Despite efforts to remedy procedural difficulties, the studies by Hess and colleagues continue to be controversial. After reexamination of Hess and Polt's original data, Nicholas Skinner (1980) has submitted a set of arguments contending that the conclusions reached by Hess and collaborators are invalid. Specifically, that only by including "aberrant" response data from *one* particular subject can the authors "justify" their conclusions that the heterosexual response to nude male pictures is a constriction in pupillary dilation, a result congruent with their predictions.

Metalis and Hess (1982) have since attempted to provide additional support for the covariance of pupillary response to a stimulus with subjects' attitudes. The subjects were shown a series of photographs portraying persons in a neutral setting, persons with grotesque skin diseases, or nude males or females in erotic positions. As a control, each picture was preceded by a slide of "comparable overall luminance." Each pair (each control–experimental pair) was presented three times, with data extracted from only two: the first and the third. A pupillary response was defined as the average change in pupil size to the control slide of the first and third pairings. In addition, the subjects were requested to complete a semantic differential scale (SDS) for each picture; the relevant dimensions of the SDS were the Attention–Interest and the Pleasantness–Evaluation subscales. They found that the responses to the slides depicting skin diseases evoked constrictions, whereas dilations occurred to the erotic photographs, with no differences between sexes evident; the neutral slides fell in the middle. In addition, subjects' ratings on the SDS differed *between* picture themes, whereas *within* themes SDS ratings differed only to the slides depicting disease. This led Metalis and Hess to conclude that both the pupil and SDS indices discriminate between affective themes.

The same concerns that Janisse and Peavler (1974), among others, had regarding Hess et al.'s earlier work are applicable to this study. Without question, a more clever paradigm that eschews the problems associated with current procedures (i.e., pictoral stimuli) must be devised. Such an attempt was launched by Green, Kraus, and Green (1979). College students either were shown or were told they would be shown pictures of a seminude male or female, a baby, and a landscape. Using the resting pupil size as the covariate, they did not find a sex difference in response to visually presented stimuli. They did find, however, that males responded more to the verbal (than to the visual) mode of presentation as well as responding more than women to verbal stimuli. Contrary to previous results, males responded as much as or more than females to verbal *or* visual presentation of baby stimuli. The authors concluded that the verbal, or anticipatory, mode seems to be at least as sensitive as the visual mode and eliminates the problems associated with the control of visual materials.

In any event, Goldwater (1972) points out that no one has satisfactorily documented a significant relationship between attitudes and pupillary oscillations when auditory, olfactory, or tactile stimuli were implemented. Furthermore, Hess and associates are alone in the demonstration of pupil constrictions to affective stimuli. Thus, the relationship of affect to pupil size is still a debatable issue.

15.4.2 *What eye movements tell us*

15.4.2.1 *Perception*

Obviously, eye movements should reflect the procedures used to "search" for information from our environment. Perception refers to the internal strategies that determine how we search our environment for "relevant" information. Vurpillot (1968) and others (Nodine & Lang, 1971) have evaluated how children go about performing the task of searching pictures to make the same or different judgments. If one presents two pictures of an object to a child and asks whether the two are identical, how does the child go about the task of arriving at a decision? Younger children (3 years of age) base their judgments on a more restricted sample of stimulus information than is true for older children (9 years of age). Boersma and Wilton (1974) compared 7-year-old conservers and nonconservers as defined by their performance on a Piagetian conservation task. Conservers engaged in more visual scanning and distributed their visual search over a larger segment of the display than nonconservers. Nodine and Lang (1971) have evaluated visual scanning strategies of expert, as compared to novice radiologists and described differences in their scan paths. Yarbus (1967) has described eye movement patterns during perception of complex objects, such as faces and scenes involving a number of people. When examining faces, one usually pays most attention to the eyes, the lips, and the nose. In other situations, viewers are most likely to spend more time looking at aspects of a picture that is unfamiliar or incomprehensible. Yarbus suggests that how we scan a picture, where we start, what particular aspect of the display we dwell on or ignore, and so on, are less determined by the nature of the display than by the question the viewers pose themselves as they look at a scene. Mackworth and Bruner (1970) had adults and young children look at a picture of a fire hydrant. Dramatic differences in both the extent of scanning of the hydrant and dwell time on particular aspects of the object discriminated between the viewing patterns of adults and children.

We have described a few of the many studies describing eye movement patterns associated with the perception of objects. It is clear from such studies that children utilize different search strategies than are characteristic of adults and that perception, as reflected in eye movements, is as much a function of the perceiver as it is of the stimulus material.

15.4.2.2 *Cognition*

We focus here on information abstraction strategies that can be inferred from eye movements recorded during reading. At the simplest level, we can evaluate the internal strategy used by the reader to find her or his way from the end of one line to the beginning of the next line, whereas at more complex levels, we can deal with the pattern of eye movements utilized in reading as the reader is required to abstract superficial as compared to "deep" information.

How do readers find their way from the end of a line to the beginning of a new line? This question, surprisingly, has not been investigated to any great extent. We can point to a set of studies by Netchine, Pugh, and Guihou (1987) that have evaluated the use of head movements in slewing the eyes from the end of a line to the beginning of a new line of text. These authors have demonstrated that children are more likely to make such head movements during reading than adults and that, for both children and adults, the likelihood of such head movements increases as a function of line length (longer lines have a greater likelihood of head movements), difficulty of the text for the reader (greater likelihood of head movements with difficult material), and when reading aloud as compared to silently. Of course, if there are head movements returning gaze from the end of a line to the beginning of a new line, there must be head movements toward the right during the reading of a line. Whether these head movements occur concurrent with saccades or during fixation pauses is a question that has not been systematically investigated.

Two major patterns of line change saccades can be identified in adult readers. The first shifts the eye from the end of a line to the beginning of the next line in a single, efficient saccade. The second utilizes two saccades: The first sweeps the eye approximately 80 percent of the distance "normally" covered followed by a short duration fixation pause, with a second saccade that moves the eyes back the remaining 20 percent of the distance. Stern (1978) reviews a doctoral dissertation by Goltz (1975) that evaluated these line change saccades in competent and less competent college student readers. The fixation pause between these two saccades was the only pause that was significantly shorter in duration for less as compared to more competent readers. These results were interpreted as suggesting that the less competent readers used the two saccades to find their way back to the beginning of a new line, whereas the more competent reader used it to abstract information. Only if that information did not make sense to them (in terms of material previously acquired), would they regress to the beginning of a line. The time taken following the major saccade to determine that you are not at the beginning of the line is shorter than the time necessary to abstract information on the basis of which the reader decides that he or she cannot integrate the new material into what has previously been read. Thus, the former makes for a shorter fixation pause than the latter.

Psychologists since the time of Javal (1879) have used eye movement patterns to make inferences about aspects of the reading process. These inferences have ranged from studying physical attributes such as optimal type style, line length, and distance between lines to optimal lighting and reflectance conditions. On the information-processing side (or abstracting information from printed text), they have dealt with issues such as the effective perceptual span (how many letter spaces can we appreciate during a single fixation) to questions dealing with the effect of speed-reading courses on eye movement patterns during reading as well as questions dealing with the patterning of saccadic eye movements that discriminate competent from less competent readers.

The interested reader is referred to Just and Carpenter (1987) and Rayner (1983) as exemplars of books that are partially (or wholly) devoted to using eye movements for drawing inferences about the reading process.

15.4.2.3 *Information-processing strategies*

A number of authors (Bakan, 1971; Galin & Ornstein, 1974; Gur & Gur, 1975) have demonstrated that when persons are asked questions requiring reflection (thought), most make a lateral eye movement to the left or right as they start to think about the answer to the question. Ehrlichman and Weinberger (1978) have reveiwed the literature dealing with this phenomenon and find that it reliably occurs in most individuals under most circumstances. If we ask a person a series of questions in a face-to-face manner, two-thirds of the people questioned demonstrate consistent eye movements to either the left or right for 70 percent of the questions to which they make lateral eye movement. One-third are less consistent in the direction of their initial eye movement. The two-thirds who are consistent divide into one-half for whom most of such eye movements are to the left and one-half for whom most such movements are to the right. Upon this, most researchers agree. There is, however, considerable debate about the interpretation of these findings. The most common (and parsimonious) rationalization suggests that left and right movers prefer to use different information-processing strategies. According to Gur, Gur, and Harris (1975), it is principally under somewhat anxiety-arousing conditions that subjects will utilize their preferred strategy. Thus, face-to-face interviewing by a somewhat threatening interviewer should elaborate the preferred processing strategy more reliably than if the "interview" does not involve face-to-face interaction. Left movers are reported to be more susceptible to hypnotic and other suggestions, are more involved with feelings and inner experience, and report more psychosomatic symptoms. They are also more likely to utilize visualization and holistic strategies in solving problems, whereas right movers are more analytic and verbal in their approach to solving problems.

Attempts at relating preferred processing strategies or direction of LEM to aspects of CNS function have, at best, come up with equivocal results. The idea that left eye and head movements are associated with greater utilization of the right hemisphere, whereas right eye and head movements are associated with greater utilization of the left hemisphere, as indexed by electroencephalographic markers, has received little support (Gevins & Schaffer, 1980).

15.4.2.4 *Pharmacological effects and psychiatric diagnosis*

Saccadic eye movements have been used to evaluate pharmacological effects as well as as an adjunct to psychiatric diagnosis. What effects do CNS depressants have on these eye movements, and are these effects more sensitive indicants of the presence of a drug than is true of behavioral effects?

A number of studies (Gentles & Llewellyn-Thomas, 1971; Stern, Bremer, & McClure, 1974) have demonstrated that peak velocity or duration of saccadic eye movements is significantly slowed by tranquilizers such as Valium as well as CNS depressants such as alcohol (Beideman & Stern, 1977). The Stern at al. study demonstrated, in addition to the preceding, that Valium not only had significant effects on the saccadic eye movement, but also affected the occurrence of long fixation pauses during reading. It is during the fixation pause that information is abstracted from the printed text and integrated with prior information. The occurrence of unusually long fixation pauses suggests that the reader either is having difficulty integrating the currently abstracted chunk of information with earlier acquired data or he or she may be taking time out from processing information or staring at the page without abstracting information. The latter was these authors' preferred interpretation to account for the effect of Valium. Whether CNS excitants lead to shorter duration or higher peak velocity saccades or whether they lead to faster information abstraction, as reflected by shorter duration fixation pauses, has not, to the best of our knowledge, been systematically investigated. It is our impression that they may lead to more rapid perceptual processes, which might be reflected in shorter duration saccades and shorter visual reaction time to simple perceptual stimuli but not to significant enhancement of cognitive processes. A drug that will make us smarter has yet to be developed.

With respect to psychiatric diagnosis, we focus on eye movement impairment in schizophrenia. Diefendorf and Dodge (1908) suggested that smooth pursuit eye movements were disrupted by saccadic eye movements to a greater extent in "insane" than normal persons. Holzman and co-workers (1972) have investigated this impairment in smooth pursuit activity in mental patients and have elaborated some important findings. Smooth pursuit eye movements were studied while subjects tracked a simple pendulum. In their earliest studies, the pendulum was a piece of string with a fishing weight attached at one end. The subject is required to track the movement of the weight. Schizophrenic patients, as compared to normal subjects, are more likely to have their smooth pursuit eye movements interrupted by saccades. In some cases, saccades predominate, and the pattern of eye movements resembles a cogwheel rather than a smooth sinusoidal wave. These saccadic intrusions appear to be characteristic of schizophrenia and occur both while patients are actively schizophrenic as well as when they are in remission. Shagass, Amadeo, and Overton (1976) suggested that these saccadic intrusions were due to patients being unable to sustain attention on the task. To increase attentional demands, they placed numbers of the faces of the weight and had subjects report the numbers as the weight swung through its sinusoidal arc. A significant improvement in eye tracking was produced by this strategy, but patients were still markedly inferior to controls with respect to the occurrence of intrusive saccades. This eye-tracking abnormality is not diagnostic in hospitalized psychiatric patients since it is seen not only in schizophrenia, but also in approximately half of all patients with affective disorders. However, with remission of symptoms, the eye track pattern of affectively disturbed patients reverts to a pattern indistinguishable from that of normal controls, whereas that of schizophrenics in remission remains abnormal (Levin, Holzman, Rothenberg, & Lipton, 1981). In twins discordant for schizophrenia (i.e., only one twin is diagnosed as schizophrenic), concordance of eye movement impairment is greater among monozygotic than dizygotic twins (Holzman et. al., 1980.) Holzman et al. (1972) also report that the majority of first-degree relatives of schizophrenics demonstrate impaired smooth pursuit eye tracking, whereas first-degree relatives of patients with affective disorders have a prevalence of abnormal eye tracking in the range of that found for normal subjects (8–12 percent).

What is of special interest is that this abnormality of tracking is not attributable to a dysfunction of the tracking or saccading system. Requiring patients to maintain fixation on a central spot while rotating their heads leads to normal pursuit movements, as reported by Lipton, Levin, and Holzman (1980). These same patients demonstrate pursuit impairment when tracking a moving target. This suggests that the abnormal pattern is only seen under conditions of attention mobilization and higher order information processing. Not only are such intrusive saccades observed when schizophrenics are required to track targets, but they are also seen when they are required to fixate a nonmoving target (Brockway, 1975; Shimazono et al., 1976).

These studies are illustrative of the utility of using oculomotor activity to index aspects of psychotic behavior and to provide clues concerning the CNS mechanisms implicated in the abnormal behavior (Levin, 1984). This suggests that saccadic intrusions during smooth pursuit tracking may be associated with impaired functioning of frontal eye field mechanisms as well as temporo-parietal mechanisms of task engagement.

15.4.2.5 *Alertness*

What can eye movements tell us about altered states of alertness? What happens to our eyes as we go from a state of alertness to sleep? As we become drowsy, our eyelids droop and assume a partially closed position. To what extent do eye movements reflect alterations in alertness? Bahill and Stark (1975) have suggested that saccadic eye movements are slowed not only by CNS-depressant drugs but by fatigue processes as well. There is a class of pursuitlike eye movement indicative of drowsiness. These eye movements are referred to as SEMs (or slow eye movements) and have been described by Lehmann and Kuhlo (1961), Stern, Goldstein, and Walrath (1984), and others. These eye movements are slow, rolling movements of the eyeball in the horizontal plane. Their frequency, as described by Kuhlo and Lehmann (1964), is in the range 0.2–0.6 Hz. It is our impression that SEMs occur before major electroencephalographic evidence of sleep is manifested. Kuhlo and Lehmann (1964) also report that these eye movements are seen in the eyes closed alert condition (as defined by the presence of normal alpha activity in this EEG). They report that SEM increases in amplitude and regularity as the person moves toward drowsiness (as indexed by a reduction of alpha frequency and amplitude in the EEG).

There is, of course, another set of eye movements seen principally during sleep, namely, REMs (or rapid eye movements). These movements occur in association with a shift from stage 4 sleep to a light level of sleep and are somewhat slower than normal saccades (Aserinsky, 1986). In humans the ability to report dreamlike activity is associated with the occurrence of REM sleep. Subjects awakened during REM sleep are significantly more likely to report dreaming than when awakened during other stages of sleep. However, unless one is willing to attribute dreaming to newborn infants or animals lower on the phylogenetic scale than man, such as cats and rats, one cannot say that dreaming is a necessary consequence of REM sleep; only that REM sleep may be necessary for the occurrence of much dreaming.

15.4.3   *What eyeblinks tell us*

The eyeblink, aside from the startle-elicited blink, has been little studied by either psychologists or physiologists. Stern, Walrath, and Goldstein (1984) reviewed much of the literature dealing with the spontaneous or endogenous eyeblink prior to 1982. Though the literature is sparse, seminal studies were performed by Ponder and Kennedy (1928), Kennard and Glaser (1964), Luckiesh (1947), and Hacker (1962); Ponder and Kennedy implicated higher nervous processes as the major determinant of blink enhancement and inhibition. Blinks, for example, occur more frequently when witnesses in a court of law are interrogated by the opposition lawyer (Ponder & Kennedy, 1928), in patients suffering from anxiety neuroses (Kanfer, 1960), and when subjects are fatigued or tired (Luckiesh, 1947). Blinking is inhibited when subjects are required to perform a visually demanding task such as reading (Ponder & Kannedy, 1928) or visual tracking (Poulton & Gregory, 1952). When studied, the variable of principal interest has been blink rate. We shall attempt to document the utility of the eyeblink in indexing aspects of information abstraction. It should be pointed out that blinking in association with perceptual or cognitive activity is not obligatory, but if a blink does occur, it will most likely occur at a definite timepoint in the information-processing chain. It has long been known that blinking is inhibited during the act of reading and other visually demanding tasks; therefore, another approach to evaluating aspects of perception and cognition is to look at periods of blink inhibition.

15.4.3.1 *Perception*

What evidence is there that the act of taking in visual or auditory information affects aspects of blinking? Studies from our laboratory have demonstrated that subjects inhibit blinking during stimulus presentation and that such inhibition occurs with both visual and auditory stimulus presentation (Stern, Walrath, & Goldstein, 1984). Blinks are most likely to occur at a fixed time following stimulus onset. Where they occur is a function of task demands. For example, requiring subjects to discriminate between a 200- and a 400-ms duration light or tone, and making a simple motor response to the longer of the two stimuli versus responding to the shorter one, produces not only differences in reaction time but also differences in blink latency (Bauer, Strock, Goldstein, Stern, & Walrath, 1985; Goldstein, Walrath, Stern, & Strock, 1985). Blinks are inhibited longer (with respect to stimulus onset) for the 400-ms duration stimulus. It is our impression that the blink signals the onset of a "rest" period: A decision has been made about the nature of the stimulus and the required response, allowing one to take "time out" and blink.

Taking time out and blinking is best seen following the termination of a visually demanding task in both laboratory as well as more natural situations. In the laboratory, as soon as subjects realize that an experimental run has been completed, one sees a flurry of blinking that may last for a minute or longer. It is our impression that this flurry of blinks is quite independent of the *amount* of blinking engaged in during task performance; it is seen following tasks that produce blink inhibition as well as following tasks where there is an actual increase over the "normal" (for the individual) blink rate. We suspect that it is the relief from inhibiting blinking during specific time periods that accounts for the increase. In more realistic environments, such as flight simulators, one sees a similar flurry of blinking after "release from blink inhibition." For example, in flying DC-9 simulators, one sees inhibition of blinking during landing approaches. Once there is touchdown and during the "roll-out" portion of the landing, there is a marked elevation of blinking.

Not only is blink rate affected by perceptual task demands, but the waveform of the blink is also task dependent. We blink differently when performing an auditory as compared to a visual vigilance task (Goldstein et al., 1985). Blink closure durations during auditory vigilance task performance are significantly longer than those that occur during visual vigilance task performance. A "principle" of shorter closure durations with greater visual demandingness of a task can also be demonstrated. More demanding visual tasks lead to shorter closure durations than less demanding tasks. What makes a task more or less demanding? One component is stimulus predictability. The less predictable, the greater the visual demandingness. For example, in a signaled reaction-time experiment with a fixed foreperiod preceding imperative stimulus presentation, one would expect blink closure durations of those blinks that occur close in time to the signaled event to be shorter in duration than those that occur at a more remote point in time. This is exactly what one finds (Bauer, Goldstein, & Stern, 1987), and concurrent with this, of course, one finds that the likelihood of blink occurrence decreases in expectation of a stimulus. Thus, it appears that if the system cannot inhibit the occurrence of a blink close to the point in time where a stimulus is expected, the system falls back on a second strategy, namely, to make closure duration short, so that the likelihood of signal onset being missed is minimized.

We thus suspect that the perceptual demandingness of visual and probably auditory tasks can be indexed by a judicious evaluation of blink timing and blink closure duration.

Although not relevant to spontaneous blinks but to startle blinks, another phenomenon deserves mention here. Startle blinks can be initiated by a variety of unexpected stimuli. The most used is a sudden, loud noise such as a pistol shot (Landis & Hunt, 1939). A number of investigators have demonstrated that if the startle-inducing stimulus is preceded by another sensory stimulus, the amplitude of the blink is significantly inhibited (Hoffman & Ison, 1980). The time window between the warning stimulus and the startle-inducing stimulus is critical for demonstrating this effect. At interstimulus intervals (ISIs) ranging between approximately 30 and 100 ms, one sees such inhibition in normal adults. As we shall see, such inhibition apparently does not occur in certain types of psychopathology or, perhaps, in patients with brain damage to specific sites.

15.4.3.2 Cognition

As alluded to earlier, cognitive variables may have profound effects on aspects of blinking. The fact that we blink significantly less frequently when actively reading has been well documented since the 1920s (Ponder & Kennedy, 1928). What is, of course, unclear is whether this inhibition in blinking is a reflection of the perceptual demands of the task or whether the "cognitive" components play a part. The answer to this question is not available as yet, but as we shall show later, cognitive components do affect where blinks occur during reading. Although the evidence is purely anecdotal and scattered throughout the literature, one finds statements suggesting that the blink rate during reading is, in part, determined by the interest the reader has in the material. The greater the interest in the content of the text, the greater the blink inhibition. Where do readers blink during text reading? One commonly finds that most such blinks occur as the reader is shifting from one page of text to another. Hall (1945) suggested (on the basis of minimal data) that readers are more likely to blink at the end of a paragraph, sentence, thought, or punctuation mark. In other words, at semantically appropriate points in the text. We have begun to investigate this question, and preliminary results[2] suggest marked individual differences in where people blink during reading. For all readers, many blinks do occur in association with page changes. Restricting the evaluation to blinks during active reading, we find that some readers do most of their blinking in association with regressive eye movements and others are more likely to blink during or shortly following line change saccades, whereas others blink predominantly during long fixation pauses. In other words, blinks are *least* likely to occur during "fluent" reading, that is, reading involving a pattern of successive right-going saccades. Thus, the pattern of blinking during reading may be somewhat more complicated and informative about the reading process than suggested by Hall (1945).

Using a task where aspects of information processing can be more tightly defined than with text reading, we find that both blink frequency and waveform are affected by cognitive task demands (Bauer et al., 1987). Bauer (1986) evaluated aspects of blinking while subjects were performing the Sternberg memory task. In this task, subjects are required to commit information in the form of discrete items (letters, figures, etc.) to memory and retain that information and are then challenged with a single stimulus that is or is not a member of the set. They are required to make a discriminative response. In the Bauer study, subjects were required to commit to memory small and large memory sets that were either letters or Japanese Katakana characters. Subjects were all non-Japanese readers; thus the Katakana characters were not meaningful figures for them. The small set size was two and one item, respectively, for letters and Katakana characters and six and two, respectively, for the large set size. Stimuli were presented for 1 s, with an interstimulus interval of 5 s between the memory set and the test item. What happens to blink timing, blink rate, and blink closure duration as a function of these manipulations?

Significant blink latency (from stimulus onset) differences were obtained as a function of set size. Blinking was inhibited significantly longer for large as compared to small set size, with no difference between letters and Katakana characters. Thus, if the blink indexes a point in time following the perception and storing (in short-term memory) of the memory set, one would except a longer delay in blinking for the large as compared to the small set size. The results are in accord with this hypothesis.

Blink rate was abstracted for consecutive half-second periods following stimulus onset. There is marked inhibition of blinking during the period of stimulus presentation, a large increase in the periods immediately preceding and following stimulus termination, and a significant reduction as one approached the presentation of the test stimulus. Blink rate during the information retention period was significantly greater for the "large" Katakana set as compared to all other stimulus sets. Is the higher blink rate during Katakana character retention a function of a different retention mode for unusual as compared to easily named characters?

Closure duration also discriminated between small and large set sizes. During memory set presentation, blink closure duration was significantly shorter for blinks occurring during large set size presentation. During the 5-s delay, the large set size led to significantly longer closure duration blinks for both letters and Katakana characters, with the effect somewhat stronger for the Japanese characters. Thus, blink closure durations provide us with information different from that obtained from analysis of blink rate only.

One other component deserves mention, the relationship of blinks to eye movements. It has long been known that blinks are more likely to occur concurrent with head movements and with large amplitude as compared to small-amplitude saccades. Concurrence of blinks with head and body movement has been documented in one study involving horses and cows (Haberich & Wittge, 1956). We know of no published study documenting this phenomenon in man. The co-occurrence of blinks with small and large saccadic eye movements was recently studied in our laboratory (Fogarty & Stern, in press) in a task requiring the detection and identification of peripherally presented stimuli at four locations (50° left, 15° left, 15° right, and 50° right). The identity conditions required the observer to compare a centrally presented letter with the peripherally presented one and signal her or his response (same, different) as rapidly as possible. A fixed time later, a new set of stimuli were presented about which the same decision had to be made. We demonstrated that blinks were more likely to ocur with large- than small-amplitude eye movements. However, these blinks were much more likely to occur in conjunction with the eyes returning from the peripheral location (98 percent) as compared to moving to the location from which letter information had to be abstracted (2 percent). This study demonstrates that blinking in association with large-amplitude saccades is not obligatory and that blinks are inhibited when information at the peripheral location has to be rapidly acquired. Since there is information intake suppression during both a blink and a saccade and since the suppression is usually longer for a blink than a saccade, it is "best" not to blink when information acquisition is important. One can observe this same phenomenon in simulators as well as in the real world. We give a real-world example based upon naturalistic observations but one that can be replicated by the inquisitive without instrumentation. Observe the driver of an automobile scan her or his rear-view mirror. If the eyes and head turn toward the mirror during a "routine" check of rear traffic and then returns to the windshield, the pattern of blinking associated with that movement is different from that if the mirror gaze is made in anticipation of passing a car. Under the latter condition, blinks will most likely be inhibited as gaze shifts toward the mirror. Blinks are more likely as gaze returns to the road ahead. Under the former condition, one is likely to blink in association with both gaze shifts. Thus, if information acquisition is critical, there is inhibition of blinking (usually) association with large-amplitude gaze shifts involving either or both eye and head movements.

15.4.3.3 Pharmacological effects and psychiatric diagnosis

What effects do pharmacological agents have on the spontaneous eyeblink? It has long been known that patients with Parkinson's disease demonstrate a marked reduction in spontaneous blinking and a marked increase in reflexive blinking. L-dopa, a drug used to relieve many of the symptoms of the Parkinsonian syndrome, produces a significant increase in blink rate while enhancing reflex blinking and reducing habituation of the glabellar reflex. Parkinson-like symptoms are also produced by neuroleptic drugs, such as the phenothiazines and butyrophenones, and are the earliest signs of extrapyramidal system damage (tardive dyskinesia) produced by these drugs (Stevens, 1978). Evaluating aspects of the eyeblink, thus, has potential diagnostic utility in regulating the use of some psychotropic medication. The neural pathways through which these effects are produced are only poorly understood. Certainly, dopaminergic centers in the brainstem and higher cerebral structures in the frontal and parietal cortex that exert inhibitory control over these dopaminergic centers are implicated. The evidence from studies of eye movement dysfunction in schizophrenia reviewed earlier in this chapter suggests that the cortical control centers, rather than those directly controlling premotor and motor activity of the eyes, are responsible for such dysfunctions in psychiatric patients, whereas extrapyramidal symptoms are more likely to be drug induced.

Disturbances in the spontaneous eyeblink and the blink reflex again are found in schizophrenia. The pioneer work of Stevens (1978), evaluating such eyeblinks in schizophrenics, concluded that abnormalities in both blink rate and the blink reflex (to glabellar taps) characterizes this patient group. She was, however, uncertain about the cause of these abnormalities. Although she studied patients who had been withdrawn from neuroleptic medication, she suggested that these symptoms could be secondary to drug-induced damage to the pyramidal system rather than being symptomatic of schizophrenia.

What effects do CNS depressants and excitants have on the waveform, frequency, and timing of blinks? This, again, is a question that has not been, but deserves to be, investigated.

15.4.3.4 *Affect*

Again, the work by Ponder and Kennedy (1928) provides us with some insights into the impact of affective processes on aspects of blinking. These authors went into courtrooms and (observationally) recorded the blink rate of persons being interrogated on the witness stand by either a friendly or adversary lawyer. They report that the blink rate was higher under conditions of being examined by the adversary lawyer. One can conclude that being examined by an opposition lawyer will arouse apprehension or anxiety and that the elevated blink rate may be taken as an index of such feelings. We know of one study (Kanfer, 1960) that evaluated the blink rate of women diagnosed as anxiety neurotics and compared it to the blink rate of normal women, finding that the neurotics blinked significantly more frequently than the normal women. Ponder and Kennedy also implicated the affect anger as leading to an increase in blinking.

15.5 SOCIAL FACTORS AFFECTING OCULOMOTOR ACTIVITY

15.5.1 *Demand characteristics*

Although it appears that ANS and CNS reactivity to environmental stimuli and to "internal" processing can be effectively and reliably measured via the oculomotor response system, other factors, too, may effectively alter the shape or magnitude of the response. For example, when recording pupillary oscillations, it is important for the subject to sit upright, keep her or his head in a constant position, fixate gaze on a single point, and inhibit blinking as much as possible, not to mention performing the task at hand as well as possible. It is obvious that these requests require some effort on the part of the subject; therefore, it is important that the subject be made as comfortable as possible and be familiarized with the experimental chamber and apparatus before the experiment begins so as to reduce any artifactual responding. In addition, temperature, air quality, and brightness are considerations that must be addressed; if not controlled for, these variables may manifest themselves through unwanted (artifactual) eyeblinks, eye movements, or pupillary oscillations.

The "ideal" subject is one who is rested, physically comfortable, and familiar with the experimental chamber and apparatus, understands the paradigm, is not overwhelmed with instructions, and is not currently taking medication (alcohol included). Although this sounds like a tall order, a well-planned experimental procedure can reduce most of these concerns. The rest is up to the subject.

15.5.2   *Social interaction*

Gaze behavior, in a general context, tells us what the viewer is observing. As any introductory texbook of psychology suggests, such gaze behavior is in part genetically determined and in part environmentally determined. Infants as young as 10 hours demonstrate preferences for visual displays, as indexed by the duration for which a display maintains their visual attention. Fantz (1961), in experiments that have been replicated many times, found that a picture of a bull's eye captured an infant's attention for about twice as long as a card painted red, yellow, or white. Infants prefer complex patterns to simple ones, patterns with curved lines to those with only straight lines, and manifest great interest in faces, and these "interests" appear to be present shortly after birth.

Gaze behavior, in a social context, generally refers to eye contact. Eye contact is established when one sees another person looking at one's eyes. Of course, one has to be looking at the other person's eyes to make that inference. Such looking behavior allows us to make a wide variety of inferences about the nature of the social interaction being played out, so to speak, before our very eyes. Personal attributes of the viewer as well as social variables determine the nature of this complex interaction. Terms such as "losing face," "keeping an eye on you," "staring one down," "tender looks," and "apprehensive glance" all attest to the importance of visual gaze interactions. That these interactions are learned rather than inborn is well demonstrated by studies of cultural differences in gaze behavior. For example, persons brought up in Arab, Latin American, and southern European cultures engage in more as well as longer periods of eye contact than Indians, Chinese, and northern Europeans. Violations of these culturally determined gaze patterns may be interpreted as signs of rudeness, dishonesty, disrespect, and threat. Thus, for northern Europeans, too long a gaze is perceived as threatening, insulting, or disrespectful, whereas for the southern Europeans, too short a gaze may be interpreted as symptomatic of dishonesty or disinterest (Watson & Graves, 1966).

Are there biological predispositions that allow animals to "interpret" gaze behavior as friendly or threatening? Exline (1974) conducted a study on staring behavior and threat responses on the part of male rhesus monkeys. Staring at an animal by the human experimenter led to either attack (47 percent of trials) or threat displays (29 percent of trials) on the part of the animal. Cutting off gaze, by looking away through eye or head movements, shutting eyes, assuming a sleeplike posture, shaking the head, and bobbing the head up and down, resulted in a marked reduction of threat or attack behavior.

Gaze behavior in the human infant can be demonstrated shortly after birth. At 1 hr postbirth, term infants orient toward visual and auditory stimuli. At about 2 weeks, they follow moving objects. At 2–3 months, stimuli that look like a pair of eyes elicit gaze behavior and smiling in the infant. A face with the eyes covered is less likely to elicit a smile than one with only the eyes uncovered. A profile face, with one eye hidden, is less likely to lead to smiling behavior. Thus, the eyes of the observed are important providers of cues to the infant observer.

That the eyes of the observed are important providers of information to adults as well as infants is demonstrated in a series of studies by Dimberg and Öhman (1983) and Dimberg (1987). Dimberg and Öhman studied the effect of directional facial cues on conditional electrodermal responses to facial stimuli. They used pictures of faces expressing anger that were either directed toward the subject or about 30° to the left of the perceiver. Conditional electrodermal responses were equally well established to either set of pictures. However, the extinction of the conditional effect was much slower for the angry face directed at the observer than that oriented away from the observer. Thus, the conditioned emotional response persists longer to a face depicting threat directed toward the observer than to a face where the threat is directed away from the observer.

Knowledge that pupil diameter conveys information has been known since antiquity. Women as well as men have used eye makeup to accentuate and focus attention on their eyes. During the middle ages, women used a drug (belladonna) that produced pupillary enlargement to make themselves appear more attractive. These are but a few examples to demonstrate the importance of the eyes and face as a source of information about the person.

15.6   RANGE OF APPLICATIONS

15.6.1   *Human factors*

It is somewhat surprising that with the importance of visual information intake, more attention is not paid to aspects of oculomotor activity. Part of the problem is the fact that the acquisition and evaluation of oculometric variables require more instrumentation and greater sophistication on the part of the user than is true of many of the tools used in engineering psychology. What advantage do we gain over other methods by collecting oculometric data in the human engineering context? Human engineers are concerned with the design of equipment that will maximize the functioning of the system. Their concern is principally with systems that have man as a component of the system. Man evaluates outputs from the system and makes decisions about its functioning, for example, how to program the system and how to subvert it when a component breaks down. What is the optimal procedure for presenting information to the observer? Are digital displays more slowly or more rapidly interrogated? Is color coding of displays a useful strategy? How much information can the viewer be expected to abstract and deal with? What are conditions that lead to degradation in the performance of man? These are the types of questions frequently asked of the human engineer. We believe that there are three ways in which such questions can be asked. For example, what is the most reasonable display of the speedometer so that the driver can maintain a speed around the speed limit? Our concern can be with location of the speedometer, whether the display is digital, analog, or a combination of the two, or whether auditory information about speed is the more useful procedure for providing such information.

The most common evaluative procedure involves the use of subjective reports of drivers required to drive under the various display conditions, or, what is even more common, asking drivers for their impression of the relative utility of these procedures. We will discount the latter procedure in this case and utilize sophisticated rating scales to answer the question.

A second procedure would involve the use of an objective output measure from the vehicle to evaluate this question. In this case, deviation from ideal speed and fuel consumption might be used to answer the question.

Using biological signals, we are concerned with the effect of such manipulations on the operator. Since our concern in this chapter is with the eye, what can it tell us that will be useful in making design decisions?

We might ask, "What is the dwell time on the visually displayed speedometer?" with our assumption being that long duration gazes on the speedometer are not as "good" as short duration gazes if the driver's task is to keep her or his eyes on the road and road signs. We might ask about somnolence-inducing characteristics of the display. Is the automatic drone of a voice synthesizer reporting vehicle speed every X seconds more likely to lead to periods of somnolence, indexed by eye closures or long closure duration eyeblinks, than the visual presentation of speed information?

It is thus readily apparent that the human factor engineer has a battery of measures available to answer related (but not identical) questions that *should* influence the design of automobiles.

A very timely question of concern to human factor specialists is the evaluation of text display devices. There is considerable push for the use of computer-controlled visual display terminals (VDTs) rather than the use of the printed word, or "hard-copy" text. Literature demonstrates that VDT-displayed text is read between 20 and 30 percent more slowly than hard-copy text. What is it about VDT-displayed text that makes reading it so much slower? The literature dealing with this issue has been reviewed by Stern and Strock (1987), with no definitive answer to the question available. We know that experience with VDTs is not a relevant variable; we know that there is no speed/accuracy trade-off. The slower reading from VDTs is not accompanied by better retention of the material, by more accurate proofreading, by less fatigue as a function of time on task, and so on. Again, we can ask what can oculometric measures contribute to the identification of the variable(s) that determine this effect. We can ask, using eye movement information, what does the reader do differently under the two conditions? Does he or she spend more time on all fixation pauses? Is the reader likely to make more regressive saccades when reading from the VDT? Is there more difficulty in finding her or his way from the end of a line to the beginning of a line? Is he or she more likely to use a combination of head and eye movements with the VDT? And so on. Again, these are questions that can be asked but have not been asked as yet.

These are but a few examples of the utility of evaluating oculometric variables in answering important applied questions.

15.6.2   *Clinical applications*

As alluded to earlier, oculometric variables should be useful in opthalmological, neurological, and psychiatric applications. We know, for example, that eye scan patterns discriminate schizophrenics from normals and that the unusual eye scan pattern is trait rather than state dependent. Schizophrenics evidence the pattern both while demonstrating symptoms as well as when they are asymptomatic. We believe oculometric measures could be useful in monitoring drug effects in the treatment of schizophrenia. Many of the drugs used, when administered for relatively long periods of time, produce irreversible neurological damage known as tardive dyskinesia. We suspect that prior to the development of readily visible symptoms of this disorder, subtle changes in the frequency and waveform of the eyeblink occur. Such measures can be routinely monitored and could be used to adjust drug dosage, change to a different drug, and so on.

Another clinical application lies in the monitoring of CNS-depressant drugs and other drugs (e.g., antihistamines) that produce drowsiness in many individuals.

Although such drugs carry recommendations suggesting that the user not drive, most users do drive. Users of these drugs might be required to wear special spectacles that identify eyelid closures. Driving with closed eyes is dangerous! Why not monitor the eyelids and provide the driver with feeback when her or his eyes remain closed for more than a specific time period, say, 1 s.

15.6.3 *Education*

How might oculometric measures be used in student evaluation and training? We know that all measures of intelligence are contaminated by the fact that cultural variables significantly affect the ability to answer many questions on such tests. What might we do to reduce cultural influence?

As described earlier when we reviewed some of the work by Beatty (1986), Kahneman (1973), and Janisse (1977), one could consider using changes in pupillary diameter while students are solving arithmetic problems to evaluate the difficulty of the task for the individual. Two persons might answer an arithmetic question equally quickly and correctly, but one may have to mobilize more "effort" in solving the problem than the other. Pupillary diameter changes should reflect the amount of effort expended in arriving at the answer to the question. We might think of defining intelligence in terms of the amount of "psychic energy" that has to be mobilized to answer a given question rather than being restricted to speed and accuracy measures. Using this and other physiological variables may allow us to develop a radically different metric for assessing intelligence, one less dependent on our cultural heritage than measures in current vogue. We should point out that our example involving an arithmetic task was selected with the assumption that viewers for cultures using a number system such as ours could be evaluated. When language variables enter the picture, the issue again becomes clouded.

A second issue might be a concern with determining how children learn to read, the question of what defines acceptable eye movement parameters during reading for specific age groups, and the question of how oculometric variables might be utilized to help children and adults become more competent readers. On the evaluation side, we have already alluded to the issue of how readers find their way from the end of one line to the beginning of the next line. With computer-displayed text assuming a more and more prominent role in our society in general and in the presentation of text in particular, it appears to us that line length and spacing between lines could be easily adjusted to conform to the visuomotor skills of the child. If teachers do not believe in using one's finger to guide the eye from the end of one line to the beginning of the next or if they object to the child using a ruler or piece of paper as a guide to help the eyes move from one line to the next, the development of such "undesirable" habits may be prevented by adjusting line length and interline spacing on computer-displayed or even computer-generated text.

Rayner (1983) and Just and Carpenter (1987) have provided excellent reviews of the literature dealing with the use of oculometric measures for evaluating aspects of the reading process ranging from perceptual to complex cognitive variables.

15.7   CONCLUDING COMMENTS

Some words of caution to the behavioral or social scientist applying oculometric measures. You should be warned that most measurements of oculometric variables have been done under highly constrained conditions, and there is at least suggestive evidence that when these constraints are removed, the system is found to operate somewhat differently. What are the constraints normally imposed by visual scientists concerned with eye movements? Since they are only interested in eye movements, they may inhibit head movements by the use of a bite-bar or head restraints. Thus, there may be some questions about generalizing from data collected under the preceding constraints to data collected under less constrained conditions. For example, the occurrence of "express saccades," those occurring with fixation pauses of less than 200 ms between them, were not observed (or perhaps they were ignored) until 5 or 10 years ago. They occur in a large variety of situations of interest to the behavioral scientist but very infrequently under the more "sterile" or controlled conditions routinely employed by visual scientists.

Similarly, the use of a bite-bar or chin rest and head restraint precludes or reduces the likelihood of a viewer using head movements to acquire visual information. In the "real" world, a combination of eye and head movements are frequently made to acquire visual information. The nature of eye movements associated with such gaze shifts may be quite different from eye movements made without head movements.

Similar comments can be made about the evaluation of eyeblinks. For example, the computer-based algorithm used in our laboratory was developed to evaluate blinks under somewhat restricted conditions, ones where the likehood of eye and head movements associated with gaze shifts were minimal. The blink detection algorithm necessary to reliably identify blinks under more complex laboratory conditions or real-world situations will be somewhat more complicated than the one initially developed.

One other caveat should be mentioned: The use of calibration procedures may alter the subject's procedure for acquiring visual information in even relatively simple experimental settings. Bartz (1966), for example, found that calibrating the eye movement system by immobilizing the subject's head significantly altered gaze shifts in subsequent experiments. Introduction of the calibration procedure significantly reduced the likelihood of head movements during the actual experiment. Instructions to acquire information "normally" does little to affect this phenomenon!

Thus, the behavioral scientist planning to use oculometric measures needs to rely on observational skills to augment conclusions drawn from the laboratory-based studies of the visual scientist.

NOTES

1 L. G. Tassinary and J. T. Cacioppo, personal communication.
2 L. Orchard and J. A. Stern, personal communication.

REFERENCES

Ahern, S. K. (1978). *Activitation and intelligence: Pupillometric correlates of individual differences in cognitive abilities.* Unpublished doctoral dissertation, University of California, Los Angeles.
Ahern, S. K., & Beatty, J. (1979). Physiological signs of information processing vary with intelligence. *Science, 205,* 1289–1292.
Ahern, S. K., & Beatty, J. (1981). Physiological evidence that demand for processing capacity

varies with intelligence. In M. Friedman, J. P. Dos, & N. O'Conner (Eds.), *Intelligence and learning.* New York: Plenum Press.

Alexandridis, E. (1985). *The pupil.* New York: Springer-Verlag.

Aserinsky, E. (1986). Proportional jerk: A new measure of motion as applied to eye movements in sleep and waking. *Psychophysiology, 23,* 340–347.

Bahill, A. T., & Stark, L. (1975). Overlapping saccades and glissades are produced by fatigue in the saccadic eye movement system. *Experimental Neurology, 48,* 95–106.

Bakan, P. (1971). The eyes have it. *Psychology Today, 96,* 64–67.

Bartz, A. G. (1966). Eye and head movements peripheral vision: Nature of compensatory eye movements. *Science, 153,* 1644–1645.

Bauer, L. O., Goldstein, R., & Stern, J. A. (1987). Effects of information processing demands on physiological response patterns. *Human Factors, 29,* 213–234.

Bauer, L. O. (1986). *Probe evoked potentials and lateralized cognitive activity. Effects of expectancy, processing demands, and time.* Ph.D. dissertation, Washington University, St. Louis, MO.

Bauer, L. O., Strock, B. D., Goldstein, R., Stern, J. A., & Walrath, L. C. (1985). Auditory discrimination and the eyeblink. *Psychophysiology, 22,* 636–641.

Beatty, J. (1982). Phasic not tonic pupillary responses vary with auditory vigilance performance. *Psychophysiology, 19*(2), 167–172.

Beatty, J. (1986). The pupillary system. In M. G. H. Coles, E. Donchin, & S. W. Porges (Eds.), *Psychophysiology: Systems, processes, and applications.* New York: Guilford Press.

Beatty, J., & Wagoner, B. L. (1978). Pupillometric signs or brain activation vary with level of cognitive processing. *Science, 199,* 1216–1218.

Beideman, L. R., & Stern, J. A. (1977). Aspects of the eyeblink during simulated driving as a function of alcohol. *Human Factors, 19,* 73–77.

Bender, W. R. G. (1933). The effect of pain and emotional stimuli and alcohol on pupillary reflex activity. *Psychological Monographs, 44,* 1–32.

Bitterman, M. E. (1945). Heart rate and frequency of blinking as indices of visual efficiency. *Journal of Experimental Psychology, 35,* 279–292.

Boersma, F. J., & Wilton, K. M. (1974). Eye movements and conservation acceleration in mildly retarded children. *American Journal of Mental Deficiency, 80,* 636–643.

Bradshaw, J. L. (1968). Pupil size and problem solving. *Quarterly Journal of Experimental Psychology, 20,* 116–122.

Brockway, L. F. (1975). *Attentional disturbance and thought disorder in schizophrenia as measured by eye movements and conceptual performance.* Unpublished doctoral dissertation, Washington University, St. Louis, MO.

Buettner-Ennever, J. A. (1977). Pathways from the pontine reticular formation to structures controlling horizontal and vertical eye movements in the monkey. *Developments in Neurosciene, 1,* 89.

Buettner-Ennever, J. A., & Henn, V. (1976). An autoradiographic study of the pathways from the pontine reticular formation involved in horizontal eye movements. *Brain Research, 108,* 155.

Buettner-Ennever, J. A., & Lang, W. (1978). Connections of a vertical eye movement are in the rostral mesencephalic tegmentum of the monkey. *Society of Neuroscience Abstracts, 4,* 161.

Bumke, O. (1903). Beitrage zur Kenntnis der Irisbewegungen. *Zentralblatt für Nervenheilkunde und Psychiatrie, 26,* 673–680.

Cacioppo, J. T., & Petty, R. E. (1986). Social processes. In M. G. H. Coles, E. Donchin, & S. W. Porges (Eds.), *Psychophysiology: Systems, processes, and applications.* New York: Guilford Press.

Darwin, C. (1872). *The expression of emotion in man and animals.* London: Murrary.

Diefendorf, A. R., & Dodge, R. (1908). An experimental study of the ocular reactions of the insane from photographic records. *Brain, 31,* 451–489.

Dimberg, U. (1987). Facial reactions, autonomic activity and experienced emotion: A three component model of emotional conditioning. *Biological Psychology, 24,* 105–122.

Dimberg, U., & Öhman, A. (1983). The effects of directional facial cues on electrodermal conditioning to facial stimuli. *Psychophysiology, 20,* 160–167.

Dunham, D. N. (1986). *The task-evoked pupillary response in a dichotic shadowing task.* Unpublished masters thesis, Ball State University, Muncie, IN.

Ehrlichman, H., & Weinberger, A. (1978). Lateral eye movements and hemispheric asymmetry: A critical review. *Psychological Bulletin, 85,* 1080–1101.

Exline, R. V. (1972). Visual interaction – The glances of power and preference. In J. K. Cole (Eds.), *Nebraska Symposium on Motivation.* Lincoln: University of Nebraska Press.

Fantz, R. L. (1961). The origin of form perception. *Scientific American, 204,* 66–72.

Feldon, S. E., & Burde, R. A. (1987). The oculomotor system. In R. A. Moses & W. M. Hart, Jr. (Eds.), *Adler's physiology of the eye.* St. Louis: Mosby.

Fischer, B., & Ramsperger, E. (1984). Human express saccades: Extremely short reaction times of goal directed eye movements. *Experimental Brain Research, 57,* 191–195.

Fogarty, C., & Stern, J. A. (in press). Eye movements and blinks: Their relationship to higher cognitive processes. *International Journal of Psychophysiology.*

Fox, S. A. (1966). The palpebral fissure. *American Journal of Ophthalmology, 62,* 73–78.

Galin, D., & Ornstein, R. (1974). Individual differences in cognitive styles: I. Reflective eye movements. *Neuropsychologia, 12,* 367–376.

Gang, K. (1945). Psychosomatic factors in the control of pupillary movements. *Journal of Clinical Psychopathology and Psychotherapy, 6,* 461–472.

Gentles, W., & Llewellyn-Thomas, E. (1971). Effects of benzodiazepines upon saccadic eye movements in man. *Clinical Pharmacology and Therapeutics, 12,* 563–574.

Gevins, A. S., & Schaffer, R. E. (1980). A critical review of electroencephalographic (EEG) correlates of higher cortical functions. *CRC Critical Reviews in Bioengineering,* October, 113–164.

Goldstein, R., Walrath, L. C., Stern, J. A., & Strock, B. D. (1985). Blink activity in a discrimination task as a function of stimulus modality and schedule of presentation. *Psychophysiology, 22,* 629–635.

Goldwater, B. C. (1972). Psychological significance of pupillary movements. *Psychological Bulletin, 77,* 340–355.

Goltz, T. H. (1975). *Comparison of the eye movements of skilled and less skilled readers.* Unpublished doctoral dissertation, Washington University, St. Louis, MO.

Green, J. L., Kraus, S. K., & Green, R. G. (1979). Pupillary responses to pictures and descriptions of sex-stereotyped stimuli. *Perceptual and Motor Skills, 49*(3), 759–764.

Gur, R. E., & Gur, R. C. (1975). Defense mechanisms, psychosomatic symptomatology and conjugate lateral eye movements. *Journal of Consulting and Clinical Psychology, 43,* 416–420.

Gur, R. E., Gur, R. C., & Harris, L. J. (1975). Cerebral activation as measured by subjects' lateral eye movements is influenced by experimenter location. *Neuropsychologia, 13,* 35–44.

Haberich, F. J., & Wittge, G. (1956). Beobachtungen ueber den Lidschlag des Rindes. *Zeitschrift für Vergleichende Physiologie, 39,* 89–96.

Hacker, W. (1962). Zur modification des sogenannten spontanen Lidschlags im Handlungsvollzug. *Probleme und Ergebnisse der Psychologie, 5,* 7–43.

Hakerem, G., & Sutton, S. (1964). *Pupillary reactions during observations of the near light threshold stimuli.* Paper presented at the annual meeting of the American Psychological Association, Los Angeles.

Hakerem, G., Sutton, S., & Zubin, J. (1964). Pupillary reactions to light in schizophrenic patients and normals. *Annals of the New York Academy of Sciences, 105,* 820–831.

Hall, A. A. (1945). The origin and purposes of blinking. *British Journal of Ophthalmology, 29,* 445–467.

Hansmann, D., Semmlow, J., & Stark, L. (1974). A physiological basis of pupillary dynamics. In M. P. Janisse (Ed.), *Pupillary dynamics and behavior.* New York: Plenum Press.

Heinrich, W. (1896). Die aufmerksamkeit und die Funktion der Sinnesorgane. *Zeitschrift für Psychologie und Physiologie der Sinnersorgane, 9,* 343–388.

Hess, E. H. (1965). Attitude and pupil size. *Scientific American, 212,* 46–54.

Hess, E. H. (1975). *The tell-tale eye.* New York: Van Nostrand Reinhold.

Hess, E. H., & Polt, J. M. (1960). Pupil size as related to interest value of visual stimuli. *Science, 132,* 340–350.

Hoffman, S., & Ison, J. R. (1980). Reflex modification in the domain of startle: I. Some empirical findings and their implications for how the nervous system processes sensory input. *Psychological Review, 87,* 175–189.

Holzman, P. S., Kringlen, E., Levy, D. L., & Haberman, S. (1980). Deviant eye tracking in twins discordant for psychosis: A replication. *Archives of General Psychiatry, 37,* 627–631.

Holzman, P. S., Proctor, L. R., Levy, D. L., Yasillo, N. J., Meltzer, H. Y., & Hurt, S. W. (1972). Eye-tracking dysfunction in schizophrenia patients and their relatives. *Archives of General Psychiatry, 31,* 143–151.

Huey, E. B. (1908). *The psychology and pedagogy of reading.* New York: Macmillan.

Janisse, M. P. (1974). *Pupillary dynamics and behavior.* New York: Plenum Press.

Janisse, M. P. (1977). *Pupillometry: The psychology of the pupillary response.* Washington, DC: Hemisphere Publishing.

Janisse, M. P., & Peavler, W. S. (1974). Pupillary research today: Emotion in the eye. *Psychology Today, 7,* 60–63.

Javal, E. (1879). Essai sur la physiologie de lecture. *Annales d'Oculistique, 82,* 242–253.

Just, M. A., & Carpenter, P. A. (1987). *The psychology of reading and language comprehension.* Newton, MA: Allyn & Bacon.

Kahneman, D. (1973). *Attention and effort.* New York: Prentice-Hall.

Kahneman, D., & Beatty, J. (1966). Pupil diameter and load on memory. *Science, 154,* 1583–1585.

Kanfer, F. H. (1960). Verbal rate, eyeblink and content in structured psychiatric interviews. *Journal of Abnormal and Social Psychology, 61,* 341–347.

Kennard, D. W., & Glaser, G. H. (1964). An analysis of eyelid movements. *Journal of Nervous and Mental Disease, 139,* 31–48.

Kuhlo, W., & Lehmann, D. (1964). Das Einschlaferleben und seine neurophysiologische Korrelate. *Archive für Psychiatrie and Zeitschrift für die Gesamte Neurologie, 205,* 687–716.

Landis, C., & Hunt, W. A. (1939). *The startle pattern.* New York: Farrar and Rinehart.

Lehmann, D., & Kuhlo, W. (1961). *EEG und subjektive Phänomene beim einschlafen und im frühen Schlafstadien.* Paper presented at the EEG Gesellschaft, Bad Nauheim.

Levin, S. (1984). Frontal lobe dysfunctions in schizophrenia I: Eye movement impairments. *Journal of Psychiatric Research, 18,* 27–55.

Levin, S., Holzman, P. S., Rothenberg, S. J., & Lipton, R. B. (1981). Saccadic eye movements in psychotic patients. *Psychiatric Research, 5,* 47–58.

Lidsky, A., Hakerem, G., & Sutton, S. (1971). Pupillary reactions to single light pulses in psychiatric patients and normals. *Journal of Nervous and Mental Disease, 153,* 286–291.

Lipton, R. B., Levin, S., & Holzman, P. S. (1980). Horizontal and vertical pursuit movements, the oculocephalic reflex, and the functional psychoses. *Psychiatric Research, 3,* 193–203.

Loewenfeld, I. E. (1958). Mechanism of reflex dilation of the pupil. *Documenta Ophthalmologica, 12,* 185–359.

Loewenfeld, I. E. (1966). Comment on Hess' findings. *Survey of Ophthalmology, 11,* 291–294.

Lowenstein, O., & Loewenfeld, I. E. (1951). Types of central autonomic innervation and fatigue. *Archives of Neurology and Psychiatry, 66,* 581–599.

Lowenstein, O., & Loewenfeld, I. E. (1962). The pupil. In H. Dawson (Ed.), *The eye* (Vol. 3). New York: Academic Press.

Luckiesh, M. (1947). Reading and the rate of blinking. *Journal of Experimental Psychology, 37,* 266–288.

Luckiesh, M., & Moss, F. K. (1942). *Reading as a visual task.* New York: Van Nostrand.

Luria, A. R. (1973). *The working brain.* New York: Basic Books.

Mackworth, N. H., & Bruner, J. (1970). How adults and children search and recognize pictures. *Human Development, 13,* 149–177.

Matin, E. (1974). Saccadic suppression: A review and analysis. *Psychological Bulletin, 81,* 899–917.

Metalis, S. A., & Hess, E. H. (1982). Pupillary response/semantic differential scale relationships. *Journal of Research in Personality, 16,* 201–216.

Moruzzi, G. (1972). Reviews of physiology: *Biochemistry and experimental pharmacology. The sleep-waking cycle.* New York: Springer-Verlag.

Moses, R. A. (1987). The eyelids. In R. A. Moses & W. M. Hart (Eds.), *Adlers physiology of the eye.* St. Louis: Mosby.

Netchine, S., Pugh, A. K., & Guihou, M. C. (1987). The organization of binocular vision in conjunction with head movements in French and English readers of 9 and 10 years. In O'Regan and Lèvy-Schoen (Eds.), *Eye movements: From physiology to cognition.* Amsterdam: North-Holland/Elsevier.

Nodine, C. F., & Lang, N. J., (1971). Development of visual scanning strategies for differentiating words. *Developmental Psychology, 5,* 221–231.

Oster, P. J., & Stern, J. A. (1980). Measurement of eye movement: Electrooculography. In I. Martin & P. H. Venables (Eds.), *Techniques in psychophysiology*. Chichester: Wiley.

Paivio, A. (1973). Psychophysiological correlates of imagery. In F. J. McGuigan & R. A. Schoonover (Eds.), *The psychophysiology of thinking: Studies of covert processes*. New York: Academic Press.

Plouffe, L., & Stelmack, R. M. (1979). Neuroticism and the effect of stress on the pupillary light reflex. *Perceptual and Motor Skills, 40*, 304.

Ponder, E., & Kennedy, W. P. (1928). On the act of blinking. *Quarterly Journal of Physiology, 18*, 89–110.

Poulton, E. C., & Gregory, E. L. (1952). Blinking during visual tracking. *Quarterly Journal of Experimental Psychology, 4*, 57–65.

Rayner, K. (Ed.) (1983). *Eye movements in reading: Perceptual and language processes*. New York: Academic Press.

Rubin, L. S., & Barry, T. J. (1972). The effect of the cold pressor test on pupillary reactivity of schizophrenics in remission. *Biological Psychiatry, 5*, 181–197.

Satterfield, J. H., & Dawson, M. E. (1971). Electrodermal correlates of hyperactivity in children. *Psychophysiology, 8*, 191–197.

Schluroff, M. (1982). Pupil responses to grammatical complexity of sentences. *Brain and Language, 17*(1), 133–145.

Shagass, C., Amadeo, M., & Overton, D. A. (1976). Eye-tracking performance and engagement of attention. *Archives of General Psychiatry, 33*, 121–125.

Shimazono, Y., Ando, K., Sakamoto, S., Tanaka, T., Eguchi, T., & Nakamura, H. (1965). Eye movements of waking subjects with closed eyes. *Archives of General Psychiatry, 13*, 537–543.

Skinner, N. F. (1980). The Hess et al., study of pupillary activity in heterosexual and homosexual males: A re-evaluation. *Perceptual and Motor Skills, 51*(3, Pt. I), 844.

Stanners, R. F., Coulter, M., Sweet, A. W., & Murphy, P. (1979). The pupillary response as an indicator of arousal and cognition. *Motivation and Emotion, 3*(4), 319–340.

Stanners, R. F., Headley, D. B., & Clark, W. R. (1972). The pupillary response to sentences: Influences of listening set and deep structure. *Journal of Verbal Learning and Verbal Behavior, 11*, 257–263.

Stern, J. A. (1978). Eye movements, reading, and cognition. In J. W. Senders, D. F. Fisher, & R. A. Monty, (Eds.), *Eye movements and the higher psychological functions*. Hillsdale, NJ: Erlbaum.

Stern, J. A., Bremer, D. A., & McClure, J. N., Jr. (1974). Analysis of eye movements and blinks during reading: Effects of Valium. *Psychopharmacologia, 40*, 171–175.

Stern, J. A., Goldstein, R., & Walrath, L. C. (1984). Phasic inattention: Electrooculographic markers. In M. G. H. Coles, J. R. Jennings, & J. A. Stern (Eds.), *Psychophysiological perspectives: Festschrift for Beatrice and John Lacey*. New York: Van Nostrand.

Stern, J. A., & Strock, B. D. (1987). Oculomotor activity and man–machine interaction in the workplace. In A. Gale & B. Christie (Eds.), *Psychophysiology and the electronic workplace*. New York: Wiley.

Stern, J. A., Walrath, L. C., & Goldstein, R. (1984). The endogenous eyeblink. *Psychophysiology, 21*, 22–33.

Stevens, J. (1978). Eyeblink and schizophrenia: Psychosis or tardive dyskinesia? *American Journal of Psychiatry, 135*, 223–226.

Vurpillot, E. (1968). The development of scanning strategies and their relation to visual differentiation. *Journal of Experimental Child Psychology, 6*, 632–650.

Watson, O. M., & Graves, T. D. (1966). Quantitative research in proxemic behavior. *American Anthropologist, 68*, 971–985.

Wilder, J. (1958). Modern psychotherapy and the law of initial values. *American Journal of Psychotherapy, 12*, 199–221.

Woodmansee, J. J. (1966a). Methodological problems in pupillographic experiments. *Proceedings of the 74th Annual Convention of the APA, 1*, 133–134.

Woodmansee, J. J. (1966b). An evaluation of pupillary response as a measure of attitude towards negroes. (Doctoral dissertation, University of Colorado, 1965). *Dissertation Abstracts, 26*, 6896–6897.

Yarbus, A. L. (1967). *Eye movements and vision*. New York: Plenum Press.

Yoss, R. E., Moyer, N. J., & Hollenhorst, R. W. (1970). Pupil size and spontaneous pupillary waves associated with alertness, drowsiness, and sleep. *Neurology, 20*, 545–554.

Young, L. R., & Sheena, D. (1975). Methods and designs: Survey of eye movement recording methods. *Behavior Research Methods and Instrumentation, 7,* 397–429.

Zahn, T. P. (1986). Psychophysiological approaches to psychopathology. In M. G. H. Coles, E. Donchin, & S. W. Porges (Eds.), *Psychophysiology: System, processes, and applications.* New York: Guilford Press.

Zahn, T. P., Little, B. C., & Wender, P. H. (1978). Pupillary and heart rate reactivity in children with minimal brain dysfunction. *Journal of Abnormal Child Psychology, 6,* 135–147.

Zuckerman, M. (1971). Physiological measures of sexual arousal in the human. *Psychological Bulletin, 75,* 297–329.

16   *The gastrointestinal system*

ROBERT M. STERN, KENNETH L. KOCH, AND MICHAEL W. VASEY

One of the most outspoken early proponents of the interaction of mind and gastrointestinal (GI) functioning was the gastroenterologist Walter Alvarez, who wrote the book *Nervousness, Indigestion and Pain* primarily for physicians. We recommend this book to all researchers and clinicians interested in the psychophysiology of the GI system and quote from the introduction:

I need hardly explain to fellow gastro-enterologists why I have chosen to discuss in one book nervousness, indigestion, and pain. Because these are the three main complaints that we commonly find associated together in one patient we must all of us be prepared to study and treat them together. We cannot very well treat a woman's indigestion while a psychiatrist treats her mind and a neurologist treats her pain. I discovered this years ago when a psychoanalyst referred to me a psychopathic woman with an irritable digestive tract. He said, "You take care of her colon and I'll take care of her mind," but this division of labor didn't work well, because on the days when her colon was "screaming at her" she couldn't listen to his psychotherapy, and when she came complaining to me about a mucous colic I hated to start any treatment until I had found out what particular mental conflict had that day thrown her nerves into an uproar. (1943, p. vii)

16.1   HISTORICAL BACKGROUND

16.1.1   *Gastric motor activity*

Until quite recently the psychophysiology of the GI system was a relatively unexplored area. This is surprising when one considers the landmark work of Wolf and Wolff (1943) in which they described the secretory and motility changes of their fistulated subject to various stress situations. A more recent report of Stern and Higgins (1969) indicated that for college-age individuals, GI symptoms are the most common bodily response to stress. However, the paucity of psychophysiology research on the GI system is not so surprising when we consider the instrumentation and measurement problems of obtaining data from far inside this constantly changing many-meter-long system.

As a consequence of these problems, no psychophysiological studies of absorption are known to the authors, and few studies of gastric acid secretion have been conducted by psychophysiologists. However, several studies of motor activity, particularly the more easily accessible two ends of the GI tract, the esophagus and rectum, but also the stomach, have been conducted. In this chapter we review psychophysiological studies that have measured gastric motor activity; the major emphasis will be on the motor activity of the stomach as measured with the electrogastrogram, or EGG. Current applications of EGG recording to psychological and health issues will be reviewed.

554

Empirical observation of human stomach motility began in earnest in 1825 with William Beaumont's observations of his patient Alexis St. Martin who had suffered an accidental gunshot wound that resulted in permanent gastric fistula (Beaumont, 1833). These observations and later experiments on fistulous patients and animals conducted primarily by German and Russian physiologists provided the bulk of the early information on gastric motility in digestion and disease. Extensive and important as they were, the observations tended to be qualitative rather than quantitative, and since they necessarily came from a very limited and always abnormal population, generalizations were difficult to make.

With the discovery of X-ray in 1895, Walter B. Cannon (1898) and (in 1904) Walter C. Alvarez (1968) began to study the movements of the stomach. At first a series of individual X-rays were used to make motion pictures. This procedure was eventually replaced by films (and today, video tapes) made directly from a fluoroscope screen. To be sure, motility can be examined by fluoroscopy for a limited period of time, although with this method quantification is also difficult, conditions are abnormal, and a definite risk to health exists.

During the first half of this century the most common method of studying gastric motility used pressure-recording systems attached to swallowed balloons. Many years passed before investigators realized that the inflated balloons stimulated the stomach and indeed brought about contractile activity (Davis, Garafolo, & Kveim, 1959). More recently, direct measures of mechanical and electrical activity associated with motility involve placing transducers or electrodes in or on the stomach and, therefore, share with the balloon method the double disadvantage of affecting the measured response and restricting the situations in which stomach activity can be examined. The same disadvantages arise, though possibly to a lesser degree, with swallowed metal balls, open-tipped catheters, tiny swallowed transducers (endoradiosones) that transmit pressure, and even fiber-optic endoscopes.

It is not surprising, then, that research on the control of stomach motility has come largely from in vitro and in vivo electrophysiological studies of animal preparations. Precontractile and contractile events in segments of guinea pig tenia coli and rat ileum and jejunum provided the data upon which models of the control of human motility were built. However, recent advances in techniques of biomedical measurement have opened the way for research on digestive and nondigestive motility in the undisturbed human gastrointestinal tract. We refer here to electrogastrography, the method of recording gastric potentials from the surface of the skin.

16.1.2 Electrogastrogram (EGG)

On October 14, 1921, Alvarez (1922) recorded what is considered to be the first EGG. Alverez described that experience as follows:

In 1921 I saw a very thin old woman who had a large bulging operative hernia in the left upper quardrant of the abdomen. The wall of the hernia, consisting as it did of almost nothing but skin and peritoneum, was so thin that the movements of the stomach could easily be seen under it. By placing electrodes on the skin over the stomach I was able to get what, as far as I know, were the first human electrogastrograms ever made. (1968, p. 1576)

In the mid-1950s R. C. Davis and co-workers began a series of exploratory studies with the EGG. They published two influential papers describing research with the EGG before Davis's untimely death in 1961. The first of these, Davis, Garafolo, and Gault (1957), described their technique for recording electrical potentials originating in the abdomen from electrodes on the skin surface. The EGG that was recorded was described and the possible role of other bodily signal generators such as respiration, bodily movements, heart, galvanic skin response, and general tissue potentials was evaluated. This initial study also included an attempt to validate the EGG using concomitant recordings from a mine detector that picked up the movements of a steel ball in the subjects' GI system. It was concluded that events in the stomach, intestines, and possibly other internal organs produce many of the waves recorded from the surface of the skin.

Davis, Garafolo, and Kveim (1959), in the second of these exploratory studies, investigated the effects of factors such as food, rest, and visual stimulation on the EGG. They also compared the EGG with records obtained from a gastric balloon, the common method of recording gastric contractions at that time. They reported that the activity of the stomach is at its lowest point when the stomach is empty, a controversial finding in light of the reports of Cannon and Carlson (e.g., Cannon & Washburn, 1912; Carlson, 1916). Davis et al. (1959) made the point that so-called hunger contractions are rather rare and seemed to be stimulated by the introduction of a balloon into the stomach, just as if the system was attempting to digest the actual recording balloon.

Although Davis et al.'s research with the EGG was certainly not the earliest, these two publications were very important in stimulating the work of other investigators, including the present authors. The probable reason why other investigators did not follow up on the work of Alvarez (1922) is that the technology was not available for obtaining stable recordings of the relatively slow, low-amplitude EGG signals. On the other hand, by the time Davis et al.'s articles appeared, improved amplifiers and recorders were available and there was a greater recognition of the need for new methods of recording the motor activity of the stomach that did not involve an invasive technique, which by its very presence would prevent the recording of normal ongoing activity. (For a more complete history of the EGG see Stern, 1985.)

16.2   ANATOMY AND PHYSIOLOGY OF THE GASTROINTESTINAL TRACT WITH PARTICULAR EMPHASIS ON THE STOMACH

The GI system extends from the mouth to the rectum and includes the mouth, esophagus, stomach, small intestine, large intestine, and rectum. The three functions of the GI system are movement of food through the alimentary tract, secretion of substances that aid in digestion or protect the alimentary tract, and absorption of the digestive end products.

The GI tract may be considered to be a series of muscular tubes that have been modified to perform region-specific digestive functions, that is, transit of food from esophagus to stomach, mixing and emptying of ingested foods from the stomach into the duodenum, and absorption of micronutrients from the small intestine. Other specialized tubes (i.e., the cecum, ascending, transverse, and descending colon, and rectum) conserve water, electrolytes, and nutrients and evacuate wastes. These functions require exquisite control and integration of relevant neural, muscular, mucosal, and hormonal systems within the GI tract.

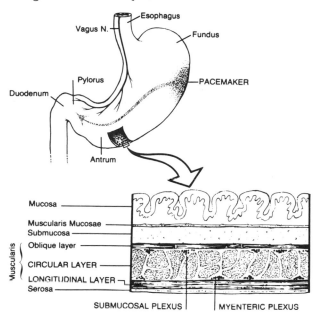

Figure 16.1. Stomach and its principal regions. Inset shows major layers of gastric wall. Origin of gastric pacesetter potentials (pacemaker signals) indicated by stippled region on gastric body. (Reprinted by permission from Stern & Koch, 1985.)

The purpose of this section is to describe briefly the anatomy and physiology of the stomach. Although basic similarities exist between the anatomy and physiology of the stomach and other regions of the GI tract, each region has its own function-specific modifications. The interested reader is referred to Johnson, Christensen, Jacobsen, and Schultz (1987) for a review of the physiology of these other regions of the GI tract.

16.2.1 *Gastric anatomy*

In most subjects the stomach lies in the left upper quadrant of the abdomen, although there is a wide range of individual variability in its shape and form (Figure 16.1; see also chapter 3 in Williams, 1956). The body and antrum, however, are rotated toward the midline such that the antrum is near the epigastric region. As is shown in Figure 16.1, the esophagus enters the stomach in the fundic region; the antrum is connected to the first portion of the duodenum, the duodenal bulb, via the pyloris.

The stomach has three major regions: the fundus, body, and antrum. The stomach wall has three layers: outermost is the serosa; innermost is the mucosa, which secretes acid and pepsin; and the thickest layer is the muscular portion, which has three layers, an outer longitudinal layer, an inner circular layer, and in some areas an oblique layer (see Figure 16.1).

The muscular wall of the stomach contains extensive neural elements, both extrinsic and intrinsic. Extrinsic nerves are pre- and postganglionic parasympathetic fibers from the vagus nerve and postganglionic neurons from the sympathetic splanchnic nerves. These extrinsic neural circuits are closely integrated with the intrinsic nervous system of the stomach and of all regions of the GI tract, the enteric nervous system.

The enteric nervous system is a collection of nerve cell bodies in plexi located between the circular and longitudinal muscle layers, that is, the myenteric plexus (Auerbach's plexus) and submucosal plexus (see Figure 16.1). The myenteric and submucosal plexi are the largest, but seven discrete plexi have been described. Postganglionic parasympathetic neurons, internuncial neurons, and sensory neurons are present within the plexi. At least 10 different types of enteric neurons have been identified by immunohistochemical methods (Furness & Costa, 1980). It has been estimated that there are 10^9 neurons in the enteric nervous system, a number similar to that in the spinal cord. Fibers from the sympathetic neurons synapse on myenteric plexus neurons and innervate the circular muscle layer. Thus, the muscular layers of the stomach, particularly the circular muscle layers, have rich neural integration that allows for fine control of muscular contraction required for normal digestive function. The interested reader may refer to review articles on neural control of gastric motility (Meyer, 1987; Roman & Gonella, 1987).

16.2.2   *Postprandial gastric physiology*

The major physiological activities of the stomach are to receive ingested foodstuffs and to mix the foodstuffs into suspensions until they are appropriate for emptying and further digestion in the small intestine.

Normal reception of ingested food requires the gastric fundus to relax and to accommodate the particular ingested volume. These muscular activities of the stomach are termed receptive relaxtion and accommodation and are accomplished via vagal efferent activity (Roman & Gonella, 1987). Moreover, because nearly 90 percent of vegal fibers are sensory, it is assumed that sensory vagal traffic modulates ongoing vagal efferent activity.

After ingestion solid foods are moved from the gastric fundus into the gastric body and antrum for mixing and emptying. This period is called the *lag phase* because it precedes actual emptying of the nutrient suspensions from the stomach into the duodenum (Lavigne, Wiley, Meyer, Martin, & MacGregor, 1978; Meyer, MacGregor, Gueller, Martin, & Cavalieri, 1976). In contrast to solids, nonnutrient liquids such as water have no lag phase. Before emptying, solids are normally mixed and reduced to 0.1–1 mm diameter particles and suspended in gastric juice (Meyer, Ohashi, Jehn, & Thompson, 1981).

The stomach accomplishes the work of mixing and emptying through a series of smooth rhythmic contractions at the rate of 3 cycles per minute (cpm). This phase in the digestive process, known as peristalsis, commences in the gastric body and moves through this region into the antrum where the waves dissipate in the prepyloric region. As a result of these wavelike contractions, small food particles already in suspension are carried through the open pyloric sphincter into the duodenum (Meyer et al., 1981; Meyer, Gu, Dressman, & Amidon, 1986). The pyloris and the duodenum may contract to create resistance to gastric emptying or may relax to promote *gastroduodenal synchrony* and enhance gastric emptying (Meyer, 1987). The hydrodynamics of the suspension itself may determine which particles are emptied and their rate of emptying (Meyer et al., 1986).

Control of the mixing and emptying of gastric content is complex. In addition to physical properties of the gastric contents and the various neural–muscular responses, the release of gastrointestinal hormones (e.g., gastrin, secretin, cholecystokinin, enteroglucagon, gastric inhibitory polypeptide, somatostatin, vasoactive intestinal polypeptide, and motilin, to name a few of the more than 20 GI hormones and candidate hormones) is believed to modulate the contractile responses of the stomach and to affect overall gastric emptying rates. However, specific actions of most GI hormones on gastric motility in humans remain to be determined.

The rate at which foodstuffs are emptied from the stomach is dependent on many factors including the volume of ingested material, caloric density (i.e., fat, protein, or carbohydrate), osmolality, temperature, acidity, and viscosity. These factors are adjusted by chemo- and mechanoreceptors in the stomach and duodenum and the variety of hormones released by the specific foodstuffs (Meyer, 1987).

Emptying of liquids is thought to be controlled by fundic tone. That is, after the ingestion of a liquid such as water fundic pressure is greater than duodenal pressure. The pressure gradient between fundus and duodenum provides the force necessary to empty the liquid from the stomach (Meyer, 1987). Other studies indicate that the antrum has a more active role in the emptying of liquids (Camilleri, Malagelada, Brown, Becker, & Zinsmeister, 1985; Stemper & Cooke, 1975).

16.2.3 *Gastric physiology during fasting*

During the interdigestive state (e.g., an overnight fast), the stomach completes its digestive function and participates in a stereotyped periodic sequence of contractile events termed the *interdigestive complex.* The complex is divided into three phases: Phase I is a period of quiescence lasting approximately 20 min; Phase II is a period of irregular contractile activity of the body and antrum lasting about 80–90 min; and Phase III is a 5–10 min period of regular and intense 3-cpm contractions of the gastric body and antrum. The antral contractions are peristaltic, moving into the duodenum and subsequently through the small bowel. Phase III activity occurs approximately every 90–110 min in humans during prolonged fasts and has been associated with bursts of pancreatic and biliary secretions and elevations in plasma motilin levels (Code & Marlett, 1975; Lee, Chey, Tai, & Yajima, 1978; Meyer, 1987; Schlegel & Code, 1975; Vantrappen et al., 1979).

From a physiological viewpoint, Phase III contractions have been shown to empty fibrous meal residue from the stomach (Schlegel & Code, 1975). The Phase III contractions may serve a similar function in the small intestine and have been termed the "intestinal housekeeper."

16.2.4 *Relationship between gastric motor activity and gastric myoelectric activity*

The gastric contractions that occur at 3 cpm during the mixing and emptying of meals are the result of coordinated electromechanical coupling of circular layer smooth muscle cells. What are the electrical and mechanical events within the smooth muscle that underlie the mechanical work performed by the stomach?

16.2.4.1 *Gastric slow waves*

Gastric slow waves are the electrical events that control gastric contractions. The slow waves result from spontaneous depolarizations of the longitudinal muscle in

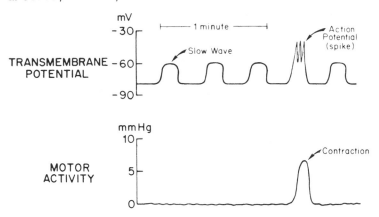

Figure 16.2. Relationship among slow waves, action (spike) potentials, and contractile or motor activity in stomach. Rhythmic slow waves are not associated with appreciable contractile activity. In contrast, when spike potentials are linked to slow waves and occur on slow wave plateaus, contraction of circular muscle occurs. (Reprinted by permission from Feldman & Schiller, 1983.)

the region of the juncture of the fundus and body on the greater curvature (see Figure 16.1). The outer layer of the circular muscle layer may participate in the genesis of slow waves. From this region, the pacemaker area, the depolarization wave front moves circumferentially and distally toward the distal antrum (see Figure 16.1). The normal slow-wave frequency in humans is 3 cpm (Abell & Malagelada, 1985; Couturier, Roze, Paologgi, & Debray, 1972; Hamilton, Bellahsene, Reichelderfer, Webster, & Bass, 1986; Hinder & Kelly, 1977; Kwong, Brown, Whittaker, & Duthie, 1970). The slow wave does not move into the fundic area, which is electrically silent. The slow wave is a spontaneous event, sodium mediated and omnipresent, and is associated with very low amplitude contractile activity (Morgan, Schmalz, & Szurszewski, 1978; You & Chey, 1984).

The slow-wave coordinates the frequency and propagation velocity of gastric contractions in the body antrum. That is, the slow wave brings the circular muscle layer near the point of depolarization, and if physical, neural, and/or hormonal signals are appropriate for contraction, the depolarization threshold is reached and circular muscle contraction occurs (Figure 16.2). Because circular muscle contractions are linked with the slow wave, the circular muscle contractions occur at the slow-wave frequency (3 cpm in humans) and the contractions propagate at the slow-wave velocity (0.8–4 cm/s). For these reasons the slow waves have also been called pacesetter potentials and electrical control activity (Meyer, 1987; Roman & Gonella, 1987).

Slow waves are considered myogenic phenomena, but extrinsic neural input may modulate the rhythmicity of depolarization. For example, after vagotomy in dogs and humans, the slow-wave frequency may be disrupted for weeks (Kelly & Code, 1969; Stoddard, Smallwood, & Duthie, 1981). The precise origins and controls of slow-wave activity are unknown.

16.2.4.2 *Gastric spike potentials*

The electrical events underlying circular smooth muscle contractions are plateau and spike potentials (see Figure 16.2). Depolarizations of the circular muscle, in contrast to the longitudinal muscle, are very fast (i.e., spikes). The spikes may or may not occur on plateau potentials, which are associated with the slow wave. The spikes reflect fluxes of calcium passing through the circular muscle membrane. Contractions of the circular muscle may increase tone and/or intraluminal pressure, particularly if they form concentric ring contractions. Such strong contractions may be recorded with strain gauges, intraluminal pressure transducers, or perfused cathers. However, gastric contractions that are not concentric may not be recorded by intraluminal devices but will be recorded by strain gauges positioned on the muscle itself (You & Chey, 1984).

In summary, gastric slow waves are present at all times and control the frequency and propagation velocity of spike potentials (i.e., circular muscle contractions) when the latter are elicited by the appropriate stimuli. Gastric slow waves and spike potentials are the myoelectric components of gastric contractions. It is these contractions that perform the work of mixing and emptying foodstuffs.

Slow waves and spike potentials from the stomach may be recorded from electrodes sewn to the serosa or from electrodes applied to the gastric mucosa. Because these slow waves occur within a conducting medium (i.e., the body), they are also recorded with fidelity from electrodes positioned on the skin (Abell & Malagelada, 1985; Brown, Smallwood, Duthie, & Stoddard, 1975; Familoni, Bowes, Kingma, & Cote, 1987; Hamilton et al., 1986). The relationship of these signals (EGGs) to gastric myoelectric and motor activity is discussed in the next section.

16.3   INFERENTIAL CONTEXT

16.3.1   *Relationship of the EGG to gastric myoelectric activity and gastric motor activity*

16.3.1.1 *EEG and gastric myoelectric activity*

Nelsen and Kohatsu (1968) simultaneously recorded the electrical activity from electrodes implanted on the serosal surface of the stomach and EGGs from 13 patients. They found an excellent correspondence between the frequency of the signals obtained from the EGG and the internal electrodes. They did not compare the amplitudes of the signals. A more recent comparison of EGG and serosal recordings from dogs by Smout, van der Schee, and Grashuis (1980b) also indicated a perfect correspondence between the frequency of the signals.

In an effort to study the relationship of the EGG to internal electrical activity of the stomach without involving surgery, several investigators have compared the EGG to simultaneously recorded mucosal signals. The mucosal signals are obtained from swallowed electrodes (i.e., electrodes inside the stomach). Hamilton et al. (1986) compared EGG and mucosal signals from 20 human subjects during fasting, after ingesting milk, and in one case, during a period of spontaneous dysrhythmia. They summarized their findings as follows:

We did find that the surface recordings were of similar visual form as those obtained directly from the mucosa simultaneously. In addition, frequency analysis determined that the two simultaneously obtained signals were of the same frequency. Finally when the rare arrhythmic events occurred, they were detected in both the mucosal and cutaneous signals. Therefore, the signal obtained from the skin does seem to accurately reflect the BER as measured directly from the stomach mucosa. (p. 37)

Abell and Malagelada (1985) used magnetic force to maintain internal electrodes in opposition with the gastric wall and compared signals obtained from the mucosal electrodes with those obtained from the EGG. They also reported that frequency analysis showed very good correspondence between the internal and EGG signals.

16.3.1.2 *EGG and gastric motor activity*

Until the mid-1960s investigators who used the EGG assumed that they were recording, from the surface of the skin, voltage changes that were due to the contractions of the smooth muscle of the stomach; that is, they assumed a one-to-one relationship between the EGG and the contractions of the stomach. However, in 1968 Nelsen and Kohatsu presented a different view of the source of the EGG signal. They stated that the EGG was a function of gastric slow-wave activity, or pacesetter potentials. Nelsen and Kohatsu and others have claimed that the surface-recorded EGG reflects the waxing and waning of pacesetter potentials of the stomach but not gastric contractions. However, they did present evidence that indicated that when contractions do occur, they are time locked to the slow wave and, therefore, to the EGG.

Beginning in 1975 Smallwood and his colleagues published a number of studies (e.g., Smallwood, 1978; Smallwood & Brown, 1983) in which they examined the frequency of the EGG and made numerous advances in techniques for analysis of the EGG signal. In some studies (e.g., Brown et al., 1975) they compared the EGG signal with intragastric pressure recordings. Their findings were the same as those of Nelsen and Kohatsu (1968). When contractions occurred, they occurred at the same frequency as the EGG signals; and whereas the EGG showed 3 cpm almost continuously for most subjects, contractions as recorded with intragastric pressure instruments did not.

It should be noted that the simultaneous presence of 3-cpm EGG and the absence of changes in intragastric pressure does not necessarily indicate that the EGG is unrelated to contractions as Nelsen and Kohatsu (1968), Brown et al. (1975), and others have suggested. The possibility exists that the EGG is a more sensitive measure of gastric contractile activity than the pressure-sensitive probes. That is, the EGG may reflect increases in electrical activity (i.e., spike activity) during contractile events that do not alter gastric intraluminal pressure. In fact, in a recent report, Vantrappen, Hostein, Janssens, Vanderweerd, and De Wever (1983) indicated that low-amplitude 5-cpm motor activity is always present in the dog. In addition, You and Chey (1984) have shown that in dogs the 5-cpm pacesetter potentials correlated well with low-amplitude contractions recorded by strain gauges sewn to serosa but correlated poorly with intraluminal pressure changes.

From 1980 to the present, published reports have appeared that not only suggest that the EGG provides information about frequency of contractions but also, indeed, that the amplitude of the EGG is related to the degree of contractile activity (Smout, 1980; Smout, van der Schee, & Grashuis 1980a; Smout et al., 1980b). The major contribution of Smout and his colleagues was to point out that the amplitude of the

EGG increases when a contraction occurs. They concluded that the pacesetter potential and the second potential, which is related to contractions, are reflected in the EGG. Abell, Tucker, and Malagelada (1985) recently conducted a study in which they compared the EGG signal from healthy human subjects with the electrical signal recorded from the mucosal surface of the stomach and intraluminal pressure. They summarized their findings as follows: "Antral phasic pressure activity, when present, was accompanied by an increase in amplitude and/or a change in shape of both the internal and external ECG" (p. 86).

Koch and Stern (1985) reported a perfect correlation of EGG waves and peristaltic antral contractions observed during simultaneous EGG–fluoroscopy recordings in four healthy subjects. Hamilton et al. (1986) reported that fluoroscopy revealed contractions in the antrum that correlated with three- and fourfold increases in amplitude of the EGG.

The relationship of the amplitude of EGG waves to contractions is complex and not totally understood at this time. However, in addition to the studies mentioned, there is considerable indirect evidence linking amplitude changes in the EGG with strength of contractile activity. For example, in situations where increased contractile activity would be expected (e.g., eating, after swallowing barium), EGG amplitude increases (Hamilton et al., 1986; Jones & Jones, 1985; Koch, Stewart, & Stern, 1987). And in patients with diabetic gastroparesis, where one would expect weak contractility activity, Hamilton et al. (1986) found no increase in the amplitude of EGG after eating.

Can EGG amplitude alone be used to infer reliably the presence or absence of GI contractions? No, not at this time. It is possible that with improved methods of measuring contractile activity we shall find that all myoelectric activity is accompanied by some contractile activity (see Morgan et al., 1978; Vantrappen et al., 1983; You & Chey, 1984) and that the amplitude of the EGG is related to the intensity or strength of contractile activity. A significant question then becomes: Can the amplitude of the EGG be used to determine whether the accompanying gastric contractile activity is of sufficient strength to do the motor work of the stomach (i.e., mixing and propelling)?

In summary, it is generally accepted that the frequency of the EGG is identical to the frequency of gastric pacesetter potentials recorded from the mucosal or serosal surface of the stomach. There is no general agreement, on the other hand, as to the sources of the amplitude of the EGG. Indirect evidence from several studies has demonstrated that amplitude increases during an increase in contractile activity; however, the amplitude of the EGG alone cannot be used reliably to determine the presence or absence of contractions.

16.3.2 *Quantification of the EGG*

16.3.2.1 *Early attempts*

R. C. Davis developed procedures for hand-scoring EGG records in 30-s segments for amplitude, frequency, and displacement (see Russell & Stern, 1967, for details). *Amplitude* was the favored measure in precomputer times because changes in it were more obvious than the other measures. We are still interested in the amplitude of the EGG today but must caution the reader that it does vary from subject to subject and within the same subject from site to site. Therefore, amplitude changes

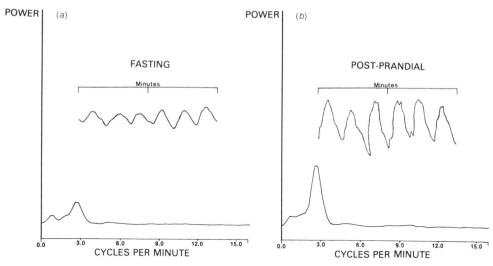

Figure 16.3. Spectral plots and corresponding EGG data from subject (a) before and (b) after eating. Note increase in power at 3 cpm after eating.

should only be considered within a session and from the same recording site. *Frequency* is of great interest to contemporary workers in this area; spectral analysis will be discussed in the next section. *Displacement* was Davis's term for very slow changes in the EGG. We now believe that some of what Davis called displacement was caused by inadequate techniques (e.g., electrode or amplifier drift) and some was ultraslow wave activity 0.5–2.0 cpm. We (Stern, Koch, Stewart, & Lindblad, 1987) have noted the presence of ultraslow wave activity in the EGG, as have others (e.g., Hölzl, Löffler, & Müller, 1985).

16.3.2.2 *Spectral analysis*

Spectral analysis typically uses the Fast Fourier Transform (FFT) to convert a signal in the time domain into a series of coefficients describing the amplitudes and phase relationships of its independent sinusoidal waveforms. A thorough description of spectral analysis techniques is beyond the scope of this chapter. The interested reader is referred to the chapter in this volume on the FFT (Porges & Bohrer, chapter 21). The output of a spectral analysis is the squared magnitude of the FFT and is typically graphed as a curve showing the strength, or power, of the frequencies into which the original signal can be decomposed. Figure 16.3 shows an example of a spectral analysis with the original EGG record. Although power has a very specific meaning in mathematics and physics, we may think of it as an index of the amplitude of the sine waves of a particular frequency that would be required in order to recreate the EGG record. In the analysis of EGG recordings we are usually interested in the power within the following three frequency bands: 0.5–2.0, 2.5–3.5, and 4.0–9.0 cpm. The first represents the often found but poorly understood ultraslow rhythm. The second encompasses the basic electric rhythm of the human gastric antrum (3 cpm), and the third includes frequencies commonly associated with nausea and is referred to as tachygastria.

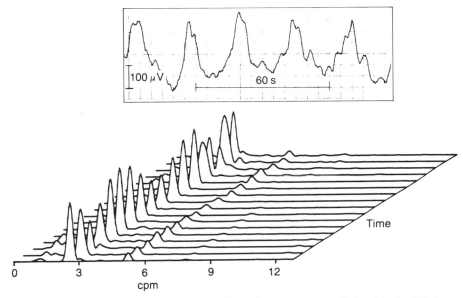

Figure 16.4. Running spectral analysis from resting control subject plotted as pseudo-three-dimensional display. Frequency is depicted on x-axis, time on y-axis, power appears to rise from page as third dimension. Note strong 3-cpm activity in portion of EGG record included in figure and in pseudo-three-dimensional display.

Spectral analysis is currently the most commonly used method of analyzing the EGG (see Smallwood & Brown, 1983) and the method favored by the authors. Van der Schee, Smout, and Grashuis (1982) have described an extension of this method that makes use of running spectral analysis to depict EGG data. Running spectral analysis, with overlapping power spectra displayed as a function of time, yields both frequency and time information. The more conventional spectral analysis provides power only as a function of frequency, not time. With this new technique, frequency, power, and time can be depicted two-dimensionally either with a pseudo-three-dimensional display or with a gray-scale plot. Figure 16.4 shows an example of a pseudo-three-dimensional display and a portion of the corresponding raw EGG record.

A brief description of the procedure used to go from raw EGG data to a pseudo-three-dimensional display follows. Because of the very slow electrical changes that are associated with the EGG, only a very slow electrically stable electrode can be used; silver-silver chloride (Ag–AgCl) electrodes are recommended. The optimal recording sites will depend on the nature of the signal desired, for example, largest possible amplitude; lowest artifact from EKG, respiration, and subject movement; and position of the subject's internal organs, particularly the antrum of the stomach and the diaphragm (Mirizzi & Scafoglieri, 1983). For single-channel recording for most subjects the greatest EGG amplitude will be obtained with bipolar electrodes: one electrode on the subject's left side approximately 6 cm from the midline and just below the lowest rib and the other on the midline just above the umbilicus. The location of the electrodes will not affect the

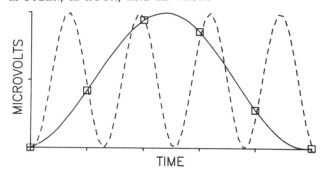

Figure 16.5. Illustration of aliasing effect. With only six samples over interval, sinusoid with frequency 4 appears identical to one with frequency 1. Thus, in waveform composed of both frequencies but sampled at this slow rate, power of frequency 4 component would leak into power of frequency 1 component.

frequency of the EGG but will affect the amplitude and waveform. The amplifying and recording system should filter out signals below 0.5 and above 15 cpm. With these filter settings one can record ultraslow rhythms (0.5–2.0 cpm) but still eliminate shifts in baseline due to DC potentials. Frequencies higher than 30 cpm are filtered out to avoid domination of the gastric signal by electrocardiographic activity. Respiration can also obscure the EGG, but its frequency range falls near that of tachygastria, and rather than remove it with analog filters at the time of recording, it is preferable to remove it later with more precise and flexible digital filters.

From the polygraph the EGG signal is channeled to an analog-to-digital (A/D) converter where it is digitized into a series of numerical values representing discrete voltage levels of the input signal. Thus the analog EGG signal is converted to a digital time series that can then be subjected to a wide range of analyses. The A/D conversion units typically allow sampling at a wide range of speeds. Given an EGG signal that has had frequencies faster than 15 cpm, or 0.25 Hz, attenuated at the time of recording, a sampling rate of at least 1 Hz is desirable. Since the FFT procedure requires a number of points equal to a power of 2, a noninteger sampling rate may be chosen to fulfill this requirement. For example, a sampling rate of 4.267 Hz yields 256 data points per minute. We recommend such a high sampling rate because of the potential for aliasing high-frequency components such as EKG that may be present in the EGG. Even when the EGG signal is subjected to a high-frequency filter with a relatively low cutoff such as 0.25 Hz, some EKG may still be present, though greatly attenuated. A high sampling rate such as 4.267 Hz allows complete resolution of all frequencies remaining in the EGG and thus prevents aliasing of these frequencies.

When several frequency components of a signal are indistinguishable after sampling, the signal is said to be aliased. Figure 16.5 illustrates the aliasing effect. With only six samples over the interval, a function of frequency 4 appears identical to one with frequency 1. In such an example, the power present at frequency 4 would be added to the true power at frequency 1. This problem is known as leakage. The power at the higher frequency leaks into the estimate representing the power at the lower frequency. Thus, one should choose a high enough sampling rate to ensure that even low-amplitude, high-frequency components of the EGG do not

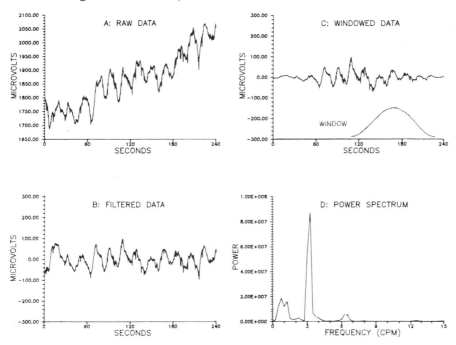

Figure 16.6. (*a*) Raw EGG segment showing slow shift in baseline. (*b*) Same segment after zero centering and removal of slow shift via high-pass filtering. (*c*) Segment after Hamming window was applied. Hamming window is shown below windowed waveform. (*d*) Power spectrum of windowed data segment.

leak into the frequency ranges of interest. As noted, we recommend a rate of 4.267 Hz, which ensures that leakage is minimal.

Once one has digitized the EGG signal, it must be preprocessed in order to best meet the assumptions of spectral analysis. The reader is referred to chapter 21 (Porges & Bohrer) and chapter 22 (Gottman) for a thorough discussion of these assumptions. Because the dominant frequency in the EGG is so slow, we recommend the use of at least 4-min data windows. Thus, at 4.267 samples per second, a 4-min segment would be composed of 1,024 data points. It is generally desirable to center data for spectral analysis around a mean of zero. This is easily accomplished by subtracting the mean of the segment from each data point. Additionally, the EGG is likely to contain some very slow components that reflect a shifting baseline or other undetermined factors. Such extremely low frequency shifts and simple linear trends should be removed to provide a clean spectrum. A high-pass digital filter that attenuates frequencies below 0.01 Hz accomplishes such trend removal. One can also remove simple linear trends by fitting a least-squares regression line and subtracting it from the data segment.

Figure 16.6 demonstrates the processing of the EGG. A raw digitized EGG segment of 4 min duration and composed of 1,024 data points is presented in Figure 16.6. This data segment shows an obvious baseline shift. First, the segment was zero centered and the baseline shift was removed using a high-pass filter (see Figure 16.6). Next, this data segment was windowed in order to reduce leakage (see Figure

16.6). Windowing is the application of a weighting function that tapers the beginning and end of the data segment to zero. Thus, the middle of the segment is unaltered, or multiplied by a weight of 1, whereas the ends are multiplied by weights gradually approaching zero. This is necessary because when a signal abruptly terminates, there is leakage in the power spectrum. The window shown in Figure 16.6 gradually tapers a signal to zero at each end of the segment and greatly reduces this leakage. The window applied in this example is a Hamming window. However, many other windows may be chosen depending on the characteristics of the signal (see Porges & Bohrer, chapter 21). Generally, such windows as the Hamming, Hanning, and Tukey–Blackman all provide compararable results when used with the EGG.

After such preprocessing, the data segment is Fourier transformed and the spectral density estimates calculated. The spectrum of our example data segment is shown in Figure 16.6. These density estimates reflect the power at the various frequency components of the data segment. In our example, this Fourier transformation provides 512 power estimates for the frequency range 0–2.134 Hz, which yields resolution of frequencies at intervals of 0.0042 Hz, or 0.25 cpm. This is the case because spectral analysis provides information on frequencies only up to half the sampling rate, which was 4.267 Hz in this example. These estimates may be averaged together to provide more stable estimates of power.

In order to produce a running spectral analysis, one overlaps consecutive data segments by 75 percent. In other words, segment 1 includes minutes 1–4, segment 2 includes minutes 2–5, and so on. Thus, 1 min of new information is provided in each consecutive power spectrum. These overlapping power spectra can be plotted in a pseudo-three-dimensional fashion to allow easy viewing of changes in power at various frequencies as a function of time (see Figure 16.4).

While such running spectral analysis does provide a useful way to view frequency and power changes over time, it is important to note that transient changes in the EGG may go unnoticed if they are small. If such transient changes are large enough, they will appear but only as a gradual change, with the peak in spectral density appearing in the pseudo-three-dimensional display several minutes after it occurred in real time. Thus, running spectral analysis may not be appropriate for experiments in which very short duration stimulus-induced changes are expected. Analysis of very short discrete data segments would be more appropriate in such a case.

Similarly, spectral analysis is useful only when the EGG signal contains a significant amount of cyclical activity. This is usually the case for 3-cpm activity. However, some gastric phenomena occur intermittently and may not appear in a spectral plot. For most studies examining only the 3-cpm activity, this is not a problem because any segment of normal EGG is likely to contain a strong cyclical component. However, for phenomena such as tachygastria the issue is less clear. We have experienced no difficulty in quantifying this phenomenon through spectral analysis. When bursts of tachygastria are seen during motion sickness, they are typically 1 or more minutes in duration and are seen quite clearly in running spectral plots of 4-min epochs (Stern, Koch, Stewart, & Lindblad, 1987). However, there may indeed be more appropriate methods of analysis for quantification of very brief duration, intermittent phenomena (see, e.g., Hölzl et al., 1985, for a discussion of so-called zoom FFTs).

16.3.3 *Current understanding of the EGG*

The publication of an edited volume devoted to the EGG (Stern & Koch, 1985), the inclusion of three chapters (Hölzl, 1983; Müller, Hölzl, & Brüchle, 1983; Stern, 1983) dealing with EGG recording in a recent book edited by Hölzl and Whitehead (1983), a chapter on the EGG (Davis, 1986) in a psychophysiology reference book edited by Coles, Donchin, and Porges (1986), and a recent review article in *Psychophysiology* by Stern, Koch, Stewart, and Vasey (1987) and in *Digestive Diseases and Sciences* by Abell and Malagelada (1988) indicate increasing interest in this measure. Individuals trained in psychology, psychiatry, physiology, gastroenterology, and bioengineering working in Canada, Germany, Holland, France, Italy, England, Russia, China, Japan, and the United States are studying EGG methodology and validation as well as using the measure to study the effects of food, drugs, psychological variables, and individual differences on gastric motility in health and disease. Stern, Koch, Stewart, and Vasey (1987) listed the following points as a summary of their current understanding of the EGG.

1 The 3-cpm frequency of the EGG reflects the frequency of pacesetter potentials occurring at the serosal and mucosal surfaces of the stomach.
2 Under many situations, increases in the amplitude of the EGG are indicators of increased gastric contractile activity.
3 Tachygastria (4–9 cpm) recorded with the EGG reflects identical frequencies recorded with mucosal electrodes from the gastric antrum.
4 Low-frequency components (approximately 1 cpm) often appear in the EGG signal, but their psychological and physiological significance is unknown at this time.
5 Some forms of stress such as that evoked by the Stroop test or motion sickness simulators as well as any condition involving nausea are accompanied by a decrease in amplitude of the EGG and/or a change in the dominant frequency of the EGG from 3 cpm to dysrhythmia, usually in the range of 4–9 cpm, or 1 cpm.

Stern et al. (1987) concluded that there is sufficient understanding of the relationship of the EGG to electrical and mechanical activity of the stomach to warrant its use in psychophysiological studies of gastric motor activity.

16.4 APPLICATIONS OF EGG RECORDING TO PSYCHOLOGY AND MEDICINE

Approximately one-half of all publications that describe the use of the EGG are technical rather than applied articles. By technical we mean papers that deal with methodology and/or validation. We would expect that as we learn more about the technical nature of the measure, a greater proportion of EGG publications will be devoted to application. Applications that have been described in the psychological and medical literature to date include the following areas: eating, stress and anxiety, motion sickness, and GI disorders.

16.4.1 *EGG and eating behavior*

Koch and Stern (1985) have shown that eating elicits high-amplitude 3-cpm EGG waves almost immediately after ingestion. Hamilton et al. (1986) have reported that after drinking 100 cm^3 of milk their subjects showed a 300–400 percent increase in the amplitude of their 3-cpm EGG waves and simultaneously recorded mucosal signals. Smout et al. (1980b) and Jones and Jones (1985) have reported finding similar increases in the amplitude of the EGG following eating.

Stern, Crawford, Stewart, Vasey, and Koch (1989) have used a sham feeding procedure to examine cephalic influences on the EGG. Following a 15-min baseline period, subjects were required to chew and expectorate a hotdog and roll. After another 10-min baseline period, subjects were given a second hotdog to eat normally. The effect on the EGG of eating the hotdog was as expected, a large increase in the amplitude of the 3-cpm EGG wave that lasted several minutes. The effect on the EGG of sham feeding was an equally large but short-lasting increase in the amplitude of the EGG. It was of interest to note that two subjects who reported after the session that the experience of chewing and expectorating the hotdog was disgusting showed a decrease rather than an increase in the amplitude of their EGG during sham feeding.

Of considerable clinical significance is the following: Do patients with anorexia nervosa or unexplained nausea and vomiting respond with an increase in the amplitude of their 3-cpm EGG following eating? Abell, Lucas, Brown, and Malagelada (1985) have reported that several of their anorexic subjects failed to show an increase in amplitude of their 3-cpm EGG following eating and some showed tachygastria (4–9 cpm). Geldof, van der Schee, Blankenstein, and Grashuis (1983) found that 48 percent of their patients with unexplained nausea and vomiting showed tachygastria and the absence of the normal increase in amplitude of the EGG after eating.

16.4.2   Stress and anxiety

Stewart (1987), working in our laboratory, studied the effects of brief exposure to two laboratory stressors on EGG activity. Forty-two fasted undergraduates were subjected to 2 days of laboratory stress testing. Laboratory sessions consisted of an initial resting baseline followed in sequence by (1) a bland control task; (2) a second rest period; (3) stress task; and (4) a final period. A computer-paced version of the Stroop color–word conflict task presented on a color computer monitor served as the stressor task for one session and was matched with reading a history essay as an innocuous control task. Viewing an industrial training film that depicted a series of three mutilating injuries served as the other stressor task. It was matched with viewing a documentary on the modern Olympics as its control task. Stroop stress produced an attenuation of EGG 2.5–3.5-cpm spectral power (referred to hereafter as 3 cpm) but no change in levels of tachygastria activity. The stress film produced no change in either 3-cpm or tachygastria power. Other than a diminution of tachygastria power during the Olympic film, control tasks produced no change in EGG activity. Subjective reports of stress, arousal, gastric, and somatic symptoms all showed marked increases following involvement with the stress but not control tasks.

We are currently looking at the effects of another stressor the cold pressor test, on EGG activity. The procedure used is similar to that used by Thompson, Richelson, and Malagelada (1982), who reported a significant decrease in gastric emptying as a response to cold stress. In our experiment subjects who had recently eaten were asked to put their hand into a container of ice water (4°C) for 1 min, take it out for 15 s, put it back for 1 min, and so on, for a total of 20 min. The results are similar to those reported by Stewart (1987) for the effects of the Stroop stress and are what would be predicted by the gastric emptying results of Thompson et al. (1982). There was a marked attenuation of EGG 3-cpm activity starting at the point in time when

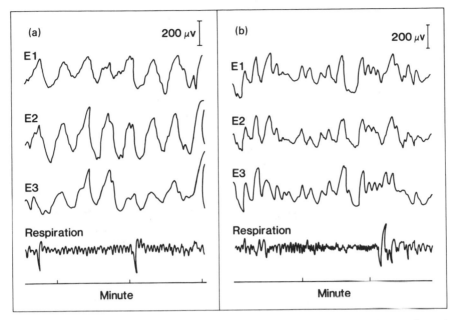

Figure 16.7. (a) EGG activity recorded from upper, middle, and lower electrodes (E1–E3) prior to drum rotation. The EGG frequency is 3 cpm. (b) EGG from same subject after start of drum rotation. Note presence of tachygastria (6 cpm). Tachygastria began at 4 min. Subject reported nausea at 6 min and requested that drum rotation be stopped at 11 min. (Reprinted with permission from Stern, Koch, Leibowitz, Lindblad, Shupert, & Stewart, 1985.)

the subjects put their hand in the ice water. At the completion of the cold stress, some subjects showed greater 3-cpm activity than they did prestress. Tachygastria was not seen as a response to the cold pressor test.

16.4.3 Motion sickness

In the first experiment that attempted to relate changes in gastric myoelectric activity to the development of symptoms of motion sickness, Stern, Koch, Leibowitz, Lindblad, Shupert, and Stewart (1985) obtained EGGs from 21 healthy human subjects who were seated within a drum, the rotation of which produced vection (illusory self-motion). Fourteen subjects developed symptoms of motion sickness during vection, and in each the EGG frequency shifted from the normal 3 to 4–9 cpm, tachygastria. An example of the EGG recording of one of these subjects is shown in Figure 16.7. In six of seven asymptomatic subjects, the 3-cpm EGG pattern was unchanged during vection. A portion of one of these EGG recordings is shown in Figure 16.8. It was concluded that the sensory mismatched created by the illusory self-motion produced tachygastria and symptoms of motion sickness in susceptible subjects.

In a follow-up study (Stern, Koch, Stewart, & Lindblad, 1987), 15 healthy subjects were exposed to the rotation of the same drum. Ten subjects showed a shift of the dominant frequency of their EGG from 3 to 4–9 cpm, tachygastria, during drum

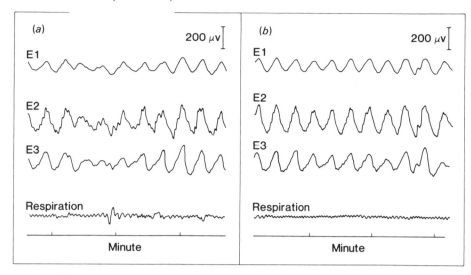

Figure 16.8. (a) The EGG activity prior to drum rotation. The EGG frequency is 3 cpm. (b) The EGG from same subject 7 min after start of drum rotation. Subject reported no symptoms of motion sickness and EGG frequency remained 3 cpm during 15 min of drum rotation. (Reprinted with permission from Stern, Koch, Leibowitz, Lindblad, Shupert, & Stewart, 1985.)

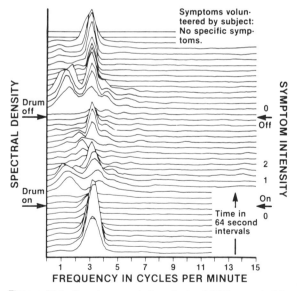

Figures 16.9. Running spectral analysis of EGG recorded from subject who reported no specific symptoms of motion sickness. Spectral density, or power, is plotted as third dimension rising from page. Symptom intensity (from 0 to 7) is indicated on right. Each time line, going from bottom to top, represents 4-s moving average shifted 1s at a time. Note absence of tachygastria and absence of specific symptoms of motion sickness. (Reprinted with permission from Stern, Koch, Stewart, & Lindblad, 1987.)

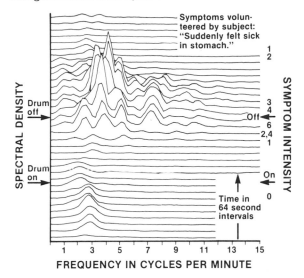

Figure 16.10. Running spectral analysis of EGG recorded from subject who reported that he suddenly felt sick in his stomach and requested that drum rotation be stopped. Note attenuation of 3 cpm power with drum onset and presence of tachygastria just prior to subject requesting termination of drum rotation. (Reprinted with permission from Stern, Koch, Stewart, & Lindblad, 1987.)

rotation and reported symptoms of motion sickness. A comparison of running spectral analyses and symptom reports revealed a close correspondence over time between tachygastria and the development of symptoms of motion sickness. Examples of an asymptomatic and a symptomatic subject are shown in Figures 16.9 and 16.10.

Rague and Oman (1987), in a preliminary report, described their use of EGG to measure gastric myoelectric activity and the symptoms of motion sickness of subjects who sat in a rotating chair and repeatedly touched their heads to their shoulders. Rague and Oman reported that subjects experiencing the symptoms of motion sickness showed a loss in power of 3-cpm activity and an increase in power in the tachygastria range but quantitatively not to the extent recently described by Stern, Koch, Stewart, and Lindblad (1987). We believe that the differences in the magnitude of the effect are largely due to differences in the stimulus situation used in the two laboratories.

We (Harm, Stern, Koch, & Vasey, 1987) recently presented preliminary results of an ongoing study aimed at measuring EGG from volunteers experiencing parabolic maneuvers in the KC-135 airplane. We are seeking to learn if there will be the same shift in the dominant frequency of the EGG in subjects who experience the symptoms of motion sickness in zero gravity as there is on the ground. To date, we have analyzed the EGG of 2 of 13 subjects. One subject was asymptomatic and his EGG showed a normal 3-cpm signal. The second subject experienced nausea and vomiting during the parabolic maneuvers, and his EGG did look similar to that recorded from subjects who experience motion sickness in our laboratory: a decrease in power at 3 cpm and an increase in power at 4–9 cpm, tachygastria.

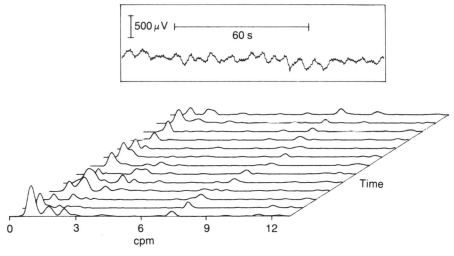

Figure 16.11. Running spectral analysis and portion of EGG record from pregnant woman suffering from nausea and vomiting. Tachygastria, 7 cpm activity, was seen in entire recording.

16.4.4   *Gastrointestinal disorders*

Walker and Sandman (1977) have reported that using the EGG they were able to differentiate between duodenal ulcer patients, rheumatoid arthritis patients, and healthy controls during a laboratory session involving the presentation of mildly stressful stimuli. Russian investigators have been using the EGG to diagnose GI disorders since the 1960s (e.g., Krapivin & Chernin, 1967; Sobakin, Smirnov, & Mishin, 1962). Recently a group of French investigators (Murat, Martin, Stevanovic, Beloncle, & Masson, 1985) reported the successful application of the EGG to the study of digestive pathology. Gaultier and Baille (1982) have used biofeedback of the EGG to increase the rate of gastric emptying. According to the authors 12 training session were necessary before the patients improved enough to be taken off of medication. In China, an electrogastrograph designed and manufactured at Anhui College of Traditional Chinese Medicine has been used in numerous hospitals and clinics and on more than 1,000 patients to diagnose GI disorders and to measure the therapeutic effects of acupuncture (e.g., Xu & Zhou, 1983).

Two areas currently being studied by our group using the EGG are the nausea of some pregnant women and the severe nausea and vomiting of some diabetics. Koch, Creasy, Dwyer, Vasey, and Stern (1987) recorded the EGG from 33 women with nausea ascribed to pregnancy. On the day of the study the women indicated their current intensity of nausea on a 300-mm visual analog scale. Gastric dysrhythmias were found in 26 of the 32 women: 15 had tachygastria and 11 had bradygastria. Figure 16.11 shows the spectral plot and a portion of the EGG record of one of the subjects who displayed tachygastria. The mean nausea score of the 26 women with dysrhythmias was significantly higher than the mean nausea score for the 6 women who did not show dysrhythmias in their EGGs on the test day. It was concluded that gastric dysrhythmias may contribute to the pathogenesis of nausea of pregnancy.

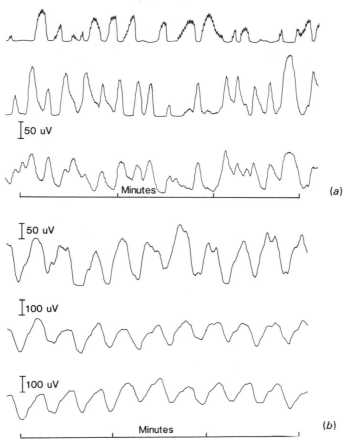

Figure 16.12. (a) The EGG of diabetic patient prior to treatment showing obvious tachygastria. (b) The EGG recorded from same patient after 4 months of treatment with domperidone. Note strong 3 cpm activity.

Koch, Stern, Stewart, and Dwyer (1986) recorded the EGG and obtained gastric emptying test results for four insulin-dependent diabetics prior to and for up to 12 months after treatment with domperidone. Domperidone is a drug that increases the contractile activity of the stomach and is thought to act directly on the smooth muscle of the stomach. Before domperidone treatment no patient showed a normal 3-cpm EGG: two showed tachygastria and two showed a flat line. By the second to the sixth month of treatment all patients showed 3-cpm activity in their EGG and all reported symptom improvement. Figure 16.12 shows tachygastria in the EGG of one of these patient's pretreatment and a normal 3-cpm EGG after 4 months of treatment with domperidone. Interestingly, after 6 months, only one of the patients showed normal gastric emptying using conventional testing procedures. We concluded that gastric dysrhythmias appear to have a pathophysiological role in the symptoms of diabetic nausea and vomiting. Control of the dysrhythmias and establishment of 3-cpm EGG activity with domperidone improved symptoms in all patients.

16.5   SUMMARY AND CONCLUSIONS

The EGG is a valid and reliable measure of gastric myoelectric activity. Frequencies recorded with the EGG are identical to the corresponding frequencies of gastric motor activity. The amplitude of the EGG increases with increases in contractile activity.

The normal frequency of the EGG is 3-cpm. Ultraslow rhythms, 0.5–2.0 cpm, are often seen, but neither their derivation nor behavioral significance is clear at this time. Tachygastria, 4–9 cpm, is usually seen in the EGG when subjects report nausea and may also be the response of some subjects to stress. The amplitude of the EGG increases following eating (or sham feeding) in normal subjects. The amplitude of the EGG decreases in response to some stressors.

In conclusion, we feel that enough is known about the relationship of the EGG to gastric motor activity to encourage its application to a great variety of areas in psychology and medicine. This completely safe, noninvasive measure can be used with humans or lower animals to study gastric responses in health or disease and to study the effects of various therapies on gastric responding.

NOTE

Portions of the research reported in this chapter were supported by grant NAG9-118 from the National Aeronautics and Space Administration.

REFERENCES

Abell, T. L., Lucas, A. R., Brown, M. L., & Malagelada, J. R. (1985). Gastric electrical dysrhythmias in anorexia nervosa (AN). *Gastroenterology, 88,* 1300. (Abstract).
Abell, T. L., & Malagelada, J. R. (1985). Glucagon-evoked gastric dysrhythmias in humans shown by an improved electrogastrographic technique. *Gastroenterology, 88,* 1932–1940.
Abell, T. L., & Malagelada, J. R. (1988). Electrogastrography: Current assessment and future perspectives. *Digestive Diseases and Sciences, 33,* 982–992.
Abell, T. L., Tucker, R., & Malagelada, J. R. (1985). Simultaneous gastric electro-manometry in man. In R. M. Stern & K. L. Koch (Eds.), *Electrogastrography* (pp. 78–88). New York: Praeger.
Alvarez, W. C. (1922). The electrogastrogram and what it shows. *Journal of the American Medical Association, 78,* 1116–1119.
Alvarez, W. C. (1943). *Nervousness, indigestion and pain.* New York: Hoeber.
Alvarez, W. C. (1968). Early studies of the movements of the stomach and bowel. In C. F. Code (Ed.), *Handbook of physiology. Section 6, Alimentary canal: Vol. 4, Motility.* Washington, DC: American Physiological Society.
Beaumont, W. (1833). *Experiments and observations on the gastric juice and the physiology of digestion.* Plattsburg: Allen.
Brown, B. H., Smallwood, R. H., Duthie, H. L., & Stoddard, C. J. (1975). Intestinal smooth muscle electrical potentials recorded from surface electrodes. *Medical Biological Engineering, 13,* 97–103.
Camilleri, M., Malagelada, J. R., Brown, M. L., Becker, G., & Zinsmeister, A. R. (1985). Relation between antral motility and gastric emptying of solids and liquids in humans. *American Journal of Physiology, 249,* G580–G585.
Cannon, W. B. (1898). The movements of the stomach studied by means of the roentgen rays. *American Journal of Physiology, 1,* 359–382.
Cannon, W. B., & Washburn, A. L. (1912). An explanation of hunger. *American Journal of Physiology, 29,* 441–454.
Carlson, A. J. (1916). *The control of hunger in health and disease.* Chicago: University of Chicago Press.
Code, C. F., & Marlett, J. A. (1975). The interdigestive myo-electric complex of the stomach and small bowel of dogs. *Journal of Physiology, 246,* 289–309.

Coles, M. G. H., Donchin, E., & Porges, S. W. (1986). *Psychophysiology: Systems, processes, and applications.* New York: Guilford Press.

Couturier, D., Roze, C., Paologgi, J., & Debray, C. (1972). Electrical activity of the normal human stomach: A comparative study of recordings obtained from serosal and mucosal sides. *Digestive Diseases and Sciences, 17,* 969–976.

Davis, C. (1986). The gastrointestinal system. In M. G. H. Coles, E. Donchin, & S. W. Porges (Eds.), *Psychophysiology: Systems, processes, and applications.* New York: Guilford Press.

Davis, R. C., Garafolo, L., & Gault, F. P. (1957). An exploration of abdominal potentials. *Journal of Comparative and Physiological Psychology, 50,* 519–523.

Davis, R. C., Garafolo, L., & Kveim, K. (1959). Conditions associated with gastrointestinal activity. *Journal of Comparative and Physiological Psychology, 52,* 466–475.

Familoni, B. O., Bowes, K. L., Kingma, Y. J., & Cote, K. R. (1987). Can transcutaneous electrodes diagnose gastric electrical abnormalities? *Digestive Diseases and Sciences, 32,* 909 (Abstract).

Feldman, M., & Schiller, L. (1983). Disorders of gastrointestinal motility associated with diabetes mellitus. *Annals of Internal Medicine, 98,* 378–384.

Furness, J. B., & Costa, M. (1980). Types of nerves in the enteric nervous system. *Neuroscience, 5,* 1–20.

Gaultier, C., & Baille, J. (1982). Cognitive mediations in biofeedback. *Agressologie, 23,* 285–297.

Geldof, H., van der Schee, E. J., van Blankenstein, M., & Grashuis, J. L. (1983). Gastric dysrhythmia; an electrogastrographic study. *Gastroenterology, 84,* 1163 (Abstract).

Hamilton, J. W., Bellahsene, B. E., Reichelderfer, M., Webster, J. H., & Bass, P. (1986). Human electrogastrograms. Comparison of surface and mucosal recordings. *Digestive Diseases and Science, 31,* 33–39.

Harm, D. L., Stern, R. M., Koch, K. L., & Vasey, M. W. (1987). Tachygastria during parabolic flight (Abstract). *Space life sciences symposium: Three decades of life science research in space.* Washington, DC: NASA.

Hinder, R. A., & Kelly, K. A. (1977). Human gastric pacesetter potentials: Site of origin and response to gastric transection and proximal vagotomy. *American Journal of Physiology, 133,* 29–33.

Hölzl, R. (1983). Surface gastrograms as measure of gastric motility. In R. Hölzl & W. E. Whitehead (Eds.), *Psychophysiology of the gastrointestinal tract* (pp. 69–121). New York: Plenum Press.

Hölzl, R., Löffler, K., & Müller, G. M. (1985). On the conjoint gastrography or what the surface gastrograms show. In R. M. Stern & K. L. Koch (Eds.), *Electrogastrography: Methodology, validation, and applications* (pp. 89–115). New York: Praeger.

Hölzl, R., & Whitehead, W. E. (Eds.) (1983). *Psychophysiology of the gastrointestinal tract: Experimental and clinical applications.* New York: Plenum Press.

Johnson, L. R., Christensen, J., Jacobsen, E. D., & Schultz, S. G. (Eds.) (1987). *Physiology of the gastrointestinal tract.* New York: Raven Press.

Jones, K. R., & Jones, G. E. (1985). Pre- and postprandial EGG variation. In R. M. Stern & K. L. Koch (Eds.), *Electrogastrography: Methodology, validation, and applications* (pp. 168–181). New York: Praeger.

Kelly, K. A., & Code, C. F. (1969). Effect of transthoracic vagotomy on canine gastric electrical activity. *Gastroenterology, 57,* 51–58.

Koch, K. L., Creasy, A., Dwyer, A., Vasey, M., & Stern, R. M. (1987). Gastric dysrhythmias and nausea of pregnancy. *Digestive Diseases and Sciences, 32,* 917. (Abstract).

Koch, K. L., & Stern, R. M. (1985). The relationship between the cutaneously recorded electrogastrogram and antral contractions in man. In R. M. Stern & K. L. Koch (Eds.), *Electrogastrography: Methodology, validation, and applications* (pp. 116–131). New York: Praeger.

Koch, K. L., Stern, R. M., Stewart, W. E., & Dwyer, A. E. (1986). Effects of long term domperidone therapy on gastric electromechanical activity in symptomatic patients with diabetic gastroparesis. *Gastroenterology, 90,* 1497. (Abstract).

Koch, K. L., Stewart, W. R., & Stern, R. M. (1987). Effects of barium meals on gastric electromechanical activity in man: A fluoroscopic-electrogastrophic study. *Digestive Diseases and Sciences, 32,* 1217–1222.

Krapivin, B. V., & Chernin, V. V. (1967). Study of the motor function of the stomach by the electrogastrographic method in patients with peptic ulcer. *Soviet Medicine, 30,* 57–60.

Kwong, N. K., Brown, B. H., Whittaker, G. E., & Duthie, H. L. (1970). Electrical activity of the gastric antrum in man. *British Journal of Surgery, 12,* 913–916.

Lavigne, M. E., Wiley, Z. D., Meyer, J. H., Martin, P., & MacGregor, I. L. (1978). Gastric emptying rates of solid food in relation to body size. *Gastroenterology, 74,* 1258–1260.

Lee, K., Chey, W., Tai, H., & Yajima, H. (1978). Radiommunoassay of motilin: Validation and studies on the relationship between plasma motilin and interdigestive myoelectric activity of the duodenum of dog. *Digestive Diseases and Sciences, 23,* 789–795.

Meyer, J. H. (1987). Motility of the stomach and gastroduodenal junction. In L. R. Johnson, J. Christensen, E. D. Jacobsen, & S. G., Schultz (Eds.), *Physiology of the gastrointestinal tract* (pp. 613–630). New York: Raven Press.

Meyer, J. H., Gu, Y. G., Dressman, J., & Amidon, G. (1986). Effect of viscosity and flow rate on gastric emptying of solids. *American Journal of Physiology, 250,* G161–G164.

Meyer, J. H., MacGregor, I. L., Gueller, R., Martin, P., & Cavalieri, R. (1976). ^{99}Tc-tagged chicken liver as a marker of solid food in the human stomach. *American Journal of Digestive Diseases, 21,* 296–304.

Meyer, J. H., Ohashi, H., Jehn, D., & Thompson, J. B. (1981). Size of liver particles emptied from the human stomach. *Gastroenterology, 80,* 1489–1496.

Mirizzi, N., & Scafoglieri, V. (1983). Optimal direction of the electrogastrographic signal in man. *Medical and Biological Engineering and Computing, 21,* 385–389.

Morgan, K. G., Schmalz, P. F., & Szurszewski, J. H. (1978). The inhibitory effects of vasoactive intestinal polypeptide on the mechanical and electrical activity of canine antral smooth muscle. *Journal of Physiology, 282,* 437–450.

Müller, G. M., Hölzl, R., & Brüchle, H. A. (1983). Conjoint gastrography: Principles and techniques. In R. Hölzl & W. E. Whitehead (Eds.), *Psychophysiology of the gastrointestinal tract* (pp. 123–159). New York: Plenum Press.

Murat, J., Martin, A., Stevanovic, D., Beloncle, M., & Masson, J. M. (1985). Electroenterography: Application to digestive pathology. In R. M. Stern & K. L. Koch (Eds.), *Electrogastrography: Methodology, validation, and applications* (pp. 215–225). New York: Praeger.

Nelsen, T. S., & Kohatsu, S. (1968). Clinical electrogastrography and its relationship to gastric surgery. *American Journal of Surgery, 116,* 215–222.

Rague, B. W., & Oman, C. M. (1987). Detection of motion sickness onset using abdominal biopotentials. (Abstract). *Space life sciences symposium: Three decades of life science research in space.* Washington, DC: NASA.

Roman, C., & Gonella, J. (1987). Extrinsic control of digestive tract motility. In L. R. Johnson, J. Christensen, E. D., Jacobsen, & S. G. Schultz (Eds.), *Physiology of the gastrointestinal tract* (pp. 507–553). New York: Raven Press.

Russell, R. W., & Stern, R. M. (1967). Gastric motility: The electrogastrogram. In P. H. Venables & I. Martin (Eds.), *Manual of psychophysiological methods* (pp. 218–243). Amsterdam: North-Holland.

Schlegel, J. F., & Code, C. F. (1975). The gastric peristalsis of the interdigestive housekeeper. In G. Vantrappen (Ed.), *Proceedings from the Fifth International Symposium of Gastrointestinal Motility* (p. 321). Belgium: Herentals.

Smallwood, R. H. (1978). Analysis of gastric electrical signals from surface electrodes using phase-lock techniques. Part 2: System performance with gastric signals. *Medical and Biological Engineering and Computing, 16,* 513–518.

Smallwood, R. H., & Brown, B. H. (1983). Non-invasive assessment of gastric activity. In P. Rolfe (Ed.), *Non-invasive physiological measurements* (Vol. 2). London: Academic Press.

Smout, A. J. P. M. (1980). *Myoelectric activity of the stomach: Gastroelectromyography and electrogastrography.* Unpublished master's thesis, Erasmus University, Rotterdam.

Smout, A. J. P. M., van der Schee, E. J., & Grashuis, J. L. (1980a). What is measured in electrogastrography? *Digestive Diseases and Sciences, 25,* 179–187.

Smout, A. J. P. M., van der Schee, E. J., & Grashuis, J. L. (1980b). Postprandial and interdigestive gastric electrical activity in the dog recorded by means of cutaneous electrodes. In J. Christensen (Ed.), *Gastrointestinal motility* (pp. 187–194). New York: Raven Press.

Sobakin, M. A., Smirnov, I. P., & Mishin, L. N. (1962). Electrogastrography. *IRE Transactions of Biomedical Electronics, BME-9,* 129–132.

Stemper, T. J., & Cooke, A. R. (1975). Gastric emptying and its relationship to antra contractile activity. *Gastroenterology, 69,* 649–653.

Stern, R. M. (1983). Responsiveness of the stomach to environmental events. In R. Hölzl & W. E.

Whitehead (Eds.), *Psychophysiology of the gastrointestinal tract* (pp. 181–207). New York: Plenum Press.

Stern, R. M. (1985). A breif history of the electrogastrogram. In R. M. Stern & K. L. Koch (Eds.), *Electrogastrography: Methodology, validation, and applications* (pp. 3–9). New York: Praeger.

Stern, R. M., Crawford, H. E., Stewart, W. R., Vasey, M. W., & Koch, K. L. (1989) Sham feeding, cephalic vagal influences on gastric myoelectric activity. *Digestive Diseases and Sciences, 34,* 521–527.

Stern, R. M., & Higgins, J. D. (1969). Perceived somatic reactions to stress. Sex, age, and familiar occurrence. *Journal of Psychosomatic Research, 13,* 77–82.

Stern, R. M., & Koch, K. L. (Eds.) (1985). *Electrogastrography: Methodology, validation, and applications.* New York: Praeger.

Stern, R. M., Koch, K. L., Leibowitz, H. W., Lindblad, I., Shupert, C., & Stewart, W. R. (1985). Tachygastria and motion sickness. *Aviation Space and Environmental Medicine, 56,* 1074–1077.

Stern, R. M., Koch, K. L., Stewart, W. R., & Lindblad, I. M. (1987). Spectral analysis of tachygastria recorded during motion sickness. *Gastroenterology, 92,* 92–97.

Stern, R. M., Koch, K. L., Stewart, W. R., & Vasey, M. W. (1987). Electrogastrography: Current issues in validation and methodology. *Psychophysiology, 24,* 55–64.

Stewart, W. R. (1987). *Stress-induced alterations in gastric myoelectric activity as measured with the electrogastrogram.* Unpublished doctoral dissertation, Penn State University, University Park, PA.

Stoddard, C. J., Smallwood, R. H., & Duthie, H. L. (1981). Electrical arrhythmias in the human stomach. *Gut, 22,* 705–712.

Thompson, D. G., Richelson, E., & Malagelada, J. R. (1982). Perturbation of gastric emptying and duodenal motility through the central nervous system. *Gastroenterology, 83,* 1200–1206.

van der Schee, E. J., Smout, A. J., Smout, A. J. P. M., & Grashuis, J. L. (1982). Applications of running spectrum analysis to electrogastrographic signals recorded from dog and man. In M. Wienbeck (Ed.), *Motility of the digest tract* (pp. 241–250). New York: Raven Press.

Vantrappen, G., Hostein, J., Janssens, J., Vanderweerd, M., & De Wever, I. (1983). Do slow waves induce *mechanical* activity? *Gastroenterology, 84,* 1341. (Abstract).

Vantrappen, G., Janssens, J., Peeters, T. L., Bloom, S. R., Christofides, N. D., & Hellemans, J. (1979). Motility and the interdigestive migrating motor complex in man. *Digestive Diseases and Sciences, 24,* 497–500.

Walker, B., & Sandman, C. (1977). Physiological response patterns in ulcer patients: Phasic and tonic components of the electrogastrogram. *Psychophysiology, 14,* 393–400.

Williams, R. (1956). *Biochemical individuality: The basis for the genotrophic concept.* New York: Wiley.

Wolf, S., & Wolff, H. G. (1943). *Human gastric function.* New York: Oxford University Press.

You, C. H., & Chey, W. Y. (1984). Study of electromechanical activity of the stomach in humans and in dogs with particular attention to tachygastria. *Gastroenterology, 86,* 1460–1468.

Xu, G., & Zhou, Y. (1983). Modulated effect of acupuncture on gastroelectrical activity. *Acupuncture Research, 8,* 1–6.

17 The pulmonary system

TYLER S. LORIG AND GARY E. SCHWARTZ

17.1 OVERVIEW

Gas exchange is one of the most fundamental operations of the functioning organism. In mammals, a complex integrated system of muscles, receptors, and central control mechanisms all work to produce the act of pulmonary ventilation. This ventilation is known to be sensitive to a variety of metabolic and psychological variables. In fact, as Woodworth and Schlosberg (1954) point out, it is such a sensitive response system related to so many different psychological variables that interpretation of changes within the system is often difficult. Why, then, measure pulmonary activity?

17.1.1 Historical context

Investigators have been intensely interested in pulmonary activity since the time of Galen (Pauly, 1957). Each country's history of medical research includes early contributions to the study of respiration that were structured within the philosophical context of their culture's approach to medicine (Dudley, 1969). Although most have been concerned with the basic anatomy and physiology of the system, researchers in the early portion of this century began to investigate the relationship between psychological variables and ventilation. Lehman (1905, cited in Stein & Luparello, 1967) studied the effects of pleasure and displeasure on respiratory rate. Attempts have been made to define different personality types on the basis of respiratory data (Nielsen & Roth, 1929). Differential patterns of respiratory activity were found when different personality groups were stressed by the recall of emotional stimuli (Ziegler & Levine, 1925). Finesinger (1939) found that the respiratory patterns of neurotic subjects varied as a function of the pleasantness of recalled stimuli. These studies as well as Feleky's (1916) investigations of the inspiration-expiration ratios formed the basis for subsequent psychophysiological studies of breathing.

Studies of the psychophysiology of respiration that took place in the middle of this century tended to be more conservative than earlier studies. Fewer attempts were made to account for all personality variables by the way in which someone breathed. Stevenson and Ripley (1952) simply attempted to correlate respiratory pattern to emotional state as subjects were interviewed. Wolf (1947) found that extension of the diaphragm changed during discussion of conflicts (see Stein & Luparello, 1967, for review). Studies such as these pointed to the value of pulmonary measurement in relation to psychological stressors. Present-day experiments that involve pulmonary measurement tend to employ the same paradigm while

580

measuring a variety of other response systems (Grossman, 1983; Hassett, 1978). Although these paradigms are useful and help us to better understand the complexity of the stress response, few modern experiments have been concerned primarily with the functional relationship between breathing and psychological variables.

The history of research in this century has indicated that pulmonary activity is exquisitely sensitive to psychological manipulation. Yet little is known of why the exchange of gases through the lungs should be so variable and so easily influenced by personality, mood, and stress. Interpretations of changes in pulmonary activity must be cautious since mechanisms that account for this system sensitivity are unknown.

17.1.2 Functions of the respiratory system

Most investigators interested in respiratory activity see this system as having a single homeostatic function related to the inspiration of oxygen and the expiration of carbon dioxide. This singular view is based on the observation that the amount of oxygen entering the system and the amount of carbon dioxide leaving is highly correlated with both metabolic and pulmonary rate (West, 1979). Thus, those variables associated with increased metabolic rate, such as exercise or fear-producing stimuli, should produce greater demand for oxygen and tend to produce an increase in the volume of air entering the lungs either by an increase in ventilation rate or by an increase in inspiratory volume or both. This relationship has been demonstrated many times (West, 1979).

Although this metabolic-rate-based model may be sufficient to explain gross changes in respiratory rate and tidal volume over relatively long periods, it is not capable of explaining more subtle, transient irregularities in the pulmonary system such as those sensitive to psychological variables. One such irregularity is the cessation of breathing upon the commencement of high-demand cognitive activity. Woodworth and Schlosberg (1954) suggest that the initial cessation in breathing during activities of increased vigilance and demand is necessary because "maximum efficiency is sought by keeping the breathing as quiet as possible while maintaining the normal supply of oxygen" (p. 171). Such an interpretation of breath cessation seems unlikely and would be a consequence of the simple functional model (Kaufman & Schneiderman, 1986; Macklem, 1978; West, 1979). An alternative explanation of this phenomenon would include a second function for the pulmonary system. This function might be information acquisition. As air is drawn into the lungs, it is most often inhaled through the nose, thereby introducing a flood of olfactory information into the nervous system. Lehmann and Knauss (1976) found a widespread decrease in integrated EEG amplitudes during the inhalation cycle of normal breathing and an increase in EEG amplitudes during exhalation. Such EEG changes are common during other types of sensory stimulation (Lorig & Isaac, 1984; Moruzzi & Magoun, 1949) and suggest that olfactory stimulation is producing an increase in EEG activity during normal breathing. Servit, Kristof, and Kolinova (1976) found that inhalation of room air through the nose rather than the mouth was significantly more likely to induce seizure activity in epileptics. Recently, Lorig, Schwartz, Herman, and Lane (1988) compared EEG alpha and theta activity during nose and mouth breathing and found that inhalation of room air through the nose produced a significant decrease in alpha activity when compared to inhalation through the mouth. These findings suggest that even "odorless" air has an effect upon central nervous system activity when inhaled through the nose and given the opportunity to stimulate the nasal mucosa. Thus, breath cessation during high-demand cognitive tasks may be the result of active exclusion of irrelevant or competing olfactory sensory cues, as has been demonstrated in other sensory modalities (Fuster, 1980; Mishkin, 1964).

Whereas this example is by no means proof of a second major function for the pulmonary system, it does point to the utility of reevaluation of the functional components of this system. Tactile stimulation of the nostrils by airflow may also be an important variable affecting the regulation of the pulmonary cycle. Given the variability of this system to psychological variables and the insufficiency of the simple functional model used to account for this variability, a broader view of the regulation of pulmonary activity is necessary. After all, how much information is lost about the gastrointestinal system if we concentrate on calories and ignore taste?

17.1.3   *Respiration and pulmonary ventilation*

The act of respiration involves the exchange of gases. Although a simple definition, this system encompasses not only the act of inhalation and exhalation with all its complexities but also the transmission of oxygen to the bloodstream and the exchange of gases across cell membranes. Psychologists have typically been more concerned with the filling and emptying of the lungs with air, also known as pulmonary ventilation, than with the exchange of gases once inside the organism. For this reason, the remainder of this chapter concentrates primarily on the act of ventilation rather than the broader respiratory system.

17.2   BIOMECHANICS OF PULMONARY ACTION

17.2.1   *The mechanics of ventilation*

The major muscle of inspiration is the diaphragm. This is a dome-shaped muscle suspended between the lower ribs and the sternum. Contraction of this muscle leads to increased volume within the rib cage, with the lower pressure causing air to flow into the lungs (Figure 17.1). Additionally, the action of the diaphragm pushes down on the top portion of the abdomen, producing a distension of the ventral surface known as "belly breathing." This type of breathing varies among individuals depending on abdominal muscle tone (e.g., Clausen, 1951; Svebak, 1975).

Associated with the action of the diaphragm are the external intercostals. These muscles interconnect the ribs and are recruited to aid in increasing lung capacity. The diaphragm and external intercostals are individually capable of producing enough of a pressure change to cause sufficient airflow into the lungs to maintain normal respiratory function. They tend, however, to act additively in normal breathing (Macklem, 1978). The action of the external intercostals is to pull the ribs up, producing a larger chest cavity, as may be seen in Figure 17.1.

Expiration is largely a passive operation. After air flows into the lungs, it must again flow out to regain an equilibrium. The passive elastic recoil of the lungs, rib cage, and diaphragm accounts for the majority of expiratory pressure in normal, nonforced breathing. The remaining volume of air may be actively expelled, especially during exertion. As the diaphragm contracts, the chest cavity is made

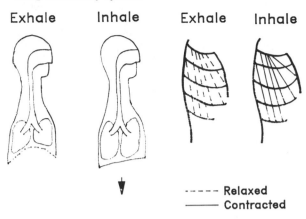

Exhale   Inhale   Exhale   Inhale

- - - - - Relaxed
————— Contracted

Figure 17.1. Action of diaphragm (left pair) and external intercostal muscles during inhalation and exhalation.

larger and air rushes into the lungs, thereby equalizing air pressure inside and outside the body. Upon relaxation of the diaphragm, the size of the chest cavity becomes smaller and air is pushed out. The air pressure, already in equilibrium, resists this change. Additionally, constriction of airways and decreased elasticity of the lungs may further oppose the outflow of air. Thus it is necessary to actively empty the lungs by contracting abdominal muscles, which flatten the rib cage. Lung capacity is further reduced by the action of the internal intercostal muscles, which act in opposition to the external intercostals and cause the ribs to be pulled down. This relationship is diagrammed in Figure 17.1.

17.2.2   Neural control of ventilation

Control of the pulmonary rhythm is maintained by a complex interaction of neural areas and peripheral feedback mechanisms. The major central nervous system structures responsible for the pulmonary rhythm are the dorsal and ventral respiratory groups located in the medulla, slightly inferior to the level of the pons. These groups represent a diffuse collection of nuclei related by function and local anatomy. Major efferents for respiration arise in the dorsal group and descend to the phrenic nucleus. Second-order fibers from this nucleus form the phrenic nerve and exit the spinal cord at the thoracic level, where they innervate the diaphragm. Afferents from the diaphragm return to the dorsal respiratory group via the vagus nerve and form a feedback loop. This loop is responsible for the Hering–Breuer reflex, a decrease in ventilation frequency produced by excessive inhalation. This reflex was once thought to be responsible for the maintenance of the pulmonary rhythm but now appears to be largely inactive in adults (Guz, Noble, Eisele, & Trenchard, 1970; West, 1979). The feedback for normal pulmonary rhythm seems to be from central carbon dioxide chemoreceptors located in the medulla near the respiratory groups (Cohen, 1970).

Although this feedback loop is the major mechanism effecting control of the diaphragm, the modulation of the loop itself appears to be a function of the ventral respiratory group and the pons. Destruction of the ventral group results in

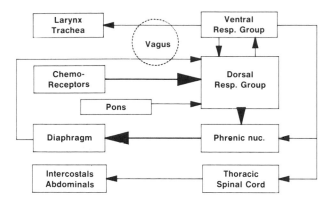

Figure 17.2. Schematic diagram of CNS origin of ventilation rhythm.

maintenance of breathing but severely impairs the cyclicity of the rhythm (Cohen, 1970). Efferents from the ventral group descend to the phrenic nucleus and also to the thoracic cord, where second-order fibers innervate the intercostal and abdominal muscles. The ventral group is also richly interconnected with the dorsal respiratory group (West, 1979). The interrelations of this system are presented in Figure 17.2.

Control of respiration may also be exerted voluntarily. The mechanisms for this type of control are apparently quite different from those necessary for the maintenance of the pulmonary rhythm. Efferents responsible for the rhythmic innervation of the diaphragm descend in the ventrolateral spinal cord; those involved in voluntary ventilation descend dorsolaterally. Thus, it is possible to dissociate the two mechanisms of control via lesions to the ventrolateral cord, producing a form of sleep apnea called *Ondine's curse* (Kaufman & Schneiderman, 1986).

The system responsible for voluntary control has not received the same degree of study as the system for maintenance of the pulmonary rhythm. Plum (1970), however, has described the major components of the voluntary ventilation system. These include efferent neurons arising in the cortex (probably frontal cortex) and descending via the dorsolateral cord to the thoracic level. Second-order fibers then arise and travel to the diaphragm. Feedback within this system is probably from somatic stretch receptors in the chest cavity by way of the thalamus. Coordination of this type of breathing is modulated by interaction of the basal ganglia nuclei. The diagram of this system's interconnections is presented in Figure 17.3.

17.2.3   Interaction with cardiovascular system

Although many studies of respiratory activity have included other physiological measures, few have been concerned with the dynamic interaction among systems. Grossman (1983) points out that cardiovascular psychophysiologists have rarely considered respiratory influences on cardiovascular activity an important area of inquiry. In his extensive review, Grossman (1983) discusses several areas of respiratory influence on the cardiovascular system. The mechanical consequences of inhalation and exhalation alter thoracic pressure and facilitate blood flow through the heart. Lung inflation receptors also influence vagal tone and thus influence heart

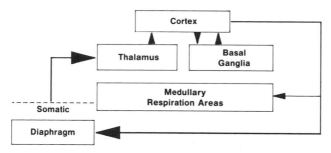

Figure 17.3. Schematic diagram of voluntary control of ventilation.

rate. Vascular chemoreceptors jointly alter cardiac and ventilatory activity and are, in turn, affected by the subsequent flux in oxygen and CO_2.

Grossman also points out that certain other respiratory activities are known to affect heart rate. Breath holding, for instance, produces a marked increase in heart rate as does an increase in tidal volume of air inspired. One of the respiratory effects most prominent in the research of psychophysiologists has been respiratory sinus arrhythymia (RSA), a phenomenon occurring during normal ventilation in which heart rate, modulated by vagal tone, accelerates during inspiration and decelerates during exhalation. It is of interest because it has been linked to hyperactivy and psychosis in children (Porges, 1976) as well as to the aging process (Hirsch & Bishop, 1981). The mechanisms for the production of RSA are poorly understood but are known to involve CNS coupling of respiratory and cardiovascular areas as well as interactions at the chemoreceptor level (Grossman, 1983).

17.3 TRANSDUCTION AND DATA REDUCTION

Questions related to pulmonary function require specific measurements of the pulmonary system. Hypotheses concerning oxygen utilization, for instance, might be tested by measuring abdominal distension since it is correlated with oxygen intake (Scheafer, 1979). This correlation is the result of increased vital capacity in the lungs and a larger volume of air, and therefore oxygen, flowing into the lungs. It is possible, however, to measure oxygen utilization directly, and this approach should be taken when the technique employed does not interfere with experimental protocols. For measurement of pulmonary activity and other psychophysiological phenomena, the selected technique should always be as directly related to the hypotheses as possible. Measurement techniques should be driven by the hypotheses themselves rather than by the available technology. A flow chart for the choice of typical ventilatory measurement techniques is presented in Figure 17.4.

The next section describes techniques historically associated with the measurement of pulmonary activity.

17.3.1 *Measure of respiratory gases*

17.3.1.1 *Spirometry*

Spirometry is one of the oldest and most widely used techniques for pulmonary analysis. Although there are many variations in features, most have similar operation. A typical spirometer is presented in Figure 17.5.

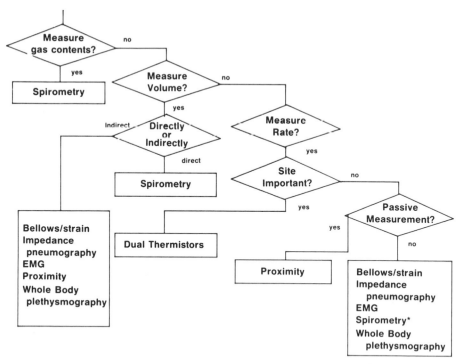

Figure 17.4. Flow chart of ventilatory measurement techniques.* Some instruments may not give rate.

A subject wearing a noseclip breathes into and out of the mouthpiece. The volume of the breathed air displaces a cylinder and causes a pen to record the volume of air on a drum or x–y recorder. Some spirometers have no clean air intake and require that subjects breathe only a few times before the oxygen in the tank is expended and the CO_2 level becomes too high. Others, like the one in the diagram, have lime in the tank to absorb CO_2.

Output of these spirometers also vary. Some provide only a breath-by-breath chart that allows for easy quantification of rate by counting inspirations per minute. Volume of respired air may be calculated by integrating the area under the inspiratory curves. Other spirometers provide a record of inspired air similar in form to the cumulative records used in operant conditioning. Volume of air may be quantified by reading the level of the recording. Rate may be identified by examining the number of inspirations (stair steps) in a given duration record. Figure 17.6 shows a typical record of this type.

Although the spirometers described thus far are adequate for the direct determination of ventilatory volume, they alone cannot provide a measure of gas content. Four techniques have typically been used for this purpose. First, a spirometer tank may be fitted with a sampling valve connected to a gas analyzer capable of recording the concentration of CO_2 and oxygen present in the breathed gases (Auchincloss, Gilbert, & Baule, 1966). Second, a Douglas bag (Astrand & Saltin, 1961) may be used. This requires a subject to breath into the Douglas bag. An

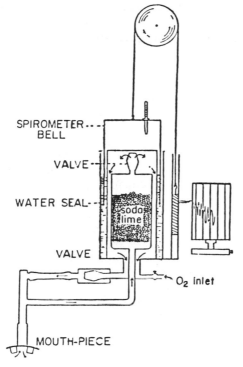

Figure 17.5. Schematic diagram of Benedict–Roth spirometer. (Reprinted from Best & Taylor, 1961.)

Spirographic Record

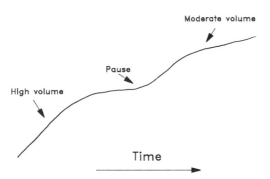

Figure 17.6. Simulation of typical spirographic record.

experimenter then empties the contents of the bag into a spirometer and gas analyzer for the resulting volume and gas content measurements. A third technique uses servo-controlled gas samplers connected to breathing tubes (Webb & Troutman, 1970) for the measurement of only gas content. The last technique is the most comprehensive and uses a full face mask coupled to automated volume and content measurement sensors (Kaufman & Schneiderman, 1986). Typically, gas content analyzers directly read out the concentration or partial pressure of respired gases and do not require data reduction before statistical analysis.

17.3.1.2 Thermal flux

Although insensitive to the content of respiratory gases, thermal measurements have also been employed to detect the inspiratory and expiratory phases of the ventilation rhythm (Kallman & Feurstein, 1977). This technique is based on the simple assumption that expired gas is warmer than inhaled gas. The information gained from this technique is generally relativistic in nature. Inspiratory and expiratory times and thus respiration rate, however, may be absolute. The technique involves the placement of one or two small temperature sensors (either thermocouples or thermistors) in the airflow of the nostrils. Thermistors change their electrical resistance as a function of temperature and may be recorded using an amplifier capable of recording very small resistive changes such as those used in electrodermal response recording. Thermocouples, on the other hand, produce a variable voltage depending upon ambient temperature and must be amplified using a high-gain DC amplifier. Both techniques have similar advantages and limitations. Because these techniques require common amplification equipment found in most psychophysiology laboratories, they are easy to implement. They also may be output continuously as a temperature fluctuation over time using a polygraph equipped with appropriate amplifiers.

Quantification of the resulting polygraph record may be done by measurement of the inspiratory and expiratory times for a given cycle. Because temperature rather than a more rapidly changing variable is being measured, thermal pulmonary recordings are less prone to be influenced by measurement artifacts than are other similar measures. Unfortunately, they may still be influenced by capacitance in the hookup cables when subjects move (although this may be reduced by using twisted cable pairs). Another advantage of this technique is the ability to record responses from the individual nostrils indicating airflow into the two nasal cavities. This variable may be of interest to a variety of investigators given the findings of Werntz and associates (Werntz, Bickford, Bloom, & Shannaloff-Khalsa, 1983), who demonstrated EEG and behavioral differences dependent upon the degree of constriction of the left and right nostrils.

Although thermistry is a reliable method for the determination of respiratory rate, it also has limitations. Primary among these limitations is the sluggishness of the temperature response. It takes time for the thermal sensor to warm and to cool, thus producing a temporal offset between the actual response and the recorded response. Although this may not be a problem for many investigators examining only respiration, it would represent a substantial limitation for those interested in the relation between respiration and other variables being recorded simultaneously. New temperature sensors promise to reduce this problem by decreasing lag time. Another potential problem with this type of measure is the nonlinearity of thermal sensors' response and its interaction with ambient temperature. Investigators should choose a sensor with a linear response across the range of ambient temperatures in which they will be collecting data. Problems also arise when the subject's mouth breathes or sneezes on the thermistors. In the former case, response of the sensor may be significantly diminished, and in the latter case, the ability of

Table 17.1. *Reduction of pulmonary activity recording techniques*

Technique	Parameters extracted	Function
Spirometry	average slope	rate
	vertical distance between breaths	volume
	blood gas analysis	metabolism
Thermal flux	interrespiratory interval	rate
Pneumotachometer	slope	rate
	direct readout	rate
Plethysmography	interrespiratory interval	rate
	integrated amplitude	volume
Strain gauge,	interrespiratory interval	rate
aneroid bellows	integrated amplitude	volume
Impedance	interrespiratory interval	rate
pneumograph	integrated amplitude	volume
Electromyography[a]	interrespiratory interval	rate
	integrated amplitude	volume
Proximity	interrespiratory interval	rate

[a] Refers to rectified and integrated EMG output.

the sensor to dissipate heat may be retarded, thereby altering the device's response characteristics.

17.3.1.3 *Pneumotachograph*

This device typically consists of a breathing tube and valves connected to a pressure-sensitive gas flowmeter. The rate of breathing may be output to a polygraph as a fluctuating signal representative of each breath or to a device similar to a cardiotachometer, which produces a signal output directly proportional to the rate of breathing. Some pneumotachograph devices have a digital readout eliminating experimenter data reduction. Others, similar to the cardiotachometer, require measurement of the amplitude of the recorded activity. By using a rate calibration signal, the pneumotachograph output may be translated into a rate measure for statistical analysis. If the tachograph outputs only a signal that fluctuates with each breath, this too may yield a direct measure of gas volume by integrating the amplitude of the inspiration curves.

17.3.2 *Measures of breathing mechanics*

17.3.2.1 *Plethysmography*

One of the oldest and presently least used techniques for the recording of pulmonary activity is the full-body plethysmograph (Table 17.1) (Woodworth & Schlosberg, 1954). This technique requires an individual to be immersed in water while measurements of the flux in the displaced water are made. As an individual inhales, water displacement increases; during exhalation, displacement is reduced. Although somewhat invasive, this technique has the advantage of accurately measuring pulmonary volume without requiring the subject to breathe through a mouthpiece or wear a noseclip.

17.3.2.2 *Strain gauges and aneroid bellows*

Two more popular methods include the use of mercury strain gauge and aneroid chest bellows. Both of these techniques involve the measurement of chest expansion and compression during breathing by a sensor placed around the subject's chest or abdomen. The mercury strain is a device that changes its electrical resistance when stretched, so that as an individual inhales, the strain gauge is stretched and resistance is increased. During exhalation the strain gauge returns to its resting resistance. The aneroid bellows may also be a resistive device but works by exerting a change in air pressure on a pressure-sensitive gauge. Typically, a nonelastic belt secured to the bellows is placed around the subject so that as the chest expands, the bellows are stretched. A rigid-walled plastic tube is used to connect the bellows to a pressure-sensitive gauge that changes resistively with increased pressure. Newer models use piezoelectric crystals that change potential with increased pressure.

Both of these sensors may be interfaced to a polygraph or computer by an amplifier capable of recording resistive changes such as those produced by a thermistor or electrodermal response. Piezoelectric crystal devices produce a small, slowly fluctuating voltage and are best measured with DC amplifiers or AC amplifiers with a low-frequency cutoff in the 0.01-Hz range.

Placement of these sensors on the subject should reflect the particular aspects of ventilation in which the investigator is interested. Diaphragmatic breathing, for instance, would probably be best measured from the abdomen if not for the variability of abdominal tone (Clausen, 1951; Svebak, 1975). Investigators concerned only with pulmonary rate should consider placement around the upper chest area just under the armpits since this area is relatively sensitive to respiratory change and is less prone to produce movement artifacts since the transducer is abutted against the subject's arms. Particular care must be taken to ensure sensitivity of this placement with a subject tending toward shallow breathing. Additionally, those investigators interested in pulmonary volume should consider placements in both **chest and abdominal areas. There are no firm guidelines for the exact placement of these transducers. The investigator must make a reasonable choice based on the variables of interest and the constraints of the experiment environment.**

Both the aneroid bellows and strain gauge have similar advantages. They are both easy to implement and use standard laboratory equipment (although certain strain gauges require a special external bridge circuit usually available from the manufacturer). Both techniques produce a relativistic measure of chest movement over time that is easily quantified. The two techniques also suffer from similar problems: The aneroid bellows is a high-quality rubber that tends to oxidize and crack. Although a large crack in the bellows will be easily noticed by the investigator, a smaller crack will produce a mildly distorted record that may go unnoticed. Oxidation of the rubber can be reduced by storing the bellows in an airtight pouch. Breakdown of the mercury strain gauge is all or none. If stretched too far, the elastic tube containing the mercury will rupture and spill mercury.

17.3.2.3 *Impedance pneumography*

Impedance pneumography has also been used to measure pulmonary activity. This technique takes advantage of the increased volume of the thorax during inhalation

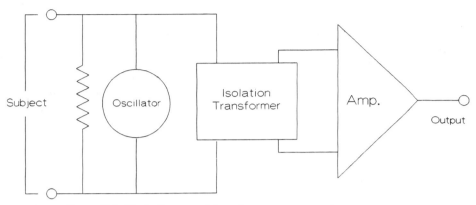

Figure 17.7. Block diagram of impedance pneumograph.

to alter electrical impedance between two electrodes. A constant, low-voltage alternating current is passed between two electrodes placed on the subject's thorax. As the volume of the chest expands during the ventilation cycle, the current passes through the subject less readily. This change in measured current may be output to an ink-writer or computer analog-to-digital converter. A schematic diagram for an impedance pneumograph is presented in Figure 17.7.

Because this impedance pneumograph makes use of alternating rather than direct current, ionic polarization does not occur in the electrode gel and thus recordings are not influenced. The technique is described in some detail by Baker and colleagues (Baker, Geddes, & Hoff, 1965) but has not found wide use in psychophysiology.

17.3.2.4 *Electromyography*

Electromyography (EMG) has also been used to a limited extent in the measurement of respiration. Pauly (1957) examined the activity of the diaphragm and intercostals using multichannel EMG. His results indicated that EMG was a reliable means for direct measurement and dissociation of the action of the internal and external intercostals.

Electromyographic recording of pulmonary action is accomplished by placing surface EMG electrodes over the muscles of interest and recording raw or integrated EMG. This technique has the advantage of relatively direct measurement of individual muscles involved in respiration. Unfortunately, because the EMG is a measure of electrical activity and because of the proximity to the heart, contamination of the recordings from heart potentials may be a problem and would suggest that the bipolar electrode pair be placed in close proximity.

Electromyography related to respiration may also be recorded from the muscle responsible for dilation of the nostrils (dilator naris) (Sasaki & Mann, 1976). The technique used by Saski and Mann employed the placement of concentric needle-type electrodes in the *alae nasi,* a procedure the authors report was "not excessively painful." Recordings from this muscle indicate an increase in activity during inspiration when the mouth is closed. Activity of the muscle also increases when air passage resistance is increased (Sasaki & Mann, 1976).

17.3.2.5 *Proximity*

A novel means of identifying pulmonary activity useful in certain restrictive environments is the proximity indicator (Casali, Wierwille, & Cordes, 1983). The indicator is attached by a metal belt to the subject's abdomen. As the subject inhales, the abdomen distends and comes closer to the proximity indicator, thus producing a discriminable change in a polygraph record. This device is small and may be placed on a subject with relative ease, thus making it an attractive means for rapid screening of pulmonary activity or for use in cramped quarters such as an airplane cockpit where it may be placed a fixed distance from the subject. Devices such as this may be easily telemetered, as may other techniques described here.

17.3.3   Data reduction

The techniques described tend to produce two types of data concerning pulmonary function. Analysis of blood gases, for instance, may produce discrete breath-by-breath measures of carbon dioxide and other blood gases. Strain gauge measurements produce a continuous readout of chest diameter over time. Quantifying these types of measurements may often be difficult. Although it is a relatively simple matter to calculate an average CO_2 level for a subject during different epochs within an experiment, it is more difficult to reduce the continuous data produced by strain gauges, bellows, spirometers, thermistors, thermocouples, or other forms of transduction.

17.3.3.1 *Pulmonary rate*

For the continuous measures described here, determination of pulmonary rate is one of the more straightforward types of analysis. Reduction of this measurement is accomplished by counting the number of inspiration–expiration cycles over an epoch within an experiment and then dividing the measure to establish the mean number of breaths within a minute. One may also measure the duration of the respiratory cycle from onset to onset to determine rate. The only concern in these types of analysis is the treatment of segments of records containing artifacts. Some artifacts in continuous records tend to be high-frequency components that "ride" on top of the signal of interest. These may be due to amplifier noise, ambient electrical noise, or irregularities in the sensors. In cases such as these, the artifacts may be reduced by filtering out high-frequency aspects of the signal. A passband of 0.01–3 Hz would be sufficient to limit most artifacts in this type of record. This can be done by the use of digital filtering algorithms after data collection if the data are acquired by a computer. Other, more typical artifacts are produced by subject movement. Unfortunately, data segments with artifacts such as these may be eliminated only by extending the epoch in question by the length of the artifact or, in the case of epochs of sufficient duration, epochs may be reduced by the length of the artifact.

17.3.3.2 *Volume measures*

Volumetric measures or measures of pulmonary amplitude may also be of interest to many investigators. For this application, spirometry is probably the best

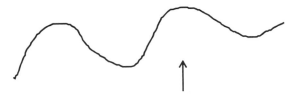

Peak Inspiration

Figure 17.8. Typical respiratory cycle recorded using strain gauge or aneroid bellows.

measurement technique if other variables in the experiment will not be adversely affected by the restricted environment (mouth breathing through a tube for the duration of the experiment). Spirometry has the advantage of producing an absolute measure of the volume of gas exchanged which may be of value for some applications. In those cases where relative, within-subject comparisons are appropriate, other techniques such as aneroid bellows, strain gauges, or proximity transducers may be used. For these types of measures, expirations and inspirations may be averaged over an epoch to determine a baseline from which inspiration peak and expiration trough measurements are made. A similar means for determination of pulmonary amplitude is to measure the peak-to-trough difference for an inspiration–expiration cycle. Measures such as these are relativistic because strain gauges and other instruments are stretched to differing degrees on different subjects.

Peak-to-trough differences give a rough estimate of inspiratory volume but may be misleading if subjects inhale over a long period of time or if the peaks are difficult to determine. In these cases, integration of inspirations and expirations may provide a better measure. If the data are digitized, integration may be accomplished simply by summing the response for its specific duration. If the data are not to be digitized, an integrating amplifier may be connected to the raw respiration channel. The write-out of this device will then provide a record of relative inspiratory or expiratory volume over a specified period. Volume measures of analog records may be determined on a breath-by-breath basis by the use of a polar planimeter.

17.3.3.3 *Measures of pulmonary cycle*

One of the most studied forms of respiratory data reduction is the inspiration–expiration ratio (*I/E*). This measure is obtained by dividing the duration of the inspiration by the duration of the expiration. A related measure is the *I* fraction. This is obtained by dividing the duration of inspiration by the duration of the entire pulmonary cycle. Figure 17.8 indicates the proper division of the inspiratory and expiratory cycles.

For greater reliability, Woodworth and Schlosberg (1954) have recommended the use of the *I* fraction rather than *I/E*. Feleky (1916) found the *I* fraction useful in discriminating emotions, and more recently, Hassett (1978) has recommended this

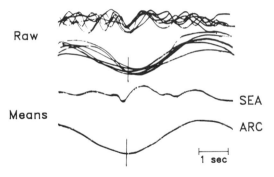

Figure 17.9. Simulation of raw waves for EEG (*top*) and chest diameter (*bottom*) contributing to ARC and SEA means.

technique as well as respiration in general as a useful and often overlooked technique in psychophysiology.

17.3.3.4 *Average repetitive cycle*

Schwartz, Whitehorn, Hernon, and Jones (1986) have recently introduced a technique particularly appropriate as a stage in the data reduction of continuous pulmonary activity. The technique is based on the averaging of successive repetitive waves and produces an average repetitive cycle (ARC). As an average, the ARC has the advantages of evoked and event-related potential techniques in terms of signal noise reduction. The ARC is produced by selecting an important and easily identifiable feature of the signal to be measured, such as peak inspiration or onset of inspiration. Data for specific intervals on either side of this feature are then averaged with data obtained around earlier features. The result is a single waveform "ARCed" around some feature of interest. Other physiological measures recorded simultaneously with the signal being ARCed may also be averaged and thus produce a synchronized event average (SEA). To produce the SEA, the same data segment in another channel that is arranged around the feature detected in the ARC is averaged. If the physiological data on the channels to be SEAed is randomly distributed with respect to the ARC channel, the result will be a flat average wave since the data in the SEA time segments will not have any synchronous elements. If, however, the ARC channel bears some relationship to the SEA data, there should be a nonflat SEA wave. Care must be taken to assure that systematic noise or error is not centered around the ARCed signal since this will also produce a nonflat SEA and contaminate any true response.

Consider the case of the inspiration of odor and its subsequent affect on the EEG. If the inspiration of an odor produces a consistent change in EEG activity, that change should follow the inspiration and should be discernable in the SEA waveform. The construction of an ARC and a SEA for pulmonary and EEG data is presented in Figure 17.9.

The advantage of this technique is that it produces a single composite wave with enhanced signal-to-noise characteristics. The addition of the SEA indicates the possible interrelation of other physiological signals with the signal being ARCed. The technique also has its disadvantages, which focus mainly on determining the point in the repetitive cycle to be ARCed. If the signal is slowly oscillating such as a pulmonary ventilation signal, it may be difficult to determine a peak since there may be many points that might qualify. The selection of this point will be very important to the analysis because if it is not synchronized with the other peaks in the analysis, it will degrade the amplitude of the resulting ARC.

The ARC waveform may be reduced using the volumetric or cycle-based measures mentioned previously. Additionally, because wave shape may be an important characteristic of certain psychological phenomena, this may be further reduced using the topographic analysis technique developed by Cacioppo and Dorfman (1987) (see Dorfman and Cacioppo, chapter 21).

17.4 SOCIAL AND INFERENTIAL CONSIDERATIONS

As mentioned previously, pulmonary activity is sensitive to a variety of metabolic and psychological variables. Many of these psychological variables pertain to social contexts. Breathing can change dramatically in interactions with others. The most obvious of these interactions includes the production of speech. Normal cyclic breathing tends to be abolished during active speech. Exhalations may last 15 s in some cases and are followed by deep, rapid inhalatory pauses (Dudley, 1967). Laughter also is highly disruptive to the typical pulmonary cycle (Svebak, 1975) and appears almost as diaphragmatic spasms.

Dudley (1969) described breathing patterns typical of a number of social situations. Prominent among these situations are conditions of anxiety and anger induced during interviews. Characteristic patterns emerge for individuals experiencing anxiety during these interviews. Their pneumographic records indicate occasional rapid and deep inspirations followed by long expiratory cycles. These are the quantified sighs of individuals experiencing anxiety. Similar sighs are induced in normal subjects simply instructed to "relax."

Anger also produces characteristic patterns of breathing. Increases in rate and decreases in depth are typical of this state. Dudley (1969), quoting Darwin, reports: "Men during numberless generations, have endeavored to escape from their enemies or danger by headlong flight, or by violently struggling with them; and such great exertions will have caused the heart to beat rapidly, the breathing to be hurried, the chest to heave, and the nostrils to be dilated" (p. 87). Evidence of our tendency to fight or flee, so often examined in cardiovascular research, is also a major component of the pulmonary response system.

Rate, depth, and the ratio of our inhalation to exhalation cycle (*I/E*) are all highly sensitive to phasic changes in psychological state. The mechanisms for this sensitivity remain unknown. Theoretical models of pulmonary response have tended to identify a single variable, typically metabolic rate, and to attribute the majority of the variability of the pulmonary response to that variable. Metabolic rate alone cannot account for the variance in this system. It is necessary to identify other contributory sources to the variance within the system and to create a more comprehensive model of the respiratory response. Until such a model is established, inferences as to the functional significance of alterations in breathing will be limited.

17.5   GENERAL CONSIDERATIONS

The particular method of pulmonary activity quantification and later reduction should be based on the information needed by the investigator coupled with how the technique will interface to the experimental protocol. Consider an experiment in which metabolic rate is a primary concern of the experimenters, as are environmental odor cues. The best method for the determination of metabolic rate is the use of blood gas analysis, which requires breathing through a mouthpiece while the nose is clamped. This clamp, of course, precludes the possibility of introducing odor cues. An alternative measure would be to infer metabolic rate from a pulmonary rate measure since these two variables have previously been highly correlated (West, 1979). Pulmonary rate may then be measured by any technique that does not interfere with ventilation through the nose.

Although pulmonary activity is often recorded in psychology, it is not often the variable of primary (or even secondary) interest (Hassett, 1978). As a result, we know relatively little about the relation of respiration to variables of psychological importance. There has been little interest in the measurement of pulmonary activity for the last 50 years, as evidenced by the limited number of recent psychological investigations cited here. Even in the 1954 edition of *Experimental Psychology*, Woodworth and Schlosberg mention that measurement of respiration has "fallen out of favor." This should not be the case. Respiration is a more complicated variable than the simple measure of rate indicates. The fact that I fractions change as a function of emotion (Feleky, 1916) should indicate a relationship of interest to psychologists, as should the fact that respiration is anticipatory to exertion (Cannon, 1932, cited in Woodworth & Schlosberg, 1954). Unfortunately, general activation theory came to "explain" these relationships, and respiration became less favored as a measure of activation phenomena. Now that psychology is once again questioning the utility of a general activation model, it seems prudent to reexamine the nature of respiration and the specificity of this system as well as its integration with other physiological and psychological processes.

NOTE

The authors wish to thank K. Herman for her editorial assistance in the review of this manuscript.

REFERENCES

Astrand, P., & Saltin, B. (1961). Oxygen uptake during the first minutes of heavy exercise. *Journal of Applied Physiology, 16,* 971–976.

Auchincloss, J. H., Gilbert, R., & Baule, G. H. (1966). Effect of ventilation on oxygen transfer during exercise. *Journal of Applied Physiology, 21,* 810–818.

Baker, L. E., Geddes, L. A., & Hoff, H. E. (1965). Quantitative evaluation of impedance spirometry in man. *American Journal of Medical Electronics, 4,* 73–77.

Best, C. H., & Taylor, N. B. (1961). *The physiological basis of medical practice.* Baltimore: Williams & Wilkins.

Cacioppo, J. T., & Dorfman, D. D. (1987). Waveform moment analysis in psychophysiological research. *Psychological Bulletin, 102,* 421–438.

Casali, J. G., Wierwille, W. W., & Cordes, R. E. (1983). Respiratory measurement: Overview and new instrumentation. *Behavior Research Methods, Instruments and Computers, 15,* 401–405.

Clauson, G. (1951). Respiration movement in normal, neurotic and psychotic subjects. *Acta Psychiatrica et Neurologica* (Supp.), 68.

Cohen, M. I. (1970). How respiratory rhythm originates: Evidence from discharge patterns of brainstem respiratory neurons. In R. Porter (Ed.), *Breathing: Hering-Breuer centenary symposium.* London: Churchill.

Dudley, D. L. (1969). *Psychophysiology of respiration in health and disease.* New York: Appleton-Century-Crofts.

Feleky, A. (1916). The influence of emotions on respiration. *Journal of Experimental Psychology, 1,* 218–222.

Finesinger, J. E. (1939). Effect of pleasant and unpleasant ideas on respiration in psychoneurotic patients. *Archives of Neurological Psychiatry, 42,* 425–490.

Fuster, J. M. (1980). *The prefrontal cortex: Anatomy, physiology and neuropsychology of the frontal lobe.* New York: Raven Press.

Grossman, P. (1983). Respiration, stress, and cardiovascular function. *Psychophysiology, 20,* 284–300.

Guz, A., Noble, M. I. M., Eisele, J. H., & Trenchard, D. (1970). The role of vagal inflation reflexes in man and other animals. In R. Porter (Ed.), *Breathing: Hering-Breuer centenary symposium.* London: Churchill.

Hassett, J. (1978). *A primer of psychophysiology.* San Francisco: Freeman.

Hirsch, J. A., & Bishop, B. (1981). Respiratory sinus arrhythmia in humans: How breathing modulates the heart. *American Journal of Physiology, 241,* H620–H629.

Kallman, W. M., & Feurstein, M. (1977). Physiological procedures. In A. Ciminero (Ed.), *Handbook of behavioral assessment.* New York: Wiley.

Kaufman, M. P., & Scheiderman, N. (1986). Physiological basis of the respiratory system. In M. G. H. Coles, E. Donchin, & S. W. Porges (Eds.), *Psychophysiology: Systems, processes, and applications.* New York: Guilford Press.

Lehmann, D., & Knauss, T. A. (1976). Respiratory cycle and EEG in man and cat. *Electroencephalography and Clinical Neurophysiology, 40,* 187.

Lorig, T. S., & Isaac, W. (1984). Quantification of cortical arousal: Correlation with locomotor activity. *Physiological Psychology, 12,* 253–256.

Lorig, T. S., Schwartz, G. E., Herman, K. B., & Lane, R. M. (1988). EEG activity during nose and mouth breathing. *Psychobiology, 16,* 285–287.

Macklem, P. T. (1978). Respiratory mechanics. *Annual Review of Physiology, 40,* 157–184.

Mishkin, M. (1964). Perseveration of central sets after frontal lesions in monkeys. In J. Warren & K. Akert (Eds.), *The frontal granular cortex and behavior.* New York: McGraw-Hill.

Morruzzi, G., & Magoun, H. W. (1949). Brainstem reticular formation activity and activation of the EEG. *Electroencephalography and Clinical Neurophysiology, 1,* 455–473.

Nielsen, J., & Roth, P. (1929). Clinical spirography. *Archives of Internal Medicine, 43,* 132–138.

Pauly, J. E. (1957). Electromyographic studies of human respiration. *Chicago Medical School Quarterly, 18,* 80–88.

Plum, F. (1970). Neurological integration of behavioral and metabolic control of breathing. In R. Porter (Ed.), *Breathing: Hering-Breuer centenary symposium.* London: Churchill.

Porges, S. W. (1976). Peripheral and neurochemical parallels of psychopathology: A psychophysiological model relating autonomic imbalances to hyperactivity, psychopathology and autism. In H. W. Reese (Ed.), *Advances in child development and behavior.* New York: Academic Press.

Sasaki, C. T., & Mann, D. G. (1976). Dilator naris function. *Archives of Otolaryngology, 102,* 365–367.

Scheafer, K. E. (1979). Respiratory pattern affecting metabolic processes and CNS function. In K. E. Scheafer, G. Hildebrandt, & N. Macbeth (Eds.), *Basis of an individual physiology.* Mt. Kisco, NY: Futura.

Schwartz, G. E., Whitehorn, D., Hernon, J., & Jones, M. (1986). The ARC method for averaging repetitive cycles: Application to respiration during stress and relaxation. *Psychophysiology, 23,* 460.

Servit, Z., Kristof, M., & Kolinova, M. (1977). Activation of epileptic electrographic activity in the human by nasal airflow. *Physiologia Bohemoslovenica, 26,* 499–506.

Stein, M., & Luparello, T. J. (1967). The measurement of respiration. In C. C. Brown (Ed.), *Methods in psychophysiology.* Baltimore: Wilkins.

Stevenson, I., & Ripley, N. (1952). Variations in respiration during changes in emotion. *Psychosomatic Medicine, 14,* 476–490.

Svebak, S. (1975). Respiratory pattern as a predictor of laughter. *Psychophysiology, 12*, 62–65.

Webb, P., & Troutman, S. J. (1970). An instrument for continuous measurement of oxygen consumption. *Journal of Applied Physiology, 28*, 867–871.

Werntz, D. A., Bickford, R. G., Bloom, F. E., & Shannahoff-Khalsa, D. S. (1983). Alternating cerebral hemisphere activity and the lateralization of autonomic nervous function. *Human Neurobiology, 2*, 39–43.

West, J. B. (1979). *Respiratory physiology: the essentials* (2nd ed.). Baltimore: Wilkins.

Wolf, S. (1947). Sustained contraction of the diaphragm, the mechanism for a common type of dyspnea and precordial pain. *Journal of Clinical Investigation, 26*, 1201.

Woodworth, R. S., & Schlosberg, H. (1954). *Experimental psychology* (rev. ed. pp. 169–173). New York: Holt, Reinhart & Winston.

Ziegler, L. H., & Levine, B. S. (1925). The influences of emotional reaction based on metabolism. *American Journal of Medical Science, 169*, 68–76.

18   *The sexual response system*

JAMES H. GEER AND SUSAN HEAD

Sexual psychophysiology can be distinguished from other branches of sex research by its use of a particular methodological approach. The approach utilizes electrophysiological measures, principally of genital responding, to assess sexual arousal and response patterns in humans. When most effectively applied, this approach entails the systematic exploration of the interdependence between cognitive, affective, and behavioral processes in association with physiological activation of the sexual response system (Rosen & Beck, 1987). In this sense sexual psychophysiology can be used to help clarify and understand the interplay of interpersonal and environmental events and their effects on the sexual response system. Conversely, it seeks to understand the effects of the response system (i.e., genital reactions and response) on the interpretation of interpersonal and environmental events.

18.1   HISTORICAL DEVELOPMENT OF SEXUAL PSYCHOPHYSIOLOGY

The early history of research on sexual arousal was dominated by the use of extragenital measures such as heart rate, respiration, blood pressure, sweat gland activity, and body temperature. In 1971, Zuckerman reviewed that literature and concluded that, due to their lack of specificity, extragenital measures of sexual responding were not very useful in assessing sexual arousal. Zuckerman's review of the literature, coupled with Master's and Johnson's (1966) report that myotonia and vasocongestion, particularly that occurring in the genitals, were the two major indicators of sexual arousal in humans, accounts for the recent trend in the field toward using direct genital measures to assess sexual arousal and response patterns. In spite of the fact that most psychophysiological studies of sexual arousal employ genital measures, we begin with a brief review of extragenital measures.

18.1.1   *Extragenital measures*

In 1937, Wilhelm Reich attempted to measure the galvanic skin response in the genitals in what was perhaps the earliest reported psychophysiological investigation of sexuality. Although skin conductance measures from nongenital sites have been shown to be successful indicators of sexual responding, they have failed to provide discriminatory data for distinguishing between sexual arousal and emotional arousal of other varieties (Zuckerman, 1971).

In experiments utilizing skin temperature as an index of sexual arousal, findings have been mixed. Hoon, Wincze, and Hoon (1976) found that forehead temperature

599

increased in the presence of erotic stimuli. On the other hand, Wenger, Averill, and Smith (1968) reported that finger temperature decreased in response to erotic stimuli, whereas facial temperature did not discriminate between erotic and control stimuli.

Several studies have utilized extragenital cardiovascular changes such as increased heart rate and blood pressure as the dependent variables in measuring sexual arousal to erotic stimuli (Bartlett, 1956; Corman, 1968; Romano, 1969; Wenger et al., 1968; Wood & Obrist, 1968). Masters and Johnson (1966) claimed that heart rate and both systolic and diastolic blood pressure elevations in the excitement phase increase correspondent with increased genital responding. Research indicates that heart rate is not a very sensitive measure of sexual arousal prior to genital manipulation (Bartlett, 1956). Also, heart rate increases were not shown to differentiate between sexual response and response to other external stimuli (Fisher & Osofsky, 1968; Romano, 1969). On the other hand, systolic blood pressure was found to increase significantly in response to an erotic motion picture (Corman, 1968).

Other investigators have studied the relationship between EEG phenomena and sexual arousal. Lifschitz (1966) reported that subjects' averaged evoked responses (AERs) differed between presentations of focused and unfocused slides of three different subject categories (indifferent scenic, repulsive medical, and nude female photographs). However, subjects' AERs, in terms of wave amplitude and frequency, did not discriminate erotic from control stimuli. Cohen, Rosen, and Goldstein (1976) examined laterality changes during masturbation and reported significant shifts in laterality during orgasm. At the present time, the relationships between central nervous system events, as measured by EEG and related techniques, and sexual arousal are not clearly understood and research in the area is scant.

In 1968, Hess reported pupil dilation as an indicator of sexual interest or arousal. However, research following from this possibility has been limited. Although Hamel (1974) found that female undergraduates exhibited significant pupil dilation when they viewed nude photographs of males and females, there were no appropriate controls for other types of emotional responses that are known to affect pupil dilation. Also, the relationship between pupil dilation and self-report of sexual arousal in this study was weak (Geer, O'Donahue, & Schorman, 1986).

As with extragenital measures, biochemical measures of sex hormone production have failed to provide specific indices of sexual arousal (Geer et al., 1986). Although urinary acid phosphate was reported to increase in response to sexual stimulation (Barclay, 1970; Gustafson, Winokur, & Reichlin, 1963), Barclay's work noted that levels were also affected by anger and previous sexual experience.

In reviewing the research utilizing extragenital measures, it seems clear that Zuckerman's assertion that extragenital measures are insufficient as specific discriminators of sexual arousal still holds. In that genital measures partially circumvent problems of nonspecificity posed by extragenital measures, genital measures appear to be the best psychophysiological indices available for studying sexual behavior and arousal. When used in concert with subjective and behavioral measures, genital measures provide a powerful set of research strategies for expanding our knowledge concerning sex in specific and, perhaps, emotion in general (Geer, 1980). With this in view the rest of this chapter will concentrate upon genital measures. We begin with a review of the historical development of the various devices. Descriptions of the more widely used measurement devices will be covered in a later section of this chapter.

18.1.2 *Genital measures*

18.1.2.1 *Male*

The earliest genital devices were developed for the monitoring of male erection. The first of these devices was a simple electromechanical transducer (Ohlmeyer, Brilmayer, & Hullstrung, 1944). The device consisted of a circular ring that fit around the subject's penis and provided a simple binary signal of the presence or absence of erection.

Current research in male sexual arousal relies primarily on the use of either circumferential measures or volumetric measures of the penis. In 1963 Freund reported on a device that involved air volumetric plethysmography. Variants of penile volumetric devices have been reported. For example, McConaghy (1967) designed a penile plethysmograph made of materials more readily accessible than those used in Freund's device. A penile plethysmograph that displaces fluid rather than air was developed by Fisher, Gross, and Zuch in 1965. In general volumetric penile plethysmographs have not proven popular due to their bulk and awkwardness in use. Fisher, Gross, and Zuch (1965) described the use of a penile circumference gauge that consisted of a hollow rubber tube filled with mercury and sealed at the ends with platinum electrodes inserted into the mercury. This device, known as a mercury-in-rubber strain gauge, was adapted from a similar transducer used in Shapiro and Cohen's (1965) study of nocturnal tumescence. Another type of mercury-in-rubber strain gauge was developed by Bancroft, Jones, and Pullan (1966). It has a plastic supporting structure that allows the device to be fitted to the individual penis. Another variant of the penile strain gauge was introduced in 1967 by Jovanovic and used graphite rather than mercury as the conducting material. Although quite sensitive to small changes, the graphite may separate when large changes occur.

A widely used penile strain gauge, which was developed by Barlow, Becker, Leitenberg, and Agros (1970), is a device made of two arcs of surgical spring material joined with two mechanical strain gauges. A description of this device along with instruction for its placement during experimental procedures are included later in this chapter.

Thermistor measurement devices have been designed to detect temperature changes that may accompany penile tumescence changes (Solnick & Berrin, 1977). In Solnick and Berrin's (1977) study, they compared thermistor measures of tumescence with circumference measures. The results showed a relatively high concordance between temperature changes and penile circumference. Webster and Hammer's results (1983) supported the Solnick and Berrin (1977) results.

Bancroft and Bell (1985) have developed a reflectance photometer for noninvasive measurement of penile arterial pulse amplitude. The essential components of this device are similar to those used in the vaginal photometer, described later in this chapter. It has recently been suggested that penile pulse amplitude may provide an index of arterial inflow related to generalizable penile tumescence (Rosen & Beck, 1987). The currently available data are insufficient to warrant a judgment on the usefulness of the penile photometer.

18.1.2.2 *Female*

The development of genital measurement devices for females has been stimulated by the Masters and Johnson (1966) report of vaginal vasocongestion being a relatively invariant concomitant of sexual arousal and by Zuckerman's (1971) report, which stated that the lack of genital measurement in women was an obstacle to research on sexuality.

In 1967, Palti and Bercovici reported that they mounted a miniature light source and photoelectric cell on a vaginal speculum to detect vaginal pulse waves. Although the device reliably yielded a record of vaginal pulse waves, the method was not developed for, nor has it been adopted for, use in sex research. Other early attempts to measure genital responding in women included a device designed to measure vaginal pH as an indicator of lubrication (Shapiro, Cohen, DiBianco, & Rosen, 1968). The attempts to measure vaginal pH or vaginal lubrication have been technically difficult and instrusive (Wagner & Levin, 1978). A mechanical strain gauge was developed to measure clitoral engorgement (Karacan, Rosenbloom, & Williams, 1970). Although it detected clitoral changes, the subjects in that study (Karacan et al., 1970) were women with congenital clitoral enlargement. It appears that the device is not applicable to the general female population. Jovanovic (1971) developed a balloonlike device that was filled with water inserted through the cervix into the uterus. This device, designed to measure uterine contractions, has many problems, including the tendency of highly anxious women to extrude the device and pain associated with placement of the device (Rosen & Beck, 1987).

A well-validated device is the vaginal blood flowmeter or vaginal thermistor probe developed by Shapiro et al. (1968) and further validated by Cohen and Shapiro (1970). The unit consists of two thermistors mounted on an individually fitted diaphragm ring that is placed in its normal position against the cervix. Fisher and colleagues (1983) have recently reported data from 10 female volunteers on patterns of female sexual arousal during sleep and waking hours using the Shapiro et al. (1968) device. The data indicated that the vaginal blood flowmeter is sensitive to the effects of erotic stimulation in the waking state. The nighttime data were complex and require further investigation. The main disadvantages are that it is a relatively delicate device and it requires custom fitting of the diaphragm by a medically trained staff.

The vaginal photometer, originally called a photoplethysmograph, was developed by Sintchak and Geer (1975). This device is made of clear acrylic plastic and is shaped like a menstrual tampon. Hoon, Wincze, and Hoon (1976) introduced an improved model of the vaginal photometer that substituted an infrared LED (light-emitting diode) for the incandescent light source and a phototransistor detector for the photocell. These innovations reduce or eliminate potential artifacts associated with blood oxygenation levels and reduce problems of hysteresis and light history effects.

Another device that offers a promising approach for the detection of sexual arousal in women is the oxygenation thermistor probe developed by Levin and Wagner (1978). This device consists of a heated oxygen electrode held against the vaginal wall by means of suction. The probe is designed to measure both blood flow and blood oxygen levels by assessing oxygen diffusion. Oxygen diffusion has been shown to be closely correlated with arterial oxygenation levels (Baumberger & Goodfriend, 1951; Rooth, Sjostedt, & Caligara, 1957, as cited in Rosen & Beck, 1987).

An advantage of this probe is that its reliability is not affected by variation in placement (Levin & Wagner, 1978). However, use of this device has been limited due, in part, to the expense of the instrumentation.

Fisher and Osofsky (1968) and Fisher (1973) used a Yellow Springs thermistor probe to measure vaginal temperature as an indicator of female sexual arousal. These studies indicated that vaginal temperature generally reflects core temperature and is relatively insensitive to changes in arousal. In contrast to the just described studies, Fuglmeyer, Sjogren, and Johansson (1984) describe a radiotelemetric method for measuring vaginal temperature using a battery-powered transducer mounted on a diaphragm ring. They reported decreases in vaginal temperature that were speculated to be due to vaginal wall edema during sexual arousal (Wagner & Levin, 1978). Advantages of the device include absence of movement artifacts and the ability to utilize the device in natural settings (Rosen & Beck, 1987). In view of the conflicting reports, replication is needed before the utility of vaginal temperature as a measure of arousal is fully ascertained.

Henson, Rubin, and Henson (1978) have described a transducer for measuring labial temperature. This device is composed of three surface temperature probes designed to measure temperature changes from an individually determined baseline. Labial temperature of 9 of the 10 subjects in Henson and Rubin's study was shown to increase in response to their viewing an erotic film. The labial thermistor clip appears to hold promise as an additional means of measuring female genital response to erotic stimuli.

18.1.2.3 *Cross-sex comparisons*

The desire to develop devices that will allow direct comparison of the sexes has been an impetus for the development of genital measurement devices. Unfortunately, it often has not been recognized that the problem is much more complex than simply developing similar measures from similar locations. In general, investigators have ignored psychometric considerations. For example, it has been shown that vaginal vascular responses continue for 15 min or so following masturbatory induced orgasm (Geer & Quartararo, 1976). Since that time course is much longer than found for penile detumescence, it appears likely that the time course for pelvic vasocongestion differs between the sexes. It then follows that simple correlations, for example, are inadequate to study sex differences or similarities. The issues of cross-sex differences in subjective ratings and possible sex differences in the nature of the relationship between physiological and subjective indices may contribute to the complexity of cross-sex comparisons. Our point is that although between-sex comparisons are crucial to the complete understanding of sexuality, we must be careful not to oversimplify the issues.

Regardless of the complexities, several investigators have worked on developing devices to facilitate cross-sex comparisons. Bohlen and Held (1979) described a device designed to monitor intra-anal pressure changes and pulse waves. The anal probe is based on the suggestion that anal changes accompanying the experience of sexual arousal are a result of increased blood volume and muscle tension throughout the pelvic area (Masters & Johnson, 1966).

A unique application of temperature measurement is thermography, which has been proposed as a methodology that can be used in cross-sex comparison (Seeley, Abramson, Perry, Rothblatt, & Seeley, 1980). Thermography is a method of detecting

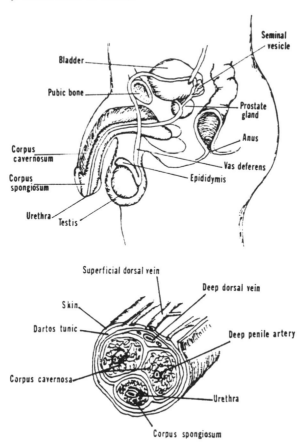

Figure 18.1. Cross section of male pelvic region and cross section of penis.

and measuring heat from various of regions of the body and transforming them into signals that can be recorded photographically. The result is a picture of heat patterns of a particular region. The principle of thermography will be described in a later section of this chapter.

18.2   PHYSICAL CONTEXT

18.2.1   *Physical/physiological basis of the response system*

Before beginning a discussion of the methodologies of measuring responses obtained from the genital devices, some background material may be of value. We begin with a brief discussion of some aspects of genital anatomy and responding, limiting our discussion to those aspects that are relevant to this chapter.

18.2.1.1   *Males*

In males, the external sex organs consist of the penis and the scrotum, which contains the sperm-producing testes. Figure 18.1 contains drawings of the male pelvic region in

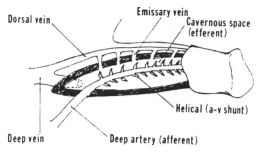

Figure 18.2. Vascular system of penis, depicting afferent, shunting, and efferent systems.

cross section and a cross section of the penis. Of particular interest to this chapter is the internal structure of the penis. There are three cylindrical spongelike bodies of erectile tissue in the penis; the two lying dorsally are called the corpora cavernosa and the one lying ventrally is called the corpus spongiosum. The structures contain small irregular compartments (vascular spaces) separated by bonds of smooth muscle tissue. These bodies become engorged with blood during erection. The function of the corpora cavernosa is purely erectile. The corpus spongiosum and glans also act as a urinary conduit and an organ of ejaculation. On erection, the corpus spongiosum and the glans develop a modest turgidity but never become rigid enough to shut off the urethral lumen. Along with its sensory function, the glans swells appreciably during arousal and ejaculation.

With the exception of several minor branches from the scrotal and epigastric arteries, the blood supply to the penis is furnished by the two internal pudendal arteries. Each pudendal artery branches off to become a complex of arteries (bulbar, penile, and urethral) that supply the penis (Figure 18.2).

Of particular interest is the deep artery of the penis, which follows the length of the penis, terminating at the glans. In its course, the deep artery gives off many branches to the corpus spongiosum and, most importantly, to the helical arteries. The numerous helical arteries provide the arteriovenous shunts that are integral to the mechanism of erection. From the helical arteries arise short-end arteries with bulbous tips that open into the cavernous spaces. Numerous anastomoses or connections are present between all the arteries of the penis.

The three major subdivisions of the veins of the penis include the superficial dorsal vein, the deep profunda dorsal vein, and the deep veins of the corpus spongiosum, which include the bulbar and urethral vessels. Important anastomotic channels unite the veins of the penis at various junctions.

Polsters appear as a split in the internal elastic lamella of certain blood vessels with the intervening space filled with longitudinal muscle and connective tissue fibers. They are present in both arteries and veins and constitute a variable amount of the lumen. Polsters are found not only in the blood vessels of the penis but also in most of the muscular arteries throughout the body.

Previous theories of erection (Conti, 1952; Weiss, 1972) implicated the polsters as important structures in the mechanism of erection. It was postulated that the contraction or relaxation of the muscle or connective tissue in the polsters, under parasympathetic control, resulted in dilating or contracting the lumen of the vessel. It was assumed that erection was effected by opening of the shunts aided by active relaxation of the polsters in the arteries leading to the cavernous spaces, coincident with active contraction of polsters within the arteries to the somatic parts of the penis and the veins draining the penis. A recent study (Newman & Northup, 1981) based on the examination of more than 75 cadavers and several human volunteers suggests that polsters exert only a passive impedance to flow. These authors further suggest that polsters apparently represent a response to aging and stress and that, due to their age distribution in the population, location, and microscopic picture, may be related to the incidence of arteriosclerosis (Newman & Northup, 1981). It appears, therefore, that increased arterial inflow, perhaps via parasympathetic vasodilation of penile arteries, and subsequent shunting of the increased arterial blood via the helical arteries is adequate to induce erection and that polsters are at best minimally involved (Newman & Northup, 1981).

From this point of view, erection is essentially a hydrodynamic manifestation, weighing arterial inflow against venous outflow. Erection is produced by the shunting of arterial blood into the cavernous spaces through arteriovenous anastomoses. The deep artery of the penis is the afferent vessel, whereas the helical arteries serve as arteriovenous shunts. The cavernous spaces lined by endothelium represent the efferent venous segment that empties directly into the emissary and deep veins of the penis.

18.2.1.2 *Females*

We present in Figure 18.3 a view of the external female genitals and a cross-sectional view of the pelvic region. The external female genital area is known as the vulva. The entire genital area has been found to be rich in nerve endings and heavily vascularized. The layer of fatty tissue covering the junction of the pubic bones at the top of this area is known as the mons pubis. The labia majora, also known as the outer lips, consist of two large folds of tissue extending downward from the mons and surrounding the genital area. The labia minora, or inner lips, lie just inside the labia majora. The labia minora enclose an area called the vestibule, which contains the clitoris, the urethral opening, and vaginal opening. The portion of the labia minora that covers the clitoris is known as the prepuce, or the clitoral hood. The clitoris is composed of the clitoral shaft, measuring about 1 in. in lengh by ¼ in. in width, the crura, which divides at the base of the shaft, and the clitoral head or glans. Erectile tissue of the clitoral shaft becomes engorged with blood during sexual arousal in much the same way as does the male penis.

The organ that has been the principal focus of psychophysiological measurement in women has been the vaginal barrel. The vaginal barrel is a collapsed canal that is more a potential than a permanent space. During sexual arousal vasocongestion occurs, and it appears that vaginal lubrication occurs as a result of changes associated with the vasocongestion (Levin & Wagner, 1978). Vascular responding of the erectile tissues of the introitus and extending to the clitoris is, as with the penis, controlled by the parasympathetic nerves that pass through the nervi erigentes from the sacral plexus (Guyton, 1971).

18.2.2   *Hormonal control of the response system*

That sexual arousal involves mediation of the central nervous system, autonomic nervous system, and hormonal system has been well documented. It has also been noted that there are species and sex differences in the dependence of sexual arousal

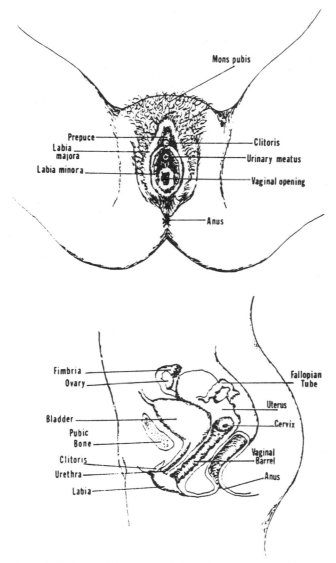

Figure 18.3. External female genitals and cross section of pelvic region.

on the neocortex and hormones (Beach, 1958). A brief description of some of the hormonal effects upon the response system is warranted.

Male hormones, often referred to as androgens, are defined as those that have masculinizing effects and female hormones as those that have feminizing effects. Although both males and females produce both types of hormones, males produce more masculinizing hormones, and females produce more feminizing hormones. In humans, sex hormones are produced throughout life with an increase beginning at puberty. At puberty the increase in sex hormones results in the lowering of the voice, development of secondary sex characteristics, and further development of the genitals.

Even though the level of sex hormones in the bloodstream has less effect on the sexual activity of humans than of other animals, the sex hormones still have an influence on sexual behavior. For males, sexual interest tends to be highest during the ages when androgen levels are highest (about 15 to 25). Also, men with low androgen levels generally have less than average frequencies of erection and sexual activity (Kalat, 1984). With females, a marked decrease in sexual response was shown in about one-third of women after removal of the sex organs (Zussman, Zussman, Sunley, & Bjornson, 1981, as cited in Kalat, 1984), presumably due to decreased levels of both estrogens and androgens. Androgen replacement has been shown to be effective in restoring sexual activity in women (Burdine, Shipley, & Papas, 1957, as cited in Kalat, 1984). Bancroft (1987) suggests that sexual interest is more variably influenced by hormone levels in women than in men. With the exception, noted later, of changes associated with the menstrual cycle, there is little evidence relating hormone levels to psychophysiological measures of sexual arousal.

18.2.3   Neurophysiology of erection

Weiss (1972) has presented a dual-innervation model of erection that relies on both psychogenic and reflexogenic control of erection. According to this model, the reflexogenic component consists of a sacral parasympathetic pathway, whereas the psychogenic pathway is sympathetic in origin. These two pathways are thought to interact such that psychogenic stimuli such as sexual fantasy can enhance genital responding by diminishing the amount of tactile genital stimulation necessary to produce an erection. By the same token, other psychogenic stimuli, such as guilt or hostility, can operate in the reverse direction to inhibit reflexive arousal (Weiss, 1972). To further complicate the matter, it has been shown that erection can occur in a purely reflexive manner on the basis of sacral innervation alone, without connections to the brain (Money, 1961).

Although the reflexive, parasympathetic component of erection has been widely accepted, recent research (Wagner & Brindley, 1980, as cited in Rosen & Beck, 1987) has raised doubts about the role of cholinergic mediation in erection. In their study, Wagner and Brindley (1980) reported little effect of atropine blockade on tumescence. Although poorly understood, adrenergic mechanisms also appear to play a part in erection. Histological examination has revealed that the penile corpora are richly endowed with alpha-adrenergic receptors (Levin & Wein, 1980, as cited in Rosen & Beck, 1987).

Brindley (1983) has produced reflex erection in the laboratory by local injection of alpha–adrenoceptor blockers (phenoxybenzamine, phentolamine). Also, injection of papaverine, a smooth muscle relaxant, has been shown to produce reflex erections (Zorgniotti & Lefleur, 1985). In a recent double-blind comparison study of phenoxybenzamine versus papaverine-phentolamine versus saline, Szasz, and colleagues (Szasz, Stevenson, Lee, & Sanders, 1987) found intracavernous injections of both phenoxybenzamine and papaverine-phentolamine to produce appreciable penile swelling in subjects with organic erection dysfunction. In studies reported by Ottesen, Wagner, Virag, and Fahrenkrug (1984, as cited in Rosen & Beck, 1987), a vasoactive intestinal polypeptide (VIP) has been implicated in the mediation of erection. It appears that VIP release is associated with relaxation of the smooth muscle tissue, decreased peripheral resistance, and increased arterial inflow.

In summary, doubts concerning the specifics of the neural mediation of erection have been raised. The exact role of sympathetic and parasympathetic pathways is unclear. Recent research has tended to focus on the effects of adrenergic mechanisms and the specific function of VIP in the neural mediation of erection.

18.2.4   *Neurophysiology of vaginal arousal*

According to Masters and Johnson (1966), the first observable response of sexual arousal in women is vaginal lubrication. The process of vaginal lubrication has been referred to as a "sweating" of the vaginal epithelium and appears simultaneous with increased blood flow to the vagina (Wagner & Levin, 1978). A model presented by Wagner and Levin (1978) suggests fluctuations in the regulation of the sodium-potassium balance of the vaginal tissue as a relevant mechanism mediating the production of vaginal lubricant. They suggest that with the vasodilation resulting from sexual arousal there is increased NaCl transduced across the vaginal wall producing the "glairy lubricating fluid on the surface of the vagina" (Wagner & Levin, 1978, p. 135).

The view that for both sexes parasympathetic innervation is dominant during moderate levels of sexual arousal and that subsequently sympathetic innervation is dominant during high levels of sexual arousal and orgasm is based upon the assumption that observed physiological changes are clear indicants of neural activity. However, research has failed to link physiological activity during sexual arousal with neural activity in the parasympathetic portion of the brainstem (Hoon, Wincze, & Hoon, 1976; Wenger et al., 1968). Therefore, the current theory of parasympathetic dominance during the initial stages of sexual arousal has little direct support. Clearly we need more basic research on this important topic.

18.2.5   *Models of sexual arousal*

18.2.5.1   *Masters and Johnson's model of the sexual response cycle*

Masters and Johnson (1966) have proposed a four-phase descriptive model of the responses that occur in humans during sexual behavior. The model is described in terms of four sequential stages or phases. The phases, in order, are (1) the excitement phase, (2) the plateau phase, (3) the orgasmic phase, and (4) the resolution phase. Masters and Johnson (1966) have described the genital and extragenital responses that they reported as being typically associated with each phase. These responses provide cues as to psychophysiological measures that might provide helpful indices of sexual arousal throughout the cycle. Masters and Johnson's description of sexual responses emphasize two generalized responses to sexual stimulation: vasocongestion and myotonia. Up to this time the former has proven more useful in research.

To return to the model, the first phase (excitement) describes the initial response to "effective" sexual stimulation. During the excitement phase there is a continuous increase in the level or intensity of arousal. If effective stimulation is continued, the individual will enter the plateau phase. This phase, which consists of high-level arousal of relatively consistent intensity, will, with continued stimulation, ultimately result in orgasm. However, cessation of stimulation during the plateau or excitement phases results in eventual return to prestimulation levels. The orgasmic phase, which signals the end of the plateau phase, is of brief duration and represents the involuntary reaching of maximal sexual tension. Males report that a period of ejaculatory inevitability develops at the beginning of the orgasmic phase. The resolution phase, which follows the orgasmic phase, is characterized by a loss of tension, which leads to an eventual return to prestimulation levels. Masters and Johnson note that there are substantial individual differences in sexual response cycles. Their model is presented here as a heuristic and not as an absolute. In particular, the evidence of a clearly identifiable plateau phase is questionable. See Masters and Johnson (1966) for a detailed description of the responses they describe as occurring during the four phases in the sexual response cycle.

Although few investigators would dispute the importance of the Masters and Johnson model, it has been subjected to serious criticism. Among these criticisms are included the fact that they failed to describe adequately the methods they used to collect their psychophysiological data, making it impossible to replicate their studies. In addition, the data reported were unquantified, and there have been conflicting findings concerning the presence of increased vasocongestion in female genitals during orgasm (Geer & Quartararo, 1976). Finally, questions have been raised concerning the universality of the model (Rosen & Rosen, 1981). Replications using standardized physiological measures and eliciting conditions are needed to resolve these discrepancies in the literature.

18.2.5.2 *Barlow's interactive model*

Several models have been proposed to explain the interactive mechanisms of sexual arousal. Barlow (1986) has recently proposed an interactive model of sexual arousal emphasizing the cognitive–affective processes in the mediation of sexual arousal. In his model Barlow (1986) focuses particularly on the perception of physiological arousal and the processing of erotic cues. He suggests that the sexual arousal experience for an individual may begin with that individual's perception of external expectations for sexual arousal. The individual responds emotionally to the external situation either positively or negatively. This emotional response influences the saliency of certain features of the erotic situation. Attentional focus on salient features, when influenced by a positive response to the erotic situation, serves to enhance sexual arousal. Salient features then serve to increase the focus upon erotic cues. The positive affective response also acts to trigger autonomic arousal. Attention to autonomic arousal results in further processing of erotic cues, thus heightening arousal in a feedback loop. Continued processing of erotic cues ultimately leads to sexual approach behavior. Conversely, when influenced by a negative response to the erotic situation, attention is focused on negative aspects of the situation, ultimately producing avoidance behavior. Under these latter conditions, sexual arousal does not occur. By combining cognitive–affective and physiological features of sexual response, consideration of this type of cognitive–affective model in concert with Masters and Johnson's (1966) physiologically based model of the sexual response cycle affords a more complete picture of the psychophysiological phenomenon of sexual arousal.

18.2.6 *Description of measurement devices for the assessment of sexual arousal*

Before describing several of the more widely used devices for the assessment of sexual arousal, we would like to mention a few guidelines concerning sterilization

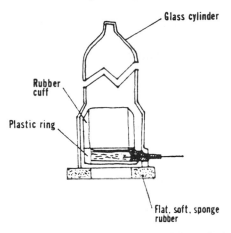

Figure 18.4. Schematic diagram of Freund's (1963) air volumetric plethysmograph.

procedures. In light of the current impact of AIDS (acquired immune deficiency syndrome) on societal concerns in general and sexual concerns in particular, the use of genital devices must include consideration of procedures that guarantee that inadvertent transmission of the AIDS virus cannot occur. Standardized sterilization procedures (use of activated gluteraldehyde) kill viruses (Geer, 1978) including the dreaded AIDS virus. Researchers must consult with infection control experts to assure that the specific procedures that they are using guarantee that AIDS transmission cannot and will not occur. We now turn our attention to a more detailed description of the most commonly used measurement devices.

18.2.6.1 *Male genital measurement devices*

Figure 18.4 presents a schematic diagram of Freund's (1963) air volumetric plethysmograph. This device used the general principle of volumetric plethysmography in which a body part is enclosed in a sealed container with air or fluid. The air-filled penile plethysmograph is positioned on the subject by the experimenter, who places a sponge-rubber ring over the penis. Next, a plastic ring with an inflatable cuff made from a condom is fitted over the penis and the ring. Finally, a glass cylinder with a funnel at the top is fitted over the other components and strapped to the subject's body. The cuff is then inflated, sealing the penis within the cylinder. Changes in the size of the body part result in displacement of air/fluid, yielding a change in the air/fluid pressure. This pressure change is detected by a pressure transducer whose output is recorded. Calibration allows precise determination of volume changes.

A diagram of the mercury-in-rubber strain gauge described by Fisher and colleagues (1965) is shown in Figure 18.5. The device consists of a hollow rubber tube filled with mercury and sealed at the ends with platinum electrodes that are inserted into the mercury. These electrodes are attached to a bridge circuit for connection to a polygraph. The operation of the mercury-in-rubber strain gauge depends upon penile circumference changes that cause the rubber tube to stretch or shorten, thus altering the cross-sectional area of the column of mercury within the tube. The resistance of the mercury inside the tube varies directly with its

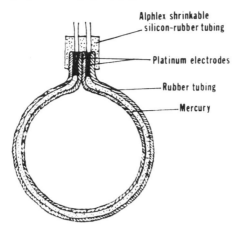

Alphlex shrinkable
silicon-rubber tubing

Platinum electrodes

Rubber tubing

Mercury

Figure 18.5. Schematic diagram of mercury-in-rubber penile strain gauge.

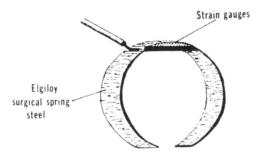

Strain gauges

Elgiloy
surgical spring
steel

Figure 18.6. Schematic representation of penile strain gauge developed by Barlow and co-workers (1970).

cross-sectional area, which in turn is reflective of changes in the circumference of the penis. This means that a display of resistance changes in the mercury reflects changes in the circumference of the penis. These circumferential changes can then be rather precisely calibrated as physical units.

The penile strain gauge, which was developed by Barlow and co-workers (1970), is depicted in Figure 18.6. This device is made of two arcs of surgical spring material joined with two mechanical strain gauges. These gauges are flexed when the penis changes in circumference, producing changes in their resistance. The resistance changes are in turn displayed, through appropriate circuitry, on the polygraph. Correct positioning of this gauge is critical. Some placements can produce artifactual decreases in circumference due to failure of the ends of the surgical steel arcs to separate. Mechanical strain gauges of this sort are quite sensitive and more rugged than their rubber counterparts. However, if improperly designed or fitted, they may yield artifacts (Geer, 1980).

In the case of both the strain gauge and the volumetric plethysmograph, penile tumescence from a laboratory subject is normally recorded on a polygraph.

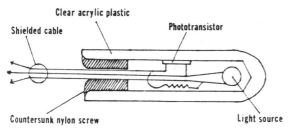

Figure 18.7. Schematic representation of vaginal photometer.

Depending on the type of transducer, signals from the gauge are either fed directly into the polygraph input coupler or through a preliminary bridge circuit.

18.2.6.2. *Female genital measurement devices*

The vaginal blood flowmeter (Shapiro et al., 1968) consists of two thermistors mounted on an individually fitted diaphragm ring that is placed in its normal position against the cervix. One thermistor is placed in contact with the vaginal wall and is heated slightly ($4°C$) above intravaginal temperature. The second thermistor is placed so as to avoid contact with the vaginal wall and thus record intravaginal temperature. The current necessary to maintain a constant temperature difference between the two thermistors reflects dissipation of heat into the vaginal wall. Change in heat dissipation being primarily a function of blood flow in the surrounding tissues, the device does not measure vaginal temperature but rather appears to measure blood flow. As noted in an earlier section, Fisher and colleagues (1983) have recently reported data indicating that the vaginal blood flowmeter detects vaginal responding during sleep, although the interpretation of those data is unclear. The main disadvantages are that it is a relatively delicate device and it requires custom fitting of the diaphragm by a medically trained staff.

The vaginal photometer, originally developed by Sintchak and Geer (1975) and improved upon by Hoon, Wincze, and Hoon (1976), is depicted in Figure 18.7. Embedded in the front end of the probe is an LED that illuminates, albeit at very low levels, the vaginal walls. Light is reflected and diffused through the tissues of the vaginal wall and reaches a photoreceptive cell surface mounted within the body of the probe and held against the vaginal wall. Changes in the resistance of the cell correspond to changes in the amount of back-scattered light reaching the light-sensitive surface. Recent research (Tahmoush & Francis, 1986) appears to establish that changes in the walls of the vascular bed in response to changes in blood pressure is the principal event influencing light reflection. The suggestion that the vaginal photometric response differs from that found elsewhere and is related to lubrication appears untenable. Until there is developed a methodology to satisfactorily measure lubrication, the issue cannot be determined with certainty. The vaginal photometer is designed so that it can be easily placed by the subject. A shield can be placed on the probe's cable so that depth of insertion and orientation of the photoreceptive surface is known (Geer, 1983). The subject can insert the probe, plug the cable from the device into the appropriate jack, and take her place in a chair or whatever else is used by the subject when recordings are made. The device is sensitive to movement.

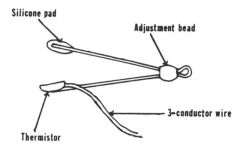

Figure 18.8. Diagram of labial thermistor clip developed by Henson, Rubin, and Henson (1978).

Figure 18.8 depicts the transducer Henson et al. (1978) designed for measuring labial temperature. This device is composed of three surface temperature probes designed to measure temperature changes from an individually determined baseline. One of the thermistors is used to monitor ambient room temperature and is positioned on a wall about 1.5 m from the subject. The other two thermistors are employed to monitor changes in surface skin temperature. One is attached to the labia minora by means of a brass clip, and the other is attached to an extragenital site (i.e., the chest) and provides a reference temperature. The labial thermistor clip holds promise as an additional means of measuring female genital response to erotic stimuli.

18.2.6.3. Cross-sex measurement devices

The anal probe described by Bohlen and Held (1979) was designed to monitor events intra-anally. The authors suggest that it can be used to directly compare sexual responses in men and women. The design of the anal probe is based on the observation that genital changes associated with the experience of sexual arousal are a result of increased blood volume and muscle tension throughout the pelvic area and does include anal responding (Masters & Johnson, 1966).

The anal probe consists of an LED–transistor photometer and pressure transducer encased within a body constructed of silicone rubber tubing. The head and base of the device are constructed of epoxy-resin. Electrical signals reflecting anal pulse wave activity and muscle tension are fed directly to the recording system. While in use, the probe maintains a fixed orientation that minimizes motion artifact and assures the comparison of a similar area of the anal mucosa from session to session and from subject to subject.

We noted that thermistors have been used to measure genital temperature in both sexes. Since the measurements are obtained from different anatomical structures, we do not include that methodology under the male–female category. We do, however, wish to consider thermography here since it has been proposed as a methodology that can be used in cross-sex comparisons (Seeley et al., 1980). The principle of thermography is based on the fact that all objects, both animate and inanimate, emit infrared radiation as a function of their temperature (Gershon-Cohen, 1964). A thermogram is a picture or temperature "map" illustrating hot and cold areas, vascular patterns, and temperature irregularities of the object under

Table 18.1 *Overview of most commonly used measures*

Male devices

I. Measures of penile volume
   A. Device
      1. Air-filled plethysmograph
      2. Water-filled plethysmograph
   B. Application considerations: most useful when sensitive data on erection is needed and interest is focused on nature of penile response; devices are not recommended when intrusiveness to subject is serious problem

II. Measures of penile diameter or circumference
   A. Devices
      1. Mercury in rubber strain gauge
      2. Mechanical strain gauge
   B. Application considerations: particularly valuable when concerned about subject reactivity since subject can place device; may prove helpful in detection of physiological problem of blood flow; mercury in rubber gauge has shortened shelf life and can be easily broken; placement may be critical for mechanical gauge

III. Measures of penile temperature and pulse waves
   A. Devices
      1. Penile thermistor
      2. Penile photometer
   B. Application considerations: photometeric evaluation may be useful in determining blood flow anomalies; penile temperature may prove useful in comparing different anatomical structures; additional validation of these devices is needed to determine their utility as measure of sexual arousal.

Female devices

IV. Measures of vaginal blood flow
   A. Device
      1. Blood flowmeter
      2. Radiotelemetric blood flowmeter
   B. Application considerations: valuable where longer-term recording is needed (e.g., sleep studies) and where movement artifacts pose serious problems; device is fragile and must be fitted by medical professionals, thus reducing its utility in many settings

V. Measures of vaginal arterial oxygen pressure
   A. Device
      1. Oxygenation thermistor probe
   B. Application considerations: valuable where detailed physiological information is needed; since it can be combined with blood flow device, a powerful combination of measures is available; expense and intrusiveness may limit scope of application.

VI. Measures of vaginal pulse waves
   A. Device
      1. Vaginal photometer
   B. Application considerations: useful where vaginal measures are important and where subject acceptance is crucial; widely used and well-validated with considerable technical improvements available; problems with movement artifacts may occur

VII. Measures of labial temperature
   A. Device
      1. Labial clip
   B. Application considerations: useful where time course of response is of reduced importance and when subjects reject intravaginal measures; device can be placed by subject in privacy

VIII. Measures of vaginal temperature
   A. Device
      1. Thermistor probe
   B. Application consideration: useful for comparison studies with other temperature measures; data conflict concerning usefulness so that further validation is needed

Table 18.1 (*cont.*)

Devices applicable to both sexes
IX. Measures of anal responses
   A. Device
      1. Anal probe
   B. Application considerations: useful where subject acceptance of anal measures is possible and direct cross-sex comparisons are crucial; device measures two variables: anal pulse waves and anal pressure
  X. Measures of infrared radiation from body surface
   A. Device
      1. Thermograph
   B. Application considerations: since subject must be unclothed, subject acceptance of intrusive procedures is crucial; valuable where there is interest in obtaining data from a number of body sites at the same time with a common measure; equipment is expensive and complex

---

consideration. By analyzing thermograms, it is possible to detect subtle elevations in temperature due to cellular and metabolic changes. Since vasocongestion accompanied by temperature change is one of the principal peripheral physiological responses associated with sexual arousal, thermography appears to provide a sensitive and specific index of sexual arousal. The methodology is seldom used because it is quite costly and extremely intrusive since subjects must be unclothed when measures are taken. Table 18.1 contains a brief overview of the various measurement devices.

18.3   INFERENTIAL CONTEXT

18.3.1   *Mensuration and quantification*

The degree to which the different genital measures can be calibrated to known aspects of physiological events varies. This creates serious problems since some of the measures use arbitrary units, such as mm of pen deflection, for scoring. The hope of investigators is that when arbitrary units are used, they can be shown, even in the face of arbitrariness, to have validity. The following discussion of how genital measures relate to physiological events will not cover all possible measures but will cover those that are most widely used. We begin our discussion with a consideration of measures obtained from male genitals.

18.3.1.1   *Male measures*

In the case of volume penile plethysmography, devices can be calibrated and scored in terms of absolute actual penile volume or penile volume changes recorded in terms of ml of volume. The devices do not, however, allow a determination of the anatomical site of change. A problem may be present in the volume change measure since one often does not know the absolute volume of the penis during baseline or prestimulation conditions. It may be that the *Law of Initial Values* holds if a negative relationship is found between volume change and absolute penile volume. A positive correlation between basal measures and change scores may well be attributable to the fact that part of the variance of change scores is determined by the basal measure. Whether or not these correlations pose a serious problem often depends upon the nature of the experimental design that is used in an investigation.

Strain gauge devices represent a circumferential approach to the measurement of penile tumescence. These devices have become increasingly popular in laboratory use due to the relative ease of their use in contrast with volumetric devices. A recent report by Wheeler and Rubin (1987) supports the use of the strain gauge over volumetric devices, noting that volumetric measures were less responsive to their experimental manipulations than were circumferential measures. As with volume, the available measure can be a known physical event such as mm of diameter or mm of change in diameter (Barlow et al., 1970). In the case of the strain gauge it is easy to obtain a baseline or resting level of the diameter of the penis.

As with the volume measurement, although the measure of the diameter of the penis and changes in that dimension may very well be quite objective, they relate only indirectly to the physiological events, both central and peripheral, that control erections. By *indirect* we mean that the measure, in this case penile circumference, measures the product of complex physiological events. The nature of those events are still under study so that the indirect measurement of them via recording of behavioral events is fraught with potential error. If our fundamental interest is in, for example, cognitive activity that accompanies sexual stimuli, the measurement of penile circumference will by the nature of its remoteness have error. We hasten to point out that in this sense much of psychophysiology suffers from similar problems.

Another methodological consideration in the use of the strain gauge is whether to use AC or DC coupling. It has been suggested (Jovanovic, 1967) that AC coupling of the strain gauge's output provides information regarding the characteristics of the penile pulse. The DC coupling provides direct circumferential data and is by far the most widely used method for obtaining strain gauge data. Figure 18.9 represents a typical recording of penile circumference as rendered by a strain gauge device using DC coupling. Perhaps, as will be noted again in pulse wave measurement, automatic back-off circuits that allow sensitive undistorted signals may prove useful when a signal contains both AC and DC components.

A potential problem in the use of circumferential measures is the suggestion that penile circumference may show a slight decrease at the onset of sexual arousal (Abel, Barlow, Blanchard, & Mavissakalian, 1975; Laws & Bow 1976; McConaghy, 1974). A brief decrease in circumference may represent a problem in that the onset of tumescence changes may be incorrectly interpreted as a decrease in sexual arousal below basal values. Further, it has also been noted that strain gauge devices may be unreliable at the upper end of the tumescence curve (Earls, Marshall, Marshall, Morales, & Surridge, 1983). This disadvantage may represent a serious limitation if the measures are to be used for determining the full range of erectile capacity.

Alternative measures of penile responding, such as temperature or photometric evaluation of pulse amplitude changes in the penis, have somewhat different concerns that will be discussed when considering women's responses where those methodologies are more widely used.

It has been suggested (Hahn & Leder, 1980; Karacan et al., 1978) that perhaps the appropriate penile response that should be evaluated is whether or not the penis is sufficiently erect to permit vaginal penetration. There have been limited attempts to determine penile rigidity. Karacan et al. (1978) have reported the use of "buckling strength" as a dependent variable in penile responding. Although this approach has

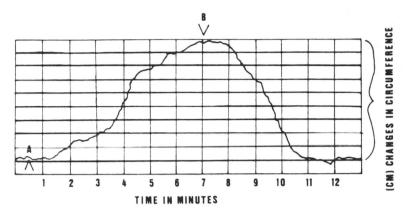

Figure 18.9. Example of typical DC-coupled recording from penile strain gauge. Elevation from point *A* to point *B* represents penile circumference changes over particular time span.

not gained acceptance, the attempt to develop a measure of how rigid the penis becomes is an interesting approach. This work represents thinking about penile measurement in terms of behaviorally relevant criteria. Time will be needed to determine if this direction of penile measurement proves useful.

We wish to note one final approach to the development of dependent variables in the measurement of penile responding. In this procedure the subject's maximum response is elicited and subsequent responding is then described as a percentage of "full erection." Percentage of full erection is determined by visual examination by either or both the subject and the investigator (Karacan et al., 1978). The attempt here is to develop a common metric against which all subjects can be compared. There are some problems with this methodology. If, as noted by Earls et al. (1983), strain gauges are nonlinear at the upper end, the use of a strain gauge during full erection may present a problem. Perhaps more importantly, how does one determine with certainty that full erection was actually obtained? Subject report or direct observation both carry potentially serious problems; yet they are necessary to determine what is full erection. Regardless of the concern just noted, the percentage of full erection measure has been successfully used (Barlow et al., 1970; Laws & Rubin, 1969). It may well be that percentage of any standardized stimulus condition, in this case the response to a highly effective stimulus, typically masturbation, works, so that whether or not full erection is obtained is unimportant. Rather, it may be that what is important is that investigators use a standard against which to make comparisons. Of course, the standard must not covary with the experimental conditions, and it must function to reduce error variance. To blindly employ a standard that does not contribute to reducing error by facilitating comparisons across subjects will decrease the power of any analysis.

18.3.1.2 *Female measures*

We now turn our attention to measures of genital responding in women. Three approaches are most widely used. First are the sophisticated measures obtained from the device developed and described by Levin and Wagner (1978) in which a heated oxygen probe is used to detect changes in oxygen pressure (pO_2) that is transduced across the walls of the vagina. It is assumed that the more blood that is present in the tissues, the greater the amount of oxygen that is perfused across the vaginal epithelium. Using this device, it is possible to determine rather precisely the level of oxygen in the blood of the tissues located beneath the device. The actual dependent variable used is pO_2 expressed in terms of millimeters of mercury. What is less clear is the relationship of those oxygen levels to the behavioral phenomena of interest to psychologists.

The device that measures pO_2 can also measure heat dissipation into the tissues under the transducer. As with the unit developed by Cohen and Shapiro (1970), this methodology uses as the actual dependent variable the amount of energy, expressed in units such as milliwatts, that is required to keep the temperature of the heated thermistor constant. Since the temperature from the thermistor in contact with vaginal tissue is heated, it will experience loss of heat into the surrounding tissue. That is, the device's energy consumption necessary to keep its temperature a constant amount above the internal vaginal temperature is a function of the heat sink properties of the contacted tissues. Changes in heat loss in the device is determined by blood flow, which can be conceptualized as transporting heat from the tissues. There is no direct conversion available by which blood flow patterns can be precisely linked to the heat sink characteristics of the tissue. Thus, as with many of the psychophysiological devices, we are left with an indirect, albeit perhaps very useful, measure, namely, energy consumption by the heated thermistor.

Some of the devices that were described as being used in the study of genital responding have used temperature-sensing units. In women such devices have been intravaginally positioned (Fisher & Osofsky, 1968; Fisher et al., 1983; Fuglmeyer et al., 1984) and some have measured temperature in the labia (Henson et al., 1978). Thus, it is possible to measure specific sites of interest or multiple sites if so desired. These devices have well established physical referents. The unit of measurement, temperature, or temperature change can be obtained with great accuracy. Temperature in the genitals also can be evaluated by thermography. In a study by Seeley et al. (1980), thermographic pictures of a male subject engaging in masturbation and pictures of a female subject engaging in masturbation were compared. Since myotonia and vasocongestion during sexual arousal are both associated with increased temperature in the genital area, thermographic measurement was used in this instance to assess sexual arousal of the subjects during masturbation. The actual dependent variable used in thermography is temperature change expressed in degrees celsius. The results of the Seeley et al. study suggested that thermography did reflect sexual arousal in the tested conditions. The relationship of temperature, regardless of the methodology by which it is obtained, to physiological events in the various genital structures is unclear, as studies have not been done to directly relate thermographic data to vascular responses.

The photometer yields two analyzable dependent variables. The main channel (DC channel) is used at low sensitivity (typically 10 mV/cm). The second channel is AC coupled, typically with a 1-s time constant, and is operated at 5–10 times the sensitivity of the main channel. The AC-coupled channel provides information on vaginal pulse wave. The typical dependent variable used is mm of pen deflection from the bottom to the top of a pulse wave. This measure, often referred to as pulse wave amplitude, is summed across several pulse waves at whatever points in time

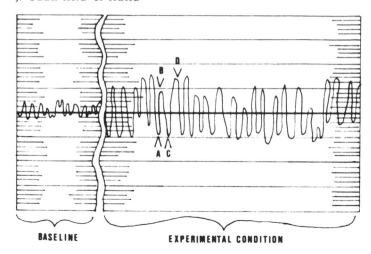

BASELINE   **EXPERIMENTAL CONDITION**

Figure 18.10. Example of AC or pulse wave component obtained from vaginal photometer. Changes are expressed in terms of millimeters of pen deflection summed and averaged across points (A, B, C, D,...) in time.

are of interest to the investigator or clinician. The second channel available from the photometer is the DC component, which is thought to provide information on pooled blood volume (Hatch, 1979). The typical dependent variable is change in the DC component expressed in millimeters of pen deflection measured from a baseline to the point of interest. Both measures have been found to reflect responses to erotic stimuli, although the AC or pluse wave component appears most useful (Geer et al. 1986). Figure 18.10 depicts the pulse wave components as rendered by the vaginal photometer under experimental conditions. As with so many other measures, pen deflection produced by the photometer is an arbitrary measure whose usefulness needs to be established and not simply accepted. Although it is possible to relate the pulse wave response to blood pressure units, it would require an indwelling arterial catheter to establish the relationship. Needless to say, such a methodology is not likely to be widely used. Perhaps the use of automatic back-off circuits will preclude the need for two channels of recordings and yet allow precise measurement.

A consideration when conducting sexual psychophysiological research with females concerns the point in the subject's ovulatory cycle. Palti and Bercovici (1967) found variations in vaginal pulse amplitude to be dependent upon the stage of the subject's menstrual cycle. The implications for laboratory confounding are obvious, and controls, including randomization, are advised.

As mentioned in the preceding, both the vaginal blood flowmeter and the vaginal photometer offer accurate read-outs, with the photometer being the less intrusive of the two. Other devices can be used as the experimental situation dictates, as for example, the labial thermistor is available when vaginal measures are precluded. Hatch (1979) details the various approaches to the assessment of sexual arousal in women and reveals a great deal of methodological variation in the extant literature. The reader should consult Hatch (1979) and Geer (1980) for additional details. Regrettably, the literature relating various devices is scant.

18.3.2 *Experimental logic establishing utility of the various measures*

We noted that some genital measures use as dependent variable units that although quite reliable are arbitrary in nature. They appear to reflect important physiological events, but the validity of such measures must be demonstrated empirically. Two general types of studies have been conducted that have had as their goal the establishment of the usefulness of genital measures. First, genital measures should reflect changes that are known to occur in the relevant situations. This can be determined by examining studies that evaluate genital change in the context of erotic stimulation or sexual arousal. This strategy has been particularly important in the case of genital changes in women. The obvious changes in penile tumescence that occur in men when sexual stimuli are present leaves even the most skeptical hard pressed to doubt the relevance of penile tumescence changes in measurement of male sexual arousal. In women, where genital changes are not as obvious and where measures tend to reflect less obvious physiological events, the requirement of demonstration that the changes in genital measures track experimentally imposed erotic stimuli has been more rigorous.

A related series of studies have sharpened this approach by examining the degree to which genital changes are either specific to erotic stimulation or "better" measures than other psychophysiological events. These studies ask whether or not the genital changes index sexual stimuli more accurately than, for example, concomitantly occurring heart rate activity, electrodermal activity, or vascular changes in structures other than the genitals. What can be reported beyond any question is that the evidence is clear that genital measures are responsive to sexual stimuli. Further, the evidence is clear that genital measures for both sexes are more responsive to erotic stimuli than are the more general systemic nongenital psychophysiological phenomena. The reader is referred to Hatch (1979); Hoon, Hoon, and Wincze (1976); Geer (1975); Rosen and Beck (1987); Rosen and Keefe (1978); and Zuckerman (1971) for extensive reviews of these issues.

In a study of vaginal responding during sleep, Fisher and colleagues (1983) have reported data from 10 female volunteers on patterns of vaginal responding during sleep and waking hours using the Cohen and Shapiro (1970) device. The data replicated the validity of the vaginal blood flowmeter in the waking state. The nighttime data were complex; however, the authors suggest that in many respects they mimic the nocturnal penile response.

The second general strategy that has been widely used to evaluate genital measures and index their validity has been to relate genital changes to the subjective experience of the individual. In the typical experiment on that question subjects are exposed to an erotic stimulus, their genital responses are measured simultaneously, and they are asked to rate their sexual experience in some manner. The data are then correlated to determine if subjective experience and genital changes are related. The results are that under most conditions genital measures do reflect the experience of sexual arousal reported by the individual. Under certain conditions the correlations may reach as high as the .80s and .90s (Korff & Geer, 1983; Speiss, Geer, & O'Donohue, 1984). The size of the correlations between the subjective experience and the genital change are, in general, greater than is typically the case in psychophysiological research. Nevertheless, in some studies the correlations have not been statistically significant for either sex (Farkas, Sine, & Evans, 1979; McConaghy, 1969; Osborne & Pollack, 1977; Wincze, Hoon, & Hoon, 1977).

There have been a series of studies that have directly examined aspects of the subjective–physiological relationship. Those studies reveal that methodological considerations play an important role in determining the size of the subjective–genital correlation. For example, providing the subject with a range of erotic stimuli and, among women, suggesting that genital responding be checked by the subject act to increase the size of the correlations (Hoon, Wincze, & Hoon, 1976; Korff & Geer, 1983; Speiss et al., 1984). It has been suggested (Korff & Geer, 1983) that the subjective–physiological correlation itself should be a variable of interest with potentially important theoretical meaning.

18.3.3   Implications for other response systems

There is little substantial information concerning the degree to which genital responding will provide data useful in understanding other response systems. As noted previously a vasoactive intestinal peptide has been shown to be involved in the mediation of erection (Ottesen, Wagner, Virag, & Fahrenkrug, 1984, and Polak & Bloom, 1984, as cited in Rosen & Beck, 1987). Thus, it appears that the neurotransmitters that affect genital vascular responses are different from those that operate in other vascular beds. This obviously restricts the generalizations that can be made at some of the most basic physiological levels. On the other hand, it may well be that generalizations can be made at a more conceptual level. It has been argued both elsewhere in this chapter and in other writings (Geer et al. 1986) that sexual responding may be particularly useful in clarifying certain general issues of interest to the psychophysiologist. We now turn our attention breifly to these opportunities.

As noted, depending upon the methodology employed, there is a high correspondence between the subjective experience of the individual and her or his genital responding. This fact may provide researchers with the opportunity to study basic phenomena that are more elusive in other psychophysiological response systems. If the variables that influence sexuality operate in the same manner as in other emotional states, an assumption not yet established, sexuality may be very useful in studying general questions that arise in emotion theory (Steinberg, 1986). Most theories of emotion note that emotions are complex phenomena that involve relationships among physiological, behavioral, and cognitive events. Given that the ties between the cognitive (i.e., subjective experience) and physiological events are strong in sexuality, the opportunity is present to use sexuality as a model to study that relationship and perhaps generalize it to the broader rubric of emotion theory. The solid beginning that has been made in applying cognitive concepts to sexual arousal (Barlow, 1986; Geer & Fuhr, 1976), provides considerable optimism that by studying sexuality broad issues in emotion theory may be addressed.

We might briefly speculate as to why sexuality is particularly well suited to study the relationships among the components of emotional states. Perhaps it is because the physiological changes in the genitals is so directly involved in the expression of sexual behavior (Geer, 1986). (The clearest example is that sexual intercourse, for all practical purposes, cannot take place without the occurrence of penile erection.) The close ties have two implications. The first is that since the physiological events are directly tied to the behavior of interest, this leads to perhaps the clearest instance of *response stereotypy* found in emotions. The long and often tortuous arguments that have surrounded response stereotypy in psychophysiology appear ludicrous when applied to sexuality. It could well be argued that the ties between genital changes and other sexual behaviors are necessary for the perpetuation of the species. That is, if males do not get erections, given the nature of human reproduction, the species would cease to exist. Although genital changes for women may not be as obviously connected to reproductive success, it may be argued that genital responding among women facilitates sexual interactions. From a strictly evolutionary perspective, if genital responding did not occur to sexual stimuli, the species would quickly disappear. Regardless of the reasons for the close ties, the fact of the close tie makes the genital response ideal for studying important emotional concepts.

The second implication of the close ties between various components of the sexual response is the potential that is offered for the study of the role of cognition in emotion. Whereas, in fact, this is a detailing of the preceding point, it merits particular emphasis. The fact that the subjective experience of the individual does relate closely to the genital responses allows a study of factors that influence the effect of either response upon the other. The study of these relationships has begun and shows great promise. It has been demonstrated that cognitive activity leads to genital change (Geer & Fuhr, 1976; Stock & Geer, 1982) and that factors that effect cognitive activity influence the relationship (Beck & Barlow, 1984; Geer & Fuhr, 1976). Hopefully, the future will result in further clarification of the cognitive–behavioral–physiological interface in sexuality and, perhaps, by generalization to emotions in general.

18.4   SOCIAL CONTEXT

18.4.1   *Social context of measurement*

18.4.1.1 *Confidentiality, informed consent, and subject welfare*

Although subject confidentiality is a major issue of concern in all areas of psychological research, it is of particular import in studies employing sexual psychophysiology. Due to the highly personal nature of the inquiry, researchers must be particularly sensitive to the individual concerns of their subjects in an endeavor to ensure both the confidentiality of the data and the comfort and well-being of research or clinical participants. Researchers concerned with subjects' welfare must recognize that because laboratory recording will be conducted on a sensitive topic, using genital devices in a setting that is very far removed from the natural setting, the subject may experience anxiety. Since researchers must be concerned with the welfare of their subjects, care must be taken to avoid negative reactions by subjects. It has been reported (Rosen, 1976) that male erection measures in the laboratory can create performance anxiety with patients under-going treatment for sexual dysfunction. It is reasonable to assume that the same would hold true for females in a similar situation. To lessen the effect of reactivity in the laboratory and to promote subject welfare, Hoon (1979) has suggested the following laboratory protocol:

Researchers should design research and clinical procedures so that performance expectations are minimally salient; establish rapport carefully and explain procedures and their rationale thoroughly; avoid coercion and allow patients and subjects to withdraw from assessment at any time; minimize mechanistic aspects of laboratory settings by the use of comfortable, friendly, and appropriately self-disclosing research assistants and experimenters. (p. 51)

Fully informed voluntary consent coupled with well-trained experimenters is the best line of defense for both confidentiality and subject welfare issues.

A problem that must be acknowledged is the fact that the need for fully informed voluntary consent means that subjects cannot be studied without their having considerable information concerning the nature of the experiment and the stimuli that will be employed. It would be inappropriate to expose individuals to explicit sexual material without their having full knowledge that such will be the case. This means that subjects in sex research are told a great deal about the nature of the stimuli to which they will be exposed. In turn, this means that they will have developed "expectations" concerning the nature of the study, and the influence of such expectations is unknown. In a related vein, Amoroso and Brown (1973) reported that demand characteristics of sex research can create artifacts in both physiological and subjective assessments of sexual arousal. Their study found that subjects attached to electrical recording devices rated stimuli more erotic than subjects outside the specific laboratory setting. In another study, Hicks (1970) showed that different experimenter mood and behavior produced different physiological records and subjective reports. It is not possible to avoid these problems and maintain the very high ethical standards that must accompany sex research.

18.4.1.2 *Volunteer biases*

Volunteer biases are reflected in the types of individuals who typically volunteer for sexual research. Wolchik, Braver, and Jensen (1985) studied the effects of increasingly intrusive measures of sexual arousal on volunteer rate and type of volunteer. They compared sexual behaviors and attitudes of volunteers and nonvolunteers across increasingly intrusive experimental conditions. They also examined gender differences in volunteer rates across these same conditions. Predictor variables included sexual experience, sexual difficulties, attitudes toward sexuality, experience with and attitudes toward pornography, and sex typing. The researchers found that female volunteers were more sexually experienced than female nonvolunteers, that volunteers of both sexes displayed more sexual curiosity than nonvolunteers, and that male volunteers experienced more sexual difficulties and were exposed to more erotica than male nonvolunteers. In addition, males were more likely to volunteer than females. It was found that the more intrusive the method of investigation, the lower the rate of volunteers. For these reasons, researchers must be aware of the limits of generalizability in studies employing genital measures.

The question, of course, is not whether there are differences between volunteers and the general population but whether or not those differences influence the outcome of research. There is no definitive answer to that question. By definition, we do not collect information on genital responding from nonvolunteers so that the question as to how they would respond is moot. What is of some interest is the fact that large numbers of subjects (10–20 percent) who are relatively unsophisticated and who are relatively inexperienced do participate in sex research measuring genital responses. That finding suggests less bias than might otherwise be expected.

Another general methodological consideration needs to be noted. Since the study of sexual psychophysiology is a relatively new field, much of the research in the field has naturally focused on the development of recording devices. As described for both males and females, there are several available devices for the recording of sexual arousal. Therefore, the choice of an appropriate transducer depends on the measurement characteristics of the device, the goals of the particular study, and the reactions of the subject to the device. Since the potential for reactive measurement effects is greatest in clinical applications, Rosen and Keefe (1978) have recommended that the transducer of choice for clinical research be one that is as comfortable as possible, lightweight, simple, and rugged. Therefore, they recommend the strain gauge. For physiological research, where precise measurement of penile tumescence may be the most important criteria in choosing a transducer, the volumetric methods may offer the greatest potential precision for tumescence measurement (Rosen & Keefe, 1978). However, since volumetric devices have considerable drawbacks in size and reactivity, Rosen and Keefe (1978) recommend their use only when data from simpler circumference transducers will not suffice. Our point is that these kinds of factors cannot be disregarded by the clinician or the researcher since they impact on both the subject and the outcome of research.

18.4.2   *Social factors*

In sexuality the social context within which research is conducted is particularly important. This flows rather naturally from the controversial nature of sexuality. Research on sexuality is often viewed with both suspicion and concern by professionals and lay persons alike. These concerns run the gamut from questions concerning the motivation of investigators and subjects to questions as to whether sexuality should not be left unstudied because such research is inappropriate or wrong. The bottom line of these widely differing issues is that the sex researcher must be particularly attentive to both subjects' attitudes and to ethical issues in research.

It is also clear that social variables influence sexuality. Ever since the pioneering work of Alfred Kinsey and his colleagues (Kinsey, Pomeroy, & Martin, 1948; Kinsey, Pomeroy, Martin, & Gebhard, 1953) the role of societal variables in sexuality have been acknowledged. The importance of such variables as religiosity, social class, and educational level on sexuality is evidence of the influence of social factors in sexuality. Further we can note that much sex research is directed at examining cultural differences to see the role of societal factors (Davenport, 1987; Kon, 1984). To the researcher these facts mean that care must be taken to evaluate or control social variables in studies. It could well be argued that cultural and societal factors are among the most interesting in the field of sexuality, and their presence adds a richness to the area of study.

18.4.3   *Range of application*

It is difficult to imagine a field of behavioral research that cannot or does not have an impact on or, in turn, may be impacted by sexuality. Although attempts to discuss each would be exhausting and not very useful, several general points may be of interest. First, a truism that is not often noted is that the study of sexuality is a discipline that has been characterized by interdisciplinary activity. The senior author of this chapter has recently been involved in editing a book that emphasizes that fact. The text, entitled *Theories of Human Sexuality* (Geer & O'Donohue, 1987), contains 14 chapters written by experts from various disciplines concerning their perspective's view of sexuality. The approaches that were selected for inclusion in that text ranged from biological to anthropological, from learning approaches to psychoanalytic, from feminist to evolutionary, with each of the varying views having something of substance to offer to sexuality. The point is that sexuality is an interdisciplinary topic that is of interest to a very wide range of scholarly as well as applied disciplines.

The second point is that within psychology there are several areas in which sexuality and research on same is particularly relevant. First is the obvious impact on psychopathology. There are many phenomena that are identified as psychopathological that are sexual in nature. In fact, there has been the development of "sex therapy" as a specific treatment area. The study of the psychopathology of sexuality from the vantage point of psychophysiology holds real promise. There already exist many investigations using the methodology of psychophysiology that look at various aspects of sexual dysfunction. These include classification and the tracking of treatment outcome as well as attempts to treat using genital measures to guide treatment procedures. The reader should consult sources such as Heiman and Hatch (1971), Geer and Messe (1982), and Rosen and Beck (1987) for both descriptions of and references to these studies.

We anticipate that there will be areas of significant growth in our understanding of sexuality, and we expect that the psychophysiologist will be integrally involved in these developments. One area that we predict will take on increasing importance is knowledge concerning biological factors in sexuality. There is increasing evidence that human sexual behavior is influenced by biological events in profound ways. As an example of this trend in sexuality, we recommend that the reader note the recent article in *Psychological Bulletin* (Ellis & Ames, 1987) that outlines a theory proposing a significant role for biological factors in the development of homosexuality. The psychophysiologist with her or his contribution to knowledge of biological events will play an important part in the increased recognition of the importance of biological events to human sexuality.

It can be anticipated that certain clinical phenomena will be seen as increasingly important and will be the focus of increased attention. For example, the societal concern over child sexual abuse will be reflected in increased activity aimed at addressing that problem. Psychophysiology's contribution to research on applied problems in sexuality has tended to focus on diagnostic issues, including the assessment of progress in therapeutic programs. Studies of child molesters and rapists have often used psychophysiological methodologies with useful outcomes (e.g., Abel et al., 1975; Freund, 1963; McConaghy, 1967). Those studies will continue and will gain increased attention from the public as well as the psychophysiologist.

Progress in the field of sexual psychophysiology has been highlighted by the development of increasingly accurate devices for the recording of sexual arousal; we fully expect this trend to continue. In particular, we expect continued work on measurement devices that permit direct comparisons between the sexes. An additional spur to methodological sophistication will be the continuing need to develop behaviorally relevant measures with minimal intrusiveness.

REFERENCES

Abel, G., Blanchard, E., Barlow, D., & Mavissakalian, M. (1975). Measurement of sexual arousal in male homosexuals: The effects of instructions and stimulus modality. *Archives of Sexual Behavior, 4*, 623–629.

Amoroso, D. M., & Brown, M. (1973). Problems in studying effects of erotic material. *Journal of Sex Research, 9*, 187–195.

Bancroft, J. (1987). A physiological approach. In J. H. Geer & W. T. O'Donohue (Eds.), *Theories of human sexuality*. New York: Plenum Press.

Bancroft, J., & Bell, C. (1985). Simultaneous recording of penile diameter and penile arterial pulse during laboratory based erotic stimulation in normal subjects. *Journal of Psychosomatic Research, 29*, 303–313.

Bancroft, J., Jones, H. G., & Pullan, B. R. (1966). A simple transducer for measuring penile erection, with comments on its use in the treatment of sexual disorders. *Behavior Research Therapy, 9*, 239–241.

Barclay, A. M. (1970). Urinary acid phospatase secretion in sexually aroused males. *Journal of Experimental Research in Personality, 4*, 233–238.

Barlow, D. H. (1986). Causes of sexual dysfunction: The role of anxiety and cognitive interference. *Journal of Counselling and Clinical Psychology, 54*, 140–148.

Barlow, D. H., Becker, R., Leitenberg, H., & Agras, W. S. (1970). A mechanical strain gauge for recording penile circumference change. *Journal of Applied Behavior Analysis, 3*, 73–76.

Bartlett, R. G. (1956). Physiologic responses during coitus. *Journal of Applied Physiology, 9*, 469–472.

Beach, F. A. (1958). Neural and chemical regulation of behavior. In H. F. Harlow & C. N. Woolsey (Eds.), *Biological & biochemical bases of behavior*. Madison: University of Wisconsin Press.

Beck, J. G., & Barlow, D. H. (1984). Current conceptualizations of sexual dysfunction: A review and an alternative perspective *Clinical Psychological Review, 4*, 363–378.

Bohlen, J., & Held, J. (1979). Anal probe for monitoring vascular and muscular events during sexual response. *Psychophysiology 16*, 318–323.

Brindley, G. S. (1983). Cavernosal alpha-blockade: A new technique for investigating and treating erectile impotence. *British Journal of Psychiatry, 143*, 332–337.

Cohen, H. D., Rosen, R. D., & Goldstein, L. (1976). Electroencephalographic laterality changes during human sexual orgasm. *Archives of Sexual Behavior, 5*, 189–199.

Cohen, H., & Shapiro, A. (1970). A method for measuring sexual arousal in the female. *Psychophysiology, 8*, 251. (Abstract).

Conti, G. (1952). L'erection du penis humain et ses bases morphologico-vasculaires. *Acta Anatomica, 14*, 217.

Corman, C. (1968). *Physiological response to asexual stimulus*. Unpublished bachelor's thesis, University of Manitoba, Canada.

Davenport, W. H. (1987). An anthropological approach. In J. H. Geer & W. T. O'Donohue (Eds.), *Theories of human sexuality*. New York: Plenum Press.

Earls, C. M., Marshall, W. L., Marshall, P. G., Morales, A., & Surridge, D. H. (1983). Penile elongation: A method for the screening of impotence. *Journal of Urology, 139*, 90–92.

Ellis, L., & Ames, M. A. (1987). Neurohormonal functioning and sexual orientation: A theory of homosexuality–heterosexuality. *Psychological Bulletin, 101*, 233–258.

Farkas, G. M., Sine, L. F., & Evens, I. M. (1979). The effects of distraction, performance demand, stimulus explicitness and personality on objective and subjective measures of male sexual arousal. *Behavior Research and Therapy, 17*, 25–32.

Fisher, C., Cohen, H. D., Schiavi, R. C., Davis, D., Furman, B., Ward, K., Edwards, A., & Cunningham, J. (1983). Patterns of female sexual arousal during sleep and waking: Vaginal thermo-conductance studies. *Archives of Sexual Behavior, 12*, 97–122.

Fisher, C., Gross, J., & Zuch, J. (1965). Cycle of penile erection synchronous with dreaming (REM) sleep. *Archives of General Psychiatry, 12*, 27–45.

Fisher, S. (1973). *The female orgasm*. New York: Basic Books.

Fisher, S., & Osofsky, H. (1968). Sexual responsiveness in women, physiological correlates. *Psychological Reports, 22*, 215–226.

Freund, K. (1963). A laboratory method for diagnosing predominance of hemo- or hetero-erotic interest in the male. *Behaviour Research and Therapy, 1*, 85–93.

Fuglmeyer, A. R., Sjogren, K., & Johansson, K. (1984). Radiotelemetry: A vaginal temperature registration system. *Archives of Sexual Behavior, 13,* 247–259.

Geer, J. H. (1975). Direct measures of genital responding. *American Psychologist, 30,* 415–418.

Geer, J. H. (1978). Sterilization of genital devices. *Psychophysiology, 15,* 385.

Geer, J. H. (1980). Measurement of genital arousal in human males and females. In I. Martin & P. H. Venables (Eds.), *Techniques in psychophysiology.* New York: Wiley.

Geer, J. H. (1983). *Measurement and methodological considerations in vaginal photometry.* Paper presented at the meeting of the International Academy of Sex Research, Harriman, NY.

Geer, J., & Fuhr, R. (1976). Cognitive factors in sexual arousal: The role of distraction. *Journal of Consulting and Clinical Psychology, 44,* 238–243.

Geer, J. H., & Messe, M. R. (1982). Sexual dysfunctions. In R. J. Gatchel, A. Baum, & J. E. Singer (Eds.), *Handbook of psychology and health. Behavioral medicine and clinical psychology/psychiatry: Overlapping disciplines,* (Vol. 1). Hillsdale, NJ: Erlbaum.

Geer, J. H., & O'Donohue, W. T. (Eds.). (1987). *Theories of human sexuality.* New York: Plenum Press.

Geer, J. H., O'Donohue, W. T., & Schorman, R. H. (1986). Sexuality. In M. G. H. Coles, E. Donchin, & S. W. Porges (Eds.), *Psychophysiology: Systems, processes and applications* (pp. 407–427). New York: Guilford Press.

Geer, J. H., & Quartararo, J. D. (1976). Vaginal blood volume responses during masturbation. *Archives of Sexual Behavior, 5,* 403–414.

Gershon-Cohen, J. (1964). Medical thermography: A summary of current status. *Annals of New York Academy of Science, 121,* 403–431.

Gustafson, J. E., Winokur, G., & Reichlin, S. (1963). The effect of psychic and sexual stimulation on urinary and serum acid phosphatase and plasma non-esterified fatty acids, *Psychosomatic Medicine, 25,* 101–105.

Guyton, A. C. (1971). *Textbook of medical physiology.* Philadelphia: Saunders.

Hahn, P. M., & Leder, R. (1980). Quantification of penile buckling force. *Sleep, 3,* 95–97.

Hamel, P. F. (1974). Female subjective and pupillary reaction to nude male and female figures. *Journal of Psychology, 2,* 171–175.

Hatch, J. P. (1979). Vaginal photoplethysmography: Methodological considerations. *Archives of Sexual Behavior, 8*(4), 357–374.

Heiman, J. R., & Hatch, J. P. (1971). Conceptual and therapeutic contributions of psychology to sexual dysfunction. In S. N. Haynes & L. Gannon (Eds.), *Psychosomatic disorders.* New York: Praeger.

Henson, D., Rubin, H., & Henson, C. (1978). Consistency of the labial temperature change measure of human female eroticism. *Behavior Research and Therapy, 16,* 125–129.

Hess, E. H. (1968). Pupillometric assessment. *Research in Psychotherapy, 3,* 573–583.

Hicks, R. G. (1970). Experimenter effects on physiological experiments. *Psychophysiology, 6* (meeting). Plymouth State Home & Training School.

Hoon, P. W. (1979). The assessment of sexual arousal in women. *Progress in Behavior Modification, 7,* 2–53.

Hoon, P. W., Hoon, E. F., & Wincze, J. P. (1976). An inventory for the measurement of female sexual arousability: The SAI. *Archives of Sexual Behavior, 5,* 291–300.

Hoon, P. W., Wincze, J. P., & Hoon, E. F. (1976). Physiological assessment of sexual arousal in women. *Psychophysiology, 13,* 196–204.

Jovanovic, U. J. (1967). Some characteristics of the beginning of dreams. *Psychologie Fortschung 30,* 281–306.

Jovanovic, U. J. (1971). The recording of physiological evidence of genital arousal in human males and females. *Archives of Sexual Behavior, 1,* 309–320.

Kalat, J. W. (1984). *Biological psychology* (2nd ed.). Hillsdale, CA: Wadsworth.

Karacan, I., Rosenbloom, A., & Williams, R. (1970). The clitoral erection cycle during sleep. *Psychophysiology, 7,* 338. (Abstract).

Karacan, I., Salis, P. J., Ware, J. C., Dervent, B., Williams, R. L., Scott, F. B., Attia, S. L., & Beutler, L. E. (1978). Nocturnal penile tumescence and diagnosis in diabetic impotence. *American Journal of Psychiatry, 135,* 191–197.

Kinsey, A., Pomeroy, W., & Martin, C. (1948). *Sexual behavior in the human male.* Philadelphia: Saunders.

Kinsey, A., Pomeroy, W., Martin, C., & Gebhard, P. (1953). *Sexual behavior in the human female.* Philadelphia: Saunders.

Kon, I. S. (1987). A sociocultural approach. In J. H. Geer and W. T. O'Donohue (Eds.), *Theories of human sexuality*. New York: Plenum Press.

Korff, J., & Geer, J. H. (1983). Relationship between subjective sexual arousal experience and genital responses. *Psychophysiology, 20*, 121–127.

Laws, D. R., & Bow, R. A. (1976). An improved mechanical strain gauge for recording penile circumference changes. *Psychophysiology, 13*, 596–599.

Laws, D. R., & Rubin, H. B. (1969). Instructional control of autonomic sexual response. *Journal of Applied Behavior Analysis, 2*, 93–99.

Levin, R. J., & Wagner, G. (1978). Haemodynamic changes of the human vagina during sexual arousal assessed by a heated oxygen electrode. *Journal of Physiology, 275*, 23–24.

Lifschitz, K. (1966). The averaged evoked cortical response to complex visual stimuli. *Psychophysiology, 3*,55–68.

Masters, W. H., & Johnson, V. E. (1966). *Human sexual response*. Boston: Little, Brown.

McConaghy, N. (1967). Penile volume changes to moving pictures of male and female nudes in heterosexual and homosexual males. *Behavior Research and Therapy, 3*, 43–48.

McConaghy, N. (1969). Subjective and penile plethysmograph responses following aversion relief and apomorphine therapy for homosexual impulses. *British Journal of Psychiatry, 115*, 723–730.

McConaghy, N. (1974). Measurements of change in penile dimensions. *Archives of Sexual Behavior, 3*, 381–388.

Money, J. (1961). Sex hormones and other variables in human eroticism. In W. C. Young (Ed.), *Sex & internal secretions* (3rd ed., Vol. 2, pp. 1383–1400). Baltimore: Williams & Wilkins.

Newman, II. Γ., & Northup, J. D. (1981). Mechanism of human penile erection: An overview. *Urology, 17*, 399–408.

Ohlmeyer, P., Brilmayer, II., & Hullstrung, H. (1944). Periodische organge im schlaf II. *Pfluegers Archiv fuer die, Gesamta Physiologic 249*, 50–55.

Osborne, C. A., & Pollack, R. H. (1977). The effects of two types of erotic literature on physiological and verbal measures of female sexual arousal. *Journal of Sex Research, 13*, 250–256.

Palti, Y., & Bercovici, B. (1967). Photoplethysmographic study of the vaginal blood pulse. *American Journal of Obstetrics and Gynecology, 97*, 143–153.

Reich, W. (1937). Experimentelle Ergebnisse uber die elektrische funktion von sexualitat and angst. Institute für sexualokonomische forschung klinische and experimentelle berichte. (Translated in *Journal of Orgonomy, 3*, 1969, 4 29.)

Romano, K. (1969). *Psychophysiological responses to a sexual and an unpleasant motion picture.* Unpublished bachelor's thesis, University of Manitoba, Canada.

Rosen, R. C. (1976). Genital blood-flow measurement: Feedback applications in sexual therapy. *Journal of Sex and Marital Therapy, 2*, 184–196.

Rosen, R. C., & Beck, J. G. (1987). *Sexual psychophysiology: Concepts and methodology in laboratory sex research*. New York: Guilford Press.

Rosen, R. C., & Keefe, F. S. (1978). The measurement of human penile tumescence. *Psychophysiology, 15*, 366–376.

Rosen, R. C., & Rosen, L. R. (1981). *Human sexuality*. New York: Knopf.

Seeley, F., Abramsen, P., Perry, L., Rothblatt, A., & Seeley, D. (1980). Thermographic measures of sexual arousal: A methodological note. *Archives of Sexual Behavior, 9*, 77–85.

Shapiro, A., & Cohen, H. (1965). The use of mercury capillary length gauges for the measurement of the volume of thoracic and diaphragmatic components of human respiration: A theoretical analysis and a practical method. *Transactions of the New York Academy of Sciences, 26*, 634–649.

Shapiro, A., Cohen, H., DiBianco, P., & Rosen, G. (1968). Vaginal blood flow changes during sleep and sexual arousal in women. *Psychophysiology, 4*(3), 349. (Abstract).

Sintchak, G., & Geer, J. H. (1975). A vaginal plethysmograph system. *Psychophysiology, 12*, 113–115.

Solnick, R., & Berrin, J. E. (1977). Age and male erectile responsiveness. *Archives of Sexual Behavior, 6*,1–9.

Speiss, W., Geer, J. H., & O'Donohue, W. (1984). A psychophysiological and psychophysical investigation of ejaculatory latency. *Journal of Abnormal Psychology, 9*, 242–245.

Steinberg, J. L. (1986). *The psychology of sexual arousal: An information processing analysis.* Unpublished doctoral dissertation. State University of New York, Stony Brook.

Stock, W., & Geer, J. (1982). A study of fantasy-based sexual arousal in women. *Archives of Sexual Behavior, 11*, 33–47.

Szasz, G., Stevenson, W. D., Lee, L., & Sanders, H. D. (1987). Induction of penile erection by intracavernosal injection: A double-blind comparison of phenoxybenzamine versus papaverine-phentolamine versus saline. *Archives of Sexual Behavior, 16*, 371–378.

Tahmoush, A. J., & Francis, M. E. (1986). In vitro studies of the pulsetile radiometric signal. *Psychophysiology, 20*, 115–115.

Wagner, G., & Levin, R. (1978). Vaginal fluid. In E. Hafez & T. Evans (Eds.), *The human vagina*. Amsterdam: Elsevier.

Webster, J. S., & Hammer, D. (1983). Thermistor measurement of male sexual arousal. *Psychophysiology, 20*, 115–115.

Weiss, H. D. (1972). The physiology of human erection. *Annals of Internal Medicine, 76*, 793–799.

Wenger, M. A., Averill, J. R., & Smith, D. D. B. (1968). Autonomic activity during sexual arousal. *Psychophysiology, 4*, 468–478.

Wheeler, D., & Rubin, H. B. (1987). A comparison of volumetric and circumferential measures of penile erection. *Archives of Sexual Behavior, 16*, 289–299.

Wincze, J. P., Hoon, E. P., & Hoon, E. F. (1977). Sexual arousal in women: A comparison of cognitive and physiological responses by continuous measurement. *Archives of Sexual Behavior, 6*(2), 121–133.

Wolchik, S. A., Braver, S. L., & Jensen, K. (1985). Volunteer bias in erotica research: Effects of intrusiveness of measure & sexual background. *Archives of Sexual Behavior, 14*, 93–107.

Wood, D. M., & Obrist, P. A. (1968). Minimal and maximal sensory intake and exercise as unconditioned stimuli in human heart-rate conditioning. *Journal of Experimental Psychology, 76*, 254–262.

Zorgniotti, A. W., & Lefleur, R. S. (1985). Auto injection of the corpus cavernosum with a vasoactive drug combination for vasculogenic impotence. *Journal of Urology, 133*, 39–41.

Zuckerman, M. (1971). Physiological measures of sexual arousal in the human. *Psychological Bulletin, 75*, 329.

J. A. SKELTON AND JAMES W. PENNEBAKER

A chapter on self-reports may seem out of place in a book on psychophysiology. Indeed, psychophysiology developed partly because investigators since the early Greeks have believed physiological measures allow us to obtain data that individuals cannot or will not report (Furedy, 1986; Stern, Ray, & Davis, 1980). But we shall show that verbal reports have an undeservedly bad reputation. When properly used, self-reports of physiological activity, mood, and other internal states can provide critical insights into individuals' psychological and physiological states.

To delineate the domain of this chapter, we adopt the distinction among symptoms, signs, and undetected bodily responses suggested by Cacioppo and Petty (1982). *Symptoms* refer to the subjective component of a physiological reaction as sensed or felt only by the affected person. *Signs* are objectively measurable physiological changes that can sometimes be detected by the affected subjects themselves and also by observers. *Undetected bodily responses* are physiological changes occurring outside subjects' awareness but that can potentially be measured objectively. For example, a headache (a symptom) might be traced by the subject or a physician to increased neck muscle tension (a sign), which in turn could be mediated by the release of norepinephrine from the adrenal medulla (undetected bodily response).

Symptoms, the primary focus of this chapter, are usually measured via oral or written self-reports and thus exemplify verbal modes of responding. Verbal measures can be used to obtain information about highly specific physical sensations (e.g., heart rate, tight stomach), emotional states (anger, guilt), or general characterization of physical state (fatigue, arousal, healthiness). The other response systems studied by psychophysiologists emphasize signs and undetected bodily responses, but verbal responses tap subjects' *perceptions* of their world. Whether this subjectively perceived world accurately reflects physiological responses as assessed by signs and undetected bodily responses is often of only secondary importance with respect to health- and illness-related behaviors or other voluntary activities based upon perceived bodily states.

19.1   HISTORICAL BACKGROUND

People's ability to report on their physical condition is highly dependent on language. By the time children reach 3 years of age, they have typically learned over 500 words (Carey, 1978). Many of these words refer to emotions (happy, sad, mad), discomfort (hurt, hungry), and body parts (head, ears, throat). The ability to report verbally on internal state is not limited to humans. Researchers who train gorillas and chimpanzees to use language indicate that apes can readily learn to report a variety of internal states, such as hunger, sadness, and pain (Patterson & Linden, 1981; Premack & Premack, 1983).

19.1.1   Origin and evolution of self-report measures

Reliance on self-reports of physiological activity has evolved from three independent traditions: clinical psychology and medicine, psychophysics, and social psychology. We briefly examine the major assumptions and findings of each tradition.

19.1.1.1   Clinical psychology and medicine

Physicians and clinical psychologists use self-reports in diagnosing and treating physical and psychological problems. Self-reports are viewed as imperfect indicators of physiological processes. In clinical interviews with a patient, for example, the extraction of self-reported physical symptoms and feelings serves as only a clue, albeit an important one, concerning the patient's "true" problem. The clinical approach is more concerned with searching for signs and covert bodily activity *implied* by symptom reports than with symptoms per se.

Clinical skepticism toward verbal measures of bodily states can be justified on the grounds that self-reports of physiological responses are only weakly correlated with their physiological referents. For example, self-reported and actual heart rates correlate only about +.30 on average. Similarly, modest relationships exist between actual and self-reported breathing rate, blood pressure, hand sweatiness, fatigue, muscle tension, and other somatic indexes (see Mihevic, 1981, and Pennebaker, 1982, for reviews). In short, if the investigator is primarily interested in veridical physiological responses – signs and covert activity – he or she should not rely on verbal reports.

19.1.1.2   Sensory psychology and psychophysics

Many of the earliest issues addressed by psychologists evolved from epistemological speculations concerning how we come to know our world (e.g., Locke 1959/1690). With the rapid growth of scientific method and statistical theory in the eighteenth and nineteenth centuries, the way was cleared for the first experimental psychologists to study the mathematical functions linking peoples' reports of their mental worlds with objective changes in the physical world. Both Fechner (1960/1860) and Wundt (1904/1874) reported numerous studies that indicated a close correspondence between physical changes in the intensity of light, sound, and touch and the verbal report of these changes.

The development of signal detection theory (SDT; Pastore & Scheirer, 1974; Stevens, 1975; Swets, 1964, 1973) and methodology allowed researchers in psychophysics to map the correspondence between sensory stimuli and subjective judgments of stimuli. Recently, SDT techniques have been adapted to measure the accuracy of people's estimates of stomach contractions (Whitehead & Drescher, 1980) and heartbeats (Jones, Jones, Cunningham, & Caldwell, 1985; Katkin, 1985) and the relationship between stimulus magnitudes and pain reports (Craig & Prkachin, 1978; Lloyd & Appel, 1976).

The psychophysical approach to *visceral perception* (the study of perceived relative to actual autonomic activity) is characterized by remarkable precision and experimental control in assessing the accuracy of verbal reports. Unfortunately, this advantage is frequently purchased at the expense of external validity because psychophysical studies usually control situational and extraneous sensory cues. Because such cues potently affect everyday symptom reporting, this requirement eliminates important sources of information that affect verbal reports of bodily activity in everyday life.

19.1.1.3 *Social psychology and attitudes*

The most intensive examination of the properties of the verbal response system has come from social psychologists interested in attitudes and attitude change. Unlike other perspectives, the social psychological view has been that verbal responses can directly tap subjects' perceptions and beliefs concerning their private worlds (e.g., Cacioppo & Petty, 1982; McGuire, 1985). Verbal responses are thus viewed as face-valid measures of what subjects believe and feel about objects, events, and aspects of themselves.

Originally, the study of verbal response systems focused on subjects' attitudes about issues, events, objects, and other people. Although many of the earlier theorists emphasized how attitudes influenced behaviors (e.g., Allport, 1935), most agreed that an adequate conceptualization of attitudes must include cognitive, affective, and behavioral components (cf. Brown, 1965; Campbell, 1947). Consequently, an attitude such as "I like apples" denotes beliefs about apples, feelings toward apples, and implicit consummatory behaviors.

Early attitude research contributed to the development of a host of self-report measurement strategies. Attitudes towards apples, for example, could be assessed by having subjects (1) rate their feelings along several dimensions (good–bad, happy–sad, relaxed–tense) using semantic differentials (Osgood, Suci, & Tannenbaum, 1957), (2) agree or disagree with specific statements about apples (e.g., strongly agree, agree, disagree, strongly disagree) using a Likert (1932) format, or (3) check a series of statements that had previously been scaled to reflect degrees of opinion about apples (I could not live in the same neighborhood with apple eaters, I could not live in the same house with apple eaters, etc.) using Guttman's (1944) procedures. Dawes and Smith (1985) provide an excellent overview of these and other measurement techniques, many of which have been adapted to verbal reports of physiological state.

A perennial criticism of attitude research is that people's attitudes are poorly correlated with attitude-relevant behaviors (Wicker, 1969). In general, attitudes and behaviors associated with prejudice (LaPiere, 1934), health seeking (Janis, 1967; Leventhal, 1970), altruism (Ajzen & Fishbein, 1980), and virtually all other domains correlate, on average, about +.30 (also see Mischel, 1968). Many of the problems of linking attitudes to behaviors are strikingly similar to the difficulties that researchers face in attempting to demonstrate a close correspondence between symptom reports on the one hand and signs and undetected bodily responses on the other.

19.1.2 *Issues in assessing and interpreting verbal responses*

19.1.2.1 *Cues for self-reports*

A common misconception is that the verbal report of a particular symptom derives primarily from internal sensory stimulation. According to this view, perceptions of heart rate "should" come from heartbeat sensations; perceptions of hunger "should" derive from specific physiological changes such as increased stomach contractions or blood glucose levels. But there is much evidence to indicate that symptoms are highly dependent on external, situational cues as well, and these are accessible not only to the subject but also to observers.

That situational cues are powerful determinants of symptom reports is not a new idea. Beecher (1959) studied pain reports and pain medication requests of injured soldiers and found that noncombat injuries were perceived as more painful than comparable injuries incurred during combat. Beecher argued that combat-related injuries were less threatening, and were thus experienced as less painful, because these allowed the soldier to escape from battle. Noncombat injuries, on the other hand, disrupted normal daily activities but, lacking the functional value of combat injuries, were experienced as more noxious. Thus, external factors such as the functional significance of injuries affected their perception and reporting.

When naturally occurring situational cues are restricted, subjects estimate physiological changes quite poorly. Visceral perception research using signal detection methods, for example, requires subjects to estimate heart rate or stomach contractions with "extraneous" visual, auditory, and proprioceptive cues tightly controlled. In such studies, subjects typically estimate heart rate and stomach activity at levels averaging about 8 percent above chance (e.g., Katkin, 1985; Ross & Brener, 1981; Pennebaker & Hoover, 1984; Whitehead & Drescher, 1980). On the other hand, in studies where subjects are encouraged to use extraneous cues, accuracy in estimating heart rate, blood pressure, and other autonomic activity can increase by a factor of between 3 and 4 (e.g., Barr, Pennebaker, & Watson, 1988; Pennebaker, 1981; Pennebaker & Epstein, 1983; Pennebaker & Watson, 1988).

19.1.2.2 *Individual differences in symptom reporting*

There are consistent individual differences in the degree to which people report symptoms, independently of variation in their physiological state. Trait measures of symptoms and bodily complaints are highly correlated with trait measures of anxiety, neuroticism, repression–sensitization, depression, and negative moods in general (Costa & McCrae, 1985, 1987; Diener & Emmons, 1984; Watson & Clark, 1984; Watson & Pennebaker, in press). The tendency to report negative moods has been termed negative affectivity (NA; Watson & Clark, 1984) or neuroticism (Costa & McRae, 1985), and dispositional symptom reporting is a consistently observed characteristic of NA and neuroticism. High NA or neuroticism individuals report greater distress and dissatisfaction at all times, across the life span, regardless of physiological state (see also Watson & Tellegen, 1985).

19.1.2.3 *Symptoms and arousal*

State and trait measures of symptom reporting are internally consistent: A person who reports a headache is also more likely to report stomach tension, fatigue, chest pains, and other sensations. Whereas measures taken from different physiological response systems often vary independently (Lacey, 1967), verbal measures of multiple symptoms tend to be unitary.

A number of psychological theories rely upon the notion of "general arousal" or "activation" as a mediating concept, for example, Schachter's cognitive labeling theory of emotions (Schachter & Singer, 1962), cognitive dissonance theory's account of attitude change (Fazio & Cooper, 1983; Festinger, 1957), and self-awareness theory (Wicklund, 1975). Intercorrelations between symptoms suggest that traditional arousal concepts may be valid for the verbal response system. But we believe that it is a mistake to regard symptom reports as substitutes for direct measures of physiological responses. Although we have already made this point, it should be reiterated because it has been subject to conceptual confusion.

Thayer (1970) found that self-reports of arousal/activation correlate more highly with composite measures of skin conductance, heart rate, blood volume, and mean arterial pressure than the individual physiological measures correlate among themselves. Such findings led some (e.g., Eysenck, 1975; Mackay, 1980) to propose that self-reports can better index arousal than can physiological measures. The correlations, however, are predictable on the basis of elementary reliability theory (e.g., Carmines & Zeller, 1979). *Any* composite measure is more internally consistent than a single-item measure; internally consistent measures correlate more highly with other measures than do measures based on only a single item. A composite of self-reported stress items *must* correlate more highly with a composite physiological measure than any single-item physiological measure correlates with another single-item physiological measure. So, Thayer's proposal has little relevance to the problem of measuring arousal per se (Cacioppo & Petty, 1986).

Proposals that self-reports may substitute for physiological measures of arousal fail to distinguish between arousal as bodily activation and arousal as perceived by the subject; the distinction between symptoms and undetected bodily responses indicates that these two types of "arousal" are not identical (cf. Hirschman & Clark, 1983; Zillman, 1983). Most importantly, if symptom reports are a joint function of internal and external cues, then such reports may lack discriminant validity (Cook & Campbell, 1979) in that they measure more than one construct. Therefore, we strongly discourage the use of verbal reports as "substitutes."

19.2 PHYSICAL CONTEXT

The symptom–sign distinction indicates that subjects can be aware of some physiological responses. In this section, we first briefly map the receptor and sensory projections involved in bodily sensations. We then point to the multiple central nervous system centers that can influence the verbal response system.

19.2.1 *Receptor and sensory projections*

Much of our awareness of bodily sensations originates in sensory receptors embedded in the skin, the joints, and organ structures of the body. Three types of somatic senses relevant to the direct perception of symptoms include mechano-receptive somatic senses, thermoreceptive senses, and pain senses. Mechano-receptive senses are stimulated by the displacement of tissue within the body and are sensitive to touch, pressure, vibration, and kinesthetic changes. The thermo-receptive senses detect heat and cold. The pain senses are usually triggered by damage to the tissues. Each of the senses in the body is associated with multiple types of receptors that differ in their speed of transmission, number of synaptic connections, and density of nerve endings (Guyton, 1976; Willis & Grossman, 1981).

All sensory nerves within the body enter the spinal cord through the posterior roots.

The spinal pathways for transmitting sensory information to the brain include the dorsal column, the spinocervical, and the spinothalamic tracts. Nerves from the lower thorax and lumbosacral regions ascend to the medulla along a dorsal column structure called the fasciculus cuneatus; those from the upper thorax and cervical areas ascend in the fasciculus gracilis (Willis & Grossman, 1981, chapter 7). Both project from nuclei in the medulla to a midbrain structure, the medial lemniscus, and thence to the ventral posterior lateral (VPL) nucleus of the thalamus and finally to the somatosensory areas of the cerebral cortex. The information transmitted along the dorsal column seems primarily to be proprioceptive (body position) and discriminative mechanoreceptive ("active touch"). The dorsal column typically transmits information extremely quickly while maintaining a high degree of localization and subtle gradations in the intensity of the stimulus.

The spinocervical tract also transmits mechanoreceptive information along a similar pathway to that used by the dorsal column. But according to Wills and Grossman (1981, pp. 285–286), it differs in two important ways from the dorsal column. First, it is not activated by proprioceptive stimuli. Second, it transmits some pain information.

The spinothalamic tract, although slower and less localized than the other pathways, transmits a broad spectrum of sensory experiences such as pain and sexual and thermal sensations. The mechanoreceptive information transmitted along the spinothalamic tract is thought to be relatively crude, for example, gross proprioceptive and nondiscriminative touch stimuli. In its pathway to the brain, this tract bypasses the medial lemniscus of the medulla, projecting directly to the VPL and/or the intralaminar nuclei of the thalamus and then to the cortex. It has been suggested that portions of the spinothalamic tract that project only to the intralaminar nuclei of the thalamus respond characteristically only to very intense stimuli and are very poor in providing information about the locus of stimulation (Willis & Grossman, 1981, p. 287).

Whereas the neural pathways subserving somatic sensations are reasonably well known, many of the symptoms with which this chapter is concerned arise from visceral stimuli. Here, the neural pathways are poorly known. One of the greatest difficulties in measuring and evaluating visceral sensations is that individuals often cannot accurately describe their location. This problem is most acute in cases of visceral pain. Many organs, such as the heart, esophagus, liver, stomach, colon, and kidneys, have relatively few pain and mechanoreceptors. Further, receptors in these areas connect with multiple pathways. Visceral pain fibers from the heart, for example, enter the spinal cord in multiple locations and synapse with fibers from other visceral areas. The net result is that individuals often report feeling pain in areas that are not, in fact, damaged. An example of this phenomenon, called referred pain, can be seen in heart attacks where damage to cardiac muscles can be perceived in the shoulders and arms rather than over the heart itself (Willis & Grossman, 1981). By the same token, chest pain, which is occasionally interpreted as a heart attack, can be the result of damage to the stomach, esophagus, or even the liver (see Melzack, 1973).

19.2.2   Brain mechanisms

As noted earlier, nerve fibers entering the dorsal columns and spinocervical tract project upwards and synapse in the medulla and again in the thalamus and are then projected to highly specific regions of the somatosensory cortex, which lies mainly in the anterior portions of the parietal lobes. The spinothalamic tract, however, projects directly to the thalamus without synapsing in the medulla and then projects to a variety of cortical and subcortical areas. This suggests that information transmitted along the spinothalamic tract is not finely organized in a particular area in the cerebral cortex, which may help to account for the problems associated with localizing visceral sensations and pain mentioned earlier.

Although virtually every part of the brain contributes to the verbal reports of internal state, those discussed in the following sections are particularly important.

19.2.2.1 *The somatosensory cortex*

The somatosensory cortex receives highly localized neural signals. Based on stimulation studies, it is believed that the primary somatosensory cortex analyzes only simple aspects of bodily sensations. As sensations are integrated and become more complex, sensory information is further processed and elaborated upon in the adjacent parietal lobes (Guyton, 1976).

19.2.2.2 *The frontal cortex*

Recent investigations by Davidson (1984), Ray and Cole (1985), and others indicate that the frontal regions are important in the awareness, integration, and expression of emotion. Both EEG and lesion studies suggest that the left frontal lobe is associated with the control of positive affect, whereas the right frontal lobe controls negative emotions. For example, destruction of the left frontal region causes individuals to perceive and report negative moods, distress, and physical symptoms to a heightened degree (Davidson, 1984; Luria, 1980).

19.2.2.3 *The speech and language centers*

The ability to report on one's internal state is, of course, dependent on language production. Sensory and affective information that is analyzed and organized elsewhere must then be converted to language. The relevant language areas, which are usually localized in the left temporal lobes, allow individuals to consciously report (and probably perceive) physical symptoms. Indeed, when language areas are blocked with drugs or even hypnosis, individuals fail to report induced pain, even though autonomic responses to pain stimulation suggest that the subjects are, in fact, processing the pain signals (see Davidson, 1984, and Kihlstrom, 1987, for reviews).

19.2.2.4 *The limbic system*

Sensory signals from the spinothalamic tract are processed to a high degree in various nuclei within the limbic system. If, as some believe (e.g., Heath, 1963), limbic structures are implicated in subjective emotions, then it is possible that spinothalamic signals relating to physical symptoms are part of the mechanism that mediates the consistently observed relationship between symptom reporting and negative moods (e.g., Watson & Pennebaker, in press). At present, however, this is only a speculation.

19.2.3   *Summary of physical context*

Our discussion in section 19.1 suggested that the perception and reporting of symptoms and moods is based on more than the simple stimulation of receptors in the body. A stomachache, for example, is partially attributable to sensory projections along various pathways. However, the *report* of a stomachache will also depend on the settings individuals are in, the degree of reinforcement they have received in the past for reporting the stomachache, and a variety of individual differences. Thus, we caution against attempting to understand verbal reports of internal states by tracing the neural pathways involved.

19.3   INFERENTIAL CONTEXT

19.3.1   *Measurement techniques*

Relative to measurements of other psychophysiological response systems, verbal reports of bodily feelings and symptoms appear simple to devise, administer, and quantify. No elaborate equipment is required. Large numbers of subjects can be run in short periods of time. Often, the response can be directly read from the self-report instrument in the form of numeric ratings, with no further data transformation needed. However, the apparent simplicity of reports from the verbal mode is deceptive and may lead the psychophysiological researcher to be less attentive to how he or she constructs verbal response measures than to obtaining bioelectric or biomechanical measures. As we show here, several classes of symptom measures can be distinguished, each relevant to different research goals.

19.3.1.1   *Immediate bodily states*

A basic question for the psychophysiologist interested in using verbal reports is whether immediately experienced states or more long-term, traitlike aspects of such reports are to be the focus of measurement. State measures are most appropriate when the concern is to assess the impact of immediate stimuli and psychological states on the representation of bodily events. State measures can be further subdivided into those that are principally concerned with the subject's representation of (1) physiological responses (e.g., heartbeats, GI contractions), (2) specific symptoms (headaches, sweating), or (3) general states (arousal, illness), which presumably are superordinate compounds of multiple symptoms.

State measures belonging to class 1 are typically used in studies of visceral perception. The central issues in these studies concern the factors that determine whether and when physiological responses are detectable (i.e., are transformed from signs to symptoms) and the functional significance of such transformation. A variety of measurement technologies exist for assessing subjects' accuracy in reporting the occurrence of discrete autonomic activity, particularly in the cardiac and gastrointestinal response systems (for reviews, see Blascovitch & Katkin, 1983; Pennebaker & Hoover, 1984; Reed, Harver, & Katkin, ch. 9).

It is often practical for reports of specific symptoms (class 2), and of general bodily states (class 3) to be obtained simultaneously. For example, Shields (1984, study 1) used the Somatic Perception Questionnaire (Landy & Stern, 1969) to determine whether anxiety and sadness are characterized by different patterns of symptom

Table 19.1. *Sample symptom checklist*

Right now, at this moment, I am experiencing:					
No headache					Headache
No watering eyes					Watering eyes
No racing heart					Racing heart
No congested nose					Congested nose
No tense muscles					Tense muscles
No upset stomach					Upset stomach
No flushed face					Flushed face
No sweaty hands					Sweaty hands
No shortness of breath					Shortness of breath
No cold hands					Cold hands
No dizziness					Dizziness
No ringing in ears					Ringing in ears

reports (class 2) and by differing degrees of overall symptom awareness (class 3). Subjects described incidents during which they felt anxious and sad. After each description, subjects rated the degree to which they experienced each of 10 symptoms using 5-point Likert scales (1 = not at all, 5 = acutely). Subjects also indicated which of the symptoms was experienced to a greater degree than all the other symptoms. By calculating the percentage of subjects endorsing each symptom as the "primary" one, Shields was able to show that anxiety and sadness have different associated symptom patterns (cf. Pennebaker, 1982, ch. 5). By summing the ratings of each symptom, she concluded that subjects were generally more aware of symptoms when anxious than when sad. This procedure can be easily adapted to studies in which physiological measures are also obtained and can thereby shed light on the relationship between perceived bodily states and objective measures of physiological responses.

In our own work, we have used various self-report measures of symptoms. An example of one of these is shown in Table 19.1. This symptom checklist measures how intensely subjects are experiencing each of 12 common symptoms (headache, watering eyes, etc.) It is an internally consistent, additive scale with Cronbach alpha coefficients averaging .75 over many subject samples (Pennebaker, 1982, Appendix A). Test–retest correlations tend to be small and to decrease over a 4-month interval. Such properties suggest that the checklist measures immediate states rather than a stable disposition to report symptoms but that at any instant there is tendency for reports of specific symptoms to covary.

Although the symptom checklist in Table 19.1 has a 7-point response scale, there

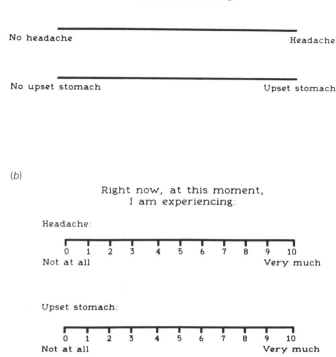

Figure 19.1. (a) Graphic response scales for immediate symptoms. (b) Numeric response scales for immediate symptoms.

is no requirement that this convention be observed. Five-, 9-, and 10-point response scales are equally usable. Indeed, we have often used a graphic response scale consisting of a 100-mm line, as shown in Figure 19.1(a); subjects indicate their response by making a slash mark or an X on the line. A score is then assigned by measuring the point at which the subject's mark crosses the line, to the nearest millimeter, yielding a 100-point scale. Two advantages of such a graphic scale are that it minimizes any tendency by subjects to mark the same blank on multiple symptom items or repeated measurements of the same symptom, and it virtually guarantees that there will be some variability in measures. This is less likely to be the case as the number of response options is reduced (e.g., from 9-point to 5-point to 3-point scales).

Figure 19.1 (b) shows yet another type of response scale. Here, subjects circle a number to indicate their rating. In general, we think there are few reasons to prefer one type of response scale (checklist, graphic, numeric) over another if the intent is to measure the intensity with which subjects are experiencing particular symptoms or their overall awareness of symptoms at a particular moment. Checklist and numeric scales that have a zero point as their anchor do have the advantage that they can be used simultaneously to measure not only symptom intensities but also symptom frequencies, that is, the number of symptoms the subject is experiencing with greater-than-zero intensity. When such a measure is theoretically relevant to the researcher, we recommend including a "Not at all" of "zero" anchor on the scale.

Obviously, any of the response scales shown here can readily be adapted to measure moods and emotions. For further information, we recommend Mackay (1980) and Pennebaker (1982).

All the scales shown here are unipolar, that is, each is constructed according to a "None" to "Very much" logic. Some symptoms, however, can be conceived in bipolar terms, for example, "Cold hands" versus "Warm hands." Likewise, changes in the intensity of many perceived symptoms ("Less" vs. "More") would seem, by definition, to be bipolar. We have sometimes used bipolar scales (e.g., Pennebaker & Epstein, 1983; Pennebaker & Skelton, 1981, experiment 1). Still, we recommend unipolar scales because bipolarity is an assumption about how subjects represent their symptoms. We believe that it is better to examine bipolarity directly, with empirical data, rather than by assuming that people conceptualize symptoms in bipolar terms. For instance, if warm and cold hands were bipolar, we would expect correlations between ratings of each symptom made at the same time to be substantially negative. In our experience, this is rarely the case: Although correlations between reports of the two symptoms are almost always negative, they rarely approach -1.00 and are sometimes not even significant. In one study, we found that self-reports of warm hands but not cold hands predicted blood pressure fluctuations for some subjects, whereas self-reports of cold but not warm hands were significant blood pressure predictors for other subjects (Pennebaker, Gonder-Frederick, Stewart, Elfman, & Skelton, 1982).

All the immediate-state measures discussed thus far focus on the magnitude or intensity of subjects' bodily feelings, but we have alluded to a somewhat different class of measures, frequency estimates. Here, the aim is to determine how many symptoms the subject experiences. As previously noted, frequency measures can be derived from intensity ratings that present a zero point. Alternatively, frequency estimates can be obtained directly by asking subjects to report how often they have experienced one or more symptoms or bodily feelings during a given time interval. Such measures may be useful in studies of the biasing effects of experimental manipulations upon recall of symptom episodes (e.g., Skelton & Strohmetz, 1986).

Finally, certain behaviors may also be used as measures of subjects' bodily experience. Coughing, self-scratching, and exercise tolerance are examples. Some are discussed in a later section.

19.3.1.2 *Individual differences*

Trait measures are appropriate when the researcher wishes to define subgroups of subjects. As already noted, some individuals are chronically more likely than others to report symptoms and bodily feelings. A number of instruments exist for measuring such individual differences. For example, in the domain of stress- and emotion-related symptoms there is the Autonomic Perception Questionnaire (APQ; Mandler, Mandler, & Uviller, 1958), which asks subjects to rate on 9-point scales how frequently they experience 18 symptoms (e.g., hot face, perspiration, muscle tension) when feeling anxious. Higher scores indicate a greater degree of "autonomic awareness" under anxiety conditions. Although APQ scores distinguish anxiety from anger and sadness (Shields, 1984, study 2) and subjects who exhibit labile physiological responses to anxiety situations from less labile subjects (Mandler et al., 1958), APQ scores do not distinguish accurate from inaccurate subjects in visceral perception tasks (Brener, 1977).

The Autonomic Response to Stress (ARS) subscale of the Perceived Somatic Response Inventory (PSRI; Meadow, Kochevar, Tellegen, & Roberts, 1978) is a similar individual difference measure. Subjects rate how likely it is that they experience 14 symptoms such as dry mouth, dizziness, and so forth when in stressful situations. The ARS subscales have an internal consistency reliability coefficient (Cronbach alphas) exceeding .8. An important feature of PSRI subscales is that these were developed so as to maximize discriminant validity. Scores on all subscales, for example, are only modestly correlated with the Hypochondriasis subscale of MMPI.

The Somatic Anxiety Questionnaire (SAQ) is seven items from Schwartz, Davidson, and Goleman's (1978) Cognitive and Somatic Anxiety Questionnaire. It is similar to the APQ and the ARS subscale in that subjects rate how much they experience various symptoms when in anxiety-provoking situations.

Other symptom inventories are primarily oriented toward measuring health problems rather than bodily responses to stressful emotions. These include the following:

1   The Hopkins Symptom Checklist (HSCL; Derogatis, Lipman, Rickels, Uhlenhuth, & Covi, 1974) Somatization subscale, 12 items (e.g., faintness trouble catching your breath) rated in terms of how intensely each was experienced during the past week.
2   The Cornell Medical Index (CMI; Brodman, Erdmann, & Wolff, 1949; see also Costa & McCrae, 1985), particularly the first 12 sections in which subjects report respiratory, cardiovascular, and other health complaints. These are summed to produce a single score representing total health complaints.
3   The Health Status Questionnaire (HSQ; Belloc, Breslow, & Hochstim, 1971) includes an 11-item symptom subscale scored by totaling the number of problems reported as occurring during the past year.

The Pennebaker Inventory of Limbic Languidity (PILL; Pennebaker, 1982, Appendix B) is the trait inventory we use most frequently. It consists of 54 common symptoms that subjects rate for frequency of occurrence using a 5-point scale ("More than once a day" to "Never or almost never"). PILL scores are derived by assigning a 1 to each symptom that is rated as occurring at least once per month and 0 to less frequently occurring symptoms. Thus, the final score represents the number of symptoms a subject experiences at least monthly, with a minimum of 0 and a maximum of 54. In college student samples, the mean PILL score is usually between 16 and 20.

Alternative scoring schemes (e.g., summing the individual item ratings) yield scores that correlate .96 with the symptoms-per-month method. PILL is internally consistent (Cronbach alphas average .88). Factor analyses of the scale tend to yield small symptom clusters (e.g., running nose and congested nose; stiff muscles and sore muscles). Test–retest correlations of .7 to .8 are common over 2-month intervals.

Pennebaker (1982, Chapter 7; see also Watson & Pennebaker, in press) has reported extensively on PILL's discriminant and concurrent validity. Not surprisingly, PILL scores are most strongly related to scores on another symptom measure, the HSCL (Derogatis et al., 1974). PILL scores correlate significantly but modestly with measures of health behavior, including use of student health facilities, aspirin use, and days lost due to sickness. Perhaps most interesting in light of our earlier discussion of the NA construct, PILL also correlates with such measures as the Self-Consciousness Scale (Fenigstein, Scheier, & Buss, 1975), the SAQ (Schwartz et al., 1978), with various self-reports of concern with self-image, and most startlingly, with self-reports of early sexual trauma.

19.3.2 *Paradigms for studying symptoms*

Prior to the 1970s, studies in which measures of symptoms and related bodily feelings served as more than a "manipulation check" were rare. Since that time, however, several identifiable classes of research have emerged that, in one way or another, regard symptoms as more than an adjunct measure. First, there are studies in which symptoms and related bodily states are treated as primary dependent variables. Such research, in general, attempts to identify factors affecting bodily experience per se, including prior expectancies, focus of attention, placebos, availability of health-relevant cognitions, degree of veridical physiological activation, personality variables, and so on.

A newly emerging class of research efforts addresses the role of symptoms in applied health problems. For example, patient beliefs concerning the symptomatic concomitants of chronic diseases such as hypertension and diabetes have come under close examination. The working hypothesis guiding research in this area is that patient beliefs concerning the causal meaning of their symptoms affect patients' attempts to treat their disease.

Finally, some studies have aimed at testing theories that postulate variations in perceived arousal as an effective intervening variable. Such studies do not measure symptoms directly but instead establish conditions from which a role for bodily experience can be inferred from subjects' performance on drive-sensitive tasks or their attitude statements following manipulations intended to affect interpretations of bodily states which, theoretically, mediate the attitude statements. We shall briefly examine examples of each type of research in turn.

19.3.2.1 *Symptoms as primary dependent variable*

Studies in which both symptom reports *and* physiological measures are obtained concurrently have been exceedingly rare in psychophysiology, where the focus has been primarily upon signs and undetected bodily responses. This situation has begun to change in the past few years, as indicated in our earlier discussion of recent research into the relationship between internal and external stimuli to symptoms.

Social psychology, on the other hand, offers many examples of studies examining effects of immediate, situational factors on verbal reports of symptom intensity or frequency. A nonexhaustive list of some of the factors investigated in these studies includes controllable versus uncontrollable stress (Pennebaker, Burnam, Schaefer & Harper, 1977), expectations concerning the physiological effects of environmental stimuli (Burnam & Pennebaker, 1977; Pennebaker & Skelton, 1981), and self-focused versus externally focused attention (Gibbons, Carver, Scheier, & Hormuth, 1979; Pennebaker & Lightner, 1980, study 2; Scheier, Carver, & Matthews, 1983). The logic of such studies is to manipulate the factor(s) of interest and then to assess its (their) impact upon self-reports of specific symptoms. It is unusual for concurrent physiological measures to be obtained in such studies. Zillmann's (e.g., 1978, 1979, 1983) work on the energization of emotional behavior consequent upon residual physiological excitation represents a significant exception, but we believe our generalization is nonetheless valid.

There have been many studies examining the relationship between subject variables (demographic and personality measures) and symptom reporting. As noted in our earlier discussion of the PILL symptom inventory, a variety of individual difference and personality measures correlate with symptom reporting; we refer the reader to Pennebaker (1982, chapter 7) for a general review and to Scheier et al. (1983) for a review of research on self-consciousness and perceived bodily states. Such paradigms, unfortunately, suffer at least two serious limitations.

First, as in the social psychology paradigms, subject variable studies that obtain both symptom and physiological measures are rare. Of course, there are exceptions (see Pennebaker, 1982, 1984). Second, the nature of subject variable studies, especially in the personality domain, is such that causal inferences are hazardous. At the most fundamental level, there always exists the question of whether the subject variable is the cause and symptom reporting the effect or vice versa. Moreover, the possibility exists that personality–symptom reporting relationships are spurious correlations mediated by higher order dispositions such as NA and neuroticism. As a result, we share Leventhal's (1987) skepticism concerning the ability of personality–symptom research to tell us much about the process of symptom reporting.

19.3.2.2 *Applications to health problem*

Symptom reports play an important role in research concerning how patients with chronic diseases conceptualize their health problems. Spurred by the work of Leventhal and his associates with hypertension and cancer patients (e.g., Leventhal, Meyer, & Nerenz, 1980; Leventhal, Nerenz, & Straus, 1982; Meyer, Leventhal, & Gutman, 1985), a growing number of researchers are examining such issues as how patients use symptoms to inform themselves of their illness status, the accuracy of patients' symptom beliefs, and the effect of symptom beliefs on self-care.

Gonder-Frederick and her associates (Gonder-Frederick, Cox, Bobbitt, & Pennebaker, 1986; Gonder-Frederick, Cox, Clarke, & Carter, 1987) have studied the symptom beliefs of diabetic patients over a 7-year period. They have found that diabetic patients rely overwhelmingly upon perceived symptoms rather than upon objective measures of blood glucose (BG) levels to monitor their condition (Gonder-Frederick, Cox, Pohl, & Carter, 1984). Patient dependence on symptoms has been observed elsewhere (e.g., Leventhal et al., 1980, 1982), but Gonder-Frederick et al.'s efforts to determine the accuracy of patients' symptom beliefs are prototypic of efforts in this area.

In this context, "accuracy" has to do with the relationship between the covariation of reported symptoms and BG levels and the covariation as perceived by patients. To assess the empirical covariation, Gonder-Frederick et al. (1986) had patients rate the intensity of 10 symptoms (including 5 standard symptoms) a total of 40 times during a hospital stay. After completing each set of ratings, patients measured their BG level with a reflectance meter. This yielded 40 symptom checklist–BG observations per patient. Six months and again 1 year after hospitalization, these patients contributed 40 more pairs of symptom and BG data. During the final at-home phase, patients also rated each symptom for the extent to which they *believed* it was related to hypo- and hyperglycemia. Pearson *r*-coefficients were then calculated between symptom intensity ratings and BG measurements for each subject ("within-subject" *r*s are calculated in the same way as any Pearson *r*, except that the data pairs are not observations from individual subjects but repeated observations from the same subject). Some symptoms were predictive of BG variations for most subjects, but the pattern of BG-predictive symptoms differed from patient to patient (cf. similar findings for blood pressure symptoms by Bauman & Leventhal, 1985, and Pennebaker et al., 1982, and an independent replication for BG by Moses & Bradley, 1985). Moreover, symptom–BG relationships weakened over time; fewer symptoms were predictive after a year than at the beginning of the study.

The accuracy of patients' beliefs about symptom–BG covariation was assessed by analyzing the four possible relationships between belief ratings and the empirical covariation between intensity ratings and BG (the terminology is borrowed from signal detection theory): *Hits* (where the patient believes a BG-predictive symptom is predictive), *misses* (where the patient fails to identify a BG-predictive symptom as predictive), *correct rejections* (where the patient believes a nonpredictive symptom is, in fact, nonpredictive), and *false alarms* (where the patient calls a nonpredictive symptom predictive). Patients' hit rates averaged only 46% at the beginning of the study and declined to less than 33% by year's end. The average rate of correct rejections was over 77% at the beginning of the study but declined slightly, to 71%. Outright misses were uncommon and stable throughout the year, but false alarms increased from less than 23% to almost 30%. Gonder-Frederick and her associates have moved on to assessing the clinical significance of patients' mistaken beliefs and are developing programs to correct these beliefs (Gonder-Frederick et al., 1987).

19.3.2.3 *Bodily feelings as intervening variable*

In addition to the research described in the preceding, where symptom-reporting served as a major variable, we should also mention studies in which subjective bodily experience has been theorized to act as an intervening variable that drives such processes as attitude change (e.g., Fazio & Cooper, 1983), aggressive behavior (Zillmann, 1979), and the facilitating versus inhibiting effects of others upon behavioral performance (Baron, 1985). In these research traditions, the focus is rarely upon specific bodily feelings and symptoms but instead upon relatively vague and diffuse perceptions of arousal. Moreover, arousal per se is less of a concern than is its theoretical status as mediator.

Cognitive dissonance research exemplifies a tradition in which arousal has played a major role as theoretical concept. Interpreters of Festinger's (1957) theory proposed that perceived inconsistencies between cognitions result in arousal the person feels motivated to eliminate (e.g., Brehm & Cohen, 1962). The arousal postulate of revised dissonance theory would probably have been of only minor importance had it not been for Bem's (e.g., 1972) challenge to its necessity. Thus ensued a host of studies attempting to verify the arousing consequences of cognitive dissonance (reviewed by Fazio & Cooper, 1983). Direct attempts to verify the arousal postulate with physiological measures met with limited success; the very act of obtaining physiological measures seemed to eliminate the attitude change effects of dissonance (Croyle & Cooper, 1983). As a result, researchers turned to less direct means of obtaining evidence for dissonance-induced arousal.

One approach has relied upon the misattribution paradigm derived from Schachter's (Schachter & Singer, 1962) two-factor theory of emotion. The misattribution model assumes that people are motivated to explain arousal feelings they experience and will ordinarily attribute such feelings to the most salient plausible cause in their phenomenal field. If this happens to be an emotional stimulus, the person will label the arousal in emotional terms; if nonemotional causes are most salient, arousal will be experienced as less emotional. An implication is that people may misattribute arousal if misleading cues are available.

Zanna and Cooper (1974) were the first to apply the misattribution paradigm to the problem of dissonance-induced arousal. They found that subjects who were induced to endorse an unpopular position and to regard the endorsement as freely chosen did *not* exhibit dissonancelike attitude change if they also received a pill (actually a placebo) described as having arousing side effects. Subjects who "chose" to endorse the unpopular position but who received an allegedly "relaxing" pill, on the other hand, showed a very large degree of attitude change. The results appeared to show that dissonance is arousing because when arousal can be attributed to a plausible alternative cause, dissonance effects are eliminated.

Another indirect method for assessing the presence of dissonance-induced arousal is by comparing the performance of subjects who do versus do not meet the theoretical conditions for dissonance on tasks that are known to be sensitive to arousal. Arousal facilitates performance on simple or well-learned tasks but undermines performance on complex or novel tasks (Spence, 1960), so dissonance-aroused subects should perform better on simple tasks, relative to nonaroused subjects, and worse on more complex tasks (Kiesler & Pallak, 1976). In a recent study testing this hypothesis, subjects wrote essays favoring the position that tooth-brushing is harmful under high-choice or no-choice conditions (Gaes, Melburg, & Tedeschi, 1986). Half the subjects in each condition completed a simple task (copying rows of one-digit numbers) after writing their essay; the other half completed a more complicated copying task requiring them to substitute numbers from a table. Subjects also completed a "health survey" that included an item concerning their agreement with the counterattitudinal position. Consistent with the dissonance prediction, high-choice subjects expressed greater agreement with the self-report item and copied more numbers when the task was simple but fewer when it was complex than did the no-choice subjects.

But there are at least three problems with viewing the results of misattribution and drive-sensitive task experiments as providing conclusive evidence for the arousing properties of dissonance. The first derives from the distinction among symptoms, signs, and undetected bodily responses made at the beginning of this chapter. There is an implicit assumption in both types of studies that dissonance arousal is consciously experienced as a symptom; an equally plausible interpretation is that dissonance arousal is an undetected bodily response. Second, the arousal postulate implies that subjects' attitude change should be proportional to their arousal. Yet Gaes et al. (1986) found only negligible correlations between self-reported attitudes and the performance measures among high-choice subjects; arousal as measured by task performance was unrelated to subjects' expressed attitudes toward toothbrushing. Finally, even if we grant symptom status to arousal, misattribution research is plagued by an ironic failure: Even when behaviors are affected by attribution manipulations, it is very difficult to find self-report evidence that the supposedly crucial attributions occurred (Wilson, 1985; Wilson & Linville, 1982). Thus, the assumption that subjects engage in a conscious, arousal attribution process may be untenable (cf. Cacioppo & Petty, 1982). We recommend Fazio and Cooper (1983) and Cooper and Croyle (1984) for reviews of further developments in the dissonance–arousal arena.

19.4   SOCIAL CONTEXT

Our discussion to this point indicates that verbal reports in psychophysiological studies should be regarded as representing subjects' *understanding* of their bodily states but not necessarily the actuality of those states. Social factors, we believe, are crucial to making sense of symptom reports and other responses from the verbal system. Hence, we turn to a consideration of some of those factors.

19.4.1   *Social context of symptom measurement*

19.4.1.1 *The problem of demand characteristics*

Demand characteristics (Aronson, Brewer, & Carlsmith, 1985; Orne, 1962) are all those aspects of a research setting that combine to make subjects aware of the research hypothesis. When subjects who are aware of the hypothesis exhibit hypothesis-consistent behavior, it then become an open question as to whether the behavior was mediated by the substantive variables manipulated in the study or, instead, is simply an attempt to behave "as expected."

The potential is relatively great for demand characteristics to affect symptom reports in any given study. At least two factors are at work here. First, because symptoms can be assessed directly only via self-reports, it is virtually impossible to conceal the fact of measurement from subjects' awareness; and if subjects know they are being measured, they must realize that the measurements are relevant to some aspect of the research setting. This is not a unique problem for symptom measurement per se; it applies to all self-report measures. But the researcher must take it into account.

The second factor is relatively unique to symptom measurement. As we have already noted, symptom reporting is at least as highly responsive to people's perceptions of situational cues and to their beliefs about how their bodies react to those cues as it is to veridical physiological activity. Thus, to the degree that the research setting presents cues subjects can link to their beliefs about bodily reactions, symptom report data may reflect these cues.

To achieve some perspective on the demand characteristics issue, we think it is useful to distinguish studies in which demand characteristics are a *problem* from those in which the elucidation of such demands is, in fact, the *point* of the research. In studies of suggestibility, for example, the important question is *not* whether subjects picked up on cues concerning the symptoms the experimenter expects them to experience. Instead, the question is whether the research allows us to see *how* such cues affect symptom reporting. Given that the nonlaboratory world is rich in information that suggests to people how they "should" feel, we believe that there is room for experimental studies that model that world so long as their purpose is not merely to demonstrate but also to explain the operation of suggestion. In short, we believe that it is valid to invoke "demand characteristics" as a criticism of a research study only if the study fails to explain the mechanisms through which demands affect symptom reporting.

19.4.1.2 *Symptom-relevant behaviors*

Attempts to control experimental demands have sometimes bypassed self-reports and, instead, observed symptom-relevant behaviors (signs) unobtrusively. Pennebaker (1980, 1982) reports several studies in which the dependent measure was coughing or self-scratching behavior. If we assume that people cough in response to tickly throat sensations and scratch in response to itching sensations, then we might infer that the symptoms caused the behavior. This inference, however, presupposes (perhaps unjustifiably) a direct relationship between symptoms and signs.

Symptom-relevant behavior may not be consistent with symptoms as experienced by the subjects. For example, Pennebaker and Lightner's (1980, study 1) subjects ran equal distances over a cross-country course and a stadium track. Subjects' running times and reports of fatigue and other symptoms at the completion of running were recorded for both types of running conditions. There were no differences in reports of fatigue and symptoms between the two conditions, but subjects ran faster on the cross-country course. To interpret these results, one must assume that subjects regulated their running pace in response to perceived (but unmeasured) variations in fatigue symptoms associated with the two types of courses (for similar inconsistencies between a performance measure and self-reported symptoms, see Snyder, Schulz, & Jones, 1974). Such assumptions may beg the entire definition of symptoms.

19.4.1.3 *Cover stories and other distractors*

It is sometimes useful to disguise the purpose of studies in which symptom reporting is a primary dependent variable. One way in which to do this is to present a "cover story" that provides a convincing rationale for the experiment. For example, Ruble (1977) studied the effects of women's beliefs about their stage in the menstrual cycle upon their reports of menstrual symptoms. When subjects arrived at the laboratory, they were connected to an impressive-looking but inoperative machine that purportedly could accurately predict the onset date of the next menstrual period. This cover allowed Ruble to manipulate her subjects' *apparent* stage in the menstrual cycle via bogus information read from the machine and to rationalize the collection of symptom data. Ruble found that women who were told they were within a few days of their period's onset reported more menstrual symptoms (water retention, appetite changes) than those told they were 2 weeks away from onset or those told nothing about their "stage" in the cycle. Other "covers" for obtaining symptom data include telling subjects that "people sometimes have different reactions to experiments, and this information helps us to control for individual differences" (Skelton & Strohmetz, 1986).

Another way to disguise a study's concern with symptom reports is to "imbed" the symptom manipulation and measures in a larger set of irrelevant events and measures. Subjects in a study concerning the effects of retrieving a prior symptom episode upon immediately experienced symptoms (Skelton, 1987b) were told that the study was a comparison of the vividness of different mental imagery modes. To reinforce this story, all subjects generated "mental images" of familiar sound and sights (e.q., a favorite tune, a friend's face) in addition to recalling a specific physical symptom; order of the imagery trials was counterbalanced. After each image, subjects completed several vividness ratings and then a list of 15 mood and symptom ratings. A postexperimental questionnaire revealed that subjects did not guess the purpose of the study; however, ratings of the specific symptom they recalled were higher immediately after it had been retrieved than on auditory and visual imagery trials and also higher than any other symptoms on the 15-items list.

19.4.2 *Social and psychological meaning of symptoms*

19.4.2.1 *Affect and symptoms*

We have already indicated the strong and pervasive link between affect and reported symptoms. Experimental manipulations that influence subjects' immediate moods will almost certainly affect the number and kinds of symptoms reported (Croyle & Uretsky, 1987; Pennebaker, 1982, chapter 5; Shields, 1984). This poses few problems in studies where subjects can be randomly assigned to experimental groups because the random assignment procedure should control for pre-experimental moods and symptoms.

But in correlational or quasi-experimental studies, where random assignment is impossible by definition, the affect–symptom relationship must be taken into account. Our earlier discussion of NA and neuroticism showed that individuals who consistently report high levels of negative emotion, stress, and so on, will also tend to report high levels of symptoms, independently of measurable signs (Costa & McCrae, 1985; Watson & Pennebaker, in press; see also Frese, 1985). Thus, when groups are composed on the basis of subject variables that have a strong affective component (anxiety, stress, self-esteem scales, etc.), subsequently measured differences in symptom reporting will likely be artifactual; the same is true when the group composition procedure is based on individual differences in symptom reporting or health status and affective measures are subsequently obtained.

For example, a psychophysiologist might conduct a study of stress effects on physiological responses and symptom reports in low- versus high-anxious subjects. The subject groups, presumably, are defined on the basis of pretest scores on an anxiety scale. If the researcher subsequently finds that high-anxious subjects are more physiologically reactive and report more symptoms following a stressful task, it would be hazardous to conclude that the physiological reactivity produced the elevated symptoms. At the very least, the researcher should also show that there is a correlation between physiological and symptom measures. In general, we recommend that researchers who wish to study symptoms and moods in settings where random assignment is not feasible should obtain repeated (pre- and post-) measures of dependent variables to control for initial NA or neuroticism levels.

19.4.2.2 *Availability of external cues*

We have repeatedly emphasized the role played by external, situational cues in people's perceptions of their bodily states. One way this has been demonstrated is by asking observers to *predict* a subject's symptoms based solely upon a description of the subject's situation. Observer-rated situational cues can account for at least as much variance in symptom reports as internal (physiological) cues. In two similar studies (Pennebaker & Epstein, 1983), subjects participated in a series of over 40 tasks, and both autonomic and symptom measures were obtained during each task. In each study, parallel samples of observer subjects simply read descriptions of tasks that actual subjects performed and rated how intensely they *believed* symptoms would be experienced during each task. Depending on autonomic channel, physiological responses accounted for about 8% of the explainable variance in actual subjects' symptom reports; external cues measured by observers' symptom ratings accounted for an additional 12% of the variance. Eight to 20% of the residual variance in self-reported symptoms was predicted by overlaps between physiological and external cues.

Results of these and other studies (e.g., Pennebaker, Gonder-Frederick, Cox, & Hoover, 1985; Pennebaker & Watson, 1988; Smith, 1986) seem to indicate that symptom reports and measurable signs of autonomic activity may correspond most strongly when subjects can freely use both internal sensory *and* external environmental cues. A further implication is that researchers need to take into account the availability of external cues to symptoms when they study the relationship between symptoms and signs and to implement studies that allow for valid generalizations about these relationships.

19.4.2.3 *Functional significance of symptoms*

Verbal reports of internal states are a form of social communication. In everyday life, statements that one is hungry, has a headache, feels tired, and so on, are not merely parenthetical comments; these often serve some purpose. We can report symptoms in order to receive medical help, attention, or emotional support from others (Zola, 1966). We can report symptoms as a way of avoiding blame for failures (Smith, Snyder, & Perkins, 1983) or to escape from unpleasant school or work obligations (Mechanic, 1978). One result of the functional value associated with symptom-reporting behaviors is that the behaviors can be reinforced when they succeed in achieving desired goals.

For example, Whitehead and his associates have shown the powerful effects of social reinforcements for symptom- and illness-related behaviors during childhood and adolescence upon adult symptom-reporting, physician visits, and absenteeism. Women whose mothers modeled and rewarded menstrual or cold complaints are more likely to complain of menstrual or cold symptoms in adulthood (Whitehead, Busch, Heller, & Costa, 1986). Irritable bowel syndrome, ulcer, and diabetes patients also exhibit symptoms and illness behaviors as a function of social reinforcements (Turkat, 1982; Whitehead, Fedoravicius, Blackwell, & Wooley, 1979; Whitehead, Winget, Fedoravicius Wooley, & Blackwell, 1982; also see Minuchin et al., 1975). Because symptoms are, by definition, accessible only to the sufferer, it is difficult to determine from such studies whether reinforcers simply lower the psychological threshold for reporting symptoms for which there exists a veridical basis in signs or, instead, actually promote symptom reporting having absolutely no physiological basis. Studies employing diagnosed patient populations suggest, at least, that the "lowered threshold" explanation is plausible; but the possibility of outright malingering cannot be wholly discounted.

A consideration in understanding verbal reports of symptoms, then, is the degree to which symptom reports have functional consequences for the individual. In correlational studies, it is important to ask how differences in the symptom reports of naturally occurring groups might have resulted from past patterns of rewards and punishments. Such individual differences are less important in laboratory studies characterized by random assignment, but the careful researcher must consider the extent to which experimental procedures provide differential reinforcement of subjects' symptom reporting. Such selective rewarding/punishing of symptom reporting, if unintended, could confound the interpretation of an experiment.

19.4.2.4 *Demographic factors*

A catalog of all the demographic factors that have been found to be related to symptom reports is beyond our scope here. Pennebaker (1982, chapter 1) provides a selective overview. The discussions by Zborowski (1969) and Zola (1966) of cultural and subcultural variations in health-related behavior, including symptom-reporting, are classics. Verbrugge's (1985) review of gender differences in health behavior is of particular value in distinguishing between symptoms and signs and in providing an up-to-date account of current hypotheses concerning the mediation of gender differences.

19.4.3 *Applications and future directions*

We began this chapter by identifying clinical psychology and medicine, sensory psychology, and social psychology as three traditions having a long-standing devotion to measuring and interpreting symptoms. To these may be added the newer fields of medical sociology and epidemiology. There is little need to belabor the value of symptom data to practitioners and scientists who work in these fields.

We have also noted that the collection of symptom data has been rather the exception in psychophysiology, no doubt partly due to the psychophysiologist's skepticism that such data can reveal anything of value. We hope we have made the case to such skeptics that it is worthwhile to obtain symptom data. Although the problems associated with mapping symptom reports onto physiological referents are frequently cited as a reason to ignore such data, we think it can be justifiably argued that it is precisely those problems (we view them as "challenges") that make it all the more important to obtain symptom data routinely. As psychophysiology adopts an increasingly cognitive orientation (e.g., McGuigan, 1978) and as links among cognitive processes, voluntary and involuntary bodily responses, and affect come under increasing scrutiny (e.g., Cacioppo & Petty, 1986; Lang, 1984; Leventhal, 1982), to overlook the processes governing people's representation of bodily activity would be a grave omission.

In the remaining paragraphs, we should like to sketch some directions we think future students of symptoms may find of interest. First and perhaps foremost is the problem of how bodily activity comes to be represented in conscious awareness. The visceral perception tradition derived from sensory psychophysics is a start, but it is clear that much more needs to be done. To cite one example, we have argued that accurate symptom reporting – verbal reports that can be related to veridical physiological responses – seems most likely to occur when cues from the external environment are permitted into the phenomenal field. But external cues (e.g., suggestions) can produce inaccurate, biased symptom reporting (e.g., Pennebaker & Skelton, 1981; Ruble, 1977). People are not infinitely suggestible regarding their bodily states; but neither are they omniscient self-observers. A specification of circumstances in which external cues help versus hinder accurate reporting of bodily states is sorely needed.

Another area requiring further study is the functional significance of symptoms in the broadest sense. Although it is certain that symptom reporting can serve socially and psychologically ulterior purposes, overemphasis of these functions may lead to needless victim blaming (Skelton, 1987a). Instead, we think it important that symptoms be studied in terms of their self-regulatory implications (e.g., Gonder-Frederick et al., 1987; Leventhal et al., 1982; Pennebaker et al., 1985). There are certainly occasions when the human ability to describe bodily experience augments our survival potential, as when the heart attack victim correctly recognizes her or his symptoms as indicators of a life-threatening condition. By increasing our understanding of the factors and conditions that govern the monitoring of symptoms and prompt people to act upon their knowledge (accurate or inaccurate) of their physical condition, we may increase individuals' prospects for survival.

NOTE

Preparation of this manuscript was made possible, in part, by grants from the National Science Foundation (BNS 86–06764) and the National Heart, Lung, and Blood Institute (HL32547) to the second author.

REFERENCES

Ajzen, I., & Fishbein, M. (1980). *Understanding attitudes and predicting behavior.* Englewood Cliffs, NJ: Prentice-Hall.

Allport, G. W. (1935). Attitudes. In C. Murchison (Ed.), *A handbook of social psychology* (pp. 798–844). Worcester, MA: Clark University Press.

Aronson, E., Brewer, M., & Carlsmith, J. M. (1985). Experimentation in social psychology. In E. Aronson & G. Lindzey (Eds.), *Handbook of social psychology* (3rd ed., Vol. 1, pp. 441–486). New York: Random House.

Baron, R. S. (1985). Distraction-conflict theory: Progress and problems. In L. Berkowitz (Ed.), *Advances in experimental social psychology* (Vol. 19). New York: Academic Press.

Barr, M., Pennebaker, J. W., & Watson, D. (1988). Improving blood pressure estimation through internal and environmental feedback. *Psychosomatic Medicine, 50,* 37–45.

Baumann, L. J., & Leventhal, H. (1985). "I can tell when my blood pressure is up, can't I?" *Health Psychology, 4,* 203–218.

Beecher, H. K. (1959). *Measurement of subjective responses: Quantitative effects of drugs.* New York: Oxford University Press.

Belloc, N. B., Breslow, L., & Hochstim, J. R. (1971). Measurement of physical health in a general population survey. *American Journal of Epidemiology, 93,* 328–336.

Bem, D. J. (1972). Self-perception theory. In L. Berkowitz (Ed.), *Advances in experimental social psychology* (Vol. 6, pp. 1–62). New York: Academic Press.

Blascovitch, J., & Katkin, E. S. (1983). Visceral perception and social behavior. In J. T. Cacioppo & R. E. Petty (Eds.), *Social psychophysiology: A sourcebook* (pp. 493–509). New York: Guilford Press.

Brehm, J. W., & Cohen, A. R. (1962). *Explorations in cognitive dissonance.* New York: Wiley.

Brener, J. (1977). Sensory and perceptual determinants of voluntary visceral control. In G. E. Schwartz & J. Beatty (Eds.), *Biofeedback: Theory and research* (pp. 29–66). New York: Academic Press.

Brodman, K., Erdmann, A. J., & Wolff, H. G. (1949). *Cornell medical index – health questionnaire.* New York: Cornell University Medical College.

Brown, R. (1965). *Social psychology,* New York: Free Press.

Burnam, M. A., & Pennebaker, J. W. (1977). *Cognitive labeling of physical symptoms.* Paper presented at the annual meeting of the Eastern Psychological Association, Boston.

Cacioppo, J. T., & Petty, R. E. (1982). A biosocial model of attitude change. In J. T. Cacioppo & R. E. Petty (Eds.), *Perspectives in cardiovascular psychophysiology* (pp. 151–188). New York: Guilford Press.

Cacioppo, J. T., & Petty, R. E. (1986). Social processes. In M. G. H. Coles, E. Donchin, & S. W. Porges (Eds.), *Psychophysiology: Systems, processes, and applications* (pp. 646–682). New York: Guilford Press.

Campbell, A. A. (1947). Factors associated with attitudes toward Jews. In T. Newcomb & E. Hartley (Eds.), *Readings in social psychology*. New York: Holt, Rinehart & Winston.

Carey, S. (1978). The child as a word learner. In M. Halle, J. Bresnan, & G. Miller (Eds.), *Linguistic theory and psychological reality* (pp. 264–293). Cambridge, MA: MIT Press.

Carmines, E. G., & Zeller, R. A. (1979). *Reliability and validity assessment*. Sage University Paper series on Quantitative Applications in the Social Sciences, series no. 07–017. Beverly Hills, CA: Sage.

Cook, T. D., & Campbell, D. T. (1979). *Quasi-experimentation: Design and analysis issues for field settings*. Chicago: Rand McNally.

Cooper, J., & Croyle, R. T. (1984). Attitudes and attitude change. In M. R. Rosenzweig & L. W. Porter (Eds.), *Annual review of psychology* (Vol. 35, pp. 395–426). Palo Alto, CA: Annual Reviews.

Costa, P. T., & McCrae, R. R. (1985). Hypochodriasis, neuroticism, and aging: When are somatic complaints unfounded? *American Psychologist, 40*, 19–28.

Costa, P. T., & McCrae, R. R. (1987). Neuroticism, somatic complaints, and disease: Is the bark worse than the bite? *Journal of Personality, 55*, 299–316.

Craig, K. D., & Prkachin, K. M. (1978). Social modeling influences on sensory decision theory and psychophysiological indexes of pain. *Journal of Personality and Social Psychology, 36*, 805–815.

Croyle, R. T., & Cooper, J. (1983). Dissonance arousal: Physiological evidence. *Journal of Personality and Social Psychology, 45*, 782–791.

Croyle, R. T., & Uretsky, M. B. (1987). Effects of mood on self-appraisal of health status. *Health Psychology, 6*, 239–253.

Davidson, R. J. (1984). Affect, cognition, and hemispheric specialization. In C. E. Izard, J. Kagan, & R. Zajonc (Eds.), *Emotion, cognition, and behavior* (pp. 320–365). New York: Cambridge University Press.

Dawes, R. M., & Smith, T. L. (1985). Attitude and opinion measurement. In G. Lindzey & A. Aronson (Eds.), *Handbook of social psychology* (3rd ed., Vol. 1, pp. 487–508). New York: Random House.

Derogatis, L. R., Lipman, R. S., Rickels, K., Uhlenhuth, E. H., & Covi, L. (1974). The Hopkins symptom checklist (HSCL): A measure of primary symptom dimensions. In P. Pichot (Ed.), *Modern problems in pharmacopsychiatry: Vol. 7. Psychological measurements in psychopharmacology* (pp. 77–110). Basel: Karger.

Diener, E., & Emmons, R. A. (1984). The independence of positive and negative affect. *Journal of Personality and Social Psychology, 47*, 1105–1117.

Eyesenck, H. J. (1975). The measurement of emotion: Psychological parameters and methods. In L. Levi (Ed.), *Emotions: Their parameters and measurement* (pp. 439–467). New York: Raven Press.

Fazio, R.H., & Cooper, J. (1983). Arousal in the dissonance process. In J. T. Cacioppo & R. E. Petty (Eds.), *Social psychophysiology: A sourcebook* (pp. 122–152). New York: Guilford Press.

Fechner, G. T. (1966). *Elements of psychophysics*. H. E. Adler, D. H. Howes, & E. G. Boring (Eds.). New York: Holt, Rinehart & Winston. (Original work published 1860).

Fenigstein, A., Scheier, M., & Buss, A. (1975). Public and private self-consciousness: Assessment and theory. *Journal of Consulting and Clinical Psychology, 43*, 522–527.

Festinger, L. (1957). *A theory of cognitive dissonance*. Stanford, CA: Stanford University Press.

Frese, M. (1985). Stress at work and psychosomatic complaints: A causal interpretation. *Journal of Applied Psychology, 70*, 314–328.

Furedy, J. (1986). Lie detection as physiological differentiation: Some fine lines. In M. G. H. Coles, E. Donchin, & S. W. Porges (Eds.), *Psychophysiology: Systems, processes, and applications* (pp. 683–701). New York: Guilford Press.

Gaes, G. G., Melburg, V., & Tedeschi, J. T. (1986). A study examining the arousal properties of the forced compliance situation. *Journal of Experimental Social Psychology, 22*, 136–147.

Gibbons, F. X., Carver, C. S., Scheier, M. F., & Hormuth, S. E. (1979). Self-focused attention and the placebo effect: Fooling some of the people some of the time. *Journal of Experimental Social Psychology, 15,* 263–274.

Gonder-Frederick, L. A., Cox, D. J., Bobbitt, S. A., & Pennebaker, J. W. (1986). Blood glucose symptom beliefs of diabetic patients: Accuracy and implications. *Health Psychology, 5,* 327–341.

Gonder-Frederick, L. A., Cox, D. J., Clarke, W. L., & Carter, W. R. (1987). Symptom perception, misattribution, and regulation of glucose levels in insulin-dependent diabetes. In J. M. LaCroix (Chair), *Illness schemas: Emerging methodological and empirical issues.* Symposium presented at the 48th annual meeting of the Canadian Psychological Association, Vancouver, B.C.

Gonder-Frederick, L. A., Cox, D. J., Pohl, S. L., & Carter, W. (1984). Patient blood glucose monitoring: Use, accuracy, adherence, and impact. *Behavioral Medicine Update, 6,* 12–16.

Guttman, L. A. (1944). A basis for scaling quantitative data. *American Sociological Review, 9,* 139–150.

Guyton, A. C. (1976). *Textbook of medical physiology.* Philadelphia: Saunders.

Heath, R. G. (1963). Electrical stimulation of the brain in man. *American Journal of Psychiatry, 120,* 571–577.

Hirschman, R., & Clark, M. (1983). Bogus physiological feedback. In J. T. Cacioppo & R. E. Petty (Eds.), *Social psychophysiology: A sourcebook* (pp. 177–214). New York: Guilford Press.

Janis, I. L. (1967). Effects of fear arousal on attitude change: Recent developments in theory and experimental research. In L. Berkowitz (Ed.), *Advances in experimental social psychology* (Vol. 3, pp. 167–225). New York: Academic Press.

Jones, G. E., Jones, K. R., Cunningham, R. A., & Caldwell, J. A. (1985). Cardiac awareness in infarct patients and normals. *Psychophysiology, 22,* 480–487.

Katkin, E.S. (1985). Blood, sweat, & tears: Individual differences in autonomic perception. *Psychophysiology, 22,* 125–137.

Kiesler, C. S., & Pallak, M. S. (1976). Arousal properties of dissonance manipulations. *Psychological Bulletin, 83,* 1014–1025.

Kihlstrom, J. (1987). The cognitive unconscious. *Science, 237,* 1445–1451.

Lacey, J. I. (1967). Somatic response patterning and stress: Of activation theory some revisions. In M. H. Appley & R. Trumbell (Eds.), *Psychological stress: Issues in research* (pp. 79–95). New York: Appleton-Century-Crofts.

Landy, F. J., & Stern, R. S. (1969). Factor analysis of a somatic perception questionnaire. *Journal of Psychosomatic Research, 15,* 179–181.

Lang, P. J. (1984). Cognition in emotion: Concept and action. In C. E. Izard, J. Kagan, & R. B. Zajonc (Eds.), *Emotions, cognition, and behavior* (pp. 192–225). New York: Cambridge University Press.

LaPiere, R. T. (1934). Attitudes versus actions. *Social Forces, 13,* 230–237.

Leventhal, H. (1970). Findings and theory in the study of fear communications. In L. Berkowitz (Ed.), *Advances in experimental social psychology* (Vol. 5, pp. 120–186). New York: Academic Press.

Leventhal, H. (1982). The integration of emotion and cognition: A view from the perceptual-motor theory of emotion. In M. S. Clark & S. T. Fiske (Eds.), *Affect and cognition: The seventeenth annual Carnegie symposium on cognition* (pp. 121–156). Hillsdale, NJ: Erlbaum.

Leventhal, H. (1987). Symptom reporting: A focus on process. In S. McHugh & T. M. Vallis (Eds.), *Illness Behavior: A Multidisciplinary Model* (pp. 219–237). New York: Plenum Press.

Leventhal, H., Meyer, D., & Nerenz, D. (1980). The common sense representation of illness danger. In S. Rachman (Ed.), *Contributions to medical psychology* (Vol. 2, pp. 7–30). New York: Pergamon Press.

Leventhal, H., Nerenz, D., & Straus, A. (1982). Self-regulation and the mechanisms of symptom appraisal. In D. Mechanic (Ed.), *Symptoms, illness behavior, and help-seeking* (pp. 55–86). New York: Prodist.

Likert, R. (1932). A technique for the measurement of attitudes. *Archives of Psychlogy, 140,* 5–53.

Lloyd, M. A., & Appel, J. B. (1976). Signal detection theory and the psychophysics of pain: An introduction and review. *Psychosomatic Medicine, 38,* 79–93.

Locke, J. (1959). *An essay concerning human understanding.* New York: Dover. (Original work published in 1890.)

Luria, A. R. (1980). *Higher cortical function in man.* New York: Basic Books.

Mackay, C. J. (1980). The measurement of mood and psychophysiological activity using self-report techniques. In J. Martin & P. H. Venables (Eds.), *Techniques in psychophysiology* (pp. 501–562). New York: Wiley.

Mandler, G., Mandler, J. M., & Uviller, E. T. (1958). Autonomic feedback: The perception of autonomic activity. *Journal of Abnormal and Social Psychology, 56,* 367–373.

McGuigan, F. J. (1978). *Cognitive psychophysiology: Principles of covert behavior.* Englewood Cliffs, NJ: Prentice-Hall.

McGuire, W. J. (1985). Attitudes and attitude change. In E. Aronson & G. Lindzey (Eds.), *Handbook of social psychology* (3rd ed., Vol. 2, pp. 233–346). New York: Random House.

Melzack, R. (1973). *The puzzle of pain.* New York: Basic Books.

Meadow, M. J., Kochevar, J., Tellegen, A., & Roberts, A. H. (1978). Perceived somatic response inventory: Three scales developed by factor analysis. *Journal of Behavioral Medicine, 1,* 413–426.

Mechanic, D. (1978). *Medical sociology* (2nd ed.). New York: Free Press.

Meyer, D., Leventhal, H., & Gutman, M. (1985). Common sense models of illness: The case of hypertension. *Health Psychology, 4,* 115–135.

Mihevic, P. M. (1981). Sensory cues for perceived exertion: A review. *Medicine and Science in Sports and Exercise, 13,* 150–163.

Minuchin, S., Baker, L., Rosman, B. L., Liebman, R., Milman, L., & Todd, T. C. (1975). A conceptual model of psychosomatic illness in children. *Archives of General Psychiatry, 32,* 1031–1038.

Mischel, W. (1968). *Personality and assessment.* New York: Wiley.

Moses, J. L., & Bradley, C. (1985). Accuracy of subjective blood glucose estimation by patients with insulin-dependent diabetes. *Biofeedback and Self-Regulation, 10,* 301–314.

Orne, M. (1962). On the social psychology of the psychological experiment: With particular reference to demand characteristics and their implications. *American Psychologist, 17,* 776–783.

Osgood, C. E., Suci, C. J., & Tannenbaum, P. H. (1957). *The measurement of meaning.* Urbana: University of Illinois Press.

Pastore, R. E., & Scheirer, C. J. (1974). Signal detection theory: Considerations for general application. *Psychological Bulletin, 81,* 945–958.

Patterson, F., & Linden, E. (1981). *The education of Koko.* New York: Holt, Rinehart & Winston.

Pennebaker, J. W. (1980). Perceptual and environmental determinants of coughing. *Basic and Applied Social Psychology, 1,* 83–91.

Pennebaker, J. W. (1981). Stimulus characteristics influencing the estimation of heart rate. *Psychophysiology, 18,* 540–548.

Pennebaker, J. W. (1982). *The psychology of physical symptoms.* New York: Springer-Verlag.

Pennebaker, J. W. (1984). Accuracy of symptom perception. In A. Baum, S. E. Taylor, & J. E. Singer (Eds.), *Handbook of psychology and health: Vol. 4. Social psychological aspects of health* (pp. 189–218). Hillsdale, NJ: Lawrence Erlbaum.

Pennebaker, J. W., Burnam, M. A., Schaefer, M. A., & Harper, D. (1977). Lack of control as a determinant of perceived physical symptoms. *Journal of Personality and Social Psychology, 35,* 167–174.

Pennebaker, J. W., & Epstein, D. (1983). Implicit psychophysiology: Effects fo common beliefs and idiosyncratic physiological responses on symptom reporting. *Journal of Personality, 51,* 468–496.

Pennebaker, J. W., Gonder-Frederick, L. A., Cox, D. J., & Hoover, C. (1985). The perception of general vs. specific visceral activity and the regulation of health-related behaviors. In E. Katkin & S. Manuck (Eds.), *Advances in behavioral medicine* (Vol. 1, pp. 165–198). Greenwich, CT: JAI Press.

Pennebaker, J. W., Gonder-Frederick, L., Stewart, H., Elfman, L., & Skelton, J. A. (1982). Physical symptoms associated with blood pressure. *Psychophysiology, 19,* 201–210.

Pennebaker, J. W., & Hoover, C. W. (1984). Visceral perception vs. visceral detection: Disentangling methods and assumptions. *Biofeedback and Self-Regulation, 9,* 339–352.

Pennebaker, J. W., & Lightner, J. M. (1980). Competition of internal and external information in an exercise setting. *Journal of Personality and Social Psychology, 39,* 165–174.

Pennebaker, J. W., & Skelton, J. A. (1981). Selective monitoring of physical sensations. *Journal of Personality and Social Psychology, 41,* 213–223.

Pennebaker, J. W., & Watson, D. (1988). Blood pressure estimation and beliefs among normotensives and hypertensives. *Health Psychology, 7,* 309–328.

Premack, D., & Premack, A. J. (1983). *The mind of an ape.* New York: Norton.

Ray, W. J., & Cole, H. W. (1985). EEG alpha activity reflects attentional demands, and beta activity reflects emotional and cognitive processes. *Science, 228,* 750–752.

Ross, A., & Brener, J. (1981). Two procedures for training cardiac discrimination: A comparison of solution strategies and their relationship to heart rate control. *Psychophysiology, 18,* 62–70.

Ruble, D. (1977). Premenstrual symptoms: A reinterpretation. *Science, 197,* 291–292.

Schachter, S., & Singer, J. E. (1962). Cognitive, social and physiological determinants of emotion. *Psychological Review, 69,* 379–399.

Scheier, M. F., Carver, C. S., & Matthews, K. A. (1983). Attentional factors in the perception of bodily states. In J. T. Cacioppo & R. E. Petty (Eds.), *Social psychophysiology: A sourcebook* (pp. 510–542). New York: Guilford Press.

Schwartz, G. E., Davidson, R. J., & Goleman, D. J. (1978). Patterning of cognitive and somatic process in the self-generation of anxiety: Effects of meditation versus exercise. *Psychosomatic Medicine, 40,* 321–328.

Shields, S. A. (1984). Reports of bodily change in anxiety, sadness, and anger. *Motivation and Emotion, B,* 1–21.

Skelton, J. A. (1987a). Legitimating second-hand symptoms: Observer judgments of illness victims. In R. T. Croyle (Chair), *Illness appraisal: Social and cognitive processes.* Symposium presented at the 59th annual meeting of the Midwestern Psychological Association, Chicago.

Skelton, J. A. (1987B). Symptom suggestibility: Somatic imagery as an underlying process? In J. M. LaCroix (Chair), *Illness schemas: Emerging methodological and empirical issues.* Symposium presented at the 48th annual meeting of the Canadian Psychological Association, Vancouver, B.C.

Skelton, J. A., & Strohmetz, D. B. (1986). Evaluating models of medical students' disease: Top-down processes in symptom perception. In J. B. Jemmott (Chair), *Self-appraisal of health status: Cognitive and social processes.* Symposium presented at the 57th annual meeting of the Eastern Psychological Association, New York.

Smith, T. W., Snyder, C. R., & Perkins, S.C. (1983). The self-serving function of hypochondriacal complaints: Physical symptoms as self-handicapping strategies. *Journal of Personality and Social Psychology, 44,* 787–797.

Smith, V. C. (1986) *Perception and estimation of blood pressure fluctuations in natural settings.* Unpublished masters thesis. Southern Methodist University, Dallas.

Snyder, M., Schulz, R., & Jones, E. E. (1974). Expectancy and apparent duration as determinants of fatigue. *Journal of Personality and Social Psychology, 29,* 426–434.

Spence, K. W. (1960). *Behavior theory and learning.* Englewood Cliffs, NJ: Prentice-Hall.

Stern, R. M., Ray, W. J., & Davis, C. M. (1980). *Psychophysiological recording.* New York: Oxford University Press.

Stevens, S. S. (1975ϯ. *Psychophysics: Introduction to its perceptual, neural, and social prospects.* New York: Wiley.

Swets, J. A. (1964). *Signal detection and recognition by the human observer.* New York: Wiley.

Swets, J. A. (1973). The relative operating characteristic in psychology. *Science, 82,* 990–100.

Thayer, R. E. (1970). Activation states as assessed by verbal report and four psychophysiological variables. *Psychophysiology, 7,* 86–94.

Turkat, I. D. (1982). An investigation of parental modeling in the etiology of diabetic illness behavior. *Behavior Research and Therapy, 20,* 547–552.

Verbrugge, L. M. (1985). Gender and health: An update on hypotheses and evidence. *Journal of Health and Social Behavior, 26,* 156–182.

Watson, D., & Clark, L. A. (1984). Negative affectivity: The disposition to experience aversive emotional states. *Psychological Bulletin, 96,* 465–490.

Watson, D., & Pennebaker, J. W. (in press). Health complaints, stress, and distress: Exploring the central role of negative affectivity. *Psychological Review.*

Watson, D., & Tellegen, A. (1985). Toward a consensual structure of mood. *Psychological Bulletin, 98,* 219–235.

Whitehead, W. E., Busch, C. M., Heller, B. R., & Costa, P. T. (1986) Social learning influences on menstrual symptoms and illness behavior. *Health Psychology, 5,* 13–23.

Whitehead, W. E., & Drescher, V. M. (1980). Perception of gastric contractions and self-control of gastric motility. *Psychophysiology, 17,* 552–558.

Whitehead, W.E., Fedoravicius, A.S., Blackwell, B., & Wooley, S. (1979). A behavioral conceptualization of psychosomatic illness: Psychosomatic symptoms as learned responses. In J. R. McNamara (Ed.), *Behavioral approaches to medicine: Application and analysis* (pp. 65–99). New York: Plenum Press.

Whitehead, W. E., Winget, C., Fedoravicius, A. S., Wooley, S., & Blackwell, B. (1982). Learned illness behavior in patients with irritable bowel syndrome and peptic ulcer. *Digestive Diseases and Sciences, 27,* 202–208.

Wicker, A. W. (1969). Attitudes versus actions: The relationship of verbal and overt behavioral responses to attitude objects. *Journal of Social Issues, 25,* 41–78.

Wicklund, R. A. (1975). Objective self-awareness. In L. Berkowitz (Ed.), *Advances in experimental social psychology* (Vol. 8, pp. 233–275). New York: Academic Press.

Willis, W. D., & Grossman, R. G. (1981). *Medical neurobiology* (3rd ed.). St. Louis: Mosby.

Wilson, T. D. (1985). Strangers to ourselves: The origins and accuracy of beliefs about one's own mental state. In J. H. Harvey & G. Weary (Eds.), *Attribution: Basic issues and applications* (pp. 9–36). New York: Academic Press.

Wilson, T. D., & Linville, P. W. (1982). Improving the academic performance of freshmen: Attribution therapy revisited. *Journal of Personality and Social Psychology, 42,* 367–376.

Wundt, W. (1904). *Principles of physiological psychology* (E. B. Titchener, Trans.). New York: Macmillan. (Original work published in 1874.)

Zanna, M. P., & Cooper, J. (1974). Dissonance and the pill: An attribution approach to studying the arousal properties of dissonance. *Journal of Personality and Social Psychology, 29,* 703–709.

Zillmann, D. (1978). Attribution and misattribution of excitatory reactions. In J. H. Harvey, W. J. Ickes, & R. F. Kidd (Eds.), *New directions in attribution research* (Vol. 2, pp. 335–368). Hillsdale, NJ: Erlbaum.

Zillmann, D. (1979). *Hostility and aggression.* Hillsdale, NJ: Erlbaum.

Zillmann, D. (1983). Transfer of excitation in emotional behavior. In J. T. Cacioppo & R. E. Petty (Eds.), *Social psychophysiology: A sourcebook* (pp. 215–242). New York: Guilford Press.

Zobrowski, M. (1969). *People in pain.* San Francisco: Jossey-Bass.

Zola, I. K. (1966). Culture and symptoms: An analysis of patients' presenting complaints. *American Sociological Review, 31,* 615–630.

PART IV

Issues in the analysis of psychophysiological data

20 Waveform moment analysis: topographical analysis of nonrhythmic waveforms

DONALD D. DORFMAN AND JOHN T. CACIOPPO

It is difficult to understand why statisticians commonly limit their inquiries to Averages, and do not revel in more comprehensive views. Their souls seem as dull to the charm of variety as that of the native of one of our flat English counties, whose retrospect of Switzerland was that, if its mountains could be thrown into its lakes, two nuisances would be got rid of at once. (Sir Francis Galton, 1889, p. 62)

Psychophysiological signals can be conceptualized as voltage–time functions. Amplitude variations in voltage across time constitute a waveform or response in the time domain; the distribution of these amplitudes within a given period of time constitutes the response in the amplitude domain; and the set of cosine curves of varying frequencies into which the voltage–time function can be decomposed constitutes that response in the frequency domain. Technological advances in bioelectronics and laboratory computing over the past two decades have made it possible to record signals from more physiological response systems with greater precision than ever before. Progress in signal representation has, however, not kept pace with advances in signal acquisition. As a result, the advances in signal acquisition have not yet had full impact on psychophysiological theory and research. For instance, multistage differential amplification, digital filtering, and sampling rates from several hertz to several kilohertz across multiple channels make detailed information available about the form of physiological events in the time, amplitude, or frequency domains; yet little of this information is captured by traditional psychophysiological measures such as mean amplitude, peak amplitude, peak latency, or power in specific frequency bands.

This chapter deals with the quantitative characterization of nonrhythmic waveforms in psychophysiology. Spectral analysis provides a useful quantitative characterization of rhythmic waveforms, with running spectral analyses revealing information about the changes in frequency across time (see Porges & Bohrer, chapter 21; Ray, chapter 12; Stern, Koch, & Vasey, chapter 16). We shall describe a general method called *waveform moment analysis,* which offers a mathematically rigorous and easily interpretable summary of nonrhythmic waveforms (Cacioppo & Dorfman, 1984, 1987). The method summarizes the waveform with a set of indicants derived from the moments of the waveform, and that is why the method is called waveform moment analysis or more succinctly, WAMA. This method performs a topographical analysis of the waveform: It describes and summarizes the size and shape of the waveform.

In general, WAMA makes two fundamental assumptions about the waveform to be analyzed. Let us denote by $f(x)$ a waveform (e.g., response) on a dimension x. The two assumptions are: (1) $f(x) \geq 0$ for all x, and (2) $f(x)$ and x are bounded. We

661

refer to waveforms that are nonnegative and bounded as *NB* waveforms. The NB waveforms are especially suited for WAMA for three important reasons: (1) all of the moments of an NB waveform exist; (2) an NB waveform is fully and uniquely characterized by the moments and total mass of the waveform; and (3) the Fourier transform of an NB waveform is fully and uniquely characterized by the moments and total mass of the waveform. (See Appendix A for a justification of these statements.)

The assumptions underlying WAMA of NB waveforms are not very restrictive to the psychophysiologist. Psychophysiological waveforms are always nonnegative and bounded in the frequency and amplitude domains. In the time domain, all nonnegative waveforms such as IEMG responses are bounded because the responses of a living organism are naturally bounded in time, amplitude, and frequency.

The first extensive use of moments to summarize the shape of probability distributions was by Karl Pearson (1895). While working on a mathematical theory of evolution in the 1890s, he found many data sets that exhibited systematic departures from the normal distribution. He developed a family of distributions called the Pearson system to deal with such departures (Ord, 1985). All of the distributions in the Pearson system are fully summarized by the first four moments. Moreover, the classical descriptors of the shape of a distribution (mean, variance, skewness, and kurtosis) are derived from the first four moments. We begin with a review of the classical shape descriptors, discussing some of their limitations and problems. We then outline our more general method of waveform moment analysis, of which the classical shape descriptors are a special case.

20.1   MOMENTS AND CLASSICAL SHAPE DESCRIPTORS: AN EXAMPLE FROM PHYSICS

Let us begin our discussion of moment analysis with a simple example from physics. Figure 20.1 presents a pile of bricks distributed along a bar. The bar is supported by a fulcrum at some arbitrary point α_x. Notice further that we have six columns of bricks, each column i ($i = 1, 2, \ldots, 6$) is centered at point x_i and each column i has a mass of $f(x_i)$. The question is: How can we characterize the size and shape of that nonrhythmic pile of bricks? If we remember some physics and some statistics, a few simple measures come to mind. We might summarize the size of that pile of bricks by its total mass, and we might try to summarize the shape with the arithmetic mean and standard deviation. The arithmetic mean should provide us with some indication of the location of the pile of bricks on the bar, and the standard deviation should give us some indication of the spread of the pile of bricks along the bar. The formulas for those measures are quite straightforward. The formula for the total mass[1] is:

$$\sum_{i=1}^{N} f(x_i) = A \tag{1}$$

Before computing the arithmetic mean and standard deviation, we must first transform the waveform to unit mass. We accomplish this by dividing the mass of each column of bricks, $f(x_i)$, by the total mass. Thus, each $f(x_i)$ is transformed to a

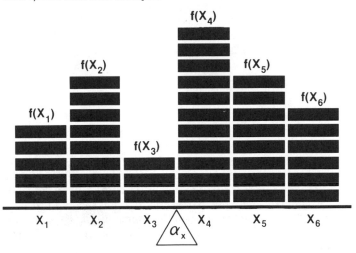

Figure 20.1. Stacks of bricks of mass $f(x_i)$ applied simultaneously at positions x_i along a bar, which is supported by fulcrum at α_x. (From "Waveform Moment Analysis in Psychophysiological Research," by J. T. Cacioppo & D. D. Dorfman, 1987, *Psychological Bulletin, 102*, p. 422.)

value $g(x_i)$ such that

$$g(x_i) = \frac{f(x_i)}{\sum_{i=1}^{N} f(x_i)} \qquad (2)$$

Notice that

$$\sum_{i=1}^{N} g(x_i) = \frac{\sum_{i=1}^{N} f(x_i)}{\sum_{i=1}^{N} f(x_i)} = 1$$

In other words, we have transformed the total mass of the waveform to a unit mass. Technically speaking, we have transformed the distribution of bricks to a probability distribution, where the probability of the event (x_i) is defined as

$$P(\{x_i\}) = \frac{f(x_i)}{\sum_{i=1}^{N} f(x_i)} = g(x_i) \qquad (3)$$

In the language of probability theory, we say that the pile of bricks has been transformed to a discrete probability density function. Now that we have converted the pile of bricks to a discrete probability density function, the computation of the arithmetic mean and standard deviation is straightforward. The formula for the arithmetic mean μ is

$$\mu = \sum_{i=1}^{N} x_i g(x_i) \tag{4}$$

and the formula for the standard deviation σ is

$$\sigma = \left[\sum_{i=1}^{N} (x_i - \mu)^2 g(x_i) \right]^{1/2} \tag{5}$$

The arithmetic mean is a measure of central tendency. In physics, it is the abscissa of the center of gravity, or more briefly the center of gravity. If the fulcrum is placed at a point equal to the center of gravity, the pile of bricks will be perfectly balanced on the bar. The standard deviation is a measure of the spread or dispersion of the pile of bricks about the center of gravity, or equivalently, about the arithmetic mean. In physics, its square is called the moment of inertia, which is a measure of the resistance of a body to angular acceleration.

The total mass provides information about the size of the waveform, and the mean and standard deviation (or its square, the variance) provide some information about the shape of the waveform. Are there additional measures we can use? Two further shape descriptors that have sometimes been computed are skewness and kurtosis. Measures of skewness are often computed to provide an index of asymmetry, and measures of kurtosis are often computed to provide an index of peakedness. A standard measure of skewness is provided by γ_1, or equivalently $\sqrt{\beta_1}$:

$$\gamma_1 = \sqrt{\beta_1} = \sum_{i=1}^{N} \left(\frac{x_i - \mu}{\sigma} \right)^3 g(x_i)$$

If the waveform is symmetrical about its mean, then $\gamma_1 = 0$. The converse, however, is not true. Thus, $\gamma_1 = 0$ does not imply that the waveform is symmetrical about its mean. Furthermore, if $\gamma_1 > 0$, the waveform is often thought to have a long tail on the right; and if $\gamma_1 < 0$, the waveform is often thought to have a long tail on the left. Those statements are a gross oversimplification. The problem is that asymmetry (or its opposite, symmetry) is too complex a property to be adequately summarized by a single number (see sections 20.1.1 and 20.2.1; see also Hoaglin, 1985a,b).

A standard measure of peakedness is provided by

$$\beta_2 = \sum_{i=1}^{N} \left(\frac{x_i - \mu}{\sigma} \right)^4 g(x_i)$$

or by a linear transformation of β_2 called γ_2:

$$\gamma_2 = \beta_2 - 3 = \sum_{i=1}^{N} \left(\frac{x_i - \mu}{\sigma} \right)^4 g(x_i) - 3$$

As γ_2 increases, the peakedness is said to increase. Thus, when $\gamma_2 = 0$, the curve is sometimes called mesokurtic or of medium peakedness. The normal curve has $\gamma_2 = 0$ and is therefore said to be mesokurtic; when $\gamma_2 < 0$, the curve is sometimes called platykurtic or less peaked than the normal curve; and when $\gamma_2 > 0$, leptokurtic or more peaked than the normal curve (Kendall & Stuart, 1963).

20.1.1 Moments and shape descriptors

A moment is always defined in terms of (1) a reference point α_x and (2) a power k. The kth moment about a reference point α_x is defined by

$$\mu_{k,x} = \sum_{i=1}^{N} (x_i - \alpha_x)^k g(x_i) \tag{6}$$

where, as before, $g(x_i) = f(x_i)/\sum_{i=1}^{N} f(x_i)$. First, notice that the waveform is converted to a unit mass before computing the kth moment. In addition, notice that if $\alpha_x = 0$ and $k = 1$, we have the arithmetic mean:

$$\sum_{i=1}^{N} (x_i - 0)^1 g(x_i) = \sum_{i=1}^{N} x_i g(x_i) = \mu$$

The arithmetic mean is therefore the first moment about the origin. Also notice that if $\alpha_x = \mu$ and $k = 2$, we have the variance:

$$\sum_{i=1}^{N} (x_i - \mu)^2 g(x_i) = \sigma^2$$

The variance is therefore the second moment about the mean. Note, too, that the root-mean-square (rms), a common measure of spread in psychophysiology, is the square root of the second moment about reference point α_x. Hence, the variance or its square root the standard deviation is a special case of the rms. More specifically, if we let $d = \mu - \alpha_x$, then

$$\sum_{i=1}^{N} (x_i - \alpha_x)^2 g(x_i) = \sum_{i=1}^{N} [(x_i - \mu) + d]^2 g(x_i)$$

$$= \sum_{i=1}^{N} [(x_i - \mu)^2 + 2(x_i - \mu) d + d^2] g(x_i)$$

$$= \sigma^2 + d^2 = \sigma^2 + (\mu - \alpha_x)^2$$

Note that in psychophysiology, the rms is generally computed about $\alpha_x = 0$. The preceding relation is useful because it allows one to relate the second moment about any arbitrary point to the variance. It is also clear from this relationship that the minimum value of the second moment is achieved when $\alpha_x = \mu$.

Now suppose we transform x to a z-score, $z = (x - \mu)/\sigma$. Whereas μ plays the role of a reference point in this transformation, σ plays the role of a scale parameter or unit of measurement. This transformed variable z is said to be standardized or in standard measure; it has mean zero and variance 1. It is now easy to see that skewness (γ_1) is a moment-based indicant:

$$\gamma_1 = \sum_{i=1}^{N} \left(\frac{x_i - \mu}{\sigma} \right)^3 g(x_i)$$

$$= \sum_{i=1}^{N} z_i^3 g(x_i)$$

In particular, γ_1 is the third moment of z about the origin. Finally, notice that kurtosis defined by β_2 or γ_2 is also a moment-based indicant:

$$\beta_2 = \sum_{i=1}^{N} \left(\frac{x_i - \mu}{\sigma} \right)^4 g(x_i)$$

$$= \sum_{i=1}^{N} z_i^4 g(x_i)$$

$$= \gamma_2 + 3$$

In particular, β_2 is the fourth moment of z about the origin. Summing up, the four classical indicants of the shape of a distribution or waveform – the mean, standard deviation (or variance), skewness, and kurtosis – are based on the moments.

20.1.2   *Limitations*

These moment-based indicants have proved to be quite useful in summarizing the shape of NB waveforms in psychophysiology. For instance, they have usefully summarized the integrated electromyographic (IEMG) responses resulting from various isometric (Cacioppo, Marshall-Goodell, & Dorfman, 1983) and mild isotonic (Grabiner, Andonian, Regnier, & Harding, 1984) muscle contractions. They have also been useful in characterizing IEMG activity recorded over superficial muscle regions in the human face and forearm in studies of information processing (Cacioppo, Petty, & Morris, 1985) and affective imagery (Cacioppo, Petty, & Marshall-Goodell, 1984). These classical moment-based indicants have also been used in the study of the electroencephalogram (EEG). For instance, they have served to characterize the amplitude density function of the EEG (Bronzino, Kelly, Cordova, Oley, & Morgane, 1981; Rieger, Krieglstein, & Schütz, 1979), the one-sided power spectral density of the EEG (one-sided power spectrum) (Saltzberg, Burton, Barlow, & Burch, 1985), and the two-sided power spectral density of the EEG (Hjorth, 1970, 1973, 1975).

Whereas moment-based indicants have been useful in summarizing and discriminating among NB waveforms in psychophysiology, there are, however, serious difficulties associated with the classical set of moment-based indicants – the mean, standard deviation (or variance), skewness, and kurtosis. These difficulties have served to limit the potential of moment-based analysis of the topography of waveforms observed in psychophysiology. The first problem noted in the preceding is that asymmetry is too complex a concept to be represented adequately by a single number. Second, the classical moment-based indicant of peakedness, kurtosis, is

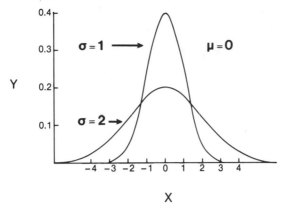

Figure 20.2. Two normal distributions with same mean ($\mu = 0$) and different standard deviations ($\sigma = 1, 2$).

not a measure of peakedness. Indeed, the meaning of kurtosis has been and continues to be debated in the statistical literature without any clear resolution (e.g., see Chissolm, 1970; Darlington, 1970; Hildebrand, 1971; Moors, 1986; Rupert, 1987). Figure 20.2 provides a simple illustration of the problem associated with interpreting kurtosis as a measure of peakedness. Figure 20.2 shows two normal distributions with the same means ($\mu = 0$) but different standard deviations ($\sigma = 1$ in one case and $\sigma = 2$ in the other). The equation for the normal distribution with mean zero is

$$f(x) = \frac{1}{\sqrt{2\pi}\,\sigma} \exp\left[-\frac{1}{2}\left(\frac{x}{\sigma}\right)^2 \right]$$

Which of these two normal distributions is more peaked? The question does not seem difficult to answer: Virtually all would agree that the normal distribution with the smaller standard deviation ($\sigma = 1$) appears more peaked. This conclusion is not surprising since the standard deviation is a well-known measure of spread, and spread is essentially the inverse of peakedness. However, the classical moment-based indicant of kurtosis leads us to a different conclusion. Since all normal distributions have the same kurtosis ($\gamma_2 = 0$, $\beta_2 = 3$), the classical measure leads us to conclude that both curves in Figure 20. 2 have the same peakedness. Hence, kurtosis is not a measure of peakedness as we would normally define that feature of a curve. In this example, the standard deviations vary.

The astute reader might suggest that although kurtosis is not a measure of peakedness for curves with unequal standard deviations, perhaps kurtosis is a measure of peakedness for curves with equal standard deviations. We now show that kurtosis is not even a measure of peakedness for curves with equal standard deviations. Figure 20.3 shows two curves, denoted by $N(x)$ and $P(x)$,

$$N(x) = \frac{1}{\sqrt{2\pi}} \exp\left(-\frac{1}{2} x^2 \right)$$

$$P(x) = \frac{1}{3\sqrt{\pi}} \left(\frac{9}{4} + x^4 \right) \exp(-x^2)$$

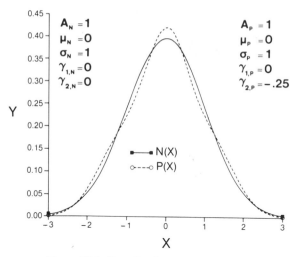

Figure 20.3. Two distributions $N(x)$ and $P(x)$ with the same area $(A = 1)$, same mean $(\mu = 0)$, same standard deviation $(\sigma_1 = 1)$, and same skewness $(\gamma_1 = 0)$ but different kurtosis $[\gamma_1 = 0$ for $N(x)$; $\gamma_1 = -0.25$ for $P(x)]$. Distribution $N(x)$ is a standard normal (Gaussian) distribution.

where $N(x)$ and $P(x)$, have the same total area or mass $(A = 1)$, the same mean $(\mu = 0)$, the same standard deviation $(\sigma = 1)$, and the same skewness $(\gamma_1 = 0)$ but different kurtosis (Kaplansky, 1945). Which curve, $N(x)$ or $P(x)$, is more peaked? Most would agree that $P(x)$ appears more peaked than $N(x)$. (Here $N(x)$ is the standard normal distribution.) What conclusions do we draw from γ_2? Since $N(x)$ is a normal distribution, $\gamma_2 = 0$ for $N(x)$. However, $\gamma_2 = -0.25$ for $P(x)$. Hence, on the basis of the classical moment-based indicant of kurtosis, $N(x)$ is more peaked than $P(x)$ since peakedness is said to increase as γ_2 increases. Thus, kurtosis is not a measure of peakedness as we would normally define that feature of a curve even in the case of equal standard deviations. Since the moment-based indicant of kurtosis is not a measure of peakedness in the case of unequal standard deviations and it is not a measure of peakedness in the case of equal standard deviations, it is not a measure of peakedness.

A third problem with the classical set of moment-based indicants is that the reference point and scale parameter are always fixed rather than open to selection by the investigator. For instance, the reference point is either set at the origin (for $k = 1$) or at the arithmetic mean (for $k = 2, 3, 4$), and the scale parameter is always set at 1 (for $k = 1, 2$) or at the standard deviation (for $k = 3, 4$). The reference point and scale parameter highlight particular features of a waveform and therefore should be open to selection by the investigator.

A fourth problem is that small fluctuations in sampling or outliers can have dramatic effects on the higher order moments and, hence, the variance associated with such measures tends to be large (Ratcliff, 1979; Yule & Kendall, 1937). Although the classical shape descriptors of skew and kurtosis have nevertheless proven informative in studies of IEMG and of EEG activity, the sensitivity to components of the waveform that are distal to the mean is particularly problematic when the number of observations constituting the waveform is small, measurement error is large, or the processes of theoretical interest are represented by the central components of the waveform.

Relatedly, Ratcliff (1979) further criticized moments and cumulants as a means of characterizing reaction-time distributions because "the measures give information about a part of the frequency curve that is of little theoretical interest" (p. 455; but see Sternberg, 1969). Of course, this assertion could change if theoretical interests were to change or if the reference point could be specified by the investigator to better weight the aspects of the waveform that are of the greatest theoretical import. Ratcliff (1979) proposed instead to represent reaction-time distributions in terms of the parameters of explicit distribution functions. For instance, he has suggested that the parameters of the convolution of a normal distribution and an exponential distribution provide a good summary of empirical reaction-time distributions (Ratcliff, 1978, 1979). Snodgrass, Luce, and Galanter (1967) have concluded, on the other hand, that the double monomial gives the best fit to reaction-time distributions. When there is agreement that a particular parametric distribution fits a particular set of waveforms, then the parameters of that distribution will provide a useful summary of the members of that set of waveforms. But such an agreement on a particular parametric distribution does not even appear to exist in Ratcliff's domain of interest—reaction time distributions. A consensus on a particular parametric function for sets of nonrhythmic waveforms in psychophysiology would be even less likely because of their relative complexity and variation with situational demands. Explicit parametric functions, therefore, are unlikely to provide a comprehensive procedure for representing nonrhythmic waveforms in psychophysiology. It should be noted, too, that the parameters of an explicit distributional form can often be expressed in terms of a few lower order moments. For instance, the parameters of the normal distribution are the mean and variance, both moment-based indicants. As mentioned earlier, the mean is the first moment about the origin, and the variance is the second moment about the mean. In contrast to the parameters of a specific distributional form, moment-based indicants provide a way of comparing and contrasting features of nonrhythmic waveforms of different distributional forms. Thus, moment-based indicants have the important advantage of being distribution free in that they do not assume a specific functional form for the waveform except for nonnegativity and boundedness.

A final problem with the classical set of four moment-based indicants is that they do not fully characterize an NB waveform. Consequently, valuable information about the shape of the NB waveform may be lost if the investigator is restricted to the classical set of indicants. This is especially the case if the waveform is irregular in shape. In the following section, we outline modifications to the classical approach for representing NB waveforms that minimize these limitations. These modifications include the following: (1) waveform-dependent and waveform-independent reference points α selected by the investigator, (2) a scaling factor β to enable comparisons across the universe of NB waveforms, (3) computation of a measure of size A of waveforms and expression of waveforms in terms of unit mass to separate size from shape of waveforms, (4) extraction of the kth root of the moments to maintain the same units of measurement for moments of all orders,[2] and (5) multidimensional indicants of asymmetry and dispersion γ_k to provide more systematic and comprehensive measures of these waveform features.

20.2   WAVEFORM MOMENT ANALYSIS: PROBING THE NB WAVEFORM

We now present a comprehensive method of characterizing the size and shape of an NB waveform. As mentioned in the introduction, we call this method waveform moment analysis. This method provides a system for probing the topography of an NB waveform. Furthermore, WAMA provides a solution to the difficulties associated with the classical set of four moment-based indicants. First, WAMA introduces a multidimensional indicant of dispersion and a multidimensional indicant of asymmetry to replace the classical unidimensional indicants of dispersion and asymmetry. Dispersion and asymmetry are features that are much too rich to be always summarized by single numbers, particularly when the investigator is confronted with complex bioelectric waveforms. Second, WAMA subsumes the misunderstood concept of kurtosis as one of a set of potential indicants within the multidimensional framework for dispersion. Third, WAMA allows the investigator to select the reference point and scale parameter for the moment-based indicants, thereby permitting the experimental question to shape the analysis. Finally, WAMA defines a set of moment-based indicants that fully characterizes the NB waveform. Computation of a particular subset of those indicants yields an approximate characterization of the NB waveform. As more indicants are computed, more information is extracted from the waveform and the characterization improves.

Let $\gamma_k(\alpha, \beta)$ denote a general moment-based indicant, where k is the order of indicant, α is the reference point, and β ($\beta > 0$) is the scale parameter. The reference point and scale parameter are selected by the experimenter. We define the general moment-based indicant of order k as follows:

$$\gamma_k(\alpha, \beta) = \left[\sum_{i=1}^{N} \left(\frac{x_i - \alpha}{\beta} \right)^k g(x_i) \right]^{1/k} \tag{7}$$

Some simple algebra shows that

$$\left[\sum_{i=1}^{N} \left(\frac{x_i - \alpha}{\beta} \right)^k g(x_i) \right]^{1/k} = \frac{1}{\beta} \left[\sum_{i=1}^{N} (x_i - \alpha)^k g(x_i) \right]^{1/k} \tag{8}$$

We now list some important theorems that provide the foundation for WAMA (see the appendix for justification of these theorems).

Theorem 1. An NB waveform is fully and uniquely characterized by the moment-based indicants and the total mass.

Theorem 2. An NB waveform of N observations is fully and uniquely characterized by the first $N-1$ moment-based indicants and the total mass.

Theorem 3. The odd moment-based indicants provide a multidimensional indicant of asymmetry about α.

Theorem 4. The even moment-based indicants provide a multidimensional indicant of dispersion about α.

Theorem 5. Suppose we have two waveforms made up of N observations with N

odd. Then the two waveforms are identical if and only if the first $\frac{1}{2}$ $(N-1)$ odd moment-based indicants, the first $\frac{1}{2}$ $(N-1)$ even moment-based indicants and the total mass are equal. If N is even, then the two waveforms are identical if and only if the first $\frac{1}{2}$ N odd moment-based indicants, the first $\frac{1}{2}$ $N-1$ even moment-based indicants, and total mass are equal.

We now review some special features of these moment-based indicants. First, the kth moment-based indicant is taken to the kth root. Consequently, all moment-based indicants have the same dimensionality and can be interpreted as distance functions when k is even. Second, asymmetry and dispersion are both multidimensional, providing more comprehensive indices of these waveform features. Third, each classical indicant reviewed in the previous section is a special case of or is a simple transformation of a general WAMA indicant. Hence, all information in the classical shape descriptors can be derived from WAMA indicants.
Thus,

$$\gamma_1(0, 1) = \left[\sum_{i=1}^{N} \left(\frac{x_i - 0}{1} \right)^1 g(x_i) \right]^1$$

$$= \sum_{i=1}^{N} x_i g(x_i) = \mu.$$

is the arithmetic mean;

$$\gamma_2(\mu, 1) = \left[\sum_{i=1}^{N} \left(\frac{x_i - \mu}{1} \right)^2 g(x_i) \right]^{1/2}$$

$$= \left[\sum_{i=1}^{N} (x_i - \mu)^2 g(x_i) \right]^{1/2} = \sigma$$

is the standard deviation;

$$[\gamma_3(\mu, \sigma)]^3 = \sum_{i=1}^{N} \left(\frac{x_i - \mu}{\sigma} \right)^3 g(x_i) = \gamma_1$$

is the skewness; and

$$[\gamma_4(\mu, \sigma)]^4 - 3 = \sum_{i=1}^{N} \left(\frac{x_i - \mu}{\sigma} \right)^4 g(x_i) - 3 = \gamma_2$$

is the kurtosis. Fourth, as noted, kurtosis is no longer interpreted as an indicant of the peakedness of an NB waveform. Rather, in WAMA, kurtosis is a measure of dispersion of order 4 with reference point μ and scale parameter σ. By contrast, the standard deviation is a measure of dispersion of order 2 with reference point μ and scale parameter 1. Fifth, the multidimensional indicant of dispersion for a specified reference point and scale parameter has the following nice properties:

(a) $$\min \left| \frac{x_i - \alpha}{\beta} \right| < \gamma_{2k}(\alpha, \beta) < \max \left| \frac{x_i - \alpha}{\beta} \right|$$

or equivalently that

$$\frac{1}{\beta} \min |x_i - \alpha| < \gamma_{2k}(\alpha, \beta) < \frac{1}{\beta} \max |x_i - \alpha|$$

where $2k$ denotes an even moment-based indicant;

(b) $\gamma_{2s}(\alpha, \beta) < \gamma_{2t}(\alpha, \beta)$ if $s < t$ unless all x_i are equal.

This means that the sequence of indicants of dispersion is strictly increasing;

(c) $$\lim_{k \to \infty} \gamma_{2k}(\alpha, \beta) = \max \left| \frac{x_i - \alpha}{\beta} \right|$$

$$= \frac{1}{\beta} \max |x_i - \alpha|$$

This means that the sequence of indicants of dispersion has the finite limit $\beta^{-1} \max |x_i - \alpha|$ for NB waveforms. Recall that $\max |x_i - \alpha|$ has a finite value in the case of NB waveforms. If, on the other hand, the $x_i's$ are unbounded, then $\gamma_{2k}(\alpha, \beta)$ goes to infinity as $k \to \infty$.

It is worth mentioning that WAMA indicants are closely related to the concept of generalized mean. A generalized mean denoted by $M(t)$ is defined as

$$M(t) = \left(\frac{1}{N} \sum_{i=1}^{N} x_i^t \right)^{1/t}$$

where $x_i \geq 0$ is $(i = 1, 2, \ldots, N)$, and $-\infty < t < +\infty$ (Abramowitz, 1965). Moreover, a generalized mean is a special case of a weighted generalized mean, which may be defined as

$$\left[\frac{\sum_{i=1}^{N} f(x_i) x_i^t}{\sum_{i=1}^{N} f(x_i)} \right]^{1/t}$$

where $x_i \geq 0$ and $f(x_i) > 0$ (Hardy, Littlewood, & Polya, 1967). If we set $t = -1$, the generalized mean equals the harmonic mean; if $t \to 0$, the generalized mean converges to the geometric mean; and if $t = 1$, the generalized mean equals the arithmetic mean. There are important differences between WAMA indicants and generalized weighted means: (1) WAMA allows $x_i - \alpha$ to be negative as well as nonnegative and (2) WAMA assumes that t is a positive integer. It might be noted that generalized means have an interesting history. The first proposal to use generalized means appears to have been by Gauss. In 1816, he proposed the use of generalized means to estimate the dispersion of errors in astronomical measurement (Norris, 1976). Generalized means were also explored in the nineteenth century by Gustav Fechner, the father of psychophysical measurement (Norris, 1976).

20.2.1 Interpretation of moment-based indicants

If we inspect the formula for the general moment-based indicant

$$\gamma_k\,(\alpha,\,\beta) = \frac{1}{\beta}\left[\sum_{i=1}^{N}(x_i-\alpha)^k g(x_i)\right]^{1/k}$$

we see that fundamental element of that formula is $(x_i-\alpha)^k\,g(x_i)$. It is useful to think of that element as a weighted Euclidean distance. In particular, if k is even, then

$$(x_i-\alpha)^k\,g(x_i) = |x_i-\alpha|^k g(x_i)$$

$$= |x_i-\alpha||x_i-\alpha|^{k-1}g(x_i)$$

Therefore, we can consider $(x_i-\alpha)^k\,g(x_i)$ as the Euclidean distance between x_i and α, $|x_i-\alpha|$, weighted by $|x_i-\alpha|^{k-1}\,g(x_i)$. Similarly, for k odd,

$$(x_i-\alpha)^k\,g(x_i) = \begin{cases} |x_i-\alpha|\,|x_i-\alpha|^{k-1}\,g(x_i), & x_i > \alpha \\[2mm] |x_i-\alpha|\,[-|x_i-\alpha|^{k-1}]\,g(x_i), & x_i < \alpha \end{cases}$$

Thus, for k odd, $|x_i-\alpha|$ is weighted by $|x_i-\alpha|^{k-1}\,g(x_i)$ when x_i is to the right of α, and $|x_i-\alpha|$ is weighted by $-|x_i-\alpha|^{k-1}\,g(x_i)$ when x_i is to the left of α. To appreciate the role of the weight $|x_i-\alpha|^{k-1}\,g(x_i)$, let k increase. We see that:

$$\lim_{k\to\infty} |x_i-\alpha|^{k-1}\,g(x_i) = \begin{cases} 0, & |x_i-\alpha|<1 \\ g(x_i), & |x_i-\alpha|=1 \\ +\infty, & |x_i-\alpha|>1 \end{cases}$$

Figure 20.4 provides a pictorial representation of these effects under the simplifying assumption that $g(x_i)=1$.

This weighting function has the effect of providing a unique probe of asymmetry for each odd k and a unique probe of dispersion for each even k. Each moment-based indicant uses all of the data, but as k increases, large deviations x_i from α tend to play an increasingly large role.

20.2.2 The reference point (α)

The specification of the reference point is an important decision for the investigator because the reference point is fundamental to the interpretation of the indicants. There are two general classes of reference points: (1) waveform-independent reference points and (2) waveform-dependent reference points. The arithmetic mean or center of gravity is a good example of a commonly used waveform-dependent reference point. Waveform-dependent reference points tend to vary across subjects and conditions. If we are interested in the shape of a waveform with reference to a fixed point common to all subjects and conditions, then a waveform-independent reference point must be used. In the physics example displayed in Figure 20.1, the beginning of the bar, the end of the bar, and the midpoint of the bar are possible choices for waveform-independent reference points.

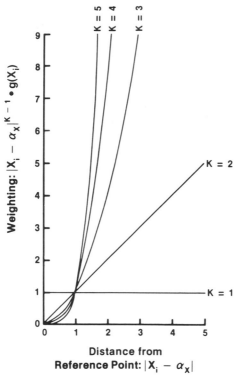

Figure 20.4. Weighting of distance of abscissa value x_i from reference point α_x as function of k, order of moment, and distance $[x_i - \alpha_x]$ under simplifying assumption that $g(x_i) = 1$. (From "Waveform Moment Analysis in Psychophysiological Research," by J. T. Cacioppo & D. D. Dorfman, 1987, *Psychological Bulletin, 102*, p. 426.)

Let us illustrate the fundamental difference between a waveform-dependent versus a waveform-independent reference point by comparing inferences derived from the arithmetic mean of the waveform as a reference point versus the midpoint of the bar as a reference point. Consider the two waveforms shown in Figure 20.5. Both waveforms are identical except for their location along the bar. It is clear from inspecting Figure 20.5 and equation (8) that if the reference point for each waveform is specified as the arithmetic mean, then the asymmetry in these waveforms would be equal and zero for all odd moment-based indicants. If, however, the reference point is defined as the midpoint of the bar, then the asymmetry in these waveforms would be different from zero, equal in absolute value, but opposite in sign for all odd moment-based indicants. Thus, although both reference points give WAMA indicants that are informative and interpretable, the particular information and interpretation derived from the waveform depends upon the reference point selected by the investigator. It is worth pointing out that in this example the WAMA indicants of dispersion – the even WAMA indicants – are identical for both waveforms irrespective of whether the reference point is the mean of the waveform or the midpoint of the bar.

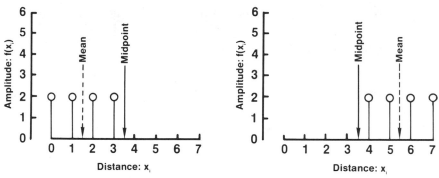

Figure 20.5. Two waveforms or responses atop identical bars. Waveforms are viewed as symmetrical if arithmetic mean is specified as reference point when calculating WAMA indicants of asymmetry and dispersion. WAMA indicants about midpoint of bar, however, indicate that waveform on left is asymmetrical with preponderance of amplitudes stacked on lower end of bar, whereas waveform on right is asymmetrical with preponderance of amplitudes stacked at upper end of bar. (From "Waveform Moment Analysis in Psychophysiological Research," by J. T. Cacioppo & D. D. Dorfman, 1987, *Psychological Bulletin, 102*, p. 428.)

20.2.3 *The scale parameter (β)*

As with reference points, there are two general classes of scale parameters: (1) waveform-independent scale parameters and (2) waveform-dependent scale parameters. If we set β equal to 1 or equal to the length of the bar, for instance, we are using a waveform-independent scale parameter. If, on the other hand, we set β equal to the standard deviation of the waveform or the length of the waveform, we are using a waveform-dependent scale parameter.

Summing up, WAMA permits the investigator to select the reference point and scale parameter. In some cases, there may be a literature or theory to guide the selection; in other cases, one may wish to conduct exploratory analyses in which the empirical utility of various choices is evaluated for the phenomena of interest. In any case, the investigator should have a good rationale for her or his choice or should cross-validate studies whose parameters are derived empirically.

20.3   ILLUSTRATIVE APPLICATIONS

We now present some illustrative applications of WAMA to the time domain, the amplitude domain, and the frequency domain.

20.3.1   *Time domain*

Suppose that we have a waveform that consists of a sequence of nonnegative amplitudes observed over some interval of time. As noted at the outset of the chapter, such a waveform is often called a response. Let t_i denote the time at which *the i*th amplitude denoted by $f(t_i)$ is recorded at some site, t_i ranges along $t_1, t_2, ..., t_N$, and $f(t_i) \geq 0$ for all t_i.

In the time domain, the formula for the moment-based indicant of order k is

$$\gamma_k(\alpha, \beta) = \frac{1}{\beta_t} \left[\sum_{i=1}^{N} (t_i - \alpha_t)^k g(t_i) \right]^{1/k} \tag{9}$$

where α_t is a reference point for the time dimension, β_t is a scale parameter for the time dimension, and

$$g(t_i) = \frac{f(t_i)}{\sum_{i=1}^{N} f(t_i)}$$

It should be pointed out that if the underlying population waveform is continuous rather than discrete, then the total mass of the waveform can be approximated by

$$\Delta \sum_{i=1}^{N} f(t_i),$$

where $\Delta = t_i - t_{i-1}$ ($i = 1, 2, \ldots, N$). If the investigator sets $\Delta = 1$, then, of course, Δ can be ignored. Note further that in the continuous case, we set

$$g(t_i) = \frac{\Delta f(t_i)}{\Delta \sum_{i=1}^{N} f(t_i)} = \frac{f(t_i)}{\sum_{i=1}^{N} f(t_i)}$$

Therefore, Δ can be ignored in the computation of the moment-based indicants when the underlying population waveform is continuous.

20.3.1.1 *Illustrative study*

To illustrate the application of WAMA to waveforms in the time domain, we present an example taken from Cacioppo and Dorfman (1987). In their study, they selected for analysis four of the seven muscle contraction tasks used by Cacioppo et al. (1983). Those tasks were chosen to generate discriminable IEMG responses. They used the data of six subjects from the original study and added data from an additional six subjects to this data set. Subjects squeezed a hand dynamometer in a prescribed fasion for 8-s epochs, the instructions differing for each task. The tasks selected for illustration here required that subject: (1) achieved and maintain a tension of 3 kg, (2) achieve and maintain a tension of 9 kg, (3) achieve a tension of 2 kg in 1 s and then increase the tension of the grip by 1 kg every second for the next 7 s, and (4) achieve a tension of 9 kg in 1 s and then decrease the tension by 1 kg every second for the next 7s. Subjects practiced each task once and then performed each task six additional times; IEMG activity, sampled once approximately every 400 ms, was recorded over the superficial forearm flexor muscle region of the preferred hand. The order in which the tasks were performed was varied between subjects and served as a between-subjects replication factor in the analysis (Cacioppo & Dorfman, 1987; Cacioppo et al., 1983). Figure 20.6 shows the

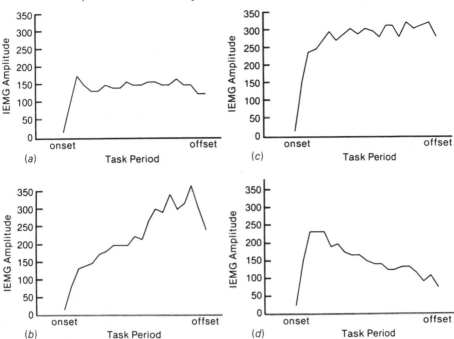

Figure 20.6. Averaged integrated electromyographic (IEMG) recordings obtained during tasks: (*a*) constant tension of 3 kg (upper left panel), (*b*) constant tension of 9 kg (upper right panel), (*c*) tension increasing from 2 to 9 kg (lower left panel), and (*d*) tension decreasing from 9 to 2 kg (lower right panel). (From "Waveform Moment Analysis in Psychophysiological Research," by J. T. Cacioppo & D. D. Dorfman, 1987, *Psychological Bulletin, 102*, p. 430.)

IEMG responses for the four tasks averaged over the 12 subjects and the six replications. It is quite apparent that there are differences in the topographies of the four waveforms. It should also be quite apparent that traditional measures of the IEMG responses based upon amplitude characteristics such as mean amplitude, peak amplitude, or peak counting are insensitive to changes in the waveform as it unfolds over time.

Each IEMG waveform was summarized by the first moment-based indicant in the amplitude domain ($\alpha = 0$, $\beta = 1$) and the first seven moment-based indicants in the time domain ($\beta = 1$). Since N is constant across all subjects, replications, and tasks, mean amplitude is proportional to total mass and therefore can be used to gauge the size of the response (cf. Cacioppo et al., 1983).

The first temporal moment about reference point zero (mean time) gauged the central tendency of the response in the time domain. The second, fourth, and sixth moment-based indicants about the mean gauged the dispersion of the response about its mean in the time domain; the third, fifth, and seventh moment-based indicants about the mean gauged the asymmetry of the response about its mean in the time domain.

Table 20.1 presents mean amplitude, mean time, dispersion time (an average of the indicants for $k = 2, 4, 6$), and asymmetry time (an average of the indicants for

Table 20.1. *Mean amplitude and means of time indicants as a function of task*

Measure	Task 1	Task 2	Task 3	Task 4
Mean amplitude[a]	126.32*	257.98**	202.12[+]	120.95*
Mean time[b]	4.46[+]	4.62[+]	5.08**	3.79*
Dispersion time[c]	2.47**	2.37*	2.35*	2.42[+]
Asymmetry time[c]	− 0.60[+]	− 0.70[+]	− 2.02*	1.55**

Note: Means in a row without a shared superscript (*,+,**) differ at $p < .05$ by the Duncan multiple-range test. From J. T. Cacioppo and D. D. Dorfman (1987).

[a] $\alpha_{f(t)} = 0$, $\beta = 1$.
[b] $\alpha_t = 0$, $\beta = 1$.
[c] $\alpha_t = \mu$, $\beta = 1$.

$k = 3, 5, 7$). Ordinarily, one would not average over the components of the vectors of dispersion and asymmetry. However, in this study, there was no interaction between tasks and components of dispersion or between tasks and components of asymmetry. Hence, to simplify this illustration, the components were averaged.

A Replication × Task (2×7) multivariate analysis of variance (MANOVA) was conducted on the data (Cacioppo & Dorfman, 1987). The main effect for Task was highly significant $[F(12, 45) = 10.82, p < .001]$, showing that these moment-based indicants discriminated among the four IEMG task-induced responses. No main effects for Replication or for Task × Replication interactions were significant, implying that the shapes of the distinctive task-induced IEMG responses were replicable. Cacioppo and Dorfman (1987) followed these analyses with Replication × Task univariate analyses of variance (ANOVAs) to determine the features on which the task-induced IEMG responses differed. Significant main effects for Task were obtained for mean time, dispersion time, asymmetry time, and mean amplitude. Again, no main effects for Replication or Task × Replication interactions were significant, implying that specific features of the shape of the task-induced IEMG responses were also replicable.

The results of pairwise comparisons by the Duncan multiple-range test are presented in Table 20.1, where means in a row with different subscripts differ significantly at $p < .05$. The pairwise comparisons tell you what particular features discriminate between pairs of waveforms. For instance, mean amplitude does not discriminate between Tasks 1 and 4, whereas mean time, dispersion time, and asymmetry time do discriminate. In summary, MANOVA, followed by ANOVAs and pairwise comparisons, provides one strategy to identify specific moment-based indicants or general features that discriminate among task-induced waveforms in the time domain (see also Russell, chapter 23). Furthermore, moment-based indicants can be easy to calculate, analyze, and interpret.

20.3.1.2 *How many moments?*

The number of moments needed to characterize the topography of a nonnegative waveform increases as the complexity of the family of waveforms under consideration increases. For instance, if all members of a family are exponential, then the first moment uniquely characterizes each member; if all members of a family are normal distributions, then the first two moments uniquely characterize each member; if all members of a family satisfy the Pearson system, then the first four moments suffice (see Johnson & Kotz, 1970). As mentioned earlier, if we have a family of discrete waveforms consisting of N points, then $N-1$ moments uniquely and fully characterize the normalized waveform (Norton & Arnold, 1985). If, on the other hand, the normalized waveform is continuous, then all of the moments are needed to uniquely and fully characterize the waveform. The lower order moments provide the most information, with increments in information decreasing as each higher order moment is added.

In the case of highly irregular, multimodal NB waveforms, the number of moments needed for an adequate characterization may be large. If one expands the Fourier transform of the NB waveform as a Taylor's series, the coefficients are proportional to the moments. One can therefore invert the Taylor's series approximation to evaluate the fidelity of the characterization (e.g., see Feller, 1966). In general, if the goal is prediction (e.g., multiple regression) or classification (e.g., discriminant analysis), use a relatively large number of moments and cross-validate. If, on the other hand, the goal is explanation or parsimonious description, a small number of moments (e.g., $k \leq 7$) should suffice.

20.3.2 Amplitude domain

The importance of amplitude measures in quantifying psychophysiological responses such as the EMG, EEG, and ERP has long been recognized. For instance, mean and peak amplitude have perhaps been the most widely used measures of the EMG in psychophysiology (see Goldstein, 1972; Lippold, 1967; McGuigan, 1978). Quantification of amplitudes has also been important in the study of EEG (Bronzino et al., 1981; Rieger, Krieglstein, & Schütz, 1979). In fact, Hans Berger, who published the first report on EEG in people, suggested that quantifications be performed on both frequencies and amplitudes (Berger, 1976/1929). Moreover, in their authoritative text on EEG technology, Cooper, Osselton, and Shaw (1980) noted that "one of the obvious features of an EEG is the amplitude of the fluctuations" (p. 235).

Suppose we observe a sequence of N amplitudes $f(t_i)$ $(i = 1, 2, ...,N)$ over some interval of time, where f is not necessarily nonnegative. Let us denote the jth distinct amplitude by f_j and the observed frequency of occurrence of f_j by N_j $(j = 1, 2, ..., p)$. Clearly, $p \leq N$. Let us now consider the observed frequency distribution of f_j. This observed frequency distribution will have a total mass of N. To convert this observed frequency distribution of amplitudes to unit mass, divide each N_j by N. Let us denote N_j/N by $g(f_j)$. Clearly,

$$\sum_{j=1}^{p} g(f_j) = \sum_{j=1}^{p} N_j/N$$

$$= N^{-1} \sum_{j=1}^{p} N_j = N^{-1} N = 1$$

Since $g(f_j) = N_j/N \geq 0$, and since $g(f_j)$ is bounded by 1, the observed amplitude distribution is an NB waveform. The population amplitude distribution will also be an NB waveform for psychophysiological responses. Moreover, under rather broad conditions, the sample moment-based indicants of the observed amplitude distribution can serve as estimates of the corresponding moment-based indicants of the underlying population amplitude distribution. We can therefore usefully perform a WAMA of the observed amplitude distribution. The formula for the amplitude moment-based indicant of order k is

$$\gamma_k(\alpha_f, \beta_f) = \frac{1}{\beta_f} \left[\sum_{j=1}^{P} (f_j - \alpha_f)^k \, g(f_j) \right]^{1/k} \tag{10}$$

where α_f is a reference point for the amplitude domain and β_f is a scale parameter for the amplitude domain. Equation (10) can be simplified. In particular,

$$\gamma_k(\alpha_f, \beta_f) = \frac{1}{\beta_f} \left[\sum_{j=1}^{P} (f_j - \alpha_f)^k g(f_j) \right]^{1/k}$$

$$= \frac{1}{\beta_f} \left[\sum_{j=1}^{P} (f_j - \alpha_f)^k \, \frac{N_j}{N} \right]^{1/k}$$

$$= \frac{1}{\beta_f} \left[\sum_{i=1}^{N} [f(t_i) - \alpha_f]^k \, \frac{1}{N} \right]^{1/k}$$

$$= \frac{1}{\beta_f} \left[\frac{\sum_{i=1}^{N} [f(t_i) - \alpha_f]^k}{N} \right]^{1/k}$$

It is important to emphasize that WAMA in the amplitude domain does *not* require that f_j be nonnegative but merely bounded. Thus, WAMA can be performed on the amplitude distribution of any psychophysiological signal recorded over time.

The WAMA of the amplitude distribution of a psychophysiological signal can often complement a WAMA of the signal in another domain such as the time domain or frequency domain (Cacioppo & Dorfman, 1987). Moreover, a WAMA in the amplitude domain should not be viewed as a rival to a WAMA in the time or frequency domain; each may contribute something to our understanding of the underlying process in question, and each may illuminate different features of the topography of the signal (Cacioppo et al., 1983). Finally, it is worth mentioning that amplitude moments are formally equivalent to probability moments in statistics (Sichel, 1949).

20.3.2.1 *Amplitude WAMA: IEMG*

To illustrate the application of WAMA to the amplitude domain, we first compute some higher order moment-based indicants of the amplitude distributions of the IEMG responses obtained in the empirical study described in the preceding. In this example, α_f was set at the mean and β_f was set at 1. Specifically, (1) indicants based on the second, fourth, and sixth moments about the mean amplitude were calculated to gauge dispersion and (2) indicants based on the third, fifth, and seventh moments about the mean amplitude were calculated to gauge asymmetry. Results of the 2 × 7 (Replication × Task) ANOVAs revealed significant task main

Table 20.2. *Means of higher order amplitude indicants as a function of task*

Measure	Task 1	Task 2	Task 3	Task 4
Dispersion amplitude	83.53*	146.76**	157.77**	108.08[†]
Asymmetry amplitude	45.38[†]	− 60.77*	103.98**	84.21[†] **

Note: Means in a row without a shared superscript (*,†,**) differ at $p < .05$ by the Duncan multiple-range test; $\alpha_{f(t)} = \mu$, $\beta = 1$. From J. T. Cacioppo and D. D. Dorfman (1987).

effects for dispersion amplitude and asymmetry amplitude (Cacioppo & Dorfman, 1987). Cell means and pairwise comparisons are summarized in Table 20.2. Notice that dispersion amplitude and asymmetry amplitude distinguish among most of the tasks. It is interesting that the IEMG responses did not differ for Tasks 1 and 4 on mean amplitude (see Table 20.1), whereas they did differ on dispersion amplitude. Thus, there is a greater variability in the amplitudes of the IEMG responses induced by Task 4. If we had restricted our probe to mean amplitude, which has often been done with IEMG responses, then we would have falsely concluded that the IEMG responses for Tasks 1 and 4 did not differ (Cacioppo & Dorfman, 1987).

20.3.2.2 *Amplitude WAMA: EEG*

Let us begin with an illustration of how to derive a set of amplitudes from a sample of EEG. Figure 20.7 presents a sample of an EEG record taken from Cooper, Osselton, and Shaw (1980, see their Figure 9.3, p. 237). Now suppose we measure the amplitudes at time points t_1, t_2, t_3, ..., t_N. This gives a set of N amplitudes $\{f(t_1), f(t_2), f(t_3), ..., f(t_N)\}$. To simplify the visual illustration, we set N equal to 8. The WAMA can be performed on such a set of N amplitudes. To aid in the interpretation of the WAMA, it is also useful to present a pictorial representation of the amplitude distribution. Since the population distribution of EEG amplitudes is apparently continuous, we present a histogram. Figure 20.8 shows a histogram of the set of eight amplitudes derived from Figure 20.7. If the width of the class intervals (bin widths) is small and N is large, then the histogram should provide a reasonable visual image of the underlying continuous amplitude density function, an amplitude domain NB waveform (cf. Hoaglin, 1985b). Empirical methods currently exist for deriving optimal bin widths for certain cases involving sequences of independent and identically distributed random variables (e.g., see Freedman & Diaconis, 1981; Scott, 1979). Such methods, however, may not apply to autocorrelated random variables such as EEG amplitudes.

The amplitude distribution for EEG is often found to be normally distributed (Cooper et al., 1980; Saunders, 1963, 1972). This is especially true when subjects are mentally idle (Elul, 1967, 1969). Elul (1967, 1969), however, found that the amplitude distribution was less likely to be normal during performance of mental arithmetic. Elul (1967) presented an interesting theory to explain why the amplitude distribution changed from normal in an idle state to nonnormal in a mentally active state. He suggested that the gross EEG is the sum of the outputs of a large number of generators. In the mentally idle state, Elul assumes that the generators are mutually independent. If all of the outputs are uniformly bounded, that is, all bounded by

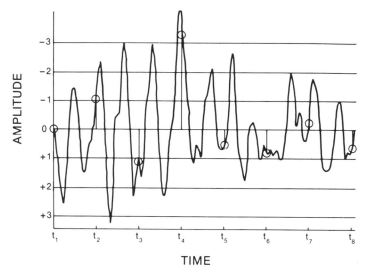

Figure 20.7. Example of EEG signal. (From *EEG Technology*, 3rd ed), by R. Cooper, J. W. Osselton, & J. C. Shaw, 1980, p. 237. Copyright 1980 by R. Cooper, J. W. Osselton, & J. C. Shaw. Reprinted by permission.)

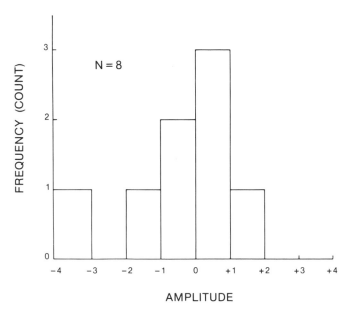

Figure 20.8. Histogram of set of eight amplitudes sampled at time points $t_1, t_2, t_3, \ldots,$ t_8 in EEG trace shown in Figure 20.7.

some fixed constant, and if mutual independence holds, then the central limit theorem applies (Feller, 1966). Therefore, in the mentally idle state, the sum of the outputs of such uniformly bounded and mutually independent generators will be approximately normally distributed. Now suppose the subject is mentally active. Then, according to Elul (1967), the generators become mutually interdependent. The central limit theorem no longer applies, and therefore the sum of the outputs of the component generators is transformed to a nonnormal distribution. Elul did not derive the effect of mutual interdependence on the amplitude distributions except to predict that they would lead to nonnormal distributions.

A similar phenomenon can be demonstrated in the area of mental testing (Lord, 1952). Suppose that a total test score (Y) is the sum of a large number of component test item scores (X_i, $i = 1, 2, \ldots, N$) so that $Y = \sum_{i=1}^{N} X_i$. Suppose further that all component test-item scores are correlated with some common underlying factor and are mutually independent if that correlation is zero. Lord (1952) showed that one can systematically modify the shape of the distribution of the total-test scores by manipulating the correlation of the component test-term scores with the common underlying factor.

Figure 20.9 shows four frequency distributions generated by manipulating that correlation. It is apparent that as the correlation increases, the moment-based indicants of dispersion increase. Hence, analysis of the moment-based indicants of dispersion provides a test of Elul's theory. Elul did not conduct a moment analysis; he merely classified amplitude distributions as normal or nonnormal. Such a dichotomous classification is much less informative than a waveform moment analysis. For one thing, his dichotomous classification scheme does not distinguish among normal distributions. Normal distributions may differ in both mean and standard deviation. For another, and perhaps most important, WAMA allows for discrimination among nonnormal distributions, whereas Elul's scheme lumps all nonnormal distributions together.

Elul, Hanley, and Simmons (1975) have also compared EEG amplitude distributions in normal children and in children with Down's syndrome. They found that normal children have nonnormal EEG amplitude distributions in the early postnatal period, which become increasingly normal before 1 year of age and remain so throughout subsequent development (Elul et al., 1975). By contrast, children with Down's syndrome exhibit highly nonnormal EEG amplitude distributions at all ages studied. The investigators argued that the brain tissue of normal children would be expected to have a much larger number of interconnections than the brain tissue of Down's syndrome children, thereby increasing the likelihood that any given cell is relatively independent of any other given cell. And it is mutual independence that results in normal distributions. If we varied the number of underlying factors mediating the component test item scores, we could perhaps simulate Elul's model of the EEG of normal children versus Down's syndrome children.

Fox and his associates (Fox, 1970; Fox & Norman, 1968) conducted some research quite relevant to Elul's theory of EEG amplitude distributions. They recorded the spontaneous EEG each millisecond from a microelectrode in the visual cortex of curarized and anesthetized cats. They computed an EEG amplitude frequency distribution from those recordings. Simultaneously, they recorded the number of times a particular nerve cell fired. They then correlated the amplitude of the microelectrode EEG (a measure of the EEG in the immediate vicinity of the

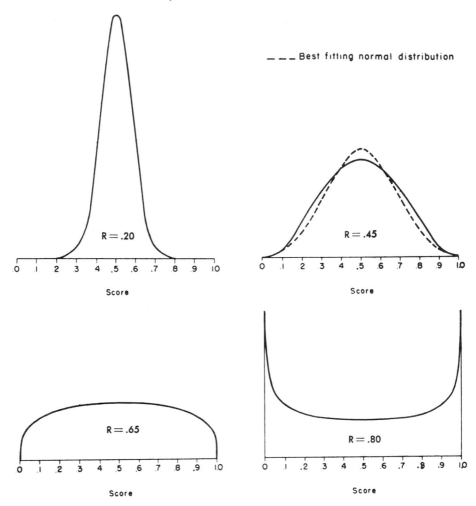

Figure 20.9. Frequency distribution of test scores as function of correlation (R) between common underlying trait and item scores. (From "A Theory of Test Scores," by F. Lord, 1952, *Psychometric Monographs*, Whole No. 7, p. 38. Copyright 1952 by F. Lord. Reprinted by permission.)

microelectrode) with the proportion of times the nerve cell fired at a given EEG voltage amplitude. Fox (1970) suggested that this correlation can serve as an index of neural homogeneity of the tissue around the microelectrode or, in the language of Elul, an index of the interdependence of the generators of the EEG. They performed their measurements and analyses under two conditions, in a spontaneous condition and in a condition in which the visual cortical nerve cell was driven by a flashing light. They found that the correlation between spike firing and EEG amplitude increased when the cells were driven by light. Figure 20.10 presents some

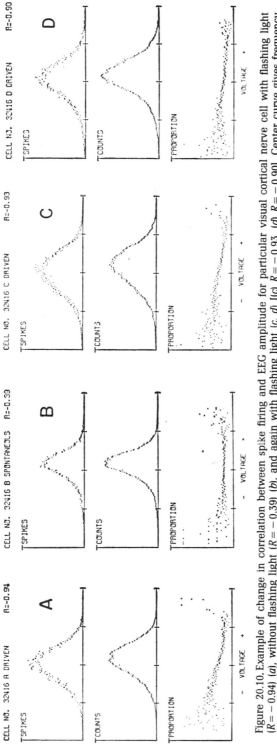

Figure 20.10. Example of change in correlation between spike firing and EEG amplitude for particular visual cortical nerve cell with flashing light ($R = -0.94$) (a), without flashing light ($R = -0.39$) (b), and again with flashing light (c, d) [(c) $R = -0.93$, (d) $R = -0.90$]. Center curve gives frequency distribution of EEG voltages, that is, EEG amplitude distribution. Top curve gives number of occurrences of cell spike at each voltage in center curve. Bottom curve gives observed conditional probability of spike firing at each voltage in center curve. (From "Functional Congruence: An Index of Neural Homogeneity and a New Measure of Brain Activity," by S. S. Fox & R. J. Norman, 1968, *Science, 159*, p. 1258. Copyright 1968 by S. S. Fox & R. J. Norman. Reprinted by permission.)

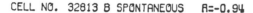

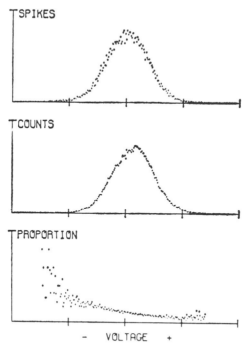

Figure 20.11. Example of high correlation between spike firing and EEG amplitude for particular visual cortical cell with no flashing light (spontaneous condition) ($R = -0.94$). Center curve gives EEG amplitude distribution. Top curve gives number of occurrences of cell spike at each voltage in center curve. Bottom curve gives observed conditional probability of spike firing at each voltage in center curve. (From "Functional Congruence: An Index of Neural Homogeneity and a New Measure of Brain Activity," by S. S. Fox & R. J. Norman, 1968, *Science, 159*, p. 1257. Copyright 1968 by S. S. Fox & R. J. Norman. Reprinted by permission.)

illustrative data on a particular nerve cell (cell no. 32416). First, we see that the absolute value of the correlation is smaller ($|R| = .39$, the sign of the correlation should be ignored) in the spontaneous case than in the driven case ($.90 \le |R| \le .94$). In conditions (a), (c), and (d), there were flashing lights; and in condition (b), there was no flashing light. We should therefore predict the smallest dispersion in condition (b), the spontaneous condition. As can be seen (middle panels), the results support this prediction derived from Lord's (1952) research. Fox and Norman (1968) also presented an example of a nerve cell with a high absolute value of the correlation with microelectrode EEG amplitude in the spontaneous condition ($|R| = .94$). The middle panel of Figure 20.11 shows the amplitude distribution for this cell (no. 32813) in the spontaneous condition. The dispersion does seem somewhat larger than in the spontaneous case for the cell with the small correlation ($|R| = .39$; see Figure 20.10). This finding also appears consistent with Elul's theory. Fox and Norman (1968) did not perform any statistical analyses of their amplitude distributions. A WAMA would allow an investigator to test formally Elul's theory, however.

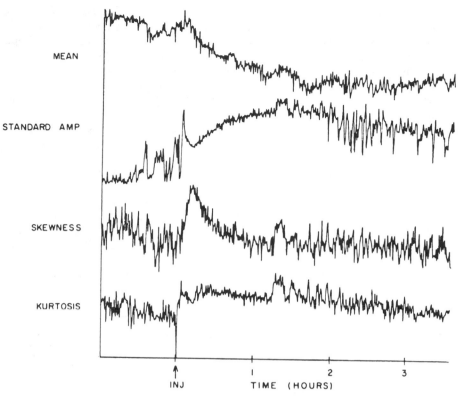

Figure 20.12. Plot of mean, standard deviation (standard amplitude), skewness, and kurtosis of amplitude distribution of cortical EEG obtained from rat. Arrow indicates when morphine sulfate (30 mg/kg) was injected. (From "Utilization of Amplitude Histographs to Quantify the EEG Effects of Systemic Administration of Morphine in the Chronically Implanted Rat," by J. D. Bronzino, M. L. Kelly, C. T. Cordova, N. H. Oley, & P. J. Morgane, 1981, *IEEE Transactions on Biomedical Engineering, BME-28*, p. 676. Copyright 1981 by J. D. Bronzino, M. L. Kelly, C. T. Cordova, N. H. Oley, & P. J. Morgane. Reprinted by permission.)

20.3.2.3 *EEG amplitude moment analysis: drug effects*

Figure 20.12 illustrates a classical moment analysis of a sequence of cortical EEG amplitude distributions on a rat before and after injection of morphine sulfate (Bronzino et al., 1981). These investigators computed the mean, standard deviation, skewness, and kurtosis of the time-varying amplitude distributions for 1 hr before and 4 hr after injection.[3] First, notice that skewness increases immediately after injection of morphine sulfate, returning to baseline after an hour. According to Bronzino et al. (1981), the increase in skewness results primarily from morphine-induced bursts of spindles. In general, moment-based indicants of asymmetry about zero or the mean are sensitive to the existence and polarity of monophasic EEG events. Also notice that kurtosis increases immediately after injection, gradually returning to baseline after about 150 min. The increase in kurtosis resulted primarily from morphine-induced high-voltage, low-frequency EEG waves (Bronzino et al.,

1981). Changes in the mean are of technical origin such as amplifier drift; changes in the standard deviation (standard amplitude) were not interpreted.[4]

Spectral analysis traditionally assumes a stationary time series. If the amplitude distribution changes over time, as illustrated in Figure 20.12, then the time series is not stationary. The Bronzino et al. (1981) study shows that moment-based indicants may be quite valuable for summarizing EEG amplitude distributions that are changing systematically over time, that is, the amplitude distributions of nonstationary time series.

Summing up, moment analyses of EEG amplitude distributions may provide valuable information to complement information extracted from traditional frequency or spectral analyses.

20.3.3 Frequency domain

There are a variety of waveforms in psychophysiology that are usefully represented in the frequency domain, for example, the EEG (e.g., Bohrer & Porges, 1982; see Coger, Dymond, & Serafetinides, 1979; Cooper et al., 1980; see also Porges & Bohrer, chapter 21).

One begins with a series of amplitudes observed sequentially in time. Such a series of observations is often called a time series. To obtain a frequency representation of that series of observations, one performs a spectral analysis; that is, one computes the power spectrum or power density spectrum of that collection of observations. The power spectrum is the Fourier transform of the autocovariance function of a stationary time series (Chatfield, 1980, p. 118). The population Fourier transform of a stationary time series is by definition a continuous function of frequency.

To estimate the power spectrum, one first detrends the means. Then the data are submitted to a Fast Fourier Transform (FFT) algorithm that efficiently computes a discrete approximation to the power spectrum. That discrete approximation is called a periodogram. One then smoothes the periodogram to obtain a continuous function that is a consistent estimate of the population power spectrum. Two points should be emphasized:

1 The power spectrum is not a reduction of the data. It is a transformation of a series of N observations to a continuous function, the power spectrum.[5] Data reduction must come after computation of the power spectrum.
2 A stationary series of observations can always be transformed to a power spectrum irrespective of whether the underlying process in rhythmic.

If the power of the spectrum is almost totally concentrated in a few very narrow frequency bands, then we can summarize the power spectrum in terms of those few frequency bands. If, on the other hand, the power spectrum is smeared over a broad spectral band in a rather smooth fashion, then the power spectrum cannot be fully characterized by a few narrow frequency bands. In that case, it may be useful to characterize the power spectrum in terms of moment-based indicants.

The power spectrum is a nonnegative waveform. If we assume that the power spectrum is band limited, then the power spectrum is an NB waveform. The power spectrum is sometimes called the *power density spectrum* (Cooper et al., 1980), the *spectral density function* (Chatfield, 1980), or the *power spectral density* (Saltzberg & Burch, 1971). Those terms make good sense because the power spectrum is a density function although not necessarily standardized to a unit mass. If we divide the

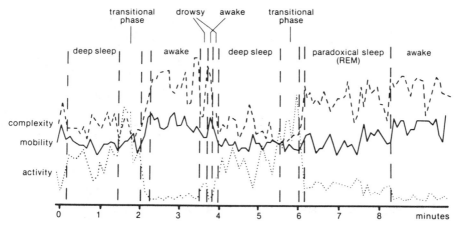

Figure 20.13. Hjorth's (1973) descriptors of activity, mobility, and complexity computed from every epoch of 5 s during a fronto-parietal recording from a rat. Descriptors display characteristic patterns, corresponding to states of sleep and waking estimated from original EEG trace. (From "The Physical Significance of Time Domain Descriptors in EEG Analysis," by B. Hjorth, 1973, *Electroencephalography and Clinical Neurophysiology, 34*, p. 322. Copyright 1973 by B. Hjorth. Reprinted by permission.)

power at each frequency by the total power, then the power spectrum is thereby transformed to a probability density function (Cacioppo & Dorfman, 1987). Hence, a moment analysis can be performed on the power spectrum (Cacioppo & Dorfman, 1984).

20.3.3.1 *Spectral moment analysis: EEG*

Psychophysiologists and neuroscientists interested in the EEG have suggested that indicants based on the moments may provide a valuable summary of the power spectrum (Hjorth, 1970, 1973, 1975; Saltzberg & Burch, 1971; Saltzberg et al., 1985). Hjorth (1970) proposed that EEG be summarized by three parameters: activity, mobility, and complexity. Those parameters are directly related to the two-sided power spectrum. Activity is the total mass of the two-sided power spectrum or equivalently the second moment of the amplitudes taken from zero baseline, often called *mean power* (Hjorth, 1970, 1975). Mobility is the standard deviation of the two-sided power spectrum normalized to a mass of 1. Note that the two-sided power spectrum is symmetrical about zero frequency with identical branches stretching into both negative and positive frequencies with mean frequency equal to zero (Hjorth, 1970). Therefore, Hjorth (1970) did not measure skewness or asymmetry because all odd moments are zero, and hence skewness is zero for the two-sided power spectrum. Hjorth's (1970) parameter complexity can be shown to equal the square root of a common measure of kurtosis, β_2, if we convert the two-sided spectrum to a unit mass (Cacioppo & Dorfman, 1987). Hjorth slightly modified his definition of complexity in later work so that a nondecaying sinusoid would give a value of zero (Hjorth, 1973, 1975).

Hjorth's (1970, 1973, 1975) three descriptors have been found to be quite useful. For instance, Figure 20.13 illustrates their utility in distinguishing among different

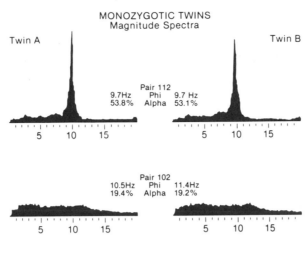

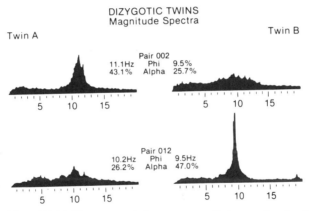

Figure 20.14 Electroencephalogram magnitude spectra (positive square root of power spectra) of monozygotic and dizygotic twins at rest, eyes closed. Magnitude spectra were standardized to mass of 1. Phi is median frequency within "alpha bump"; alpha is proportion of total spectrum contained within a 3-Hz band centered on φ. (From "Genetic Determination of EEG Frequency Spectra," by D. T. Lykken, A. Tellegen, & K. Thorkelson, 1974, *Biological Psychology, 1,* pp. 252, 254. Copyright 1974 by D. T. Lykken, A. Tellegen, & K. Thorkelson. Adapted by permission.)

states of sleeping and waking (Hjorth, 1973). Hjorth's descriptors have proved to be a valuable complement to conventional EEG scoring of sleep stages (Kanno & Clarenbach, 1985). They have also been used to distinguish between eyes open versus eyes closed and EEG reactions to performance on arithmetic and vocabulary tests (Chavance & Samson-Dollfus, 1978); they have also been used to assess the effects of hemodialysis on visual discrimination, memory, and tapping speed (Spehr et al., 1977) as well as to provide a topographical display of localized EEG abnormalities (Persson & Hjorth, 1983). Thus, Hjorth's (1970, 1973, 1975) approach suggests that a

Table 20.3. *WAMA indicants of magnitude spectra[a]*

Indicant	Monozygotic twins				Dizygotic twins			
	Pair 112		Pair 102		Pair 002		Pair 012	
	A	B	A	B	A	B	A	B
Mean frequency								
Dissimilarity[b]	0.01		0.03		0.87		0.15	
$\gamma_{1,0}$	9.48	9.47	8.43	8.46	9.93	9.06	9.50	9.65
Dispersion about mean frequency								
Dissimilarity[c]	0.14		0.06		0.75		1.47	
γ_{2,γ_1}	3.66	3.59	4.81	4.85	4.27	4.59	4.53	3.68
γ_{4,γ_1}	5.34	5.29	5.98	5.97	5.58	5.78	5.68	5.29
γ_{6,γ_1}	6.34	6.32	6.84	6.83	6.35	6.58	6.43	6.20
Asymmetry about mean frequency								
Dissimilarity[c]	0.26		0.10		16.32		0.53	
γ_{3,γ_1}	2.82	2.96	3.45	3.40	-2.73	2.60	2.75	2.57
γ_{5,γ_1}	5.12	5.19	5.76	5.73	-3.66	5.06	4.93	
γ_{7,γ_1}	6.35	6.40	6.97	6.95	4.11	6.38	6.12	5.96

[a] From J. T. Cacioppo and D. D. Dorfman (1987).
[b] Dissimilarity indices calculated using WAMA indicants, $\alpha = 0$, $\beta = 1$.
[c] Dissimilarity indices calculated using WAMA indicants, $\alpha = \mu$, $\beta = 1$.

moment-based representation of the power spectrum is of some value. There is a weakness in Hjorth's approach in that three descriptors may not adequately characterize the power spectrum (Denoth, 1975). Moreover, Hjorth (1970, 1973, 1975) used time domain approximations to the spectral moments, and practical limitations (signal-to-noise ratio) make it difficult to compute higher order spectral moment-based indicants in the time domain with sufficient accuracy (Hjorth, 1975). A more fruitful approach would involve computation of spectral moments directly from the power spectrum (Cacioppo & Dorfman, 1984; Saltzberg et al., 1985).

As another illustration of the utility of spectral moment-based indicants, let us look at a representation of the physically realistic one-sided power spectrum by moment-based indicants. In particular, consider some one-sided power spectra reported by Lykken, Tellegen, and Thorkelson (1974). Power spectra were computed from EEG samples with an FFT algorithm. The power spectrum was converted to a magnitude spectrum by taking the positive square root of power and was then standardized to unit mass.

Figure 20.14 presents four pairs of magnitude spectra, two pairs for monozygotic twins and two pairs for dizygotic twins. Monozygotic twins come from the same fertilized egg and are therefore identical genetically, whereas dizygotic twins come from different fertilized eggs and are no more alike genetically than brother and sister. All spectra were obtained under a rest condition, eyes closed. Lykken et al. (1974) were interested in the heritability of EEG. On the basis of genetic similarity, one should expect the monozygotic twin pairs to have more similar spectra than the dizygotic twin pairs. In accord with the genetic hypothesis for the inheritance of

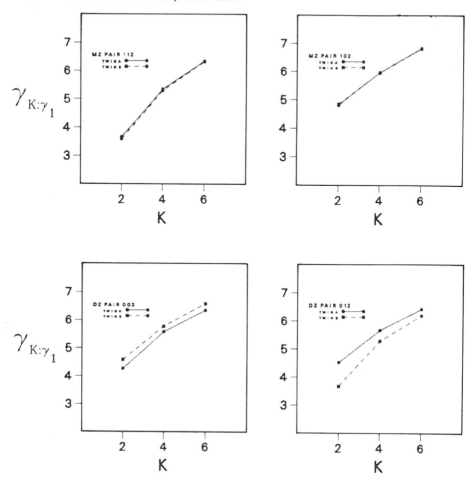

Figure 20.15. WAMA analysis of dispersion for monozygotic and dizygotic twin pairs.

EEG, the magnitude spectra for the monozygotic pairs do seem more alike than the magnitude spectra for the dizygotic pairs.

The results of a WAMA of the magnitude spectra are presented in Table 20.3. No statistical tests were performed because of the illustrative nature of this example. For each magnitude spectrum, the mean frequency $\gamma_{1,0}$ was computed, three WAMA indicants of dispersion about mean frequency (γ_{2,γ_1}, γ_{4,γ_1}, γ_{6,γ_1}) were computed, and three WAMA indicants of asymmetry were computed (γ_{3,γ_1}, γ_{5,γ_1}, γ_{7,γ_1}). Figure 20.15 presents the WAMA analyses of dispersion for the four twin pairs, and Figure 20.16 presents the WAMA analyses of asymmetry for the four twin pairs. The results shown in Figures 20.15 and 20.16 show that the monozygotic twin pairs are virtually identical on both dispersion and asymmetry, suggesting very high heritability of EEG magnitude spectra.

To gauge the dissimilarity between each twin spectra pair, we formed moment-based indexes of dissimilarity in mean frequency, in dispersion about mean

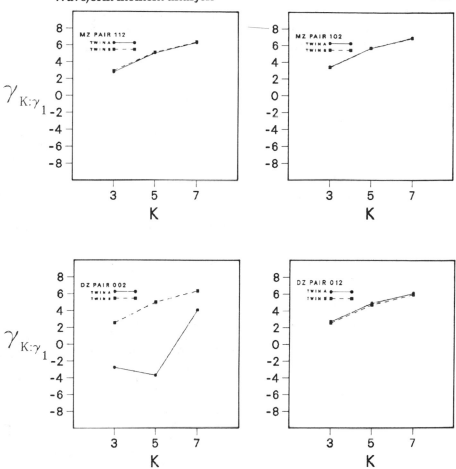

Figure 20.16. WAMA analysis of asymmetry for monozygotic and dizygotic twin pairs.

frequency, and in asymmetry about mean frequency. Let $\gamma_{k,\alpha}^{(m)}$ denote the moment-based indicant of order k taken about reference point α for twin m ($m=1$, 2) and let $n+1$ denote the number of indicants calculated. For instance $\gamma_{1,0}$ is the mean. The index of dissimilarity in mean was defined as

$$|\gamma_{1,0}^{(1)}-\gamma_{1,0}^{(2)}|;$$

the index of dissimilarity in dispersion was defined as

$$\sum_{k=1}^{n/2}|\gamma_{2k,\gamma_1}^{(1)}-\gamma_{2k,\gamma_1}^{(2)}|;$$

and the index of dissimilarity in asymmetry was defined as

$$\sum_{k=2}^{n/2+1}|\gamma_{2k-1,\gamma_1}^{(1)}-\gamma_{2k-1,\gamma_1}^{(2)}|.$$

As n increases, the moment-based indicants capture an increasing amount of the information in the NB waveform. In this example, $n+1=7$.

Table 20.3 presents the scores on dissimilarity for the four pairs of twins. Clearly, the EEG spectra of monozygotic twins were more similar than the EEG spectra of dizygotic twins on mean frequency, on dispersion about mean frequency, and on asymmetry about mean frequency. Such data are consistent with a genetic hypothesis for the inheritance of EEG (Lykken et al., 1974; Lykken, Tellegen, & Iacono, 1982).

Summarization of one-sided power spectra by moment-based indicants (mean, variance, skewness, kurtosis) has also been proposed for lengthy, nonstationary EEG records (Saltzberg et al., 1985). They compute the moments of the power spectrum from weighted samples of the autocorrelation to reduce the computational requirements of first generating power spectra. They are quite enthusiastic about moment-based summaries of power spectra:

> Of major significance in clinical applications, these parameters provide easily interpretable measures of change in basic stochastic properties of complex time series and therefore offer an efficient and mathematically rigorous approach to the analysis and monitoring of complex biological signals such as the EEG. (Saltzberg et al., 1985, p. 93)

As illustrated, these classical shape descriptors are a special case of WAMA.

20.3.3.2 Interpretation of spectral moments

The spectral moments have a simple interpretation in the time domain. If the time domain waveform has mean equal to zero baseline and if the time domain waveform is normalized to unit power, then the variance of the nth-order derivative of the normalized time domain waveform equals the $2n$th even moment of the two-sided power spectrum (Denoth, 1975) and twice the $2n$th even moment of the one-sided power spectrum.

There is also a simple relation between zero crossings per second and the power spectrum. The square of the number of crossings per second of the $(n-1)$th derivative of the time domain waveform equals the $2n$th even moment of the normalized two-sided power spectrum and twice the $2n$th even moment of the one-sided normalized power spectrum (Saltzberg & Burch, 1971; Saltzberg et al., 1985). This important result allows one to compute even moments of the power spectrum by counting zero crossings (Saltzberg, 1973; Saltzberg & Burch, 1971).

One sometimes summarizes the EEG power spectrum by presenting the relative power in four frequency bands (Ray, chapter 12): delta (0.5–3.5 Hz), theta (4–7.5 Hz), alpha (8–12 Hz), and beta (13–30 Hz). There are problems with that method of summarizing the power spectrum. First, it does not fully characterize the spectrum. Second, inspection of the spectra shown in Figure 20.14 shows that those four frequency bands can be arbitrary, except perhaps for the alpha band. The decomposition of the power spectrum into four frequency bands appears to be predicated upon the theory that a small number of frequency generators produce the EEG and a few factor-analytic studies have provided limited support in favor of this particular decomposition (e.g., see Ray, chapter 12). A power spectrum, however, is merely a transformation of a series of observations, and every series of observations can be transformed to a power spectrum. Therefore, the existence of a power spectrum is not evidence for the existence of frequency generators that operate exclusively within those frequency bands. A moment analysis, on the other hand, may shed light on aspects of the EEG power spectrum that are not readily captured by a frequency band representation. Thus, WAMA may serve as a valuable complement to the frequency band analysis.

20.3.4 *Statistical analysis*

Waveform moment analyses reduce an NB waveform to a vector of observations. Replications within subjects provide for estimation of within-subject variability and replications between subjects provide for estimation of between-subjects variability (e.g., see Cacioppo et al., 1983).

Under the assumption of the robustness of Gaussian statistics, statistical tests derived from classical univariate and multivariate normal distribution theory should be appropriate. On the other hand, there are methods for interval estimation and hypothesis testing that are distribution free–that is, they are not based upon classical Gaussian distribution theory–and yet are powerful. One such technique, the jackknife technique, can be applied to the moment-based indicants if one wishes to avoid classical Gaussian distribution theory (Arvesen & Salsburg, 1975; Efron, 1982; Rey, 1978; Tukey, 1969). Two very readable introductions to the jackknife technique written for psychologists can be found in Mosteller and Tukey's (1968) chapter and in Tukey's (1969) article.

20.4   CONCLUDING REMARKS

As R. A. Fisher (1922) noted, the purpose of statistical representations is to accomplish a reduction of a large quantity of data:

A quantity of data which by its mere bulk may be incapable of entering the mind is to be replaced by relatively few quantities which shall adequately represent the whole, or which, in other words, shall contain as much as possible, ideally the whole, of the relevant information contained in the original data. (p. 309)

Each form of quantitative representation achieves its economy by highlighting unique features of the data. Hence, although a waveform moment analysis may shed light on aspects of psychophysiological responses that are not readily captured by other representations, the moment-based representation of a waveform outlined in this chapter is not a rival to other representations.

The potential complementarity across forms of numeric representation in psychophysiology can be seen in the use of WAMA to represent the power spectrum of the EEG. The spectral analysis of the EEG has proven to be a breakthrough in the study of spontaneous cortical events and behavior (for a historical review, see Brazier, 1980; Ray, chapter 12). Ray organizes his discussion of the literature on the EEG in terms of delta (0.5–3.5 Hz), theta (4–7.5 Hz), alpha (8–12 Hz), and beta (13–30 Hz) activity. Recent research, however, has demonstrated that: (1) the amount of EEG activity within any given frequency band is often unrelated to the amount in other frequency bands (e.g., Ray & Cole, 1985) and (2) the pattern of EEG activity across the frequency domain rather than the simple amount within a given frequency band tends to be important (e.g., Tucker, Dawson, Roth, & Penland, 1985). Heretofore, it has been difficult to rigorously characterize the size and form of the EEG power spectrum, whereas WAMA provides both a powerful and sensitive means of accomplishing this characterization.

Finally, research in psychophysiology has repeatedly revealed that frequency and amplitude representations of bioelectrical signals provide unique and important information (e.g., Bronzino et al., 1981; Cacioppo et al., 1983). Glaria and Murray (1985), for instance, reported a study to determine the optimal method of EEG analysis to track changes in patient status during surgery. Electroencephalographic activity was recorded from 25 patients undergoing cardiac surgery, and the EEG recordings were subjected to a variety of frequency and amplitude analyses. Results revealed that changes in the EEG were usually apparent in both domains but that some cases were found in which an amplitude-only representation showed no changes whereas a frequency representation revealed changes and that some cases were found in which a frequency-only representation showed no changes whereas an amplitude representation revealed changes. The authors concluded that "to avoid missing these more subtle changes, techniques which inherently use both an amplitude and frequency approach should be used" (Glaria & Murray, 1985, p. 329). The features of the data that were extracted in the amplitude and frequency analyses conducted by Glaria and Murray (1985) were not directly comparable, however, making rigorous comparisons across domains difficult. On the other hand, WAMA has the advantage of providing systematic and comparable analyses of complex waveforms across domains of representation.

In sum, waveform moment analysis offers a unique and significant reduction of NB waveforms in the time domain, in the frequency domain, and of arbitrary bounded waveforms in the amplitude domain. It permits interindividual and intraindividual comparisons, and the moment-based indicants can provide precise descriptions regarding the manner in which the waveforms of interest differ. Hence, if, as Fisher (1922) suggested, one major purpose of statistics is to summarize as much as possible the useful information contained in a data set, then we believe that a waveform moment analysis appears to have a good chance of accomplishing this goal in a wide variety of applications in psychophysiology.

APPENDIXES

The theorems and proofs presented in these appendixes are, for the most part, straightforward adaptations of classical results of theoretical statistics. Unfortunately, the relevant theorems and proofs in theoretical statistics were usually not in exactly the form we needed for direct application to psychophysiological waveforms. For purposes of completeness, the appendixes present all theorems and proofs in exactly the way they are needed for fruitful application to psychophysiology.

Appendix A: The NB waveform, the moments, and the Fourier Transform

Assume that we have an NB waveform $f(x)$ with $|f(x)| \le B < \infty$ and $|x| \le C < \infty$. To simplify the exposition, we restrict our analysis to two simple but fundamental cases of broad interest: (1) the waveform is continuous except perhaps for a countable number of discontinuities and (2) the waveform is discrete. In case 1, we define the kth moment about an arbitrary point α as

$$v_{k,\alpha} = \int_{-c}^{c} \frac{(x-\alpha)^k f(x) \ dx}{A}$$

where

$$A = \int_{-c}^{c} f(x) dx.$$

In case 2 we define the kth moment about α as

$$v_{k,\alpha} = \sum_{j} \frac{(x_j - \alpha)^k f(x_j)}{A}$$

where the summation may be over a finite or countably infinite set and where

$$A = \sum_{j} f(x_j) < \infty.$$

Let $g(x) = f(x) / A$, so that $g(x)$ is $f(x)$ converted to unit mass and is therefore a density function. We shall call an NB waveform converted to unit mass a unitized NB waveform.

Theorem A.1. Moments of all orders exist for an NB waveform.

Proof. First, consider case 1. By assumption, $|x| \leq C < \infty$. Therefore,

$$|x - \alpha| \leq |x| + |\alpha| \leq C + |\alpha| < \infty$$

so that $|x - \alpha|$ is bounded. Let the bound be $D = C + |\alpha|$.
Hence,

$$\int_{-c}^{c} |x - \alpha|^k g(x) \, dx \leq \int_{-c}^{c} D^k g(x) \, dx = D^k < \infty$$

and therefore all moments exist. Now consider case 2. By a like argument.

$$\sum_{j} (x_j - \alpha)^k g(x_j) \leq \sum_{j} D^k g(x_j) = D^k \sum_{j} g(x_j) = D^k < \infty$$

Thus, all moments exist in the discrete case. That completes the proof.

For any fixed α, knowledge of the moments about α of a unitized NB waveform is equivalent to knowledge of the Fourier Transform of that waveform. This major fact is embodied in the next theorem.

Theorem A.2. For any fixed α, the sequence of moments about α of a unitized NB waveform is in one-to-one correspondence with the Fourier Transform of the unitized NB waveform.

We define the Fourier Transform of the unitized NB waveform $g(x)$ as

$$\phi_g(u) = \int_{-c}^{c} e^{iux} g(x) \, dx$$

or

$$\phi_g(u) = \sum_{j} e^{iux} g(x_j)$$

for cases 1 and 2, respectively, where $i = \sqrt{-1}$. Note that since $g(x)$ has unit mass, its Fourier Transform can be called a characteristic function (Feller, 1966).

Proof. We first show that the Fourier Transform of $g(x)$ uniquely determines the moments of $g(x)$ taken about the origin. From Theorem A.1, we know that all of the moments of an NB waveform exist. Therefore,

$$\frac{d^k \phi_g (0)}{du^k} = i^k v_{k,0}$$

for all k, where $v_{k,0}$ denotes the kth moment of $g(x)$ taken about the origin (Burrill, 1972, Theorem 12–3B, p. 263). Hence, the Fourier Transform of $g(x)$ uniquely determines the moments of $g(x)$ taken about the origin. We now show that for any fixed α, the Fourier Transform of $g(x)$ uniquely determines the moments of $g(x)$ taken about α. According to binominal theorem,

$$(x - \alpha)^k = \sum_{i=0}^{k} \binom{k}{i} x^i (-\alpha)^{k-i}$$

It immediately follows that

$$v_{k,\alpha} = \sum_{i=0}^{k} \binom{k}{i} v_{i,0} (-\alpha)^{k-1}$$

Therefore, for any fixed α, the moments of $g(x)$ taken about the origin uniquely determine the moments of $g(x)$ taken about α. Since the Fourier Transform of $g(x)$ uniquely determines the moments of $g(x)$ taken about the origin, for any fixed α it also uniquely determines the moments of $g(x)$ taken about α.

We now show that for any fixed α, the moments of $g(x)$ taken about α uniquely determine the Fourier Transform of $g(x)$. Since all of the moments of $g(x)$ exist, its Fourier Transform can be represented as the power series.

$$\phi_g (u) = \sum_{k=0}^{\infty} \frac{v_{k,0} (iu)^k}{k!}$$

in the interval of convergence of the series (Burrill, 1972, Corollary, p. 264). Now the radius of convergence R of a power series is given by the root test (Rudin, 1974) so that

$$\frac{1}{R} = \lim_{k \to \infty} \sup \ |v_{k,0}|^{1/k} / (k!)^{1/k}$$

It is not difficult to show that the radius of convergence is infinity. Clearly

$$|x|^k \leq C^k \leq \infty$$

This implies that

$$v_{k,0} \leq C^k \leq \infty$$

Hence,

$$\lim_{k \to \infty} \sup |v_{k,0}|^{1/k} \leq C$$

Furthermore,

$$(k!)^{1/k} \to \infty$$

as $k \to \infty$. It therefore follows that

$$\lim_{k \to \infty} \sup |v_{k,0}|^{1/k}/(k!)^{1/k} = 0$$

and therefore the radius of convergence is infinity. Thus, the interval of convergence is $-\infty < u < +\infty$. Hence, the sequence of moments of $g(x)$ about the origin uniquely determines the Fourier Transform of $g(x)$ (see Feller, 1966, Appendix, p. 487). We now show that for a fixed α the sequence of moments about α uniquely determines the Fourier Transform of $g(x)$. It follows from the binomial theorem that

$$v_{k,0} = v_{k,\alpha} - \sum_{i=0}^{k-1} \binom{k}{i} v_{i,0}(-\alpha)^{k-i}$$

and therefore for any fixed α the moments about α uniquely determine the moments about the origin of $g(x)$. Hence, they also uniquely determine the Fourier Transform of $g(x)$. That completes the proof.

Corollary 1. For any fixed α, the moments about α of $g(x)$ and A are in one-to-one correspondence with the Fourier Transform of $f(x)$.

Proof. The Fourier Transform of $f(x)$ is easily shown to equal $A\phi_g(u)$. Moreover, the moments about α of $g(x)$ uniquely determine $\phi_g(u)$. Therefore, A and the moments about α of $g(x)$ uniquely determine $A\phi_g(u)$, the Fourier Transform of $f(x)$.

We now show that the Fourier transform of $f(x)$ uniquely determines the moments about α of $g(x)$. The Fourier Transform of $f(x)$, denoted $\phi_f(u)$, equals $A\phi_g(u)$. Moreover,

$$\phi_f(0) = A$$

Therefore, the Fourier Transform of $f(x)$ uniquely determines A and $\phi_g(u)$. Since $\phi_g(u)$ uniquely determines the moments about α of $g(x)$, $\phi_f(u)$ also uniquely determines the moments about α of $g(x)$. That completes the proof.

Corollary 2. For any fixed α, the moments about α of $g(x)$ and A are in one-to-one correspondence with $f(x)$.

Proof. From Corollary 1, we know that the moments about α of $g(x)$ and A are one-to-one correspondence with the Fourier Transform of $f(x)$. But the Fourier Transform of $f(x)$ is in one-to-one correspondence with $f(x)$ since waveforms and their Fourier Transforms are in one-to-one correspondence (Bracewell, 1978). It therefore follows that the moments about α of $g(x)$ and A are in one-to-one correspondence with $f(x)$.

The finite case

Suppose we have an NB waveform $f(x_j)$ where $j = 1, 2, \ldots, N$. In other words, suppose we have an NB waveform defined by a finite set of points. In that case, a very nice theorem applies.

Theorem A.3. An NB waveform defined by a finite set of points and its Fourier Transform are fully characterized by the first $N-1$ moments and the total mass of the NB waveform.

Proof. It readily follows from results presented in Norton and Arnold (1985) that the first $N-1$ moments suffice to give the finite sequence of points $[x_j, g(x_j), j = 1, 2, ..., N]$, where $g(x_j) = f(x_j)/A$. Hence, we have the NB waveform. Moreover, if we have the NB waveform, we have the Fourier Transform of the NB waveform. That completes the proof.

Thus, if we have an NB waveform defined by N points $[x_j, f(x_j) \ j = 1, 2, ..., N]$, that waveform is fully characterized by N numbers: the first $N-1$ moments and the total mass given that we specify the domain of the waveform $(x_1, x_2, ..., x_N)$.

Appendix B: Moment similarity and waveform similarity

We should expect that if the moments of two waveforms are similar, the waveforms should be similar. We now show that this is the case under rather broad and practical conditions. Let $g_1(x)$ and $g_2(x)$ represent two unitized NB waveforms with Fourier Transforms ϕ_{g_1} and ϕ_{g_2}, respectively, and let $v^{(1)}_{k,\alpha}$ and $v^{(2)}_{k,\alpha}$ represent the kth moment about α of $g_1(x)$ and $g_2(x)$, respectively. Assume that x is a lattice variable with $x_j = a + hj$, where j runs through $0, 1, 2, ..., N$ or through $0, 1, 2, ...,$ and where h is any positive constant representing the difference between x_{j+1} and x_j.

Theorem B.1. The distance between $g_1(x)$ and $g_2(x)$ diminishes as the distance between $(v^{(1)}_{1,\alpha}, v^{(1)}_{2,\alpha}, ...)$ and $(v^{(1)}_{1,\alpha}, v^{(2)}_{2,\alpha}, ...)$ diminishes, where the distance between the two moment sequences is defined as

$$\sum_{k=1}^{\infty} |v^{(1)}_{k,\alpha} - v^{(2)}_{k,\alpha}| \frac{(\pi/h)^k}{(k+1)!}$$

Note that this distance function is a weighted city-block distance function (Coombs, Dawes, & Tversky, 1970).

Proof. According to the inversion theorem for lattice variables (Feller, 1966, p. 484),

$$g_1(x) = \frac{h}{2\pi} \int_{-\pi/h}^{\pi/h} e^{-iux} \ \phi_{g_1}(u) du$$

$$g_2(x) = \frac{h}{2\pi} \int_{-\pi/h}^{\pi/h} e^{-iux} \ \phi_{g_2}(u) du$$

Let $y = x - \alpha$. The Fourier Transform of $g_1'(y) = g_1(y + \alpha)$ is

$$\phi'_{g_1} = e^{-i\alpha u} \phi_{g_1}$$

and the Fourier Transform of $g_2'(y) = g_2(y + \alpha)$ is

$$\phi'_{g_2} = e^{-i\alpha u} \phi_{g_2}.$$

Hence,

$$|g_1(x) - g_2(x)| = \frac{h}{2\pi} \left| \int_{-\pi/h}^{\pi/h} e^{-iu(x-\alpha)} [\phi'_{g_1}(u) - \phi'_{g_2}(u)] du \right|$$

$$\leq \frac{h}{2\pi} \int_{-\pi/h}^{\pi/h} |e^{-iu(x-\alpha)}| \, |\phi'_{g_1}(u) - \phi'_{g_2}(u)| \, du$$

$$= \frac{h}{2\pi} \int_{-\pi/h}^{\pi/h} |\phi'_{g_1}(u) - \phi'_{g_2}(u)| \, du$$

since $|e^{-iu(x-\alpha)}| = 1$. Since $x - \alpha$ is bounded, it follows that (Burrill, 1972)

$$\phi'_{g_1}(u) = \sum_{k=0}^{\infty} v^{(1)}_{k,\alpha} \frac{(iu)^k}{k!},$$

$$\phi'_{g_2}(u) = \sum_{k=0}^{\infty} v^{(2)}_{k,\alpha} \frac{(iu)^k}{k!}.$$

Hence,

$$|g_1(x) - g_2(x)| \leq \frac{h}{2\pi} \int_{-\pi/h}^{\pi/h} \sum_{k=0}^{\infty} |v^{(1)}_{k,\alpha} - v^{(2)}_{k,\alpha}| \frac{u}{k!}|^k du$$

$$= \frac{h}{2\pi} \sum_{k=0}^{\infty} |v^{(1)}_{k,\alpha} - v^{(2)}_{k,\alpha}| \frac{2(\pi/h)^{k+1}}{(k+1)!}$$

$$= \sum_{k=0}^{\infty} |v^{(1)}_{k,\alpha} - v^{(2)}_{k,\alpha}| \frac{(\pi/h)^k}{(k+1)!}.$$

Thus,

$$\sup_x |g_1(x) - g_2(x)| \leq \sum_{k=0}^{\infty} |v^{(1)}_{k,\alpha} - v^{(2)}_{k,\alpha}| \frac{(\pi/h)^k}{(k+1)!}.$$

That completes the proof. By setting h small, the waveform of a lattice variable can be used to approximate the waveform of a continuous variable.

Appendix C: Odd and even moments

Odd moments and asymmetry

Theorem C.1. The unitized NB waveform is symmetrical about a point α if and only if all of the odd moments about α are zero.

Let us denote by $g(x)$ the unitized NB waveform. Since $g(x)$ is a density function, we can define a probability space (Ω, F, P). In the discrete case, Ω is the set of possible x_j's, F is the family of all subsets of Ω, and P is a probability measure determined by the distribution function:

$$G(x) = \sum_{x_j \leq x} g(x_j)$$

In the continuous case, $\Omega = \{x: x \in R\}$, where R is the set of reals, F is a σ-field of subsets of R, and P is the probability measure determined by the distribution function

$$G(x) = \int_{\infty}^{x} g(t)\,dt$$

Proof. We first prove that if all of the odd moments about α are zero, then the unitized NB waveform is symmetrical about α. Let X and Y be random variables such that $X(x) = x$ and $Y = X - \alpha$. The Fourier Transform of Y is:

$$\phi_Y(u) = \sum_{k=0}^{\infty} v_{k,\alpha} \frac{(iu)^k}{k!}$$

$$= \sum_{k=0}^{\infty} v_{2k,\alpha} \frac{(iu)^{2k}}{(2k!)} + \sum_{k=0}^{\infty} v_{2k+1,\alpha} \frac{(iu)^{2k+1}}{(2k+1)!}$$

where v_k is the kth moment about α.
If all of the odd moments $v_{2k+1,\alpha}$ are zero, then

$$\phi_Y(u) = \sum_{k=0}^{\infty} v_{2k,\alpha} \frac{(iu)^{2k}}{(2k!)} = \sum_{k=0}^{\infty} (-1)^k v_{2k,\alpha} \frac{u^{2k}}{2k!}$$

Thus, $\phi_Y(u)$ is real. If the Fourier Transform is real, then the density of Y, denoted $h(y)$, is symmetrical about zero (Feller, 1966, p. 474).

Hence

$$h(y) = h(-y)$$

But

$$g(\alpha + y) = h(y) = h(-y) = g(\alpha - y)$$

which means that g is symmetrical about α. We now prove the converse. If the unitized NB waveform is symmetrical about α, then $X - \alpha$ and $-(X - \alpha)$ have the same distribution. Hence, for all k, where E denotes expectation,

$$E(X - \alpha)^k = E[-(X - \alpha)]^k$$

But for k odd,

$$E[-(X - \alpha)]^k = -E(X - \alpha)^k$$

Therefore, for k odd,

$$E(X - \alpha)^k = -E(X - \alpha)^k$$

which implies that for k odd,

$$E(X - \alpha)^k = 0$$

Therefore, if the waveform is symmetrical about α, all odd moments are zero. The proof is complete.

Even moments and dispersion

Theorem C.2. Each kth positive root of the kth even moment about a point α of a unitized NB waveform is a distance function.

Proof. We begin with a probability space (Ω, F, P). Let X, Y, and Z be random variables such that $X(x) = x$. Let us define $d(X, Y)$ by:

$$d(X, Y) = E^{1/k}(X - Y)^k$$

where k is even. Note that E denotes expectation. First, we see that $d(X, Y) \geq 0$, so that d satisfies the first condition of a distance function (Coombs et al., 1970, p. 372). Second, we see that for k even,

$$d(X, Y) = E^{1/k}(X - Y)^k = 0$$

if and only if $X = Y$ with probability 1. Thus, the second condition of a distance function is satisfied in a probabilistic sense. Third, we see that

$$d(X, Y) = E^{1/k}(X - Y)^k = E^{1/k}(Y - X) = d(Y, X)$$

Thus, the function d is symmetric as a distance function should be. Finally, we see that the triangle inequality is satisfied:

$$d(X, Y) = E^{1/k}[(X - Z) + (Z - Y)]^k$$

$$\leq E^{1/k}(X - Z)^k + E^{1/k}(Z - Y)^k$$

$$= d(X, Z) + d(Z, Y)$$

by the Minkowski inequality (Burrill, 1972, p. 175). Now, let $Y = \alpha$.

Thus,

$$d(X, \alpha) = E^{1/k}(X - \alpha)^k$$

is a distance function. It is a measure of the distance of the random variable X from α. That completes the proof.

The measure of the distance of a random variable from a fixed point is a measure of the dispersion of the random variable about the fixed point.

For example, if $k = 2$, we have

$$d(X, \alpha) = E^{1/2}(X - \alpha)^2$$

which is the standard deviation if $\alpha = E(X)$. Finally, it should be apparent that $E(X - \alpha)^k$ is an order-preserving transformation of the distance function $E^{1/k}(X - \alpha)^k$.

NOTES

Preparation of this book chapter was supported in part by National Science Foundation Grant No. BNS-8414853.

1 Recall that the total mass of a body is equal to its total weight when the body is at sea level and 45° latitude.

2 It is worth mentioning that the standard error of a moment-based indicant of order k taken to the kth root is much smaller than the standard error of the original moment-based indicant. Specifically, if SE (θ) denotes the standard error of a statistic, then the standard error of that statistic taken the kth root is:

$$\frac{\theta^{1/k}}{k\theta} \text{ SE } (\theta).$$

Thus, higher order WAMA indicants are probably much less susceptible to small fluctuations in sampling or to outliers.

3 Bronzino, Kelly, Cordova, Oley, and Morgane (1981) used centile coefficients of skewness and kurtosis rather than moment-based coefficients in order to optimize speed and ease of computation in real time. They reported that centile and moment-based coefficients gave very similar results.

4 It is worth mentioning that the standard deviation of the amplitude distribution equals the square root of the total mass of the power spectrum.

5 The estimated power spectrum is bounded above by $S/2$ hertz, where S is the number of observations per second (see Chatfield, 1980, p. 165).

REFERENCES

Abramowitz, M. (1965). Elementary analytical methods. In M. Abramowitz & I. Stegun (Eds.), *Handbook of mathematical functions* (pp. 9–64). New York: Dover.

Arvesen, J. N., & Salsburg, D. S. (1975). Approximate tests and confidence intervals using the jackknife. In R. M. Elashoff (Ed.), *Perspectives in biometrics* (Vol. 1, pp. 123–147). New York: Academic Press.

Berger, H. (1976). On the electroencephalogram in man. In S. W. Porges & M. G. H. Coles (Eds.), *Psychophysiology* (pp. 9–14). Stroudsburg, PA: Dowden, Hutchinson, & Ross. (Original work published 1929.)

Bohrer, R. E., & Porges, S. W. (1982). The application of time-series statistics to psychological research: An introduction. In G. Keren (Ed.), *Statistical and methodological issues in psychology and social sciences research*. Hillsdale, NJ: Erlbaum.

Bracewell, R. N. (1978). *The Fourier transform and its applications* (2nd ed.). New York: McGraw-Hill.

Brazier, M. A. B. (1980). The early developments of quantitative EEG analysis: The roots of modern methods. In R. Sinz & M. Rosenzweig (Eds.), *Psychophysiology 1980* (pp. 283–290). Amsterdam: Elsevier.

Bronzino, J. D., Kelly, M. L., Cordova, C. T., Oley, N. H., & Morgane, P. J. (1981). Utilization of amplitude histograms to quantify the EEG effects of systemic administration of morphine in the chronically implanted rat. *IEEE Transactions on Biomedical Engineering, BME-28*, 673–678.

Burrill, C. W. (1972). *Measure, integration, and probability*. New York: McGraw-Hill.

Cacioppo, J. T., & Dorfman, D. D. (1984). Moments in psychophysiological research: Topographical analysis of non-negative bounded waveforms. *Psychophysiology, 21*, 571. (Abstract).

Cacioppo, J. T., & Dorfman, D. D. (1987). Waveform moment analysis in psychophysiological research. *Psychological Bulletin, 102*, 421–438.

Cacioppo, J. T., Marshall-Goodell, B., & Dorfman, D. D. (1983). Skeletomuscular patterning: Topographical analysis of the integrated electromyogram. *Psychophysiology, 20*, 269–283.

Cacioppo, J. T., Petty, R. E., & Marshall-Goodell, B. (1984). Electromyographic specificity during simple physical and attitudinal tasks: Location and topographical features of integrated EMG responses. *Biological Psychology, 18*, 85–121.

Cacioppo, J. T., Petty, R. E., & Morris, K. J. (1985). Semantic, evaluative, and self-referent processing: Memory, cognitive effort, and somatovisceral activity. *Psychophysiology, 22*, 371–384.

Chatfield, C. (1980). *The analysis of time series: An introduction* (2nd ed.). New York: Chapman and Hall.

Chavance, M., & Samson-Dollfus, D. (1978). Analyse spectrale de l'EEG de l'enfant normal entre 6 et 16 ans: Choix and validation des parametres les plus informationnels. *Electroencephalography and Clinical Neurophysiology 45*, 767–776.

Chissolm, B. S. (1970). Interpretation of the kurtosis statistic. *The American Statistician 24*(4), 19–22.

Coger, R. W., Dymond, A. M., & Serafetinides, E. A. (1979). Methods of electrophysiological research. In E. A. Serafetinides (Ed.), *Methods of biobehavioral research* (pp. 111–122). New York: Grune & Stratton.

Coombs, C. H., Dawes, R. M., & Tversky, A. (1970). *Mathematical psychology: An elementary introduction.* Englewood Cliffs, NJ: Prentice-Hall.

Cooper, R., Osselton, J. W., & Shaw, J. C. (1980). *EEG technology* (3rd ed.). London: Butterworths.

Darlington, R. B. (1970). Is kurtosis really peakedness? *The American Statistician, 24*(2), 19–22.

Denoth, F. (1975). Some general remarks on Hjorth's parameters used in EEG analysis. In G. Dolce & H. Kunkel (Eds.), *CEAN: Computerized EEG analysis* (pp. 9–18). Stuttgart: Gustav Fischer Verlag.

Efron, B. (1982). *The jackknife, the bootstrap, and other resampling plans.* Philadelphia: Society for Industrial and Applied Mathematics.

Elul, R. (1967). Statistical mechanisms in generation of the EEG. In L. J. Fogel & F. W. George (Eds.), *Progress in biomedical engineering* (pp. 131–150). Washington, DC: Spartan Books.

Elul, R. (1969). Gaussian behavior of the electroencephalogram: Changes during performance of mental task. *Science, 164*, 328–331.

Elul, R., Hanley, J., & Simmons, III, J. Q. (1975). Non-Gaussian behavior of the EEG in Down's syndrome suggests decreased neuronal connections. *Acta Neurologica Scandinavica, 51*, 21–28.

Feller, W. (1966). *An introduction to probability theory and its applications* (Vol. 2). New York: Wiley.

Fisher, R. A. (1922). On the mathematical foundations of theoretical statistics. *The Philosophical Transactions of the Royal Society, 222*, 309–368.

Fox, S. S. (1970). Evoked potential, coding, and behavior. In F. O. Schmitt (Ed.), *The neurosciences; Second study program.* New York: Rockefeller University Press.

Fox, S. S., & Norman, R. J. (1968). Functional congruence: An index of neural homogeneity and a new measure of brain activity. *Science, 159*, 1257–1259.

Freedman, D., & Diaconis, P. (1981). On the histogram as a density estimator: L_2 theory. *Zeitschrift für Wahrscheinlichkeitstheorie und Verwandte Gebiete, 57*, 453–476.

Galton, F. (1889). *Natural inheritance.* London: Macmillan.

Glaria, A. P., & Murray, A. (1985). Comparison of EEG monitoring techniques: An evaluation during cardiac surgery. *Electroencephalography and Clinical Neurophysiology, 61*, 323–330.

Goldstein, I. B. (1972). Electromyography: A measure of skeletal muscle response. In N.S. Greenfield and R. A. Sternbach (Eds.), *Handbook of psychophysiology* (pp. 329–366). New York: Holt, Rinehart and Wintson.

Grabiner, M., Andonian, M., Regnier, M., & Harding, V. (1984). *Topographical analysis of surface EMG before and after isometrically induced fatigue.* Paper presented at the American College of Sports Medicine Annual Meeting, San Diego, CA.

Hardy, G. H., Littlewood, J. E., & Pólya, G. (1967). *Inequalities.* Cambridge: Cambridge University Press.

Hildebrand, D. K. (1971). Kurtosis measures bimodality? *The American Statistician, 25*(1), 42–43.

Hjorth, B. (1970). EEG analysis based on time domain properties. *Electroencephalography and Clinical Neurophysiology, 29*, 306–310.

Hjorth, B. (1973). The physical significance of time domain descriptors in EEG analysis. *Electroencephalography and Clinical Neurophysiology, 34*, 321–325.

Hjorth, B. (1975). Time domain descriptors and their relation to a particular model for generation of EEG activity. In G. Dolce and H. Kunkel (Eds.), *CEAN: Computerized EEG analysis* (pp. 3–8). Stuttgart: Gustav Fischer Verlag.

Hoaglin, D. C. (1985a). Summarizing shape numerically: The *g*- and *h*-distributions. In D. C. Hoaglin, F. Mosteller, & J. W. Tukey (Eds.), *Exploring data tables, trends, and shapes* (pp. 461–513). New York: Wiley.

Hoaglin, D. C. (1985b). Using quantiles to study shape. In D. C. Hoaglin, F. Mosteller, & J. W. Tukey (Eds.), *Exploring data tables, trends, and shapes* (pp. 417–460). New York: Wiley.

Johnson, N. L., & Kotz, S. (1970). *Continuous univariate distributions–1: Distributions in statistics.* New York: Wiley.

Kanno, O., & Clarenbach, P. (1985). Effect of clonidine and yohimbine on sleep in man: Polygraphic study and EEG analysis by normalized slope descriptors. *Electroencephalography and Clinical Neurophysiology, 60,* 478–484.

Kaplansky, I. (1945). A common error concerning kurtosis. *Journal of the American Statistical Association, 40,* 259.

Kendall, M. G., & Stuart, A. (1963). *The advanced theory of statistics* (2nd ed., Vol. 1). London: Hafner.

Lippold, O. C. J. (1967). Electromyography. In P. H. Venables & I. Martin (Eds.), *Manual of psychophysiological methods* (pp. 245–298). New York: Wiley.

Lord, F. M. (1952). A theory of tests scores. *Psychometric Monographs* (Whole No. 7).

Lykken, D. T., Tellegen, A., & Iacono, W. G. (1982). EEG spectra in twins: Evidence for a neglected mechanism of genetic determination. *Physiological Psychology, 10,* 60–65.

Lykken, D. T., Tellegen, A., & Thorkelson, K. (1974). Genetic determination of EEG frequency spectra. *Biological Psychology, 1,* 245–259.

McGuigan, F. J. (1978). *Cognitive psychophysiology: Principles of covert behavior.* Englewood Cliffs, NJ: Prentice-Hall.

Moors, J. J. A. (1986). The meaning of kurtosis: Darlington reexamined. *The American Statistician, 40*(4), 283–284.

Mosteller, F., & Tukey, J. W. (1968). Data analysis including statistics. In G. Lindzey and E. Aronson (Eds.), *Handbook of social psychology* (Vol. 2, pp. 80–203). Reading, MA: Addison-Wesley.

Norton, R. M., & Arnold, S. (1985). A theorem on moments. *American Statistician, 39*(2), 106.

Norris, N. (1976). General means and statistical theory. *The American Statistician, 30*(1), 8–12.

Ord, J. K. (1985). Pearson system of distributions. In S. Kotz & N. L. Johnson (Eds.), *Encyclopedia of statistical sciences* (Vol. 6, pp. 655–659). New York: Wiley.

Pearson, K. (1985). Contributions to the mathematical theory of evolution. II. Skew variation in homogeneous material. *Philosophical Transactions of the Royal Society of London, 186,* 343–414.

Persson, A., & Hjorth, B. (1983). EEG topogram–An aid in describing EEG to the clinician. *Electroencephalography and Clinical Neurophysiology, 56,* 399–405.

Ratcliff, R. (1978). A theory of memory retrieval. *Psychological Review, 85,* 59–108.

Ratcliff, R. (1979). Group reaction time distributions and an analysis of distribution statistics. *Psychological Bulletin, 86,* 446–461.

Ray, W. J., & Cole, H. W. (1985). EEG alpha activity reflects attentional demands, and beta activity reflects emotional and congnitive processes. *Science, 228,* 750–752.

Rey, W. J. J. (1978). *Robust statistical methods.* New York: Springer-Verlag.

Rieger, H., Krieglstein, J., Schütz, H. (1979). Amplitude histography of the EEG in psychopharmacological research. *Pharmakopsychiatria, 12,* 94–101.

Rudin, W. (1974). *Real and complex analysis* (2nd ed.). New York: McGraw-Hill.

Rupert, D. (1987). What is kurtosis? An influence function approach. *The American Statistician, 41*(1), 1–5.

Saltzberg, B. (1973). Period analysis. In A. Remond (Ed.), *Handbook of electroencephalography and clinical neurophysiology* (Vol. 5a, pp. 67–78). Amsterdam: Elsevier.

Saltzberg, B., & Burch, N. R. (1971). Period analytic estimates of moments of the power spectrum: A simplified EEG time domain procedure. *Electroencephalography and Clinical Neurophysiology, 30,* 568–570.

Saltzberg, B., Burton, W. D., Jr., Barlow, J. S., & Burch, N. R. (1985). Moments of the power spectral density estimated from samples of the autocorrelation function (a robust procedure for monitoring changes in the statistical properties of lengthy non-stationary time series such as the EEG). *Electroencephalography and Clinical Neurophysiology, 61,* 89–93.

Saunders, M. G. (1963). Amplitude probability density studies on alpha and alpha-like patterns. *Electroencephalography and Clinical Neurophysiology, 15,* 761–767.

Saunders, M. G. (1972). The genesis of the EEG. *International Review of Neurobiology, 15,* 227–272.

Scott, D. W. (1979). On optimal and data-based histograms. *Biometrika, 66,* 605–610.

Sichel, H. S. (1949). The method of frequency-moments and its application to Type VII populations. *Biometrika, 36,* 404–425.

Snodgrass, J. G., Luce, R. D., & Galanter, E. (1967). Some experiments on simple and choice reaction time. *Journal of Experimental Psychology, 75,* 1–17.

Spehr, W., Sartorius, H., Berglund, K., Hjorth, B., Kablitz, C., Plog, V., Wiedekkmann, P. H., & Zapf, K. (1977). EEG and haemodialysis. A structural survey of EEG spectral analysis, Hjorth's EEG descriptors, blood variables and psychological data. *Electroencephalography and Clinical Neurophysiology, 43,* 787–797.

Sternberg, S. (1969). The discovery of processing stages: Extensions of Donder's method. In W. G. Koster (Ed.), *Attention and performance II* (pp. 276–315). Amsterdam: North-Holland.

Tucker, D. M., Dawson, S. L., Roth, D. L., & Penland, J. G. (1985). Regional changes in EEG power and coherence during cognition: Intensive study of two individuals. *Behavioral Neuroscience, 99,* 564–577.

Tukey, J. W. (1969). Analyzing data: Sanctification or detective work? *American Psychologist, 24,* 83–91.

Yule, G., & Kendall, M. G. (1937). *An introduction to the theory of statistics* (11th ed.). London: Charles Griffin.

21 *The analysis of periodic processes in psychophysiological research*

STEPHEN W. PORGES AND ROBERT E. BOHRER

21.1 GENERAL ISSUES

21.1.1 *Why study periodic physiological activity*

Periodic physiological activity has been observed and interpreted since antiquity when physicians assessed health by listening to heart rhythms and breathing rhythms. In more contemporary models of physiology, the concept of periodic activity has been associated with life-defining processes such as homeostasis. In spite of this interest, there is a paucity of research evaluating periodic physiological activity.

It is perplexing to try to understand why the study of periodic physiological activity has been neglected in psychophysiological research. The history of psychophysiology, with its interest in accurately monitoring central nervous system function, would seem to provide the appropriate motivation. For example, researchers for approximately 100 years have justified the placement of electrodes on the surface of the body (scalp, chest, palms etc.) as a method to provide information regarding central mediation of emotional or cognitive states. Yet the measurement of physiological activity in these studies has seldom measured periodic processes.

Quantification of physiological activity, even in the physiology literature, has generally consisted of counting events or evaluating a mean level of activity within a time period. The study of periodic physiological activity seems to be lacking. This is remarkable because the study of living systems has always emphasized temporal and periodic characteristics. There are numerous reasons for this lack of research. Perhaps the most imposing factor has been the statistical sophistication necessary to accurately quantify periodic activity. This chapter has been written in response to this need.

The chapter has been written to serve as a two-way bridge between the psychophysiologist and the statistician. We have intended this chapter to aid the psychophysiologist by introducing time-series concepts without mathematical jargon and to aid the statistician by introducing the unique problems associated with physiological data.

Periodicities in physiological activity convey important information regarding central nervous system regulation. This is true not only for the study of electrocortical activity like the EEG, but also for peripheral systems such as heart rate and EMG. In our research the amplitude of heart rate rhythms has provided reliable diagnostic information regarding the status of the central nervous system. Similarly, there have been clinical reports that muscle tone changes (i.e., EMG)

708

following brain insult. These changes in periodic activity are not an epiphenomenon but are a direct manifestation of the peripheral component of a peripheral–central–peripheral feedback system. In the healthy individual this feedback system has a characteristic frequency and gain that is reflected by a periodicity with a relatively stable duration and amplitude. When brain function is compromised by a variety of insults including tissue damage, hemorrhage, increased intracranial pressure, drugs, anoxia, severe exercise, or even psychological stress, the feedback system is disrupted and there are changes in the periodic nature of these measures.

21.1.2   *One researcher's data is another researcher's error*

With the exception of the EEG literature, which historically has emphasized rhythmicity, psychophysiological research usually has treated oscillations in physiological activity as recording error or irrelevant background physiological activity. This decision is based upon two interdependent assumptions: (1) oscillations in physiological activity reflect homeostatic activity and (2) event-related physiological responses are manifest as short latency trends.

Physiological systems are continuously changing, reflecting the dynamic regulatory function of the nervous system. It would be naive to believe that these systems are sensitive solely to the variables we choose to manipulate in our experiments. Paradoxically, the physiological systems that may be the most sensitive to psychological processes also may manifest neurophysiological regulation. Thus, we are faced with a problem of how to quantify the component of physiological activity related to the experimental manipulation, when the same physiological system is also indexing the continuous neural modulation of primary homeostatic function.

In the study of short-latency event-related responses (e.g., evoked potentials, directional heart rate responses, and stimulus-specific electrodermal activity) the spontaneous oscillations characteristic of most physiological systems are bothersome and need to be removed. In the conceptual models underlying this style of research, oscillations or "jitter" are treated as experimental error and can be removed through a variety of averaging and smoothing procedures.

These averaging procedures are insensitive both to the possibility that the signal is encoded in a parameter other than level and to the possibility that the signal is encoded in the background noise. In contrast to methods that minimize background activity, this chapter will identify problems, provide an overview of methods, and propose a series of rules for analyzing and interpreting rhythmic physiological data.

21.1.3   *Problems in the quantification of periodic processes*

There are three basic statistical problems in quantification of the periodic components of physiological processes. First, physiological data are *nonstationary*. Nonstationarity implies that the expected values of the mean and variance are not constant throughout the data set. In physiological data this is characterized by aperiodic components and slow trend shifts in level. All traditional time-series methods for quantifying periodicities assume that the data are stationary. When data are nonstationary and aperiodic, the analyses will distort the values for frequency and amplitude of the periodicity of interest. Second, physiological periodicities are *nonsinusoidal*. Most of the methods for describing periodicites assume that the periodic process may be fit with a sine or cosine wave. When periodic activity cannot be fit with a sine or cosine function, the analyses produce harmonic variances at frequencies higher than the true periodic process. This confounds the interpretation of the analyses by distributing harmonic variances at frequencies higher than the true periodic process. Third, physiological data are complex and consist of numerous *periodic* and *aperiodic* components. The researcher must not only be cognizant of the nonstationary component, but when there is more than one periodic component, the researcher must also be aware that the nonsinusoidal characteristic of slow periodic processes inflates the estimates of faster periodic activity. Later in this chapter we elaborate on the statistical characteristics of these problems and describe methods for minimizing their impact on data analyses.

There are a number of other problems associated with the description of specific periodic processes within complex physiological patterns. Based upon the preceding statistical problems, it is difficult to quantify a low-amplitude signal when it is embedded within a complex signal. Not only are there statistical problems, but amplification equipment and filters used to enhance low-amplitude signals may influence the amplitude and frequency components of the periodic process being studied.

The quantification of rhythmicity is confounded by the complexity of some physiological response systems. Obviously, it is easiest to quantify periodic activity when most of the variance of the physiological process may be described by one sinusoid. For example, recordings of respiration using measures of chest circumference or nasal airflow exhibit a predominant rhythmicity, synchronously waxing and waning with inhalation and exhalation. Unfortunately, not all physiological processes exhibit an observable periodicity that accounts for most of the variance.

In many response systems the periodic component of interest may account for a very small proportion of the variance of the process. In these situations the experimenter is attempting to accurately quantify a low-amplitude periodic process embedded in a complex signal composed of other periodic and aperiodic components. Examples of this problem can be seen in the monitoring of EEG rhythmicity or fetal heart rate. In the analyses of the periodic components of the EEG, it is important to note that the amplitude of alpha and other periodic activity is in the microvolt range, although the background skin potential from the scalp is in the millivolt range. Similarly, in the human fetus, vagal influences on the heart are modulated by central respiratory drive and manifested as an oscillation of heart period. This oscillation, fetal respiratory sinus arrhythmia, is embedded in a very complex signal of high beat-to-beat variability with identifiable contributions from blood pressure, thermoregulation, metabolic demands, and reactivity to uterine contractions. In many situations the fetal respiratory sinus arrhythmia may have an amplitude between 2 and 5 msec, and the heart period reaction to uterine contractions may at times be as great 500 or 600 msec. In these two examples, the rhythmicity of interest (i.e., alpha in the EEG study; respiratory sinus arrhythmia in the fetal heart rate study) represents an extremely small proportion of the variance of the process.

The characteristics of amplifiers contribute to difficulties in the analysis and interpretation of physiological signals. In early EEG research it was necessary to use high gain-AC amplifiers to achieve the necessary amplification to observe the low-amplitude rhythmicity emanating from the scalp. The AC amplifier provided a method for filtering slow periodic and aperiodic influences associated with skin potential and allowed the observation and quantification of low-amplitude oscillations characteristic of the EEG. Although solid-state electronics provide contemporary amplifiers with higher gain and greater stability, the basic methods used in this field have changed little over the past 50 years.

Researchers modify the signal for their research objectives by using a combination of hardware (e.g., amplifier characteristics and filter settings) and software manipulations (e.g., statistical procedures). For example, the same input signal is used for both evoked potential and EEG research. Evoked potential research emphasizes the low-frequency influence of the voltage shifts associated with stimulus processing by expanding the low frequencies passed by the amplifier via longer time constants. In contrast, EEG research emphasizes the high-frequency content by attenuating the low-frequency activity via short time constants.

In most situations, the time constants on AC amplifiers do not perform their assumed task of removing the variance of physiological processes below or above a specific frequency. Since physiological activity is composed of periodic and aperiodic components and the periodic components are never a perfect sine wave, the time constant filters pass variance of the processes in the frequencies assumed to be filtered. Therefore, AC amplifiers may distort the specific output characteristics of interest: frequency and amplitude of the EEG or latency and magnitude of evoked potential.

21.2 TIME SERIES: OVERVIEW

21.2.1 *Definitions*

Although most psychophysiological data are presented in terms of mean levels within or across subjects, the sequential pattern on which the mean is based may contain important information. Time-series statistics provide methods to describe and evaluate these patterns. A set of sequential observations, such as the circumference of the chest sampled twice a second or the time intervals between sequential heartbeats, constitutes a time series. Although there are various types of time series, the unifying dimension is that they are all indexed by time. Mathematically, a time series may be described as a string of variables that are sequentially indexed, for example, $X_t, X_{t+1}, X_{t+2}, \ldots, X_{t+n}$. In this example, the index t represents time.

A time series is *continuous* when observations are made continuously in time. An analog signal that changes over time, characteristic of many physiological processes, is a continuous process. The term continuous is used for series even when the measured variable can only take a fixed set of values. A time series is *discrete* when the observations are taken only at specific times, usually equally spaced. Most time-series methods assume that data represent discrete samples of a continuous time series sampled at equally spaced intervals. In practice, researchers are usually dealing with discrete time series, although the underlying physiological process is continuous. For example, the analog-to-digital converter in a laboratory computer transforms a continuous analog signal into digital representations at discrete time intervals. Problems often arise with discrete time series, like interbeat intervals, which are not equally spaced in time. To deal with the problem of equally spaced samples, one may assume that sequential heart periods are a discrete manifestation of a continuous process (e.g., neural inputs to the heart). Thus, interpolations are possible to adjust sampling into equal time intervals.

Time series have other characteristics. For example, a time series may be characterized by observations that can take one of only two values (e.g., 0 and 1). This type of time series is known as a *binary process*. Binary processes are common in communication theory and in the modeling of neuronal activity. In these examples, a neuron is viewed as a switch that may be either on or off and can be coded as a 1 or a 0. Other time series are characterized by the sequential time intervals between events. Unlike the EEG and EKG, which are clearly continuous processes, or the binary process, which has two states, the heart period series is a series of interevent intervals triggered by the heartbeat. This type of time series is known as a *point process*. Point processes are time series in which a series of events occur randomly in time and the duration of the event is assumed to be instantaneous.

21.2.2   *Statistical characteristic of physiological time series*

Much of statistical theory is concerned with random samples of independent observations. The special feature of time-series analysis is that sequential observations are usually not independent and the analysis must take into account the time order of the observations. This time-ordered dependency may be assessed by calculating an autocorrelation (see what follows). There is a very special case of a time series in which the sequential observations are independent. This is a string of identically and independently distributed (IID) random variables. In the IID case, knowledge of any one random variable does not influence the distribution of any other. Thus, the expected value for any one time sample is the same as any other sample. Physiological time series of healthy alert subjects are never IID. Physiological time series may approach IID in situations when the nervous system input to peripheral organs is removed via surgery or drugs.

Random variables in most time series take on other probabilities and may be viewed on a continuum of dependency. When sequential observations are dependent, future values may be predicted from past observations. If a time series can be predicted exactly from past observations, it is said to be *deterministic*. Since all physiological and behavioral processes are influenced by unknown factors, it may not be possible to describe behavioral and biobehavioral processes with a totally deterministic model. Most time series are *stochastic* and the future is only partly determined by past values. In fact, time series actually may be expressed as the sum of two uncorrelated processes, one purely deterministic and one purely nondeterministically stochastic. This theorem is known as the *Wold Decomposition Theorem*.

21.2.3   *Parameters of a time series*

Figure 21.1*a* illustrates a sine wave indexed by time. Note that the duration of one complete cycle of the sine wave is 5 s. The duration of a sine wave defines the *period*. The reciprocal of the period defines the *frequency*. In our example, the sine wave with a 5-s period has a frequency of 0.2 cycles per second, or 0.2 Hz. This frequency was selected because it is similar to the frequency of spontaneous breathing in adult subjects. In this example, the *sampling interval* was 500 ms.

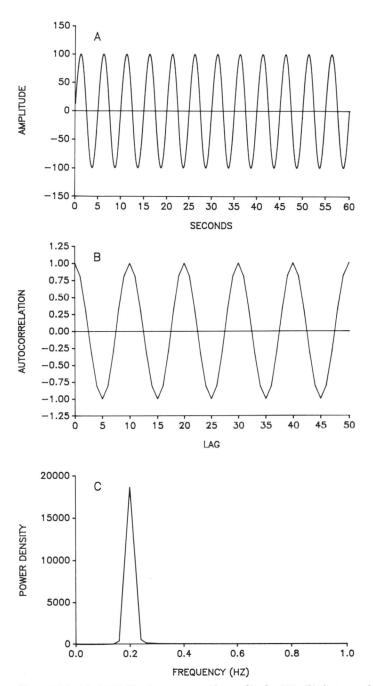

Figure 21.1. (a) A 0.2-Hz sine wave with amplitude 100. (b) Autocorrelogram of 0.2-Hz sine wave illustrated in (a). Data were sampled 2.0 Hz (lag is equivalent to sequential 500 ms sampling interval). (c) Spectral analysis of 0.2-Hz sine wave illustrated in (a).

This could be stated as a *sampling rate* of 2 Hz. Thus, if we sample twice a second (i.e., 2 Hz), a 0.2-Hz sine wave would require 10 of these samples for one complete cycle.

A number of parameters are necessary to describe a periodic process. In Figure 21.1a the sine wave takes on values from − 100 to + 100. The peak of the periodic process is called the *amplitude*. In Figure 21.1a the amplitude is 100. In psychophysiological research we are often interested in quantifying the variance of the signal. In conceptualizing variance of a periodic process, it is useful to recall the arithmetic relationship between amplitude and variance. The square of the amplitude divided by 2 is equivalent to the variance [var $= A^2/2$]. Thus, decomposition of physiological processes into sine waves would provide a method of describing component variances of the different periodic processes. This method of decomposition is the basis for spectral analysis and will be described in the section on frequency domain analyses.

The *phase* of a periodic process relates the onset of the process to the time at the origin. If the process starts at the origin (i.e., 0 on the ordinate and 0 on the abscissa), the phase is zero. The phase can be described in degrees (from 0 to 360), in radians (from 0 to 2π), or in proportion of the sinusoid temporally displaced from the origin (e.g., a half-cycle). The same temporal displacement could be described as a phase shift of 180°, π radians, or a half-cycle. In most situations the periodic process does not originate at the origin and exhibits some displacement.

21.2.4   *Methods to analyze periodic activity*

There are two basic approaches that may be used to describe and analyze the periodic components of a time series. A time series may be represented and analyzed in the time domain or in the frequency domain. Time domain representations plot data as a function of time. The time domain methods that are most relevant to the study of periodic processes are based on the *autocorrelation function*. Autocorrelation techniques are mathematical extensions of traditional correlation techniques. An autocorrelation is the correlation of one time series with a time-shifted version of itself. Frequency domain techniques are those based on the *spectral density function*. The procedure for estimating the spectral densities at various frequencies is called *spectral analysis*. Spectral analysis decomposes a time series into sinusoidal components at different frequencies and different amplitudes. Both time domain and frequency domain methods have provided valuable tools to describe periodic phenomena. In the following sections, examples of time domain and frequency domain methods will be described and evaluated.

21.3   TIME DOMAIN METHODS

Time domain statistical procedures can be used to describe periodicity. The autocorrelation function is extremely useful in detecting periodicities when the time series is characterized by a relatively pure sinusoid uncontaminated by other random influences. Inspection of the autocorrelogram for the 0.2-Hz sine wave illustrated in Figure 21.1b reflects the periodicity of the waveform. In Figure 21.1b the autocorrelations oscillate between + 1.0 and − 1.0 every 10 lags. The term *lag* represents the displacement of the time series in terms of time-sampled sequential data points. Thus, the pattern of the 0.2-Hz sine wave would be correlated 1.0 with a time-shifted version of itself when the time lag is equivalent to the period of the sine wave (i.e., 10 data points or 5 sec). The magnitude of the autocorrelation remains 1.0 every 10 lags and does not attenuate even when the time series is correlated with a time-shifted version that is displaced by 50 data points! This is a characteristic of a deterministic time series that is not representative of physiological and behavioral periodic processes.

Similarly, a cross-correlation is the correlation of one time series with a time lagged version of a second time series. The cross-correlation function provides information regarding the statistical dependence of one series on another. If the two time series are identical, the peak value of the cross-correlation function will be unity at the lag that makes the two series identical and less than unity at all other lags. In most cases, since the second series is not simply a time-shifted version of the first series, the peak value of the cross-correlation will be less than unity. Cross-correlation techniques lose their effectiveness and sensitivity to assess the communality between two series when the difference between the series is more than a temporal displacement.

We can evaluate the limitations of the autocorrelation method in detecting periodicities when we inspect the autocorrelation functions of various time series. For example, with a perfect sine wave, it is clear that the method provides an accurate description of the periodicity, although the method is merely an alternative approach of describing an obvious periodicity. However, when this method is applied to psychophysiological variables such as respiration and heart rate, its utility is more dubious.

Figure 21.2a illustrates the chest circumference changes associated with respiration. The amplitude of chest circumference was sampled at 2.0 Hz (every 500 ms). Visual inspection of the time series indicates a relatively stable breathing pattern of approximately one breath every 6 or 7 s. As illustrated in Figure 21.2b, the autocorrelation function supports this observation with the greatest magnitude correlation at 12 lags and at multiples of 12. Visual inspection of Figures 21.1b and 21.2b illustrates the differences between the autocorrelation function for a deterministic sine wave and a stochastic process of respiration. Recall that if the past history of a signal totally determines its future behavior, it is said to be deterministic. Since the wave form in Figure 21.1a depicts a pure sine wave, the process is totally predictable and, therefore, deterministic. In contrast, physiological signals are neither simple sine waves nor totally determined by their past history. The respiration signal described in Figure 21.2 is periodic, although its past behavior does not totally predict the future values in terms of amplitude, period, and phase of the signal. As the time shift gets longer, the autocorrelations of stochastic periodic processes become smaller. In the respiration example in Figure 21.2b, the peaks of the autocorrelation function decrease from approximately .6 when time shifted one cycle of the sine wave to approximately .3 when time shifted five cycles.

The preceding examples demonstrate the effectiveness of the autocorrelation method for quantifying the periodicity and stochastic nature of the process. However, these examples are limited to processes with a clearly observable rhythmic component. The characteristics of physiological processes depart from these examples. Physiological processes are complex and often are composed of multiple components, some of which are not sinusoidal. The autocorrelogram of physiological processes is therefore difficult to interpret. A time series of sequential heart period values provides an example. Unlike respiration data, heart period

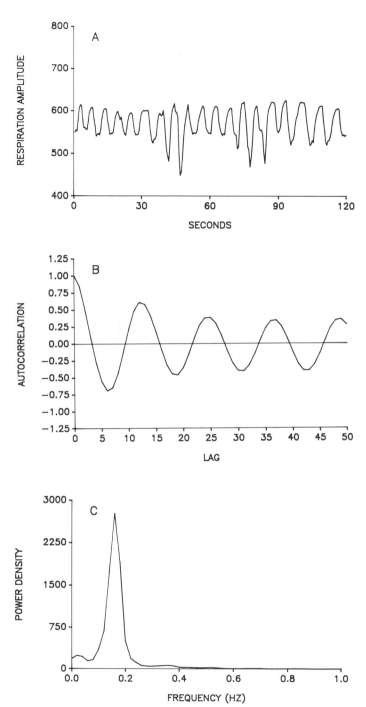

Figure 21.2. (a) Chest circumference sampled 2.0 Hz. (b) Autocorrelogram of data illustrated in (a). (c) Spectral analysis of data illustrated in (a).

reflects a number of periodic influences including respiratory (i.e., respiratory sinus arrhythmia) and blood pressure (i.e., Traube–Hering–Mayer wave) and aperiodic influences including metabolic demands (see Kitney & Rompelman, 1980).

Figure 21.3a illustrates the heart period of a subject with high heart period variability including a prominent rhythmicity associated with respiration (i.e., respiratory sinus arrhythmia). In contrast, Figure 21.4a illustrates a subject with low heart period variability. Note that the periodicity in the autocorrelogram in Figure 21.3b is not as prominent as in Figure 21.2b and in Figure 21.4b there is no apparent periodicity at lags that would be associated with either the Traube–Hering–Mayer wave (i.e., approximately 10–15 s or 20–30 lags) or respiratory sinus arrhythmia (i.e., approximately 2.5–8.0 s or 5–15 lags). From these two examples it becomes clear that as the signal becomes more complex, time domain methods of assessing and describing rhythmicity become increasingly difficult.

In spite of the obvious complexity of physiological time series, some periodicities may become obvious during visual inspection when the data are plotted over a long period of time. For example, in the study of circadian rhythms, descriptive time domain methods have been useful. One *rhythmometric* method, *cosinor analysis,* has been frequently applied. This method is based on two assumptions: (1) the circadian rhythm accounts for a major source of the variance of the process being studied and (2) the periodicity is relatively symmetrical and can be approximated by a cosine wave. Cosinor (group-mean cosine-vector) analysis was developed by Halberg (e.g., Halberg, Johnson, Nelson, Runge, & Sothern, 1972) to describe the time series with a number of operationally defined parameters. In this analysis a cosine curve is fitted to the data by least squares and a number of parameters are extracted. The rhythm-adjusted mean is called the mean level, or mesor, and is defined as a value midway between the peak and trough of the fitted cosinusoidal wave. The amplitude is quantified as half the difference between maximal and minimal values of the fitted cosinusoidal wave. Acrophase is a measure of peak time relative to some reference time described as a phase angle.

21.4 FREQUENCY DOMAIN

21.4.1 *Spectral analysis*

Based upon the preceding discussion, we can see that time domain methods are extremely useful if and only if the periodicity of interest has a relatively high amplitude (i.e., represents a large proportion of the variance of the signal). The physiological response systems that psychophysiologists study seldom meet this criterion. We are therefore forced to identify other statistical methods that might be more amenable to our needs. An alternative approach to the study of periodicities is to apply frequency domain methods.

In contrast to the time domain techniques, frequency domain techniques are those based upon the spectral density function. Spectral analysis is a mathematical technique that decomposes a time series into constituent frequencies or periodicities. The amplitude or variance associated with each frequency component is known as the spectral density estimate. There is a mathematical relationship between the time domain autocorrelation procedures and spectral analysis. The spectral density function is the *Fourier transform* of the autocovariance (unstandardized autocorrelation) function. The Fourier transform is an algebraic method of

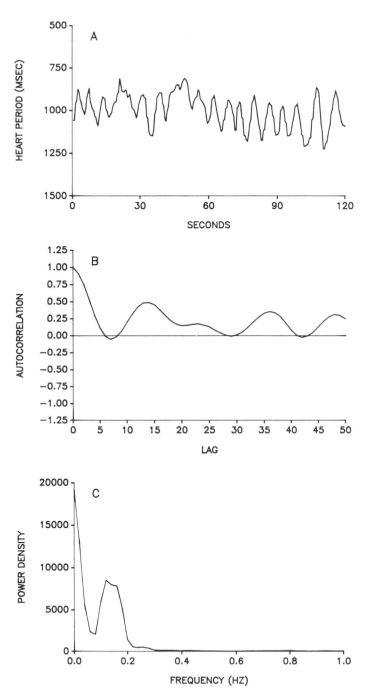

Figure 21.3. (a) Heart period sampled 2.0 Hz from subject with prominent respiratory sinus arrhythmia. (b) Autocorrelogram of data illustrated in (a). (c) Spectral analysis of data illustrated in (a).

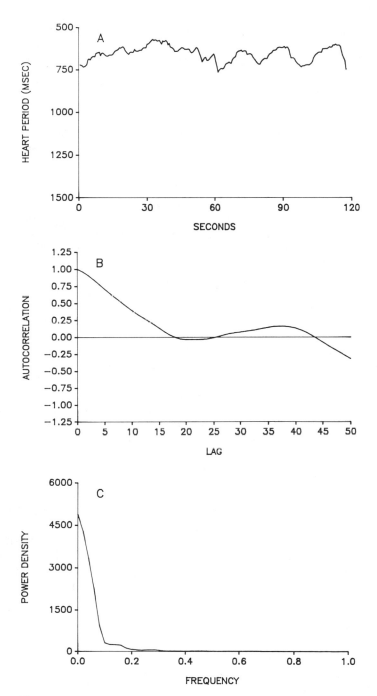

Figure 21.4. (*a*) Heart period sampled 2.0 Hz from subject with little respiratory sinus arrhythmia. (*b*) Autocorrelogram of data illustrated in (*a*). (*c*) Spectral analysis of data illustrated in (*a*).

decomposing any time series into a set of pure sine waves of different frequencies, with a particular amplitude and phase angle for each frequency. The algebraic sum of the sinusoidal components adjusted for phase angle will accurately reproduce the original time series. Moreover, the inverse Fourier transform of the spectral densities will reproduce the autocovariances.

In its strictest sense, however, the Fourier analysis of a time series is the decomposition of the series into the sum of sine and cosine terms. This decomposition is called the *periodogram*. The periodogram is the finite Fourier transform of the autocovariance function. Although the periodogram is relatively easy to calculate, it does not provide consistent estimators for the spectral densities. Thus, methods are required to smooth the periodogram to provide spectral density estimates that have less bias and variance. Spectral analysis includes methods of smoothing, or *windowing*, to enhance the description of stable estimators with stochastic processes. Recall that deterministic processes are totally predictable and that physiological processes contain probabilistic components and are therefore stochastic. This means that the parameters of the periodic process (i.e., amplitude, phase, and frequency) cannot be totally predicted by the past history of the signal.

Figure 21.1c illustrates the power spectrum of the sine wave illustrated in Figure 21.1a. Note the dominant peak at 0.2 Hz in the spectrum of power densities. This means that a major source of variance in the time series may be characterized by a sine wave with a period of 5s (i.e., 0.2 Hz). Note that the power spectrum attributes spectral densities to frequencies adjacent to the dominant frequency. If spectral analysis accurately decomposed the time series of a pure sine wave, why does the spectrum illustrated in Figure 21.1c have spectral density (i.e., variance) estimates at frequencies other than 0.2 Hz?

The answer is based upon an understanding of the application of spectral technology to stochastic processes. If we performed a Fourier transform on the deterministic sine wave plotted in Figure 21.1a, then the corresponding spectrum would distribute all the variance at 0.2 Hz. However, Figure 21.1c represents the results of a technology that has been developed to deal with stochastic processes. This analysis includes procedures to deal with the stochastic nature of the data. One of these procedures is called windowing.

Windowing is a technique for smoothing the spectral density function derived from the Fourier transform. The objective is to minimize the bias and variance of the spectral density estimates. Windowing may be implemented in either the time or frequency domain. In the frequency domain this may be accomplished by summing the weighted spectral density estimates on both sides of a specific frequency of interest. By stepping this weighted function across the spectrum (i.e., periodogram), abrupt shifts in the spectrum will be smoothed that may have represented unstable estimates. The number of frequencies included in the window is often determined by the investigator, and the coefficients are a function of the specific window selected. A simple frequency domain window may be generated by calculating a moving average two points to the left and two points to the right of a target frequency and stepping this through the spectrum. This unweighted moving average is called the Daniell window. The expected value of the new spectral density estimate becomes less biased as the duration of the time series increases. As more points are added to the moving average in the frequency domain, the variance decreases. Other frequency domain windows such as the Tukey–Hanning, Hamming, and Parzen use more complex coefficients. Windowing may also occur in the time domain. For example, the Bartlett window is often used with the Fast Fourier Transform (FFT). This procedure consists of performing the FFT on segments of the data and summing the spectra to provide one smoothed spectrum. More detailed discussion of windows may be obtained in time-series textbooks (see Chatfield, 1975; Gottman, 1981).

There are a variety of methods to calculate spectral density estimates. A common technique is the FFT. This technique greatly reduces the time required to perform a Fourier analysis on a computer. A limiting feature of most FFT algorithms is that they require data sets to be in powers of 2 (128, 256, 512, 1024, etc.). A discrete spectral analysis can be calculated with any number of data points by transforming the autocovariance function. The statistical properties of both the discrete Fourier transform and the FFT can be enhanced through frequency domain windowing. For a more mathematically based discussion of these issues see Bohrer and Porges (1982) or a recent time-series text such as Chatfield (1975) or Gottman (1981).

The value of spectral analysis becomes obvious when it is used to describe the parameters of periodicities in a complex wave. Spectral analysis provides a method to extract information about periodicities even when they are embedded in a complex pattern and may represent only a small proportion of the total variance of the time series. Figure 21.5a illustrates a complex pattern composed of the sum of three sine waves of equal amplitude. The sinusoidal components of this waveform are illustrated in Figure 21.5b. The frequencies in this example have been selected to be similar to those found in the heart rate pattern and have been associated with thermoregulation (0.04 Hz), blood pressure (0.1 Hz), and respiratory influences (0.26 Hz). For our data analyses we have sampled this complex signal every 500 ms. Figure 21.5c illustrates the confusing autocorrelogram of this complex process. In our example a "lag" is equivalent to the 500-ms sampling interval, and the three sine waves in the signal have periods of 25, 10, and approximately 4 s. If the autocorrelogram is of use in detecting periodicities in a complex signal, it should exhibit periodicity every 50 lags for the 0.04-Hz sine wave, every 20 lags for the 0.1-Hz sine wave, and approximately every 8 lags for the 0.26-Hz sine wave. Although the autocorrelogram exhibits periodicities, it is difficult to accurately identify underlying periodicities in these data. The corresponding spectral analysis illustrated in Figure 21.5d decomposes the variance of the process into constituent frequency components between zero and 1.0 Hz. Note the easily identified frequencies and the similarity of the spectral density estimates of the three peaks reflecting the similar amplitudes of the component sine waves. The effect of frequency domain smoothing is also evident in the width of the peaks and the overlapping of the spectral density estimates for the 0.04- and 0.1-Hz signals. Recall that the frequency domain windows are employed to deal with the stochastic characteristics of the signal even though in this example we used a deterministic simulation.

A more appealing example is provided by the spectral analysis of the data illustrated in Figure 21.6a. As illustrated in Figure 21.6b, these data are composed of the three frequencies used in Figure 21.5 with different amplitudes. The 0.04-Hz sine wave has an amplitude of 100, the 0.1-Hz sine wave has an amplitude of 50, and the 0.26-Hz since wave has an amplitude of 25. Figure 21.6c illustrates the autocorrelogram that is dominated by a periodicity of approximately 50 lags, reflecting the impact of the high-amplitude 0.04-Hz sine wave that has a period of 25 s, or 50 lags.

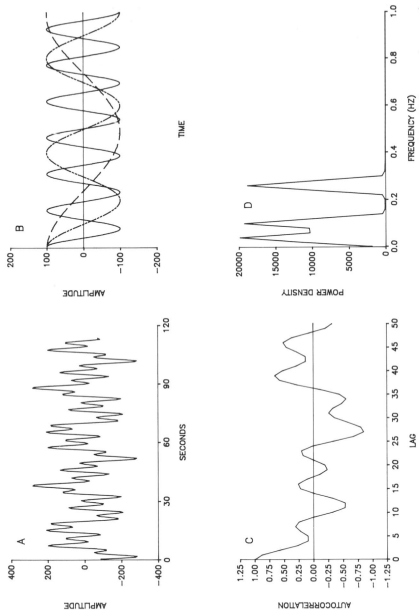

Figure 21.5. (a) Sum of three pure sine waves of equal amplitude. (b) Constituent periodicities of data illustrated in (a). (c) Autocorrelogram of data illustrated in (a). (d) Spectral decomposition of data illustrated in (a).

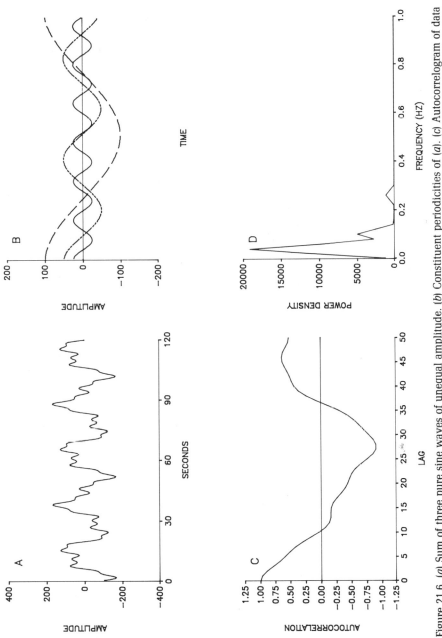

Figure 21.6. (a) Sum of three pure sine waves of unequal amplitude. (b) Constituent periodicities of (a). (c) Autocorrelogram of data illustrated in (a). (d) Spectral decomposition of data illustrated in (a).

Figure 21.6*d* demonstrates the effectiveness of the spectral procedure in extracting estimates of the amplitude and frequency of the three frequency components even when one component represents a small proportion of the variance. Closer inspection illustrates that the power density estimates for each of the three frequencies reflect their relative variances. Recall that amplitude squared divided by 2 is equivalent to variance. Thus, amplitudes in the ratio of 4:2:1 would produce variances in the ratio of 16:4:1. Since power density estimates are a linear transformation of variance, the three peaks in the power density spectrum reflect this ratio.

We can now inspect the spectral decomposition of the respiration and heart period data presented in Figures 21.2*c*, 21.3*c*, and 21.4*c*. Figure 21.2*c* illustrates the spectrum for the respiration signal. The spectrum is characterized by one dominant frequency at approximately 0.18 Hz (i.e., approximately 5.6 s per breath, or 11.8 breaths per minute). Very little of the variance from the respiration recording is attributed to other frequencies. In contrast, when we inspect the spectral densities for the heart period patterns, a different picture emerges. Figure 21.3*a* illustrates the heart period pattern recorded simultaneously with the respiration data illustrated in Figure 21.2*a*. Inspection of Figure 21.3*c* identifies a prominent peak associated with the respiratory frequency, although most of the variance (i.e., spectral densities) of the heart period process has been attributed to frequencies slower than respiration. Figure 21.4*c* illustrates the spectrum for the heart period pattern displayed in Figure 21.4*a*. Note that most of the heart period variance is associated with extremely low frequencies, whereas the peak at the respiratory frequency is low.

As illustrated in Figure 21.8*a*, the heart period data and the respiration data illustrated in Figures 21.2*a* and 21.3*a* are superimposed to emphasize the covariation of the two processes. The impact of the respiratory system on heart period (i.e., respiratory sinus arrhythmia) is characterized generally by a decrease in heart period (i.e., heart rate acceleration) with inhalation and increase in heart period with exhalation. In our example, respiration was monitored by quantifying the changing chest circumference associated with breathing. Inspiration produces an increase in chest circumference and an increase in our measure of respiration amplitude. When the two processes are superimposed, the rhythmic respiratory process is clearly manifested as respiratory sinus arrhythmia in the heart period process. The heart period is systematically attenuated during inhalation (i.e., increases in chest circumference or respiration amplitude in our example) and increased during exhalation. In our example, the amplitude of respiratory sinus arrhythmia appears to be more variable than the relatively constant amplitude of the respiratory process.

Although the spectral decomposition theorem is quite straightforward, its application to physiological data is extremely complicated. The spectral decomposition function decomposes all time series into constituent sine waves, each sine wave with an amplitude proportional to the variance the sine wave accounts for in the process. With pure sine waves the spectral decomposition is not ambiguous and functions to perfection. When time series are the sum of pure sine waves whose periodicities are hard or impossible to decipher from a graphic representation of the time series or from the autocorrelogram, the Fourier transform perfectly identifies the frequency and amplitude of the periodic components. Although spectral analyses will decompose any time series into constituent sinusoidal components, physiological activity is a composite of aperiodic and periodic components.

Moreover, the periodic activity is not sinusoidal and is seldom stationary. Therefore, spectral decomposition will distribute variance at low frequencies for the trends and slow aperiodic activity and at high frequencies for the harmonics of the periodic processes and high-frequency components of the aperiodic process. Thus, the peak frequencies identified in the spectral analysis of physiological data may not correspond to periodic physiological processes.

The preceding paragraph describes a situation in which spectral analysis does not provide consistent spectral density estimates. When the data are not stationary, no inference can be made regarding the characteristics of the spectrum. If, however, the time series is stationary, it is possible to obtain consistent estimates of the processes from a single finite sample of data. This important point has been mathematically proven by the *ergodic theorems*, which show that, for most stationary processes, the sample moments (i.e., mean, variance, autocovariance, etc.) of an observed record converge to the corresponding population moments.

The preceding characteristics of physiological time series make the application of spectral technology to psychophysiological research difficult. Figures 21.2c, 21.3c, 21.4c, and 21.8b provide appropriate examples to discuss three major concerns about spectral analysis of heart period patterns.

1. When the greatest power density occurs at the lowest frequency of the spectrum, the data are nonstationary and violate a primary assumption underlying spectral analysis. Spectral analysis always works. It always decomposes the variance of the process into sine wave components. Thus, regardless of potential violations of assumptions, spectral analysis will always provide descriptive information. However, the designation of a peak in the spectrum as being statistically significant implies that the underlying assumptions have not been violated. The spectral decomposition of an aperiodic nonstationary process will distribute a large amount of variance in the lowest frequency band. To deal with this problem, many researchers detrend the original data with low order (e.g., linear) regression fits across the entire data set prior to analysis. This method functions well if and only if the data have a linear or low-order trend. Although these trends often account for a significant proportion of the variance, the residual series are seldom stationary. In section 21.5 we describe methods developed to remove the nonstationary components of time series. The only other sources for variance in the lowest frequency are if the researcher failed to remove the mean level from the data prior to analysis or if there is a real periodicity at a frequency slower than the slowest defined frequency band. If the latter is the case, there may still be problems in the interpretation of faster periodicities in the spectrum. Since physiological processes are not perfect sine waves, extremely slow periodic processes might contribute variances to faster frequencies in the spectrum.

2. The spectra of physiological processes do not always reflect the multiple periodic processes theoretically assumed to be present. For example, in the literature it has repeatedly been stated that there are three periodicities in the heart rate spectrum. These rhythms have been theoretically associated with respiratory influences (i.e., respiratory sinus arrhythmia) at approximately $0.12-0.40$ Hz, blood pressure feedback (i.e., Traube–Hering–Mayer wave) at approximately $0.08-0.10$ Hz, and thermoregulation at approximately 0.04 Hz (see Kitney & Rompelman, 1980). It is hard to identify any peaks in Figure 21.4c. In Figure 21.3c the 0.04- and 0.1-Hz periodicities are not represented. However, with some imagination one can identify a periodicity of approximately $10-12$ s and another periodicity of approximately

20–30 s with careful visual inspection of Figures 21.3a and 21.4a. The ability to study these rhythms is greatly influenced by the aperiodic characteristics of the heart period pattern. Appropriate filtering might enhance the possibility of confirming whether these signals exist and the ability to study their behavior during psychophysiological experimentation. However, there are instances when these rhythms do not exist. These rhythms, which reflect neural modulation of the heart, may be greatly attenuated or blocked due to individual differences in neural control, pharmacological treatments, disease states, or physiological stress (Porges, 1986; Porges, 1988; Porges, McCabe, & Yongue, 1982).

3. The dominant frequency in one physiological response spectrum is not necessarily the dominant frequency in another physiological response spectrum even when both variables have common mechanisms. In our example in Figure 21.8b, the peak of the respiration spectrum is at a slightly faster frequency than the peak of the heart period spectrum. Yet our observations of the two processes in Figure 21.8a would lead us to believe that the rhythmicity of the breathing and the manifested respiratory sinus arrhythmia would be at the same frequency. The peaks may differ because the periodicities in the heart period pattern are less sinusoidal than the periodicities in the respiratory data. The heart period pattern includes more low-frequency and aperiodic influences. It is possible that the "respiratory" peak in the heart period spectrum is, in part, influenced by variances associated with low-frequency and aperiodic influences and is, thus, not reflecting the frequency and amplitude associated with an accurate measure of respiratory sinus arrhythmia. To assess whether this is truly happening, in a subsequent section we attempt to filter from the heart period pattern all aperiodic influences and periodicities slower than breathing. If our speculation is correct, the appropriately filtered data will have a peak frequency more similar to the peak of the respiration series.

21.4.2   Bivariate time series

Often there is interest in evaluating the covariation of two time series. Psychophysiological constructs such as *response fractionation* (Lacey, 1967) and *cardiac-somatic coupling* (Obrist, Webb, Sutterer, & Howard, 1970) have been defined in terms of the statistical relationship among physiological response systems. Similarly, arousal theory has been tested by assessing multiple variables. However, it is possible that the descriptive statistics of mean and variance used to define these constructs are not sensitive to all the underlying organizational characteristics of the nervous system. Specifically, mean and variance statistics are insensitive to rhythmic co-occurrence (i.e., coherence). Thus, the conclusions of earlier research (e.g., Lacey, 1967) may have been a function of an insensitive statistical methodology rather than of the underlying principles of neural and behavioral organization.

The cross-correlation function is a bivariate time domain method that is useful in describing covariation of two response systems when each is characterized by the same predominant periodicity. In Figure 21.7a the cross-correlogram is illustrated for the simultaneously recorded respiration and heart period illustrated in Figure 21.8a. Note that the periodic nature of the respiratory rhythm is reflected in the cross-correlogram. The magnitude of these correlations oscillates and dampens from approximately ±.50 to approximately ±.25 at lags representing multiples of a time displacement of approximately 12 lags, or 6 s.

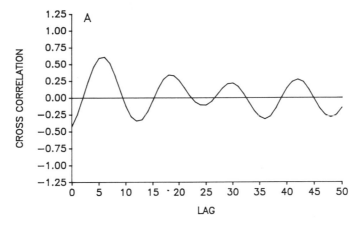

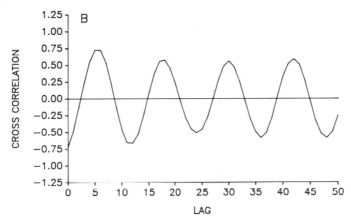

Figure 21.7. (a) Cross-correlogram of respiration and heart period data illustrated in Figure 21.8a. (b) Cross-correlogram of data illustrated in Figure 21.8a transformed with moving polynomial filter.

Since physiological time series are seldom characterized by a single periodicity, the bivariate time domain methods like the cross-correlation suffer from the same weaknesses attributed to the autocorrelation. A more effective method of describing the covariation of two physiological processes is the frequency domain technique of cross-spectral analysis.

Refer back to our example of simultaneously recorded respiration and heart period illustrated in Figure 21.8a. Note that there appears to be a synchronous pattern of decreases in heart period associated with inhalation and increases in heart period associated with exhalation. In Figure 21.8b the spectra are super-imposed, and there is a peak in heart period spectrum approximately at the peak of the respiration spectrum. Figure 21.8b does not provide the relevant information regarding covariation of the two processes. The figure merely describes their similarity in the spectral decomposition. It is possible to have similar spectra for both processes during states in which the processes are totally unrelated.

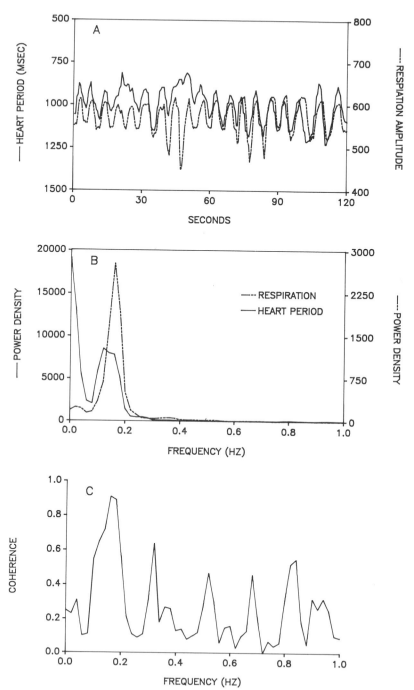

Figure 21.8. (a) Simultaneously recorded heart period and respiration data. (b) Spectral decomposition of data illustrated in (a). (c) Coherence spectrum of data illustrated in (a).

Crosss-spectral analysis is the appropriate frequency domain method of assessing the covariation of respiration and heart period at the breathing frequencies.

Cross-spectral analysis generates a coherence function that is a measure of the best linear association of each observed rhythm in one variable on the same rhythm in the second variable. Coherence is the square of the correlation between the two processes at a specific frequency. The coherence at any specific frequency is the square of the cross-spectral density divided by the product of the spectral densities of each series at the specific frequency. Note the similarity of this relationship with the calculation of the squared correlation coefficient. The cross-spectral density parallels the squared cross-products and the spectral densities parallel the variances. Conceptually, the coherence may be thought of as a time-series analog of eta or the proportion of variance accounted for by the influence of one series on the other at each specific frequency. For a more detailed discussion of coherence and a relevant modification of the procedure for psychophysiological data, see Porges et al. (1980).

Figure 21.8c illustrates the coherence spectrum for the heart period and respiration data illustrated in Figure 21.8a. Coherence scores are generated for all frequencies in the spectrum. Coherence, similar to the squared correlation coefficient, varies from zero to 1.0. Note that the coherence is not constant across all frequencies and there is a peak in the coherence spectrum in the general area that the dominant respiratory frequencies occur. Careful inspection of Figure 21.8c suggests that the coherence spectrum is exhibiting peaks at the dominant frequency of breathing and at integer multiples of this frequency (i.e., *harmonics*). These harmonic peaks do not represent important or interpretable data. Rather they are caused by the fact that both respiration and heart period processes are not perfectly sinusoidal and the sine wave fit to the periodicity leaves variances at higher frequencies. These small variances (note in Figure 21.8b that the spectral densities are extremely small at frequencies faster than respiration) are associated with the respiratory process and its manifestation on heart period and therefore should exhibit a high degree of covariation. The relatively high coherence at the harmonic frequencies confirms this point.

When the coherence in high, it is possible to interpret the phase relationship between the two series. Figure 21.9a illustrates the phase spectrum for the cross-spectral analyses conducted on the respiration and heart period data illustrated in Figure 21.8a. The frequency in the phase spectrum associated with the high coherence between respiration and heart period is identified by an arrow. Note that the phase varies between $\pm \pi$ (i.e., with π equal to 180° or one half-cycle). The phase at the frequency of peak coherence suggests that the heart period oscillations are approximately one half-cycle delayed from the respiration. However, inspection of Figure 21.8a demonstrates that the oscillations are virtually in phase. This contradiction is cause by the scaling of variables. When respiration amplitude increases during inspiration, heart period decreases. If we were to plot respiration amplitude and heart period on similar axes (i.e., larger numbers higher on the ordinate), the two series would appear to be temporally displaced by approximately one half-cycle and thus be consistent with the analysis.

Since physiological rhythms are never a perfect sine wave and occur over a band of frequencies, the calculation of a summary statistic that describes the proportion of shared variance of the two systems would be useful. In previous publications (see Bohrer & Porges, 1982; Porges et al., 1980) We have described a method of modifying

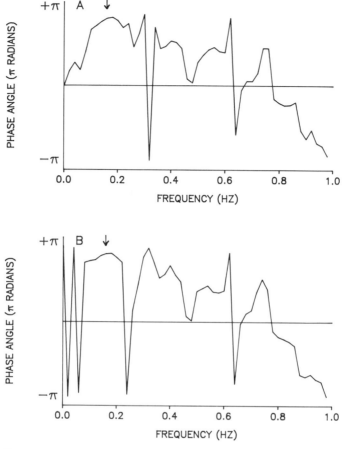

Figure 21.9. (a) Phase spectrum from cross-spectral analysis of respiration and heart period data illustrated in Figure 21.8a. (b) Phase spectrum of data illustrated in Figure 21.8a transformed with moving polynomial filter.

the coherence function that would enable one number to describe the general relationship or coupling between two time series. In our example, we have selected a frequency band between 0.12 and 0.4 Hz to calculate the summary statistic for the coherence spectrum, the *weighted coherence* (C_w).

If the spectral densities were equally distributed, an unweighted mean coherence (for all frequencies) would accurately described the relationship. For any other situation, it is necessary to calculate a weighted coherence, which provides an exact measurement of the proportion of the variance of one series that is shared between the two processes. In our example, the C_w between heart period and respiration has been defined as the proportion of total variance of the heart period process that is shared with the respiration process within the frequency band defined between 0.12 and 0.4 Hz. This frequency band has been selected because it is most representative of the spontaneous respiratory rhythms in human adults. During various experimental conditions it might be functional to shift this band to accurately describe the respiratory behavior of the subjects. In our example, we have weighted each of the coherence estimates within the 0.12–0.40 Hz frequency band by the spectral density for the heart period process at that frequency. This procedure assumes that respiration is driving the heart period process. If we assumed that heart period was driving respiration, we would weight the same coherence estimates by the spectral densities for the respiration process. In our example $C_w = .76$.

21.4.3 *Vulnerabilities of spectral analysis*

Spectral analysis decomposes the variance of the time series into constituent sine waves of various frequencies and amplitude. For spectral analysis to appropriately function, it is necessary that the data are *stationary* and that the data are *not aliased*. If the data do not possess these two properties, the spectral analysis may not be meaningful.

Stationarity implies that the expected value of the mean and variance are independent of the segment sampled and that the autocovariance function is solely a function of lag. Stationarity assumes that statistical properties of the time series do not change over time. Implicit in the property of stationarity is the assumption that time of initiation of an experimental manipulation is irrelevant. Thus, the application of spectral analysis that assumes stationarity would be inappropriate to many psychophysiological manipulations in which the experimental manipulation violates the stationarity property by creating a change in mean heart rate or heart rate variance.

Aliasing is a problem associated with selecting an inappropriate sampling rate. Spectral analysis decomposes the signal into component variances associated with frequencies from zero to one-half the sampling rate. Thus, if respiration were sampled every 500 ms (i.e., 2.0 Hz), spectral analysis as illustrated in Figure 21.2c would decompose this signal into frequencies from zero to 1.0 Hz. The fastest frequency we can detect in any spectrum is the *Nyquist frequency*. The Nyquist frequency for any data set, assuming equal sampling intervals, is the frequency of a sinusoid whose period is twice the time interval between successive samples. In our examples in Figures 21.1c, 21.2c, 21.3c, and 21.4c, the data were sampled at 2.0 Hz (i.e., sampling interval 500 ms) and the Nyquist frequency is 1.0 Hz (i.e., period is 1,000 ms). If there are oscillations faster than 1.0 Hz, then sampling at 2.0 Hz is too slow and the spectral analysis of the time series would be insensitive to these faster periodicities. The consequences of sampling too slowly are twofold. First, it would be impossible to visually identify rhythms whose period is less than the distance between time-sample observations. Second, the variance of the faster process is not totally lost or "filtered" from the data but is "folded back" on the slower frequencies in the spectrum. Thus, it is possible for high frequencies to be aliased as low frequencies.

Figure 21.10a illustrates a sine wave and Figure 21.10b illustrates the time series derived from the sine wave when the data are sampled too slowly. Assume that Figure 21.10a represents a 3-Hz sine wave and Figure 21.10b illustrates data sampled from the sine wave in Figure 21.10a at the rate of 5 Hz. Note the difference in number of oscillations between the two figures: The original sine wave has three oscillations and the sampled data exhibit two oscillations. In this example, the Nyquist frequency is 2.5 Hz and the variance associated with the 3-Hz sine wave would be aliased as frequencies below 2.5 Hz.

If we know the frequencies embedded in the physiological signal, we can avoid

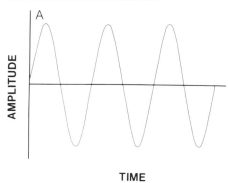

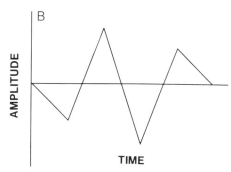

Figure 21.10. (a) Underlying rhythmic process to be sample. (b) Data generated by sampling process illustrated in (a) too slowly (example of aliasing).

the problems associated with aliasing by increasing the sampling rate. Unfortunately, in many electrophysiological response systems we are not aware of the entire range of periodic activity. In fact, one application of spectral technology has been to describe this range. Without an appropriate a priori physiological knowledge base, this approach might provide inexplicable epiphenomena. In addition, inappropriate alectrode application may, in itself, produce high-frequency artifacts in the signal that may be aliased as slower frequencies.

21.5   DETRENDING METHODS AND FILTERS

21.5.1   *The impact of detrending and filters*

From the preceding sections it is clear that spectral analysis is dependent upon the statistical characteristics of the data being analyzed. If the data are aperiodic and nonstationary, major problems are encountered. In this section, we assess the effectiveness of a variety of detrending and filtering methods to remove low-frequency and aperiodic nonstationary components from the physiological time series.

Throughout this chapter we have assumed that the time series being analyzed accurately represents the highest frequency components imbedded in the signal. Of course, if the data were sampled too slowly, then high-frequency components will be aliased on lower frequencies. Similarly, analog low-pass filters are frequently used to remove the impact of unwanted sources of variance (e.g., 60 Hz) associated with line voltage. The analog low-pass filter will not have serious quantitative consequences if the variances of the frequency components being filtered are small relative to the signal being studied. However, in some situations analog low-pass filters will distort high-frequency processes and transform them into slower processes. The concept of a polygraph integrator functionally employs this procedure in dealing with very high frequency components like EMG.

Filters transform one time series into another. The frequency domain modification of the time series by the filter is called a *transfer function*. The transfer function provides information regarding the filter's ability to block, attenuate, and amplify specific frequencies within the spectrum.

An ideal filter would remove the sources of variance that confound the assessment of the periodicities of interest to the researcher. Our discussions of filters will be limited to detrending methods that remove nonstationary influences and perform other high-pass functions. A detrending filter needs to have a number of characteristics to successfully perform. First, the filter must be able to remove nonstationary trend from the time series. Second, the filter should have a sharp cutoff so the nonstationary and low-frequency variations are completely removed without distorting the frequency and amplitude components of the periodicity being studied. Third, since periodic physiological activity seldom can be described by a single sine wave, the filter should have the ability to remove the influences of slow processes that although periodic may have component variances in the frequency band of the periodicity of interest. Fourth, the transfer function of the filter should be predictable for all applications.

Filtering can occur in the time domain or in the frequency domain. In this section we deal only with time domain filters. Frequency domain filters do not appear to be useful for many psychophysiological applications. Frequency domain filters perform their filtering after the data have been transformed into the frequency domain. In the frequency domain it is impossible to determine which proportion of a spectral density estimate represents the real signal and which part is a function of a nonstationary series or a slower periodic process that is not a perfect sine wave. Thus, frequency band rejection does not ensure that all the variances associated with nonstationary and slow periodic (but not perfect) sine waves will be removed.

One practical way of assessing the transfer function of a filter is to observe the impact of the filter on a white-noise time series. Since white noise is defined as a time series with the expected value of the spectral densities being the same for all frequencies, the spectrum of white noise should theoretically be flat. With the knowledge of the spectral characteristics of a white-noise time series, we can evaluate the transfer function of the filter on the spectrum by comparing the filtered spectral densities to the white-noise spectrum. If we divide the original white-noise spectrum into the filtered spectrum, we will be able to estimate the transfer function. If the numbers at specific frequencies approximate 1.0, the filter provides an accurate description of periodicity. If the numbers are less than 1.0, the filter attenuates the spectral densities. If the numbers approach zero, the filter rejects specific frequencies. If the numbers are greater than 1.0, the filter amplifies specific frequencies.

In Figure 21.11 spectra are illustrated for three detrending methods and the original white-noise series. Figure 21.11*a* illustrates the spectrum of the white-noise

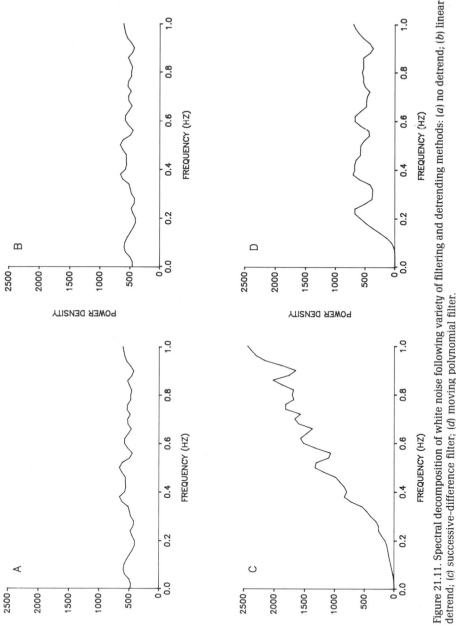

Figure 21.11. Spectral decomposition of white noise following variety of filtering and detrending methods: (a) no detrend; (b) linear detrend; (c) successive-difference filter; (d) moving polynomial filter.

series. Note that across frequencies, spectral densities are relatively uniform and approximate the theoretical flat spectrum. The values are not identical because the white-noise series is a sample of finite duration. If we increased the number of data points or averaged over a number of spectra, the spectrum would be flatter.

21.5.2 Linear detrending

Since heart rate patterns often exhibit trends, a common method of detrending is to remove the linear influence. This is done by fitting a linear regression to the data. This method removes linear influences and transforms the data set into a series with mean of approximately zero. Linear detrending has little impact on the spectrum of white noise. However, if we had superimposed the white-noise series on a large linear trend, the spectral decomposition of this series would distribute most of the variance at 0 Hz in the spectrum. A spectrum with a relatively large proportion of the variance at 0 Hz is a characteristic time series with nonstationary components. If the nonstationarity is caused by a linear trend, linear detrending will remove the nonstationary influence and provide an interpretable spectrum. Unfortunately, the nonstationary influences in physiological times series are seldom fit with a linear regression. Routine application of linear and other low-order polynomial fits (quadratic, cubic, etc.) to the entire data set seldom achieves the anticipated goal of removing nonstationary influences.

21.5.3 Successive-difference filters

In the psychophysiological literature, it has been proposed that successive-difference statistics such as the successive-difference mean square (see Heslegrave, Ogilvie, & Furedy, 1979) are useful in removing linear trends and other slow sources of variation. All measures of successive differences, like other filters, have a transfer function. When the data are sampled at equal time intervals (i.e., second by second and not beat by beat), the transfer function will be consistent across all subjects and conditions. However, if this family of statistics is calculated on the sequential heartbeat measures of period or rate, the transfer function is unreliable due to the variance of the sampling rate between and within subjects. The successive differencing of slow heart rate passes lower frequencies than the successive differencing of fast heart rate. Thus, the component variances of the complex heart rate pattern that are partially determined by the temporal characteristics of neural feedback are not treated consistently across subjects and conditions.

With data sampled at equal time intervals, it is interesting to observe the dramatic impact of successive differencing on the spectrum of white noise. In our example, we have sampled from the white-noise process at rates of 2 Hz. All spectra decompose the time series in frequencies from zero to π or in Figure 21.11 from zero to 1.0 Hz. Inspection of Figure 21.11c illustrates an important phenomenon. The low frequencies in the spectrum are greatly attenuated, demonstrating the success that the successive-difference filter has with low frequencies. However, the successive-difference filter amplifies higher frequency components. The 1.0-Hz component of the white-noise series has been amplified by a factor of 5. Knowledge of this transfer function is extremely important in interpreting data that have been successively differenced. At frequencies approximately one-sixth the sampling rate ($\pi / 3$), the spectral densities are relatively accurate. At frequencies slower than one-sixth the sampling rate, the spectral densities are greatly attenuated. At frequencies faster than one-sixth the sampling rate, the spectral densities are amplified.

21.5.4   *Summary of problems with traditional methods*

As we have repeatedly discussed, detrending and filtering procedures need to be capable of removing nonstationary components and rejecting low periodic nonsinusoidal activity that may have higher frequency harmonics. The commonly employed methods of linear and successive-difference filtering do not succeed. Statisticians do not have standard tools to deal with these problems. Most available time series statistical packages merely ritualize and exacerbate the existing problems by lulling the researcher into believing that he or she had adequately manipulated the data. Given these problems, what can the researcher do to ensure that the data are appropriately analyzed?

Being most familiar with heart rate patterns, we describe the problems and solutions associated with the extraction of an accurate measure of respiratory sinus arrhythmia. If the baseline trend is a complex function that cannot be mathematically described by a linear or low-order polynomial or by a sum of sine waves slower than the frequencies characteristic of respiratory sinus arrhythmia, the spectral composition of the baseline trend will include faster frequency components. The higher frequencies associated with the trend will "leak" through the detrending techniques and be superimposed on the spectral representation of the amplitude of respiratory sinus arrhythmia. Since the amplitude of the faster frequency components of the baseline trend are not known a priori and cannot be estimated a posteriori from the spectrum because they change over time when the baseline is not constant (i.e., nonstationary), high-pass filters do not eliminate all of the variance of baseline trend; a traditional high-pass filter cannot discriminate between the component variances associated with trend and the amplitude of respiratory sinus arrhythmia if both coexist in the same frequency band.

21.5.5   *A solution to the problem: the moving polynomial filter*

These points focus on the problems of applying spectral technology to accurately describe rhythmic physiological processes. In some situations it may be possible to minimize the impact of a complex baseline trend on the periodic activity by analyzing relatively short epochs and fitting the remaining trend with a linear fit. This approach is based on the assumption that a complex trend may be approximated by a series of adjacent linear trends. This method will be effective if and only if the trend component in each epoch is primarily linear. It is, however, possible to model the complex aperiodic baseline with a series of localized polynomials (see Porges, 1985). These short-duration polynomials may be stepped through the data set. The *moving polynomial filter* smooths the data set by conforming to the shifting levels of the baseline. When the smoothed baseline is subtracted from the original data set, the residual time series is free from the influence of the baseline and slow periodic activity.

Figure 21.12 illustrates how the moving polynomial procedure functions. The top panel illustrates 60 s of heart period data sampled every 500 ms from a healthy adult. Note the rhythmic oscillations occurring approximately 20 times within the 60-s data set. This oscillation is respiratory sinus arrhythmia. A graph of

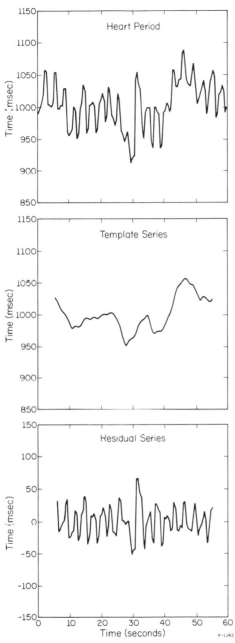

Figure 21.12. Moving polynomial procedure. *Top.* Unfiltered heart period series. *Middle:* Smoothed template series fit to changing baseline and slow periodic processes. *Bottom:* Filtered heart period series illustrating respiratory sinus arrhythmia.

simultaneously recorded respiration (e.g., see Figure 21.8a) would reflect the same periodicity.

The heart period data were collected while the subject was seated quietly and not involved in an experimental task. However, the pattern of the heart period data, even during these conditions, exhibited a complex trend that included contributions of slower periodic activity (e.g., Traube–Hering–Mayer wave) and aperiodic activity (e.g., acceleratory trend). A simple way of estimating the relative contributions of the various components to the total variance of the heart period pattern is to approximate the range of each component. In the example plotted in Figure 21.12, respiratory sinus arrhythmia has a range of about 50 ms, the Traube–Hering–Mayer wave has a range of about 50 ms, and the trend has a range of about 100 ms. Thus, even in an example in which respiratory sinus arrhythmia is visually apparent, respiratory sinus arrhythmia contributes far less than 50 percent of the total variance of the time series. There are situations, such as with the fetus, when heart period oscillations in the respiratory frequencies account for less than 1 percent of the total heart period variance (Donchin, Caton, & Porges, 1984).

The complex trend cannot be fit accurately with a linear regression over the entire data set. Moreover, the Traube–Hering–Mayer wave cannot be fit with a perfect sine wave. If spectral analysis is used to describe respiratory sinus arrhythmia, the amplitude of respiratory sinus arrhythmia may be inflated because linear detrending and frequency domain filtering would pass variance unrelated to respiratory sinus arrhythmia into the respiratory frequency band. Thus, traditional filtering strategies will inflate respiratory sinus arrhythmia amplitude. This presents the possibility that estimates of respiratory sinus arrhythmia amplitude derived from spectral density analyses may be modulated not by changes in the cardio-vagal tone mediated by respiration but by changes in trend and Traube–Hering–Mayer wave profiles.

It is possible that harmonics from the Traube–Hering–Mayer wave distort efforts to quantify respiratory sinus arrhythmia. The Traube–Hering–Mayer wave, associated with blood pressure feedback, has been reported in the heart period spectrum at frequencies between 0.07 and 0.10 Hz. This periodic process is far from sinusoidal and theoretically should have higher frequency harmonics at integer frequencies in the band from 0.14 to 0.20 Hz. Coincidentally, the 0.14–0.20-Hz band represents normal respiration for may healthy resting adults. Thus, the quantification of respiratory sinus arrhythmia is potentially inflated by the harmonics of the slower periodic heart period activity. Since the appropriateness of the sinusoidal fit to the Traube–Hering–Mayer wave is not known prior to data collection and the shape of the wave is far from reliable within a subject, it is impossible to determine how much of the variance attributed to the respiratory frequency band is a function of respiratory sinus arrhythmia and how much is a function of the Traube–Hering–Mayer wave.

The Traube–Hering–Mayer example understates the problem of harmonics in the heart period spectrum. The heart period pattern is very complicated. The spectral densities in the frequency bands associated with both the Traube–Hering–Mayer wave and respiratory sinus arrhythmia are confounded by even slower periodic nonsinusoidal processes that reflect thermoregulatory, ultradian, and circadian influences.

The moving polynomial procedure functions as a high-pass filter and partitions the time series into two uncorrelated components: a smoothed template series (see middle panel) containing the slow periodic and aperiodic activity (i.e., trends) that occurs at frequencies slower than breathing and a residual series (see bottom panel) generated by subtracting the template series from the unfiltered data that now conforms to the requirements of weak stationarity. Note how effectively the template series fits the complex aperiodic baseline and the quasi-periodic Traube–Hering–Mayer wave. The residual series clearly and accurately passes the frequency components associated with respiratory sinus arrhythmia.

The moving polynomial filter has unique performance characteristics as a filter since it does not make specific assumptions regarding the spectral characteristics of the trend prior to detrending. The number of coefficients and order of the polynomial are critical. In the example illustrated in Figure 21.12, a filter was designed to pass variance associated with frequencies above 0.12 Hz. With knowledge of the transfer function of the moving polynomial procedure and the sampling rate of the time series, it was possible to design a sensitive filter that dynamically fit the changing base level (see Porges, 1985). The residual series may then be analyzed with spectral analysis to extract the variance associated with the respiratory frequency band.

The order and duration of the polynomial are selected to bend into slow-moving trends without distorting the frequency band of interest. In our research on respiratory sinus arrhythmia we have selected a cubic order polynomial with a duration of 10.5 s for the research with human adults and a cubic order polynomial with a duration of 4.2 s for the research with human neonates. Other duration cubic polynomials have been used when we have studied other subject populations and other physiological rhythms. Figure 21.12a illustrates the original heart period signal of an adult subject, Figure 21.12b illustrates the smoothed series, and Figure 21.12c illustrates the residual filtered series.

Figure 21.11d illustrates the impact of a cubic moving polynomial filter with a duration of 10.5 s on the white-noise time series. Note that the spectral densities at the low frequencies are totally rejected and the high frequencies are not amplified. The theoretical transfer function for this filter indicates slight attenuation at the low end of the respiratory frequency band (i.e., 0.12 and 0.14 Hz) and fidelity at frequencies above 0.16 Hz. Although longer duration polynomials would provide greater fidelity of a sine wave at the slow repiratory frequencies, it would compromise the analysis by passing influences of slower periodic processes such as the Traube–Hering–Mayer wave. In fact, it has been demonstrated that with extremely slow breathing, respiratory sinus arrhythmia and the Traube–Hering–Mayer wave merge and become extremely difficult to interpret (Kitney, 1986). The attenuation of respiratory sinus arrhythmia at the slowest respiratory frequencies is of little concern and has only negligible impact on estimates of respiratory sinus arrhythmia because respiratory sinus arrhythmia occurs over a band of frequencies and the spectral densities are windowed.

We can now evaluate the influence of the moving polynomial filter on our respiratory and heart period data presented in Figure 21.8a. Recall that in Figure 21.8b the peak of heart period spectrum within the respiratory frequencies did not match the peak of the respiratory spectrum although the periodicity seems synchronous in Figure 21.8a. We speculated that this difference could be an example of how frequency components of aperiodic and slow periodic nonsinusoidal influences could distribute variance in higher frequencies and distort the

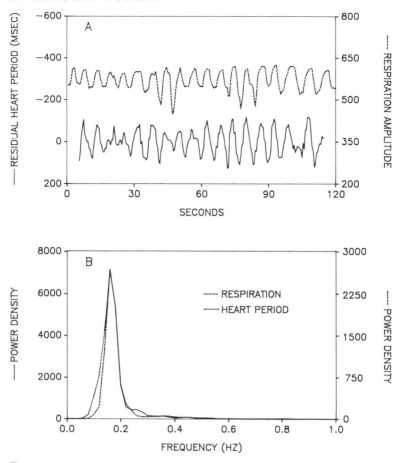

Figure 21.13. (a) Heart period transformed by moving polynomial filter and simultaneously recorded respiration. (b) Spectral analyses of data illustrated in (a).

estimate of respiratory sinus arrhythmia. In Figure 21.13a the detrended times series of the heart period data are presented with synchronously monitored respiration. Note that the removal of trend in the heart period also changes the values of the heart period series. Now the series has a mean of approximately zero, and the values of the residual series reflect deviations in milliseconds from the moving baseline trend that was subtracted from the data. In Figure 21.13b the spectrum of the filtered heart period data now exhibits a peak coincidental with the peak of the respiration data. The filter has successfully rejected the low frequencies and removed most of the aperiodic influences that had distorted, in Figure 21.8b, the peak of heart period spectrum in the respiratory frequency band. Linear detrending of the heart period data would also have produced a spectrum similar to that in Figure 21.8b with a distorted peak within the respiratory frequencies.

The moving polynomial filter can also be used to enhance bivariate methods. For example, when the simultaneously recorded respiration and heart period data illustrated in Figure 21.8*a* are transformed by the moving polynomial filter, the cross-correlogram becomes more regular. As illustrated in Figure 21.7*b*, the cross-correlations now oscillate between ±.75 and ±.50. Moreover, the moving polynomial filter appears not to influence the phase of highly coherent processes. As illustrated in Figure 21.9*b*, the phase between respiration and heart period at the dominant respiratory frequency is virtually identical to the phase of the unfiltered time series.

We could also assess the impact of a filter by applying it to a time series consisting of a sine wave of known amplitude superimposed on a periodic nonsinusoidal pattern. We could simulate two processes: one periodic but nonsinusoidal at a frequency similar to the Traube–Hering–Mayer wave and the other a perfect sine wave at a frequency similar to respiration. In our example, we use a 0.16-Hz sine wave superimposed on a 0.08-Hz periodic nonsinusoidal pattern. The 0.08-Hz pattern was generated by transforming values of a simulated sine wave to zero when they were negative. This procedure will produce harmonics at integer multiples of 0.08 Hz. This periodic nonsinusoidal pattern in illustrated in Figure 21.14*a*. The sine wave is illustrated in Figure 21.14*b*. The combined process is illustrated in Figure 21.14*c*. We know the real spectral characteristics of the sine wave by calculating a spectrum separately on the sine wave.

In Figure 21.15*a* the spectrum of the 0.08-Hz periodic nonsinusoidal process is illustrated. Note that the nonsinusoidal characteristics of this periodic process result in component variances being distributed to the first harmonic, 0.16 Hz. In Figure 21.15*b* the spectrum of the 0.16-Hz sine wave is illustrated. In Figure 21.15*c* the spectrum of the combined signal is illustrated. Inspection of this figure without knowledge of the underlying components would result in overestimating of the spectral densities associated with 0.16 Hz.

Figure 21.16 illustrates the relative impact on the spectrum of three filtering procedures. Linear detrending, illustrated in Figure 21.16*a*, produces a spectrum similar to the nondetrended spectrum in Figure 21.15*c*. Since there was no linear trend, this was expected. The successive-difference filter removed most of the variance at 0.08 Hz and greatly attenuated the variance estimates at 0.16 Hz. These results would have been anticipated with knowledge of the transfer function for the successive-difference filter. In contrast to the linear detrending and successive-difference filtering (see Figure 21.16*b*), the moving polynomial filter illustrated in Figure 21.16*c* removed the variances associated with the periodic activity at 0.08 Hz and also removed the harmonic variances associated with this process. The variance estimates at 0.16 Hz are very similar to the actual variances produced when the 0.16-Hz sine wave is analyzed by itself (see Figure 21.15*b*).

Similar to the preceding example, we can apply the various filtering procedures to the heart period data illustrated in Figures 21.3*a* and 21.8*a*. In Figure 21.17*a* the spectrum of the undetrended data are characterized by spectral densities at the lowest frequency and by the broad peak in the respiratory frequency band. In Figure 21.17*b* the spectrum for the linear detrended data are characterized by an attenuation of the deterministic component at the lowest frequency confirming that the data were nonstationary and had a major linear trend. The respiratory peak remains broad. In Figure 21.17*c* the spectrum for the successive-difference data demonstrate the impact of the filter's transfer function. The low frequencies have been totally rejected and although the peak frequency is more similar to the peak of the respiratory spectrum illustrated in Figures 21.2*c* and 21.8*c*, the amplitude of the

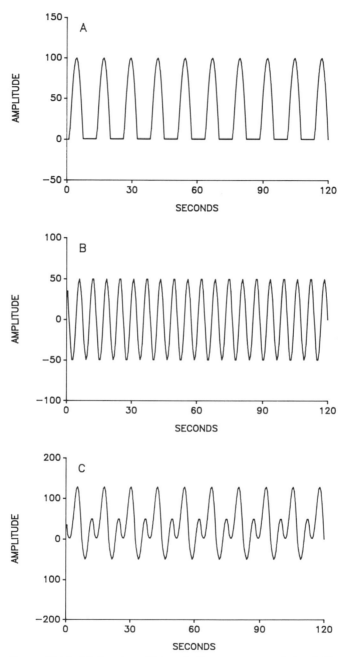

Figure 21.14. (a) Nonsinusoidal periodic component of signal illustrated in (c).
(b) Sinusoidal component of signal illustrated in (c). (c) Complex periodic process.

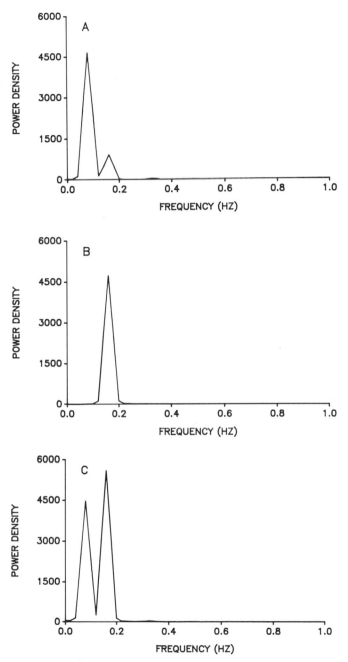

Figure 21.15. (a) Spectral decomposition of nonsinusoidal periodic signal illustrated in Figure 21.14a. (b) Spectral decomposition of sine wave illustrated in Figure 21.14b. (c) Spectral decomposition of complex periodic process illustrated in Figure 21.14c.

743

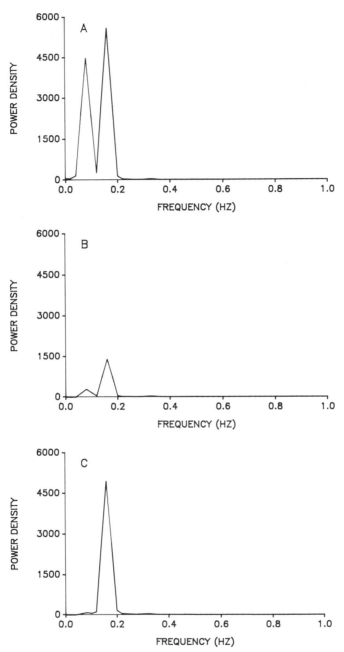

Figure 21.16. Spectral decomposition of complex periodic process illustrated in Figure 21.14c following a variety of filtering and detrending methods; (a) linear detrending; (b) successive-difference filter; (c) moving polynomial filter.

744

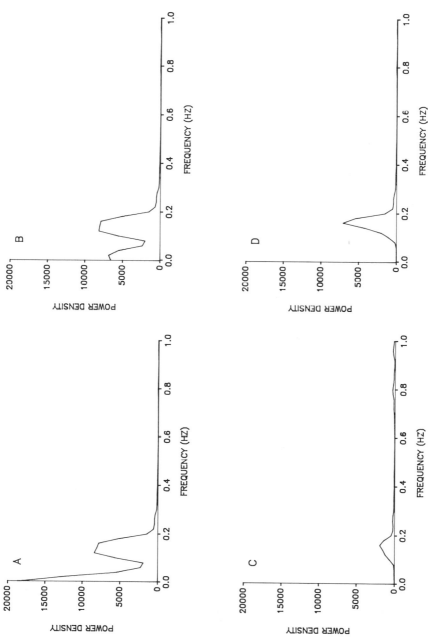

Figure 21.17. Spectral decomposition of heart period data illustrated in Figure 21.3*a* following a variety of filtering and detrending methods; (*a*) no detrending; (*b*) linear detrending; (*c*) successive-difference filter; (*d*) moving polynomial filter.

peak has been greatly attenuated. In Figure 21.17d the spectrum for the moving polynomial filter data is illustrated. Note the rejection of low-frequency components and the accurate manifestation of the amplitude and frequency of the higher frequency components.

21.5.6   *Alternative methods to describe amplitude of periodicities*

In many physiological and psychophysiological experiments descriptive methods have been used to quantify the amplitude of oscillations. For example, respiratory sinus arrhythmia has been quantified with a variety of heart rate variability measures including peak-to-trough calculation and differencing methods (e.g., beat-to-beat variability, short-term variability) as well as the spectral techniques previously described. In virtually all of these cases the problems associated with aperiodicity, nonstationarity, and periodic nonsinusoidal patterns have been totally neglected.

One of the most common methods is the peak-to-trough measure (Grossman & Wientjes, 1986; Hirsch & Bishop, 1981; Katona & Jih, 1975). Although this method has been successful in demonstrating systematic changes in the amplitude and frequency of respiratory sinus arrhythmia due to breathing maneuvers and vagal manipulations, the method has severe quantitative vulnerabilities.

In employing the peak-to-trough measure to quantify respiratory sinus arrhythmia, the researcher measures the difference between a maximum and a minimum point associated with a specific respiratory cycle. Or the researcher may employ a trough-to-peak measure. In this case the change is evaluated during the "up-phase" of the cycle rather than during the "down-phase" of the cycle. The researcher assumes that the peak-to-trough measure accurately reflects the instantaneous influence of the cardiac vagus on the heart (i.e., parasympathetic tone).

If the variability of the heart period activity were solely determined by respiratory sinus arrhythmia, measurement of either the up-phase or down-phase would provide an extremely accurate measure of respiratory sinus arrhythmia. However, respiratory sinus arrhythmia is usually superimposed on a complex trend and other slower periodic processes that are not perfect sine waves (e.g., Traube–Hering–Mayer wave).

The peak-to-trough method is a poor measure of both average and instantaneous parasympathetic tone because of two critical quantitative problems. First, the impact of nonstationarity associated with the complex trends will stretch and compress the peak-to-trough measure, amplifying and attenuating the measure when the amplitude of the underlying process is not changing. Second, the impact of slow periodic processes that are not perfect sine waves such as the Traube–Hering–Mayer wave will result in different durations in which the peak-to-trough measure would be stretched and compressed. Thus, the trend and slower periodic processes would significantly contribute variance to the peak-to-trough measure.

Although there are problems with many of the detrending methods used in the application of spectral analyses (see the preceding), the literature on peak-to-trough measurements is devoid of attempts to remove trends. As described the presence of trends would stretch the peak-to-trough measure during periods when the trend is ascending and compress the peak-to-trough measure during periods when the trend is descending.

To illustrate this problem, we have selected a sine wave with an amplitude of 50 (e.g., ± 50 ms) oscillating at a fequency of 0.16 Hz (Figure 21.18*a*). This sine wave is similar in amplitude and frequency to respiratory sinus arrhythmia in the healthy human adult and is identical to the sine wave used in our earlier example demonstrating the effectiveness of the moving polynomial filter (See Figure 21.14). The peak-to-trough measure for this sine wave is 100 ms. In our examples, to realistically approximate physiological characteristics, the trend has linear and higher order components. When the sine wave is superimposed either on an ascending trend (See Figure 21.18*b*) or a descending trend (see Figure 21.18*c*), the amplitude characteristics of the sine wave are changed. When the trend is relatively stable, the sine wave is accurately represented. When the trend is ascending, the peak-to-trough measure is compressed from 100 ms to approximately 73 ms. When the trend is descending, the peak-to-trough measure is stretched from 100 ms to approximately 134 ms. Note that not only is the peak-to-trough measure stretched or compressed by the trend, but also the trend contributes instability (i.e, increased variance) to the peak-to-trough measure.

If the amplitude of the sine wave were lowered and superimposed on the trend illustrated in Figure 21.18*b*, the trend would contribute even a greater percentage of the measured variance of the time series. The trend would also contribute more to the relative variability of the peak-to-trough measure. Thus, when the underlying periodic process accounts for only a small percentage of the total variance, the peak-to-trough method provides a greatly distorted estimate of the amplitude of the periodic process. In contrast, when the underlying periodic process accounts for most of variance, the peak-to-trough method will provide an accurate measure. Special populations who have low-amplitude respiratory sinus arrhythmia, such as diabetics, head injury patients, human fetuses, heart transplant patients, and high risk infants, are extremely vulnerable to these methods.

To illustrate the impact of detrending on the peak-to-trough measure, we have applied various methods to the ascending time series illustrated in Figure 21.18*b*. Figure 21.19*a* represents the time series with the linear trend removed. Although a major influence of trend is removed, the impact of the trend is still visible and is reflected in the variability in the peak-to-trough measures, which range between 127 and 88 ms. Figure 21.19*b* depicts the time series detrended by successive differences. Note the massive attenuation and variability of the peak-to-trough measure. Figure 21.19*c* illustrates the time series detrended by the moving polynomial filter. Note the stable and accurate representation of the peak-to-trough characteristics of the original sine wave (see Figure 21.18*a*).

The peak-to-trough method is not inherently a poor technique. It is accurate when applied to a time series consisting of a single oscillatory process. It is a useful method when applied to a complex time series that has been appropriately filtered (see Figure 21.18*c*). When the complex trends and slower periodic activity are effectively filtered, the method will provide an extremely accurate estimate of average or instantaneous parasympathetic tone by quantifying respiratory sinus arrhythmia. However, the method is severely compromised when time series reflect complex processes. Similar to the spectral technology described in the preceding, the problem with the peak-to-trough measure is not with the method but with the inappropriate application of the method to complex time series.

High correlations among various methods of measuring heart rate variability do not confirm that the measures behave the same. For example, in our research we investigated the influence of sleep state on measures of heart rate variability in

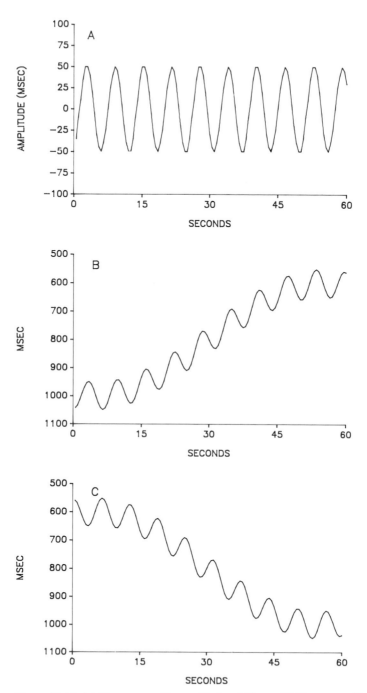

Figure 21.18. (*a*) Sine wave with amplitude of 50 ms. (*b*) Sine wave illustrated in Figure 21.18*a* superimposed on ascending trend. (*c*) Sine wave illustrated in Figure 21.18*a* superimposed on descending trend.

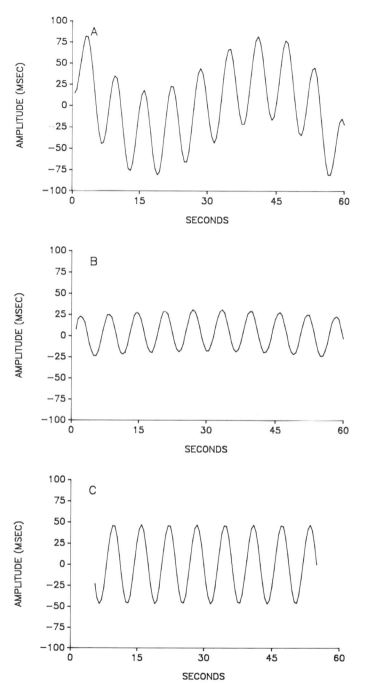

Figure 21.19. Ascending trend with sine wave illustrated in Figure 21.18*b* detrended with different methods: (*a*) linear regression fit: (*b*) successive differences; (*c*) moving polynomial filter.

healthy full-term neonates. The amplitude of respiratory sinus arrhythmia derived from the moving polynomial filter (i.e., vagal tone) was highly correlated with the standard deviation of the heart period during quiet sleep ($r = .88$) and active sleep ($r = .78$). However, the measures behaved differently across the sleep states. During active sleep the overall heart period variability was higher than during quiet sleep. In contrast, the amplitude of respiratory sinus arrhythmia derived from the moving polynomial filter reflected the hypothesized increase in parasympathetic tone associated with quiet sleep relative to active sleep. The magnitude of the sleep state effect in the analysis of variance, although in different directions for the two variables, was large, accounting for 29 percent of the variance in the moving polynomial measure and 43 percent in the standard deviation measure. This analysis demonstrates that high within-condition correlations do not provide information regarding the behavior of the derived variables. Also, it demonstrates that a component of the total variance (i.e., respiratory sinus arrhythmia) behaves differently than he composite standard deviation measure.

In the same study we successive differenced our data and calculated the mean successive difference. Successive differencing removes the impact of slow frequencies and amplifies the variances of fast frequencies. In this example, the mean successive difference behaved like the moving polynomial respiratory sinus arrhythmia measure. It was higher during quiet sleep than during active sleep. However, the effect size was much smaller, accounting for only 15 percent of the variance. In the preceding examples, we can see that successful filtering of our data provides the possibility of extracting physiological variables that closely parallel theoretical constructs of variables like cardiac vagal tone.

21.6   CONCLUSION

21.6.1   *Summary points regarding physiological response systems*

This chapter has addressed some of the major issues involved in the use of time-series analyses to detect and quantify periodicities in physiological response systems. The points described will be reviewed, and we conclude with a strategy to quantify periodic rhythms that attempts to overcome some of the problems inherent in psychophysiological research.

1. Physiological data may be described conveniently as time series. The hardware that psychophysiologists commonly use, the polygraph and the computer, readily lend themselves to the production of time-series data. The polygraph provides a continuous analog signal indexed by time. The computer with an analog-to-digital converter transforms the analog physiological signal into a digital representation at equally spaced intervals. This produces a discrete time series that is a manifestation of a continuous time series. The normal collection of physiological data satisfies many of the sampling requirements for time-series analyses. With minor modifications interevent series, such as heart period, may conform to these sampling requirements.

2. Many physiological response systems exhibit periodicities. These periodic processes tend to be of great interest to psychophysiologists because physiological rhythmicity in general is a manifestation of neural modulation of peripheral processes.

3. The accurate quantification of periodic physiological activity is difficult

because physiological data do not conform to the underlying assumptions necessary for most time-series analyses. Physiological data are not stationary, and the nonstationary components must be removed prior to the analyses of periodic activity.

4. Periodic physiological activity is generally not sinusoidal and cannot be fit by one sine wave at the frequency of the periodic activity. Therefore, periodic physiological processes have higher frequency components. These higher frequency components are often observed at integer multiples of the dominant frequency and are harmonics. These harmonics do not indicate that the high-frequency activity represents unique physiological activity. Rather, the harmonics reflect the nonsinusoidal nature of the main periodic component.

5. Many periodicities are manifested in more than one physiological system. For example, respiratory activity is manifested in heart period, blood pressure, vasomotor, and skin potential patterns. Thus, the problems described in the quantification of heart period oscillations will be similar to those encountered in other physiological response systems.

6. Measurement of the covariation of periodic processes in pairs of physiological response systems can be evaluated with cross-spectral analysis. Since physiological systems do not produce a constant periodicity, a weighted coherence can be calculated that expresses the shared variance of two processes across a band of frequencies.

21.6.2 — *Quantification strategies*

As we have argued the major problem in quantifying the periodic components of physiological activity is that physiological time series are nonstationary and the periodic components are not sinusoidal. The application of spectral methods to physiological response patterns is extremely limited because spectral methods were developed to work with stationary times series. Moreover, the spectral decomposition theory assumes that the sinusoidal components are statistically independent. In our examples, it has become clear that since periodic physiological processes are not sinusoidal, the spectral decomposition of physiological processes often produces harmonic variances that are highly correlated with the dominant "fundamental" frequency.

Adherence to the following guidelines will minimize some of the problems described.

1. The sampling rate must be fast enough to prevent aliasing. Aliasing may be avoided by sampling faster than twice the frequency of the highest frequency potentially present in the signal.

2. The nonstationary component of the process must be removed before the periodic components can be evaluated. This may be accomplished by the moving polynomial filter procedure, which successfully removes aperiodic components from the data set. Other methods of detrending such as the successive-difference and linear regression methods do not function as well as the moving polynomial filter procedure.

3. It is necessary to know the transfer function of a detrending or filtering method. As discussed earlier, some filtering procedures do not produce the assumed fidelity within the frequency band of interest. Moreover, procedures such as the moving polynomial filter can be designed to reject different low-frequency bandwidths.

Selection of a detrending and filtering method is a function of the frequency band of interest.

4. To accurately quantify various periodic components in the same time series, multiple filtering strategies have to progress from low to higher frequencies. Because periodic physiological activity is not sinusoidal, the variance of a periodic physiological process is distributed not only on the fundamental frequency of the process but also at whole-number integers of the fundamental frequency (i.e., harmonics). These harmonic variances distort the estimates of faster periodic processes. By developing moving polynomial filters that fit into the nonsinusoidal characteristics of slow periodic physiological activity, it becomes possible to quantify more accurately the higher frequency physiological activity. For example, in studying the multiple rhythms in the heart period process, a moving polynomial filter passing frequencies above 0.06 Hz might be used to study the Traube–Hering–Mayer wave and a second filter passing only frequencies above 0.12 Hz might be used to study respiratory sinus arrhythmia.

5. The twice modal duration rule should be used in designing the moving polynomial filter. This rule states that the duration of the polynomial should be twice the period of the modal frequency being evaluated. This rule has been developed as a guideline to deal with the shape of the transfer function of the filter and the fact that the frequency of periodic physiological processes is not constant but varies within a predictable band of frequencies.

This chapter has briefly described in nonmathematical terms methods to quantify periodic physiological activity. For a number of years progress toward this goal was slowed by the absence of appropriate statistical and hardware methods to deal with nonstationary trends and nonsinusoidal periodicities characteristic of physiological response systems. The method described as the moving polynomial filter works well in many situations. No method is perfect, and we have identified problems in simulated situations when we apply this filter to trends or slow periodic processes that have rapid transitions (i.e., step functions or square waves). The moving polynomial cannot fit rapid transitions because the slope of the transition mimics the frequency band of interest. Attempts to redesign the moving polynomial to fit rapid transitions change the transfer function and greatly attenuate the variances in the frequency band of interest. In spite of this limitation, we believe that the application of the moving polynomial method to detect and quantify periodic physiological activity is a significant advancement over other existing time-series methods.[1]

NOTES

The preparation of this chapter was supported, in part, by grant HD22628 from the National Institute of Child Health and Human Development awarded to Stephen W. Porges. The authors are grateful to Evan A. Byrne for his diligent work in developing the examples and illustrations. A special thanks is offered to Carol Sue Carter for editorial comments.

1 The application of the moving polynomial procedure to evaluate the amplitude of periodic physiological processes is protected by a U.S. patent. Individuals interested in applying this methodology independent of the commercial products currently available (i.e., the Vagal Tone Monitor and the Vagal Tone Analysis Program manufactured and distributed by Delta-Biometrics, Inc., 9411 Locust Hill Road, Bethesda, MD 20814) should contact the patent holder (SWP) for guidelines.

REFERENCES

Bohrer, R. E., & Porges, S. W. (1982). The application of time-series statistics to psychological research: An introduction. In G. Keren (Ed.), *Psychological statistics*. Hillsdale, NJ: Erlbaum.

Chatfield, C. (1975). *The analysis of time series: Theory and practice*. London: Chapman and Hall.

Donchin, Y., Caton, D., & Porges, S. W. (1984). Spectral analysis of fetal heart rate in sheep: The occurrence of respiratory sinus arrhythmia. *American Journal of Obstetrics and Gynecology*, 148, 1130–1135.

Gottman, J. M. (1981). *Time-series analysis*. Cambridge: Cambridge University Press.

Grossman, P., & Wientjes, K. (1986). Respiratory sinus arrhythmia and parasympathetic cardiac control: Some basic issues concerning quantification, applications and implications. In P. Grossman, K. Janssen, & D. Vaitl (Eds.), *Cardiorespiratory and cardiosomatic psychophysiology* (pp. 117–138). New York: Plenum Press.

Halberg, F., Johnson, E. A., Nelson, W., Runge, W., & Sothern, R. (1972). Autorhythmometry procedures for physiological self-measurements and their analysis. *Physiology Teacher, 1,* 1–11.

Heslegrave, R. J., Ogilvie, J. C., & Furedy, J. F. (1979). Measuring baseline-treatment differences in heart rate variability: Variance versus successive difference mean square and beats per minute versus interbeat intervals. *Psychophysiology, 16,* 151–157.

Hirsch, J. A., & Bishop, B. (1981). Respiratory sinus arrhythmia in humans: How breathing pattern modulates heart rate. *American Journal of Physiology, 241,* H620–629.

Katona, P. G., & Jih, R. (1975). Respiratory sinus arrhythmia: A non-invasive measure of parasympathetic cardiac control. *Journal of Applied Physiology, 39,* 801–805.

Kitney, R. I. (1986). Heart rate variability in normal adults. In P. Grossman, K. H. Janssen, & D. Vaitl (Eds.), *Cardiorespiratory and cardiosomatic psychophysiology* (pp. 83–100). New York: Plenum Press.

Kitney, R. I., & Rompelman, O. (Eds.), (1980). *The study of heart-rate variability*. Oxford: Clarendon Press.

Lacey, J. I (1967). Somatic response patterning and stress: Some revisions of activation theory. In M. H. Appley & R. Trumbell (Eds.), *Psychological stress: Issues in research*. New York: Appleton-Century-Crofts.

Obrist, P. A., Webb, R. A., Sutterer, J. R., & Howard, J. L. (1970). Cardiac deceleration and reaction time: An evaluation of two hypotheses. *Psychophysiology, 6,* 695–706.

Porges, S. W. (1985). *Method and apparatus for evaluating rhythmic oscillations in aperiodic physiological response systems*. (Patent number: 4,510,944). Washington, DC: U.S. Patent Office.

Porges, S. W. (1986). Respiratory sinus arrhythmia: Physiological basis, quantitative methods, and clinical implications. In P. Grossman, K. Janssesn, & D. Vaitl (Eds.), *Cardiac respiratory and cardiosomatic psychophysiology* (pp. 101–115). New York: Plenum Press.

Porges, S. W. (1988). Neonatal vagal tone: Diagnostic and prognostic implications. In P. N. Vietze & H. G. Vaughn (Eds.), *Early identification of infants at risk for mental retardation* (pp. 147–159). Philadelphia: Grune & Stratton.

Porges, S. W., McCabe, P. M., & Yongue, B. (1982). Respiratory–heart rate interactions: Psychophysiological implications for pathophysiology and behavior. In J. Cacioppo & R. Petty (Eds.), *Perspectives in cardiovascular psychophysiology* (pp. 223–264). New York: Guilford Press.

Porges, S. W., Bohrer, R. E., Cheung, M. N., Drasgow, F., McCabe, P. M., & Keren, G. (1980). New time-series statistic for detecting rhythmic co-occurrence in the frequency domain: The weighted coherence and its application to psychophysiological research. *Psychological Bulletin, 88,* 580–587.

22 *Time-series analysis applied to physiological data*

JOHN GOTTMAN

22.1 INTRODUCTION

What kinds of statistics might one wish to obtain from time-series analysis? This chapter will refer to three kinds of statistics. The first involves detecting cycles of interest, and the statistic is derived from the spectral density function; it assesses the amount of variance in the data that can be attributable to a given frequency compared to what this variance would have been if the series were white noise (the null hypothesis that there are really no cycles of interest in the data). The second involves assessing if a time series has changed significantly following a baseline. The method here is called the interrupted time-series experiment. The third involves statistics that assess relationships between two time series. This chapter will discuss time and frequency domain statistics for the study of bivariate relationships.

This chapter is concerned with a selected set of techniques of time-series analysis that are useful for the analysis of physiological data collected (or summarized) at intervals, such as the EKG and other cardiovascular time series, the EEG, the EMG, and the electrodermal response (EDR). This chapter will not review aspects of data preparation and signal conditioning since those topics have been covered in Part III of this book.

This chapter is designed to introduce the reader to general concepts in time-series analysis and to illustrate its application for psychophysiological data. Readers who wish additional information on time-series analysis can consult several readily available sourcebooks (Anderson, 1975; Box & Jenkins, 1970; Brillinger, 1975; Chatfield, 1975; Glass; Willson, & Gottman, 1975; Gottman, 1981; Koopmans, 1974; Williams & Gottman, 1981). A variety of computer programs for time-series analysis are available from standard packages such as SPSS, BMDP, and ASYST. A computer package written by the author specifically for beginners is available (Williams & Gottman, 1981) as well as the accompanying book (Gottman, 1981). This package consists of 10 computer programs that can be run on a personal computer compatible with an IBM-XT (with 640 kb of random-access memory [RAM], with a math coprocessor chip). These 10 programs were written for the beginner, so they are interactive and easy to use. They also give visual (and numeric) confidence intervals for the rapid summary of appropriate statistical tests. Table 22.1 is a summary of what these programs do.

22.1.1 *The selected topics*

This chapter discusses (1) stationarity and what must be done if the data violate this critical assumption; (2) the interrupted time-series experiment; (3) linear filtering of

754

Table 22.1. *Overview of programs in Gottman–Williams package for time-series analysis*

IF YOU WANT TO	YOU WILL NEED
1. Assess the effects of an intervention, i.e., do an interrupted time-series analysis.	1. Program ITSE. It would be useful to employ the univariate model-fitting programs for examining and removing trend and seasonal components (programs DETRND, LINFIL, DESINE, ARFIT, and SPEC).
2. Examine one time series for component cyclicities.	2. Program SPEC (also can be used to compute the periodogram).
3. Forecast data (limited to one step ahead).	3. Program FORCST.
4. Examine two series for cyclical covariation, i.e., synchronicity and cyclic lead–lag relationships.	4. Program CRSPEC.
5. Perform bivariate time-series analysis, controlling for autocorrelation in each series (Gottman–Ringland procedure).	5. Program BIVAR.
6. Do regression from a set of predictor time series to a criterion time series.	6. Program TSREG.

the data and the fundamental theorem; (4) Fourier estimation and other forms of estimation, including the Projection Theorem; (5) univariate spectral time-series analysis using the periodogram and the spectral density function; (6) bivariate spectral time-series analysis; and (7) time-series regression and other multivariate extensions, including the Gottman – Ringland procedure for controlling autocorrelation in inferring cross-correlation.

22.2   STATIONARITY

The central assumption of time-series analysis concerns notions of stationarity, which essentially can be translated for practical purposes into the idea that the mean, variance, and autocovariance structure of the time series are independent of historical time. The notion of "autocovariance" is generally not well known and will be briefly reviewed here. If a time series is denoted $x(t)$, where t is time, a lagged version can be created, say, $x(t+1)$ for lag 1, and a covariance computed between $x(t)$ and $x(t+1)$; in a similar way a lag-k autocovariance can be computed between $x(t)$ and $x(t+k)$. The notion of autocorrelation involves a similar extension.

This assumption of stationarity can be violated in many ways with various consequences. The violations of stationarity almost always have serious consequences for statistical tests, and it is therefore necessary for people who would use time-series techniques to pay careful attention to their data. Violations of stationarity in psychophysiological data will involve a change in level or slope of the data or a more profound change in underlying autocorrelational structure, which would occur if, for example, a new cycle were added to the series or an underlying cyclicity changed its frequency. This means that it is unlikely that a set of data in a study can all be analyzed in exactly the same automatic way because different treatments will be required for different series depending on stationarity.

What can one do if the data are not stationary? There are four general options when the data are not stationary: (1) break the data into chunks that are stationary; (2) model the time series into the sum of three components – trend (defined quite generally), deterministic cycles, and a stochastic, stationary time series; (3) transform the data, or (4) combinations of these three options. Transforming the data (e.g., by filtering or differencing) has easily computable consequences only when the transformation (filter) is linear. However, the consequences of even a linear transformation may be very powerful in ways that will be surprising to the uninitiated. For example, successive differencing of a series [transforming a series $x(t)$ into $[x(t+1) - x(t)]$ eliminates *local* as well as overall trend. This means that if there is a brief slope to the data (say, lasting 15 observations), it will be flattened; if there is a later brief (say, 15 observations) slope in a different direction, it will also be flattened; there will only be a jump between the change in slopes. The difference transformation will also amplify high-frequency signals. Thus, a successive-difference transformation does far more than remove an overall trend in the time series (see also Porges & Bohrer, chapter 21).

The notion of transformation introducing complex changes in a time series has an important historical lesson. At one time (before 1930) economists were freely transforming their data, but an important theorem by a Russian named Slutzky put a stop to all that. Slutzky proved that it is quite possible to introduce new patterns not originally in the data by filtering, and in fact, this was the basis of Slutzky's (1937) models and Yule's (1971) models in the early 1930s. Slutzky's initial results were that it was possible to create any kind of pattern by suitable averaging of white noise. This includes any set of cycles one desires. As noted here, this finding shocked his contemporaries, who were doing this averaging freely to reduce noise, never thinking that they might be introducing new and spurious patterns and cycles based on the noise itself. The same error could apply to unexamined components in the creation of an evoked potential; it is not possible to determine the extent of this methodological problem without detailed statistical study. The Fundamental Theorem of Filtering now makes it possible to estimate these effects. Perhaps an intuitive discussion will make this clear. White noise, like white light or white acoustical sound, contains all frequencies with equal expected amplitude. They are also independent of one another, and thus, by suitable selected averaging of noise with various lags, any "color" or frequency of oscillation can be deleted or enhanced. If noise is represented by the series $e(t)$, a moving average model is a weighted sum of the series lagged, that is, $e(t-s)$, where $s = 0, 1, 2, \ldots, q$. For further discussion, see Box and Jenkins (1970).

22.2.1 *Modeling*

In many cases it will be useful to develop a mathematical model for a time series. How can one know that a model is appropriate? The answer is that with a proper fit, the residual of the modeled or transformed series should be white noise. Statistical tests for whether a time series is essentially white noise exist (e.g., the Box–Pierce test). Perhaps the most useful approach to modeling a time series is to break it into deterministic and nondeterministic components. These are actually relative terms (i.e., components are more or less deterministic). Deterministic components have predictability over long time periods without too much increase in the confidence intervals of forecasts as one moves away from the prediction point. For example, a sine wave at a fixed frequency of oscillation would be determinstic; if the frequency and amplitude of the sine wave were each a random variable with a distribution, the sine wave would be nondeterministic. Economists are quite interested in modeling a time series. In physiology, modeling in a particular experimental context would be interesting if it had some theoretical meaning. For example, the particular range of the interbeat interval spectrum related to respiration (the respiratory sinus arrhythmia) has its own meaning and neurophysiological significance as vagal tone (Porges, 1984). A variety of computer packages can be used to assist in this modeling. For example, the first four computer programs of the Williams–Gottman package are designed to remove linear trend (program DETRND), for linear filtering (LINFIL), to remove deterministic cycles (DESINE), and to fit autoregressive models to the stochastic component.

22.3 THE INTERRUPTED TIME-SERIES EXPERIMENT (ITSE)

The interrupted time-series experiment is a general procedure used to scan for changes in a time series at some particular class of event. For example, does an angry facial expression create a statistically significant increase in heart rate compared to the baseline? Interrupted time-series analyses employ a particular stationary model (e.g., an autoregressive model whose order might be specified by the user) to perform the assessment of whether the series has changed. As an example, in the Gottman–Williams package, program ITSE is designed to do only one kind of analysis of the effects of planned or unplanned events on a time series, one based on autoregressive models that vary around one straight line in the baseline and a different straight line after intervention. Statistical tests are provided for change in level and slope of the two chunks of the time series, the one before and the one after the critical event. There are advantages to using autoregressive models in terms of their ease, but there are also disadvantages. The disadvantage is that autoregressive models do not change rapidly; they change gradually, so they would not be very good at modeling an intervention effect that had a sudden onset. Much more complex models and modeling procedures exist. The general class of nonlinear models introduced by Box and Jenkins (1970) is called the ARIMA models (autoregressive integrated moving average models). These models and procedures are available in time-series packages (e.g., the BMDP series). The disadvantage of these procedures is that model fitting has been described as an art form; it is difficult to fit moving average parameters once the number of these parameters increases beyond about 2 because the equations to be solved for fitting these parameters are nonlinear. An alternative procedure has been invented by Pandit and Wu (for a review, see Gottman, 1981).

22.3.1 *Algorithm of the Gottman–Williams ITSE program*

The data before the supposed "intervention" are represented as one straight line with slope and intercept plus an autoregressive model, and the data after the intervention are represented as a different straight line with different slope and

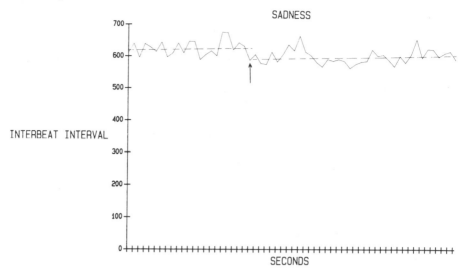

Figure 22.1. Changes in IBI of 5-year-old child after spontaneously elicited facial expression of sadness.

intercept but with the same autoregressive model added. This is the representation in the "big model"; in the little model, which is the null hypothesis .model, the straight line is presumed to have stayed the same, with the same slope and intercept. The general linear model is set up, and *t*-tests are provided for change in slope and level.

22.3.2   *Example*

In Figure 22.1 we can see the graph of a 5-year-old female child's interbeat interval (denoted IBI, the time between R-waves of the EKG) average over 1-sec intervals. There is a baseline that precedes her first expression of sadness [coded by Ekman and Friesen's (1978) EMFACS system] during a filmed induction of sadness. The interrupted time-series experiment here tests whether there has been a statistically significant reduction in IBI (increase in heart rate) following the sadness facial expression. Program ITSE was employed with a first-order autoregressive model. The *t*-test for change in level was 2.50, with 38 degrees of freedom, and the *t*-test for change in slope was 0.27, with 38 degrees of freedom. Hence, there was a significant change in level but not slope in these data. This result of a heart rate increase with a sadness facial expression is consistent with Ekman, Levenson, and Friesen (1983). It is also consistent with the notion that emotion is associated with increased autonomic activity. However, Ekman et al. found that heart rate decreases during the emotion of disgust.

22.4   LINEAR FILTERING AND THE FUNDAMENTAL THEOREM

Filtering is used quite often with physiological data, for example, to eliminate artifact or to smooth a noise series such as an EMG signal. Often this is done by equipment prior to the signal being stored in the computer, but at times the full signal is available for analysis. The equation of a linear filter defines an operator that shows how, precisely, the spectral density function of the filtered series will relate to the spectral density function of the original series. For example, for a first-order moving average filter (usually, $-1 < b < +1$),

$$x'(t) = x(t) + bx(t-1)$$

the spectral density function of x, $p(x; f)$, will be multiplied by

$$1 + b^2 + 2b \, \cos \, (2\pi f)$$

times a constant (sigma noise squared divided by 2π). Depending on the value of b, this can be a low-pass or a high-pass filter (negative b are high pass, positive b are low pass).

It is wise to compute the shape of the filter before applying it because it is possible for a filter to introduce new spurious patterns into the spectrum (this can also happen with some spectral windows). Hamming's (1977) book is a good resource for seeing what linear filters will do to the spectrum. The Fundamental Theorem of Filtering is a generalization of the relationship shown in the preceding; it gives the exact mathematical relationship between the spectral density functions of the two series. Linear filters can be designed to amplify or attenuate any band of cycles in a time series.

22.5 FOURIER ESTIMATION AND THE PROJECTION THEOREM

In this section the notion of why sines and cosines enter into time-series analysis will be discussed as well as those situations in which one may wish to generalize beyond sines and cosines. In 1822 Fourier showed that the best least-squares approximation to a wide class of functions was to be obtained by employing a subclass of sines and cosines whose weights were determined and computable from the function itself. Actually, Fourier proved this theorem incorrectly, and it took the best mathematical minds of a century to do it correctly, and the product was to be known in mathematics as *modern analysis*. One exciting result from modern analysis is a theorem called the *Projection Theorem*, which will be discussed here. To simplify matters, consider what is known as the *overtone series*, and assume that there are an odd number of data points in the series, $x(0)$, $x(1),...,x(T)$.

22.5.1 *The overtone series*

Once we know how many data points there are in the series, we automatically have available to us only a selected set of sine and cosine waves for our estimation, and these are determined by a specific set of frequencies (cycles per unit) called the overtone series. The more data points we have, the finer the grid we have available for our estimation. But note that the actual cycles are very likely to fall in between the grid given by the overtone series. These cycles are

$$W_j = 2\pi j/T$$

where $j = 1, 2, 3,..., (T-1)/2$. Hence, for $T = 31$, we have 15 cycles to use for our estimation. Had we collected 131 data points, we would have had 65 cycles for our estimation. For $T = 31$, w_j would go from $2\pi (1/31) = 0.202$ in multiples of up to 2π $(15/31) = 3.040$. Our frequency grid is divided into j/T units, starting from $1/T = 0.032$, to $2/T = 0.065$, up to $15/T = 0.484$. This means that the more data points in the time series, the finer our grid is for estimating the true cycles in the data.

We are limited to these cycles because estimation cannot proceed without the use of a set of functions that have a property called *orthogonality*; that is, the covariances of the set of estimator functions must be zero. The set of functions we use for our estimation is called our *orthogonal basis*. This basis can be represented as a set of axes in our $[(T-1)/2]$-dimensional space for our estimation. The time series we wish to estimate can be represented as a line in this space. The generalization of the notion of covariance is the *projection*, or the shadow cast by the function we are trying to estimate on each of the functions in our orthogonal basis. A more detailed discussion of these concepts can be found in most books on Hilbert spaces.

22.5.2   Why this is good news

The Projection Theorem is good news because there are certain kinds of data for which sines and cosines are not very good estimators even if they are best in a least-squares sense. This is true for several reasons. First, it is true if the data come close to violating the assumptions that must be satisfied by Fourier's theorem. For example, Fourier approximation becomes very complex if there are outliers, in which case it is necessary to give substantial weights to many of the cycles in the overtone series. The result will be that the interpretation of the frequency content of our data will be very misleading; all these frequencies' are not actually *in* the data, but they must be employed to approximate the series and the outlier. However, other orthogonal bases exist for strange data. For example, one orthogonal basis that has seen a lot of application in engineering is an orthogonal basis made up of functions with lots of little discrete boxy steps called Walsh functions. They are like sines and cosines except they are boxy, not smoothly changing in the circular fashion of sines and cosines.

We start with the *periodogram*, which is the Fourier estimate of the spectral density function. If the time series is $x(t)$, the periodogram is denoted $I(f)$: The equation of the periodogram is

$$I(f) = \frac{1}{2\pi T} \left[\left(\sum_{t=0}^{T-1} x(t) \cos 2\pi ft \right)^2 + \left(\sum_{t=0}^{T-1} x(t)' \sin 2\pi ft \right)^2 \right]$$

This function loses the important phase information in the component cycles used to estimate the observed time series. In this case phase tells us how the sines and cosines used in the overtone series of functions are to be combined so that they will add and cancel in the right places. Phase refers to the location on the y-axis where the sine or cosine waves cross at zero time. All we have left with the periodogram is the square of the amplitudes of the sine and cosine components at each frequency. To be precise, if $x(t)$ is a sum of $A_j \cos(2\pi f_j t) + B_j \sin(2\pi f_j t)$, then at each frequency the value of the periodogram will be

$$I(f_j) = \left(\frac{T}{4\pi} \right) \tfrac{1}{2}[(A_j)^2 + (B_j)^2]$$

One way of thinking about this in simplified terms is to think of each oscillation in

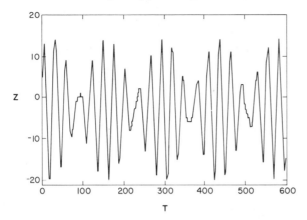

Figure 22.2. Whittaker and Robinson data on brightness fluctuations of variable star.

the overtone series as a pendulum. If a pendulum is shoved harder, it will have a larger amplitude. In fact, the square of the amplitude is proportional to the energy with which the pendulum was shoved. This is an important metaphor. It equates *variance* with *energy*. The phase of the component cycle has to do with when in its swing the pendulum is shoved. Adding cycles amounts to attaching one pendulum onto the bottom of another; the resultant oscillation is what the bottom of all these pendula is doing, with all the pendula above swinging at different phases and with different amplitudes.

The weights of each member of the overtone series are derived from the time series itself. The time series $x(t)$ is represented in the Fourier approximation as

$$x(t) = \sum_j (a_j \cos w_j t + b_j \sin w_j t) + e(t)$$

In this case, we can estimate (least squares) the a_j and the b_j by A_j and B_j:

$$A_j = \frac{2}{T} \sum_{t=0}^{T-1} x(t) \cos w_j t$$

$$B_j = \frac{2}{T} \sum_{t=0}^{T-1} x(t) \sin w_j t$$

Before we discuss the periodogram, we consider a nineteenth-century approach to its computation called the Buys–Ballot tables, which make the notion of the periodogram intuitively understandable.

22.5.3 *The dream of the periodogram*

In the nineteenth-century Whittaker and Robinson (1924) collected a famous data set of the brightness of a variable star. They observed the star for 600 consecutive days and obtained the time series shown in Figure 22.2. These data turned out to have two cycles, and this led them to conclude that they were in fact observing a binary star, not one star, and that these two stars rotated around a common focus. To conclude that there were two component cycles, they used an approach called the

Table 22.2. *Illustration of computation of periodogram using Buys–Ballot table*

	T = 5					T = 4			
	1	2	3	4	5	1	2	3	4
	.00	.95	.59	− .59	− .95	.00	.95	.59	− .59
	.00	.95	.59	− .59	− .95	− .95	.0	.95	.59
	.00	.95	.59	− .59	− .95	− .59	− .95	.0	.95
	.00	.95	.59	− .59	− .95	.59	− .59	− .95	.0
						.95	.59	− .59	− .95
Means	.00	.95	.59	.59	− .95	.0	.0	.0	.0

Buys–Ballot table, which is a simple computational procedure for computing the periodogram.

An assumed period is tested for by arraying the data in columns. For example, suppose the data follow a period $T = 1/f = 5$. Say that $x(t)$ is consecutively equal to 0.00, 0.95, 0.59, −0.59, −0.95, 0, and so on. If we are fortunate enough to guess that $T = 5$, we would array our data as shown in Table 22.2 (left side). We would notice that the means of these columns are indeed the series, and so the ratio of the two variances, the variances of the means divided by the variance of the series, would be 1 if we guessed the period correctly. If we guess incorrectly, say $T = 4$, the data are arrayed as shown in the table (right side) and the variance of the means is zero. This is the situation when we have no noise in the data. When we have noise, the variance at the incorrect period is not zero, and we need to be able to compute confidence intervals around the estimated periodogram to see if our values are statistically significant compared to the null hypothesis that the whole series is noise (i.e., without any cycles).

22.5.4   The failure of the periodogram

Unfortunately, the periodogram turned out to be an unusable statistic because the variance of the periodogram does not decrease as the sample size T increases. Thus we have no way of narrowing the confidence intervals around each spectral estimate as we collect more data. The solution is to create a moving average of the periodogram; by varying this moving average, confidence intervals can be created around the new spectral density estimate that decrease as T increases. These moving averages are called *spectral windows*.

22.5.5   Example

The data presented in Figure 22.3 are the spectral analysis of 60 observations from a diary record of the severity of migraine headaches recorded by a patient in a headache clinic. The data were analyzed with program SPEC. They show graphically how to do the test of statistical significance for a peak. The line represents the estimated spectral density function, and the asterisks represent the confidence bands around this estimate. The vertical line is what the spectral density function

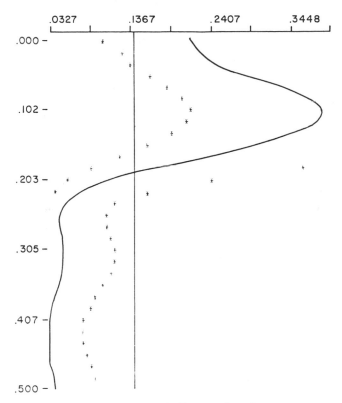

Figure 22.3. Spectral analysis of self-report data of severity of migraine headaches of one patient.

should (theoretically) look like if the data were actually perfect white noise. This vertical line should be below the confidence band's lower limit for the peak to be significant.

Unfortunately, there are problems with this solution of averaging the periodogram. The problem is that moving averages of the periodogram can obscure peaks that may be real. It is important to note that a moving average of the periodogram is not the same as a moving average of the original time series. In fact, a moving average of the time series will act as a low-pass filter, smoothing or filtering out high-frequency oscillations. Here we are talking about averaging the periodogram, not the series. Figure 22.4 shows how the periodogram suggests the presence of a very low frequency (long-period) peak that is smoothed over by the averaging. The only solution is to employ a range of smoothing options. It is wise to always also compute the periodogram. In this manner the investigator can determine if there are cycles of interest in the data that there may not be enough power to detect at this point in the research. As a rule of thumb, the periodogram gives the least power and probably the most spurious peaks; various smoothing options will maximize power but be conservative with regard to peak determination.

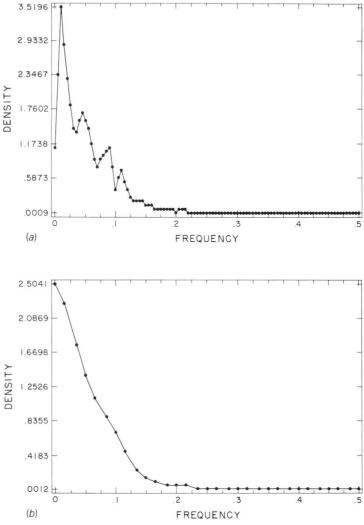

Figure 22.4. Importance of selecting range of bandwiths for smoothing periodogram. Figure shows low-frequency peak, which is obscured by averaging in creating spectral density function from periodogram.

22.6   NINETEENTH- AND TWENTIETH-CENTURY DIFFERENCES IN CONCEPTUALIZATION

A major conceptual change took place between the nineteenth and twentieth centuries. The nineteenth-century view was that a data set was composed of deterministic cycles plus noise and the function of time-series analysis was to reduce noise so that the signal could be detected. The twentieth-century view is that the cycles themselves have amplitudes and frequencies that are random variables so that the notion of periodic functions has been replaced by the notion of *almost periodic functions.* An almost periodic function has a period that is sometimes 15 s, sometimes 16 s, sometimes 14 s. The implication of this view is that a *band* of frequencies will be significant, in general, rather than a particular spike. One result of this fact is that there is only local prediction, confidence intervals increase as we move away from the present. This is, in fact, the dilemma of all forecasting; most forecasters employ a method of *one-step-ahead* forecasting that involves predicting only the next point in a time series and then updating the prediction once the data are available and repeating the process. This is not the case with deterministic cycles. In place of the sharp spikes in the periodogram or spectral density function that we find when analyzing periodic functions, we find broad peaks when analyzing the spectrum of almost periodic functions such as those obtained with the headache data. What makes this such an art form is that the notion of "deterministic" is not all or none; rather, real data have, to varying degrees, components that are more or less deterministic or nondeterministic. This state of affairs makes the process of building a model for a time series an extremely challenging and creative process. Wherever possible, psychophysiologists should be guided by theory (e.g., physiology).

22.7 BIVARIATE SPECTRAL ANALYSIS

In bivariate spectral analysis we require two functions, the *coherence spectrum*, which is a measure of the amount of covariance between the two series of each frequency component in the overtone series, and the *phase spectrum*, which gives us an indication of the lead and lag of each cycle. To examine these two functions of frequency, we first examine the statistical significance of the coherence and, if it is significant at a frequency, we can examine the phase spectrum at that frequency. One problem with interpreting the phase spectrum in terms of lead or lag is that it is invariant to shifts of $\pm 2\pi$ so that lead and lag are interchangeable in this phase spectrum. Hence it can only be used in this regard for speculation. We need to leave the frequency domain and enter the time domain for inferences about lead and lag.

Consider a metaphor for understanding bivariate spectral analysis. We have two series with the same number of observations. This is important because it gives us the same overtone series to use in approximating each time series. Think of these functions as the strings of two pianos that are in the same room. The strings each vibrate at precisely the same frequencies; for example, there is a string on both pianos for middle C. However, the first piano will not resonate to the second piano's middle C perfectly because its string may be duller than that of the first piano. Several possibilities exist. There may not be enough energy in the first piano's middle C to get any response from the second piano's middle C. In that case there will be zero coherence at that frequency. Or there may be a partial transfer, and the percentage of energy transfer is the coherence. Or there may be a time delay and a transfer. The time delay is the phase at this frequency. In actuality, the strings of both pianos only *approximate* the intricate melodies of each time series with the same crude overtone series.

22.7.1 *Example*

In this example, a constant time lag between two series was created. The phase spectrum in this case follows a straight line (Figure 22.5), which is the phase divided

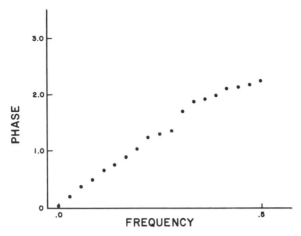

Figure 22.5. Phase spectrum for constant time lag.

by $2\pi f$, the constant time lag. It is only possible to examine the phase when the coherence is statistically significant. This is the case because if the coherence is R^2, the variance of the phase spectrum is proportional to $(1 - R^2)/R^2$. Thus, the confidence interval for the phase will be very large if the coherence is small. This state of affairs can be assessed by examining if the coherence is above the vertical line. Then the phase spectrum can be examined; the graph gives its confidence intervals. Details of these computations are given in Gottman (1981, chapter 23).

22.8   MULTIVARIATE TIME DOMAIN APPROACHES

22.8.1   *Gottman–Ringland*

In a bivariate analysis, the closest we can come to a causal inference is to assess the extent to which there is cross-correlation once we control for autocorrelation. For example, suppose we wish to assess the relationship between a mother's behavior $M(t)$ and a baby's behavior $B(t)$ during face-to-face social interaction. To assess one direction of influence, from the baby to the mother, we want to assess the extent to which the baby's past behavior adds information to the prediction of the mother's behavior over and above what we can *predict* from the mother's past. Stated mathematically, we compare a big model,

$$M(t) = \sum a_i^* M(t - i) + \sum b_i^* B(t - i) + e^*(t)$$

to a smaller, null hypothesis model,

$$M(t) = \sum a_i M(t - i) + e(t)$$

The likelihood ratio procedure yields a test statistic, Q, which, if the smaller model is true, is distributed as χ^2 with degrees of freedom equal to the difference in the number of parameters in the two models. The procedure is done in stepwise fashion, adding on first the smallest autoregressive model and then smallest cross-regressive model.

The analysis is then done in the other direction, predicting from the mother to the baby. Four possibilities exist: (1) $M \to B$ and $B \to M$ (bidirectionality); (2) $M \to B$ but not the other way around; (3) $B \to M$ but not the other way around; and (4) neither $M \to B$ nor $B \to M$.

22.8.2 *Transfer functions*

Transfer functions are ways of transforming one time series into another through a linear filter. In other words, they provide the best linear estimate of one time series that one can obtain from another time series. This is thus the equivalent of linear regression. The estimation of a transfer function can have meaning in terms of underlying physiology. For example, if two sites of EEG recording were generated by the same set of underlying oscillators, then they would be strongly related. The set of weights relating the two series, called the *impulse response function*, can provide information about lead or lag as well. If we want to predict one series $y(t)$ from another series $x(t)$, we can use a linear filter to do this prediction, predicting $y(t)$ from the past of $x(t)$:

$$y(t) = \sum_s x(t-s) + e(t)$$

where we assume that $e(t)$ is uncorrelated with $x(t)$. The h_s plotted against s is called the impulse response function. An easy way to obtain estimates of the impulse response function is to *prewhiten* the input, by which it is meant to use a transformation that converts $x(t)$ to white noise. To find this transformation, we need to compute the coefficients of an autoregressive model to fit $x(t)$. For example, if it turns out that $x(t)$ can be written as

$$x(t) = 0.5\, x(t-1) + e(t)$$

where $e(t)$ is the white-noise residual, then the transformation that prewhitens $x(t)$ is $x(t) - 0.5x(t-1)$. Call this transformation L. If we apply L to the transfer function equation, we get

$$Ly(t) = h_s Lx(t-s) + Le(t)$$

Because the $Lx(t)$ becomes white noise, it becomes easy to solve for the impulse response weights (for details, see Gottman, 1981, p. 321).

22.8.3 *Time-series regression*

In this case we have one dependent variable time series, $Y(t)$, and a set of independent variable time series, $X_1(t)$, $X_2(t),\dots,$ $X_k(t)$. The independent variable series can be lagged versions of one series. To solve this equation, we have to employ a procedure called *two-stage least squares*, which corrects for the problem of correlated residuals. This procedure is followed by the program TSREG.

22.9 EXAMPLES

This section will present a worked example of the time-series analysis of brief segments of the IBIs of a distressed married couple's interaction. There is a

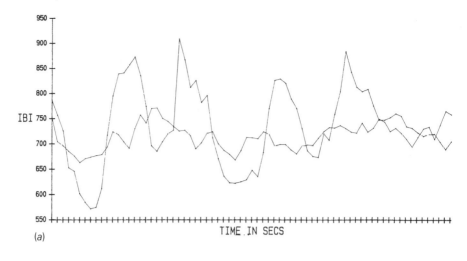

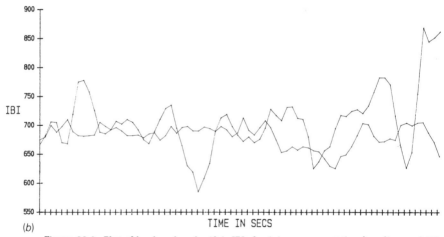

Figure 22.6. Plot of husband and wife's IBIs for (a) preconversation baseline and (b) high-conflict marital discussion of an unhappily married couple (IBI in ms).

preconversation baseline that preceded their discussion of the major issue in their marriage. This marital interaction is characterized by her expressions of contempt for her husband followed by his fear. This contempt-to-fear pattern is characteristic of many unhappy marriages in which there is a dominance pattern. In this marriage we had been able to study their interaction when they were first married, in which the husband was contemptuous of the wife's weight and she was self-deprecating. At that time the husband was starting a new business. Five years later, when these data were collected, his business was failing and the contempt pattern had reversed. In the interaction he is asking her about requesting a loan from her mother and she is very critical and disdainful of the idea. Figure 26.6 is a graph of the IBIs of 73 s of baseline (preconversation) and high-conflict interaction.

22.9.1 *Spectral and cross-spectral analyses*

The spectral analyses of the IBI data for both the baseline and the interaction are quite similar in the shape of the spectral density function across frequency (Figure 22.7). In these plots program SPEC was used with an averaging window of 10 lags. We see more power at lower frequencies for the wife. Also note that in examining the coherence spectrum it makes sense to look at the ranges of *both* spectra that are statistically significant. To do this, note the frequency where the asterisks cross the vertical line in each spectral density function. Next, examine the *overlap* of these intervals for the husband and wife in each period. In the baseline period this cutoff would be at $f = .096$; in the interaction it would also be at 0.096. We would then look at the coherence spectra from $f = 0$ to $f = 0.096$. In the baseline we can see that the coherence in this range of frequencies is statistically significant (above the vertical line), whereas this is not the case during the interaction segment. Thus, it makes no sense to examine the phase spectrum for the interaction segment. The phase spectrum for the baseline segment, however, is of interest in the range of frequencies discussed. Within this range, we can see what resembles a constant time lead–lag relationship, with a positive slope indicating that the time series entered second (the wife's in this case) leads at a constant time lag given by the phase slope divided by 2π. The slope is about 12, which is then divided by 2π, or an estimated lead by the wife of 1.9 s. As a piece of time-series esoterica, it is interesting to note that the general slope of this phase spectrum is repeated three times on this plot; this repeating is a function of the fact that the phase wraps itself around a cylinder in three dimensions; the steeper the slope, the more often it will repeat in this fashion.

Still, the slope is determined to $\pm 2\pi$, so lead can be lag, and the interpretation that the wife leads the husband is questionable. To deal with this problem, we employ the BIVAR program, which controls for autocorrelation in each series in turn.

22.9.2 *Bivariate time domain analysis*

In these analyses, we began with a low number of terms in the equations that relate husband and wife time series because we have only a few degrees of freedom with which to work with 74 points and so many parameters to fit. Recall that we begin by testing whether we gain any information in predicting the first series entered (the husband's) over and above a knowledge of his past IBIs by entering the wife's IBI data. This analysis tests the extent to which $W \rightarrow H$; in our case $\chi^2 = 15.335$ with $df = 1$; converting this to a z-score gives $z = 10.137$, which is quite significant. It is also consistent with the cross-spectral analysis of the baseline data. Next we examine the second set of equations to test the $H \rightarrow W$ hypothesis. In this case we find $\chi^2 < 0.001$, so the answer here is a resounding no. This is a case of unidirectional and not bidirectional influence. For the interaction segment, the χ^2 for $W \rightarrow H$ was 16.289 with $df = 1$, or $z = 10.811$; for the $H \rightarrow W$ effect $\chi^2 = 2.954$ with $df = 1$, or $z = 0.477$, not significant again. Here we see that the time domain analyses have given us far more consistent results than the frequency domain results. Recall that this type of analysis is the closest thing we can come to with two time series for making causal inferences.

The interpretation of these results is that the IBI data of the dominant person (the wife) in the interaction serves as a lead indicator of her partner's IBI data, possibly

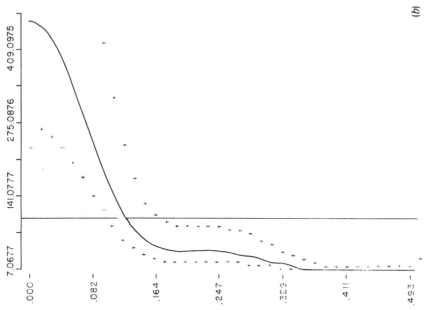

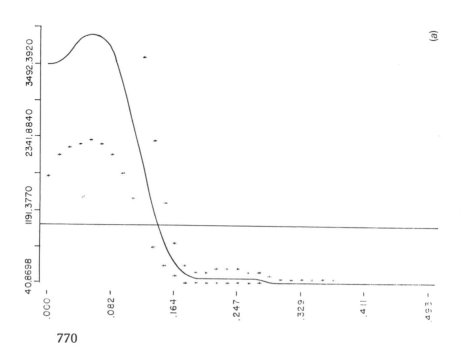

770

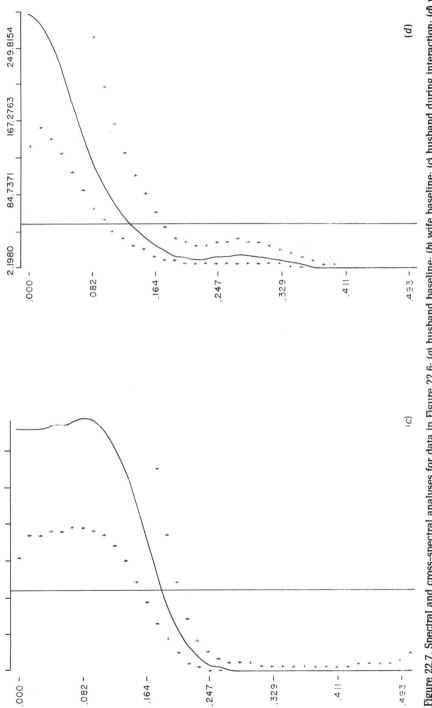

Figure 22.7. Spectral and cross-spectral analyses for data in Figure 22.6: (*a*) husband baseline; (*b*) wife baseline; (*c*) husband during interaction; (*d*) wife during interaction; (*e*) coherence spectrum during baseline; (*f*) coherence spectrum during interaction; (*g, h*) phase spectrum during baseline and interaction.

771

Figure 22.7 (cont.)

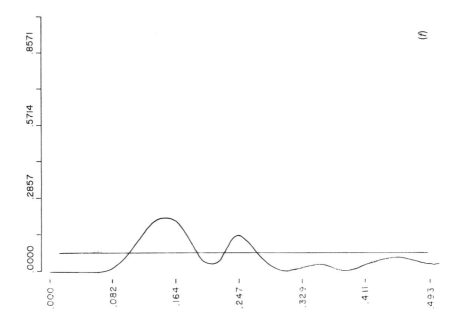

(f)

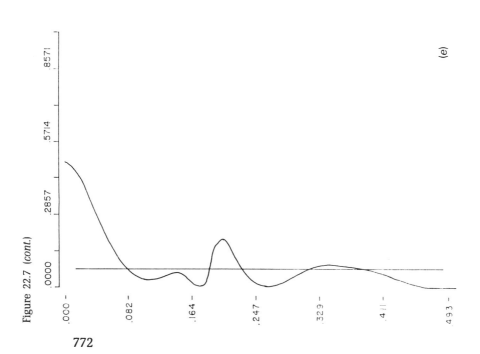

(e)

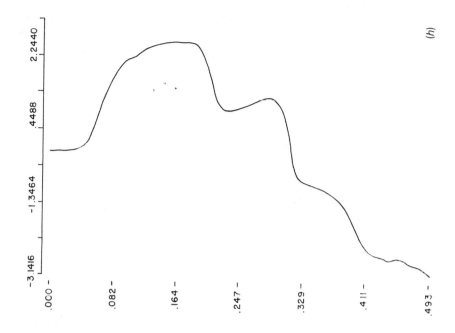

(h)

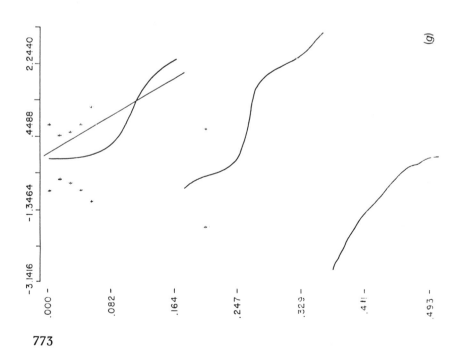

(g)

773

through dispensing emotional messages of contempt to her anxious husband.

More complex models are possible with more time series. See Gottman (1981, p. 376ff) for the use of "bedspring models." The program TSREG can also be used to create more complex models. As noted in the discussion of transfer function models, prewhitening the input is another approach.

REFERENCES

Anderson, O. D. (1975). *Time series and forecasting: The Box–Jenkins approach.* London: Butterworths.

Box, G. E. P., & Jenkins, G. M. (1970). *Time-series analysis: Forecasting and control.* Francisco: Holden-Day.

Brillinger, D. R. (1975). *Time series data analysis and theory.* New York: Holt, Rinehart & Winston.

Chatfied, C. (1975). *The analysis of time series: Theory and practice.* London: Chapman & Hall.

Ekman, P., & Friesen, W. V (1978). *The facial action coding system.* Palo Alto, CA: Consulting Psychologists Press.

Ekman, P., Levenson, R. W., & Friesen, W. V. (1983). Autonomic nervous system activity distinguishes among emotions. *Science, 221,* 1208–2210.

Glass, G. U., Wilson, V. C., & Gottman, J. M. (1975). *Design and analysis of time series experiments.* Boulder, CO: Colorado Associated University Press.

Gottman, J. M. (1981). *Time-series analysis: A comprehensive introduction for social scientists.* New York: Cambridge University Press.

Hamming, R. W. (1977). *Digital filters.* Engelwood Cliffs, NJ: Prentice-Hall.

Koopmans, L. H. (1974). *The spectral analysis of time series.* New York: Academic.

Porges, S. W. (1984). Heart rate patterns in neonates: A potential diagnostic window to the brain. In T. Fields & A. Sostek (Eds.), *Infants born at risk: Physiological, perceptual, and cognitive processes.* New York: Grune & Stratton.

Slutzky, E. (1937). The summation of random causes as the source of cyclic processes. *Econometrica, 5,* 105–246.

Whittaker, E. T., & Robinson, G. (1924). *The calculus of observation.* New York: Van Nostrand.

Williams, E. A., & Gottman, J. M. (1981). *A user's guide to the Gottman–Williams time-series analysis computer programs for social scientists.* New York: Cambridge University Pres.

Yule, G. U. (1971). On a method of studying time series based on their internal correlations. In A. Stuart & M. Kendall (Eds.), *Statistical papers of George Udny Yule.* New York: Hafner.

23 The analysis of psychophysiological data: multivariate approaches

DANIEL W. RUSSELL

With the advent of large mainframe computers and readily available statistical software, increasing use is being made of multivariate statistics in the conduct of psychophysiological research. Given the large number of psychophysiological parameters that are typically assessed in such research, multivariate approaches to the data appear most appropriate. A number of advantages of multivariate procedures over more traditional univariate approaches are apparent. For example, one is able to examine patterns of change that may occur across parameters in a multivariate analysis. Multivariate approaches may also reveal an effect of an experimental treatment that is not apparent from univariate analyses of the dependent variables by taking into account the association between measures. For example, the difference between two psychophysiological parameters may serve to differentiate experimental conditions, a pattern of results that would be missed in a univariate analysis of the variables. Finally, multivariate approaches to repeated-measures analyses may assist psychophysiological researchers in overcoming problems associated with the univariate approach to such data (see discussion by Vasey & Thayer, 1987).

Although multivariate approaches to data analysis hold great promise for psychophysiological research, there appear to be a number of misconceptions regarding these analytic procedures. The purpose of this chapter is to provide a nontechnical discussion of multivariate analysis, focusing on methods that are most relevant to psychophysiological research. An overview of multivariate methods is first presented, with a discussion of relevant statistical issues. Multivariate analysis of variance (MANOVA) is discussed, and an example from a study of facial EMG activity is presented. Problems presented by research designs that involve repeated assessments of subjects are discussed, and a multivariate approach to the analysis of data from such designs is described. Analyses of the facial EMG data are presented to illustrate this approach. Finally, the chapter concludes with a discussion of issues that arise in analyzing change in psychophysiological parameters over time.

More technical presentations of these issues can be found in textbooks on multivariate statistics (Bock, 1975; Finn, 1974; Harris, 1985; Overall & Klett, 1972; Tatsuoka, 1988). The reader may also want to consult the recent books by Bray and Maxwell (1985) and Barker and Barker (1984) or the paper by O'Brien and Kaiser (1985) for other less technical discussions of multivariate statistics.

23.1 OVERVIEW OF MULTIVARIATE METHODS

Multivariate statistics is a term that refers to a group of closely related statistical methods. Typically included among these methods are multivariate analysis of variance, discriminant function analysis, and canonical correlation analysis. These statistical methods are all variations on the general linear model and, although not commonly viewed in this manner, fundamentally represent the same statistical procedure. For example, in a MANOVA the analysis attempts to form a weighted composite of the dependent variables that maximally differentiates between the groups. The goal of a discriminant function analysis is identical. A discriminant function or functions (which is a weighted composite or composites of the dependent variables) is formed to maximally differentiate between the groups. The results of a MANOVA and a discriminant function analysis are the same. Thus, there is little reason to perform both types of analyses on the same data set, as some investigators have done. Canonical correlation analysis is performed when both the independent and dependent variables are assessed on some continuous scale (typically assumed to be at least ordinal in nature). In contrast to a multiple regression analysis, there are multiple independent and multiple dependent variables in a canonical correlation analysis. New canonical variables are formed on both the independent and dependent variable sides of the equation to maximize the relations between the two sets of variables. Of course, it is possible to perform a canonical correlation analysis where the independent variables reflect group membership, in which case the results would be identical to those derived from a MANOVA or a discriminant function analysis. Indeed, statistical programs for performing MANOVA or discriminant function analysis will commonly report canonical correlation coefficients to represent the overall degree of association between the independent and dependent variables.

Given these similarities among the statistical procedures, the following discussion will focus on MANOVA since that procedure is most commonly used in psychophysiological research.

23.2   MULTIVARIATE ANALYSIS OF VARIANCE

The present discussion will focus on several issues where there appears to be a great deal of misunderstanding regarding the use of MANOVA in analyzing psychophysiological data. It should be noted that the points to be raised are also applicable to discriminant function or canonical correlation analysis.

23.2.1   *Assumptions of MANOVA*

A first assumption of MANOVA is that the dependent variables are distributed in a multivariate normal manner. This assumption is, of course, a natural extension of the normality assumption for univariate analysis of variance (ANOVA). As is true in the case of ANOVA, Monte Carlo studies have indicated that MANOVA is robust to violations of the assumption of multivariate normality (Ito, 1969; Mardia, 1971; Olson, 1974).[1]

A second assumption made by MANOVA concerns the equality of within-group variances and covariances. This assumption is also a natural extension of the equality-of-variance assumption made by ANOVA, adding the stipulation that the correlations among the dependent variables be similar across groups. The Box M test was developed to evaluate this assumption and is typically reported by statistical packages as part of the MANOVA ouput. However, it should be noted that the Box M test is also affected by violations of multivariate normality (Olson, 1974).

Fortunately, Monte Carlo studies have indicated that MANOVA is robust to violations of the homogeneity-of-variance-and-covariance assumption if the sample size is equal across groups and the differences in the variances and covariances between groups are not large (Ito, 1969; Ito & Schull, 1964).

Given the nonnormal distributions of many psychophysiological parameters, it is important for investigators to carefully examine the distributions of their data prior to analysis. Although MANOVA appears to be robust to violations of these distributional assumptions, extreme violations of the assumptions may occur when analyzing psychophysiological data. Transformations of the data to meet the distributional assumptions may be necessary [see Weisberg (1985) for a useful discussion of data transformations to address different types of distributional problems and Levey (1980) for a discussion of transformations typically applied to psychophysiological data].

23.2.2   Significance tests

One confusing aspect of MANOVA and related multivariate procedures concerns the significance tests that are reported by statistical packages in evaluating the overall differences between groups. In order to understand fully the statistics that are reported, however, it is important to first understand the computational processes involved in conducting a MANOVA. As mentioned earlier, the goal of a MANOVA is to form an optimal combination of the dependent variables in terms of maximizing differences between groups and then evaluate whether or not the groups differ significantly on that optimum combination of the variables. Thus, just as is true in the case of discriminant function analysis, MANOVA forms a new variate or variates from the dependent variables. The number of functions that are formed is equal to p (the number of dependent variables) or $k-1$ (the number of groups minus 1), whichever is smaller. Although the mathematical computations that are involved will not be discussed here, several aspects of the statistical procedure should be noted. First, each variate is designed to maximize the proportion of between-group variation on the dependent variables that is explained. Second, each succeeding variate is formed with the constraint that it be orthogonal or uncorrelated with the preceding variates. As a consequence, the outcome of a MANOVA is in many ways similar to the results of a factor analysis: Each succeeding variate accounts for a smaller portion of the between-group differences, and the variates are uncorrelated with one another.

Another similarity between factor analysis and MANOVA involves the computation of how much variation is explained by each variate. Each dependent variable receives a weight when forming the variates in a MANOVA; these weights are conceptually similar to factor loadings. By squaring these weights and summing them for a particular variate, we can compute an eigenvalue. As is true of factors from a factor analysis, the eigenvalue for each variate represents the proportion of the variation in the dependent variables that is accounted for by the variate. If we further summed these eigenvalues across the variates that are formed by the MANOVA, then we would have a value that reflects the total between-group variation that is explained by the variates. This value is a multivariate extension of the measures of association or effect size estimates (i.e., ω^2) that are computed in the case of a univariate ANOVA.

These eigenvalues for the discriminant variates are employed in testing the

Table 23.1. *Significance tests reported by MANOVA*[a]

Wilks lambda	$= \prod_{i=1}^{s} \dfrac{1}{1-\lambda_i}$
Pillai–Bartelett trace	$= \sum_{i=1}^{s} \dfrac{\lambda_i}{1-\lambda_i}$
Hotelling–Lawley trace	$= \sum_{i=1}^{s} \lambda_i$
Roy's GCR	$= \dfrac{\lambda_1}{1+\lambda_1}$

[a] In these formulas, S represents the number of new variates that are formed by the MANOVA and λ the eigenvalue associated with each of the variates.

statistical significance of the MANOVA. Table 23.1 presents the formulas for the various significance tests that are commonly reported by MANOVA programs. Wilk's lambda represents a product of the between-group variation that is not explained by each variate. Thus, low values of lambda indicate that the groups differ on the variates. Both the Pillai–Bartlett trace and the Hotelling–Lawley trace represent a sum of the between-group variation that is explained by the variates. One advantage of the Pillai–Bartlett trace is the simple computation of a multivariate effect size estimate found by dividing the trace value by s, where s represents the number of variates that are formed by the MANOVA (see Maxwell, Arvey, & Camp, 1981).[2] As mentioned earlier, this effect size estimate is a multivariate extension of ω^2 described by Hays (1973) and represents the proportion of the variation in the dependent variables that is accounted for by the experimental conditions. So, for example, a multivariate effect size estimate of .20 would indicate that 20 percent of the variation across the dependent variables was explained by differences between the groups.

The final significance test is Roy's GCR (greatest characteristic root), which is based on the between-group variation explained by the first variate. This statistic has been controversial. Harris (1985) is a strong advocate of employing Roy's GCR in testing the statistical significance of a MANOVA, noting its utility in conducting follow-up tests. However, by focusing on the first variate, this significance test does not take into consideration possible differences between the groups on subsequent variates found by the MANOVA.

For all of these statistics except Roy's GCR, formulas have been developed for converting the values to a quasi-F-statistic, which is then used in evaluating the statistical significance of the differences between groups (see Bray & Maxwell, 1985). The statistical significance of Roy's GCR is evaluated by reference to tables that are commonly available in multivariate statistics texts (e.g., Harris, 1985). In the case where only a single discriminant variate is formed (e.g., where there are only two groups of subjects), the F-values are exact and are identical for the different significance tests. In other cases, however, the resultant F-values will vary, raising a question regarding which statistic to report. Monte Carlo studies have compared the sensitivity of each test to between-group differences as well as the robustness of the test statistic to violations of the assumptions underlying MANOVA. In terms of statistical power comparisons, all of the tests except Roy's GCR appear to be very similar in their sensitivity to between-group differences. Roy's GCR is more powerful than the other tests when group differences are concentrated on the first variate, whereas the other three significance tests are more powerful when group differences are present on the other variates that are formed by the MANOVA (Olson, 1976, 1979; Stevens, 1979). The Pillai–Bartlett trace appears to be most robust to violations of the homogeneity of the variance-and-covariance assumption (Olson, 1979; Stevens, 1979). Therefore, it appears that the Pillai–Bartlett trace is the statistic of choice, particularly in analyzing psychophysiological data that may violate the homogeneity of the variance-and-covariance assumption.

23.2.3   Follow-up tests

One area of controversy concerning the use of MANOVA has involved the interpretation of a statistically significant result. A primary reason for conducting a MANOVA in many studies has involved a belief that the multivariate analysis would guard against making a Type I error in conducting subsequent univariate analyses on each dependent variable (Bock, 1975). According to this protected-*F* perspective, finding an overall difference between groups from the multivariate test would permit the investigator to conduct follow-up univariate tests for each dependent variable without concern about possible inflation of the Type I error rate due to the number of statistical tests that would be conducted. In such a situation, the investigator has no substantive interest in the multivariate results from the MANOVA (i.e., in the new variates that are formed in maximizing group differences). Instead, the MANOVA was conducted as a means of controlling the overall error rate associated with the subsequent univariate ANOVAs.

This strategy of employing the multivariate analysis to guard against inflation of the overall error rate from subsequent univariate analyses is incorrect. Conducting subsequent univariate ANOVAs following a statistically significant MANOVA can result in an overall Type I error level that exceeds the alpha level of the multivariate test (see discussion by Bray & Maxwell, 1982; Strahan, 1982). To understand this point, consider what is tested in conducting the initial multivariate analysis. A statistically significant multivariate result indicates that the groups differ from one another on some weighted combination of the dependent variables. Thus, we can reject the null hypothesis in terms of an optimal combination of the dependent variables. The statistically significant multivariate effect implies that there may also be a "true" difference between groups on one or more of the dependent variables.[3] For these dependent measures, conducting the subsequent univariate ANOVAs presents no problem. However, for other dependent variables involved in the mutlivariate analysis, there may not be a true difference between the groups (i.e., the null hypothesis is correct). By conducting the univariate tests for these latter dependent measures, the possibility of making a Type I error is increased above the alpha level.

As should be apparent from the preceding discussion, it is impossible to determine in an actual research setting to what extent the alpha level is increased by using this protected-*F* procedure. In essence, one would need to know whether or not the null hypothesis was true for the individual dependent variables in order to estimate the impact on the overall alpha level of using this procedure. Therefore, some writers have recommended assuming that the null hypothesis may be true for all of the dependent variables and using the Bonferroni procedure to set the Type I error rate for the set of univariate ANOVAs at a particular alpha level (Bray & Maxwell, 1985; Harris, 1985). In the Bonferroni procedure, the overall alpha level is divided by the number of statistical tests to be performed. So, for example, if the overall alpha level was .05 and there were three dependent variables, then the alpha level for each univariate test would be set at .017. The Bonferroni procedure assumes that the statistical tests to be performed are independent of one another. In the case where the dependent variables are correlated (as is typically true in conducting a MANOVA), the Bonferroni procedure will overadjust for the number of comparisons. Thus, when the dependent variables are intercorrelated, the actual Type I error level for the set of comparisons would be less than alpha.

In a situation where a number of dependent variables have been employed in a study (as is true in many psychophysiological investigations), use of the Bonferroni procedure may result in a very low alpha level being employed to evaluate the statistical significance of each comparison. Furthermore, high correlations among the dependent variables may result in a serious overcorrection for the number of comparisons that are conducted. These two factors serve to increase the probability of making a Type II error (i.e., affirming the null hypothesis when it is incorrect). Two approaches to addressing these problems in psychophysiological research are recommended. First, researchers should examine the intercorrelations among the dependent variables that have been assessed. Variables that are highly correlated (i.e., above .60) should be standardized and combined together to form a single composite variable since little information will be gained by treating the variables separately in an analysis.

Second, investigators should consider employing a less stringent overall alpha level for the comparisons. In this regard, Keppel (1982, pp. 147–150) suggests the use of a modified Bonferroni procedure. Specifically, this procedure involves setting the overall alpha level by multiplying the number of planned comparisons that the investigator is willing to conduct at the alpha level being used for the investigation and then dividing this value by the actual number of comparisons that are conducted. As suggested by Keppel, suppose an investigator decides he or she is willing to conduct $n-1$ (where n equals the number of groups) planned contrasts, with the alpha level for each contrast set at .05. If the investigator had five groups of subjects, the overall or experimentwise alpha level would be .20. In conducting the Bonferroni correction, this overall alpha level would be used in setting the specific alpha level for each comparison. So, for example, if the investigator conducted 10 comparisons, the individual alpha level would be set at .02 (i.e., .20/10), versus an individual alpha level of .005 (i.e., .05/10) that would be employed on the basis of the unmodified Bonferroni correction. In using the modified Bonferroni procedure, the investigator needs to justify the overall alpha level that is chosen since the likelihood of a Type I error is increased by altering the overall alpha level that is employed.

As noted in the preceding, the MANOVA procedure seeks to find one or more weighted combinations of the dependent variables that significantly differentiate between the groups. Another approach to interpreting a statistically significant multivariate result is to focus on the meaning of these weighted combinations of the variables. Finding a statistically significant multivariate F indicates that one or more of these new variates is accounting for a significant portion of the between-group variation. MANOVA programs also report significance tests for each of the individual variates as part of what is termed a dimension reduction analysis. A statistically significant result from this analysis indicates that the variate adds significantly to the explained between-group variation.

Interpretation of the meaning of these variates can be based on the relative weights associated with each dependent variable. An issue that arises concerns which set of weights to employ in interpreting the meaning of the variate. Several sets of discriminant function weights are reported by MANOVA programs. Raw discriminant function weights are the values one would use to actually compute scores for subjects on this new variate. The raw discriminant function weight for each dependent variable is affected by the variability of that measure and the extent of correlation among the dependent variables, creating problems for interpretation. Standardized discriminant function weights remove the problem of differential variability across the dependent variables by converting each measure to a z-score. However, correlations among the dependent variables affect these values. Most MANOVA programs also report simple correlations between each dependent variable and the discriminant functions, which appear to be most useful for interpretative purposes.

Another interpretive issue concerns group differences on these variates. Harris (1985) advocates the use of the Roy–Bose Simultaneous Confidence Interval (SCI) approach to testing group differences, which relies on Roy's GCR to evaluate the statistical significance of differences on the variates. However, two problems are apparent with this procedure. First, since this approach employs Roy's GCR in conducting the significance test, it is only appropriate for evaluating differences between groups on the first variate formed by the MANOVA. Second, Monte Carlo studies have indicated that use of the SCI procedure in interpreting group differences is very conservative (Hummel & Sligo, 1971). Therefore, use of this procedure in evaluating group differences following a significant multivariate result is not recommended.

Instead, a more reasonable approach to differences on these new variates involves the computation and comparisons of group means or centroids. The raw discrimininant function weights for each dependent variable reported by the MANOVA procedure can be used to compute scores for each subject on the variates. From these scores, group centroids can be computed and analyses conducted to test the statistical significance of differences between the groups. Due to the post hoc nature of these comparisons, a procedure such as the Bonferroni or Scheffé should be used to correct the alpha level used to evaluate the statistical significance of group differences on these variables.

23.2.4 *Example of a MANOVA analysis*

To illustrate the use of MANOVA, analyses were conducted on data from a study examining facial EMG activity (Tassinary, Cacioppo, & Geen, 1989).[4] A sample of 15 subjects was asked to pose a number of different facial expressions. For the purposes of these analyses, three different poses (neutral, smile, and anger) were examined. While subjects engaged in these poses, EMG activity was recorded at four different sites on the face: depressor supercilii/procerus, corrugator supercilii, lower zygomaticus major, and upper zygomaticus major muscle regions.[5]

Table 23.2. *Multivariate significance tests and dimension reduction analysis*

Statistics	Value	Approximate F^a
Wilks lambda	0.098	21.33 [b]
Pillai–Bartelett trace	1.343	20.44 [c]
Hotelling–Lawley trace	4.679	22.22 [d]
Roy's GCR	0.769[a]	

Function	Eigenvalue	Percentage of variance	Approximate F^a
1	3.332	71.23	21.33 [b]
2	1.346	28.77	17.95[c]

[a] $p < .001$.
[b] $df = 8{,}78$.
[c] $df = 8{,}80$.
[d] $df = 8{,}76$.
[e] $df = 3{,}40$.

A one-way MANOVA was conducted on these data comparing the EMG activity from the four different electrode placements during the three poses.[6] The first step in interpreting the results of the MANOVA involved the test of the homogeneity of variance and covariance assumption. The Box M statistic was 420.02, which was found to be highly significant, $F(20, 6331) = 18.07$, $p < .001$. This result indicates that the variance and covariance of the dependent variables differed across groups. As discussed earlier, MANOVA is robust to violations of this assumption, particularly (as is true in this case) when there are equal numbers of subjects in each group. Therefore, this difference in variance/covariance across groups is not of concern. However, as suggested by Barker and Barker (1984), examination of the group differences can be useful in understanding how these differences may affect the results of the MANOVA. The determinants of the variance–covariance matrices for the three groups were examined to evaluate whether one outlier group was responsible for this result. Inspection of these determinants indicated that one group, corresponding to the neutral expression condition, was clearly an outlier, with a determinant (9.86) that was much smaller than the smile (21.47) or anger (24.91) groups. These results indicate that, as might have been expected, there was much less variability across subjects in facial EMG activity during the neutral expression than during the other two expressions. Since the neutral expression group was less variable than the other groups, the effect of this outlier was to decrease the error term associated with the MANOVA, thereby making the test for group differences more liberal. Therefore, one should interpret the results of the MANOVA cautiously, by employing a more stringent alpha level (e.g., .01) for the multivariate test of significance.

Results of the MANOVA are presented in Table 23.2. As can be seen in the top half of Table 23.2, all four of the multivariate significance tests indicated that the differences between poses on the dependent variables were highly significant, although the magnitude of the quasi-F-values varied. In conducting the multivariate test of group differences, two new variates (equal to the number of groups minus 1)

Table 23.3. *Correlation between dependent variables and variates and results of the univariate ANOVAS*

	Variate		
Dependent variable	1	2	Univariate $F^{a,b}$
Depressor supercilii/procerus	0.478	−0.575	25.32
Corrugator supercilii	0.662	−0.715	45.14
Lower zygomaticus major	−0.744	−0.665	51.27
Upper zygomaticus major	−0.313	−0.346	10.25

[a] $p < .001$.
[b] $df = 2,42$.

were formed by assigning weights to the dependent variables. The bottom half of Table 23.2 presents the results of a dimension reduction analysis that evaluated the statistical significance of each variate. As can be seen, both variates accounted for a statistically significant proportion of the between-group variance, although the first variate predominated.

Based on the Pillai–Bartlett trace, the multivariate effect size was calculated by dividing the trace (1.343) by the number of variates (2), resulting in an effect size estimate of .672. Using the formula presented by Serlin (1982; see note 2), the population effect size was estimated to be .656.[7] From this result, we conclude that these three different poses accounted for approximately 66 percent of the variability in EMG activity across the four recording sites.

Table 23.3 provides information relevant to interpreting the MANOVA results. Correlations between each of the dependent variables and the two variates formed by the MANOVA are presented. Variate 1 appears to contrast EMG activity in the brow region (i.e., depressor supercilii/procerus and corrugator supercilii) with EMG activity in the cheek area (i.e., zygomaticus major). The second variate reflects the lack of EMG activity across the four recording sites given the negative association with all of the dependent measures.

Also reported in Table 23.3 are the results of univariate ANOVAs that were conducted on each of the individual dependent variables. Setting the overall alpha level for these univariate analyses at .05 and using the Bonferroni correction, the alpha level employed in evaluating the statistical significance of each *F*-value was .0125. As can be seen in Table 23.3, statistically significant differences between the groups were found on all four of the dependent variables following the Bonferroni correction.

A final interpretative issue concerns group differences on the variates formed by the MANOVA. As noted in the preceding, the results suggest that variate 1 may reflect a differentiation in EMG activity between the brow and cheek regions, whereas variate 2 appears to reflect a general lack of facial EMG activity. To examine how the three posed expressions were related to these two variates, group centroids were computed on each variate on the basis of the discriminant function coefficients reported by the MANOVA (see Table 23.4). For the first variate, anger elicited the highest scores followed by the neutral and smile poses. Post hoc analyses using the Bonferroni correction for the number of comparisons indicated that these group differences were statistically significant. Consistent with the second

Table 23.4. *Group means on the variates*

Pose	Variate 1	Variate 2
Neutral	0.200*	−0.291*
Smile	−2.425[†]	−2.471[†]
Anger	1.858**	−2.826[†]

Note: Differences between means with different superscripts (*, †, **) were statistically significant ($p<.05$) following the Bonferroni correction for the number of comparisons (6) that were conducted.

variate representing general facial activity, scores on this variate separated the neutral pose from the other two poses. These latter results indicate there was greater EMG activity across all recording sites associated with the smile and anger poses than the neutral pose.

23.2.5 *Summary*

Use of MANOVA in psychophysiological research would appear to be particularly appropriate when the investigator has a substantive interest in the variate or variates that are formed by the procedure in differentiating among groups. Conducting a MANOVA to guard against Type I errors that would result from univariate analyses on each psychophysiological parameter is an inappropriate use of the procedure. In such situations, conducting the univariate analyses and using the Bonferroni procedure to set the overall alpha level at a particular value is more appropriate.

Two other characteristics of MANOVA should be noted. First, the preceding discussion and example of a MANOVA analysis has focused on a one–way design, where only a single independent variable was examined. The issues discussed also apply to factorial designs, where several independent variables (and corresponding interaction terms) are examined. In analyzing factorial designs, researchers should keep in mind that the variates formed by the MANOVA in maximizing group differences may vary greatly depending on the effect that is being tested. So, for example, a particular weighting of the dependent variables may serve to differentiate among groups that represent the main effect of an independent variable, whereas a completely different weighting of the dependent variables may be formed to maximize group differences associated with an interaction between that independent variable and another independent variable. These differential weightings of the dependent variables depending on the effect being examined need to be considered carefully in interpreting the results of a multivariate factorial design.

A second characteristic of MANOVA derives from the similarity to discriminant function analysis. In the literature on discriminant function analysis, the phenomenon of "shrinkage" of results when applied to new samples of cases and the need for cross-validation of findings have been well-documented. This problem occurs when one attempts to use a discriminant function equation derived from an analysis on one sample to predict group membership in a second sample. Since discriminant function analysis and MANOVA are designed to derive optimal weightings of the dependent variable to maximize group differences, both statistical procedures may capitalize on chance characteristics of the sample being analyzed in developing weights for the predictor variables. As a consequence, the resulting variates formed may not be as predictive of group membership (or, in the case of MANOVA, differentiate among the groups as well) in a new sample.

Researchers should therefore be cautious in interpreting the weighting of variables from a MANOVA. Ideally, the reliability of the findings should be examined by attempting to cross-validate the results in a new sample. For example, data could be collected from a second sample of subjects and scores on the variates found from the initial multivariate analysis computed. Analyses could then be conducted that evaluate group differences on these variates in the new sample, employing a priori comparisons to examine the reliability of group differences found in the original sample. Alternatively, data could be gathered from a larger sample of subjects in the initial investigation and a hold-out sample randomly selected. The multivariate analyses would first be conducted on the remaining cases and cross-validated on the hold-out sample. This latter strategy would permit an examination of the replicability of the findings in the context of a single investigation, with the cost being the need to gather data from a larger sample of subjects.

23.3 REPEATED-MEASURES ANALYSIS

A very common type of research design in psychophysiological research involves the repeated assessment of subjects over time. Typically, this adds a trial factor to the design. For example, participants in a study may be randomly divided into two (or more) groups that receive different experimental treatments. A number of psychophysiological parameters are then assessed repeatedly over time, with the time periods separated into trials. This represents a condition × trials design. Alternatively, the trials factor may involve the manipulation of additional independent variables. So, for example, rather than simply assessing subjects under the same conditions over time, additional experimental conditions (e.g., stimuli) may be presented to subjects on each trial as part of the repeated assessment to gauge their effect.

In the context of univariate ANOVA, this type of design is commonly referred to as a split-plot, or repeated-measures, design. Within-subject factors represent experimental conditions (such as a trials factor) that all subjects experience as part of the study. The problem presented by this design for univariate ANOVA involves the possible correlation that may exist between the repeated assessments of the same variable across the within-subjects conditions. A basic assumption of ANOVA is that all observations are independent. Violation of this assumption requires modification to the traditional univariate ANOVA in terms of the error terms that are employed in evaluating the statistical significance of the within-subjects effects (see discussion in textbooks on univariate ANOVA, such as Keppel, 1982; Kirk, 1982; Winer, 1971).

Use of the univariate approach to analyzing data from repeated-measures designs is based on restrictive assumptions about the variances and covariances of the dependent measure across the repeated assessments. This is typically referred to as the sphericity assumption. Huynh and Feldt (1970) have shown that a necessary and sufficient condition for sphericity is that the variation in subject response to the repeated treatment levels are homogeneous.[8] This is termed homogeneity of treatment deviations (h. o. t. d. v.). So, for example, consider a simple design where there are three trials that represent the within-subjects factor. The sphericity assumption would be met if the differences in subject responses to trial 1 versus trial 2 were similar to the differences in subject responses to trial 1 versus trial 3 and to trial 2 versus trial 3.

In most research settings it is unlikely that the data would conform to this assumption, particularly if the study involves a number of trials over time. For example, consider the repeated assessment of a psychophysiological parameter over time. One would expect to find less change in the parameter for adjacent trials (e.g., from trial 1 to trial 2) than for trials that are separated by a greater length of time (e.g., from trial 1 to trial 3). Having a large number of trials over fairly long periods of time as part of the experiment would appear to increase the likelihood of violating this assumption. If in addition to the repeated assessment of subjects over time additional variables are manipulated as within-subject factors (i.e., stimuli that are presented to subjects during each trial), then it would appear even more likely that the data would not meet the sphericity assumption.

Although these assumptions underlying repeated-measures analysis of variance have been known for a number of years, it appears from published studies that few investigators have examined whether or not their data conform to this assumption. In a review of studies that appeared in the journal *Psychophysiology* during 1975, Jennings and Wood (1976) found that 84 percent of the investigations that employed a repeated-measures design did not test whether or not the data met the sphericity assumption. After reviewing studies that appeared in *Psychophysiology* during 1984 and 1985, Vasey and Thayer (1987) indicated that the situation had improved, although 50 percent of the investigations still did not test whether the data met the assumptions of the univariate repeated-measures analysis.

One reason for concern about this practice by researchers derives from the effect that violations of the sphericity assumption has on the results of a repeated-measures analysis. If data do not meet the assumption, then the resulting Type I error rate is increased above the alpha level (Huynh & Feldt, 1980). Due to this inflation of the Type I error rate, Huynh and Feldt (1970, 1976) and Greenhouse and Geisser (1959) have developed correction factors ε to be used in reducing the degrees of freedom associated with the F-value. One of these correction factors should be applied before conducting significance tests when data do not meet the sphericity assumption.[9]

An explanation for why researchers have not routinely evaluated whether or not their data meet the sphericity assumption has been the lack of available statistical software to test this assumption. In recent years, two of the most widely available statistical packages (SPSS–X MANOVA and BMD programs P2V and BMDP4V, in mainframe and microcomputer versions) have incorporated a test of the sphericity assumption. In addition to testing whether or not the data meet the assumption underlying the repeated-measures analysis, these packages also report the correction factors ε to be used in adjusting the degrees of freedom for the F-value.

In a recent paper, O'Brien and Kaiser (1985) have argued persuasively for a different approach to analyzing repeated-measures designs based on MANOVA. Although this method of analyzing repeated-measures designs has been described previously (e.g., Cole & Grizzle, 1966; Harris, 1985; Timm, 1980), their paper presents a nontechnical description of how to conduct such a multivariate analysis. O'Brien and Kaiser contend that the adjustment to the degrees of freedom associated with the univariate repeated-measures analysis may greatly reduce statistical power. The multivariate approach to repeated-measures designs makes no restrictive assumptions about the relationships among the repeated measures over time and therefore is more powerful in cases where the data do not meet the sphericity assumption.

To illustrate this multivariate approach, consider a simple design where two groups of subjects are assessed repeatedly on the same psychophysiological parameter over a series of five trials. Each subject would therefore have five scores on the dependent variable. The first step in a multivariate analysis of this repeated-measures design would involve converting these five scores into four new variables that represent the difference between scores on adjacent trials. So, for example, the first difference score would be created by subtracting the score on trial 1 from trial 2, the second difference score by subtracting the score on trial 2 from trial 3, and so forth. These four difference scores would then be entered into a MANOVA as four dependent variables, with group membership as the independent variable. Two multivariate significance tests would be produced by the MANOVA program. The first test, for the constant effect, evaluates whether or not these four difference scores are significantly greater than zero. Although it may not appear to be the case at first inspection, this provides us with a test for an overall trial effect. If there are no differences on the psychophysiological parameter across trials, then we should find that these four difference scores do not differ significantly from zero. Univariate tests of the constant effect for each of the four difference scores would also be computed by the MANOVA program. These univariate analyses provide information concerning whether or not there are significant differences between scores on the adjacent trials. Results from these latter analyses are identical to pairwise or correlated *t*-tests. A multivariate test for the group membership variable is also conducted by the MANOVA, which provides a test for the group × trial interaction. Different patterns of change on the psychophysiological parameter from trial to trial for the two groups of subjects is tested by this effect, which would reflect an interaction between the group and trial factors. Once again, the univariate tests for each difference score would provide information concerning group differences in changes over adjacent trials.

Although it is possible to construct contrast variables and conduct multivariate analyses as described by O'Brien and Kaiser (1985), these procedures are too unwieldy for most researchers. Fortunately, the SPSS-X MANOVA and BMDP4V programs (in mainframe and microcomputer versions) have recently been modified to allow analysis of repeated-measures designs using both univariate and multivariate approaches. To illustrate these two approaches to the analysis of repeated-measures designs, the following section will present an example.

23.3.1 *Example of a repeated-measures analysis*

The data for this example are drawn from the study of facial expression described earlier (Tassinary et al., 1989). The previous analysis of these data treated the observations as being derived from independent samples of subjects for illustrative purposes. Analyses to be reported here will treat the data as being derived from repeated observations of the same 15 subjects.

Average EMG scores for subjects from the four recording sites (i.e., depressor

Table 23.5. *EMG activity from the four recording sites following each pose*

	Neutral	Smile	Anger
Depressor supercilii/procerus	8.92	8.82	104.65
Corrugator supercilii	13.28	6.61	121.03
Lower zygomaticus major	1.65	128.14	81.51
Upper zygomaticus major	1.73	69.68	17.18

Table 23.6. *Results of the univariate repeated–measures analysis of variance*

Source	SS	df	MS	F
Pose	91,729.47	2	45,864.74	26.92[a]
Error	47,701.85	28	1,703.64	

[a] $p < .001$.

supercilii/procerus, corrugator supercilii, lower zygomaticus major, and upper zygomaticus major muscle regions) following the three different poses (i.e., neutral, smile, and anger) are presented in Table 23.5. To illustrate the differences between the univariate and multivariate approaches to repeated measures, the first analyses that were conducted focused on EMG activity recorded at the depressor supercilii/procerus muscle region.[10] These data were first analyzed using a traditional univariate repeated-measures approach. Results for the test of sphericity indicated that the data did not meet the assumption, χ^2 (2, $N = 15$) = 42.32, $p < .001$. Consistent with this result, the Huynh–Feldt ε was equal to .512 and the Greenhouse–Geisser ε was equal to .510. Both of these ε-values indicate that a sizeable adjustment in the degrees of freedom associated with the univariate ANOVA is necessary. Results of the univariate ANOVA are shown in Table 23.6. As can be seen, the main effect for pose was highly significant. However, these results have not been adjusted for the preceding values of ε shown. Adjusting for ε reduces the degree of freedom for the F-value shown in Table 23.6 to approximately 1 and 14. Although the F-value remains statistically significant at $p < .001$ even after this adjustment, making this correction to the degrees of freedom clearly lessens the power of the univariate test.

These data were also analyzed according to the multivariate approach described by O'Brien and Kaiser (1985). As discussed in the preceding, this procedure creates contrast variables to represent the repeated-measures factor. The program will automatically create these contrast variables or the users of the program can create their own orthogonal contrasts to test specific comparisons of interest. In the present analysis, two orthogonal contrast variables were created. The first contrast variable compared EMG activity at the depressor supercilii/procerus muscle region during the neutral pose to EMG activity during the smile and anger poses, whereas the second contrast variable compared EMG activity during the smile and anger poses. Thus, the first contrast variable tests for the impact of the two posed expressions on the depressor supercilii/procerus muscle region, whereas the second contrast variable compares the two posed expressions to one another.

Consistent with the univariate results, a highly significant multivariate effect for pose was found, $F(2, 13) = 14.09$, $p = .001$. The MANOVA program also conducted univariate tests for the two contrast variables. These tests provide useful information concerning the source of the differences that were found for the pose main effect. Consistent with the earlier discussion of conducting univariate follow-up tests with MANOVA, the Bonferroni procedure was employed to set the alpha level at .05 for the set of univariate analyses. Since two univariate ANOVAs were conducted, the alpha level for interpreting the statistical significance of each individual test was set at .025. The univariate test for the first contrast variable, which compared the neutral pose to the other two poses, was highly significant, $F(1, 14) = 26.11$, $p < .001$. Results for the second contrast variable, which compared EMG activity following the two posed expressions, was also highly significant, $F(1, 14) = 29.70$, $p < .001$. On the basis of these findings, we can conclude that the source of variation in EMG activity at the depressor supercilii/procerus muscle region was the anger pose, as is clearly indicated in Table 23.5.

23.3.2   Doubly multivariate analysis of variance

Although the preceding analysis employed a multivariate approach, the focus was on a single dependent variable (depressor supercilii/procerus) that had been assessed following the three poses. An extension of this analysis to multiple dependent variables involving EMG activity from additional recording sites is possible. This type of design, termed a *doubly multivariate analysis*, involves the repeated assessment of multiple dependent variables. Although this type of analysis has seldom appeared in the literature, it represents a simple extension of the multivariate analysis of a single dependent variable that has been assessed over time.

In conducting a doubly multivariate analysis, contrast variables are formed for each of the dependent variables. To illustrate this process, consider the four dependent variables employed in the facial EMG study. Two contrast variables were formed for each of the four recording sites (i.e., the depressor supercilii/procerus, corrugator supercilii, lower zygomaticus major, and upper zygomaticus major muscle regions) to represent the influence of pose on these measures. As was done in the earlier analysis, the first contrast variable compared the neutral pose to the smile and anger poses, whereas the second contrast variable compared the smile and anger poses. To test for an overall effect of pose, a multivariate analysis of variance was conducted on these eight dependent variables. As was done in the earlier analysis on the single dependent variable, the hypothesis was tested that these eight variables did not differ significantly from zero. The multivariate test of differences between the poses was statistically significant, $F (8, 7) = 9.45$, $p < .01$.

Univarite analyses of variance were also conducted for each of the eight dependent variables. In evaluating the statistical significance of these univariate tests, the Bonferroni correction to the alpha level was employed. Thus, the overall alpha level was divided by the number of comparisons (8), resulting in an alpha level of .006 that was used to evaluate each individual F-value. These results are presented in Table 23.7. As can be seen, three of the four recording sites were found to differentiate among the poses. For the fourth recording site, involving the upper zygomaticus major, statistically significant differences were found between the smile and anger poses only.

Table 23.7. *Results of the univariate analyses for the contrast variables*

Dependent variable	Contrast	F^a
Depressor supercilii/procerus	1	26.11^b
	2	29.70^b
Corrugator supercilii	1	53.43^b
	2	59.18^b
Lower zygomaticus major	1	50.42^b
	2	67.49^b
Upper zygomaticus major	1	8.09
	2	19.31^b

[a] $df = 2,14$.
[b] $p < .006$.

23.3.3   Summary

To summarize this discussion of repeated-measures analysis, the general recommendation is that investigators routinely evaluate whether or not their data meet the sphericity assumption underlying the traditional univariate approach. As O' Brien and Kaiser (1985) note, the univariate approach remains the most powerful analytic strategy when the data meet the sphericity assumption. However, applying the univariate approach when the data do not meet this assumption increases the probability of a Type I error. Thus, researchers should be required to demonstrate that their data meet the sphericity assumption. If their data do not meet this assumption, then investigators should adjust the degrees of freedom associated with the *F*-value based on ε or conduct a multivariate test of their hypotheses.[11]

Researchers interested in applying the multivariate approach to analyzing repeated-measures data may also want to examine the examples given by O'Brien and Kaiser (1985). As already noted, the SPSS-X MANOVA and BMDP4V programs will conduct multivariate repeated-measures analyses of variance. However, the programs are very complex. The reader therefore may also want to acquire the volumes by Barcikowski (1983a,b), which contain sample computer runs for conducting various types of analyses of variance using SPSS-X and BMD.

One problem posed by the multivariate approach to repeated-measures design should be noted. In order to conduct such an analysis, the number of subjects must exceed the number of dependent variables. Otherwise, the data matrix will be singular (i.e., the error degrees of freedom will be zero or negative), and the multivariate model cannot be estimated. In the case of a multivariate repeated-measures analysis of a single dependent variable, this restriction means that the number of repeated conditions (e.g., trials) minus 1 must be less than the sample size. For a doubly multivariate analysis, the total number of dependent variables (i.e., the number of dependent variables times the number of repeated conditions minus 1) must be less than the sample size.

These sample size requirements clearly constrain the applicability of the multivariate approach to repeated-measures analysis in many psychophysiological investigations. When the number of dependent variables equals or exceeds the sample size, the investigator may still employ the univariate approach to repeated measures, after making any necessary adjustments to the degrees of freedom that may be required due to violations of the sphericity assumption. The researcher may also want to employ the univariate approach to repeated measures when the number of subjects does not exceed the number of dependent measures by a sufficient number. Monte Carlo studies have compared the relative power of the univariate and multivariate approaches to repeated-measures analysis when the number of subjects exceeds the number of dependent variables by a small number (i.e., < 20; see review by Vasey & Thayer, 1987). On the basis of this research, Vasey and Thayer (1987) recommend using the univariate approach whenever the difference between the number of subjects and the number of dependent variables is less than 6.

It should be noted that the multivariate approach to repeated-measures analyses can be generalized to more complex designs involving a number of within-subjects factors. For example, consider a within-subjects factorial design. In such designs, the repeated measure is assessed under varying experimental conditions, such as different stimulus conditions. The effect of these within-subject conditions is estimated by constructing contrast variables that reflect the variation in conditions. For example, assume that a 2×2 within-subjects design is employed. Each subject would have a total of four measures, one for each experimental condition. The two main effect terms and an interaction term would be tested by forming orthogonal contrast variables that correspond to these effects. Assuming that such a design has been correctly specified in the program, the SPSS–X MANOVA or BMDP4V programs will automatically create the contrast variables for such a design.

23.4   ANALYSIS OF CHANGE IN PSYCHOPHYSIOLOGICAL PARAMETERS

The final data analysis issue to be addressed concerns how one should analyze change in psychophysiological parameters over time. According to the Law of Initial Values (Wilder, 1950, 1965), the physiological response of a subject to a stimulus is in part determined by the initial level of the parameter. As the baseline level of the parameter increases, the response to the stimulus decreases, resulting in a negative correlation between the baseline and response measures of the physiological parameter. Thus, it is important to incorporate information concerning the subject's baseline level of the parameter into the analysis in order to eliminate the influence of the baseline value on the subject's response to the stimulus.

Psychophysiological researchers have employed two different approaches to this problem (see discussion by Johnson & Lubin, 1972). One approach involves the computation of a change or difference score that is derived by subtracting the subject's baseline score from her or his score following the presentation of the stimulus. A problem with this approach concerns the reliability of change scores. As discussed by Cronbach and Furby (1970), change or difference scores are often less reliable than the component scores that are employed in their computation. Specifically, change scores will be less reliable than the baseline and response scores when the two component scores are positively correlated.[12] When the baseline and response scores are negatively correlated (as should be true given the Law of Initial Values), the change or difference score would be expected to be more reliable than the two component scores used in the computation. However, as Johnson and Lubin (1972) note, physiological parameters do not necessarily conform to the Law of Initial Values, suggesting the need for psychophysiological researchers to evaluate the reliability of change scores.

To illustrate the computation of reliability coefficients for change scores, consider the data presented previously from the study of posed facial expressions.[13] Using the formula presented by Nunnaly (1978), the reliability of a change score represented by the difference between EMG activity recorded at the depressor supercilii/procerus muscle region during the neutral and posed (i.e., smile vs. anger) expressions was calculated.[14] The first step in these calculations involved the computation of reliability estimates for the neutral and posed expression data. Since subjects engaged in the neutral and posed (i.e., smile and anger) expressions twice, test—retest correlations were employed as reliability estimates. As might be expected these values were very high ($r = .934$ for the neutral expression; $r = .915$ for the posed [smile vs. anger] expressions). In contradiction to the Law of Initial Values, EMG activity during the neutral and posed expression was found to be positively correlated, $r = .186$. Despite this positive correlation, the change score based on these measures was found to be very reliable, $\rho = .909$. Although the reliability of the change score was not as high as that of the two component scores, the measure of change was sufficiently reliable to justify further analysis.

An analysis of variance was therefore conducted that compared the smile and anger poses in terms of changes in EMG activity at the depressor supercilii/procerus muscle region. Differences between the two poses were found to be statistically significant, $F(1, 28) = 26.01$, $p < .001$. The smile pose evoked a slight decline in EMG activity in contrast to the neutral pose ($M = -.010$), whereas the anger pose evoked a substantial increase in EMG activity in contrast to the neutral pose ($M = 95.73$).

A second approach to the problem of initial values that has been recommended by psychophysiological researchers is based on analysis of covariance (ANCOVA; Benjamin, 1967; Johnson & Lubin, 1972). This approach employs the baseline measure of the parameter as a covariate in the context of an analysis of variance that evaluates the effect of the experimental treatment on the dependent variable. In conducting an ANCOVA, the baseline score is used to predict scores on the parameter following the experimental manipulation. This serves to remove the influence of individual differences between subjects on the baseline measure of the parameter when examining the effect of the experimental condition. In contrast to the change score approach, the dependent variable in an ANCOVA is a residualized score that represents variation in the parameter that cannot be accounted for by the baseline value.[15]

One effect of employing the baseline score as a covariate in the analysis is to increase the statistical power of the ANOVA. That is, assuming the baseline measure is predictive of scores on the parameter following the experimental manipulation, the error term for testing the effect of group membership should be less after controlling for the influence of the baseline measure. To illustrate this point, an ANCOVA was conducted on depressor supercilii/procerus scores following the posed expressions (i.e., smile and anger) using scores from the neutral expression as the covariate. The ANCOVA results were compared to an ANOVA that did not control for EMG activity during the neutral expression. The results of the ANCOVA indicated that scores following the neutral expression represented a nonsignificant covariate, $F(1, 27) = 1.92$, $p < .20$. After controlling for baseline scores, the difference between the two posed expressions in EMG activity at the depressor supercilii/procerus muscle region was highly significant, $F(1, 27) = 26.87$, $p < .001$. Consistent with the change score analysis, less EMG activity at the depressor supercilii/procerus muscle region occurred following the smile ($M = 8.82$) in contrast to the anger ($M = 104.65$) expressions. Controlling for depressor supercilii/procerus scores following the neutral expression did serve to reduce the error term that was employed in testing the effect of the posed expressions. The MS_{error} from ANOVA was 2647.00, whereas the MS_{error} from the ANCOVA was 2562.73. Thus, the latter analysis provided a more powerful test of the hypothesis.[16]

Two issues need to be considered in conducting an analysis of covariance.[17] First, an assumption of ANCOVA that is often not tested by investigators concerns homogeneity of covariance. In simple terms, this assumption is met if the correlation between the covariate and the dependent variable is the same across groups. For the preceding example, the correlation between depressor supercilii/procerus scores following the neutral and posed (i.e., smile and anger) expressions should be similar for the two groups of subjects in order for the data to meet this assumption.

To test this assumption, it is necessary to evaluate whether or not there is a statistically significant interaction between the covariate and the variable representing group membership (i.e., smile vs. anger pose) in predicting scores on the dependent variable (i.e., depressor supercilii/procerus scores following the posed expressions). Since most ANOVA programs do not permit such a test, it is usually necessary to conduct a multiple regression analysis to determine whether or not the data meet the homogeneity-of-covariance assumption (see Pedhazur, 1982). In conducting this regression analysis, the independent variables are the covariate, a categorical variable reflecting group membership, and an interaction term that is created by multiplying the covariate by the group membership variable. A statistically significant interaction would indicate that the correlation between the covariate and dependent variable is significantly different across the experimental groups.

To illustrate this test for homogeneity of covariance, a multiple regression analysis was conducted that predicted depressor supercilii/procerus scores following the posed expressions from neutral expression scores, pose (i.e., smile vs. anger), and the interaction between the neutral expression scores and the pose condition. The interaction term was found to be nonsignificant, $F(1, 26) < 1$. This result indicates that the correlation between depressor supercilii/procerus scores following the neutral and posed expressions was similar for subjects in the smile and anger conditions. Thus, the data meet the homogeneity of covariance assumption.

A second issue that arises in conducting an analysis of covariance concerns the reliability of the covariate. Random error in the covariate tends to attenuate the estimate of the relationship between the dependent variable and the covariate. As a result, the ANCOVA underadjusts for the baseline scores of subjects, and the effects of individual differences in the parameters being assessed are not entirely removed from the analysis (see discussion by Reichardt in Cook & Campbell, 1979). A general recommendation in the literature is that ANCOVA not be performed unless the covariate has a reliability greater than .70. However, it should be noted that even that level of random measurement error can seriously affect the results.

23.4.1   *Summary*

According to Reichardt (in Cook & Campbell, 1979), analysis of covariance will typically provide a more powerful test of the hypothesis than an analysis of change scores. This point was illustrated in the present example in that, despite the reliability of the change score measure and the relatively low correlation between the covariate and the dependent variable, slightly stronger effects for the pose variable were found for the ANCOVA in contrast to the change score analyses. Even larger differences between the two methods of assessing change over time can be expected in other research settings where the change score measure is less reliable.

It therefore appears that ANCOVA is the preferred method of analysis to be used in examining change over time in psychophysiological parameters. This does not mean, however, that there are not issues to be considered prior to conducting an ANCOVA. Investigators need to evaluate whether or not their data meet the homeogeneity-of-covariance assumption and should also establish that the covariate is a reliable measure prior to conducting an ANCOVA. In examining the reliability of the covariate, investigators can employ the test–retest procedure employed in the example here or, in the case where multiple assessments of the covariate during the baseline period are available, compute coefficient alpha (Nunnaly, 1978). This latter procedure could be applied when there are multiple samples of the psychophysiological parameter taken during the baseline assessment and an average value computed to represent the baseline level. These multiple observations of the parameter could be viewed as "items" and coefficient alpha computed based on the covariance among these observations of the parameter. The SPSS–X RELIABILITY program will compute coefficient alpha and a number of other reliability estimates and is available in both microcomputer and mainframe versions of the statistical package.

A problem that arises concerns what should be done by an investigator when the baseline measure proves to be unreliable (i.e., a reliability coefficient below .70). In that situation, employing the baseline measure as a covariate will underestimate the relation between the baseline and response measures. As a result, the ANCOVA will not completely equate subjects in terms of the baseline measure, and some relationship between the two measures will remain. Computation of change scores in that situation would also be problematical. Since the baseline measure is unreliable, it is doubtful that the change score would be sufficiently reliable to justify analysis.

In that situation, the investigator is left with two choices. First, he or she can attempt to improve the reliability of the baseline assessment either by improvements in recording techniques or by employing a longer time interval for the baseline assessment. Use of this latter procedure would be synonymous to increasing the number of items on a measure and thereby increasing reliability (see Nunnaly, 1978). A second approach to solving the problems presented by the reliability of the covariate involves estimation of an ANCOVA model using latent variable methods, such as the LISREL (Jöreskog & Sörbom, 1985) or EQS (Bentler, 1985) computer programs (see discussion by Bentler, 1980). Both of these programs are available as stand-alone packages in mainframe and microcomputer versions, with LISREL now being distributed by SPSS and EQS by MBD.

To illustrate the use of these procedures, Figure 23.1 presents an example of a latent variable ANCOVA model examining the impact of pose (i.e., smile vs. anger) on EMG activity in the brow area, controlling for the level of brow EMG activity during the neutral expression. In order to estimate this model, two or more indicators of the latent variables reflecting EMG activity are necessary. Therefore, the depressor supercilii/procerus and corrugator supercilii measures were used as two indicators of brow EMG activity during both the baseline and pose periods. The level of brow

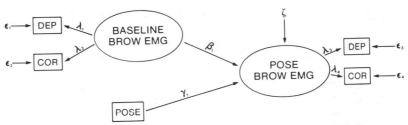

Figure 23.1. ANCOVA latent variable model for facial EMG data; DEP, Depressor Supercilii; COR, Corrugator Supercilii.

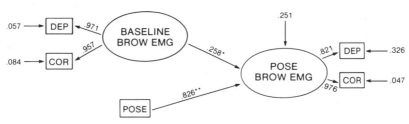

Figure 23.2. Results for ANCOVA latent variable model; abbreviations as in Figure 23.1; $^*p<.05;^{**}p<.01$.

activity during the baseline period was estimated based on the covariance between these two EMG measures. Lambda values in Figure 23.1 reflect the association between the two latent variables (enclosed in ovals) and the measured variables (i.e., depressor supercilii/procerus and corrugator supercilii). These values are equivalent to factor loadings in factor analysis. Error variation in each of these measures was estimated on the basis of residual variation in each EMG measure that was not shared with the other indicator of brow activity. These values are represented by the epsilons in Figure 23.1, corresponding to each of the measured EMG variables. By estimating these error terms, the latent variable procedure is able to remove the effects of random measurement error from the analysis.[18] The path from baseline to pose brow EMG in Figure 23.1, symbolized by beta, represents the relation between the covariate and the dependent variable. In the present model, this path is equal to the simple correlation between the two latent variables. The pose variable was represented in the model by a dummy-coded variable, where $0 =$ smile pose and $1 =$ anger pose. This variable is enclosed in a rectangle in Figure 23.1 to indicate that it is not a latent variable. Finally, residual variation in the dependent variable that is not explained by the two predictor variables (i.e., baseline brow EMG and pose) is indicated by zeta in Figure 23.1. This latter value is equivalent to the residual term in a regression equation.

This model was estimated using the maximum-likelihood methods of LISREL VI (Jöreskog & Sörbom, 1985). The results are presented in Figure 23.2. This model was found to provide an excellent fit to the data, χ^2 (4, $N = 30$) = 4.36, $p = .36$.[19] As indicated in Figure 23.2, both the baseline level of brow EMG activity and the pose were found to be statistically significant predictors of brow EMG activity during the pose. Overall, these two predictor variables accounted for approximately 75 percent of the variation in brow EMG activity following the pose, with the pose explaining 68 percent of the variation.

For comparative purposes, an ANCOVA was also conducted on these data. A composite score representing brow EMG activity was constructed by standardizing the depressor supercilii/procerus and corrugator supercilii measures and summing them together to represent the baseline and response measures. In contrast to the results from the latent variable analysis, the baseline measure of brow EMG activity was not a statistically significant covariate, $F(1, 27) = 3.69$, $p = .07$. As expected, the correlation between the baseline and response measures of EMG activity was lower from the ANCOVA analyses ($r = .213$) than was found from the latent variable analysis ($r = .258$). The removal of measurement error in the variables also increased the estimate of the pose effect in the latent variable analysis. As noted, the difference between the two poses accounted for 68 percent of the variation in brow EMG activity following the pose in the latent variable analysis, whereas pose accounted for 62 percent of the variation in ANCOVA analysis. These results clearly indicate an additional benefit of latent variable analyses: increased statistical power due to the estimation and removal of random measurement error from the analysis.

Although use of latent variable procedures would clearly enhance the power of the analysis and accuracy of the results, such an analysis requires a large number of subjects relative to the sample sizes that are typically employed in psychophysiological studies. Bentler (1985) recommends a minimum of five cases per parameter in conducting a latent variable analysis. For the analysis reported here, a minimum of 55 cases would be required to test the ANCOVA model. Thus, the findings from these analyses cannot be considered reliable.

To conclude the discussion of ANCOVA, it should be noted that covariates can also be used in the context of the multivariate procedures that were discussed previously. For example, it is possible to employ baseline scores as covariates in MANOVA either with or without repeated assessments of the parameters as part of the experiment. Thus, one can also examine patterns of change across a number of psychophysiological parameters while simultaneously controlling for baseline levels of the parameters through a multivariate analysis of covariance (MANCOVA).

23.5   CONCLUSION

This chapter has presented an overview of issues to be considered by the psychophysiological researcher in employing multivariate statistical procedures. These methods provide a number of advantages over traditional univariate approaches. Among these advantages are the ability to examine patterns of change in psychophysiological parameters in response to experimental conditions and to address problems associated with univariate approaches to repeated-measures designs.

It should be noted that a number of important multivariate procedures that are widely used in other areas of psychological research have either not been discussed (i.e., factor analysis, multidimensional scaling) or just briefly mentioned (i.e., multiple regression analysis, structural equation analysis with latent variables). The emphasis on the MANOVA model in this chapter derives primarily from a common characteristic of psychophysiological research. Such investigations typically involve small samples of subjects, which preclude the use of many multivariate procedures. This is not to say, however, that psychophysiological research might not be improved by use of such procedures. Indeed, multivariate procedures such as LISREL have the potential to greatly enhance the conceptualization and measurement of psychophysiological variables and would permit more powerful tests of theoretical predictions. However, use of these complex multivariate procedures would require psychophysiological researchers to employ much larger samples in their investigations. As these procedures become more widely used throughout psychology, psychophysiological researchers need to carefully consider whether gathering larger amounts of data may not be warranted in order to improve the quality of the multivariate analyses that can be conducted.

NOTES

1 Although MANOVA is robust to violations of the multivariate normality assumption, psychophysiological researchers may want to directly evaluate whether or not their data meet this assumption given the badly skewed nature of many psychophysiological parameters. An issue that arises involves how to test this assumption since statistical tests of multivariate normality are not provided in most statistical packages. Recently, however, the EQS program developed by Bentler (1985) has been released by BMD, in both mainframe and microcomputer versions. Although developed for other purposes, this program does provide the means for testing the multivariate normality assumption on the basis of the multivariate kurtosis parameter developed by Mardia (1970).

2 This estimate of the effect size is sample specific. A population estimate of the effect size can be found by taking the effect size estimate (call it e) and entering this value into the following formula:

$$1 - (1 - e)\frac{N-1}{N-s-1},$$

where N equals the sample size and s represents the number of variates (Serlin, 1982). For an example of the computation of the population estimate, see note 7.

3 It is possible for the results of the multivariate test to be statistically significant, with the groups found not to differ significantly from one another on any of the individual dependent variables. An example where this pattern of findings might occur would involve a situation where the difference between scores on two dependent variables served to differentiate the groups.

4 I would like to thank the authors for making these data available for analysis.

5 To simplify the presentation of this and other examples, only a subset of the data that were collected in the investigation will be presented. Subjects engaged in 12 additional poses as part of the investigation, and EMG activity was also recorded at two additional sites on the face (i.e., zygomaticus minor and buccinator/risorius; see Tassinary, Cacioppo, & Geen, 1989, for details).

6 This investigation did, in fact, involve a within-subjects design, where all of the subjects engaged in each of the poses. However, for purposes of illustration this nonindependence of the data will be ignored here. Subsequent analyses to be presented will employ a repeated-measures approach to these data.

7 Based on the formula presented in note 2, the following procedure was used to calculate the population estimate of the effect size. The value for e (effect size) derived from the Pillai–Bartlett trace was .672. To compute the population estimate, e was entered into the formula

$$1 - (1 - e)\frac{N-1}{N-s-1},$$

where N equals the sample size (45 in this case, since the data were treated as being from a between-subjects design) and s equals the number of variates that are formed by the MANOVA (2 in this example). For this example, the population effect size estimate was .656.

8 Many writers, such as Kirk (1982), have contended that the data employed in a repeated-measures analysis of variance meet the sphericity assumption of the univariate test if the repeated assessments possess *compound symmetry*. Compound symmetry is present if the repeated assessments (1) have the same variance and (2) have the same

covariance or correlation with one another. So, for example, the correlation between the measures taken during trials 1 and 2 would have to equal the correlation between the measures taken during trials 1 and 3. However, Huynh and Feldt (1970, 1976) have demonstrated that compound symmetry is a sufficient but not necessary condition for the data to meet the sphericity assumption. Thus, it is possible for data to meet the sphericity assumption even if the correlations among the repeated assessments of the dependent variable are not equal over time, as would be true if the data possessed compound symmetry.

9 An issue that arises concerns which of the two estimates of ε to employ in adjusting the degrees of freedom if the data do not meet the sphericity assumption. Comparisons of the Huynh–Feldt and Greenhouse–Geisser adjustments indicate that the Huynh–Feldt statistic is more accurate when violations of sphericity are mild, whereas the Greenhouse–Geisser statistic is more accurate when violations of sphericity are severe (Mendoza, Toothaker, & Nicewander, 1974; Rogan, Keselman, & Mendoza, 1979). Since the Greenhouse–Geisser adjustment to the degrees of freedom is greater than that based on the Huynh–Feldt statistic, a conservative approach would argue for employing the Greenhouse–Geisser adjustment.

10 It should be noted that this dependent variable was randomly selected for analysis from the data set. Thus, employing this variable in the analyses was not meant to imply anything regarding the sensitivity of the depressor supercilii/procerus to emotional expression.

11 This recommendation has recently been formally adopted as part of the editorial policy of the journal *Psychophysiology*. Partly on the basis of the article by Vasey and Thayer (1987), Jennings (1987) argues for the importance of testing the sphericity assumption in analyzing psychophysiological data from repeated-measures designs and either correcting the degrees of freedom employed in conducting the univariate test in light of any violations of assumptions that are found or conducting a multivariate test of the hypotheses. Clearly, researchers interested in publishing in *Psychophysiology* should heed these recommendations, and one would assume that other journals would develop similar standards for the analysis of psychophysiological data from repeated-measures designs.

12 To understand why this is the case, consider the formula for computing the reliability of a change score presented by Nunnaly (1978; see note 14). The error variation in the change score is calculated by first computing the error variance in the baseline and response scores and summing these values together. This error variance estimate is then divided by the total variation in the change score to derive an estimate of the proportion of the variation in the change score that represents random measurement error. The resulting estimate of the error variation is therefore affected by the total variation in the change scores, which will vary depending on the correlation between the baseline and response scores. Upon reflection, it should become apparent that the variation in the change scores will be larger than the variation in the component scores when the baseline and response scores are negatively correlated and smaller than the variation in the component scores when the baseline and response scores are positively correlated. Thus, the reliability of the change score relative to the reliability of the baseline and response scores depends in part on the nature of the relation between the two component scores.

13 For the purpose of this and the subsequent example, the data from the study were treated as if the two posed expressions (i.e., smile and anger) were done by distinct groups of subjects. Thus, pose was treated as a between-subjects variable.

14 The formula for the reliability of a change score is

$$\rho_{x_1 - x_2} = 1 - \frac{\sigma^2_{x_1}\ (1 - \rho_{x_1}) + \sigma^2_{x_2}\ (1 - \rho_{x_2})}{\rho^2_{x_1 - x_2}},$$

where $\sigma^2_{x_1}$ and $\sigma^2_{x_2}$ represent the variance of the two measures from which the difference score is being computed, ρ_{x_1} and ρ_{x_2} represent the realiability of the two original scores (based on coefficient alpha), and $\sigma^2_{x_1 - x_2}$ represents the variance of the resulting difference scores.

15 Although not typically recognized as such, the covariance approach provides results that are identical to findings based on the computation of the Autonomic Lability Score (ALS) advocated by Lacey (1956). In computing the ALS, one first performs a regression analysis where the response measure of a parameter is regressed upon the baseline measure. A

residual score is then calculated by subtracting the actual response measure from the predicted value based on the baseline measure. This procedure is, of course, identical to that employed in an analysis of covariance to remove the effects of the baseline measure on the response measure. Therefore, one need not go through the process of actually calculating ALS scores.

16 In this example, it should be noted that the correlation between the covariate and the dependent variable was fairly small in magnitude (i.e., .186). As a result, the reduction in the MS_{error} was relatively small. In situations where the relation between the covariate and dependent variable is larger in magnitude, a much greater reduction in the error term from the ANCOVA will occur, resulting in a greater increase in statistical power.

17 Other issues also arise when employing analysis of covariance with nonexperimental data (see Reichardt, in Cook & Campbell 1979; Woodward & Goldstein, 1977). These issues include the underadjustment for group differences on the covariate due to random error in the covariate and the possibility that the covariate may be causally related to the treatment. However, these issues are relevant only in the case where subjects have not been randomly assigned to condition.

18 ANCOVA models would also typically include the possibility of correlated or systematic measurement error in the model, reflecting biases in the assessment due to employing the same measure repeatedly over time (see Bentler, 1980). However, these correlated error terms were found to be nonsignificant for the present model and therefore were not included among the parameters that were estimated.

19 The chi-square test represents a goodness-of-fit test, evaluating to what extent the model can reproduce the variance and covariances of the variables. Thus, a nonsignificant chi-square indicates that the model fits the data (see discussion by Bentler, 1980).

REFERENCES

Barcikowski, R. S. (Ed.) (1983a). *Computer packages and research design: Vol. 1, BMDP.* New York: University Press of America.

Barcikowski, R. S. (Ed.) (1983b). *Computer packages and research design: Vol. 3. SPSS and SPSSX.* New York: University Press of America.

Barker, H. R., & Barker, B. M. (1984). *Multivariate analysis of variance (MANOVA): A practical guide to its use in scientific decision making.* University, AL: University of Alabama Press.

Benjamin, L. S. (1967). Facts and artifacts in using analysis of covariance to undo the law of initial values. *Psychophysiology, 4,* 556–566.

Bentler, P. M. (1980). Multivariate analysis with latent variables: Causal modeling. *Annual Review of psychology, 31,* 419–456.

Bentler, P. M. (1985). *Theory and implementation of EQS: A structural equations program.* Los Angeles: BMDP Statistical Software.

Bock, R. D. (1975). *Multivariate statistical methods in behavioral research.* New York: McGraw-Hill.

Bray, J. H., & Maxwell, S. E. (1982). Analyzing and interpreting significant MANOVAs. *Review of Educational Research, 52,* 340–367.

Bray, J. H., & Maxwell, S. E. (1985). *Multivariate analysis of variance.* Beverly Hills, CA: Sage.

Cole, J. W. L., & Grizzle, J. E. (1966). Applications of multivariate analysis of variance to repeated measures experiments. *Biometrics, 22,* 810–828.

Cook, T. D., & Campbell, D. T. (1979). *Quasi-experimentation: Design and analysis issues for field settings.* Boston: Houghton Mifflin.

Cronbach, L. J., & Furby, L. (1970). How we should measure "change" – or should we? *Psychological Bulletin, 74,* 68–80.

Finn, J. D. (1974). *A general model for multivariate analysis.* New York: Holt, Rinehart & Winston.

Greenhouse, S. W., & Geisser, S. (1959). On methods in the analysis of profile data. *Psychometrika, 24,* 95–112.

Harris, R. J. (1985). *A primer of multivariate statistics* (2nd ed.). New York: Academic Press.

Hays, W. L. (1973). *Statistics for the social sciences* (2nd ed.). New York: Holt, Rinehart & Winston.

Hummel, T. J., & Sligo, J. R. (1971). Empirical comparison of univariate and multivariate analyses of variance procedures. *Psychological Bulletin, 75,* 49–57.

Huynh, H., & Feldt, L. S. (1970). Conditions under which mean square ratios in repeated measurements designs have exact *F*-distributions. *Journal of the American Statistical Association, 65,* 1582–1589.

Huynh, H., & Feldt, L. S. (1976). Estimation of the Box correction for degrees of freedom from sample data in the randomized block and split-plot designs. *Journal of Educational Statistics, 1,* 69–82.

Huynh, H., & Feldt, L. S. (1980). Performance of traditional *F* tests in repeated measures designs under variance heterogeneity. *Communications in Statistics: Series A, 9,* 61–74.

Ito, K. (1969). On the effect of heteroscedasticity and nonnormality upon some multivariate test procedures. In P. R. Krishnaiah (Ed.), *Multivariate analysis II.* New York: Academic Press.

Ito, K., & Schull, W. (1964). On the robustness of the T^2 test in multivariate analysis of variance when variance-covariance matrices are not equal. *Biometrika, 51,* 71–82.

Jennings, J. R. (1987). Editorial policy on analyses of variance with repeated measures. *Psychophysiology, 24,* 474–475.

Jennings, J. R., & Wood, C. C. (1976). The epsilon-adjusted procedure for repeated measures analyses of variance. *Psychophysiology, 13,* 277–278.

Johnson, L. C., & Lubin, A. (1972). On planning psychophysiological experiments: Design, measurement, and analysis. In N. S. Greenfield & R. A. Sternbach (Eds.), *Handbook of psychophysiology* (pp. 125–158). New York: Holt, Rinehart & Winston.

Jöreskog, K. G., & Sörbom, D. (1985). *LISREL VI user's guide.* Mooresville, IN: Scientific Software.

Keppel, G. (1982). *Design and analysis: A researcher's handbook* (2nd ed.). Englewood Cliffs, NJ: Prentice-Hall.

Kirk, R. E. (1982). *Experimental design: Procedures for the behavioral sciences* (2nd ed.). Belmont, CA: Wadsworth.

Lacey, J. I. (1956). The evaluation of an autonomic response: Toward a general solution. *Annals of the New York Academy of Sciences, 67,* 123–164.

Levey, A. B. (1980). Measurement units in psychophysiology. In I. Martin & P. H. Venables (Eds.), *Techniques in psychophysiology* (pp. 597–628). New York: Wiley.

Mardia, K. V. (1970). Measures of multivariate skewness and kurtosis with applications. *Biometrika, 57,* 519–530.

Mardia, K. V. (1971). The effects of nonnormality on some multivariate tests and robustness to nonnormality in the linear model. *Biometrika, 58,* 105–121.

Maxwell, S. E., Arvey, R. D., & Camp, C.J. (1981). Measures of strength of association: A comparative examination. *Journal of Applied Psychology, 66,* 525–534.

Mendoza, J. L., Toothaker, L. E., & Nicewander, W. A. (1974). A Monte Carlo comparison of the univariate and multivariate methods for the groups by trials experimental design. *Multivariate Behavioral Research, 9,* 165–177.

Nunnaly, J. C. (1978). *Psychometric theory* (2nd ed.). New York: McGraw-Hill.

O'Brien, R. G., & Kaiser, M. K. (1985). MANOVA method for analyzing repeated measures designs: An extensive primer. *Psychological Bulletin, 97,* 316–333.

Olson, C. L. (1974). Comparative robustness of six tests in multivariate analysis of variance. *Journal of the American Statistical Association, 69,* 894–908.

Olson, C. L. (1976). On choosing a test statistic in multivariate analysis of variance. *Psychological Bulletin, 83,* 579–586.

Olson, C. L. (1979). Practical considerations in choosing a MANOVA test statistic: A rejoinder to Stevens. *Psychological Bulletin, 86,* 1350–1352.

Overall, J. E., & Klett, C. J. (1972). *Applied multivariate analysis.* New York: McGraw-Hill.

Pedhazur, E. J. (1982). *Multiple regression in behavioral research: Explanation and prediction* (2nd ed.). New York: Holt, Rinehart & Winston.

Rogan, J. C., Keselman, H. J., & Mendoza, J. L. (1979). Analysis of repeated measurement. *British Journal of Mathematical and Statistical Psychology, 32,* 269–286.

Serlin, R. C. (1982). A multivariate measure of association based on the Pillai–Bartlett procedure. *Psychological Bulletin, 91,* 413–417.

Stevens, J. P. (1979). Comment on Olson: On choosing a test statistic in multivariate analysis of variance. *Psychological Bulletin, 86,* 355–360.

Strahan, R. I. (1982). Multivariate analysis of variance and the problem of Type I error. *Journal of Counseling Psychology, 29,* 175–179.

Tassinary, L. G., Cacioppo, J. T., & Geen, T. R. (1989). A psychometric study of surface electrode placements for facial electromyographic recording: I. The brow and cheek muscle regions. *Psychophysiology, 26,* 1–16.

Tatsuoka, M. M. (1988). *Multivariate analysis: Techniques for educational and psychological research* (2nd ed.). New York: Macmillan.

Timm, N. H. (1980). Multivariate analysis of variance of repeated measures. In P. R. Krishnaiah (Ed.), *Handbook of statistics. Vol. 1. Analysis of variance* (pp. 41–87). New York: Elsevier/North-Holland.

Vasey, M. W., & Thayer, J. F. (1987). The continuing problem of false positives in repeated measures ANOVA in psychophysiology: A multivariate solution. *Psychophysiology, 24,* 479–486.

Weisberg, S. (1985). *Applied linear regression* (2nd ed.). New York: Wiley.

Wilder, J. (1950). The law of initial values. *Psychosomatic Medicine, 12,* 392.

Wilder, J. (1965). Pitfalls in the methodology of the law of initial values. *American Journal of Psychotherapy, 19,* 577–584.

Winer, B. J. (1971). *Statistical principles in experimental design* (2nd ed.). New York: McGraw-Hill.

Woodward, J. A., & Goldstein, M. J. (1977). Communication deviance in the families of schizophrenics: A comment on the misuse of analysis of covariance. *Science, 197,* 1096–1097.

A glossary of technical terms and general concepts in psychophysiology

ACETYLCHOLINE (ACh)   A simple organic compound ($C_7H_{17}NO_3$) that is released from the axonic terminals (i.e., the bouton) of certain nerve cells into the synaptic cleft upon receipt of an electrical impulse. The presence of this compound is instrumental in the transmission of the action potential.

ACTIVATION   A psychophysiological concept usually associated with the work of Duffy, Hebb, Lindsley, and Malmo that refers to a fundamental change within the organism that is necessary for all actions and reactions. In general, an organism is said to exhibit increasing degrees of activation as it exhibits relative increases in the intensity of responding in sympatheticlike directions. The related concept of *arousal* is often used interchangeably.

AC-TO-DC CONVERTER   An electronic unit that rectifies and smooths the flow of an alternating current, thus converting it into a direct current.

ADAPTATION   In psychophysiology, a decrease in physiological responsivity that occurs with repeated presentation of the same stimulus. See *Habituation*.

ADMITTANCE (Y)   The generic term for the property of any component of a system that is susceptible to current flow. It includes both simple conductance and susceptance and is expressed in mhos or siemens. Mathematically, it is the reciprocal of electrical impedance.

ADRENERGIC   A term applied to those nerve fibers that liberate norepinephrine at a synapse upon receipt of an action potential, e.g., the fibers constituting the sympathetic nervous system, or to an agent that stimulates such fibers. Also known as *sympathicomimetic*.

AFFERENT   Centripetal; conveying toward a center. The term is typically used to refer to sensory nerve fibers.

AFTER-LOAD   The resistance against which the ventricles of the heart contract. Factors contributing to after-load include aortic or pulmonary arterial impedance, peripheral vascular resistance, as well as the mass and viscosity of the blood.

AGNOSIA   A neuropsychological term that refers to an impairment of an organism's ability to recognize the functional significance or meaning of sensory stimuli in the absence of other sensory impairments.

ALGORITHM   A term derived from the root *algorism*, which means "the art of computing with Arabic numerals." The term now refers to any method of computing, whether algebraic or numerical, or to any method of computation

802

specifically adapted to the solution of a problem of some particular type that consists of a comparatively small number of steps taken in a preassigned order. Broadly, the term connotes any effective procedure for solving a problem or accomplishing some end.

ALIASING   The reflection of frequency values with respect to half the sampling frequency or with respect to frequency zero. The effect is termed aliasing since unwanted high-frequency components appear under the alias of wanted low-frequency components. See *Folding Frequency*.

ALPHA-MOTONEURON   A neural structure whose cell body is located in the anterior horn of the spinal cord and, through its relatively large-diameter axon and terminal branches, innervates a group of striated muscle fibers.

AMINO ACIDS   Any organic acid that incorporates one or more amino groups. Most of the biological study of these acids has centered around the relatively small group of alpha-amino acids that are combined in amide linkage to form proteins. With few exceptions, these compounds possess the general structure NH_2CHRCO_2H, where the amino group occupies a position on the carbon atom alpha to that of the carboxyl group and where the side chain R may be of diverse composition and structure.

AMPERE   The amount of current that flows when one volt of electromotive force is applied across one ohm of resistance.

AMPLIFIER   A device for increasing the strength of a signal without appreciably altering signal characteristics within a specified amplitude/frequency range. Examples of the amplifier classifications referred to in psychophysiology include *capacitance coupled* (*AC*) and *direct coupled* (*DC*). The *AC amplifiers* strengthen the difference between two electrical potentials such that low frequencies are attenuated in the output relative to their size in the input signal. Typical AC amplifiers include user-adjustable *bandpass* filters. In contrast, *DC amplifiers* have a frequency response that extends to 0 Hz. Typical DC amplifiers include user-adjustable *low-pass filters*. See *Filters*.

AMPLITUDE   In general, a quantity that expresses the value of a waveform at any point along its length. In psychophysiology, the term has two additional, distinct meanings. First, it can be used to denote the size of a response (typically the arithmetic mean) calculated over all occasions on which a response is actually present. However, it is also occasionally used to refer to the maximum value that a waveform obtains within a specified length. Compare *Magnitude*.

ANALOG   Pertaining to data in the form of continuously variable quantities. Contrast with *Digital*.

ANALOG-TO-DIGITAL CONVERTER   An electronic device designed to transform continuous varying analog quantities into a series of discrete numerical values coded in binary form.

ANGIOTENSIN   A polypeptide present in the blood and formed by the catalytic action of renin on angiotensinogen in the blood plasma. Angiotension I, the inactive form, is in turn acted upon by a converting enzyme, chiefly in the lungs, to form the hormone angiotension II, a powerful vasopressor and a stimulator of aldosterone secretion by the adrenal cortex. By its vasopressor action, this hormone raises blood pressure and diminishes fluid loss in the kidney by restricting flow. Angiotensin II is hydrolyzed to form angiotensin III, which has limited vasopressor properties but has pronounced effects on the output of the adrenal cortex.

ANTI-ALIASING FILTER   A high-quality, low-pass analog filter used to eliminate any frequencies higher than the *Nyquist,* or *folding frequency.* See *Filter.*

AORTIC VALVE   The valve between the left ventricle of the heart and the ascending aorta.

APOCRINE   One of two types of sweat glands. These particular glands are typically associated with hair follicles distributed primarily throughout the axilla and are generally believed to be of minimal importance in the measurement of electrodermal activity. The sweat produced by these glands includes the apical portion of the secreting cell along with the secretary products that have accumulated therein. It is this organic material that, upon bacterial decomposition, produces a strong characteristic odor. Contrast with *Eccrine.*

APRAXIA   A neuropsychological term that refers to an impairment of an organism's ability to perform familiar, purposeful movements in the absence of paralysis or other sensory impairment.

AROUSAL   See *Activation.*

ARTIFACT   Unwanted signals that may mimic the signal of interest. One common source of artifacts arises from the AC power mains; another is high electrode impedance. When artifacts are caused by movement of the subject, this usually results from a fluctuation in voltage due to the mechanical disturbance of the skin–electrolyte–electrode surface interface. See *Noise.*

ASSOCIATION CORTEX   Those areas of the neocortex that are neither primary input (sensory) nor specific output (motor) projection areas. The function of an association area may be unknown, or it may mediate complex functions associated with basic psychological processes such as perception, memory, and/or emotion.

ATRIOVENTRICULAR VALVE   The valves separating the atria and ventricles of the heart. The atrioventricular valve of the right heart is known as the *tricuspid valve* and that of the left heart is known as the *mitral valve.*

ATROPINE   An alkaloid ($C_{17}H_{23}NO_3$) that is a cholinergic-blocking agent. It is used primarily as either a muscle relaxant or a cardiovascular disinhibitor (i.e., it increases heart rate by blocking the tonic inhibitory action of the vagus nerve).

ATTENUATION   The decrease in amplitude of a wave or wave component as it travels through any transmitting medium. Attenuation factors are typically expressed as a ratio or as the logarithm of a ratio (e.g., decibels).

AUSCULTATORY TECHNIQUE   In general, any technique in which sounds originating from within the body are used in diagnosis. In reference to the cardiovascular system, this term refers specifically to a technique used to measure blood pressure involving the use of a blood pressure cuff, stethoscope, and manometer. See *Sphygomanometer.*

AUTOCORRELATION   The correlation between a waveform and itself shifted in time for all possible units of time. When expressed as a function of the time shift, the resulting waveform is known as the autocorrelation function. By definition, this function will be symmetrical about the zero time shift axis and have unit value at zero time.

AUTONOMIC BALANCE   A concept introduced to the psychophysiological literature by Wegner and associates in the 1940s that refers to the extent to which the autonomic responses of an individual tend to be dominated by either the sympathetic or parasympathetic branches of the autonomic nervous system. This is related to the earlier concepts of *vagotonia* and *sympathicotonia* introduced by Eppinger and Hess in the early part of the 20th century.

AUTONOMIC NERVOUS SYSTEM (ANS)   The portion of the nervous system concerned with the regulation of the activity of cardiac muscle, smooth muscle, and glands. Includes the parasympathetic nervous system (PNS), the sympathetic nervous system (SNS) and the enteric nervous system (ENS).

AUTORECEPTOR   A biochemical receptor typically found on the presynaptic neuron that, when activated by a neurotransmitter, inhibits the release of the same transmitter from the cell. If these receptors are located on the axon terminal, they serve to regulate the amount of neurotransmitter released into the synapse with each action potential. If they are located on the cell body or dendrites, they help to regulate the firing rate of the neuron by controlling the relative refractory period of the neuron.

AUTOREGRESSION   A statistical technique used in time-series analysis to construct a model of a set of sequential observations with respect to time. An autoregressive model expresses the current observations in terms of both the current observations and all of the past observations.

AVERAGING   The process whereby the sum of many measurements (or sets of measurements) is divided by the number of measurements in order to form the mean value or average. This technique can be used to distinguish a small signal that is unrecognizable in other activity if the following conditions approximately hold: (1) The specified signal and noise nearly sum together to produce the recorded waveform, (2) the evoked signal wave shape attributable solely to the stimulus is the same for each repetition of the stimulus, and (3) the noise contributions to the observed data appear sufficiently irregular so that they can be considered to constitute statistically independent samples of a random process.

AXON   The relatively elongated part of a neuron that conducts impulses away from the cell body.

BACKING OFF   The process of opposing a potential (possibly representing another value, such as conductance) by an equal and opposite potential so as to suppress a tonic level and hence enable phasic responses to be measured with greater resolution (synonymous with bucking).

BANDWIDTH   The difference between the upper and lower limits of a given band of frequencies expressed in hertz. See *Filters*.

BARORECEPTOR REFLEX   A neural reflex mechanism involving receptors (i.e., baroreceptors) sensitive to pressure variation that functions to quickly stabilize blood pressure.

BEL (B)   A dimensionless unit for expressing the ratio of two values of power. It is defined as the logarithm to the base 10 of the power ratio.

BIAS POTENTIAL   Potentials inherent in electrodes that confound the recording of low-level bioelectric signals and thus increase measurement error.

BLOOD–BRAIN BARRIER   A protective encapsulation of blood vessels in the brain that prevents many substances in the blood, particularly those with large molecules, from diffusing into the brain and thereby directly affecting neural activity.

BLOOD PLASMA   The natural liquid medium in which cellular elements of blood are suspended.

BLOOD PRESSURE   The pressure of the blood on the arterial walls. It is primarily a function of the energy of heart action, the elasticity of the arterial walls, the resistance of the arterioles and capillaries, and the volume and viscosity of the blood. The maximum pressure occurs near the end of the stroke output of the left ventricle of the heart and is termed maximum, or *systolic,* pressure. The minimum pressure occurs late in ventricular diastole and is termed minimum, or *diastolic* pressure. *Mean blood pressure* refers to the average of blood pressure levels, *basic blood pressure* to the pressure during quiet rest or basal conditions, and *pulse pressure* to the difference between systolic and diastolic pressures.

BLOOD VOLUME   The total quantity of blood in the body, usually expressed in liters or liters per kilogram of body weight. In psychophysiology, the term typically refers to the overall engorgement of a particular body part (limb, finger, etc.) and is often used as an index of tonic blood flow.

BRADYCARDIA   A slow heart rate, usually defined as less than 60 bpm.

BRADYGASTRIA   Periodic gastric myoelectric activity slower than the normal 3 cpm.

BUCKING   See *Backing off.*

CALIBRATION   A generic term for any method of defining an accurate and known relationship between the input and output of a system. Usually involves applying a known quantity (e.g., a 10 Hz, 5 μV sine wave) and noting the response of the system.

CAPACITANCE   The property of a *dielectric* material between conductors that permits the storage of electricity when a difference of potential exists between the conductors. The unit of measurement is the farad.

CAPACITOR   An electronic component that is capable of storing an electric charge. A capacitor exists whenever two conducting surfaces are separated by a *dielectric* material. Capacitance is a function of the area of the surfaces, type of dielectric, spacing between the conducting surfaces, and size of the electrical potential between the two conducting surfaces.

CARDIAC CYCLE   In medicine, a complete cycle of cardiac systole and diastole with the intervals between. In psychophysiology, this term typically refers to the time period extending from any event in the heart's action to the moment when that same event is repeated.

CARDIAC OUTPUT   The quantity of blood discharged by the ventricle (left or right) per unit time.

CARDIAC SOMATIC HYPOTHESIS   Part of a theory associated with P. Obrist and his associates regarding the behavioral significance of cardiovascular changes. According to this hypothesis, cardiovascular changes are seen as primarily reflecting changing metabolic requirements during the preparation for action. Contrast *intake rejection hypothesis.*

CARDIOTACHOMETER   A device for measuring heart rate and/or heart period. Strictly, an accurate measure of heart rate in units of beats per minute (bpm) can only be obtained by actually counting the number of beats produced in 1 min. However, a cardiotachometer measures the interbeat interval (i.e., interval between R-wave components), and this time (i.e., heart period) is either displayed directly as a voltage level proportional to heart period or its reciprocal, heart rate. In a hardware cardiotachometer, the current level of the output voltage is always proportional to the previous beat since the level can only change once a beat has occurred.

CARRIER FREQUENCY   The frequency upon which a signal is impressed for transmission in a coherent fashion to a receiver. It is then stripped of its carrier frequency, amplified, and reproduced.

CARTESIAN COORDINATES   Coordinates from any N-dimensional space such that the absolute values of any unit length are the same. When the surfaces are mutually perpendicular, the system is *curvilinear* or *orthogonal*; when the surfaces are orthogonal planes, the system is *rectangular*; if the surfaces do not intersect at right angles, the system is said to be *affine* or *nonorthogonal*. The term *Cartesian coordinate system* can refer to either a rectangular system or a system of planes not at right angles to each other (i.e., an oblique coordinate system). However, Cartesian typically means rectangular Cartesian. The familiar XY plane is Cartesian if one unit along the X-axis is the same as one unit along the Y-axis.

CASCADE   Any connected arrangement of separable elements whose result is to multiply the effect, such as filtering or amplifying, created by the individual elements.

CATECHOLAMINES   One of a group of similar organic compounds with endocrine and transmitter functions, primarily having an *adrenergic* action. Such compounds include dopamine, norepinephrine, and epinephrine.

CAUDAL   An anatomical term denoting a position more toward the tail than some specified point of reference. In human anatomy, the term *inferior* is more often used.

CENTRAL VENOUS POOL   The small volume of blood concentrated in the great veins of the thorax. The pressure difference between the central venous pool and the right atrial volume plays an important role in determining venous return.

CEREBRAL CORTEX   The thin outer layer of gray matter (i.e., cell bodies) that covers the entire folded surface of the cerebral hemispheres. It has been estimated that the average adult cortex contains approximately 9 billion individual nerve cells.

CHANNEL   A path along which signals can be sent.

CHOLINERGIC   A term applied to those nerve fibers that liberate acetylcholine at a synapse upon receipt of an action potential, e.g., the fibers constituting the parasympathetic nervous system, or to an agent that stimulates such fibers. Also known as *parasympathicomimetic*.

CHOLINESTERASE   A complex organic compound that, acting as the principal enzyme in the decomposition of *acetylcholine* present in the synaptic cleft into choline and an anion, limits the time that this neurotransmitter can effect electrical and chemical changes in the postsynaptic membrane.

CIRCUIT   A system of conducting mediums designed to pass an electric current.

CLAMP   The process of giving an AC signal a specific DC level.

CLUSTER ANALYSIS   A class of statistical techniques for allocating objects into groups such that all objects in a given group have similar properties and all objects with similar properties are in the same group. Although generally considered to be a form of classification, it is somewhat limited in that it typically does not take into account such considerations as biological lines of descent (as in Linnean classification) or varying criteria at different levels (as in libraries).

COACTIVATION   In electromyography, the term has two distinct meanings. It may either refer to the simultaneous activation of alpha- and gama-motoneurons within a muscle or to the simultaneous activation of agonist and antagonist muscle groups.

CODE   A set of unambiguous rules specifying the manner in which elements in one set may be represented by elements in another set.

COLLIMATED LIGHT   Light composed of parallel rays.

COMMON-MODE REJECTION   A fundamental aspect of differential amplification that refers to the attenuation of in-phase (e.g., unwanted 60/50 Hz interference) over antiphase (e.g., biological) signals. The efficiency of the common-mode rejection is given by the equation $CMRR = V_{cm}/V_e$, where CMRR is the common-mode rejection ratio, V_{cm} is input amplitude of the common-mode voltage, and V_e is the output amplitude of the common-mode voltage (also known as the common-mode error voltage).

CONCOMITANT   A term recently proposed by Cacioppo and Tassinary (see chapter 1) to refer to a particular class of psychophysiological relationships. More specifically, the term refers to any many-to-one, context-free relationship between psychological and physiological events or constructs.

CONDUCTANCE (G)   The susceptibility of any component of a system to the flow of constant current. It is expressed in units of mhos or siemens. Mathematically, it is the reciprocal of electrical resistance.

CONDUCTOR   A material capable of transmitting energy.

CONSTANT-CURRENT METHOD   A method of measuring skin resistance where the current through the skin between two electrodes is maintained at a constant value. By Ohm's Law, the voltage output from electronic devices using this method is directly proportional to skin resistance.

CONSTANT-VOLTAGE METHOD   A method of measuring skin conductance where the potential across electrodes on the skin surface is maintained at a constant value. By Ohm's Law, the current output from electronic devices using this method is directly proportional to skin conductance.

CONSTRICTION   Reduction in the size of a blood vessel or other opening. The act of constricting or reducing the size of the lumen of a hollow structure.

CONTINGENT NEGATIVE VARIATION (CNV)   A slow negative shift of cortical potential observed when subjects are told that they must respond to an event some time after a warning signal is given. Compare *Readiness potential.*

CONTRACTILITY   The ability or property of a substance, especially muscle, of shortening, becoming reduced in size, or developing tension in response to a suitable stimulus. Because the ventricles of the heart are innervated primarily by the sympathetic branch (beta-adrenergic) of the autonomic nervous system, measures of *left-ventricular contractility* have been used to index change in sympathetic influences on the heart.

CORPUS CALLOSUM   The major tract of nerve fibers that connects the two cerebral hemispheres and allows for interhemispheric communication.

COULOMB (C)   The quantity of electric charge that passes any cross section of a conductor in one second when the current is maintained at a constant one ampere.

COUPLING   The transfer of energy between two or more components of a system.

COVARIANCE   A condition where a change in one variable is associated with a change in another. Where x and y are the deviations from the means of the paired values in the series, covariance is given by the formula $\Sigma xy/N$, where N is the number of paired values.

CROSS-CORRELATION   In general, any correlation between series ordered in time and space with or without a lag between the series. Typically, however, the term is used to denote the correlation between two signals occurring at different times.

CROSS-TALK   A type of interference caused by signals from one source appearing as signals from another source.

CUE   A generic term used in psychology and psychophysiology to refer to any signal or stimulus enabling the organism to make a discrimination that is used in the guidance or control of behavior and experience. *External cues* refers to stimuli orginating in the environment or social setting (e.g., facial expressions of conspecifics), whereas *internal cues* refers to stimuli originating within the subject (e.g., physiological reactions).

CURRENT (I)   The rate of transfer of electric charge from one point to another measured in amperes. The term *alternating current (AC)* refers to an electric current that periodically reverses direction of electron flow. The rate at which a full cycle occurs in a given unit of time (generally a second) is called the frequency of the current. The term *direct current (DC)* refers to an electric current whose electrons flow in one direction only. It may be constant or pulsating as long as their movement is in the same direction.

CURRENT LIMITING   A method of protecting the power converter from excessive current as the load approaches becoming a short circuit. Two types of current limiting are commonly employed. *Foldback limiting* decreases the output current as the load increases from its rated level to short circuit. At a predetermined maximum overload, the output current will decrease to considerably less than rated current and thus prevent overheating. *Constant-current limiting* simply limits the output current to some specified value by breaking the circuit once that limit has been surpassed.

CYTOARCHITECTURE   The three-dimensional organization of cells in the structure of an organ or tissue. The term usually refers to the way different types of cells are arranged and distributed in various parts of the nervous system, especially in the cerebral cortex.

DALE'S PRINCIPLE (DALE'S LAW)   The concept, first suggested by Sir Henry Dale in the 1930s, that if a particular neurotransmitter is released by one of a neuron's synaptic endings, the same chemical is released at all of the synaptic endings of that neuron. Recent evidence suggests that this principle is in need of revision.

DAMPING   The progressive reduction or active suppression of the oscillation of a system in response to a stimulus with respect to time. A system is said to be *underdamped* when the system continues to respond after changes in the value of the stimulus (a condition also known as *overshoot*), *overdamped* when the response of the system lags after changes in the value of the stimulus, and *critically damped* when the response of the system to stimulus changes is as fast as possible without overshoot. See *Hysteresis.*

DATA   A representation of facts, concepts, or instructions in a formalized manner suitable for communication, interpretation, or processing by human or automatic means.

DECIBEL (dB)   One-tenth of a bel. It is a relational unit equal to one-tenth the common logarithm of the ratio between two powers. It is also equal to one-twentieth the common logarithm of a ratio between two voltages or two currents. In psychological terms, one decibel is the amount by which the pressure of a pure sine wave of sound must be varied in order for the change to be detected by the average human ear. The decibel can express an actual level only when compared to a definite reference level that is assumed to be 0 dB. For example, the unit abbreviated dBspl refers to the number of decibels a signal is above or below a standard sound pressure level (typically, 0.0002 dynes/cm^2).

DECOUPLING CAPACITOR   A capacitor that provides a low-impedance path to ground to prevent common coupling between circuits.

DENDRITE/DENDRON   Large and often complex branches of postsynaptic neural fibers that convey action potentials toward the cell body. Sensory neurons typically have single dendrites, whereas motoneurons may have many.

DEOXYRIBONUCLEIC ACID (DNA)   An extremely complex molecule composed of substructures of phosphates, bases, and sugars organized as a single double helix. The particular sequence of these subunits determines the genetic information that is carried by the chromosomes and regulates all metabolic processes.

DEPOLARIZATION   The breakdown of the ionic equilibrium across a cell membrane such that negative ions flow outward across the membrane. The propagated depolarization of the neuron is the electrical sign of the passage of the action potential.

DEPRESSOR RESPONSE   Any response that tends to decrease blood pressure. A good example of a depressor response is the decrease in heart rate and ventricular contractility triggered by a increase in blood pressure. This response pattern, mediated by the baroreceptor reflex, results in a compensatory decrease in blood pressure and thus forms one part of the negative-feedback system involved in the regulation of blood pressure.

DETERMINANT   The generalized variance of elements in a matrix. Applications of determinants in multivariate statistics typically involve variance–covariance matrices, in which the determinant represents the product of the variances of the variables minus the product of the covariances of the variables. Multiplying the elements of a matrix by the reciprocal of the determinant serves to invert (i.e., reverse the order of) the matrix. The determinant of a matrix is zero if it includes variables that are linearly dependent upon each other; a condition known as *singularity*. In such a situation the matrix cannot be inverted, thereby preventing the application of most multivariate statistical procedures to date.

DIASTOLE   The period in the heart cycle, especially of the ventricles, during which the muscle fibers lengthen, the heart dilates, and the cavities fill with blood. It coincides with the interval between the second (S2) and first (S1) heart sounds and represents the period of muscle relaxation that alternates with *systole*.

DIASTOLIC PRESSURE   The point of least pressure in the arterial vascular system occurring late in ventricular diastole.

DICROTIC NOTCH   A small oscillation on the falling phase of the arterial pulse wave. It is due to vibrations generated by closure of the aortic valve.

DIELECTRIC   An insulating (i.e., nonconducting) medium.

DIELECTRIC BREAKDOWN   Any change in the properties of dielectric that causes it to become conductive. Normally a catastrophic failure because of excessive voltage.

DIELECTRIC CONSTANT   Also known as *permittivity*. It is the property of a dielectric that determines the amount of electrostatic energy that can be stored by the material when a given voltage is applied to it. Specifically, it is the ratio of the capacitance of a capacitor using the dielectric to the capacitance of an identical capacitor using a vacuum as a dielectric.

DIGITAL   Refers to the process whereby continuous information is transformed into an ordered sequence of numbers that are typically represented by discrete (usually binary) characters. Contrast *Analog*.

DILATION   The act of stretching the lumen of a hollow structure beyond normal dimensions, e.g., the enlargement of a blood vessel.

DIPOLE   A source of electrical potential whose length is small relative to the extent of the medium in which it is enclosed and whose poles are of equal magnitude but of opposite polarity. An *alternating dipole* is one in which these polarities are constantly reversing. When such a dipole is embedded in a conducting medium, it causes an alternating current to flow in it.

DIRECTIONAL FRACTIONATION   A psychophysiological term that refers to the phenomenon where different components of a bodily response pattern (e.g., heart rate and electrodermal activity) respond in opposite directions to the same stimulus.

DISCRIMINANT ANALYSIS   A class of statistical methods used to address empirical problems of classification. By specifying the number of possible groups or populations and assuming that each individual is a member of one such group, the major problem remaining is to correctly assign each individual to the correct population with a minimum of error. This is done on the basis of multiple measurements on each individual whose origin is unknown and a prior set of similar measurements on individuals whose origin is known. A *discriminant function* is a linear weighting of the values of each measurement that maximizes the correct classification and minimizes the incorrect classification of individuals of known origin.

DISINHIBITION   The temporary removal or reduction of background inhibition as a result of introducing an outside or irrelevant stimulus. It is functionally equivalent to a direct excitation.

DISTAL   A general term defined simply as farther from any point of reference. In control theory, this term refers to variables or processes that can be conceptualized as regulated endpoints. For example, blood pressure is a function of heart rate, stroke volume, and regional blood flow in each vascular bed. Thus, blood pressure is distal to heart rate, stroke volume, and regional blood flow. In electromyography, the term usually refers to the point of insertion of a muscle. Compare *Proximal*.

DISTORTION   An undesired change in wave form as the signal passes through a device.

DOPPLER EFFECT   A physical phenomenon, first predicted by Christopher Doppler in 1842, where the frequencies of received waves are dependent on the motion of the source or observer relative to the propagating medium. As a result, the observed frequencies increase or decrease according to the speed at which the distance between the point of observation and the source is decreasing or increasing. This phenomenon is exploited in recent technological advances in the measurement of blood flow. For example, the pulsed Doppler flowmeter is a device used to measure relative changes in the rate of blood flow through vascular beds by comparing the frequency characteristics of emitted and received high-frequency signals.

DORSAL SPINOCEREBELLAR TRACT   The main neural pathway for conveying proprioceptive information through the spinal cord to the cerebellum.

EARTH   A British term for a zero-reference ground.

ECCRINE/EXOCRINE SWEAT GLAND   One of two types of sweat glands. These particular glands are distributed throughout the surface of the body but with maximum density on the palms of hands and soles of feet and assume major importance in electrodermal measurement as the presumed proximal mechanism of action. The sweat produced by these glands is clear with a faint characteristic odor and contains water, sodium chloride, and traces of albumin, urea, and other compounds. Its composition varies as a function of both organismic and environmental factors such as fluid intake, external temperature, humidity, and hormonal activity. Compare *Apocrine*.

ECHOCARDIOGRAPHY The use of ultrasound techniques to record the size, motion, and composition of various cardiac structures. Also known as *ultrasonic cardiography*.

EDEMA An abnormal accumulation of watery fluid in connective tissue or in a cavity remaining after coagulation.

EEG FREQUENCY BANDS Conventionally divided into alpha (8–12 Hz), beta (13–30 Hz), delta (0.5–3.5 Hz), spindling activity (12–14 Hz), and theta (4–7.5 Hz); also gamma, kappa, and lambda waves and K complexes.

EFFERENT Centrifugal; conveying away from a center. The term is typically used to refer to motor nerve fibers.

EFFICIENCY Ratio of output power to input power, expressed as a percentage, generally measured at full load and nominal levels. The higher the efficiency, the less the amount of energy that is dissipated as heat.

EIGENVALUES Also known as *latent roots* or *characteristic roots*. In multivariate statistical procedures such as factor analysis, MANOVA, discriminant analysis, and canonical correlation analysis, the variables being analyzed are given weights that permit the computation of new variables (e.g., factors, discriminant functions) to meet some criterion. For example, in MANOVA and discriminant analysis, these new variates are formed so as to maximize the differences between groups in terms of average scores on these new variates. These new variates are referred to as *eigenvectors*. In this context, the eigenvalue represents the sum of the squared weights assigned to variables on the eigenvectors. Consequently, the size of the eigenvalue is proportional to the variation in the dependent measures accounted for by the eigenvector (i.e., $\%V_{ev} = ev/m$, where $\%V_{ev}$ is the percentage of variance accounted for in the set of dependent measures by the eigenvector, ev is the eigenvalue, and m is the number of dependent measures). In more formal terms, an eigenvalue is the value λ of a square matrix $\mathbf{A}$ such that $|\mathbf{A} - \lambda \mathbf{I}| = 0$, where $\mathbf{I}$ is the identity matrix. For a $p \times p$ matrix there are, in general, p such roots or values. The corresponding row vectors $\mathbf{u}$ or column vectors $\mathbf{v}$ for which $\mathbf{uA} = \lambda \mathbf{u}$ or $\mathbf{Av} = \lambda \mathbf{v}$ are called eigenvectors.

ELASTOMER Any material that will return to its original dimensions after being stretched or distorted.

ELECTROCARDIOGRAM/ELECTROCARDIOGRAPHY (EKG, ECG) A continuous record of the variations in electrical potential generated by the contraction of the myocardium and detected at the body surface.

ELECTRODE A term introduced by the English physicist Michael Faraday (1791–1867) from the Greek words meaning "route of the electricity." It refers to any probe that allows the passage of electrical activity and may be used for either recording or stimulation. In psychophysiology, it typically refers to a device/medium (e.g., a cup, disk, needle, or pad) used in the transmission of electrical activity from a biological source to amplification and display instruments.

ELECTRODERMAL ACTIVITY (EDA) The general term for the electrical activity of the skin which supersedes the terms *galvanic skin response* (GSR) and *psychogalva-*

nic skin response (PGR). It typically refers to variations in skin conductance but can also refer to variations in skin potential as well.

ELECTRODES, BIPOLAR   Electrodes placed over two electrically active sites.

ELECTRODES, REVERSIBLE   Electrodes consisting of a metal in contact with a solution containing its own ions.

ELECTRODES, SILVER–SILVER CHLORIDE (Ag/AgCl)   The most commonly used reversible electrode currently in use by psychophysiologists. The contact surface of these electrodes is an amalgam of pure silver and silver chloride, which results in a very stable and relatively bias-free electrode that is suitable for both AC and DC recording. Most commercially available electrodes are manufactured using a sintermetallic process, whereas custom-made electrodes are typically manufactured in individual laboratories using an electrolytic process.

ELECTRODES, 10–20 SYSTEM   A standardized guide to locating EEG electrodes on the scalp, based upon measurements from nasion to inion and from right to left preauricular depressions. This system is designed to ensure equivalent interelectrode spacings proportional to skull/brain size along any anteroposterior or transverse line.

ELECTROENCEPHALOGRAM/ELECTROENCEPHALOGRAPHY (EEG)   A continuous record of the electrical potentials recorded from the surface of the brain or scalp that are generated by activity in the brain.

ELECTROGASTROGRAM/ELECTROGASTROGRAPHY (EGG)   A continuous record of gastric myoelectric activity recorded with cutaneous electrodes.

ELECTROLYTE(S)   In physics and chemistry, any element capable of existing in ionized form, principally sodium, potassium, chloride, and calcium. It may also refer to any substance (usually a salt, acid, or base) that in solution dissociates wholly or partly into electrically charged particles known as ions. In psychophysiology, the term is commonly used to denote the solution itself, which has a higher electrical conductivity than the pure solvent.

ELECTROLYTE MEDIUM   A substance used to make an electrolyte viscous, or pastelike.

ELECTROMAGNET   Any device that exhibits magnetism only while an electric current flows through it.

ELECTROMAGNETIC   Referring to the combined electric and magnetic fields caused by electron motion through conductors.

ELECTROMAGNETIC COUPLING   The transfer of energy by means of a varying magnetic field. Also known as *inductive coupling*.

ELECTROMYOGRAM/ELECTROMYOGRAPHY (EMG)   A continuous record of the intrinsic electrical activity associated with muscle contraction by means of surface or needle electrodes.

ELECTROMECHANICAL SYSTOLE (EMS)   The period of time encompassing all electrical and mechanical events associated with the systolic phase of the cardiac cycle.

ELECTROSTATIC   Pertaining to static electricity, or electricity at rest.

ELECTROSTATIC COUPLING   The transfer of energy by means of a varying electrostatic field. Also known as *capacitive coupling*.

ELECTROSTATIC POTENTIALS   Nonphysiological electrical potentials induced in a subject by such things as friction. This source of electrical noise is greatly reduced through the use of appropriate grounding techniques.

END DIASTOLIC VOLUME (EDV)   The quantity of blood remaining in each ventricle at the end of diastole. It is usually about 120–130 ml, but sometimes reaches 200–250 ml in the normal heart.

ENDOCRINE SYSTEM   The system of glands and other structures that manufacture chemical substances that have a regulatory effect on particular target structures and glands. These substances (hormones) are released directly into the circulatory system and have both direct and indirect influences on metabolism and other physiological processes.

ENDORPHIN   A class of endogenous brain polypeptides that bind to opiate receptors in various areas of the brain and thereby have analgesic effects. These polypeptides occur naturally in various forms, including α-, β-, and γ-endorphins (β-endorphin being the most potent) and the enkephalins.

ENDOSOMATIC   A general term that refers to the measurement of electrodermal activity by recording intrinsic changes in potential between two points on the skin surface. Normally, one of these points is designated the *active site* and the other the *reference site*. These designations are not arbitrary and have implications for their location and preparation. The active site is typically located on a palmar or plantar surface (anatomical sites that have a high concentration of eccrine sweat glands) and is cleaned with a mild detergent. The reference site is located on a nearby nonpalmar or nonplantar surface (e.g., the forearm) and is vigorously abraded to provide a high conductance–low resistance path to the interior of the body. See *Skin potential*. Contrast *Exosomatic*.

END SYSTOLIC VOLUME (ESV)   The quantity of blood remaining in each ventricle at the end of *systole*. It is usually about 50–60 ml, but it can sometimes be as little as 10–20 ml in the normal heart.

ENERGY   The ability or capacity to operate or do work. This is a broadening of the traditional definition in terms of Newtonian mechanics where energy was simply defined as a property of moving masses.

ENERGY DISSIPATION   Loss of energy from a system due to the conversion of work into undesirable forms. An example of this is the heat loss due to friction in a mechanical system.

ENTERIC NERVOUS SYSTEM (ENS)   A collection of nerve cell bodies organized into seven discrete plexi located between the circular and longitudinal muscle layers of the stomach. It has been estimated that there are as many neurons in the ENS as there are in the entire spinal cord.

EPIDERMIS   The outermost and nonvascular layer of the skin, varying in thickness from 0.07 to 0.12 mm, except on the palms and soles, where it may be 0.8 and 1.4

mm, respectively. On the palmar and plantar surfaces, it exhibits maximal cellular differentiation and layering and is comprised of five distinct layers. The electrical properties of these distinct cellular layers constitute the proximal basis of the electrodermal response.

EPINEPHRINE   A hormone, $C_9H_{13}NO_3$, secreted by the adrenal medulla in response to splanchnic stimulation as well as in response to hypoglycemia. It is a potent stimulator of the sympathetic nervous system (adrenergic receptors) and a powerful vasopressor, increasing blood pressure, accelerating heart rate, and increasing cardiac output. Also known as adrenalin.

EPSILON CORRECTION   Refers to a set of statistical techniques used in the analysis of variance (ANOVA) when repeated observations from the same subject have been obtained. This situation typically gives rise to unequal variance–covariance matrices that may violate the *compound-symmetry* and *homogeneity-of-treatment-deviation* assumptions underlying the ANOVA. These techniques provide a correction factor (i.e., *epsilon*) for the number of degrees of freedom associated with significance testing of the repeated-measures factors.

ERYTHROCYTES   Nonnucleated red blood cells responsible for oxygen/carbon dioxide transport.

EVENT-RELATED POTENTIALS (ERPS)   Changes in electrical activity most frequently recorded from the surface of the scalp and occurring in response to discrete stimuli. Topographical features of the ERP are typically referred to as *components* whose classification most commonly involves the identification of *peaks* in the waveform. These peaks have been classified: (1) according to sequence and polarity, (2) according to polarity and peak latency, and (3) through Principal Component Analysis. A common functional classification further defines components based on their relationship to external stimuli. These are *exogenous, endogenous*, and *mesogenous* responses, referring to either an entire ERP or components thereof which are a function of physical characteristics of external stimuli, psychological demands of a situation, or a combination of the two, respectively.

EXCITATORY POSTSYNAPTIC POTENTIAL (EPSP)   The membrane potential developed by the partial depolarization of neural cell bodies and dendrites resulting from the release of an excitatory transmitter substance from the presynaptic axon terminals.

EXCITATORY SYNAPSES   Synapses in which the neurotransmitter normally acts to depolarize the postsynaptic membrane and so excite the postsynaptic cell body.

EXOSOMATIC   A general term that refers to the measurement of electrodermal activity by recording changes in resistance/conductance between two points on the skin surface by applying either a constant current or a constant voltage. Normally, both of these points are designated active sites. Both sites are typically located on the palmar or plantar surface (anatomical sites that have a high concentration of eccrine sweat glands) and are prepared by cleaning the skin with a mild detergent. See *Skin conductance* and *Skin resistance*. Contrast *Endosomatic*.

EXTRAFUSAL FIBERS   Pertaining to the striated muscle fibers outside of the muscle spindle.

FACIAL-FEEDBACK HYPOTHESIS Part of a theory of the functional significance of facial expressions in the generation of emotion that derives from the work of Charles Darwin. In its most general form, this hypothesis states that sensory feedback due to the activation of the facial musculature in particular temporal and spatial patterns modulates the physiological, phenomenological, and behavioral components of emotional states.

FARAD A unit of capacitance. In DC circuits, it is defined as the capacity of a condensor which, charged with one coulomb, provides a difference potential of one volt. In AC circuits, one farad is defined as the capacitance value that will permit one ampere of current to flow when the voltage across the capacitor changes at a rate of one volt per second. This unit is so large that the microfarad (10^{-6} F) is typically adopted as the practical unit.

FAST FOURIER TRANSFORM A digital signal-processing that dramatically reduces the amount of time required to perform a Fourier transform on a set of data. The data length must be 2^N, where N is a positive integer, for maximum efficiency. The speed advantage for the Fast Fourier Transform when this condition is met is roughly 30:1.

FEEDBACK Energy that is extracted from a later point in a system and applied to an earlier point. Positive feedback reduces the stability of a device and is used to increase the sensitivity or produce oscillation in a system. Negative feedback, also known as *inverse feedback*, increases the stability of a system and is used to maintain constant relationships between a system's output and its environment.

FIGURE OF MERIT Any number or function that expresses quantitatively the performance of a measuring device.

FILTER(S) A device or material for suppressing or minimizing waves or oscillations of certain frequencies (as of electricity, light, or sound). The functional classification of filters includes: (1) *bandpass*, ability to pass a specific range of frequencies; (2) *band reject*, ability to reject a specific range of frequencies; (3) *high pass*, ability to pass only high frequencies (also known as a *low-frequency cutoff*); (4) *low pass*, ability to pass only low frequencies (also known as a *high-frequency cutoff*); (5) *single frequency*, ability to pass only a single frequency, and (6) *notch*, ability to pass all but a single frequency.

FLOATING Referring to a circuit that has no connection to ground.

FLUX The flow of physical entities, e.g., the flow of charge or radiation across a given area. The term *incident flux* refers to the flow of energy from a source of electromagnetic radiation. Radiant flux and radiant power are synonymous terms in radiometric measurement where the energy unit is watts. The term *steady-state flux* refers to the constant average value of radiant flux over the time interval of interest. In electroencephalography, this term refers to a conceptualization of electrical brain activity as a mixture of frequencies, each having a specified amplitude, center frequency, and phase delay with reference to an epoch of time bounded by specific reference points.

FOLDING FREQUENCY The principal folding frequency is equal to half the sampling rate, but other folding frequencies appear at the zero-frequency axis and at all multiples of the principal folding frequency. The term suggests a useful visual metaphor for the effect of *aliasing* as a "folding" of the frequency spectrum of a waveform about the folding frequency. For example, sampling a 300-Hz sine wave at a sampling rate of 500 Hz will produce a single fold and an alias frequency of 200 Hz. Sampling a 600-Hz sine wave at the same rate will produce a double fold and an alias frequency of 100 Hz. See *Nyquist frequency*.

FOREARM VASCULAR RESISTANCE (FVR)   A measure of flow resistance in the forearm obtained by dividing blood pressure by the forearm blood flow (FVR = BP/FBF). By knowing the FVR, it is possible to determine whether observed changes in FBF are due to active or passive vasoconstriction/vasodilation.

FOURIER ANALYSIS   The theory of representing functions of a variable t as the sum of a series of sine and cosine terms of types $a_j \cos(2\pi_j/\lambda_j)$, where $j = 0, 1, \ldots$.

FREQUENCY   The number of times a periodic action occurs in a unit of time; typically expressed in hertz.

FREQUENCY DOMAIN   When waveforms are analyzed in terms of their spectra, the analysis is said to be in the frequency domain. Compare *Time domain*.

FREQUENCY MODULATION   A process in which the information in an original signal is encoded as frequency changes in a second signal.

FREQUENCY RANGE/RESPONSE   The band of frequencies from the highest to the lowest frequency that a device is capable of processing without distortion. All physical devices, both natural and artificial, have limits to the range of frequencies to which they can respond; for instance, the frequency range of audible signals for humans is between 20 and 20,000 Hz.

FREQUENCY/SPECTRAL ANALYSIS   In general, the process of decomposing a signal into its periodic components. The result is that the original signal in which amplitude is expressed as a function of time is converted into an amplitude spectrum, a graph of amplitude as a function of frequency. The term *Fourier series analysis* refers to the analysis of signals that repeat themselves exactly at regular intervals. Periodic signals of this type can be uniquely expressed as the sum of a series of sine waves whose frequencies are harmonically related to the repetition frequency of the signal. The components have amplitudes and phases determined by the signal pattern. The term *Fourier integral analysis* refers to a mathematical technique for describing nonperiodic transients that recur with the same size and shape. These signals cannot be represented by a harmonically related series of components, but they can be uniquely expressed as a continuous function of frequency. *Frequency analysis* can also be applied to signals that are basically rhythmical but never recur exactly, signals that characterize the bulk of the empirical bioelectrical signals investigated in psychophysiology. These signals are known as random or stochastic signals. Because the aperiodic nature of these signals violates fundamental assumptions of *Fourier analysis*, various transformations are performed on the original signal (e.g., detrending and smoothing) prior to performing the actual analysis.

GAIN   The amount of signal amplification. It is usually expressed in decibels and thus denotes the relative strength of a given signal.

GALVANIC SKIN RESPONSE (GSR)   A general term, now superseded by *electro-*

dermal activity (EDA), that denotes both *exosomatically* and *endosomatically* measured electrical properties of the skin. Synonomous with *Psychogalvanic response (PGR)*.

GAMA-AMINOBUTYRIC ACID (GABA) An amino acid that functions as the primary inhibitory neurotransmitter in many neural systems within the brain.

GAMA-MOTONEURONS The small motoneurons that innervate intrafusal muscle fibers (i.e., the muscle spindles).

GANGLION In general, any knotlike mass. In anatomy and physiology, it is a general term for a small group of nerve cell bodies and fibers located outside of the central nervous system. Occasionally this term is applied to certain nuclear groups within the brain or brainstem, e.g., the basal ganglia.

GASTRIC MYOELECTRIC ACTIVITY Electrical activity of the gastric musculature, including both slow periodic waves and spike potentials.

GASTRIC PLATEAU POTENTIALS A cluster of spike potentials superimposed on the plateau of a slow-wave potential that precedes contraction of the intrinsic musculature of the stomach.

GASTRIC SLOW WAVES The omnipresent 3-cpm waxing and waning of electrical potentials originating in the intrinsic musculature of the stomach. These particular waveforms are also referred to in the literature as electrical control activity, gastric pacesetter potentials, and basic electrical rhythm.

GASTRIC SPIKE POTENTIALS The punctate electrical event responsible for the contraction of the intrinsic circular muscle of the stomach. The occurrence of these spikes is not necessarily time locked to any particular phase of the gastric slow waves.

GLIA/GLIAL CELLS Nonneuronal specialized supporting cells within the central nervous system that perform a multitude of ancillary functions.

GLUCOSE The end product of carbohydrate metabolism and the principal source of energy for the living organism. It is found in certain foods, especially fruit, as well as in the normal blood of all organisms. Also known as dextrose.

GROUND A highly conductive pathway to the earth. Also, a common return to a point of zero potential such as the metal chassis in electronic equipment. See *Earth*.

GROUND LOOPS Alternative paths through which current can flow between system components and either a 0 V reference or the zero potential of the earth. This creates an undesirable condition because interference in the signal path(s) can be generated by ground currents when mutliple grounds are connected at more than one point.

GROUND POTENTIAL Strictly speaking, the zero potential of the earth. However, a circuit, terminal, or chassis is said to be at ground potential when it is used as a reference point for other potentials in the system.

HABITUATION The relatively permanent decrement in a response as a result of repeated stimulation that is not contingent upon reinforcement. This decrement is specific to the stimulus and is distinct from simple fatigue or sensory adaptation. See *Adaptation*.

HEART PERIOD (HP)   Also known as the *interbeat interval*. The term refers to the time between successive QRS complexes of the cardiac cycle.

HEART RATE (HR)   The reciprocal transformation of the interbeat interval (i.e., heart period), typically expressed in units of beats per minute (bpm).

HENRY (H)   A unit of inductance. An inductance of one Henry will induce a counter-electromotive force of one volt when the current is changing at the rate of one ampere per second.

HERTZ (HZ)   A unit of frequency equal to one cycle per second.

HIGH-IMPEDANCE STATE   A state in which the output of a device is effectively isolated from the circuit.

HOMEOSTASIS   A tendency to stability in the normal internal environment of an organism. This stability is achieved by a system of control mechanisms activated by negative feedback. This concept was first clearly articulated in the mid-1800s by the physician Claude Bernard and was known then as the constancy of the *Milieu interior*. The term *homeostasis* was coined by Walter B. Cannon in his seminal article entitled "Organization for Physiological Homeostasis" in 1929. For example, Cannon explained the regulation of body temperature by the mechanisms such as perspiring when the body is too hot and shivering when it is too cold as maintaining the body's equilibrium by signals based on the discrepancy between the desired state and the actual state fed back to mechanisms for minimizing this discrepancy.

HORMONE   A chemical substance produced in the body by an organ that has a specific regulatory effect on the activity of a target organ.

HYDROSTATIC PRESSURE   Pressure arising from the gravitational pull on a liquid at a certain position in space.

HYPERGLYCEMIA   Excess glucose in the blood.

HYPERTENSION   Persistently high arterial blood pressure. Criteria ranging from 140 mm Hg systolic and 90 mm Hg diastolic to as high as 200 mm Hg systolic and 110 mm Hg diastolic have been suggested. Hypertension may have no known cause (*essential*, or *idiopathic*, *hypertension*) or be associated with other primary diseases (*secondary hypertension*).

HYPOTENSION   Abnormally low blood pressure. *Orthostatic postural hypotension* refers to a fall in blood pressure associated with dizziness, cerebral ischemia, and blurred vision occurring upon standing or when standing motionless in a fixed position. It can be acquired or idiopathic, transient or chronic, and occur alone or secondary to a disorder of the central nervous system. *Vascular hypotension* refers to a condition of severe hypotension resulting from dilation of the blood vessels.

HYPOTHALAMUS   A well-defined small group of cell bodies in the thalamus near the base of the cerebrum that are generally involved in homeostatic regulation of visceral functions such as control of body temperature as well as in the neural control of emotional expression.

HYPOTHENAR EMINENCE   The pad of flesh on the palm directly below the base of the little finger. In psychophysiological applications this area is often used as an electrode site in the measurement of electrodermal activity. Compare *Thenar eminence.*

HYSTERESIS   In general, the phenomenon exhibited by a system whose state depends on its previous history. In physics, the term usually refers to a retardation of the effect when changing forces are applied to a body (as if from viscosity or internal friction).

IMPEDANCE (Z)   The generic term for the property of any component of a system that suppresses or opposes current flow. It includes both simple resistance and reactance and is expressed in ohms.

IMPEDANCE, HIGH   Generally, the area of 25,000 Ω or higher.

IMPEDANCE, LOW   Generally, the area of 1–600 Ω.

IMPEDANCE CARDIOGRAPHY   A technique used for estimating cardiac output and other cardiodynamic parameters based on the measurement of changes in thoracic impedance during the heartbeat.

IMPEDANCE MATCH   A situation where the impedance of a system component is the same as the impedance of the system, cable, or device to which it is connected.

INDUCTANCE (L)   A property of an electric circuit by which an electromotive force is induced by a variation of current either in the circuit itself or in a neighboring circuit. It is expressed in Henrys.

INFLECTION   The point or points at which the tangent of a curve changes direction, e.g., positive to zero or negative to positive.

INHIBITORY POSTSYNAPTIC POTENTIALS (IPSPs)   The membrane potential developed by the partial hyperpolarization of neural cell bodies and dendrites resulting from the release of an inhibitory transmitter substance from the presynaptic axon terminals.

INPUT RESISTANCE (or IMPEDANCE)   The resistance that a measuring device (e.g., an amplifier) presents to the measured input potential.

INSULATOR   A material with good dielectric properties that is used to isolate closely spaced electrical components such as cable conductors and integrated circuits.

INTAKE-REJECTION HYPOTHESIS   Part of a theory associated with the Laceys and their associates regarding the cognitive significance of cardiovascular changes. According to this hypothesis, cardiovascular changes are seen as primarily facilitating or inhibiting the processing of information. Contrast with *Cardiac-somatic hypothesis.*

INTERDIGESTIVE COMPLEX   A specific form of gastric contractile activity during a fast that occurs in the following sequence: (1) quiescence (Phase I), (2) irregular contractions (Phase II), and (3) intense contractions (Phase III).

INTERFERENCE   Unwanted signals or random noise entering a signal path.

INTERNEURON/INTERNUNCIAL   In general, any excitatory or inhibitory nerve cell within the central nervous system that usually has a narrow range of primary influence. However, the use of these terms is typically restricted to any excitatory or inhibitory nerve cell that functions as the interface between sensory and motoneurons within the spinal cord.

INTRACELLULAR BODY FLUIDS   Fluids compartmentalized within body cells.

INVARIANT   A term recently proposed by Cacioppo and Tassinary (see chapter 1) to refer to a particular class of psychophysiological relationships. More specifically, the term refers to any one-to-one, context-free relationship between particular psychological and physiological events or constructs.

IONIZATION   The formation of ions. Ions are produced when polar compounds are dissolved in a solvent and when a liquid, gas, or solid is caused to lose or gain electrons due to the passage of an electric current.

IONIZATION VOLTAGE   The potential at which the atoms in a relatively stable material give up electrons.

ISOLATION   The ability of a circuit or component to reject interference, usually expressed in decibels.

ISOTONIC   In general, any physiological solution that has the same osmotic pressure as normal extracellular bodily fluids. In electromyography, the term refers specifically to any muscle contraction in which the muscle shortens, as in flexing the arm, but the force exerted remains relatively unchanged throughout the shortening.

ISOVOLUMIC CONTRACTION PERIOD   The interval between closure of the mitral valve and opening of the aortic valve. During this interval, no change in ventricular volume occurs. The rate of rise of ventricular pressure (i.e. dP/dT) is maximum during this period.

ISOVOLUMIC RELAXATION PERIOD   The interval between closing of the semilunar valves and the opening of the atrioventricular valves. During this interval, ventricular pressure falls rapidly while ventricular volume remains constant.

KLUVER–BUCY SYNDROME   A neuropsychological disorder following extensive bilateral damage to both the temporal lobes and many limbic structures. It is characterized by visual agnosia, excessive attentiveness to visual stimuli, a tendency to examine objects orally, a general depression of drive and emotional reactions, and a lack of sexual inhibitions.

KOROTKOFF-SOUNDS (K-SOUNDS)   Distinct sounds that can be heard through a stethoscope placed distally to a deflating occlusion cuff that are used in the measurement of blood pressure. The sounds vary in quality as the pattern of blood flow under the cuff changes and criterial acoustic characteristics of the systolic and diastolic pressure can be identified.

LATENCY   In general, the state of seeming inactivity occurring between the instant of stimulation and the beginning of a response. *Onset latency* refers to the time from the onset of a stimulus to the beginning of a detectable change in ongoing activity. *Peak latency* refers to the time from the onset of a stimulus to the maximum amplitude of a phasic response. A *latency window* refers to a defined temporal epoch into which latency values normally fall so that apparent responses having latency values outside this window may be considered to be "outliers" or "nonspecific" responses.

LAW OF INITIAL VALUES (LIV)   As originally proposed by Wilder, the LIV states that the magnitude of a physiological response to a stimulus is negatively correlated with its immediate prestimulus level. The "law" is actually slightly more complicated than the previous statement implies since if the prestimulus level is sufficiently high, the response either may not occur or a paradoxical reversal of responses may be observed. The expression of this law is highly context specific, being dependent not only on the response system observed but also on the immediate physiological and psychosocial environment.

LEFT-VENTRICULAR EJECTION TIME (LVET)   The period of time during which the blood is being ejected from the ventricles into the circulatory system. This time period can be determined as the difference between the opening and closing of the semilunar valves. Because of the difficulty in determining the precise timing of the opening of the semilunar valves, LVET is often calculated as the time difference between the dicrotic notch and the foot of the upstroke of a peripherally recorded pulse wave.

LEVEL   A measure of the difference between a quantity or value and an established reference. In psychophysiology, it is sometimes used in conjunction with the term tonic, as in tonic level. See *Tonic.*

LIGHT-EMITTING DIODE (LED)   Semiconductor device that produces light when an electrical current is passed through it. As light sources, this class of diodes is characterized as inefficient (i.e., they will produce only small quantities of light relative to the amount of input current), yet the light intensity they do produce is roughly proportional to the input current. In addition, they are capable of being reliably switched at high speeds, and their light output is restricted to well-defined narrow bandwidths.

LOAD   A device that consumes or converts the power delivered by another device.

LOSS   The portion of energy applied to a system that is dissipated and performs no useful work.

LUMEN   The cavity or channel within a tubular structure such as an artery. In physics, it also refers to the standard unit of luminous flux defined as the amount of light emitted in a unit solid angle by a standard candle.

MAGNITUDE   A generic term that refers to a quantity that expresses the value of a waveform at any point along its length. In psychophysiology, the term is used to denote the size of a response (typically the arithmetic mean) calculated over all the occasions when a response might have been given, i.e., over all times when an external stimulus is presented or a particular internal state is inferred. Compare *Amplitude.*

MARKER   A term recently proposed by Cacioppo and Tassinary (see chapter 1) to refer to a particular class of psychophysiological relationships. More specifically, the term refers to any one-to-one, context-bound relationship between psychological and physiological events or constructs.

MERCURY STRAIN GAUGE   A transducer used in plethysmographic measurements that consists of a column of mercury sealed in an elastic tube. Because the resistance of the mercury is a function of the length of the tube, it can be interfaced to special-purpose electronic circuitry (e.g., a Wheatstone bridge) to provide a voltage output proportional to changes in length.

METABOLIC HOMEOSTASIS   The physiological state in which the needs of the body for energy (i.e., oxygen, nutrients, and other vital substances) are appropriately met.

METABOLITE   Any substance resulting from the modification of an original substance due to the physical and chemical processes that sustain life.

MHO   The unit of conductance (and of admittance) most commonly used in psychophysiological work. This term is now superseded by the siemen. Both the mho and the siemen are equal to the reciprocal of a unit resistance (ohm). In psychophysiological applications, conductance is usually expressed in terms of micro-mho or microsiemen.

MICRONEUROGRAPHY   The technique of inserting microelectrodes into peripheral nerve fibers. It is used in psychophysiological research to directly record the activity of efferent sympathetic nerve fibers that innervate muscles and the skin.

MIND–BODY PROBLEM   An important philosophical and scientific problem that concerns three intimately related fundamental questions. First, there is the question of whether a valid distinction can be made between the mind and the brain/body. Second, if such a distinction can be made, there is the question of whether in fact any things exist to which we can apply either term or both terms. Finally, if there are things to which both terms can be applied, there is the question of what the relation is between the mind and the brain/body. Disagreements among and between philosophers and scientists can and do occur on the answers to each of these questions.

MISATTRIBUTION PARADIGM   Experimental social psychological technique in which subjects are led to attribute symptoms to nonveridical causes.

MODE   A method of operation; for example, the binary mode, the interpretive mode, the alphanumeric mode. In statistics, it is defined as the most frequent value in a distribution.

MODULATION   In psychophysiology, the process by which a characteristic of one signal or response varies in accordance with variations in another signal or response. For example, the respiratory sinus arrhythmia (RSA) is a phenomenon where heart rate is modulated by respiratory processes. In engineering terminology the former is known as the *carrier* and the latter as the *information*.

MODULATION RATE   In engineering and computer science, the reciprocal of the measure of the shortest nominal time interval between successive significant instants of the modulated signal. If this measure is expressed in seconds, the modulation rate is expressed in baud.

MODULE   A self-contained unit; generally connected with others to make a complete system.

MOMENT   The product of a quantity and a distance from some significant point connected with that quantity.

MOTOFACIENT   A term applied to the phase of muscular activity during which the contraction of the muscle produces actual movement. The term *nonmotofacient,* in contrast, refers to the phase of muscular activity during which the muscle is contracting without producing any movement.

MOTONEURON/MOTOR NEURON   Relatively large nerve cells or neurons whose axons innervate extrafusal muscle fibers or glands.

MOTOR CORTEX (PRIMARY)   A portion of the cerebral cortex, approximately enclosed by the precentral gyrus, that contains the cells of origin for the pyramidal tract. It was once believed to be the source of all voluntary movements but is now known to be principally involved in the production of simple, circumscribed movements. Also known as the *agranular cortex* and *Brodmann's area 4.*

MOTOR UNIT (MU)   The single smallest controllable muscular unit by the central nervous system. The motor unit consists of a single alpha-motoneuron, its neuromuscular junction, and the muscle fibers it innervates.

MOVING AVERAGE   A method of data smoothing whereby each data point in a series is replaced by a linear combination of adjacent data points and the original data point. It is, in effect, a digital low-pass filter.

MUCOSAL   Pertaining to or composed of membrane that produces free glandular secretions. When used in electrogastrography, the term refers to the innermost muscle layer of the stomach.

MUSCLE SPINDLES   A type of sensory receptor composed of encapsulated specialized filaments of afferent neurons that are wrapped around muscle fibers. Their output is proportional to the contraction of the muscle fibers relative to a dynamically defined reference point. Muscle spindles are part of the kinesthetic system.

MYOCARDIUM   The middle and thickest layer of the heart wall, composed of cardiac muscle.

MYOTONIA   A generic term to describe increased muscular irritability and contractility associated with a decrease in the ability of the muscle(s) to relax. The term was used extensively by Masters and Johnson in their classic description of the human sexual response.

NEGATIVE CHRONOTROPIC EFFECT   In general, a decrease in the rate of a process. In reference to the cardiovascular system, the term refers to a decrease in heart rate (increased interbeat interval or heart period) resulting from either a decrease in the release of norepinephrine (via sympathetic fibers) or an increase in the release of acetylcholine (via parasympathetic fibers) on cells of the sinoatrial node (NA) of the heart.

NEOCORTEX   The most recently developed part of the cerebral cortex composing the cerebral hemispheres.

NERVE FIBER   Any of the processes of a neuron, including axons with their myelin sheaths (when present) and dendrites, that may extend for long distances in tracts or in peripheral nerves.

NEUROMODULATOR   A neuronal release product that fails to meet the defining criteria for a neurotransmitter yet reliably alters the efficacy of other substances (such as actual neurotransmitters) and/or exerts neuronal effects that last orders of magnitude beyond the effects of neurotransmitters (i.e., minutes or days as opposed to milliseconds).

NEUROTRANSMITTER   A substance that is released from the axon terminal of a presynaptic neuron on excitation and that travels across the synaptic cleft to either excite or inhibit the target cell. Also called transmitter substance.

NEURON DOCTRINE/NEURON THEORY   A set of five postulates derived primarily from the work of the great neuroanatomist Santiago Ramon y Cajal in the latter part of the nineteenth century. These are: (1) the nerve cell and its processes (i.e., the neuron) form the cellular units of the nervous system that are directly involved in its function; (2) all nerve fibers are neuronal processes; (3) the neuron and all its extensions develop embryologically from a single neuroblast; (4) the neuron and all its processes are dependent upon the nucleated cell body for their maintenance and regeneration; and (5) the functional unit of cellular communication within the nervous system is the neuron; that is, the nervous system is composed of individual neurons metabolically independent but informationally linked through the chemical synapse.

NOISE   Any unwanted and interfering variation in the size of an observed quantity produced by a process or an aspect of a process that is not of present interest. Such unwanted variations can be due either to a component malfunction that is part of the information path or to an extraneous, external signal that tends to interfere with the variations normally present in or passing through a system. Compare *Signal*.

NOMOGRAM   A chart or diagram on which a number of variables are plotted, forming a computation chart for the solution of complex numerical formulas.

NONSPECIFIC RESPONSES   Changes in physiological activity that may have the appearance of elicited responses but cannot be associated with an identifiable stimulus. Also known as *spontaneous fluctuations*.

NOTCH FILTERING   A type of highly restrictive selective filtering used to reject energy occurring over a very narrow bandwidth (e.g., a single frequency). Notch filtering is most commonly used to reject energy at the powerline frequency and its harmonics.

NYQUIST FREQUENCY   The frequency of a sine or cosine term with a period double the interval t given that data are sampled at equal time intervals t. Also known as the *folding frequency* because frequencies higher than the Nyquist frequencies can be conceptualized as being "folded" back into the range from 0 Hz to the Nyquist frequency. See *Folding frequency*.

NYSTAGMUS   The general term for a large class of eye movements of an oscillatory or unstable nature that includes both smooth and saccadic components. However, it typically refers to a repetitive eye motion comprised of a slow-moving progression followed by a rapid return period. This type of movement may be elicited by a stimulus moving with respect to the head (whether the observer is rotated or the object is moved) or by direct stimulation of the vestibular system.

OFF-LINE, ON-LINE   These terms denote whether data analysis does (on-line) or does not (off-line) proceed in parallel with data acquisition. *On-line analysis* means that data are analyzed as they are recorded. On-line analyses are typically used in biofeedback paradigms requiring immediate reduction of data in order to provide the subject with feedback based on analysis of a last response or last series of responses. *Off-line* analysis means that data are analyzed at some point in time subsequent to recording, but this term is generally used only when the data analysis being described could conceivably have been carried out on-line.

OHM (Ω)   A unit resistance (and impedance). The value of resistance through which a potential difference of one volt will maintain a current of one ampere.

OHM'S LAW   Stated $V = IR$, $I = V/R$, or $R = V/I$, the current I in a circuit is directly proportional to the voltage V and inversely proportional to the resistance R. Named in honor of George Simon Ohm (1787–1854).

OPEN CIRCUIT   A discontinuous circuit unable to conduct current. This term can refer either to a circuit physically broken at one or more points or simply to a no-load condition (e.g., the open-circuit voltage of a power supply).

OPTOELECTRONIC   A term used to describe a device that either emits or detects light when used in an appropriate electronic circuit.

OSCILLOSCOPE   An instrument in which variations in fluctuating electrical quantities are displayed as a visible waveform.

OUTCOME   A term recently proposed by Cacioppo and Tassinary (see chapter 1) to refer to a particular class of psychophysiological relationships. More specifically, the term refers to any many-to-one, context-bound relationship between psychological and physiological events or constructs.

PARALLEL   Pertaining to the concurrent or simultaneous operation of two or more devices or to the concurrent performance of two or more related activities in multiple devices or channels. Contrast *Serial.*

PARALLEL CIRCUIT   A circuit in which the identical voltage is presented to all components and the current divides among the components in proportion to their impedances.

PARASYMPATHETIC NERVOUS SYSTEM (PNS)   The craniosacral portion of the autonomic nervous system that primarily acts in the service of homeostatic functions.

PAROXYSMAL TACHYCARDIA   Sudden attack of excessive heart rate.

PEAK   The maximum value of a waveform during a defined interval.

PEAK-TO-PEAK   A measure of amplitude determined by subtracting the minima from the maxima of a waveform.

PERIOD   The distance between specific amplitude points usually measured off a baseline. More formally, it is the number k that does not change the value of a periodic function f when added to the independent variable: $f(x + k) = f(x)$, especially the smallest such number. The reciprocal of period is frequency.

PERIOD ANALYSIS (EEG)   A graphical display of the number of completed waveforms during an epoch per unit of time. The number of baseline crossings in the EEG is used to determine the periods of each waveform. The *major period* is the time relationship between points of inflection and baseline crossings, the *intermediate period* is derived from the first derivative of the primary EEG signal, and the *minor period* is derived from the second derivative of the primary EEG signal.

PERIPHERAL VENOUS POOL   The relatively large, diffuse pool of blood contained within the venous system of the systemic circulation. The interplay between the peripheral and central venous pools is an important factor in determining venous return.

pH   A standard measure of the acidity or alkalinity of a solution expressed as the logarithm of the reciprocal of the hydrogen ion concentration in moles per liter. The values range from 0 to 14, with those lying below 7.0 [excess hydrogen ions (H^+)] being acidic and those above 7.0 [excess hydroxyl ions (OH^-)] being alkaline.

PHALANGES   The divisions of the fingers (i.e., distal, medial, and proximal). In psychophysiological applications these areas are sometimes used as electrode sites in the measurement of electrodermal activity. See *Hypothenar* and *Thenar eminence*.

PHASE   In general, the relative timing of a signal in relation to another signal; if both signals occur at the same instant, they are referred to as *in phase*; if they occur at different instants, they are referred to as *out of phase*. When measured in degrees, one cycle corresponds to a change of 360°. In some applications, it refers specifically to the location of a position on a waveform of an alternating quality in relation to the start of a cycle.

PHASE SHIFT   The displacement of a waveform in time measured in degrees (or radians) as phase lag or lead. The measurement of phase implies a comparison between two waveforms, with one serving as a reference. The sign given to the phase shift (lag or lead) is determined by which waveform is chosen as the reference. If t is the displacement of a waveform in time and T is the period of the waveform, phase shift $(T°)$ in degrees is calculated as $T° = (t/T) \times 360°$. For example, if a 5 Hz sinusoidal waveform were displaced 0.05 s forward in time relative to a reference waveform, the phase lead would be $(0.05 \text{ s}/0.20 \text{ s}) \times 360° = 90°$.

PHASIC   In psychophysiology, the term *phasic response* usually refers to a short-term change in physiological activity, often following an identifiable stimulus, which can be distinguished against a background, ongoing "tonic level" of activity. The response would typically have a relatively rapid onset and a return to baseline within a period that is characteristic for different response systems. Compare *Tonic*.

PHONOCARDIOGRAPHY   The recording of sounds and murmurs originating in the heart and major structures of the cardiovascular system (e.g., carotid artery).

PHOTOCONDUCTOR   Any device that permits the flow of an electrical current corresponding to varying light input.

PHOTODETECTOR (RECEIVER) Any device that transduces light energy into electrical energy. The silicon photodiode is most commonly used for relatively fast speeds and good sensitivity in the 75–95 nm wavelength region. Avalanche photodiodes combine the detection of optical signals with internal amplification of photocurrent. The internal gain is realized through avalanche multiplication of carriers in the junction region. The advantage to using an avalanche photodiode is its higher signal-to-noise ratio, especially at high transmission rates.

PHOTODIODES Bipolar semiconductor devices in which photic irradiation of the $p-n$ junction liberates electrons from the material of which it is composed and makes them available for conduction.

PHOTOMETER A generic term for devices that measure changes in light falling upon a receptive surface; specifically, any instrument that measures changes in luminous intensity, luminous flux, illuminance, or luminance.

PHOTOMETRY Quantification of physical properties by the study of the incident light absorbance reflectance characteristics of object surfaces.

PHOTOTRANSISTOR A transistor whose switching action is controlled by light shining on it.

PILOCARPIN An alkaloid ($C_{11}H_{16}N_2O_2$) obtained from the leaves of the *Pilocarpus jaborandi* or *P. microphyllus*, which is used as a general stimulant for the parasympathetic nervous system.

PITUITRIN A sterile solution in water of extracts from the posterior pituitary gland of domestic animals that are used for food by humans. The main component of this extract is *vasopression* and is used medically primarily in the treatment of *diabetes insipitus*. Its primary physiological effects include the stimulation of smooth muscle tissue and the reabsorption of water, which result in increases in both blood pressure and urine concentration. Also known as *antidiuretic hormone* or *beta-hypophamine*.

PLASMA CORTISOL The principal adrenal glucocorticoid. It is a steroid hormone having major effects on carbohydrate metabolism, salt and water balance, and inflammation.

PLETHYSMOGRAPHY Any of a number of techniques used to measure changes in the size or volume of some organ or structure (e.g., respiration, penile engorgement, etc.).

PLEXUS A general term for a network of lymphatic vessels, nerves, or veins.

POISEUILLE'S LAW A quantitative function that relates the volume flow of a fluid through a cylindrical tube to the pressure difference between the ends of the tube and to the tube dimensions. It is named in honor of the French physician Jean Louis Marie Poiseuille (1799–1869), who in 1843 was the first to study viscosity in a quantitative manner. Poiseuille was primarily interested in the manner in which blood moved through the narrow blood vessels. The law states that the volume flow in a tube (e.g., a blood vessel) is directly proportional to the pressure drop along the length of the tube and to the fourth power of the radius of the tube and inversely proportional to the length of the tube and to the viscosity of the fluid (e.g., blood).

POLARITY The positive or negative orientation of a signal relative to a reference signal or ground. In physiology and psychophysiology, negative-going signals (gain of electrons) are conventionally displayed as rising and positive-going signals (loss of electrons) are displayed as falling. In physics and engineering, this convention is reversed.

POLARIZATION POTENTAILS   Voltage sources that develop due to the passage of current and arise at the interface between electrode and electrolyte.

POLSTER   A generic anatomical term for a small bulge. In sexual psychophysiology this term refers to a specific anatomical structure that appears in the vascular beds in muscular arteries that are found in the interface between arteries and veins. They increase in number with the aging process and had previously been thought to be part of the physical basis for erection.

POSITIVE CHRONOTROPIC EFFECT   In general, an increase in the rate of a process. In reference to the cardiovascular system, the term refers to an increase in heart rate (decreased heart period) resulting from either an increase in the release of norepinephrine (via sympathetic fibers) or a decrease in the release of acetylcholine (via parasympathetic fibers) on cells of the sinoatrial node (NA) of the heart.

POSITIVE INOTROPIC EFFECT   In general, any increase in the strength of muscular contraction. In reference to the cardiovascular system, the term refers to the increased strength of ventricular contraction due either to an increase in ventricular volume or to an increase in the activity of sympathetic innervation of the ventricular myocardium.

POSTSTIMULUS TIME HISTOGRAM (PSTH)   A frequency plot of responses that are averaged in intervals of time after the presentation of a stimulus.

POTENTIOMETER (POT)   A variable resistor with three terminals, one at each end and one on a slider (wiper), used as an analog control device.

POWER   The amount of work per unit of time. Usually expressed in watts and equal to $I \times R$ in a DC circuit. With a periodic signal, power refers to the electrical energy of a signal spectrum computed by multiplying frequency times amplitude. The terms *intensity* or *magnitude* are sometimes used as synonyms for power.

POWER LOSS   The difference between the total power delivered to a circuit, cable, or device and the power delivered by that device to a load.

PREAMPLIFIER   An electronic circuit that maintains or establishes a low-amplitude signal at a predetermined signal strength prior to that signal being amplified for reproduction through a monitor, speaker, strip-chart recorder, or analog-to-digital converter.

PREINJECTION PERIOD (PEP)   A systolic time interval representing the period of time commencing with the onset of ventricular depolarization (ECG Q-wave) and ending with the opening of the semilunar valves. In practice, PEP is measured as the difference in time between electromechanical systole and left-ventricular ejection time.

PRELOAD   The load to which a muscle is subjected before shortening. As applied to ventricular muscle, preload refers to the blood volume in the ventricular chamber prior to its contraction. See *End diastolic volume.*

PRESSOR RESPONSE Any response that tends to increase blood pressure. For example, the increase in heart rate, ventricular contractility, and subsequently, blood pressure triggered by a decrease in blood pressure. See *Baroreceptor reflex.*

PROPAGATION DELAY The time delay between a signal change at an input and the corresponding change at an output.

PROSTAGLANDINS A family of naturally occurring compounds derived from arachidonic acid having a wide variety of hormonelike actions (regulate blood pressure, control inflammation, etc.) as well as being able to affect the action of certain hormones.

PROXIMAL A general term defined simply as closer to any point of reference. In control theory, this term refers to variables or processes that underlie or determine the state of other variables. For example, cardiac output is a function of heart rate and stroke volume. Thus heart rate and stroke volume are proximal to cardiac output. In electromyography, the term usually refers to the point of origin of a muscle. Compare *Distal.*

PSYCHOGALVANIC RESPONSE (PGR) See *Galvanic skin response.*

PSYCHOPHYSIOLOGY (ΨΦ) The scientific study of social, psychological, and behavioral phenomena as related to and revealed through physiological principles and events. In terms of levels of scientific inquiry, anatomy is concerned with bodily structure, physiology with bodily functions, and psychophysiology with organismic–environmental transactions.

PULMONARY VALVE One of the two semilunar valves of the heart. The pulmonary valve is located at the exit of the right ventricle and opens toward the pulmonary circulation.

PULSE A term used to describe one particular variation in the shape of a waveform. Specifically, a signal that changes abruptly from one value to another and back to the original value in a very short length of time.

PULSE CODE MODULATION A process by which one or more analog signals are converted into binary numbers and recorded as the presence or absence of a pulse representing 1 or 0. This method of communication is characterized by a high-noise immunity.

PULSE-TRANSIT TIME A measure of the time it takes for a pulse wave to travel from heart to a peripheral site (e.g, brachial or radial artery), or alternatively, between two peripheral sites. See *Pulse wave velocity.*

PULSE WAVE VELOCITY (ARTERIAL) The rate of propagation of the pressure pulse through the arterial system. This rate is roughly proportional to the resting dimensions of the vessel and varies inversely with arterial distensibility. By making simplifying assumptions, it has been argued that the measurement of pulse wave velocity can provide a noninvasive estimate of arterial blood pressure with each cardiac cycle. See *Pulse-transit time.*

PULSE WIDTH MODULATION A process by which the logic states to which an analog signal is converted are represented by alteration in pulse width. See *Pulse code modulation.*

PURKINJE SYSTEM   A specialized conduction system composed of immature muscle fibers in the subendocardial tissue of the ventricles of the heart that plays a vital role in coordinating the passage of electrical impulses from the atria to the ventricles. Named in honor of the Bohemian anatomist, physiologist, and microscopist Johannes Evangelista von Purkinje (1787–1869).

PYRAMIDAL TRACT   A term applied to two groups of nerve fibers (corticobulbar and corticospinal) originating primarily in the sensorimotor regions of the cerebral cortex. These fibers descend through the medulla oblongata, with the corticobulbar fibers synapsing at this level with motor nuclei throughout the brain stem. The rest of the fibers continue downward to synapse with interneurons and motoneurons of the spinal cord. Approximately 80 percent of the corticospinal fibers cross at the decussation of the pyramids and then continue to descend in the spinal cord as the *lateral corticospinal tract.* Most of the uncrossed fibers form what is known as the *anterior corticospinal tract.*

QRS COMPLEX   A term that refers to the part of the ECG waveform that represents ventricular depolarization and contraction. It corresponds to the passage of electrical activity originating in the sinoatrial node (NA) through the ventricles.

RAPID EJECTION PHASE   Following the opening of the atrioventricular valves, the expulsion of blood from the ventricles is maximal due to the large pressure difference between the ventricular chamber and the ascending aorta.

REACTANCE (X)   The part of the opposition offered an alternating current that is due to capacitance or inductance or both and that is expressed in ohms. The amount of such opposition varies with the frequency of the current such that the reactance due to capacitance decreases with an increase in frequency and the current flow leads the voltage by 90°, whereas the reactance due to inductance decreases with a decrease in frequency and the current flow lags the voltage by 90°. *Capacitive reactance* X_c is expressed in ohms and has a value $\frac{1}{2}\pi fC$, where f is the frequency in hertz and C is the capacitance in farads. *Inductive reactance* X_l is expressed in ohms and equals $2\pi fL$, where f is the frequency in hertz and L is the inductance in Henrys.

READINESS POTENTIAL (RP)   A slow negative shift of cortical potential occurring just before a self-initiated movement in the absence of any concurrent external stimulus. Also known as the *Bereitschaftspotential.* Compare *Contingent negative variation.*

REBOUND   In psychophysiology, the overshooting of prestimulus levels in a direction opposite to that produced by an intense stimulus. See *Damping.*

RECRUITMENT   In medicine, the term refers to the gradual increase in the amplitude of a reflex when a stimulus of constant intensity is prolonged. In electromyography, the term refers to the increasing number of active motor units or motoneurons as a function of increasing the force of muscle contraction. The most parsimonious explanation of the observed orderly progression in the number of active motor units during muscle contraction is that the recruitment order within a motoneuronal pool progresses from the smallest to largest motoneuron. This is refered to in the literature as the *size principle*. In electrodermal research, this term refers to a particular quantitative parameter extracted from individual skin conductance responses (SCRs). See *Skin conductance*.

RECTIFICATION   A means of obtaining a direct (unidirectional) flow of current either in the positive or negative direction from an alternating source of current relative to a zero reference, i.e., a current flow that traverses a zero point. When current is permitted to flow only during unidirectional half-cycles of the AC source, the process is known as *half-wave rectification*. When, in addition, one half-cycle is inverted so that each half-cycle of the AC wave becomes unidirectional, the process is known as *full-wave rectification*.

REDUCED EJECTION PHASE   An event during the cardiac cycle that immediately follows the rapid ejection phase. It refers specifically to the reduction in the volume of blood ejected from the ventricular chamber once the pressure gradient existing between the ventricle and aorta begins to equalize.

REFERRED PAIN   Pain caused by potential tissue damage at a particular body site but that is perceived as originating from a different site.

REFLEX   A functional unit of behavior that includes five elementary components: receptor, sensory system, interneuron, effector system, and effector. These components are chained together to form a series circuit that has the following stimulus–response characteristics: (1) the response to a punctate stimulus rises to a single peak and fades away, (2) the duration and amplitude of the response is determined solely by the strength of the eliciting stimulus and the properties of the intervening synapses, and (3) feedback from the effectors does not modify the effector system output.

REFRACTORY PERIOD   A brief period of time following stimulation when a system is either completely unresponsive (*absolute refractory period*) or requires a stronger than normal stimulus (*relative refractory period*) to respond. In physiology and psychophysiology, the "system" usually refers to either a neuron or a muscle fiber. In this context, the absolute refractory period is coextensive with the passage of the nervous impulse and lasts only a few tenths of a millisecond, whereas the relative refractory period follows immediately afterward and is much longer, is more variable, and depends primarily upon the condition of the tissue.

RENIN   An enzyme synthesized, stored, and secreted by the kidney that plays a role in the regulation of blood pressure by catalyzing the conversion of angiotensinogen to the pressor substance, angiotensin I. Its secretion is induced by lowered renal blood pressure.

RESISTANCE (R)   The generic term for the property of any component of a system that suppresses or opposes the flow of constant current. The measure of the resistance of a given conductor is the electromotive force required per unit current and is usually expressed in ohms.

RESONANCE   An AC circuit condition in which inductive and capacitive reactances interact to cause a minimum or maximum circuit impedance.

RESPIRATORY SINUS ARRHYTHMIA (RSA)   The cyclical variation in heart rate linked to the inspiratory (HR acceleration) and expiratory (HR deceleration) phase of the respiratory cycle. This cyclic activity may also be observed in blood pressure.

RESPONSE SPECIFICITY   A psychophysiological concept that refers to the relationship between independent variables and response patterns. *Stimulus-response (SR) specificity* refers to the tendency of a stimulus or situation to evoke a relatively invariant pattern of physiological changes. *Individual-response (IR) specificity* refers to the tendency for an individual to exhibit a relatively invariant pattern of physiological responses across a variety of stimuli or situations. Finally, *motivational-response (MR) specificity* refers to a consistent interaction of SR and IR specificity.

RESPONSE STEREOTYPY   See *Response specificity.*

RINGING FREQUENCY   The frequency of the damped oscillation that can be generated when a step function is applied to some mechanical or electrical systems. It can also be considered as a frequency where the proximity to a resonance can create a rise in electrical output in a system that is less than critically damped.

ROOT-MEAN-SQUARE (RMS)   In statistics, the root-mean-square of n numbers x_1, $x_2, \ldots, x_n$, is the square root of the arithmetic mean of their squares: $\mathrm{rms} = \sqrt{\Sigma(x_i^2)/n}$, where i varies $1, \ldots, n$. x_1 may represent the arithmetic difference of the n numbers from any value α. For example, the rms of the deviations of a set of numbers from their mean is known as the *standard deviation,* or *root-mean-square deviation,* of those numbers. In most psychophysiological applications, the value α is set equal to zero.

ROSTRAL   An anatomical term denoting a position more toward the beak (oral or nasal region) than some specified point of reference. In human anatomy, the term may mean superior (relative to the spinal cord) or anterior (relative to the brain).

SACCADES   Quick ($20-70°/s$) eye movements that function to change the locus of fixation, i.e., to shift the gaze between two points in the field of view. Saccadic movement is nearly conjugate, i.e., the direction, amplitude, and latency of each eye's movement are nearly identical. Saccades occur whenever we explore our environment or read and are one of the most common types of eye movements.

SALTATION   The action of leaping, especially: (1) chorea or the dancing that sometimes accompanies it; (2) conduction along myelinated nerves, specifically the manner in which an action potential jumps from one node of Ranvier to the next as it propagates down a myelinated axon; and (3) in genetics, an abrupt variation in a species, a mutuation.

SAMPLING RATE   Any quantity that varies with time must have a value at all times, but measurements of it can only be made at specific points in time. Consequently, such measurements represent only a sample from the infinite number of possible values, and the number of measurements made per unit of time is the sampling rate. The unit of time will typically be seconds, in which case the sampling rate will be expressed in hertz.

SCALE   An ordered series of measurement units expressing degrees of difference within a range of quantities. Examples of different types of scales include *nominal* (units reflect typological differences; e.g., gender); *ordinal* (units reflect only the relative rank order of a series of observations, e.g., dominance); *interval* (units express equal degrees of difference between adjacent quantities, without reference to an absolute zero point; e.g., temperature in degrees centigrade); *ratio* (units express equal differences between adjacent quantities referred to an absolute zero point, e.g., temperature in degrees kelvin); *logarithmic* (units express proportional differences between adjacent quantities referred to an absolute zero point, e.g., sound pressure in decibels).

Schmitt trigger A device for converting an analog input voltage into a two-level digital signal. If the input voltage is above some chosen value, the "upper trigger point," the output is at logic 1. If the input voltage is below a second value, the "lower trigger point," the output is at logic 0. Between the upper and lower trigger points the device exhibits hysteresis and provides a degree of noise immunity.

Scotoma An area of impaired vision within the visual field surrounded by an area of less impaired or normal vision.

Semilunar valve The heart valves located at the exits of the right (pulmonary valve) and left (mitral valve) hearts. These valves open and close passively in response to variations in the pressure gradient existing between the ventricular chamber and the major arteries leading from the heart. The closure of the semilunar valves produces the second heart sound (S2).

Serial Pertaining to the sequential or consecutive occurrence of two or more related activities in a single device or channel. Contrast *Parallel*.

Serosal Pertaining to or composed of a membrane that produces or contains serum. When used in the context of electrogastrography, it refers to the outermost muscle layer of the stomach.

Serum The supernatant, cell-free portion of the blood remaining following coagulation.

Sham feeding Any of several experimental techniques of giving food to organisms in which the food is actually chewed and swallowed but is not allowed to enter the stomach, e.g., by diverting the food to the exterior by an esophageal fistula.

Shield A sheet, screen, or braid of highly conductive material placed around or between electrical components to contain any unwanted radiation and/or keep out any unwanted interference.

Short circuit A conductive path of comparatively low resistance between points on a circuit in parallel to the intended resistive path through the circuit components.

Siemen (S) The unit of conductance (and of admittance) now endorsed by the International System of Units that supersedes the mho; equal to the reciprocal of a unit of resistance (ohm). In psychophysiological applications, conductance is usually expressed in terms of micromho or microsiemen.

Sign A general term for a publicly observable, overt indication of the existence of something. In psychophysiology the term specifically refers to that class of voluntary or involuntary behaviors that indicate that a physiological response has occurred that is potentially detectable both to the affected person and to observers. Contrast *Symptom*.

Signal In information theory, a signal is simply the information about a variable that can be transmitted. In psychophysiology, the term refers to any variation in the amplitude and polarity of an observed quantity produced by a process whose mechanism is under experimental investigation.

SIGNAL DETECTION THEORY (SDT)   A mathematical psychophysical theory of human judgment in which errors are given equal consideration to correct responses in the determination of independent sensitivity (d') and response bias (β) indices. The former index is assumed to be an unbiased indicator of the subject's ability to detect particular stimuli.

SINGLE ENDED   Unbalanced, such as grounding one side of a circuit or transmission line.

SINGLE GENERATOR   A device that produces calibrated signals of known waveform and amplitude. Used for testing instrumentation or for generating a stimulus of known properties.

SIGNAL-TO-NOISE RATIO   The ratio of signal amplitude to noise amplitude. The higher the signal-to-noise ratio (the more signal, the less noise), the better the quality of the resulting representation of the signal.

SINK   A device or ciruit into which current drains. The point toward which negative charges would flow.

SINOATRIAL NODE (NA)   A microscopic collection of atypical cardiac muscle fibers at the superior end of the sulcus terminalis, at the junction of the superior vena cava and the right atrium. The cardic cycle normally takes its origin from this node. Also known as nodus sinuatrialis and the *pacemaker* of the heart.

SINTERING   The thermal treatment of an assembly of particulate material in which a dispersed system or porous body becomes a coherent mass through forming and reinforcing particle contacts and changing particle and pore geometry. This process is performed with the system or body in a partially solid state and is governed intrinsically by thermally activated atomic scale mass transport nearing-to-equilibrium processes.

SKIN ADMITTANCE   Exosomatic electrodermal activity measured as the admittance of the skin to an applied alternating voltage. The use of an alternating voltage allows the measurement to reflect the susceptive as well as simple conductive elements within the skin.

SKIN CONDUCTANCE   Exosomatic electrodermal activity measured as the conductance of the skin to applied constant voltage. In psychophysiology, this is the most common measurement of electrodermal activity (EDA). The resulting waveform is typically decomposed into tonic [skin conductance level (SDL)] and phasic [skin conductance response (SDR) components. Some typical parameters that are extracted from the phasic component include *amplitude, magnitude, half-recovery time* (the time taken for the amplitude value of an SCR to return to half the peak amplitude value), *recovery time constant* (the time taken for the amplitude value of an SCR to return to 36.8 percent of its peak value), *rise time* (the time from the onset of an SCR to its peak amplitude), *recruitment* (microsiemens gained per second during the rise time of an SCR), and *recovery rate* (microsiemens lost per second during the half-recovery time of an SCR). See *Constant-voltage method.*

Skin impedance   Exosomatic electrodermal activity measured as impedance of the skin to an applied alternating current. The use of an alternating current allows the measurement to reflect the reactive as well as simple resistive elements within the skin.

Skin potential   Endosomatically measured electrodermal activity, usually appearing as a tonic level negative at the palm with respect to a neutral reference point. It is primarily a phasic response having one, two, or sometimes three components.

Skin resistance   Exosomatic electrodermal activity measured as resistance of the skin to an applied constant current. See *Constant-current method.*

Smoothing   The effect produced by a low-pass filter, e.g., a moving average.

Smooth movements (of the eyes)   Slow (1–30°/s) sweeping rotations of the eye that serve to maintain fixation on an object moving with respect to the head. They are known as *pursuit movements* if elicited by movement of the object and *compensatory movements* if elicited by head or body movement.

Soma   In general, the body or all cells of the body with the exception of the germ or sex cells. In psychophysiology, the term typically refers specifically to the expanded part of the nerve cell immediately surrounding the nucleus and from which the dendrites and axons originate.

Somatic nervous system   The portion of the peripheral nervous system concerned with the transmission of information to and from the nonvisceral components of the body, such as the skeletal muscles, bones, and skin.

Somnogram   A compressed spectral array used to portray the power or amplitude of the EEG at the various frequencies throughout the sleep cycle.

Source resistance (or impedance)   The resistance inherent in the measurement of a potential. At the skin surface this appears as a constant resistance in series with the source of potential.

Spectrum   Frequencies or radiations that exist in a continuous range and have a common characteristic. A spectrum may be inclusive of many spectrums; e.g., the electromagnetic radiation spectrum includes the light spectrum, radio spectrum, infrared spectrum, etc. Some common examples are *autospectrum* (a spectrum reflecting signal periodicity obtained by correlating different parts of the same curve, which leads to extraction of periodic signals sometimes referred to as autocorrelation analysis); *bispectrum* (the degree of interaction of component waves making up the composite trace; contrast with the cross- and coherence spectra where the comparison is between two simultaneously recorded traces); *coherence spectrum* (the representation of the linear relationship between two time series at various frequencies); *cross-spectrum* (the representation of the in-phase and out-of-phase relationship between two time series at various frequencies; generally not of interest in itself but is used to calculate coherence and phase shifts between time series); and *power spectrum* (the representation of how the variance of a time series varies as a function of frequency). If the power spectrum is represented by a graph, the abscissa represents frequency and the ordinate represents spectral intensity. In addition to the quantitative analysis of brief epochs, the spectra over long time periods can be compressed to highlight changes in spectral components over time. See *Somnogram*.

SPHERICITY   In statistics, a fundamental assumption of univariate approaches to split-plot or repeated-measures analysis of variance that involves particular characteristics of the variances and covariances of the repeated measures. Specifically, sphericity will be present when the response to adjacent trials of conditions are homogeneous, a condition termed the *homogeneity-of-treatment deviations*. This condition should not be confused with a related condition known as *compound symmetry*. This condition refers specifically to a situation where the variances and covariances of the repeated measures are equal.

SPHYGMOMANOMETER   A device for measuring arterial blood pressure consisting of an inflatable bag connected to a pressure monitor (usually a mercury manometer). The bag is enclosed within a nondistensible cuff so that the air pressure (measured by the manometer) compresses the limb. As air is released from the system, changes in the blood flow under the cuff can be detected, and the blood pressure can be read directly from the manometer.

STATIC CHARGE   A stationary electrical charge that is bound to an object.

STATIONARY (STATIONARITY)   A property of a time series when the mean and the variance remain constant with respect to time.

STEP-DOWN TRANSFORMER   An electronic device that can change electric current from one voltage to another. The most common transformer of this type steps down voltage from 220 to 120 V. A step-down transformer does not change the frequency of the current.

STRAIN GAUGE   A device for measuring the mechanical strain in a material resulting from the application of mechanical stress. Often a semiconductor device that when pushed, pulled, bent, or twisted produces an output proportional to the applied stress.

STRATUM CORNEUM   The outer layer of the epidermis composed of nonliving cells. These cells function as a sponge for the retention of water and electrolytes.

STRATUM LUCIDUM   An intrinsic layer of the palmar and plantar epidermis that possibly acts as an active membrane involved in the determination of tonic electrodermal activity.

STRESS   In psychophysiology, this term refers to the sum of the biological reactions to any adverse stimulus that tends to disturb the organism's *homeostasis* as well as to the stimuli that elicit these reactions. In physics, this term is reserved for the stimulus, and the term *strain* refers to the reactions of the system to the applied stress.

STROKE VOLUME   The quantity of blood ejected from a ventricle during each heartbeat.

SUBJECT VARIABLE   A stable attribute of an individual or group of individuals that cannot be manipulated in a particular experimental context (e.g., a personality trait).

SUSCEPTANCE (B)   The imaginary component of admittance that includes both resistance and reactance components. It is expressed in mhos or siemens.

SYMPATHETIC NERVOUS SYSTEM (SNS)   The thoracolumbar portion of the autonomic nervous system that primarily acts in the service of preparing the body for action.

SYMPTOM   A general term referring to any subjective evidence of a person's physical condition. In psychophysiology, the term specifically refers to the conscious awareness of bodily feelings and sensations, often (but not invariably) arising from physiological responses. Contrast *Sign*.

SYMPTOM BELIEFS   A set of subjective expectancies concerning the covariation between particular symptoms and particular physiological reactions.

SYMPTOM SPECIFICITY   A concept introduced by Malmo and his associates in the 1950s to describe the tendency for psychiatric patients with a somatic symptom to display strong responses to stressful stimuli in the physiological systems presumably underlying the reported symptom. This concept is now also used to describe this tendency in nonpsychiatric patients.

SYNAPSE   A specialized structure through which neurons communicate. This communication can be mediated through chemical transmission as well as through direct electrical transmission when there is an especially close apposition of pre- and postsynaptic membranes.

SYNAPTIC CLEFT   The narrow space between the pre- and postsynaptic membranes of a chemical synapse.

SYNCYTIAL   Refers to the nature of the interconnections among the cardiac muscle fibers. Cardiac muscle fibers interconnect with each other to form a latticelike network called a syncytium. Two separate muscle syncytia surround the heart; one wraps around the atria and one wraps around the ventricles. The syncytial nature of cardiac muscle fibers facilitates the spread of cardiac muscle action potentials and thus contributes to the synchronization of heart muscle contraction.

SYSTEMIC FILLING PRESSURE   The mean pressure within the circulatory system as measured from the root of the aorta to the right atrium.

SYSTOLE   That portion of the cardiac cycle in which the heart, especially the ventricles, is contracting (i.e., the myocardial fibers are tightening and shortening). It occurs in the interval between the first (S1) and second (S2) heart sounds during which blood is surging through the aorta and pulmonary artery. It is the period of muscle contraction that alternates with *diastole*.

SYSTOLIC PRESSURE   Maximum blood pressure occurring near the end of the stroke output of the left ventricle of the heart.

SYSTOLIC TIME INTERVALS (STISs)   Based on the temporal aspects of various cardiac events during *systole*, the STIs provide noninvasive measures of several important cardiodynamic parameters. The three major STIs are electromechanical systole (EMS), left-vetricular ejection time (LVET), and the *preejection period (PEP)*.

TACHYCARDIA   Excessively rapid beating of the heart. The term is usually reserved for heart rates of over 100 bpm and may be qualified as atrial, junctional, or ventricular and as *paroxysmal*.

TACHYGASTRIA   Periodic gastric myoelectric activity faster than the normal 3 cpm (i.e., usually 4–9 cpm) that typically occurs in the absence of muscle contractions and is often associated with nausea.

TEMPERATURE COEFFICIENT   A measure of the average change in output voltage for each 1°C change in ambient temperature, expressed as a percentage of rated output.

THENAR EMINENCE   The pad of flesh on the palm at the base of the thumb. In psychophysiological applications this area is often used as an active electrode site in the measurement of electrodermal activity. Compare *Hypothenar eminence*.

THERMISTER   A device whose conductive properties are lawfully altered as a function of temperature.

TIME CONSTANT (TC)   Mathematically, the constant T in the exponential equation $Y = Ae^{-t/T}$. In simple RC circuits it represents the time taken for the voltage or charge in a capacitor to either fall to 36.8% of its initial value or rise to 63.2% of its final value. The time constant T measured in seconds is equal to the product of the resistance R in ohms and the capacitor value C in farads. For time constant T, the equivalent high-pass filter measured in hertz is equal to $\frac{1}{2}\pi T$.

TIME DOMAIN   Systems of analysis that abstract and emphasize a description of time series based on the temporal sequence of the data. No assumptions are made concerning the nature of the underlying process.

TIME SERIES   A set of ordered observations on a quantitative characteristic of an individual or collective phenomenon taken at different points in time. It is common, though not essential, for these points to be equidistant in time.

TONIC   In psychophysiology, a very general term that refers to ongoing physiological activity that may show slow changes. Compare *Phasic*.

TOPOSCOPE   A graphical variation on the conventional display of the EEG that emphasizes the phase relationships between two or more voltage derivations. This kind of display, first developed by J. C. Lilly in the 1940s (called the Bavatron), directly displays the topology and spreading of EEG potentials across time and space and thus presaged modern imaging techniques of the intact functioning brain.

TOTAL PERIPHERAL RESISTANCE   The total resistance presented to the passage of blood as it travels through the small blood vessels, especially the arterioles.

TRACER   See *Marker*.

TRACT/TRACTUS   A collection or bundle of nerve fibers having the same origin, function, and termination or a number of organs, arranged in series, subserving a common function.

TRANSDUCER   A device that functions to convert energy in one form to energy in another form, frequently into electrical signals that vary as a function of variation in input energy. Common applications include microphones, loudspeakers, and strain gauges, all of which transduce changes in applied force into electrical signals that can be measured.

TRANSIENT RECOVERY TIME   The time required for an output parameter to settle to within specified limits after a sudden step change in input. See *Damping*.

TRANSISTOR–TRANSISTOR LOGIC (TTL)   A popular logic circuit family that uses multiple-emitter transistors.

T-WAVE AMPLITUDE   The ECG waveform component representing the repolarization of the ventricles of the heart.

UNIBASE   A proprietary substance used as an electrolyte medium in the measurement of electrodermal activity (EDA).

URTICARIA   A vascular skin reaction characterized by the transient appearance of smooth, slightly elevated reddish patches that often itch severely.

VALSALVA'S MANEUVER   A respiratory exercise in which inspiration is followed by forced expiration against a closed glottis. It is thought to reduce the venous return to the heart, thereby leading to rapid and dramatic changes in both heart rate and blood pressure.

VASCULAR BED   A complex network of small blood vessels including arterioles, capillaries, and venules.

VASOCONSTRICTION   The narrowing of the diameter of blood vessels.

VASODILATION   The expansion of the diameter of blood vessels.

VASOMOTOR TONE   The degree of constriction/dilation of the blood vessels. It is determined by neural (e.g., sympathetic), local, and hormonal influences.

VECTION   The illusory sensation of self-movement.

VENOUS-OCCLUSION PLETHYSMOGRAPHY   A measurement technique in which the rate of arterial inflow into an organ or limb segment is estimated by recording the initial rate of increase in volume when its venous outflow is suddenly occluded. In psychophysiology, this technique is frequency used to measure changes in blood flow to skeletal muscle or the skin during the manipulation of global psychological variables such as mental stress.

VENOUS RETURN   The blood returned to the heart from the great veins.

VERGENCE (OF THE EYES)   A disjunctive movement involving slow (6–15°/s) rotation of the ocular axes in opposite directions to maintain binocular fixation on an object approaching or moving away from the eyes.

VISCERAL PERCEPTION   An organism's ability to detect its own internal physiological changes. Also known as interoception.

VOLT (v)   A unit of electrical potential. One volt is defined as the electromotive force required to cause one ampere of current to flow in a circuit offering one ohm of resistance.

VOLTAGE   Electrical potential or electromotive force expressed in volts.

VOLTAGE DROP   The voltage developed across a component or conductor by the current in the resistance or impedance of the component or conductor.

VOLT-AMPERE (VA)   A designation of power in terms of volts and amperes.

WATT (w)   A unit of electrical power. One watt is defined as the amount of power required to maintain a current of one ampere under the pressure of one volt in a DC circuit.

WAVEFORM   All aspects of the excursion of a value associated with a signal as it varies over time. It is inclusive of all descriptive parameters.

WAVELENGTH   The "space period" of a wave, i.e., the least translation distance that leaves the waveform invariant. It is typically defined in experimental contexts as the distance between the peak of one wave and the identical peak of the succeeding one. See *Period*.

WIENER FILTER   A statistical technique that derives optimal filter weights for signal detection based on evaluating the signal-to-noise ratio between the signal and noise spectrum.

WOODY ADAPTIVE FILTER   A particular cross-correlation technique in which the filter weights for signal detection are extracted from the original data by means of an iterative procedure.

ACKNOWLEDGMENTS

The editors extend their gratitude to Tom Geen, Beverly Marshall-Goodell, Melanie Ihrig, Kristen Klaaren, Mary Losch, Jeff Martzke, Sam Putnam, and Pat Rourke for their helpful comments and suggestions on previous versions of this glossary and to Louise Rudkin and Kathlene Merendo for secretarial assistance. We also thank the authors who provided us with lists of entries relevant to their respective chapters. Published sources for the information in this glossary include:

Andreassi, J. (1980). *Psychophysiology: Human behavior and physiological response*. New York: Oxford.
Asimov, I. (1985). *The history of physics*. New York: Walker. (Original work published 1966.)
Basmajain, J. V., & DeLuca, C. J. (1985). *Muscles alive: Their functions revealed by electromyography* (5th ed.). Baltimore: Williams & Wilkins.
Bullock, T. H. (1959). Neuron doctrine and electrophysiology. *Science, 129*, 997–1002.
Chaplin, J. P. (1975). *Dictionary of psychology* (rev. ed.). New York: Dell.
Considine, D. M. (1976). *Van Nostrand's scientific encyclopedia* (5th ed.). New York: Van Nostrand Reinhold.
Cooper, R., Osselton, J. W., & Shaw, J. C. (1980). *EEG technology* (3rd ed.). London: Butterworths.
Dorland's illustrated medical dictionary (25th ed.) (1985). Philadelphia: Saunders.
Eccles, J. C. (1977). *The understanding of the brain* (2nd. ed.) New York: McGraw-Hill.
Edwards, P. (Ed.) (1967). *The encyclopedia of philosophy*. New York: Macmillan & Free Press.
Geldard, F. A. (1972). *The human senses* (2nd ed.). New York: Wiley.
Glaser, E. M., & Ruchkin, D. S. (1976). *Principles of neurobiological signal analysis*. New York: Academic.
Gregory, R. L. (1987). *The Oxford companion to the mind*. Oxford: Oxford University Press.
Groves, P. M., & Rebed, G. V. (1988). *Introduction to biological psychology* (3rd ed.). Dubuque, IA: Brown.
Hausner, H. H., Duzevic, D. (1980). The definition of term "sintering." *Science of Sintering, 12*, 137–142.
Kendall, M. G., & Buckland, W. R. (1986). *A dictionary of statistical terms* (4th ed.). Singapore: Longman Scientific and Technical.
Martin, I., & Venables, P. H. (1980). *Techniques in psychophysiology*. Chichester: Wiley.
Reitz, H. L. (1924). *Handbook of mathematical statistics*. Boston: Houghton Mifflin.
Runes, D. D. (Ed.) (1961). *Dictionary of philosophy*. Paterson: Littlefield & Adams.
Stern, R. M., Ray, W. J., & Davis, C. M. (1980). *Psychophysiological recording*. New York: Oxford.
Sternbach, R. A. (1966). *Principles of psychophysiology: An introductory text and readings*. New York: Academic.
Technical reference personal computer AT (#1502494). (1984). Boca Raton: IBM.
Webster's ninth new collegiate dictionary (1986). Springfield: Merriam-Webster.
Young, C. (1988). *The Penguin dictionary of electronics* (2nd ed.). New York: Viking Penguin.

Abbreviations and symbols

A	Ampere
Å	Angstrom (1 Å $= 10^{-10}$ m)
ABP	Arterial blood pressure
AC	Alternating current; capacitance coupled
ACh	Acetylcholine
ACL	Adjective checklist
ACTH	Adrenocorticotrophic hormone
ADACL	Activation–deactivation adjective checklist
ADC	Analog-to-digital converter
ADH	Antidiuretic hormone
Ag/AgCl	Silver–silver chloride
ANCOVA	Analysis of covariance
ANOVA	Analysis of variance
ANS	Autonomic nervous system
APQ	Autonomic Perception Questionnaire
AV	Atrioventricular
b	Byte (1 kb $= 1,024$ b; 1 Mb $= 1,048,576$ b; 1 Gb $= 1,073,741,824$ b)
B	Bel; susceptance
BAL	Blood alcohol level
BP	Blood pressure
bpm	Beats per minute
C	Capacitance; coulomb
°C	Degrees centigrade
Ca	Calcium
CAT	Computerized axial tomography
CBF	Cerebral blood flow
CFP	Corneofundal potential
Cl	Chlorine
CLEMS	Conjugate lateral eye movements
CMOS	Complementary metal oxide semiconductor
CNS	Central nervous system
CNV	Contingent negative variation
cpm	Cycles per minute
CO	Cardiac output
CSF	Cerebrospinal fluid
D	Diode
DAC	Digital-to-analog converter
dB	Decibel
DBP	Diastolic blood pressure
DC	Direct current; direct coupled

843

DF	Degrees of freedom
ECF	Extracellular fluid
ECG	Electrocardiogram; electrocardiography
ECR	Evoked cardiac response
EDA	Electrodermal activity
EDL	Electrodermal level
EDR	Electrodermal response
EDV	End diastolic volume
EEG	Electroencephalogram; electroencephalography
EGG	Eletrogastrogram; electrogastrography
EKG	Electrocardiogram; electrocardiography
EMF	Electromotive force; electromagnetic frequency
EMG	Electromyogram; electromyography
EMS	Electromechanical systole
ENS	Enteric nervous system
EOG	Electrooculogram; electrooculography; electroolfactogram; electroolfactography
EPSP	Excitatory postsynaptic potential
ERF	Event-related field
ERP	Event-related potential
ESV	End systolic volume
eV	Electron-volt
F	Farad; frequency
°F	Degrees fahrenheit
FBF	Forearm blood flow
FFT	Fast Fourier Transform
FVR	Forearm vascular resistance
G	Conductance
GaAs	Gallium arsenide
GABA	Gamma-aminobutyric acid
GAS	General Adaptation Syndrome
GND	Ground
GSR	Galvanic skin response
H	Henry
HEX	Hexadecimal
HP	Heart period
HR	Heart rate
Hz	Hertz
I	Current
IBI	Interbeat interval
IC	Integrated circuit
ICF	Intracellular fluid
IID	Identically and independently distributed
IPSP	Inhibitory postsynaptic potential
ISI	Interstimulus interval
K	Degrees kelvin; potassium
l	Liter
L	Inductance
LED	Light-emitting diode

LVT	Left-ventricular ejection time
LIV	Law of Initial Values
m	Meter
MACL	Mood adjective checklist
MANOVA	Multivariate analysis of variance
MAP	Muscle action potential; mean arterial pressure
MAS	Manifest anxiety scale
MEG	Magnoencephalogram; magnoencephalography
mm Hg	Millimeters of mercury
NA	Sinoatrial node (nodus sinuatrialis); negative affinity
Na	Sodium
NaCl	Sodium chloride
NMR	Nuclear magnetic resonance
NS	Nonspecific response
NsSCR	Nonspecific skin conductance response
Ω	Ohm
$\Psi\Phi$	Psychophysiology
PCM	Pulse code modulation
PDF	Probability density function
PEP	Preinjection period
PET	Positron emission tomography
PGR	Psychogalvanic response
POMS	Psychiatric outpatient mood scale
POT	Potentiometer
PPT	Pulse wave propagation time
PR	Pulse rate
PSTH	Poststimulus time histogram
PTT	Pulse-transit time
PWV	Pulse wave velocity
R	Resistance
REA	Radioenzymatic assay
rec.t	Recovery time
rec.t/2	Recovery half-time
rec.tc	Recovery time constant
REM	Rapid eye movement
RFI	Radio frequency interference
RIA	Radioimmunoassay
ris.t	Rise time
rms	Root-mean-square
RP	Readiness potential
RR	Respiration rate
RSA	Respiratory sinus arrhythmia
RT	Reaction time
s	Second
S	Siemen
SA	Sinus arrhythmia; sinoatrial
SACL	Stress arousal checklist
SBP	Systolic blood pressure
SCL	Skin conductance level
SCR	Skin conductance response

SD	Standard deviation
SDT	Signal detection theory
SI	International System of Units
SN	Signal-to-noise ratio
SNS	Sympathetic nervous system
SPL	Skin potential level; sound pressure level
SPR	Skin potential response
SQUID	Superconducting quantum interference device
SRL	Skin resistance level
SRR	Skin resistance response
STI	Systolic time interval
SYL	Skin admittance level
SYR	Skin admittance response
SZL	Skin impedance level
SZR	Skin impedance response
T	Period; transformer
TC	Time constant
TLC	Thin-layer chromatography
TPR	Total peripheral resistance
TR	Transistor
TSF	Transcellular fluid
TSH	Thyroid-stimulating hormone
TT	Transit time (short for pulse-transit time)
TTL	Transistor–transistor logic
V	Volt
VA	Volt-ampere
VIP	Vasoactive intestinal polypeptide
W	Watt
X	Reactance
Y	Admittance
Z	Impedance

METRIC PREFIXES

Prefix	Abbreviation	Log_{10}	Numeral
Tera	T	12	1,000,000,000,000.0
Giga	G	9	1,000,000,000.0
Mega	M	6	1,000,000.0
Kilo	k	3	1,000.0
Hecto	h	2	100.0
Deka	da	1	10.0
Deci	d	-1	0.1
Centi	c	-2	0.01
Milli	m	-3	0.001
Micro	μ	-6	0.000001
Nano	n	-9	0.000000001
Pico	p	-12	0.000000000001
Femto	f	-15	0.000000000000001
Atto	a	-18	0.000000000000000001

Name Index

849

Subject Index